Oxford Textbook of

Neurologic and Neuropsychiatric Epidemiology

OXFORD TEXTBOOKS IN CLINICAL NEUROLOGY

Published

Oxford Textbook of Neurological and Neuropsychiatric Epidemiology
Edited by Carol Brayne, Valery Feigin, Lenore Launer, and Giancarlo Logroscino

Oxford Textbook of Neurorehabilitation 2nd edition
Edited by Volker Dietz and Nick Ward

Oxford Textbook of Epilepsy and Epileptic Seizures
Edited by Simon Shorvon, Renzo Guerrini, Mark Cook, and Samden Lhatoo

Oxford Textbook of Movement Disorders
Edited by David Burn

Oxford Textbook of Stroke and Cerebrovascular Disease
Edited by Bo Norrving

Oxford Textbook of Neuromuscular Disorders
Edited by David Hilton-Jones and Martin Turner

Oxford Textbook of Neuroimaging
Edited by Massimo Filippi

Oxford Textbook of Cognitive Neurology and Dementia
Edited by Masud Husain and Jonathan M. Schott

Oxford Textbook of Clinical Neurophysiology
Edited by Kerry R. Mills

Oxford Textbook of Sleep Disorders
Edited by Sudhansu Chokroverty and Luigi Ferini-Strambi

Oxford Textbook of Neuro-Oncology
Edited by Tracy T. Batchelor, Ryo Nishikawa, Nancy J. Tarbell, and Michael Weller

Oxford Textbook of Headache Syndromes
Edited by Michel Ferrari, Joost Haan, Andrew Charles, David Dodick, and Fumihiko Sakai

Forthcoming

Oxford Textbook of Neuro-ophthalmology
Edited by Fion Bremner

Oxford Textbook of Clinical Neuropathology
Edited by Sebastian Brandner and Tamas Revesz

Oxford Textbook of Vertigo and Imbalance 2nd edition
Edited by Adolfo Bronstein

Oxford Textbook of

Neurologic and Neuropsychiatric Epidemiology

EDITED BY

Carol Brayne

Professor of Public Health Medicine, Cambridge Institute of Public Health, University of Cambridge, UK

Valery L Feigin

Professor of Neurology and Epidemiology, National Institute for Stroke and Applied Neurosciences, Auckland University of Technology, Auckland, NZ

Lenore J Launer

Neuroepidemiologist, Washington, DC, USA

Giancarlo Logroscino

Professor of Neurology, Director Centre for Neurodegenerative Diseases and the Ageing Brain, Department of Clinical Research in Neurology, University of Bari Aldo Moro, Pia Fond. "Card. G. Panico", Tricase, Lecce, Italy

OXFORD
UNIVERSITY PRESS

OXFORD
UNIVERSITY PRESS

Great Clarendon Street, Oxford, OX2 6DP,
United Kingdom

Oxford University Press is a department of the University of Oxford.
It furthers the University's objective of excellence in research, scholarship,
and education by publishing worldwide. Oxford is a registered trade mark of
Oxford University Press in the UK and in certain other countries

First Edition published in 2021

Impression: 1

Published in the United States of America by Oxford University Press
198 Madison Avenue, New York, NY 10016, United States of America

British Library Cataloguing in Publication Data

Data available

Library of Congress Control Number: 2020938152

ISBN 978–0–19–874949–3

Printed and bound by
CPI Group (UK) Ltd, Croydon, CR0 4YY

This book is dedicated to the people suffering from neurological and neuropsychiatric disorders.

Foreword

In an age of increasing reliance on the electronic record, textbooks are paradoxically of increasing value. They provide the condensation of a topic into a focussed whole while also offering a breadth of topic usually not available to server-based searches. As such they are a boon to the interested. The ***Oxford Textbook of Neurological and Neuropsychiatric Epidemiology*** is no exception. The editors and authors of this text have applied their work to the definition of epidemiology given by A. S Evans in 1979 as "*the quantitative analysis of the circumstances under which disease processes, including trauma, occur in population groups, factors affecting their incidence, distribution, and the host response and use of this knowledge in prevention and control*". In doing so they have produced a comprehensive and current reference source dealing with the major noncommunicable neurological disorders, psychiatric disorders and less common neurological disorders, drawing on both the epidemiology and current disease understanding to highlight how in some areas disease mitigation strategies can be applied on a population basis to reduce the burden of disease.

The essence, however, of this text is in the breadth of the topics and the expertise displayed in each chapter. From Alzheimer's disease and other common neurodegenerations to stroke, amyotrophic lateral sclerosis, prion diseases, epilepsies, neuropathies, multiple sclerosis, the topics broaden to include a plethora of important topics such as end of life dementia, epidemiology of apathy, behavioural and psychological symptoms of dementia, epidemiology of schizophrenia, neuroinfections, neurotrauma, effects of magnetic fields, and metals and neurodegenerations. Throughout there are critical chapters which not only inform on neuropsychiatric epidemiology, but also reflect the utility of epidemiology in current practice.

It is no easy task to bring a work of this dimension together but the authors and editors have, in my view, succeeded. They have produced a text which balances the principles of neuropsychiatric epidemiology with that of specific disorders and illustrates the potential of epidemiological research in their management. It will prove an indispensable reference for all those with an interest neuropsychiatric epidemiology as well as in neurology.

William M Carroll, AM, MB, BS, FRACP, FRCP(E)
President, World Federation of Neurology

Preface

The epidemiological approach to study disease lies at the core of any scientific endeavour—appropriate study design, standardized implementation, quantitative analyses, and considerations of factors that may distort the interpretation of results. As a broad field of enquiry, epidemiology draws on methods from many other scientific fields, including biostatistics and informatics, medicine, biology, economics, and the behavioural sciences. As a translational science, epidemiological data are critical for developing and testing aetiological hypotheses of disease; providing information on the frequency of people with existing (prevalence) and newly developed (incidence); understanding natural history; evaluating the social, economic, and health-care consequences of disease burden, and designing interventions to lessen this burden. Epidemiology also contributes to the current focus on precision medicine, by providing the data for risk scores, and evidence to assess the value of targeting risk groups susceptible to specific diseases, as well as disorders and whole health and wellbeing.

Epidemiology methods of inquiry rely on a systematic and unbiased approach to the collection, analysis, and interpretation of data. A central concept in epidemiological research is the recognition of, and if possible, reduction in, bias. Systematic bias affects the internal validity of a study, can change the direction and magnitude of association, and can lead to the wrong interpretation of the data, for instance, concluding there is an association of two factors, when there is none.

The aim of this textbook is to review our current state-of-the-art understanding of neurological and neuropsychiatric conditions, and to highlight the underlying scientific architecture of epidemiology to be applied in future studies. The chapters also highlight the challenges that the study of the epidemiology of neurological/neuropsychiatric conditions presents beyond those posed by other health conditions. To meet these challenges research is advancing rapidly with researchers developing new approaches and new tools to provide contemporary insights including the changing context in which we live across the globe.

Lenore J Launer, Valery L Feign,
Gianocarlo Logroscino, and Carol Brayne

Contents

SECTION 4
Vascular disorders

SECTION 5
Neurology, neuropsychiatry, and phenomenology

SECTION 6
Other key neurological conditions

SECTION 7
Infections, exposures, injuries, and the brain

SECTION 8
Global health and public health

Abbreviations

AACD	ageing-associated cognitive decline
AAMI	age-associated memory impairment
ABI	ankle-brachial index
ABM	acute bacterial meningitis
ABMI	Agitated Behaviour Mapping Instrument
ACE	Addenbrooke's clinical examination
AChEI	acetylcholinesterase inhibitors
ACHIEVE	Aging and Cognitive Health Evaluation in Elders (USA)
AChR	acetylcholine receptor
AD	Alzheimer's disease
ADAS	Alzheimer Disease Assessment Scale
AED	anti-epileptic drug
AES	Apathy Evaluation Scale
AESOP	Aetiology and Ethnicity in Schizophrenia and Other Psychoses
AF	atrial fibrillation
AFHSB	Armed Forces Health Surveillance Branch
AGES	Age, Gene/Environment Susceptibility
AIDS	immune-deficiency syndrome
ALDS	Academic Medical Centre Linear Disability Scale
ALS	amyotrophic lateral sclerosis
ALSPAC	Avon Longitudinal Study of Parents and Children
A-MCI	amnestic mild cognitive impairment
AMD	age-related macular degeneration
AMPP	American Migraine Prevalence and Prevention
AMSA	Army Medical Surveillance Activity
AMSARA	Accession Medical Standards Analysis and Research Activity
Anti-MOG	anti-myelin oligodendrocyte
ANU_ADRI	Australian National University AD Risk Index
aOR	adjusted odds ratio
APOE	Apolipoprotein E
APP	amyloid precursor protein
AQP-4	aquaporin-4
ARCD	age-related cognitive decline
ARIC	Atherosclerosis Risk in Communities
ARR	absolute risk reduction
ASIA	American Spinal Injury Association
ASL	arterial spin labelling
AUC	area under the curve
Aβ	amyloid β
BBB	blood brain barrier
BDNF	brain derived neurotrophic factor
BEHAVE-AD	Behavioural Pathology in Alzheimer's Disease scale
BIOMARKAPD	Biomarkers for AD and Parkinson's disease
BMDS	Behaviour and Mood Disturbance Scale
BME	black and minority ethnic groups
BMI	body mass index
BOLD	blood oxygen level dependent
BPS	behavioural and psychological symptoms
BPSD	behavioural and psychological symptoms of dementia
BSE	bovine spongiform encephalopathy
BSF	benign senescent forgetfulness
CA	cerebral aspergillosis
CAG	cytosine adenine guanine
CAIDE	Cardiovascular risk factors, Ageing and Dementia
CAMDEX	Cambridge examination for mental disorders of the elderly
CaMEO	Chronic Migraine Epidemiology and Outcomes
CBD	corticobasal degeneration
CBF	cerebral blood flow
CBS	corticobasal syndrome
CCT	central corneal thickness
CDC	Centers for Disease Control and Prevention (USA)
CDH	chronic daily headache
CDR	clinical dementia rating scale
CERAD-BRSD	Behaviour Rating Scale for Dementia of the Consortium to Establish a Registry for Alzheimer's Disease
CFAS	Cognitive Function and Ageing Study
CFC	cognitive-functional composite
CGRP	calcitonin gene related peptide
CHD	coronary heart disease
CHESS	Comprehensive Health and Epidemiological Surveillance System
CHI	central hearing impairment
cho	choline
CI	confidence interval
CIDI	Composite International Diagnostic Interview
CIDP	chronic inflammatory demyelinating polyneuropathy
CIND	cognitive impairment without dementia
CJD	Creutzfeldt-Jakob disease
CM	cerebral malaria
CM	chronic migraine
CMT	Charcot-Marie-Tooth

CMT1	Charcot-Marie-Tooth demyelinating form
CMT2	Charcot-Marie-Tooth axonal form
CMV	cytomegalovirus
CNS	central nervous system
COBRA	Cost and Outcome of Behavioural Activation
CODEm	Cause of Death Ensemble model
CODR	C-Path online data repository
COMT	cathecol-O methyl transferase
CONSORT	Consolidated Standards for Reporting of Trials
COPD	chronic obstructive pulmonary disease
Cr	creatine
CRF	cardiovascular risk factors
CrM	cryptococcal meningitis
CSF	cerebrospinal fluid
CT	computerized tomography
CTE	chronic traumatic encephalopathy
CUSPAD	Columbia University Scale for Psychopathology in Alzheimer's disease
CVD	cardiovascular disease
CWD	chronic wasting disease
DA	dopamine activity
DALY	disability adjusted life year
DBDS	Dementia Behaviour Disturbance Scale
DBS	deep brain stimulation
DBS-STN	deep brain stimulation in the subthalamic nucleus
DCL	diagnostic confidence level
DECT	Digital Enhanced Cordless Telecommunications
DIS	Diagnostic Interview Schedule
DLB	dementia with Lewy bodies
DMED	Defense Medical Epidemiology Database (USA)
DMSS	Defense Medical Surveillance System (USA)
DoD	Department of Defense (USA)
DoDSR	Department of Defense Serum Repository (USA)
DOHaD	developmental origins of health and disease
DSD	delirium superimposed on dementia
DSM	Diagnostic and Statistical Manual
DSMMD	Diagnostic and Statistical Manual for Mental Disorders
DTI	diffusion tensor imaging
DVBIC	Defense and Veterans Brain Injury Center (USA)
Dw-MRI	diffusion-weighted magnetic resonance imaging
EBNAS	Epidemiologically Based Needs Assessment
EBV	Epstein-Barr virus
ECA	Epidemiological Catchment Area
ECD	^{99m}Tc-bicisate
EDDS	Expanded Disability Status Scale
EEG	electroencephalogram
EF	electric field
EITB	immunoelectrotransfer blot
ELF	extremely low frequency
EM	episodic migraine
EMF	electromagnetic fields
EN	enteral nutrition
EOAD	early onset Alzheimer's disease
EOD	early onset dementia
EOD	early onset depression
EOFAD	early onset familial Alzheimer's disease
EPAD	European Prevention of Alzheimer's Dementia
EPIC	European Prospective Investigation into Cancer and Nutrition
ET	essential tremor
EU-GEI	European Network of National Schizophrenia Networks Studying Gene-Environment Interactions
FA	fractional anisotropy
FDA	Food and Drug Administration
FDG	fluorodeoxyglucose
FEP	first episode of psychosis
FFI	fatal familial insomnia
FINGER	Finnish Geriatric Intervention Study to Prevent Cognitive Impairment and Disability
fMRI	functional MRI
FOAD	foetal origins of adult disease
FTD	frontotemporal dementia
FTLD	frontotemporal lobar degeneration
GAP	Global Alzheimer's Platform
GBA	β-glucocerebrosidase
GBD	Global Burden of Disease and Injuries
GBS	group B streptococcus
GBS	Guillain-Barre syndrome
GMS AGECAT	Geriatric Mental State Examination (GMS) Automated Geriatric Examination for Computer Assisted Taxonomy (AGECAT)
GMS-A	Geriatric mental state schedule
GNI	gross national income
GP	general practitioner
GSM	Global System for Mobile Communications
GSS	Gerstmann-Sträussler-Scheinker syndrome
GWA	genome-wide association
GWAIS	Genome-Wide Association and Interaction Study
HADS	Hospital Anxiety and Depression Scale
HAND	HIV-Associated Neurocognitive Disorders
HCP	healthcare professional
HD	Huntington's disease
HDSS	health and demographic surveillance site
HealthABC	Health, Aging, and Body Composition (USA)
HFEM	high frequency episodic migraine
HICs	high-income countries
HIV	human immunodeficiency virus
HL	hearing level
HLA	human leukocyte antigen
HMPAO	^{99m}Tc-exametazime
HMSN	hereditary motor and sensory neuropathy
HPA	hypothalamic-pituitary-adrenal
HR	hazard ratio
HRS	Health and Retirement study
HS	hippocampal sclerosis
HSE	Health Survey for England
HSE	herpes simplex encephalitis
HSV	herpes simplex viruses
IA	intermediate allele
IARC	International Agency for Research on Cancer
ICD	International Statistical Classification of Diseases
ILAE	International League Against Epilepsy

IOP	intraocular pressure
IPA	International Psychogeriatric Association
IQ	intelligence quotient
IQR	interquartile range
ISGEO	International Society for Geographical and Epidemiological Ophthalmology
IWG	International Working Group
JCV	JC virus
JEM	job-exposure-matrix
JEV	Japanese encephalitis virus
JPND	joint programme-neurodegenerative disease research
JTTR	Joint Theater Trauma Registry (USA)
LB	Lewy body
LCS	Longitudinal Cohort Study
LFEM	low frequency episodic migraine
LICs	low income countries
LMICs	low-middle-income countries
LOAD	late onset Alzheimer's disease
LOD	late-onset depression
LPA	logopenic progressive aphasic
LQ	longevity quotient
LTE	long-term evolution
MA	migraine with aura
MAO-B	monoamine oxidase B
MAPT	microtubule-associated protein tau
MAPT	Multidomain Alzheimer Prevention Trial
MAS	Maracaibo ageing study
MBI	mild behavioural impairment
MBM	meat bone meal
MCD	mild cognitive disorder
MCI	mild cognitive impairment
MD	mean diffusivity
MDD	major depressive disorder
MDS	Movement Disorder Society
MDT	multi-drug therapy
MF	magnetic field
MG	myasthenia gravis
MHD	mental health disorders
MHS	Military Healthcare System
mI	myo-Inositol
MICs	middle-income countries
M-MCI	mixed mild cognitive impairment
MMN	multifocal motor neuropathy
MMSE	Mini Mental Status Examination
MMT	methylcyclopentadienyl manganese tricarbonyl
MNCD	mild neurocognitive disorder
MNO	neuromyelitis optica
MO	migraine without aura
MOS	military occupational specialties
MPTP	1-methyl-4phnyl-1,2,3,6-tetrahydropyridine
MR	Mendelian randomization
MRC CFAS	Medical Research Council Cognitive Function and Ageing Study
MRI	magnetic resonance imaging
MRM	menstrual related migraine
MRS	magnetic resonance spectroscopy
MS	multiple sclerosis
MSA	multiple system atrophy
MSA-C	multiple system atrophy cerebellar
MSA-P	multiple system atrophy parkinsonian
MSMR	Medical Surveillance Monthly Report
MSON	multiple sclerosis associated optic neuritis
MSP	multiple system atrophy
MT	mutant type
MTA	material transfer agreement
MTHFR	5,10-methylenetetrahydrofolate reductase
MTL	medial temporal lobe
NAA	N-acetylaspartate
NCC	neurocysticercosis
NCD	neurocognitive disorder
NCD	non-communicable disease
NCS	National Comorbidity Surveys
NDD	neurodegenerative disease
NDE	neuronal derived exosomes
NFL	neurofilament light
NFT	neurofibrillary tangles
NGPSE	National General Practice Study of Epilepsy
NGRN	neurogranin
NIA-AA	National Institute on Aging and Alzheimer's Association (USA)
NINCDS-ADRDA	National Institute of Neurological and Communicative Disorders and Stroke and the Alzheimer's Disease and Related Disorders Association
NINDS/NIMH	National Institute of Neurological Disorders and Stroke and National Institute of Mental Health
NIV	non-invasive ventilation
N-MCI	non-memory impairment mild cognitive impairment
NMDA	N-methyl-D-aspartic acid
NMHD	neurological and mental health disorders
NMO	neuromyelitis optica
NMOSD	neuromyelitis optica spectrum disorder
NNT	number needed to treat
NPI	Neuropsychiatric Inventory
NS	nodding syndrome
NSAID	non-steroidal anti-inflammatory drug
OCT	optical coherence tomography
OHT	ocular hypertension
OR	odds ratio
OSA	obstructive sleep apnoea
PACG	primary angle-closure glaucoma
PAF	population attributable fraction
PAR	population attributable risk
PAR	predictive adaptive response
PBA	Problem Behaviours Assessment
PCA	posterior cortical atrophy
PD	Parkinson's disease
PDD	Parkinson's disease dementia
PDN	paraproteinemic demyelinating neuropathy
PDSBB	Parkinson's Disease Society Brain Bank
PET	positron emission tomography
PiB	Pittsburgh Compound B
PIGD	postural instability/gait difficulty

PML	progressive multifocal leukoencephalopathy
PMM	pure menstrual migraine
PMR	proportional mortality ratio
POAG	primary open-angle glaucoma
PoC	Proof of Concept
preDIVA	Prevention of Dementia by Intensive Vascular care trial
PRGN	progranulin
PRNP	prion protein
PRO-ACT	Pooled Resource Open-Access ALS Clinical Trials Database
PROBE	Prospective Open Label Blinded Endpoint
PRS	polygenic risk score
PSEN1	presenilin 1
PSEN2	presenilin 2
PSP	progressive supranuclear palsy
PSP	progressive supranuclear palsy parkinsonism
PSP-RS	progressive supranuclear palsy Richardson's syndrome
PTA	post-traumatic amnesia
PTA	pure tone average
P-tau	phosphorylated tau
pTBI	prior traumatic brain injury
PTSD	post-traumatic stress disorder
PVC	polyvinyl chloride
PWV	pulse wave velocity
QALY	quality of life years
QoL	quality of life
RAS	Ryden Aggression Scale
RBD	REM-behaviour disorder
rCBF	regional cerebral blood flow
RCT	randomized controlled trials
ReDeGi	Registry of Dementia of Girona
REP	Rochester Epidemiological Project
RF	radiofrequency
rho	intra-cluster correlation coefficient
RLS	restless legs syndrome
RMBPC	Revised Memory and problems checklist behaviour
RNFL	retinal nerve fibre layer
ROC	receiver operating characteristic
RR	relative risk
RRR	relative risk reduction
SAE	serious adverse events
SAR	specific absorption rate
SARA	Scale for the Assessment and Rating of Ataxia
SCENIHR	Scientific Committee on Emerging and Newly Identified Health Risks
SCI	spinal cord injury
SD	standard deviation
SDG	sustainable development goals
SDI	sociodemographic index
SE	status epilepticus
sFI	sporadic fatal insomnia
SIR	standardized incidence ratio
SMR	standardized mortality ratio
SMs	military service members
SNP	single nucleotide polymorphism
SPECT	single positron emission computed tomography
STN	subthalamic nucleus
STROBE	Strengthening the Reporting of Observational studies in Epidemiology
STROND	Standards of Reporting of Neurological Disorders
SUDEP	sudden unexplained death in epilepsy
SVD	small vessel disease
tAD	typical Alzheimer's disease
TBE	tick-borne encephalitis
TBI	traumatic brain injury
TBM	tuberculosis meningitis
TD	tremor dominant
TFC	total functional capacity score
TIA	transient ischaemic attack
TMD	temporomandibular joint disorder
TMS	total motor score
TOT	training of trainers
TSP	tropical spastic paraparesis
T-tau	total tau
UHDRS	Unified Huntington's Disease Rating Scale
UI	uncertainty interval
UMTs	Universal Mobile Telecommunications System
UN	United Nations
UPDRS	Unified Parkinson's Disease Rating Scale
VA	verbal autopsy
VA	Veterans Administration
VBM	voxel-based morphometry
VCI	vascular cognitive impairment
vCJD	variant Creutzfeldt-Jakob disease
VEP	visual evoked potentials
VPSPr	variably protease sensitive prionopathy
VZV	Varicella-Zoster virus
WHO	World Health Organization
WHS	Women's Health Study
W/kg	Watt per body mass
W/m^2	Watt per unit area
WMH	World Health Organization Mental Health
WMHs	white matter hyperintensities
WT	wild type
YLD	years lived with disability
YLL	years of life lost
YOPD	young onset Parkinson's disease
ZIKV	Zika virus

Contributors

Salmane Amidou INSERM, University Limoges, CHU Limoges, IRD, U1094 Tropical Neuroepidemiology, Institute of Epidemiology and Tropical Neurology, GEIST, Limoges, France

Lisanne J Balk Neuro-ophthalmology Expertise Centre, Departments of Neurology and Ophthalmology & Amsterdam Neuroscience, VU University Medical Centre, Amsterdam, the Netherlands

Ettore Beghi Head, Laboratory of Neurological Diseases, Department of Neuroscience, Istituto di Ricerche Farmacologiche Mario Negri IRCCS, Milan, Italy

Derrick A Bennett Statistical Group Leader and University Research Lecturer, Clinical Trials Service Unit and Epidemiological Studies Unit, Nuffield Department of Population Health, University of Oxford, Oxford, UK

Yoav Ben-Shlomo Professor of Clinical Epidemiology, Population Health Sciences, University of Bristol, Bristol, UK

German E Berrios University of Cambridge, UK

Amy R Borenstein Professor of Epidemiology in the Department of Family Medicine and Public Health, Division of Epidemiology, University of California, San Diego School of Medicine, USA

Carol Brayne Professor of Public Health Medicine, Department of Public Health and Primary Care, Cambridge Institute of Public Health, Forvie Site, University of Cambridge, School of Clinical Medicine, Cambridge Biomedical Campus, Cambridge, UK

Elisabeth Gulowsen Celius Professor and Senior Neurologist, Department of Neurology, Oslo University Hospital and University of Oslo, Oslo, Norway

Honglei Chen Professor, Department of Epidemiology and Biostatistics, College of Human Medicine, Michigan State University, East Lansing, Michigan, USA

Adriano Chiò Rita Levi Montalcini, Department of Neurosciences, University of Turin, Turin, Italy, Azienda Ospedaliero Univeritaria Città della Salute e della Scienza di Torino, Torino, Italy

Yi-Fang Chuang Assistant Professor, Institute of Public Health, National Yang-Ming University, Taipei, Taiwan

María M Corrada Departments of Neurology and Epidemiology, Institute for Memory Impairments and Neurological Disorders, University of California, Irvine, California, USA

Ian TS Coyle-Gilchrist Department of Clinical Neurosciences, University of Cambridge, Cambridge, UK

Eileen M Crimmins AARP Professor of Gerontology, Davis School of Gerontology, University of Southern California, Los Angeles, California, USA

SJ Crutch UCL Institute of Neurology and the National Hospital for Neurology and Neurosurgery, Queen Square, London, UK

Daniel Davis Senior Clinical Researcher (Honorary Consultant) in Ageing, Institute of Epidemiology & Health, University College London, UK

Tom Dening Professor of Dementia Research, Division of Psychiatry and Applied Psychology, University of Nottingham, UK

Fergus N Doubal Senior Lecturer and Consultant Stroke Physician, Centre for Clinical Brain Sciences, University of Edinburgh Royal Infirmary of Edinburgh, Edinburgh, UK

Juliana R Dutra Department of Neurology, Division of Aging and Dementia, Columbia University, New York, NY, USA

Ratnavalli Ellajosyula Consultant Neurologist and Specialist in Cognitive Neurology, Manipal Hospital, Bangalore, India, Annasawmy Mudaliar General Hospital, Bangalore, India

Valery L Feigin Professor of Neurology and Epidemiology, National Institute for Stroke and Applied Neurosciences, Auckland University of Technology, Auckland, NZ

Maria Feychting Professor Institute of Environmental Medicine, Karolinska Institutet, Stockholm, Sweden

Paul J Foster Professor of Ophthalmic Epidemiology, NIHR Biomedical Research Centre, Moorfields Eye Hospital & UCL Institute of Ophthalmology, London, UK

Laura Fratiglioni Ageing Research Centre, Department of Neurobiology, Care Sciences and Society, Karolinska Institutet, Stockholm University, Stockholm, Sweden

Valentina Gallo Senior Lecturer in Epidemiology, Blizard Institute, Queen Mary University of London, UK

Tanya P Garcia Associate Professor, Department of Statistics, Texas A&M University

Mirjam I Geerlings Associate Professor, Neuroepidemiology Department of Epidemiology, Julius Centre for Health Sciences and Primary Care, University Medical Centre Utrecht and Utrecht University, Utrecht, the Netherlands

Nils Erik Gilhus Department of Clinical Medicine, University of Bergen, Bergen, Norway

Giorgia Giussani Laboratory of Neurological Diseases, Department of Neuroscience, Istituto di Ricerche Farmacologiche Mario Negri IRCCS, Milano, Italy

Adele M Goman Johns Hopkins Cochlear Center for Hearing and Public Health; Department of Epidemiology, Johns Hopkins Bloomberg School of Public Health, Baltimore, USA

Maëlenn Guerchet Epidemiologist, Centre for Global Mental Health, Institute of Psychiatry, Psychology and Neuroscience, King's College London, UK

Bradleigh Hayhow Visiting Professor Edinburgh Dementia Prevention Research Group, Centre for Clinical Brain Sciences, University of Edinburgh, UK, Director INSERM Unit 1061 Neuropsychiatry, Montpellier, France

Mark D Hayward Centennial Commission Professor, Department of Sociology and the Population Research Center, University of Texas, Austin, Texas, USA

Anne Taraldsen Heldal Department of Clinical Medicine, University of Bergen, Bergen, Norway

Assen Jablensky Centre for Clinical Research in Neuropsychiatry, University of Western Australia, Crawley, Australia

Catherine Johnson Institute for Health Metrics and Evaluation, University of Washington, Seattle, WA, USA

Kelly M Jones National Institute for Stroke and Applied Sciences, AUT University, Auckland, NZ

Peter B Jones Department of Psychiatry, University of Cambridge, Cambridge, UK

Hannah E Jongsma Department of Psychiatry, University of Cambridge, Cambridge, UK

Claudia H Kawas Departments of Neurology and Neurobiology & Behavior, Institute for Memory Impairments and Neurological Disorders, University of California, Irvine, California, USA

Anthony Khawaja NIHR Biomedical Research Centre at Moorfields Eye Hospital & UCL Institute of Ophthalmology, London, UK, Glaucoma Service, Moorfields Eye Hospital, London, UK, Integrative Epidemiology & Visual Function, UCL Institute of Ophthalmology, London, UK

Marianthi-Anna Kioumourtzoglou Department of Environmental Health Sciences, Columbia University Mailman School of Public Health, New York, USA

James B Kirkbride Division of Psychiatry, University College London, UK

Rita Krishnamurthi National Institute for Stroke & Applied Neurosciences, Auckland University of Technology, Auckland, NZ

Kenneth M Langa Cyrus Sturgis Professor of Medicine, Department of Medicine, University of Michigan, Michigan, USA

Frank R Lin Director of the Johns Hopkins Cochlear Center for Hearing and Public Health; Professor of Otolaryngology, Medicine, Mental Health, and Epidemiology, Johns Hopkins University, Baltimore, USA

Rianne van der Linde Department of Public Health and Primary Care, Institute of Public Health, University of Cambridge, Cambridge, UK

Richard B Lipton Edwin S Lowe Professor and Vice Chair of Neurology, Professor of Epidemiology and Population Health, Albert Einstein College of Medicine, New York, USA

Giancarlo Logroscino Professor of Neurology Director, Centre for Neurodegenerative Diseases and the Ageing Brain, Department of Clinical Research in Neurology, University of Bari Aldo Moro, Pia Fondazione Cardinale G. Panico, Tricase, Lecce, Italy

Elan D Louis Division of Movement Disorders, Department of Neurology, Yale School of Medicine, Yale University, New Haven, Connecticut, USA

Jaime Luna INSERM, University Limoges, CHU Limoges, IRD, U1094 Tropical Neuroepidemiology, Institute of Epidemiology and Tropical Neurology, GEIST, Limoges, France

Karen Marder Sally Kerlin Professor of Neurology, Department of Neurology, Columbia University, New York, USA

Ivana S Marková Centre for Health and Population Sciences, Hull York Medical School, Allam Medical Building, University of Hull, UK

Rosie Mayston Centre for Global Mental Health, Health Service and Population Research Department, Institute of Psychiatry, Psychology and Neuroscience, King's College London, UK

Anna M Molesworth Senior Epidemiologist & Deputy Director, National CJD Research & Surveillance Unit, University of Edinburgh, Edinburgh, UK

Graciela Muniz-Terrera Senior Lecturer in Biostatistics, Edinburgh Dementia Prevention Research Group, Centre for Clinical Brain Sciences, University of Edinburgh, UK

Zaynah Muthy NIHR Biomedical Research Centre at Moorfields Eye Hospital & UCL Institute of Ophthalmology, London, UK, Glaucoma Service, Moorfields Eye Hospital, London, UK, Integrative Epidemiology & Visual Function, UCL Institute of Ophthalmology, London, UK

Mohsen Naghavi Professor, Department of Health Metrics Sciences, Institute for Health Metrics and Evaluation, School of Medicine, University of Washington, Seattle, Washington, USA

Charles R Newton Professor, KEMRI-Wellcome Collaborative Programme, Kilifi, Kenya, and Department of Psychiatry, University of Oxford, UK

David W Niebuhr Department of Preventive Medicine and Biostatistics, Uniformed Services University, Bethesda, USA

Bo Norrving Lund University, Skåne University Hospital, Department of Clinical Sciences Lund, Neurology, Lund, Sweden

Adesola Ogunniyi Department of Medicine, College of Medicine, University of Ibadan, University College Hospital, Ibadan, Nigeria

Leonardo Pantoni Full Professor, "Luigi Sacco" Department of Biomedical and Clinical Sciences, University of Milan

Neil Pearce Professor, Department of Medical Statistics, London School of Hygiene and Tropical Medicine, London, UK

Susan Peters Environmental Epidemiology Division, Institute for Risk Assessment Sciences, Utrecht University, Utrecht, the Netherlands

Axel Petzold The National Hospital for Neurology and Neurosurgery, Queen Square, London, UK, Expert Centre for Neuro-ophthalmology, Amsterdam UMC, Amsterdam, NL Consultant Neuro-ophthalmologist, Moorfields Eye Hospital NHS Foundation Trust, London, UK

Anna Poggesi Associate Professor of Neurology, Neurofarba Department, Neuroscience Section, University of Florence, Stroke Unit, Florence, Italy

Marco Poloni Laboratory of Neurological Diseases, Department of Neuroscience, Istituto di Ricerche Farmacologiche Mario Negri IRCCS, Milan, Italy

Pierre-Marie Preux Neuroepidemiologist, Head Inserm UMR 1094, IRD, Institute of Epidemiology and Tropical Neurology, University of Limoges, Limoges, France

A Matthew Prina Senior Lecturer, Epidemiology Health Service and Population Research Department, Institute of Psychiatry, Psychology & Neuroscience, King's College London, London, UK

Chengxuan Qiu Ageing Research Centre, Department of Neurobiology, Care Sciences and Society, Karolinska Institutet, Stockholm University, Stockholm, Sweden

Edo Richard Neurologist, Department of Neurology, Donders Institute for Brain, Cognition and Behaviour, Radboud University Medical Centre, Nijmegen, the Netherlands

Sarah Richardson NIHR Academic Clinical Lecturer, Translational and Clinical Research Institute, Faculty of Medical Sciences, Newcastle University, Newcastle upon Tyne, UK

Craig W Ritchie Professor of Old Age Psychiatry, Edinburgh Dementia Prevention Research Group, Centre for Clinical Brain Sciences, University of Edinburgh, UK

Karen Ritchie Visiting Professor Edinburgh Dementia Prevention Research Group, Centre for Clinical Brain Sciences, University of Edinburgh, UK, Director INSERM Unit 1061 Neuropsychiatry, Montpellier, France

Gregory Roth Division of Cardiology, Institute for Health Metrics and Evaluation, University of Washington, Seattle, WA, USA

James B Rowe Department of Clinical Neurosciences, University of Cambridge, Cambridge, UK

Tom C Russ Director, Alzheimer Scotland Dementia Research Centre, University of Edinburgh, UK

Stina Saunders PhD Researcher, Edinburgh Dementia Prevention Research Group, Centre for Clinical Brain Sciences, University of Edinburgh, UK

Rodolfo Savica Department of Neurology, Mayo Clinic, Rochester, Minnesota, USA

Ann I Scher Department of Preventive Medicine and Biostatistics Uniformed Services University Bethesda, USA

JM Schott UCL Institute of Neurology and the National Hospital for Neurology and Neurosurgery, Queen Square, London, UK

Joachim Schüz Head, Section of Environment and Radiation, International Agency for Research on Cancer (IARC/WHO), Lyon, France

Esteban Sepulveda Psychiatrist, Institut Pere Mata. Associate Professor, Universitat Rovira i Virgili Reus, Spain

Darrell Singer Department of Preventive Medicine and Biostatistics, Uniformed Services University, Bethesda, USA

Sergio Starkstein Associate Professor of Psychiatry, School of Medicine, The University of Notre Dame, Fremantle, Western Australia, School of Psychiatry and Clinical Neurosciences, The University of Western Australia, Crawley, Western Australia, Department of Neurology, Fiona Stanley Hospital, Murdoch, Western Australia

Madhav Thambisetty National Institute on Aging, National Institutes of Health, Baltimore, MD, USA

Alice Theadom Associate Professor of Psychology and Rutherford Discovery Fellow, National Institute for Stroke and Applied Neurosciences, Auckland University of Technology, Auckland, NZ

Torbjorn Tomson Department of Clinical Neuroscience, Karolinska Institutet, Stockholm, Sweden

Rosanna Tortelli Centre for Neurodegenerative Diseases and the Ageing Brain, Department of Clinical Research in Neurology, University of Bari Aldo Moro, Pia Fondazione Cardinale G. Panico, Tricase, Lecce, Italy

Thomas Truelsen Department of Neurology, Copenhagen University Hospital Rigshospitalet, Copenhagen, Denmark

Pierpaolo Turcano Department of Neurology, Mayo Clinic, Rochester, Minnesota, USA

Patrick JM Urwin Neurology Research Registrar, University of Edinburgh, UK

Vijay R Varma National Institute on Aging, National Institutes of Health, Baltimore, MD, USA

Roel Vermeulen Environmental Epidemiology Division, Institute for Risk Assessment Sciences, Utrecht University, Utrecht, the Netherlands

Davide Liborio Vetrano Ageing Research Centre, Department of Neurobiology, Care Sciences and Society, Karolinska Institutet, Stockholm University, Stockholm, Sweden

Julio R Vieira Assistant Professor of Neurology, Albert Einstein College of Medicine, Health Quest Medical Practice, Division of Neurology, New York, USA

Anne E Visser Department of Neurology, University Medical Centre Utrecht, Utrecht, the Netherlands

Theo Vos Institute for Health Metrics and Evaluation, University of Washington, Seattle, Washington, USA

Joanna M Wardlaw Professor Applied Neuroimaging, Honorary Consultant Neuroradiologist, Foundation Chair, UK Dementia Research Institute, Head of Division, Neuroimaging Sciences, Centre for Clinical Brain Sciences, Director, Edinburgh Imaging, College of Medicine and Veterinary Medicine, University of Edinburgh, UK

Marc Weisskopf Departments of Environmental Health and Epidemiology, Harvard School of Public Health, Boston, Massachusetts, USA

Pierre Wibawa Neuropsychiatry Unit, Royal Melbourne Hospital, Parkville, Victoria, Australia, Department of Psychiatry, University of Melbourne, Parkville, Victoria, Australia

Keir XX Yong Senior Research Fellow Dementia Research Centre, Department of Neurodegenerative Disease, Queen Square Institute of Neurology, University College London, UK

Inès Yoro-Zohoun INSERM, University Limoges, CHU Limoges, IRD, U1094 Tropical Neuroepidemiology, Institute of Epidemiology and Tropical Neurology, GEIST, Limoges, France

SECTION 1

Concepts, designs, and methods

1

A historical perspective on neurological and neuropsychiatric definitions

German E Berrios and Ivana S Marková

Introduction

Neurology, neuropsychiatry, neuro-ophthalmology, neuropsychology, neuroethics, neuropsychoanalysis, neuroimaging, neuro-ontology, neuroconstructivism, neuroepistemology, neuroaesthetics, neurohistory, etc. constitute a growing family of terms of varied usefulness where 'neuro' refers to the brain and the rest of the word to an activity or discipline seeking a relation to, or explanation in terms of, cerebral anatomy or function. It may even be that in some cases what is sought is prestige via the 'neuro' association.

The usefulness of a neuro-term determines its shelf life. Neurology, neuropsychiatry, neuro-ophthalmology and neuropsychology seem to be wearing well. Neuroethics, neuroaesthetics, neuro-ontology, or neuroepistemology are still on probation.

Historiography

Historical accounts are not always helpful. For example, one based on the assumption that current 'knowledge' is truest by definition (called presentistic, linear, progressist, Whig) will evaluate earlier ideas anachronistically and produce narratives flattering to the present, but unhelpful in terms of understanding the past. On the other hand, if past and present narratives are treated contextually and in a non-evaluative manner then the resulting historical account may be illuminating.[1] This chapter will adopt the second approach.

Historical Epistemology

'Historical epistemology' names a method of studying knowledge based on the idea that cultural objects (whether concepts, institutions, ideologies, or disciplines) owe their meaning to their historical context. This provides them with the material out of which they are constructed and the warrants (social, political, and economic) for their duration.[2] For example, medicine names a longevous discipline deeply inscribed in western and other cultures whose survival has resulted from its: (1) keeping up with the official sciences of the day; (2) good predictive power; (3) social approval; and (4) protection by powerful social institutions (medical profession, patient associations, etc.). Over the years, medicine has given rise to many specialisms. This chapter will explore the history of two of these, neurology and neuropsychiatry.

Neurology

Clinical neurology is currently defined as a branch of clinical medicine 'concerned with the diagnosis and treatment of disorders of the nervous system' (p1266).[3] In historical terms neurology has resulted from the 'convergence'[4] of a: (1) word (neurology); (2) cluster of concepts; and (3) list of 'disorders' which eventually achieved critical mass. Once constructed by means of a historical convergence, new specialisms themselves trigger social change, for example the development of professional accoutrements such as colleges, learned societies, new vocabularies, examinations, rites of passage, journals, textbooks, etc.

The word 'neurology'

Since the 17th century, the terms 'neurology' and '*névrologie/neurologie*' have been used in English and French respectively to name the study of 'nerves' (whatever the term 'nerve' actually meant at the time).[5,6] In classical Greek 'neuros' actually meant 'sinew' as attested by common terms such as 'neuronosos' (disease of sinews) and 'neuropectatos' (bow-stringing).[7] Observing the functional deficits that followed injury to nerves and sinews, Galen suggested that they might be different structures but continued using 'neuros' to refer to both.[8] 'Cephale' named the head and its contents and for centuries was unrelated to the term 'neuros'.[7] It is therefore an interesting philological quirk that later in history it was 'neuros' rather than 'cephale' that was to be used as the generic term to name all things related to the brain.

The concepts of 'neurology'

The cognitive backbone of all disciplines, concepts obtain their meaning from the historical context in which they are in service and hence can help to date a convergence. Primary concepts are directly linked to objects and functions; secondary concepts are designed to manage the primary ones and carry with them explanatory and historical information. In the case of neurology, the primary concepts are associated with its many 'neurological diseases' and the secondary ones ('neurosis', 'lesion', 'disease', 'brain', 'mind', etc.) provide the mesh of ideas and assumptions supporting the primary concepts. There is space in this chapter to deal only with 'neurosis' (a secondary concept).

The concept of neuroses

The concept of 'neurosis' presided over: (1) the construction of neurology as a medical specialism; (2) the separation of neurology from Alienism (now psychiatry); and (3) the transformation of the notion of madness into that of 'psychosis'. Only the first two headings will be touched upon in this chapter.

The word neurosis was coined and defined by William Cullen: '*Sensu et motus laesi, sine pyrexia et sine morbo locali*' (p274)[9] and redefined six years later as: '*Sensu et motus laesi, sine pyrexia idiopathica, et sine morbo locali*' (p182). By the late 18th century this was translated as: 'An injury of the sense and motion, without an idiopathic pyrexia or any local lesion' (p27).[10] Early in the 19th century Thomson[11] retranslated it as: 'Sense and motion injured, without idiopathic pyrexia, and without local disease' (p31).

Under 'neuroses' Cullen listed conditions such as dyspepsia, belching, asthma, pertussis, cholera, diarrhoea, diabetes, insanity, etc. Given that the current (post-Freudian) concept of neurosis is unhelpful to understand Cullen's notion, it is essential to delve into its historical epistemology. As attested by the work of Jorden, Sydenham, and Willis,[12] the idea that pathological changes in the 'nervous system' could cause bodily diseases had been commented upon since the early 17th century. The problem here is to try to understand how 'nervous system' was defined during that historical period when even the distinction between sinews and nerves was still being disputed. For example, Blancard wrote: 'A Nerve is a fibrous, round, long, white, porous substance like an Indian cane, which conveys the animal spirits to make the parts of the body moveable and sensible ... all the nerves below the scull proceed from the spinal marrow ... a nerve, a tendon, and a ligament are impertinently taken for one and the same thing by Chirurgeons' (p207).[13]

Equally difficult to understand is the notion of 'lesion'. Currently it means: 'Any pathological or traumatic discontinuity of tissue or loss of function of a part' (p1025),[3] that is, it includes both anatomical or physiological change. Because during the 17th century the conceptual differentiation between structure and function had not yet been completed, 'lesion' only referred to a structural discontinuity. Under the influence of Vitalism[14] medics were still using the term 'vital' to refer to functions as in the case of 'irritability'.[15] Even at the beginning of the 19th century, lesions were still being defined as: 'altérations qui surviennent par une cause quelconque, dans les propriétés vitales ou la texture de nos parties: de là la distinction de ces lésions, qui constituent toutes les maladies dont le corps humain est susceptible, en deux classes très tranchées, en organiques et en vitales' (p485).[16] After vitalism became obsolete, 'vital lesions' were redefined as 'functional lesions': 'Lesion, derangement, disorder; any morbid change, either in the exercise of functions or in the texture of organs. Organic lesion is synonymous with organic disease' (p417).[17]

Cullen subscribed to a medical theory called 'neuralpathology', which nowadays is difficult to understand. According to López Piñero:

> Cullen's system can be considered as a version of vitalism, a doctrine developed during the Enlightenment as an offshoot of the Hallerian concept of 'irritability'. He was the best representative of the school of so-called 'neuropathology' (or neuralpathology) whose main postulate was the identification of the vital principle with the activity of the nervous system ... Vitalist writers, even those not interested in 'neuralpathology', gave a great deal of attention to the nervous system ... For example, during the period immediately prior to Cullen, the followers of Stahl emphasized the role played by the nervous system as the instrument of the 'anima' ... 'irritability' led to a form of vitalism which considered the nervous system as the physiological foundation of the body and of life itself; all diseases therefore could be reduced to being 'nervous' alterations.
>
> Reproduced with permission from López Piñero J M. *Historical Origins of the Concept of Neurosis*: 12. Copyright (1983) with permission from Cambridge University Press (p12)[18]

This explains why Cullen's concept of 'neurosis' was so broad and why it needed to undergo a major semantic metamorphosis before it became the Freudian concept of neurosis.

Listed as 'Class II' in Cullen's nosology, the 'neuroses' included four orders: *Comata* (e.g. apoplexia, paralysis, hysteria); *Adinamiae* (e.g. syncope, dyspepsia, hypochondriasis, tetanus, chorea); *Spasmi* (e.g. epilepsy, diabetes, asthma); and *Vesaniae* (e.g. amentia, melancholia, mania, paraphrosyne, oneirodynia).[10] These disorders were members of the neuroses class as long as they did not have a localized anatomical lesion ('morbus locali'). During the 19th century, two factors caused the class of the neuroses to become smaller. On the one hand, many conditions were found to be associated with localized lesions; on the other, vitalism was abandoned and with it the need to link all diseases to the central nervous system. By the 1880s, Axenfeld classified the neuroses as those concerning: sensibility (e.g. neuralgias, migraine, vertigo, angor pectoris); motility (convulsions, tics, dysphagia, palpitations, ischaemic paralysis, Parkinson's disease (PD)); and complex neuroses (such as chorea, epilepsy, neurasthenia, catalepsy, hysteria).[19]

Changes in the conceptualization of 'lesion' were also important to explain such attrition. By the end of the 19th century the concept of 'physiological lesion' had given rise to that of 'psychological lesion' (in regards to the functions of the mind). In the event, the Freudian neuroses only included hypochondriasis, hysteria, anxiety disorders, neurotic depression, obsessive compulsive disorder and, for a time, Raynaud's disease (p19;[20] p30;[21] p19[22]). By the interbellum period Raynaud's disease itself had been taken out, and the remaining five neuroses gained wide acceptance even by non-Freudian writers.[23,24,25] Indeed, the concept of neuroses was written out of existence only during the 1980s.[26]

The construction of neurology as a medical specialism occurred during the 19th century. Historians of neurology vary in their views, some conflating such history with: (1) the history of what currently are called 'neurological diseases';[27] (2) the biography of medics interested in such diseases;[28] and (3) the history of ideas about the brain.[29] However, historical data indicate that the construction of 'neurology' (as a medical specialism) was only possible during the 19th century when: (1) a view of the central nervous system had developed that was able to explain the multiple symptomatology of the neurological diseases; (2) vitalism had been abandoned and electrical and chemical transmission models of the central nervous system had become available; (3) neuropathology had for the first time achieved sufficient stability and coherence to generate credible descriptions; and (4) the sociology of the medical profession permitted for a new specialism to be formed.

All these developments interacted with the concept of neurosis. As diseases of sensation, motility, and cognition became described in association with 'focal lesions', the list of neurological disorders grew to achieve critical mass. Most had no treatment and required long-term management. In England, this need was met by the foundation of the *National Hospital for the Paralysed and Epileptic* in 1860.[30] Similar developments occurred in other European countries.

Neuropsychiatry

The *Oxford English Dictionary* defines neuropsychiatry as: 'Psychiatry which relates mental or emotional disturbance to disordered brain function; neurology and psychiatry as a single discipline'.[5] The origins of the term are not clear. The French term *Neuropsychiatrie* appears in 1910[31] to name the: 'aspects physiologiques et aux impacts du fonctionnement nerveux dans les perturbations psychologiques'.[6] In German it appears somewhat earlier: 'Im 19. Jahrhundert Bezeignung für die Disziplin, die sich mit Ursachen und Behandlungen psychischer Störungen organischen un nichorganischen [sic] (nervösen) Ursprungs befaßt' (p350)[32]. By 1918 the word was already in use in English. It is not clear whether it was just a transliteration of the French word.

To be of any use the word 'neuropsychiatry' must have a stable and recognizable referent. Currently, this tends to be what is called 'organic' or 'biological' psychiatry (whatever those terms may mean).[29] If thus, all these terms become synonymous and choice would depend upon social need, for example one could use neuropsychiatry because of its convenient neuroassociation.

Others define neuropsychiatry as the study of the 'mental symptoms' occurring in the context of neurological (as opposed to psychiatric) disease, that is, as the psychiatry of neurology and inner ear pathology. All manner of mental symptoms can be seen in the context of neurological disease and the job of the neuropsychiatrist would be to study such phenomena in comparison with their counterparts as seen in psychiatric disorders.[33] The assumption behind this definition of neuropsychiatry is that the mental symptoms seen in psychiatry and in neurology are not necessarily the same phenomena.[34] 'Behavioural neurology', a sub-specialism developed within neurology, tends to overlap somewhat with this second version of neuropsychiatry.[35]

Some cultural historians conceive of neuropsychiatry as a package of ideologies and social practices loosely woven around the foundational claim that 'all mental disorders are disorders of the brain'.[36,37] There is space in this chapter only to explore the history of this foundational claim.

Foundational claim

A foundational claim or assumption is a belief posited as the starting point for an argument, action, or research programme. 'All mental diseases are diseases of the brain', 'the brain houses the mind', and 'brain lesions cause mental disease' are the foundational claims of neuropsychiatry. In epistemological terms these three claims are only partially related; in historical terms they are known to have originated in different historical periods.

For example, during the early 19th century it was generally accepted that brain and mind were closely related but there was resistance to the idea that the mind was divisible[38] and hence the notion of partial insanity was rejected (p243).[39] Be that as it may, claims that some forms of madness are related to the body, and accounts of how they might be produced can be already found in the 17th century. Thus, Willis stated:

> Melancholy is commonly defined, a *raving without a fever or fury, joyn'd with fear and sadness*; whence it follows to be a complicated affect of the brain and of the heart; for, that melancholick persons rave, it proceeds from the fault of the brain, and the disorder of the animal spirits residing in it; but that they are *sad* and *timorous*, this is attributed to the passion of the heart.
>
> (p460)[40]

Sydenham, in turn, chose blood as an explanatory medium: 'this arises from too vivid and exalted crasis of the blood. There is also another sort of mania, which succeeds long-continued intermittent fevers, and at last degenerates into idiocy. This comes from weakness and vapidity of blood, brought on by over-long fermentation' (p94).[41]

David Hartley entertained a combination of post-Newtonian views of matter and Lockean associationism.[42] Mental disorders were related to distortions in the vibration pattern of brain fibres. A normal thought and a delusion were differentiable:

> Thus suppose a person, whose nervous system is disordered, to turn his thoughts *accidentally* to some barely possible good or evil. If the nervous disorder falls in with this, it increases the vibrations belonging to its ideas so much, as to give it a reality, a connection with self. For we distinguish the recollection and anticipation of things relating to ourselves, from those of things relating to other persons, chiefly by the difference of strength in the vibrations, and in their coalescences with each other.
>
> (p401)[43]

The pattern of vibrations was always determined by external stimuli. William Battie also explained insanity in terms of vibratory mechanisms. Insanity was preceded by 'nervous over-excitation' and followed by 'nervous insensitivity'.[44] 'Original' madness occurred when without any *external* stimulus the subject 'saw' fire or 'heard' sounds (i.e. experienced hallucinations). 'Consequential' madness occurred when a recognizable anomalous *internal* stimulus to the nerves caused similar experiences (e.g. an infection). This has been interpreted as an early differentiation between psychiatric and organic hallucinations.[45]

Towards the end of the 18th century, and based on a combination of associationism, materialism, and vitalism, Pierre Cabanis proposed a new approach to the relationship between 'matter' and 'mind'.[46] Matter included a vital energy that could trigger the emergence of a mind.[47] In order to understand this phenomenon a future science of man, language, and hermeneutics needed to be created.[48] Bodily organs generated complex feeling patterns and meanings: these constituted what was then called coenesthesia and could form the basis of hypochondriacal complaints.[49 50]

By the early 19th century, a new form of materialism developed within Alienism, as illustrated by the work of Georget.[51] His theoretical views were reinforced by the findings of AJ Bayle who claimed that dementia and mental disorder were features of the same disease, namely general paralysis of the insane.[52] Bayle's work has been considered by some as an early demonstration that mental disease was physical disease.[53]

Important in this context is the work of Wilhelm Griesinger, to whom the quotation that all mental diseases are diseases of the brain has been often attributed. A physician (the concept of psychiatrist did not exist at the time) interested in infectious disease, public health, mental disorder, and the therapeutic aspects of asylum care, Griesinger worked in Cairo for a time.[54–59] His contribution to Alienism is limited to one textbook, few papers, and the foundation of the *Archiv für Psychiatrie und Nervenkrankheiten*. His work was influenced by materialist biologism, vitalism, and romanticism. Griesinger was 28 in 1845 when he published his *Textbook of Mental Pathology and Therapeutics* and needed to borrow most of the clinical cases he used as illustrations. However, his philosophical maturity and imagination led him to suggest a new way of analysing mental disorders by introducing the concept of 'elementary' units of analysis which formed the epistemological basis of the new concept of mental symptom.

Uttered in 1845, the claim 'all mental disorders are disorders of the brain' is not easy to understand. Influenced by the metaphysical physiology of Wunderlich and others, Griesinger's concepts of 'disorder' and of 'lesion' were physiological and so he placed 'mental disorders' in a new explanatory space.[60] Hence his views have been open to multiple interpretations, for example, his claim that 'psychological events' may occur in some non-conscious space has made him into a 'pioneer' of psychodynamic psychiatry.[61] Griesinger wrote at the time when concepts such as the 'organic' and the 'physiological' were both still tinged by vitalism and hence cannot be translated into their 21st century counterparts. Thus, from the fact that he called a clinical phenomenon (e.g. a hallucination) 'organic' it does not follow that he expected it necessarily to leave a footprint in the brain.[62] In other words, mental disorders happen in the brain but do not necessarily have permanent representation.

Influenced by Darwinian evolution and by the new physiology, Meynert sought to correlate development, function, and form. Associationism, localizationism, top-to-bottom inhibition, regional cerebrovascular variations, and neuronal nutritional status determined the nature and localization of mental disorders.[63] Changes in the supply of cerebral blood explained physiological states (e.g. sleep), symptoms (e.g. obsessions and hallucinations), and diseases (e.g. mania, melancholia). Nutritional changes at cellular level, resulting from haemodynamic changes or from congenital defects, were the ultimate causal mechanism.

Opinions on the merit of Meynert's views were divided from the start.[64] As opposed to his neuro-histological work, his clinical writings (e.g. the concept of 'Amentia')[65,66] have been considered as speculative. Portrayed as a 'brain mythologizer', it is often neglected that he added a number of new metaphors and analogies to the neuroscientific narrative. His *Psychiatrie* is a textbook of neuroanatomy[63] with only *in passim* references to concepts such as ego or memory.[57] The second (clinical) volume was never published.

Karl Wernicke was one of the most original neuropsychiatrists of the late 19th century,[67] and had he not died young we would now be living in a Wernickian (and not Kraepelinian) world. His *pathophysiological model* to explain all brain-related diseases (whether 'psychiatric' or 'neurological') had enough power to link psychopathology with neuropsychology. The brain was constituted by a system of projection and (transcortical) association fibres which provided anatomical support to consciousness and the highest intellectual functions.[68] Lesions of the projection system gave rise to focalized pathology and neurological disease; lesions of the association system generated mental illness. Wernicke's organ of association is redolent of the later concept of neural network.[69]

JH Jackson's interest in mental disorders is expressed in *The Factors of Insanities*.[70] The central nervous system consisted in a structural hierarchy with upper functional layers inhibiting lower ones. Driven by evolution, the system had gained complexity at the expense of stability, that is, it was opened to dissolution. Jackson's model was not meant to be mapped onto the real central nervous system despite the attempts of some to do so.[71,72] Insanity was a generic term for all departures from stable mentation, from physiological states like sleep to temporary toxic states and to chronic brain diseases. Insanity was therefore dimensional rather than categorical. Indeed, Jackson wondered why alienists did not consider post-epileptic coma (which he called acute temporary dementia) as a form of insanity.[73]

Jackson proposed that four factors converged to cause insanity. Factor 1 concerned the 'depth' of dissolution; factor 2 'the *person* who has undergone dissolution'; factor 3 the rate of dissolution (how slow or fast the 'removal of control' was); and factor 4 included personal variables and themes around which positive mental symptoms may be formed.[74] The factors model cannot explain the formation of specific symptoms (e.g. hallucinations, delusions, imperative ideas, depressions, retardation, etc.). Jackson's views on mind and matter did not cohere with his dualism or with the concept of 'concomitance' which he borrowed from Clifford.[75] Jackson's stance vis-à-vis the foundationalist claim is unclear. Given his dimensional model (which was physiological rather than structural) and his belief in a continuity between temporal brain states such as sleep and insanity, it is not altogether clear whether the conventional concept of mental disease had any meaning to him.[76,77]

Introduction Biologique a L'étude de la Neurologie et de la Psychopathologie is one of the most neglected books on neuropsychiatry in the 20th century.[78] To be able to communicate their original insights Monakow and Mourgue introduced some neologisms. *Horme* named the 'tendency of all living beings to develop all their genetic potential'. This tendency was governed by *Syneidesis*, that is, by a principle that regulates and balances all instincts in the interest of the given individual. By modulating both function and structure such principles gave rise to a 'dynamo-morphological' model.[79] Neuropsychiatry was a subfield of biology governed by 'chronogenetic localization', that is, like music, all neuropsychiatric phenomena could only find full expression in a temporo-spatial frame. Functions (e.g. movement) were redefined as processes unfolding in time according to a specific 'kinetic melody'. This meant that brain processes (and the mental symptoms that their pathology might generate) could be localized *seriatim* in different brain sites. Chronogenetic localization was a late acquisition in evolutionary time, and hence it was complex and unstable.[80] One implication of this view was that standard cross-sectional and longitudinal clinical studies were *inadequate* to capture mental symptoms in their entirety.

Conclusions

The prefix 'neuro' has become fashionable and fulfils more than one function in the construction of neuro-neologisms. It can be a genuine scientific marker but often enough it is little more than a rhetorical device. In the case of neurology, neuropsychology, neuroimaging, neuropsychiatry, etc., the association with the neurosciences is likely to be warranted and will endure.

This short chapter has only dealt with the construction of neurology and neuropsychiatry. The former is currently a medical specialism and shows a stable epistemology and social basis. Neurology resulted from the convergence of the (recycled) word neurology, of a set of primary and secondary concepts and of a list of disorders.

The word neuropsychiatry appeared in European countries at different times and in each is likely to have meant something different. For example, in France it started by referring to the combined activity of Alienists and neurologists and it is only in 1968 that the French government officially separated the two specialisms. In the UK, neuropsychiatry has had different meanings and even today there is no agreed definition. In this chapter we support the view that it should name the psychiatry of neurology.

The foundational claim of neuropsychiatry is that mental diseases are diseases of the brain. This claim has been around since the 17th century and has changed meaning *pari passu* with changes in the meaning of concepts such as brain, disease, mind, etc. There is no reason to believe that the current meanings will last for ever. This means that neuropsychiatry is but the fluid name for a fluid activity. Whether it has any advantage over psychiatry, as such, remains to be seen.

REFERENCES

1. Berrios GE. Historiography of mental systems and diseases. History of Psychiatry. 1994; 5: 175–90.
2. Rheinberger HJ. On Historicizing Epistemology. Stanford: Stanford University Press, 2010.
3. Anderson DM. Dorland Illustrated Medical Dictionary (32nd edition). New York: Saunders, 2011.
4. Berrios GE. Convergences that are no more. History of Psychiatry. 2011; 22: 133–6.
5. Oxford English Dictionary (2nd edition). Oxford: Oxford University Press, 1992.
6. Rey A. Dictionnaire Historique de la Langue Française. Paris: LeRobert, 2011.
7. Liddell HG, Scott R. A Greek-English Lexicon. Oxford: Clarendon Press, 1996.
8. Goss CM. On anatomy of nerves by Galen of Pergamon. American Journal of Anatomy, 1966; 118: 327–36.
9. Cullen W. Synopsis Nosologiæ Methodicæ. Edinburgh (no publisher or printer), 1769
10. Cullen W. Synopsis and Nosology (2nd edition). Translated from Latin to English, Hartford: Springfield, 1793.
11. Cullen W. Synopsis of Nosology. Translated by John Thompson. Philadelphia: Dobson, 1816.
12. Hare E. The history of 'nervous disorders' from 1600 to 1840. British Journal of Psychiatry. 1991; 159: 37–45.
13. Blancard S. A Physical Dictionary in Which Terms Relating to Anatomy Chirurgery, etc. are Very Accurately Explained. London: Samuel Crouch, 1684.
14. Wheeler LR. Vitalism: its History and Validity. London: Whitherby, 1939.
15. Rey AL. Metaphysical problems in Francis Glisson's Theory of Irritability. In: Nachtomy O, Smith JEH (eds). The Life Sciences in Early Modern Philosophy. Oxford: Oxford University Press, 2014. pp85–98.
16. Nacquart (no initial). Lésion. In: Dictionnaire des Sciences Médicales. Vol 27, Paris: Panckoucke, 1818. pp485–545.
17. Dunglison R. Dictionary of Medical Sciences (5th edition). Philadelphia: Lea and Blanchard, 1845.
18. López Piñero JM. Historical Origins of the Concept of Neurosis. Cambridge: Cambridge University Press, 1983.
19. Axenfeld S. Traité des Névroses (2nd edition). Paris: Baillière, 1883.
20. Leveillé G. Syndrome de Maurice Raynaud. Paris: Vigot, 1900.
21. Belinky E. Syndrome de Raynaud. Lyon: A Rey, 1915.
22. Parodi M. Contribution a l'étude de la pathogénie de l'asphyxie locale et de la gangrène symétrique des extrémités. Alger: Carbonel, 1920.
23. Core DE (1922) Functional Nervous Disorders. Bristol: John Wright, 1922.
24. Ross TA. The Common Neuroses (2nd edition). London: Arnold, 1937.
25. Culpin M. The conception of 'nervous disorder'. Lancet. 1930; 1383–7.
26. Gossop M. Theories of Neurosis. Berlin: Springer, 1981.
27. Finger S, Boller F, Tyler KL. History of Neurology. Vol 95 of Handbook of Clinical Neurology. London: Elsevier, 2010.
28. Rose FC. History of British Neurology. London: Imperial College Press, 2012.
29. Trimble MR. The Intentional Brain. Baltimore: Johns Hopkins Press, 2016.
30. Critchley M. The Beginnings of the National Hospital Queen Square (1859–1850). BMJ, 1960: 1829–37.
31. Coutier M. Matériaux pour l'histoire du vocabulaire française. Pathologie mentale et disciplines connexes (1895–1930). Paris: Klincksieck, 1986.
32. Peters UH. Wörterbuch der Psychiatrie un medizinischen Psychologie. München: Urban & Schwarzenberg, 1990.
33. Berrios GE. What is neuropsychiatry? Revista Colombiana de Psiquiatria. 2007; (Suplemento 1): 9S–14S.
34. Berrios GE, Dening TR. Biological and quantitative issues in neuropsychiatry. Behavioural Neurology. 1990; 3: 247–59.
35. Benson DF. The history of behavioural neurology. Neurological Clinics. 1993; 11: 1–7.
36. Berrios GE, Marková IS. The concept of neuropsychiatry: a historical overview. Journal of Psychosomatic Research. 2002; 53: 629–38.
37. Berrios GE, Marková IS. Assessment and measurement in neuropsychiatry: a conceptual history. Seminars in Clinical Neuropsychiatry. 2002; 7: 5–10.
38. Hagner M. The soul and the brain between anatomy and Naturphilosophie in the early nineteenth century. Medical History. 1992; 36: 1–33.
39. Berrios GE. The history of mental symptoms. Cambridge: Cambridge University Press, 1996.
40. Willis T. The London Practice of Physick. London: Thomas Basset, 1685.

41. Sydenham T. The works of Thomas Sydenham MD. Vol 1. Translated by RG Latham. London: Sydenham Society, 1848.
42. Allen RC. David Hartley on Human Nature. New York: State University of New York Press, 1999.
43. Hartley D. Observations on Man, his Frame, his Duty and his Expectations. London: Thomas Tegg and Son, 1749.
44. Battie W. A Treatise on Madness. London: J Whiston and B White, 1758.
45. Leigh D. The Historical Development of Psychiatry. Vol 1, 18th and 19th Centuries. Oxford: Pergamon Press, 1961.
46. Staum MS. Cabanis. Enlightenment and Medical Philosophy in the French Revolution. Princeton: Princeton University Press, 1980.
47. Cabanis PJG. On the Relations between the Physical and Moral Aspects of Man. 2 Vols, Mora G (ed.). Baltimore, The Johns Hopkins University Press, 1981.
48. Besançon S. La philosophie de Cabanis. Paris: Les Empècheurs de penser en rond, 1997.
49. Barsky AJ. Patients who amplify bodily symptoms. Annals of Internal Medicine. 1979; 91: 63–70.
50. Berrios GE. Hypochondriasis: history of a concept. In: Starcevic V, Lipsitt DR (eds). Hypochondriasis: Modern Perspectives on an Ancient Malady. Oxford: Oxford University Press, 2001. pp3–20.
51. Georget E. De la Folie. Paris: Crevot, 1820.
52. Bayle ALJ. Traité des Maladies du cerveau et de ses membranes. Paris: Gabon, 1826.
53. Berrios GE. 'Depressive Pseudodementia' or 'Melancholic Dementia': A 19th Century View. Journal of Neurology, Neurosurgery, and Psychiatry. 1985; 48: 393–400.
54. Lasègue (no initial). Études psychologiques sur les hommes célèbres: Guillaume Griesinger. Annales Médico-Psychologiques. 1872; 30: 15–23.
55. Walser HH. Wilhelm Griesinger—von der Inneren Medizin zur Psychiatrie. Gesnerus. 1986; 43: 197–204.
56. Westphal C. Nekrolog für Griesinger. Archiv für Psychiatrie und Nervenkrankheiten. 1868; 1: 760–74.
57. Marx O. Nineteenth century medical psychology: theoretical problems in the work of Griesinger, Meynert, and Wernicke. Isis. 1970; 61: 355–70.
58. Marx O. Wilhelm Griesinger and the history of psychiatry: a reassessment. Bulletin of the History of Medicine. 1972; 46: 519–44.
59. Wahrig-Schmidt B. Der junge Wilhelm Griesinger in Spannungsfeld zwischen Philosophie und Physiologie. Tübingen, Gunter Narr, 1985.
60. Schiller J. Physiology struggle for independence in the first half of the nineteenth century. History of Science. 1968; 7: 64–89.
61. Dietze HJ, Voegele GE. Wilhelm Griesinger's contribution to Dynamic psychiatry. Diseases of the Nervous System. 1965; 26: 579–82.
62. Berrios GE. Griesinger. In: Porter R (ed.) Dizionario Biografico della Storia della Medicina delle Scienze Naturali (Liber Amicorum) Vol. 2, Florence: Franco Maria Ricci, 1987. pp129–130.
63. Meynert T. Psychiatry. A Clinical Treatise on Diseases of the Fore-Brain. New York: GP Putnam, 1885.
64. Whitehouse PJ. Theodor Meynert: foreshadowing modern concepts of neuropsychiatric pathophysiology. Neurology. 1985; 35: 389–91.
65. Pappenheim E. On Meynert's amentia. International Journal of Neurology. 1975; 9: 311–26.
66. Lévy-Friesacher CH. Meynert-Freud 'Amentia'. Paris: Presses Universitaires de France, 1983.
67. Lanczik M. Der Breslauer Psychiater Carl Wernicke. Sigmaringen: Jan Thorbecke, 1988.
68. Wernicke C. Grundriß der Psychiatrie in klinischen Vorlesungen, Leipzig: Thieme, 1906.
69. Stein DJ, Ludik J (eds.). Neural Networks and Psychopathology. Cambridge: Cambridge University Press, 1998.
70. Jackson JH. The factors of insanities. Medical Press and Circular. 1894; 108: 615–19.
71. Kennard C, Swash M. Hierarchies in Neurology. A reappraisal of a Jacksonian Concept. London: Springer, 1989.
72. Dubrovsky B. Evolution of nervous system and psychiatry. Consequences of the vertical and horizontal duality of the evolutionary process. Journal of Psychiatry & Neuroscience. 1993; 18: 245–59.
73. Berrios GE. Introduction to the 'factors of insanities'. History of Psychiatry. 2001; 12: 353–73.
74. Berrios GE. Positive and negative symptoms and Jackson: A conceptual history. Archives of General Psychiatry. 1985; 42: 95–7.
75. Berrios GE. Introduction to body and mind by CK Clifford. History of Psychiatry. 2000; 11: 311–17.
76. Dewhurst K. Hughlings Jackson on Psychiatry. Oxford: Sandford Publications, 1982.
77. Critchley M, Critchley EA. John Hughlings Jackson. Father of English Neurology. Oxford: Oxford University Press, 1998.
78. Monakow Von C, Mourgue R. Introduction Biologique a L'Étude de la Neurologie et de la Psychopathologie. Paris: Alcan, 1928.
79. Guiraud P. Psychiatrie Générale. Paris, Le François, 1950.
80. Mourgue R. L'Œvre et la personnalité du Professeur Constantin von Monakow (1853–1930). L'Encephale. 1931; 26: 417–28.

2

Neuroimaging and fluid biomarkers of Alzheimer's disease

Implications for definition, diagnosis, and treatment

Vijay R Varma, Yi-Fang Chuang, and Madhav Thambisetty

Introduction

The global cost of Alzheimer's disease (AD) and dementia is $818 billion and is expected to reach $1 trillion by 2018.[1] There are currently no interventions that delay the onset or progression of AD.[2] It is therefore imperative to develop treatments that can increase the number of disability-free life years for older adults.

Over the past decades, biomarkers have played a significant role in a shift in AD research. AD biomarkers, including imaging and cerebrospinal fluid (CSF) markers—and increasingly blood markers—are becoming essential indicators of health and disease, markers of pathogenic processes and of pharmacological responses to interventions. The most recent diagnostic criteria for AD, mild cognitive impairment (MCI), and preclinical AD provide guidelines for the use of such biomarkers in both research and clinical settings.[3,4] As treatment efforts shift towards targeting individuals in the prodromal and preclinical stages of AD, biomarkers are becoming the primary means of identifying at-risk individuals. However, a cautionary note that must be considered here is that the individuals presenting to the types of studies that require detailed biomarker measures may be unrepresentative of those who eventually develop dementia. It is possible, therefore, that the generalizability of findings from the research discussed here will be limited in relation to those at greatest risk of dementia both within high-income countries (HICS) as well as low and middle-income countries (LMICs). Nevertheless this, rather purer and younger, dementia type still represents a substantial proportion of dementia 'burden' within populations around the world.

Below we provide a summary of AD clinical and research criteria, and describe the main biomarker modalities in AD: imaging, CSF, and blood plasma/serum. We discuss in the detail the development and use of each in clinical and research studies.

Alzheimer's Disease Clinical and Research Criteria

AD is a progressive neurodegenerative disorder characterized by memory loss and cognitive decline that interferes with activities of daily living. The definitive diagnosis of AD requires histopathological evidence of AD pathology in the brain via autopsy or biopsy.[5] However, given the inability to definitively diagnose the disease until post-mortem examination, the routine diagnosis of AD in clinical practice is still largely based on clinical evaluation and neuropsychological testing showing progressive impairment of memory and decline in at least one other cognitive domain, meeting standardized criteria such as the International Statistical Classification of Diseases and Related Health Problems, 10th revision (ICD-10),[6] the Diagnostic and Statistical Manual for Mental Disorders, fourth edition (DSM-4),[7] and National Institute of Neurological and Communicative Disorders and Stroke and the Alzheimer's Disease and Related Disorders Association (NINCDS-ADRDA).[5]

After the first NINCDS-ADRDA clinical criteria were published in 1984,[5] biomarkers have become increasingly important in identifying incipient pathology during the evolution of AD. Over the past 20 years, the prevailing theory pertaining to pathogenesis of AD is the amyloid hypothesis, which postulates that Aβ deposition in the brain triggers a cascade of events leading to neuronal and synaptic loss, and neurofibrillary degeneration, finally resulting in dementia.[8] Biomarkers of AD that characterize neuropathological processes *in vivo* are useful in distinguishing AD from other dementias, detecting presymptomatic pathological changes, and/or monitoring disease progression and response to treatment.

In 2007, the International Working Group (IWG) proposed research specific criteria for the diagnosis of AD that included 'distinctive and reliable biomarkers of AD'.[9] In 2011, the NINCDS-ADRDA work group developed revised clinical criteria for the diagnosis of AD that incorporated biomarkers within two

Table 2.1 Staging categories for preclinical AD research

Stage	Description	Aβ (PET or CSF)	Markers of neuronal injury (tau, FDG, sMRI)	Evidence of subtle cognitive change
Stage 1	Asymptomatic cerebral amyloidosis	Positive	Negative	Negative
Stage 2	Asymptomatic amyloidosis + 'downstream' neurodegeneration	Positive	Positive	Negative
Stage 3	Amyloidosis + neuronal injury + subtle cognitive/behavioural decline	Positive	Positive	Positive

AD, Alzheimer's disease; Aβ, Amyloid beta; PET, positron emission tomography; CSF, cerebrospinal fluid; ^{18}F-FDG, ^{18}F-fluorodeoxyglucose; sMRI structural magnetic resonance imaging.
Reproduced with permission from Sperling R.A., Aisen P.S., Beckett L.A., Bennett D.A., Craft S., Fagan A.M., et al. Toward defining the preclinical stages of Alzheimer's disease: recommendations from the National Institute on Aging-Alzheimer's Association workgroups on diagnostic guidelines for Alzheimer's disease. *Alzheimers Dement*, 7(3): 280–292. DOI: https://doi.org/10.1016/j.jalz.2011.03.003.

main areas into associated research criteria: (1) Amyloid β (Aβ) accumulation, measured by low CSF Aβ and abnormal tracer retention on PET (positron emission tomography) and (2) neuronal degeneration, measured by high CSF tau and decreased ^{18}F-fluorodeoxyglucose (^{18}F-FDG) uptake on PET.[4,10] While CSF- and PET-based assessments of Aβ and tau are yet to be used in the routine clinical diagnosis of AD, FDG-PET has been used to help distinguish AD from other dementias such as frontotemporal dementia (FTD) and Lewy body dementia.[11] Ongoing research into their validation, comparison, and standardization may eventually lead to their use as part of the diagnostic work up for AD in clinical settings.[12]

In countries outside the USA, including the EU, AD biomarkers are increasingly being used in the clinic for the diagnostic evaluation of dementia. In 2014, the IWG-2 included measures of CSF $A\beta_{42}$ and tau as part of diagnostic criteria for AD; this was a revision of the 2007 IWG criteria.[3] Recent recommendations from the Biomarkers for AD and PD (BIOMARKAPD), funded by the EU joint programme—neurodegenerative disease research (JPND), additionally found sufficient evidence to support the use of biomarkers, including imaging and CSF, to supplement clinical evaluations and measure/monitor disease progress.[13]

Since the 1984 NINCDS-ADRDA criteria were published, there has been broad recognition that the prodrome of AD begins years, if not decades, prior to the onset of clinical symptoms.[14] The diagnosis of MCI was first defined in 1991,[15] and clinically characterized in 1999,[16] to describe subjects who show memory declines with preserved independent function. In 2011 the National Institute on Aging-Alzheimer's Association workgroup refined the diagnosis,[17] and recommended the use of Aβ and tau biomarkers to increase diagnostic accuracy of MCI individuals who will progress to AD (i.e. MCI due to AD). This included a 'positive' marker of Aβ and tau, indicating high likelihood that the MCI syndrome is due to AD, a 'positive' marker of Aβ only, or tau only (where Aβ has not or cannot be tested), indicating intermediate likelihood that the MCI syndrome is due to AD, and a 'negative' marker of Aβ and tau indicating that the MCI syndrome is unlikely to be due to AD.[17] A recent paper reported that the National Institute on Aging-Alzheimer's Association criteria using both amyloid and neuronal injury markers provided the most accurate prognosis in clinical settings.[18]

In 2011, the National Institute on Aging-Alzheimer's Association work group developed criteria for Preclinical AD.[19] Preclinical AD is conceptualized as the first (non-clinical) stage of AD where individuals who are cognitively normal show progression of AD pathophysiology as assessed by biomarker assessments of Aβ and tau in the CSF. The hypothetical biomarker model of the preclinical stage reflects staging proposed by Jack et al.,[20] and suggests that abnormal CSF markers of Aβ and abnormal PET-based amyloid imaging are the first indications of AD pathophysiology, preceding the appearance of markers of neuronal injury (see Table 2.1).[19]

Imaging Biomarkers

Neuroimaging presents an invaluable opportunity for developing reliable AD biomarkers, enabling neuropathological features to be visualized, either directly or indirectly, in the living brain. This is best illustrated in the use of amyloid-labelling PET tracers to quantify amyloid plaques *in vivo*, which correlates strongly with *in vitro* measures of $A\beta_{42}$ burden in post-mortem AD brains.[21] In the case of neurodegeneration in AD, routine pathological examination at autopsy shows atrophy, neuronal loss, and gliosis. Imaging correlates of these features include atrophy in vulnerable brain regions such as the hippocampus and entorhinal cortex, which can be detected by high-resolution magnetic resonance imaging (MRI).[22] These changes are also reflected at the cellular level by alternations in metabolites detected by magnetic resonance spectroscopy (MRS).[23] Further changes are evident with functional imaging using functional MRI (fMRI),[24] single positron emission computed tomography (SPECT), and FDG-PET.[25] Functional abnormalities are surrogates of synaptic dysfunction in early AD and of neuronal loss with disease progression. In this section, we provide an overview of currently available neuroimaging biomarkers, with a particular focus on their roles in distinguishing AD from other neurodegenerative diseases and prediction of disease progression.

Neuroimaging Biomarkers of Aβ42 Amyloid Deposition: Amyloid PET Imaging

PET imaging allows for non-invasive quantification of cerebral blood flow, metabolism, and receptor binding. PET imaging involves the introduction of a radioactive tracer usually through an intravenous injection. A tracer is essentially a biological compound of interest that is labelled with a positron-emitting isotope, such as carbon-11 (^{11}C), fluorine-18 (^{18}F), or oxygen-15 (^{15}O).

Quantitative PET studies using diverse Aβ radiotracers have demonstrated significantly elevated retention in the brains of AD patients compared to age-matched controls.[26] The regional distribution of high amyloid retention is in frontal, posterior cingulate, precuneus, striatum, parietal, and lateral temporal cortices, in concordance with the regional distribution of amyloid pathology previously documented in post-mortem studies.[27] This regional pattern allows differentiation of AD from FTD and PD, though significant retention and a similar pattern may also be seen in dementia with Lewy bodies (DLB).[28] In a two-year longitudinal study in AD patients, there was no significant change in Aβ deposition over time, despite a decline in cerebral glucose metabolism and cognition.[29] This dissociation between PiB retention and disease progression suggests that amyloid levels in the brain may reach a plateau early in the course of disease and preceding a decline in brain function.

Approximately 50–70% of patients presenting to clinical research settings with imaging facilities, and receiving a diagnosis of MCI, show significantly elevated cortical [^{11}C]PiB retention with intermediate levels compared to AD patients and normal controls.[26,30] This high Aβ burden in MCI patients is found to correlate with lower episodic memory performance.[31,32] Furthermore, in longitudinal studies assessing the effect of Aβ deposition on disease progression, MCI patients with high [^{11}C]PiB retention at baseline have a higher rate of progression to AD than those with low Aβ burden, with sensitivity ranging from 83.3% to 100% and specificity from 41.1% to 100%, respectively.[33] Intriguingly, about 25–35% of cognitively normal elderly individuals present with high cortical [^{11}C]PiB retention with a similar regional pattern to AD patients.[30,34] These findings are consistent with results from autopsy studies reporting that about 25% of non-demented older individuals over the age of 75 have Aβ plaques in their brains.[35] Indeed, the association between the presence of neuritic plaques in the brain with dementia is weaker with increasing age, and in those over 90 years of age, multiple pathologies may contribute to dementia prevalence.[36,37]

Subsequent to the US Food and Drug Administration (FDA) approval of amyloid PET imaging for clinical use, the Amyloid Imaging Task Force of the Alzheimer's Association and Society for Nuclear Medicine and Molecular Imaging proposed appropriate-use criteria for amyloid imaging in clinical practice. In summary, these guidelines recommend that amyloid PET is appropriately used for patients with a persistent or progressive unexplained MCI; patients satisfying main clinical criteria for possible AD; and patients with early onset AD.[38,39]

Neuroimaging Biomarkers of Neurodegeneration: Fluorodeoxyglucose-PET

FDG-PET measures glucose metabolism by labelling glucose with [^{18}F] FDG and measuring its uptake in the brain, which is highly correlated with post-mortem measures of the synaptic structural protein synaptophysin.[40] Therefore, reduced brain metabolism measured by FDG-PET may be an indicator of impaired synaptic function. ^{18}FDG-PET studies in patients with AD show a specific topographic pattern of hypometabolism in the lateral temporoparietal, posterior cingulate cortices, and the precuneus. FDG-PET is closely linked to progression of clinical symptoms, supported by the observation that greater decreases in FDG uptake correlate with greater cognitive impairment along the continuum from normal cognitive status to MCI to AD. Together, these data indicate that FDG-PET uptake may be a valid indicator of the synaptic dysfunction that accompanies neurodegeneration in AD.[20]

Single-Photon Emission Computed Tomography (SPECT)

SPECT imaging uses direct photon-emitting isotopes rather than radioisotopes, and is less expensive, but has a lower resolution compared to PET. SPECT imaging is most commonly used to assess regional cerebral blood flow (rCBF) by using lipophilic and neutral tracer agents such as ^{99m}Tc-bicisate (ECD) and ^{99m}Tc-exametazime (HMPAO). In early AD and MCI patients, reduced CBF has been observed in the parietal, posterior temporal lobes, posterior cingulate, and precuneus, similar to the topological pattern of hypometabolism in ^{18}FDG-PET studies.[41,42] Prospective studies with histological confirmation in demented patients and controls have shown that the sensitivity and specificity of rCBF SPECT imaging for the differentiation of patients with AD from control subjects is 89% and 80%, respectively.[43]

Magnetic Resonance Imaging

The evolution of MRI techniques has provided important new perspectives for the development of neuroimaging biomarkers in AD.

Quantitative structural MRI studies demonstrate that volume loss in the medial temporal lobe, namely entorhinal cortex and hippocampus, is a significant and early marker of disease development in AD.[44] Volumetric or voxel-based studies show a strong correlation between the severity of atrophy and the severity of cognitive impairment. In particular, hippocampal volume is reduced in MCI patients by 10–15%, while in mild and moderate AD it is reduced by 15–30% and 30–40% respectively.[44] Longitudinal studies have shown decreased volume in the medial temporal lobe at baseline to be predictive of progression from MCI to AD, with sensitivity of 79% and specificity of 82%.[45]

Magnetic Resonance Spectroscopy

MRS is an imaging technique measuring biochemical changes that can be related to neuronal loss in AD by quantification of metabolites including myo-Inositol (mI), choline (Cho), N-acetylaspartate (NAA), and creatine (Cr). The most extensively studied biomarker using MRS in AD is decreased NAA/Cr ratio. Studies show that there is a decrement in NAA/Cr ratio in the whole brain, posterior cingulate, and superior temporal lobe between AD, MCI, and cognitively normal controls. Furthermore, lower NAA/Cr in MCI patients predicts progression to AD.[46]

Functional MRI

While neuronal loss is an obvious endpoint resulting from the progression of AD pathology and can be measured by cortical atrophy on structural MRI, there is accumulating evidence that it is preceded by neuronal dysfunction.[47] Therefore, functional neuro-imaging techniques, such as fMRI and arterial spin labelling (ASL)-MRI, are especially useful to measure neuronal activity and connectivity in AD. These imaging techniques are based either on changes in cerebral blood flow and cerebral blood volume or changes revealed by the blood oxygen level dependent (BOLD) effect.

In AD patients, fMRI studies utilizing episodic memory tasks consistently report decreased hippocampal or parahippocampal activity during the encoding of new information. However, task-based fMRI studies in individuals at risk for AD, including MCI patients and genetically at-risk individuals, have yielded somewhat inconsistent findings, including both decreased and increased medial temporal lobe (MTL) activation.[48] Longitudinal studies suggest that MTL hyperactivity at baseline may be a predictor of MCI conversion to AD, presumably reflecting functional compensation to accumulating AD pathology.[24] In resting state fMRI studies, the most consistent finding is decreased functional connectivity in AD patients compared to healthy older controls within the posterior default mode network region comprising the precuneus and posterior cingulate cortex.[49]

Diffusion Tensor Imaging

Pathological studies have revealed various types of white matter alterations in AD, such as altered myelin and oligodendrocytes, axonal degeneration, and vascular pathologies.[50–52] Diffusion tensor imaging (DTI) is an MRI technique that assesses white matter integrity by measuring the non-random movement of water molecules. In DTI, two frequently employed parameters are fractional anisotropy (FA) measuring directionality of fibre tracts and mean diffusivity (MD) determining the magnitude of overall water diffusion.[53,54]

Increased MD was consistently found in brain regions vulnerable to neurofibrillary pathology in AD, such as the hippocampus, entorhinal cortex, parahippocampal gyrus, temporo-parietal association cortex, and posterior cingulate gyrus.[53] A meta-analysis of 41 DTI studies in AD and MCI patients indicates a large effect size of white matter damage in the posterior cingulum, as well as other major white matter bundles connecting the prefrontal cortex with the medial temporal lobe and parietal cortex.[55]

Tau Imaging

The time course of tau aggregation and its dynamic relationship to other pathophysiological features in AD remain unclear. Hypothetical models of disease progression including tau pathology have been derived mainly from CSF-based measures of tau.[20,56] The development of tau-specific PET tracers is therefore a major breakthrough and allows us to measure tau deposition *in vivo* in the brain for the first time. Based on both *in vitro* and *in vivo* results, three families of radiotracers have so far shown promise as tau-specific PET tracers: the aryquinoline derivatives THK5117, THK5317, and THK5351, the pyrido-indole derivative AV-1451 (also known as ^{18}F-T807 and ^{18}F-flortaucipir), and the phenyl/pyridinyl-butadienyl-benzothiazole/benzothiazolium derivative, PBB3.

Since the advent of tau PET imaging, a growing number of studies have assessed the retention of tau PET tracers in patients with AD, in comparison to normal controls. Although different tracers may have distinct characteristics and limitations, these studies consistently found higher tau retention in AD patients compared to controls in several brain areas, especially in the medial temporal regions, in agreement with the distribution of tau deposits reported from histopathological studies.[57–59] In AD patients, increased tau retention, either globally or in the temporal cortex, is related to severity of cognitive impairment.[60] Exciting as the development of *in vivo* tau imaging is, there are also technical challenges that need to be overcome before large-scale application. The recent observation that ^{18}F-THK5351 retention in the brain is confounded by the widespread distribution of monoamine oxidase B (MAO-B) is particularly illustrative of this important consideration.[61]

Cerebrospinal Fluid Biomarkers

CSF is produced mainly from arterial blood by the choroid plexuses in the ventricles of the brain. The CSF represents one of the most direct means of studying pathology that accumulates in the brain because it is one of the only accessible fluids (*in vivo*) not separated from the brain by the blood brain barrier, it is in direct contact with the extracellular space in the brain, and it crosses interstitial fluid drainage pathways.[62] The CSF is therefore most likely, relative to other fluids including blood, to reflect biomarker profiles of normal brain physiology as well as disease pathology related to neurological disorders such as AD.

Clinical and Research Criteria for CSF Biomarkers in AD

Since the first NINCDS-ADRDA clinical criteria for AD were published,[6] CSF has become the primary ante-mortem means of identifying the central pathogenic processes, that is, the aggregation of Aβ and tau in AD. The prevailing explanation for the AD pathologic process, that is, the amyloid hypothesis, suggests that deposition of Aβ is followed by tau pathology, neurodegeneration, clinical symptoms, and dementia.[63] CSF biomarkers figure prominently in hypothetical models as the earliest biomarkers reflecting AD-related changes in Aβ and tau, relative to amyloid PET and MRI/FDG PET respectively.[56]

In 2007, IWG criteria for the diagnosis of AD included available and reliable CSF markers of pathology. In 2011, the NINCDS-ADRDA incorporated CSF biomarkers for measuring Aβ (i.e. CSF $A\beta_{42}$) and tau accumulation.[10] In 2014, IWG-2 revised criteria also included CSF $A\beta_{42}$ and elevated CSF tau as part of diagnostic criteria for AD,[3] emphasizing, however, that evidence did not indicate CSF biomarkers outperformed imaging biomarkers, or suggest that the use of CSF biomarkers improved patient well-being or reduced healthcare costs.

Below we provide an overview of the use of CSF to measure Aβ and tau concentrations as markers of AD pathophysiology.

Amyloid β

Over the past 25 years, low CSF $A\beta_{42}$ concentration has become one of the most established markers of amyloid plaque burden in the brain. In addition to clinical and epidemiologic studies exploring its diagnostic utility, post-mortem studies have clearly shown correlations between CSF levels of $A\beta_{42}$ and fibrillar $A\beta_{42}$ levels in the brain.[64,65] The seemingly counterintuitive finding that *low* levels of CSF $A\beta_{42}$ indicate greater plaque burden in the brain may be explained by reduced availability of Aβ to diffuse into the CSF due to its aggregation as insoluble plaques in the brain.[66]

The diagnostic accuracy of CSF $A\beta_{42}$ to discriminate between AD and controls has been reviewed by a number of studies. A recent meta-analysis by Olsson et al. aggregated studies from 1984–2014

Table 2.2 Summary of meta-analysis of CSF and blood biomarkers of AD

	AD: CON			MCI progress: MCI stable		
	N; cohorts	ratio (95% CI)	p-value	N; cohorts	ratio (95% CI)	p-value
Aβ						
CSF	N: 9949 AD/6841 CON Cohorts: 142 AD/134 CON	0.56 (0.55–0.58)	p<0.0001	352 MCI-AD/610 MCI Cohorts: 12 MCI-AD/12 MCI	0.67 (0.63–0.73)	p<0.0001
serum/ plasma	N: 1872 AD/3855 CON Cohorts: 22 AD/20 CON	1.04 (0.96–1.12)	p = 0.32	308 MCI-AD/379 MCI Cohorts: 3 MCI-AD/3 MCI	0.81 (0.53–1.24)	p = 0.32
t-tau						
CSF	N: 11341 AD/7086 CON Cohorts: 164 AD/143 CON	2.54 (2.44–2.64)	p<0.0001	307 MCI-AD/570 MCI Cohorts: 12 MCI-AD/12 MCI	1.76 (1.64–1.89)	p<0.0001
serum/ plasma	N: 271 AD/394 CON Cohorts: 6 AD/5 CON	1.95 (1.12–3.38)	p = 0.02		NSD	
p-tau						
CSF	N: 7498 AD/5126 CON Cohorts: 96 AD/ 91 CON	1.88 (1.79–1.97)	p<0.0001	251 MCI-AD/501 MCI Cohorts: 9 MCI-AD/9 MCI	1.72 (1.46–2.02)	p<0.0001
serum/ plasma		NSD			NSD	

AD, Alzheimer's disease; CON, Control; MCI, mild cognitive impairment; CI, confidence interval; NSD, not sufficient data.

Results indicate whether tissue-specific (i.e. CSF, serum/plasma) biomarkers of Aβ, t-tau, and p-tau may discriminate between AD vs CON samples and MCI progressors (to dementia) vs MCI stable samples.

Source: data from Olsson B., Lautner R., Andreasson U., Ohrfelt A., Portelius E., Bjerke M., et al. CSF and blood biomarkers for the diagnosis of Alzheimer's disease: a systematic review and meta-analysis. *Lancet neurology*. 2016; 15(7):673–84.

and indicated a significant difference in CSF $A\beta_{42}$ concentration in AD vs controls (Table 2.2).

The sensitivity and specificity of CSF $A\beta_{42}$ to discriminate between AD and control groups was 80% (95% CI 78–82) and 76% (95% CI 74–78) respectively.[6] The sensitivity and specificity of the Innogenetics ELISA method, the most commonly used assay for CSF $A\beta_{42}$, has a specificity and sensitivity of 86% and 90% respectively, to discriminate between AD and controls.[69] Generally, $A\beta_{42}$ is less useful in discriminating AD from non-AD dementias[70] and to measure AD severity.[71]

CSF $A\beta_{42}$ levels are also significantly different between MCI subjects who progress to dementia vs MCI subjects who remain stable (Table 2.2). Studies have consistently shown moderate to high sensitivity and specificity in the range of 55–91% and 56–96% respectively in discriminating MCI subjects who progress to dementia vs MCI subjects who remain stable.[72]

As indicated above, CSF $A\beta_{42}$ is a required component of staging categories for preclinical AD according to the National Institute on Aging-Alzheimer's Association criteria.[19] Recent studies have begun to explore the utility of CSF-defined preclinical criteria in estimating the approximate prevalence of non-symptomatic individuals at risk for AD, exploring the diagnostic value of using CSF $A\beta_{42}$ and PET imaging,[73] and testing the utility of measuring longitudinal changes in CSF $A\beta_{42}$ during the preclinical stages of AD.[74]

Tau (total and phosphorylated; t-tau, p-tau)

Tau is a microtubule-associated protein that stabilizes neuronal microtubules and is essential for neurite outgrowth.[75] Hyperphosphorylation of tau results in its detachment from microtubules and disruption of its physiological function as a stabilizer of microtubules, resulting in a breakdown of axonal structure, disruption of axonal transport, and eventual aggregation into intracellular paired helical filaments, constituting neurofibrillary tangles.[76]

Similar to $A\beta_{42}$, the diagnostic utility of t-tau and p-tau to discriminate between AD and controls has been reviewed by multiple studies. In the largest meta-analysis to date, Olsson et al. reported a significant difference in the CSF t-tau and p-tau concentration in AD vs controls (Table 2.2). Sensitivity/specificity of CSF t-tau and p-tau in discriminating AD from controls ranges between 73–85%/86–93% and 70–87%/75–91% respectively.[77,78] Similar to $A\beta_{42}$, CSF t-tau and p-tau are less useful in discriminating AD from non-AD dementias.[79]

CSF t-tau and p-tau levels are also significantly different between MCI subjects who progress to dementia vs MCI subjects who remain stable (Table 2.2). A recent meta-analysis from the Cochrane Database of Systematic Reviews reported sensitivity/specificity ranges for t-tau and p-tau in discriminating MCI due to AD between 51–90%/48–88% and 40–100%/22–86%.[80] Ritchie et al. concluded that the heterogeneity in diagnostic utility across the studies reviewed suggested uncertainty in the use of either CSF t-tau or p-tau for the diagnosis of AD in clinical practice.[80]

CSF t-tau and p-tau are key components of the staging definitions in preclinical AD and are significant in particular to the stage immediately preceding, or most proximal to MCI (i.e. Stage 3).[19] Recent research suggests that tau may be a more robust predictor or marker of risk during the early preclinical AD stages compared to $A\beta_{42}$.[81] The recent development of tau imaging[82] will help better elucidate the role of tau, particularly in the preclinical stages of AD.

There is a consensus that that the combination of CSF Aβ and tau (e.g. t-tau/Aβ ratio) provides better diagnostic utility, and greater sensitivity and specificity than any of the biomarkers alone in discriminating AD subjects from controls as well as MCI subjects progressing to AD vs stable MCI subjects.[83,84]

Experimental CSF Biomarkers

As our understanding of the underlying biology of AD pathogenesis expands, a number of novel and promising CSF biomarkers are being explored, particularly in the area of neurodegeneration. Neurofilament light (NFL) protein is a major component of the axonal cytoskeleton, which maintains axon calibre, size, and shape. A number of studies have shown that NFL may be a marker of neuronal degeneration associated with dementia comorbidities, including white matter lesions and other cerebrovascular diseases.[85–88] Recently, Zetterberg et al. found that CSF NFL was associated with AD progression, and may be a useful biomarker, in combination with imaging, to track non- Aβ and non-tau aspects of neurodegeneration.[89]

Neurogranin (NGRN) is a postsynaptic brain protein expressed in dendritic spines. Prior studies have shown that NGRN is decreased in AD subjects compared to controls,[90,91] and a recent publication by Kester et al. showed that CSF NGRN predicted progression from MCI to AD and may be a useful marker within the preclinical AD stages.[92]

Blood Biomarkers

Blood-based biomarkers offer the potential for non-invasive and inexpensive diagnosis of AD and monitoring disease progression. Unlike CSF and imaging biomarkers, blood biomarkers can be easily and routinely implemented in community settings,[93] and generally allow for repeated sampling in large cohorts. One of the main challenges to identifying AD blood biomarkers is the lack of a direct interaction between peripheral blood and the brain because of the blood brain barrier (BBB). This is one of the major physiological challenges to the development of blood biomarkers.[94] The BBB, however, has been shown to increase in permeability with ageing and AD,[95] suggesting that blood may reflect pathology as disease progresses.

Another major challenge to the development of blood biomarkers for AD is that similar to other late onset and gradually progressive diseases, there are many non-disease related alterations in cellular processes due to chronic conditions and medications that may be reflected in peripheral blood.[93]

Clinical and Research Criteria

Currently, blood biomarkers are not included in standard clinical and research criteria across the disease stages, including preclinical AD, MCI, and AD. However, a number of recent reviews have highlighted promising advances in the field, suggesting the potential for their clinical use.[96–98]

While CSF and imaging biomarkers have been highlighted in diagnostic criteria as increasingly critical to diagnosing individuals with AD or MCI that will progress to AD, blood biomarkers may also have the potential to identify individuals at greatest risk of incident AD, progressing from MCI to AD, or rapid progression within AD.[97] Recent blood biomarker studies,[93,94] have also begun to move away from binary discrimination of established AD/MCI from control samples toward exploring endophenotypes, or specific patholologic or clinical markers of AD that are relevant to the long preclinical prodrome of the disease.[98] These studies have the potential to identify crucial biological changes that occur prior to clinical symptom onset,[99] and also suggest that blood biomarkers may be a potential screening tool for efficiently identifying individuals within large samples who have a higher likelihood of testing positive for either CSF or neuroimaging markers.

Broadly, research exploring blood biomarkers for AD test the diagnostic or prognostic utility of: (1) one or a few analytes that reflect specific pathologic features of the disease (e.g. Aβ and/or tau) or (2) a panel of molecules reflecting a disease signature.

β-amyloid

As outlined previously, the predominant AD hypothesis suggests that Aβ accumulation in the brain is the first of a series of events leading to neurodegeneration and clinical symptoms. Therefore, plasma Aβ markers, including $A\beta_{42}$ (as well as $A\beta_{40}$, and the ratio of $A\beta_{42}$:$A\beta_{40}$) have been the most studied blood biomarkers for AD. The majority of studies and reviews generally indicate that plasma Aβ is not a reliable diagnostic marker of AD or MCI subjects who will progress to AD.[100–103] A recent meta-analysis by Olsson et al.[67] showed that AD subjects compared to normal controls, as well as MCI subjects who progressed to dementia compared to MCI subjects who remained stable, did not significantly differ in concentration of plasma/serum $A\beta_{42}$ (Table 2.2). There was however, a small, significant association for $A\beta_{40}$.[67]

While numerous studies have shown that the correlation between CSF Aβ/PET amyloid plaque imaging and plasma Aβ is weak,[103–105] a recent report using immunoprecipitation coupled with mass spectrometry received considerable attention as it demonstrated that plasma amyloid-β precursor protein $(APP)_{669-711}$/amyloid-β $(A\beta)_{1-42}$ and $A\beta_{1-40}/A\beta_{1-42}$ ratios could accurately predict brain amyloid-β burden measured through PiB-PET imaging.[106] One plausible explanation for the lack of correlation between blood-derived Aβ concentrations and brain amyloid burden reported in prior studies, may be the differing origins of Aβ in blood compared to the brain. While Aβ in the CSF and the ISF has been shown to originate predominantly in the CNS, Aβ from the CNS may only be reflected in low concentrations in the blood due to the BBB. Aβ in the blood has been shown to also originate from APP metabolism in skeletal muscle, pancreas, and other peripheral cells, as well as platelets.[101,107] Prior work has additionally indicated that assays for blood Aβ have high measurement variability and often lack sensitivity and reliability.[94,97,100,101]

While cross-sectional studies have generally indicated that plasma Aβ may not provide reliable diagnostic utility, longitudinal studies have shown that plasma Aβ may reflect risk during the preclinical stages.[108,109]

Tau

Tau, the primary marker of neurodegeneration, is in low abundance in the blood; ultrasensitive assays are therefore required in order to sensitively and accurately measure plasma or serum concentration of tau.[110] Exploring serum and plasma markers of tau in AD has been a relatively recent research focus; these studies, albeit in small samples, have generally shown that blood markers of tau are associated with clinical and cognitive outcomes relevant to brain injury.[111–113] Olsson et al. reported a significant difference in plasma/serum t-tau concentration in AD vs controls (Table 2.2). Generally, assays for plasma and serum p-tau levels have not been shown to be useful as AD biomarkers. One exception is recent work by Winston et al., using plasma neuron-derived exosomes (NDE) that showed that p-tau and $A\beta_{1-42}$ measured in NDE may be of utility in predicting conversion of MCI to AD dementia.[114]

Zetterberg et al. recently explored plasma tau levels in AD and MCI samples using a new ultrasensitive tau assay and found significantly elevated levels in AD patients compared to controls. However, ranges of tau levels in the AD group overlapped with both controls and MCI. Moreover, plasma tau levels in MCI patients progressing to AD were similar to stable MCI individuals.[115] It is important to note that this study did not find a significant correlation between plasma t-tau and CSF t-tau, suggesting that—similar to plasma Aβ—blood and CSF levels of t-tau may be differentially regulated. Using a similarly sensitive assay, Dage et al. recently found that plasma tau levels were higher in MCI subjects compared to cognitively normal controls, and that levels were associated cross-sectionally with cortical thickness and memory performance.[116]

Biomarker Panels

With the advancement of standardized, reliable, and cost-efficient mass spectrometry methods to measure multiple proteins and other metabolic products simultaneously, panels of proteins or metabolites are being explored as potential biomarkers for AD.

Metabolomics, a relatively newer 'omics' methodology compared to proteomics, has recently generated excitement because of the potential to capture the complex and multifactorial physiological pathways that may be altered in AD.[117,118] Metabolomics measures the biochemical products of cell processes downstream of genomic, transcriptomic, and proteomic systems, and therefore may closely reflect disease related endophenotypes.[119] Many recent studies have explored the potential for developing AD biomarkers through metabolomic profiling in blood. Mapstone et al., in particular, generated excitement in 2014 with their study identifying ten lipids from blood plasma[120] that predicted conversion to MCI or AD with 90% accuracy.[121] These findings were, however, not replicated in subsequent studies.[122,123]

A significant issue in AD blood biomarker studies is the lack of replication across different cohorts. As discussed by Thambisetty and Lovestone, adequately powered studies that aim to validate index findings using alternative approaches in independent cohorts is critical, as is independent replication of such findings by other groups.[93]

Ongoing research focusing on alternative study designs using standardized platform and assay methodologies where endpoints are established endophenotypes of AD pathology, as well as a merging of methodologies and expertise from diverse fields, including epidemiology, network biology, and data science to analyse large and longitudinal cohorts, will continue to move blood biomarkers closer towards clinical utility.

Limitations and Implications

A number of evaluation criteria have been developed and utilized across fields, including most recently, personal genomics,[124] to evaluate biomarkers in chronic diseases. Broad criteria include reproducibility, stability over time, wide availability, and whether the biomarker is a direct reflection of the disease process.[125] Considering clinical utility of the common neuroimaging modalities, only structural MRI—specifically atrophy of the medial temporal lobe—is considered useful in routine clinical practice in the diagnosis of AD.[44] Thus, the rather positive framing of the research evidence as summarized within the body of this chapter does require tempering with the realities of performance in more representative populations at risk in different cultural and socioeconomic settings. The evidence base relating to amyloid and ^{18}FDG-PET imaging has been systematically reviewed and these Cochrane reviews have not supported the routine clinical use of either amyloid-PET[126] or ^{18}FDG-PET[127] to predict conversion to dementia in individuals diagnosed with MCI. It is therefore important that further translational studies are performed to test the clinical utility of these biomarkers that show promise in tertiary referral centres before their deployment in routine clinical practice.

CSF biomarkers of t-tau, p-tau, or p-tau/Aβ ratio are deemed to be of limited clinical utility in routine practice due to risk of misdiagnosis or over diagnosis of dementia.[67]

For research and clinical trials, however, biomarkers broadly are becoming increasingly essential for enrolling preclinical subjects and tracking the biological effects of drugs.[128,129] Recent FDA regulations have even allowed biomarkers as the primary endpoints and can serve as the basis for accelerated approval of novel therapeutics.[130]

Summary and Future Directions

The discovery of novel biomarkers reflecting the pathophysiology of AD has raised the possibility that they may be used in relation to dementia outcomes in individuals at high risk. This has facilitated a long anticipated shift in the way we will think about treating AD in the future.[12,131] The use of CSF and imaging biomarkers to define the early stages of AD progression have been critical in recognizing that the key molecular events triggering the eventual development of AD dementia begin decades before the appearance of symptoms. These biomarkers have already had far-reaching impacts on clinical practice as aids in both diagnosis of AD as well as in prognosis in individuals with mild symptoms. However, it is likely that the greatest influence of AD biomarkers will be in the design of clinical trials targeting early/presymptomatic stages of disease progression. Ongoing clinical trials like the 'Anti-Amyloid Treatment in Asymptomatic Alzheimer's' (A4) study testing the efficacy of Aβ immunization as a disease-modifying treatment in preclinical AD, thus require biomarker evidence of Aβ accumulation in the brain as a criterion for enrolment.[132] The incorporation of biomarkers both to identify patients likely to benefit from experimental treatments as well as to monitor the response to such interventions are likely to become routine in the design of AD clinical trials. As research into AD biomarkers expands, the identification of biomarkers associated with distinct molecular features of AD such as neuroinflammation, perturbations in energy metabolism, lipid homeostasis, and abnormalities in specific neurotransmitter systems are in turn, likely to spur the development of novel classes of disease-modifying treatments.

REFERENCES

1. Prince M, Wimo A, Guerchet M, Ali G, Wu Y, Prina M. World Alzheimer Report 2015: The Global Impact of Dementia, an Analysis of Prevalence, Incidence, Cost and Trends. London: Alzheimer's Disease International, 2015.
2. Daviglus ML, Bell CC, Berrettini W, Bowen PE, Connolly ES, Jr, Cox NJ, et al. National Institutes of Health State-of-the-Science Conference statement: preventing Alzheimer disease and cognitive decline. Annals of Internal Medicine. 2010; 153(3): 176–81. PubMed PMID: 20547888. eng.
3. Dubois B, Feldman HH, Jacova C, Hampel H, Molinuevo JL, Blennow K, et al. Advancing research diagnostic criteria for Alzheimer's disease: the IWG-2 criteria. Lancet Neurology. 2014; 13(6): 614–29. PubMed PMID: 24849862.
4. McKhann GM, Knopman DS, Chertkow H, Hyman BT, Jack CR, Jr, Kawas CH, et al. The diagnosis of dementia due to Alzheimer's disease: recommendations from the National Institute on Aging-Alzheimer's Association workgroups on diagnostic guidelines for Alzheimer's disease. Alzheimer's Dementia. 2011; 7(3): 263–9. PubMed PMID: 21514250. Pubmed Central PMCID: PMC3312024.
5. McKhann G, Drachman D, Folstein M, Katzman R, Price D, Stadlan EM. Clinical diagnosis of Alzheimer's disease: report of the NINCDS-ADRDA Work Group under the auspices of Department of Health and Human Services Task Force on Alzheimer's Disease. Neurology. 1984; 34(7): 939–44. PubMed PMID: 6610841.
6. World Health Organization. International Statistical Classification of Diseases and Related Health Problems Vol. 1. Geneva: WHO, 2004.
7. American Psychiatric Association. Task Force on D-I. Diagnostic and Statistical Manual of Mental Disorders: DSM-IV-TR. Washington, DC: American Psychiatric Association, 2000.
8. Villemagne VL, Cappai R, Barnham KJ, Cherny RA, Opazo C, Novakovic KE, et al. The Aβcentric pathway of Alzheimer's disease. In: Barrow CJ, Small DH (eds). Aβeta Peptide and Alzheimer's Disease: Celebrating a Century of Research. London: Springer London; 2007. pp5–36.
9. Dubois B, Feldman HH, Jacova C, Dekosky ST, Barberger-Gateau P, Cummings J, et al. Research criteria for the diagnosis of Alzheimer's disease: revising the NINCDS-ADRDA criteria. Lancet Neurology. 2007; 6(8): 734–46. PubMed PMID: 17616482.
10. Jack CR, Jr, Albert MS, Knopman DS, McKhann GM, Sperling RA, Carrillo MC, et al. Introduction to the recommendations from the National Institute on Aging-Alzheimer's Association workgroups on diagnostic guidelines for Alzheimer's disease. Alzheimer's Dementia. 2011; 7(3): 257–62. PubMed PMID: 21514247. Pubmed Central PMCID: PMC3096735.
11. Marcus C, Mena E, Subramaniam RM. Brain PET in the diagnosis of Alzheimer's disease. Clinical Nuclear Medicine. 2014; 39(10): e413–422; quiz e23–26. PubMed PMID: 25199063. Pubmed Central PMCID: 4332800.
12. Goate A, Holtzman DM. Biomarkers will revolutionize the way we diagnose and treat Alzheimer's disease. Biomarkers in Medicine. 2010; 4(1): 1–2. PubMed PMID: 20387300.
13. Simonsen AH, Herukka SK, Andreasen N, Baldeiras I, Bjerke M, Blennow K, et al. Recommendations for CSF AD biomarkers in the diagnostic evaluation of dementia. Alzheimer's Dementia. 2017; 13(3): 274–84. PubMed PMID: 28341065.
14. Sperling R, Mormino E, Johnson K. The evolution of preclinical Alzheimer's disease: implications for prevention trials. Neuron. 2014; 84(3): 608–22. PubMed PMID: 25442939. Pubmed Central PMCID: 4285623.
15. Flicker C, Ferris SH, Reisberg B. Mild cognitive impairment in the elderly: predictors of dementia. Neurology. 1991; 41(7):1006–9. PubMed PMID: 2067629.
16. Petersen RC, Smith GE, Waring SC, Ivnik RJ, Tangalos EG, Kokmen E. Mild cognitive impairment: clinical characterization and outcome. Archives of Neurology. 1999; 56(3): 303–8. PubMed PMID: 10190820. eng.
17. Albert MS, DeKosky ST, Dickson D, Dubois B, Feldman HH, Fox NC, et al. The diagnosis of mild cognitive impairment due to Alzheimer's disease: recommendations from the National Institute on Aging-Alzheimer's Association workgroups on diagnostic guidelines for Alzheimer's disease. Alzheimer's Dementia. 2011; 7(3): 270–79. PubMed PMID: 21514249. Pubmed Central PMCID: 3312027.
18. Vos SJ, Verhey F, Frolich L, Kornhuber J, Wiltfang J, Maier W, et al. Prevalence and prognosis of Alzheimer's disease at the mild cognitive impairment stage. Brain. 2015; 138(Pt 5): 1327–38. PubMed PMID: 25693589. Pubmed Central PMCID: 5013930.
19. Sperling RA, Aisen PS, Beckett LA, Bennett DA, Craft S, Fagan AM, et al. Toward defining the preclinical stages of Alzheimer's disease: recommendations from the National Institute on Aging-Alzheimer's Association workgroups on diagnostic guidelines for Alzheimer's disease. Alzheimer's Dementia. 2011; 7(3): 280–92. PubMed PMID: 21514248. Pubmed Central PMCID: 3220946.
20. Jack CR, Jr, Knopman DS, Jagust WJ, Shaw LM, Aisen PS, Weiner MW, et al. Hypothetical model of dynamic biomarkers of the Alzheimer's pathological cascade. Lancet Neurology. 2010; 9(1): 119–28. PubMed PMID: 20083042. eng.
21. Rabinovici GD, Jagust WJ. Amyloid imaging in aging and dementia: testing the amyloid hypothesis in vivo. Behavioural Neurology. 2009; 21(1): 117–28. PubMed PMID: 19847050. Pubmed Central PMCID: PMC2804478.
22. Johnson KA, Fox NC, Sperling RA, Klunk WE. Brain imaging in Alzheimer disease. Cold Spring Harbor Perspectives in Medicine. 2012; 2(4): a006213. PubMed PMID: 22474610. Pubmed Central PMCID: 3312396.
23. Wang H, Tan L, Wang HF, Liu Y, Yin RH, Wang WY, et al. Magnetic resonance spectroscopy in Alzheimer's disease: systematic review and meta-analysis. Journal of Alzheimer's Disease. 2015; 46(4): 1049–70. PubMed PMID: 26402632.
24. Sperling R. Potential of functional MRI as a biomarker in early Alzheimer's disease. Neurobiology of Aging. 2011; 32(Suppl 1): S37–43. PubMed PMID: 22078171. Pubmed Central PMCID: PMC3233699.
25. Coimbra A, Williams DS, Hostetler ED. The role of MRI and PET/SPECT in Alzheimer's disease. Current Topics in Medicinal Chemistry. 2006; 6(6): 629–47. PubMed PMID: 16712496.

26. Villemagne VL, Chetelat G. Neuroimaging biomarkers in Alzheimer's disease and other dementias. Ageing Research Reviews. 2016; 30: 4–16. PubMed PMID: 26827785. Epub 2016/02/02. eng.
27. Klunk WE, Engler H, Nordberg A, Wang Y, Blomqvist G, Holt DP, et al. Imaging brain amyloid in Alzheimer's disease with Pittsburgh Compound-B. Annals of Neurology. 2004; 55(3): 306–19. PubMed PMID: 14991808.
28. Villemagne VL, Rowe CC. Amyloid imaging. International Psychogeriatrics. 2011; 23(Suppl 2): S41–9. PubMed PMID: 21729418.
29. Engler H, Forsberg A, Almkvist O, Blomquist G, Larsson E, Savitcheva I, et al. Two-year follow-up of amyloid deposition in patients with Alzheimer's disease. Brain. 2006; 129(Pt 11): 2856–66. PubMed PMID: 16854944.
30. Small GW, Kepe V, Ercoli LM, Siddarth P, Bookheimer SY, Miller KJ, et al. PET of brain amyloid and tau in mild cognitive impairment. New England Journal of Medicine. 2006; 355(25): 2652–63. PubMed PMID: 17182990.
31. Pike KE, Savage G, Villemagne VL, Ng S, Moss SA, Maruff P, et al. Beta-amyloid imaging and memory in non-demented individuals: evidence for preclinical Alzheimer's disease. Brain. 2007; 130(Pt 11): 2837–44. PubMed PMID: 17928318.
32. Ong K, Villemagne VL, Bahar-Fuchs A, Lamb F, Chetelat G, Raniga P, et al. (18)F-florbetaben Aβeta imaging in mild cognitive impairment. Alzheimer's Research & Therapy. 2013; 5(1): 4. PubMed PMID: 23324163. Pubmed Central PMCID: PMC3580329.
33. Ma Y, Zhang S, Li J, Zheng DM, Guo Y, Feng J, et al. Predictive accuracy of amyloid imaging for progression from mild cognitive impairment to Alzheimer disease with different lengths of follow-up: a meta-analysis. [Corrected]. Medicine (Baltimore). 2014; 93(27): e150. PubMed PMID: 25501055. Pubmed Central PMCID: PMC4602781.
34. Rowe CC, Ellis KA, Rimajova M, Bourgeat P, Pike KE, Jones G, et al. Amyloid imaging results from the Australian Imaging, Biomarkers and Lifestyle (AIBL) study of aging. Neurobiology of Aging. 2010; 31(8): 1275–83. PubMed PMID: 20472326.
35. Bennett DA, Schneider JA, Arvanitakis Z, Kelly JF, Aggarwal NT, Shah RC, et al. Neuropathology of older persons without cognitive impairment from two community-based studies. Neurology. 2006; 66(12): 1837–44. PubMed PMID: 16801647.
36. Kawas CH, Kim RC, Sonnen JA, Bullain SS, Trieu T, Corrada MM. Multiple pathologies are common and related to dementia in the oldest-old: The 90+ Study. Neurology. 2015; 85(6): 535–42. PubMed PMID: 26180144. Pubmed Central PMCID: 4540246.
37. Savva GM, Wharton SB, Ince PG, Forster G, Matthews FE, Brayne C, et al. Age, neuropathology, and dementia. New England Journal of Medicine. 2009; 360(22): 2302–9. PubMed PMID: 19474427.
38. Johnson KA, Minoshima S, Bohnen NI, Donohoe KJ, Foster NL, Herscovitch P, et al. Appropriate use criteria for amyloid PET: a report of the Amyloid Imaging Task Force, the Society of Nuclear Medicine and Molecular Imaging, and the Alzheimer's Association. Alzheimer's Dementia. 2013; 9(1): e1–16. PubMed PMID: 23360977. Pubmed Central PMCID: PMC3733252.
39. Johnson KA, Minoshima S, Bohnen NI, Donohoe KJ, Foster NL, Herscovitch P, et al. Update on appropriate use criteria for amyloid PET imaging: dementia experts, mild cognitive impairment, and education. Amyloid Imaging Task Force of the Alzheimer's Association and Society for Nuclear Medicine and Molecular Imaging. Alzheimer's Dementia. 2013; 9(4): e106–109. PubMed PMID: 23809369.
40. Rocher AB, Chapon F, Blaizot X, Baron JC, Chavoix C. Resting-state brain glucose utilization as measured by PET is directly related to regional synaptophysin levels: a study in baboons. Neuroimage. 2003; 20(3): 1894–8. PubMed PMID: 14642499.
41. Binnewijzend MA, Kuijer JP, Benedictus MR, van der Flier WM, Wink AM, Wattjes MP, et al. Cerebral blood flow measured with 3D pseudocontinuous arterial spin-labeling MR imaging in Alzheimer disease and mild cognitive impairment: a marker for disease severity. Radiology. 2013; 267(1): 221–30. PubMed PMID: 23238159.
42. Dai W, Lopez OL, Carmichael OT, Becker JT, Kuller LH, Gach HM. Mild cognitive impairment and Alzheimer disease: patterns of altered cerebral blood flow at MR imaging. Radiology. 2009; 250(3): 856–66. PubMed PMID: 19164119. Pubmed Central PMCID: 2680168.
43. Jobst KA, Barnetson LP, Shepstone BJ. Accurate prediction of histologically confirmed Alzheimer's disease and the differential diagnosis of dementia: the use of NINCDS-ADRDA and DSM-III-R criteria, SPECT, X-ray CT, and Apo E4 in medial temporal lobe dementias. Oxford Project to Investigate Memory and Aging. International Psychogeriatrics. 1998; 10(3): 271–302. PubMed PMID: 9785148.
44. Frisoni GB, Fox NC, Jack CR, Jr, Scheltens P, Thompson PM. The clinical use of structural MRI in Alzheimer disease. Nature Reviews. 2010; 6(2): 67–77. PubMed PMID: 20139996. Pubmed Central PMCID: PMC2938772.
45. Landau SM, Harvey D, Madison CM, Reiman EM, Foster NL, Aisen PS, et al. Comparing predictors of conversion and decline in mild cognitive impairment. Neurology. 2010; 75(3): 230–38. PubMed PMID: 20592257. Pubmed Central PMCID: PMC2906178.
46. Graff-Radford J, Kantarci K. Magnetic resonance spectroscopy in Alzheimer's disease. Neuropsychiatric Disease and Treatment. 2013; 9: 687–96. PubMed PMID: 23696705. Pubmed Central PMCID: PMC3658533.
47. Roth Kas JJ. Apoptosis in neurodegenerative disease. In: Hof P, Mobbs C (eds). Handbook of the Neuroscience of Aging. Cambridge, MA: Academic Press, 2009. pp139–46.
48. Dickerson BC, Sperling RA. Functional abnormalities of the medial temporal lobe memory system in mild cognitive impairment and Alzheimer's disease: insights from functional MRI studies. Neuropsychologia. 2008; 46(6): 1624–35. PubMed PMID: 18206188. Pubmed Central PMCID: 2760288.
49. Vemuri P, Jones DT, Jack CR, Jr. Resting state functional MRI in Alzheimer's disease. Alzheimer's Research & Therapy. 2012; 4(1): 2. PubMed PMID: 22236691. Pubmed Central PMCID: PMC3471422.
50. Brun A, Englund E. A white matter disorder in dementia of the Alzheimer type: a pathoanatomical study. Annals of Neurology. 1986; 19(3): 253–62. PubMed PMID: 3963770.
51. Englund E, Brun A, Alling C. White matter changes in dementia of Alzheimer's type. Biochemical and neuropathological correlates. Brain. 1988; 111 (Pt 6): 1425–39. PubMed PMID: 3208064.
52. Sjobeck M, Haglund M, Englund E. Decreasing myelin density reflected increasing white matter pathology in Alzheimer's disease—a neuropathological study. International Journal of Geriatric Psychiatry. 2005; 20(10): 919–26. PubMed PMID: 16163742.
53. Oishi K, Mielke MM, Albert M, Lyketsos CG, Mori S. DTI analyses and clinical applications in Alzheimer's disease. Journal

of Alzheimer's disease. 2011; 26(Suppl 3): 287–96. PubMed PMID: 21971468. Pubmed Central PMCID: PMC3294372.
54. Alexander AL, Lee JE, Lazar M, Field AS. Diffusion tensor imaging of the brain. Neurotherapeutics. 2007; 4(3): 316–29. PubMed PMID: 17599699. Pubmed Central PMCID: 2041910.
55. Sexton CE, Kalu UG, Filippini N, Mackay CE, Ebmeier KP. A meta-analysis of diffusion tensor imaging in mild cognitive impairment and Alzheimer's disease. Neurobiology of Aging. 2011; 32(12): 2322 e5–18. PubMed PMID: 20619504.
56. Jack CR, Jr, Knopman DS, Jagust WJ, Petersen RC, Weiner MW, Aisen PS, et al. Tracking pathophysiological processes in Alzheimer's disease: an updated hypothetical model of dynamic biomarkers. Lancet Neurology. 2013; 12(2): 207–16. PubMed PMID: 23332364. eng.
57. Cho H, Choi JY, Hwang MS, Kim YJ, Lee HM, Lee HS, et al. In vivo cortical spreading pattern of tau and amyloid in the Alzheimer disease spectrum. Annals of Neurology. 2016; 80(2): 247–58. PubMed PMID: 27323247.
58. Johnson KA, Schultz A, Betensky RA, Becker JA, Sepulcre J, Rentz D, et al. Tau positron emission tomographic imaging in aging and early Alzheimer disease. Annals of Neurology. 2016; 79(1): 110–19. PubMed PMID: 26505746. Pubmed Central PMCID: PMC4738026.
59. Hansson O, Grothe MJ, Strandberg TO, Ohlsson T, Hagerstrom D, Jogi J, et al. Tau pathology distribution in Alzheimer's disease corresponds differentially to cognition-relevant functional brain networks. Frontiers in Neuroscience. 2017; 11: 167. PubMed PMID: 28408865. Pubmed Central PMCID: PMC5374886.
60. Tosun D, Landau S, Aisen PS, Petersen RC, Mintun M, Jagust W, et al. Association between tau deposition and antecedent amyloid-beta accumulation rates in normal and early symptomatic individuals. Brain. 2017. PubMed PMID: 28334939.
61. Ng KP, Pascoal TA, Mathotaarachchi S, Therriault J, Kang MS, Shin M, et al. Monoamine oxidase B inhibitor, selegiline, reduces 18F-THK5351 uptake in the human brain. Alzheimer's Research & Therapy. 2017; 9(1): 25. PubMed PMID: 28359327. Pubmed Central PMCID: 5374697.
62. Agamanolis D. Chapter 14: Cerebrospinal Fluid 2016. Available from: http://neuropathology-web.org/chapter14/chapter14CSF.html.
63. Karran E, Mercken M, De Strooper B. The amyloid cascade hypothesis for Alzheimer's disease: an appraisal for the development of therapeutics. Nature Reviews Drug Discovery. 2011; 10(9): 698–712. PubMed PMID: 21852788.
64. Tapiola T, Alafuzoff I, Herukka SK, Parkkinen L, Hartikainen P, Soininen H, et al. Cerebrospinal fluid {beta}-amyloid 42 and tau proteins as biomarkers of Alzheimer-type pathologic changes in the brain. Archives of Neurology. 2009; 66(3): 382–89. PubMed PMID: 19273758.
65. Strozyk D, Blennow K, White LR, Launer LJ. CSF Aβeta 42 levels correlate with amyloid-neuropathology in a population-based autopsy study. Neurology. 2003; 60(4): 652–6. PubMed PMID: 12601108.
66. Weller RO. How well does the CSF inform upon pathology in the brain in Creutzfeldt-Jakob and Alzheimer's diseases? Journal of Pathology. 2001; 194(1): 1–3. PubMed PMID: 11329133.
67. Olsson B, Lautner R, Andreasson U, Ohrfelt A, Portelius E, Bjerke M, et al. CSF and blood biomarkers for the diagnosis of Alzheimer's disease: a systematic review and meta-analysis. Lancet Neurology. 2016; 15(7): 673–84. PubMed PMID: 27068280.
68. Mo JA, Lim JH, Sul AR, Lee M, Youn YC, Kim HJ. Cerebrospinal fluid beta-amyloid1-42 levels in the differential diagnosis of Alzheimer's disease–systematic review and meta-analysis. PLOS One. 2015; 10(2): e0116802. PubMed PMID: 25710596. Pubmed Central PMCID: 4339391.
69. Blennow K, Hampel H. CSF markers for incipient Alzheimer's disease. Lancet Neurology. 2003; 2(10): 605–13. PubMed PMID: 14505582.
70. Holtzman DM. CSF biomarkers for Alzheimer's disease: current utility and potential future use. Neurobiology of Aging. 2011; 32(Suppl 1): S4–49. PubMed PMID: 22078172. Pubmed Central PMCID: 3233690.
71. Blennow K, Dubois B, Fagan AM, Lewczuk P, de Leon MJ, Hampel H. Clinical utility of cerebrospinal fluid biomarkers in the diagnosis of early Alzheimer's disease. Alzheimer's Dementia. 2015; 11(1): 58–69. PubMed PMID: 24795085. Pubmed Central PMCID: 4386839.
72. Ferreira D, Perestelo-Perez L, Westman E, Wahlund LO, Sarria A, Serrano-Aguilar P. Meta-review of CSF core biomarkers in Alzheimer's disease: the state-of-the-art after the new revised diagnostic criteria. Frontiers in Aging Neuroscience. 2014; 6: 47. PubMed PMID: 24715863. Pubmed Central PMCID: 3970033.
73. Adamczuk K, Schaeverbeke J, Vanderstichele HM, Lilja J, Nelissen N, Van Laere K, et al. Diagnostic value of cerebrospinal fluid Aβ ratios in preclinical Alzheimer's disease. Alzheimer's Research & Therapy. 2015; 7(1): 75. PubMed PMID: 26677842. Pubmed Central PMCID: 4683859.
74. Sutphen CL, Jasielec MS, Shah AR, Macy EM, Xiong C, Vlassenko AG, et al. Longitudinal cerebrospinal fluid biomarker changes in preclinical Alzheimer disease during middle age. JAMA Neurology. 2015; 72(9): 1029–42. PubMed PMID: 26147946. Pubmed Central PMCID: 4570860.
75. Mandelkow EM, Mandelkow E. Tau in Alzheimer's disease. Trends in Cell Biology. 1998; 8(11): 425–7. PubMed PMID: 9854307.
76. Ballatore C, Lee VM, Trojanowski JQ. Tau-mediated neurodegeneration in Alzheimer's disease and related disorders. Nature Reviews Neuroscience. 2007; 8(9): 663–72. PubMed PMID: 17684513.
77. Bloudek LM, Spackman DE, Blankenburg M, Sullivan SD. Review and meta-analysis of biomarkers and diagnostic imaging in Alzheimer's disease. Journal of Alzheimer's Disease. 2011; 26(4): 627–45. PubMed PMID: 21694448.
78. Mitchell AJ. CSF phosphorylated tau in the diagnosis and prognosis of mild cognitive impairment and Alzheimer's disease: a meta-analysis of 51 studies. Journal of Neurology, Neurosurgery, and Psychiatry. 2009; 80(9): 966–75. PubMed PMID: 19465413.
79. van Harten AC, Kester MI, Visser PJ, Blankenstein MA, Pijnenburg YA, van der Flier WM, et al. Tau and p-tau as CSF biomarkers in dementia: a meta-analysis. Clinical Chemistry and Laboratory Medicine. 2011; 49(3): 353–66. PubMed PMID: 21342021.
80. Ritchie C, Smailagic N, Noel-Storr AH, Ukoumunne O, Ladds EC, Martin S. CSF tau and the CSF tau/Aβeta ratio for the diagnosis of Alzheimer's disease dementia and other dementias in people with mild cognitive impairment (MCI). Cochrane Database of Systematic Reviews (Online). 2017; 3: CD010803. PubMed PMID: 28328043.
81. Brier MR, Gordon B, Friedrichsen K, McCarthy J, Stern A, Christensen J, et al. Tau and Aβeta imaging, CSF measures, and cognition in Alzheimer's disease. Science translational medicine.

2016; 8(338): 338ra66. PubMed PMID: 27169802. Pubmed Central PMCID: 5267531.

82. Saint-Aubert L, Lemoine L, Chiotis K, Leuzy A, Rodriguez-Vieitez E, Nordberg A. Tau PET imaging: present and future directions. Molecular neurodegeneration. 2017; 12(1): 19. PubMed PMID: 28219440. Pubmed Central PMCID: 5319037.
83. Blennow K, Hampel H, Weiner M, Zetterberg H. Cerebrospinal fluid and plasma biomarkers in Alzheimer disease. Nature Reviews. 2010; 6(3): 131–44. PubMed PMID: 20157306.
84. Shaw LM, Vanderstichele H, Knapik-Czajka M, Clark CM, Aisen PS, Petersen RC, et al. Cerebrospinal fluid biomarker signature in Alzheimer's disease neuroimaging initiative subjects. Annals of Neurology. 2009; 65(4): 403–13. PubMed PMID: 19296504. Pubmed Central PMCID: 2696350.
85. Hoglund K, Fourier A, Perret-Liaudet A, Zetterberg H, Blennow K, Portelius E. Alzheimer's disease—recent biomarker developments in relation to updated diagnostic criteria. Clinica Chimica Acta; International Journal of Clinical Chemistry. 2015; 449: 3–8. PubMed PMID: 25668231.
86. Hu YY, He SS, Wang XC, Duan QH, Khatoon S, Iqbal K, et al. Elevated levels of phosphorylated neurofilament proteins in cerebrospinal fluid of Alzheimer disease patients. Neuroscience Letters. 2002; 320(3): 156–60. PubMed PMID: 11852185.
87. Pijnenburg YA, Janssen JC, Schoonenboom NS, Petzold A, Mulder C, Stigbrand T, et al. CSF neurofilaments in frontotemporal dementia compared with early onset Alzheimer's disease and controls. Dementia and Geriatric Cognitive Disorders. 2007; 23(4): 225–30. PubMed PMID: 17290105.
88. Rosengren LE, Karlsson JE, Sjogren M, Blennow K, Wallin A. Neurofilament protein levels in CSF are increased in dementia. Neurology. 1999; 52(5): 1090–3. PubMed PMID: 10102440.
89. Zetterberg H, Skillback T, Mattsson N, Trojanowski JQ, Portelius E, Shaw LM, et al. Association of cerebrospinal fluid neurofilament light concentration with Alzheimer disease progression. JAMA Neurology. 2016; 73(1): 60–7. PubMed PMID: 26524180.
90. Thorsell A, Bjerke M, Gobom J, Brunhage E, Vanmechelen E, Andreasen N, et al. Neurogranin in cerebrospinal fluid as a marker of synaptic degeneration in Alzheimer's disease. Brain Research. 2010; 1362: 13–22. PubMed PMID: 20875798.
91. Kvartsberg H, Duits FH, Ingelsson M, Andreasen N, Ohrfelt A, Andersson K, et al. Cerebrospinal fluid levels of the synaptic protein neurogranin correlates with cognitive decline in prodromal Alzheimer's disease. Alzheimer's Dementia. 2015; 11(10): 1180–90. PubMed PMID: 25533203.
92. Kester MI, Teunissen CE, Crimmins DL, Herries EM, Ladenson JH, Scheltens P, et al. Neurogranin as a cerebrospinal fluid biomarker for synaptic loss in symptomatic Alzheimer disease. JAMA Neurology. 2015; 72(11): 1275–80. PubMed PMID: 26366630. Pubmed Central PMCID: 4694558.
93. Thambisetty M, Lovestone S. Blood-based biomarkers of Alzheimer's disease: challenging but feasible. Biomarkers in Medicine. 2010; 4(1): 65–79. PubMed PMID: 20387303. Pubmed Central PMCID: 2863057.
94. Henriksen K, O'Bryant SE, Hampel H, Trojanowski JQ, Montine TJ, Jeromin A, et al. The future of blood-based biomarkers for Alzheimer's disease. Alzheimer's Dementia. 2014; 10(1):115–31. PubMed PMID: 23850333. Pubmed Central PMCID: 4128378.
95. Rosenberg GA. Blood-brain barrier permeability in aging and Alzheimer's disease. Journal of Prevention of Alzheimer's Disease. 2014; 1(3): 138–9. PubMed PMID: 26301207. Pubmed Central PMCID: 4543304.
96. O'Bryant SE. Introduction to special issue on advances in blood-based biomarkers of Alzheimer's disease. Alzheimer's Dementia (Amst). 2016; 3: 110–2. PubMed PMID: 27453933. Pubmed Central PMCID: 4949589.
97. O'Bryant SE, Mielke MM, Rissman RA, Lista S, Vanderstichele H, Zetterberg H, et al. Blood-based biomarkers in Alzheimer disease: current state of the science and a novel collaborative paradigm for advancing from discovery to clinic. Alzheimer's Dementia. 2017; 13(1):45–58. PubMed PMID: 27870940. Pubmed Central PMCID: 5218961.
98. Shi L, Baird AL, Westwood S, Hye A, Dobson R, Thambisetty M, et al. A decade of blood biomarkers for Alzheimer's disease research: an evolving field, improving study designs, and the challenge of replication. Journal of Alzheimer's Disease. 2018; 62(3):1181–98. PubMed PMID: 29562526. Pubmed Central PMCID: 5870012.
99. Varma VR, Varma S, An Y, Hohman TJ, Seddighi S, Casanova R, et al. Alpha-2 macroglobulin in Alzheimer's disease: a marker of neuronal injury through the RCAN1 pathway. Molecular Psychiatry. 2017; 22(1): 13–23. PubMed PMID: 27872486.
100. Mehta PD, Pirttila T, Mehta SP, Sersen EA, Aisen PS, Wisniewski HM. Plasma and cerebrospinal fluid levels of amyloid beta proteins 1-40 and 1-42 in Alzheimer disease. Archives of Neurology. 2000; 57(1): 100–105. PubMed PMID: 10634455.
101. Toledo JB, Shaw LM, Trojanowski JQ. Plasma amyloid beta measurements—a desired but elusive Alzheimer's disease biomarker. Alzheimer's Research & Therapy. 2013; 5(2): 8. PubMed PMID: 23470128. Pubmed Central PMCID: 3706955.
102. Song F, Poljak A, Valenzuela M, Mayeux R, Smythe GA, Sachdev PS. Meta-analysis of plasma amyloid-beta levels in Alzheimer's disease. Journal of Alzheimer's Disease. 2011; 26(2): 365–75. PubMed PMID: 21709378.
103. Koyama A, Okereke OI, Yang T, Blacker D, Selkoe DJ, Grodstein F. Plasma amyloid-beta as a predictor of dementia and cognitive decline: a systematic review and meta-analysis. Archives of Neurology. 2012; 69(7): 824–31. PubMed PMID: 22451159. Pubmed Central PMCID: 3772635.
104. Le Bastard N, Aerts L, Leurs J, Blomme W, De Deyn PP, Engelborghs S. No correlation between time-linked plasma and CSF Aβ levels. Neurochemistry International. 2009; 55(8): 820–5. PubMed PMID: 19695299.
105. Baird AL, Westwood S, Lovestone S. Blood-based proteomic biomarkers of Alzheimer's disease pathology. Frontiers in Neurology. 2015; 6: 236. PubMed PMID: 26635716. Pubmed Central PMCID: 4644785.
106. Nakamura A, Kaneko N, Villemagne VL, Kato T, Doecke J, Dore V, et al. High performance plasma amyloid-beta biomarkers for Alzheimer's disease. Nature. 2018; 554(7691): 249–54. PubMed PMID: 29420472.
107. Roher AE, Esh CL, Kokjohn TA, Castano EM, Van Vickle GD, Kalback WM, et al. Amyloid beta peptides in human plasma and tissues and their significance for Alzheimer's disease. Alzheimer's Dementia. 2009; 5(1): 18–29. PubMed PMID: 19118806. Pubmed Central PMCID: 2663406.
108. van Oijen M, Hofman A, Soares HD, Koudstaal PJ, Breteler MM. Plasma Aβ (1-40) and Aβ (1-42) and the risk of dementia: a prospective case-cohort study. Lancet Neurology. 2006; 5(8): 655–60. PubMed PMID: 16857570.
109. Graff-Radford NR, Crook JE, Lucas J, Boeve BF, Knopman DS, Ivnik RJ, et al. Association of low plasma Aβ42/Aβ40

ratios with increased imminent risk for mild cognitive impairment and Alzheimer disease. Archives of Neurology. 2007; 64(3): 354–62. PubMed PMID: 17353377.
110. Rosen C, Hansson O, Blennow K, Zetterberg H. Fluid biomarkers in Alzheimer's disease—current concepts. Molecular Neurodegeneration. 2013; 8: 20. PubMed PMID: 23800368. Pubmed Central PMCID: 3691925.
111. Randall J, Mortberg E, Provuncher GK, Fournier DR, Duffy DC, Rubertsson S, et al. Tau proteins in serum predict neurological outcome after hypoxic brain injury from cardiac arrest: results of a pilot study. Resuscitation. 2013; 84(3): 351–6. PubMed PMID: 22885094.
112. Kavalci C, Pekdemir M, Durukan P, Ilhan N, Yildiz M, Serhatlioglu S, et al. The value of serum tau protein for the diagnosis of intracranial injury in minor head trauma. American Journal of Emergency Medicine. 2007; 25(4): 391–5. PubMed PMID: 17499655.
113. Bulut M, Koksal O, Dogan S, Bolca N, Ozguc H, Korfali E, et al. Tau protein as a serum marker of brain damage in mild traumatic brain injury: preliminary results. Advances in Therapy. 2006; 23(1): 12–22. PubMed PMID: 16644603.
114. Winston CN, Goetzl EJ, Akers JC, Carter BS, Rockenstein EM, Galasko D, et al. Prediction of conversion from mild cognitive impairment to dementia with neuronally derived blood exosome protein profile. Alzheimer's Dementia (Amst). 2016; 3: 63–72. PubMed PMID: 27408937. Pubmed Central PMCID: 4925777.
115. Zetterberg H, Wilson D, Andreasson U, Minthon L, Blennow K, Randall J, et al. Plasma tau levels in Alzheimer's disease. Alzheimer's Research & Therapy. 2013; 5(2): 9. PubMed PMID: 23551972. Pubmed Central PMCID: 3707015.
116. Dage JL, Wennberg AM, Airey DC, Hagen CE, Knopman DS, Machulda MM, et al. Levels of tau protein in plasma are associated with neurodegeneration and cognitive function in a population-based elderly cohort. Alzheimer's Dementia. 2016; 12(12): 1226–34. PubMed PMID: 27436677. Pubmed Central PMCID: 5148697.
117. Trushina E, Mielke MM. Recent advances in the application of metabolomics to Alzheimer's Disease. Biochimica et Biophysica Acta. 2014; 1842(8): 1232–9. PubMed PMID: 23816564. Pubmed Central PMCID: 3842412.
118. Barba I, Fernandez-Montesinos R, Garcia-Dorado D, Pozo D. Alzheimer's disease beyond the genomic era: nuclear magnetic resonance (NMR) spectroscopy-based metabolomics. Journal of Cellular and Molecular Medicine. 2008; 12(5A): 1477–85. PubMed PMID: 18554316. Pubmed Central PMCID: 3918063.
119. Patti GJ, Yanes O, Siuzdak G. Innovation: metabolomics: the apogee of the omics trilogy. Nature Reviews Molecular Cell Biology. 2012; 13(4): 263–9. PubMed PMID: 22436749. Pubmed Central PMCID: 3682684.
120. Tibshirani R. Regression shrinkage and selection via the lasso. Journal of the Royal Statistical Society Series B (Methodological). 1996; 58(1): 267–88.
121. Mapstone M, Cheema AK, Fiandaca MS, Zhong X, Mhyre TR, MacArthur LH, et al. Plasma phospholipids identify antecedent memory impairment in older adults. Nature Medicine. 2014; 20(4): 415–18. PubMed PMID: 24608097.
122. Casanova R, Varma S, Simpson B, Kim M, An Y, Saldana S, et al. Blood metabolite markers of preclinical Alzheimer's disease in two longitudinally followed cohorts of older individuals. Alzheimer's Dementia. 2016; 12(7):815–22. PubMed PMID: 26806385. Pubmed Central PMCID: 4947451.
123. Li D, Misialek JR, Boerwinkle E, Gottesman RF, Sharrett AR, Mosley TH, et al. Plasma phospholipids and prevalence of mild cognitive impairment and/or dementia in the ARIC Neurocognitive Study (ARIC-NCS). Alzheimer's Dementia (Amst). 2016; 3:73–82. PubMed PMID: 27408938. Pubmed Central PMCID: 4925799.
124. Khoury MJ, McBride CM, Schully SD, Ioannidis JP, Feero WG, Janssens AC, et al. The Scientific Foundation for personal genomics: recommendations from a National Institutes of Health-Centers for Disease Control and Prevention multidisciplinary workshop. Genetics in Medicine: Official Journal of the American College of Medical Genetics. 2009; 11(8): 559–67. PubMed PMID: 19617843. Pubmed Central PMCID: 2936269.
125. Ahmed RM, Paterson RW, Warren JD, Zetterberg H, O'Brien JT, Fox NC, et al. Biomarkers in dementia: clinical utility and new directions. Journal of Neurology, Neurosurgery, and Psychiatry. 2014; 85(12): 1426–34. PubMed PMID: 25261571. Pubmed Central PMCID: PMC4335455.
126. Martinez G, Vernooij RW, Fuentes Padilla P, Zamora J, Bonfill Cosp X, Flicker L. 18F PET with florbetapir for the early diagnosis of Alzheimer's disease dementia and other dementias in people with mild cognitive impairment (MCI). Cochrane Database of Systematic Reviews (Online). 2017; 11: CD012216. PubMed PMID: 29164603.
127. Smailagic N, Vacante M, Hyde C, Martin S, Ukoumunne O, Sachpekidis C. (1)(8)F-FDG PET for the early diagnosis of Alzheimer's disease dementia and other dementias in people with mild cognitive impairment (MCI). Cochrane Database of Systematic Reviews (Online). 2015; 1:CD010632. PubMed PMID: 25629415.
128. Mattsson N, Carrillo MC, Dean RA, Devous MD, S., Nikolcheva T, Pesini P, et al. Revolutionizing Alzheimer's disease and clinical trials through biomarkers. Alzheimers Dementia (Amst). 2015; 1(4): 412–419. PubMed PMID: 27239522. Pubmed Central PMCID: 4879481.
129. Thal LJ, Kantarci K, Reiman EM, Klunk WE, Weiner MW, Zetterberg H, et al. The role of biomarkers in clinical trials for Alzheimer disease. Alzheimer Disease and Associated Disorders. 2006; 20(1): 6–15. PubMed PMID: 16493230. Pubmed Central PMCID: 1820855.
130. Fillit HM. FDA's updated standards remove an unnecessary barrier to testing Alzheimer's drugs 2018. Available from: https://http://www.statnews.com/2018/03/05/alzheimers-disease-drugs-fda/.
131. Lyketsos CG, Szekely CA, Mielke MM, Rosenberg PB, Zandi PP. Developing new treatments for Alzheimer's disease: the who, what, when, and how of biomarker-guided therapies. International Psychogeriatrics. 2008; 20(5):871–89. PubMed PMID: 18498669. Pubmed Central PMCID: 2688723.
132. Sperling RA, Rentz DM, Johnson KA, Karlawish J, Donohue M, Salmon DP, et al. The A4 study: stopping AD before symptoms begin? Science Translational Medicine. 2014; 6(228): 228fs13. PubMed PMID: 24648338. Pubmed Central PMCID: 4049292.

3

Life course, exposure, and ageing populations

Yoav Ben-Shlomo

Introduction

The 21st century faces many challenges, but one of the most pressing is the increasing life expectancy seen across both HIC and LMIC countries. This, with a declining fertility rate, puts pressure on how individuals, families, communities, and health and social care systems will care for the growing segment of older people in the population. The macro-economic challenges associated with this demographic change are particularly worse in LMIC settings, but may be potentially mitigated by various actions.[1] A key factor is around disease prevention or postponement of disability, which can have a large impact. For example, it has been estimated that an intervention with a 25% reduction in risk and a mean delay in onset of around two years would reduce the projected increase in the prevalence of dementia in the USA over the next 40 years from 5.75 million to 4.38 million.[2] Non-communicable diseases such as cardiovascular disease, cancer, and chronic respiratory disease continue to contribute a major burden of disease, yet have modifiable factors in earlier life as well as increasingly effective treatments. These often reduce case fatality and paradoxically can increase prevalence, leading to the common phenomenon of multiple morbidity.[3,4] Multi-morbidity results in loss of functional capacity and often involves both physical and cognitive deficits, requiring holistic approaches to care rather than uncoordinated specialist care highlighting the centrality of geriatric syndromes.[5] As Bloom notes: 'population ageing during the coming decades will naturally lead to and need changes in labour and capital markets, retirement policies and pensions and the organization and financing of health systems.'[1]

The key question is as populations continue to live longer, will they stay in good health for more years ('compression of morbidity hypothesis'[6]) or live longer with disability and poor quality life? The current evidence on this remains ambiguous and uncertain.[7] This chapter will examine how understanding the process of ageing and age-related disorders using life course models can enhance our understanding of the ageing process. Describing phenotypic trajectories, in turn, can highlight the relative importance of exposures acting at different time periods and through different exposure profiles. These concepts will be illustrated, where appropriate, using neurological exemplars around cognitive decline, dementia and PD, all of which show marked increases in incidence with greater age.[8,9] Greater life course understanding should guide policy formulation to maximize the health of future cohorts of older people.

Life Course Epidemiology

Life course epidemiology has been defined as 'the study of long-term biological, behavioural, and psychosocial processes that link adult health and disease risk to physical or social exposures acting during gestation, childhood, adolescence, earlier in adult life, or across generations'.[10] Whilst the fundamental concept behind life course epidemiology, that exposures acting in early life can have long-term consequences, is not new (see review by Kuh and Davey Smith for a historical perspective[11]) the more structured formulation of these ideas into testable hypotheses has only been recognized in the epidemiological literature for around the last two decades.

Models of trajectories

The stimuli behind the original work around life course influences was understanding the aetiology of chronic diseases such as coronary heart disease, stroke, and diabetes. Early studies were predominantly led by Professor David Barker's team, who initially observed that babies with lower birth weight had greater risk of these chronic diseases in later life. This effect was not restricted to the extreme left side of the distribution but was observed across the whole range of birth weights. This resulted in the foetal origins of adult disease (FOAD[12]) hypothesis, which argued that the period of foetal development was 'critical' and any adverse impact on the developmental trajectory in this pre-natal period resulted in an increased risk for many non-communicable diseases (NCDs) which were carried with individuals for the rest of their life. These ideas were subsequently modified to the 'developmental origins of health and disease' (DOHaD) hypothesis,[13,14] thereby extending the time period of interest to the post-natal, childhood, and adolescent years.

One of the limitations in clinical medicine is the need to dichotomise phenomena into disease versus non-disease categories. This is a sensible pragmatic approach when having to decide on individual management, to treat or not to treat, but simplifies the biological reality and is less helpful when one takes a population-based approach. When Geoffrey Rose was a medical registrar in the 1950s, he, like others, was shocked by the proposal put forward at the time by Professor George Pickering that: 'the sharp distinction between health and disease is a medical artefact for which nature, if consulted, provides no support.'[15] Pickering was to win the infamous 'Platt-Pickering' debate as to whether hypertension actually existed, and subsequent downward redefinitions of high blood pressure illustrate the arbitrary nature of earlier definitions. However, it was Rose who truly understood the implications of this idea by arguing that often, but not always, the greatest public health benefits arise from shifting the whole distribution to the left (in the case of blood pressure) thereby reducing the risk of the majority of people who lie in the middle of the distribution rather than screening and targeting high-risk individuals at the tail of the distribution.[16]

Whilst Rose only considered the cross-sectional nature of a risk factor like blood pressure, a similar concept can be applied to longitudinal changes in a risk factor by considering its trajectory. For many phenotypes, but not all, one can conceptualize a generic model that involves a developmental phase of growth, followed by a plateau phase of maintenance, and then a degenerative decline phase (see Fig. 3.1). At some phenotypic level, individuals may be classified as either having disease, functional impairment, and/or disability. The same disease endpoint can be attained through either suboptimal development, accelerated decline, or a combination of both pathways. The initial example proposed by Strachan[17] was in relation to lung function, with chronic obstructive airways disease being the clinical endpoint.

The simplicity of the figure underlines several important messages: (1) that to understand the origin of diseases, one should consider continuous traits, such as lung, cognitive, or muscle function and complex phenotypes such as ageing, as well as binary phenotypes and (2) ignoring the underlying trajectories that lead to a disease or disability endpoint in later life will attenuate risk factor associations if they are only of causal relevance for some subgroups but not others ('disease heterogeneity'). For many traits and diseases, we are limited by the available data around life course trajectories, but a growing body of research is starting to emerge. For example, it has been recently demonstrated that around half of all cases of chronic obstructive pulmonary disease occur in individuals with suboptimal adult lung function but normal age-related decline, whilst the other half occur after normal development of lung function with an accelerated decline phase.[18] A similar argument has been made for genetic association studies where the failure to understand phenotypic heterogeneity may obscure relationships.[19]

There are other advantages of using functional or performance measures, such as gait speed. This allows one to study pre-clinical disease, thereby identifying high-risk subgroups and enabling risk stratification for potential intervention studies. Trajectories are variable and dynamic, with periods of recovery as well as loss. Being able to detect early markers of suboptimal development and/or an accelerated trajectory of functional decline before it is clinically manifest is fundamental to a life course perspective because it offers an opportunity to delay the rate of decline and/or the onset of functional impairments through preventive strategies. How these trajectories differ by sociodemographic factors such as gender or socioeconomic status, geographical variability, and by birth cohorts may all provide important mechanistic clues for further investigation.[20] The idea of shifting the degenerative trajectory to the right in this longitudinal context would be equivalent to delaying the chronological effects of time so that the plateau phase was maintained for longer and the decline phase started at an older age. Thus, a 70-year-old might have the phenotype of an average 60-year-old. Alternative preventative strategies will also exist, such as maximizing the potential of the developmental phase or slowing the rate of the degenerative phase (e.g. usually referred to as a disease modifying or neuroprotective effect in the context of medications but could equally apply to lifestyle factors such as physical activity). Older populations are known to show greater inter-individual functional variability than younger populations. As Beard and Bloom comment: 'This diversity is not random. Roughly 25% of the heterogeneity in health and function in older age is genetically determined, with the remainder strongly

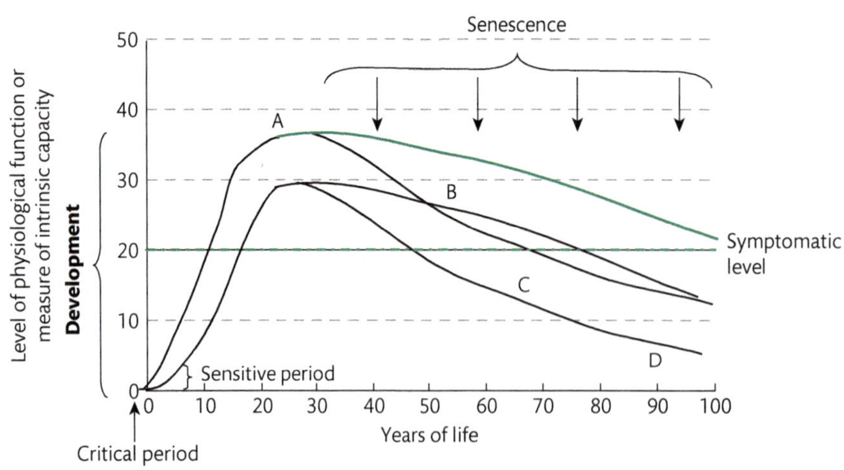

Fig. 3.1 How life course models act over different time windows on the potential trajectories of a physiological trait or intrinsic capacity.
Adapted with permission from Kuh D, Karunananthan S, Bergman H, Cooper R. A life-course approach to healthy ageing: maintaining physical capability. *Proc Nutr Soc.* 73(2): 237–48. © The Authors 2014. DOI: https://doi.org/10.1017/S0029665113003923.

affected by the cumulative effect of health behaviours and inequities across the life course.'[5]

Understanding the patterns of 'normative trajectories' is a fundamental first step in elucidating if there are certain periods of life when any adverse exposure is likely to have a disproportionate effect (see below in relation to exposure models). This is challenging as it requires repeat and sometimes frequent measures (may be clustered in more informative bursts, e.g. around puberty) which may be burdensome on participants and potentially biased by selective attrition. Such descriptive epidemiology is also frequently unappealing to funding bodies, who prefer to test specific aetiological hypotheses. Frequently, cross-sectional age differences are used to infer longitudinal age-related changes. In a large cross-sectional study of 1100 healthy adults aged between 18 to 94 years with MRI imaging, it was possible to describe how brain structure over 13 different areas altered with age using both linear and non-linear models.[21] In eight areas, such as the thalamus, accumbens, and amygdala, the best fit regression line suggested fairly linear declines in volume across age, whilst other areas such as the hippocampus, cerebral white matter, and cerebellum suggested accelerated decline after a turning point between the ages of 40–60 years. These patterns were generally supported in a smaller sample (142 subjects) with longitudinal data. The authors proposed a hypothetical model where brain volume increases in the first part of life, presumably due to myelination and axonal growth, but, before the maturational changes are complete, degeneration due to selective loss of small-diameter myelinated axons (primary degenerative event) and demyelination of larger connections (secondary degenerative event) occur, leading to a variable decline phase. How these trajectories are influenced by genetic, environmental, and neuropathological factors is unclear, but the non-linear effects suggest potential time periods whereby an intervention may have greater potential to slow down the rate of structural loss, often decades before disease onset or a more rapid acceleration phase where interventions may be too late. This may partially explain the poor results seen in trials of patients with early dementia and the move to treating high-risk individuals or those with MCI before dementia onset.[22]

Our understanding of normative trajectories for a wide variety of traits is often poor and limited to cross-sectional studies or short follow-ups. This is particularly problematic for a trait such as cognition where there may be marked cohort effects that will bias any inference based on cross-sectional data (i.e. if more recent cohorts have better cognition than their older counterparts then the age-related differences will be exaggerated). However, longitudinal data may also biased by the well-recognized 'practice effect' so that short-term changes in cognition are obscured by enhanced performance on repeat testing; then, if anything, participants actually show on average better scores despite being older. Sufficiently long-term follow-up is required to overcome any short-term benefits from retesting. A review comparing cross-sectional and longitudinal studies suggested that: 'age-related changes from age 20 to 60 tend to be small or non-existent, with speed of processing showing the largest change, whereas changes after the age of 60 have a slope that is roughly equivalent to that found in cross-sectional data. In some cases, the age-related slope is curvilinear, with a more rapid decline at older ages.'[23]

The stability of cognitive function in midlife, as suggested above, has been more recently challenged by evidence from a long-term occupational cohort. The Whitehall-II study of middle-aged civil servants has demonstrated, over ten-year follow-up, that average performance in all cognitive domains, except vocabulary, declined over follow-up in all age groups, even in those aged 45–49 years.[24] Cross-sectional and longitudinal comparisons showed interesting gender differences. Cross-sectional data considerably overestimated cognitive decline among women but not in men, a probable consequence of cohort differences in education. Age-related decline was larger in almost all cases for older subjects, but the tests themselves differed in sensitivity. For example, tests of reasoning showed a far stronger age-related dose-response pattern than tests of phonemic fluency. These results will be particularly relevant to cross-sectional studies in LMIC settings where contemporary access to education has been much improved.

The Role of Exposures Acting on Life Course Trajectories

Exposures may be genetic and/or environmental and can act at an individual or societal level, though the latter must have a biological intrinsic impact, a concept referred to by Krieger as embodiment: 'how we literally incorporate, biologically, the material and social world in which we live, from conception to death'.[25] Exposure assessment usually involves measurement of intensity and duration but often ignores timing. A classic example in epidemiology is the classification of cigarette smoking. In the seminal British doctors' study, smoking was classified into lifelong non-smoker, former, current (1–14, 15–24, ≥25 cigarettes per day).[26] Frequently, intensity and duration are combined into pack-years (20 cigarettes a day for one year is equal to one pack year). Further refinement can be obtained by stratifying intensity and duration by years, since quitting for ex-smokers, thereby enables one to establish whether the risk of certain diseases for ex-term smokers ever reaches that of never smokers even after quitting for a long period. In the Whitehall-I study, a persistent residual elevated risk of cancer was observed for ex-smokers even after 30 years cessation, indicating that carcinogenesis may occur relatively early and have a long latency period.[27] In general, most smokers initiate their habit within a fairly narrow time window, between their early and late teens and it is rare for non-smokers to start smoking after their twenties. This probably explains why few studies have examined the age of smoking initiation as a determinant of disease risk after accounting for intensity and duration. However, one notable example is a case-control study of breast cancer, which noted that smoking initiation within five years of menarche was associated with an increased risk of pre-menopausal breast cancer (OR 1.77, 95% CI 1.22, 2.57, $p = 0.002$) as compared to post-menopausal breast cancer (OR 0.81, 95% CI 0.60, 1.09, $p = 0.16$).[28] The authors postulated that polycyclic aromatic hydrocarbons, found in tobacco smoke, have greater carcinogenic effects when metabolized by breast tissue during a period of rapid cellular proliferation around puberty. Assuming this association is robust to adjustment by duration, then this example illustrates how timing as well as intensity and duration can be important.

Life Course Exposure Models

Several life course exposure models have been proposed and have been usually grouped into two subgroups: (1) Critical or sensitive period; critical period is defined as 'a limited time window in which an exposure can have adverse or protective effects on development and subsequent disease outcome. Outside this developmental window there is no excess disease risk associated with exposure.'[29] The foetal origins hypothesis that a nutritional insult during foetal life has a permanent effect on, for example, arterial smooth wall tissue leading to future hypertension would be an example of a critical period effect.[30] A sensitive period is 'a time period when an exposure has a stronger effect on development and subsequent disease risk than it would at other times. Outside the time period any excess risk will be weaker.'[29] (2) Accumulation of risk—this concept assumes that life-course exposures or insults gradually accumulate through episodes of illness and injury, adverse environmental conditions, and health damaging behaviours. A simple pack-years model would fit into an accumulation model, though in this case we are only considering a single exposure, smoking, rather than the accumulation of multiple different exposures that may be correlated due to the influence of poor socioeconomic status. However, if timing of smoking initiation is also important, for example during or after puberty, then the data may be more consistent with a sensitive period model.

As Alwin has noted[31] it is more sensible to view critical or sensitive period models as special subsets of an accumulation model when considering the effects of an exposure over time—hence the effects of exposures over different time periods do not add up in a simple additive fashion, but differ in the strength of effect in a quantitative sense (sensitive period) or in a qualitative sense, so that they can only be observed in one time period (critical period).

Exposures may have different dose patterns, such as acute, chronic, and acute on chronic. For example, when considering a neuro-toxic exposure such as pesticides, which may have an aetiological role for PD,[9] one can envisage at least three different exposure patterns: (1) high-dose acute exposure due to poisoning or an ad-hoc exposure; (2) low disease chronic exposure, for example as part of an occupation such as farming; (3) combinations of acute on chronic exposure with periodic high-level exposures against a relatively constant background low-level exposure. The biological implications of these different patterns will differ depending on whether there is a threshold effect for neurotoxicity or a continuous dose-response effect with appropriate up or down regulation of other biochemical systems in response to chronic exposure. The timing of such exposures may also have an impact on the life course trajectories of intrinsic capacity. So exposure in early life may lead in suboptimal development and hence reduced structural or functional capacity

The issue of effect modification by age is of relevance for neurodegenerative disorders that increase with age. For example, animal experiments with combinations of the herbicide paraquat and fungicide maneb have highlighted far greater neurotoxic effects in older rodents.[32] In this case exposure at 6 weeks, 5 months, and 18 months showed differences in phenotypic expression so that locomotor activity was most affected at 18 months. The number of nigrostriatal dopaminergic neurons were reduced at all ages, but these losses were progressive in the 18-month group. Whether this reflects greater sensitivity to toxicity (e.g. reduced protective effect of the BBB), diminished detoxification mechanisms, or less effective repair mechanisms is unclear, but these would all be consistent with greater susceptibility in older life. In the rodent experiment above, increased compensatory tyrosine hydroxylase enzyme activity was only observed at 6 weeks and 5 months and not in the 18-month animals.

On the other hand, if the latency period between exposure and disease onset is long as it merely triggers a sequence of pathological events which then operate independently of exposure, it is more likely that exposure in earlier life will be more relevant as the individual is more likely to live long enough to present phenotypically whilst they will probably die of another unrelated cause if only exposed in later life. If the inverse association between smoking and PD is genuinely causal, a controversial topic, then starting smoking in late life could be advantageous as the latency period for the development of cancer is relatively long and may never present clinically.

Understanding Ageing

How one defines and measures ageing remains debated, though there is a clear distinction between 'biological' as opposed to 'chronological' age. The WHO report defined biological ageing as: 'the gradual accumulation of a wide variety of molecular and cellular damage. Over time, this damage leads to a gradual decrease in physiological reserves, an increased risk of many diseases, and a general decline in the capacity of the individual. Ultimately, it will result in death.'[33] Healthy ageing, an aspiration for all societies, involves three components: (1) survival to an old age; (2) delay in the onset of chronic disease or disability; and (3) optimal functioning for the maximal period of time.[34] Functioning is operationalized by measures of physical and cognitive capability providing the capacity to undertake activities of daily living and maintaining independence in the community. In addition, it is possible to study the life course trajectories of the underlying physiological functioning of body systems such as lung function, which in turn will impact on mobility and the underlying functioning of molecules and cells. The latter has led to great interest in developing 'objective' biomarkers of a cellular process, for example telomere length or epigenetic clock,[35,36] but are more often composite markers that aggregate determinants and/or consequences of ageing.[37] The value of such biomarkers is that they may be appropriate at younger ages when it may be harder to detect variability in other measures due to ceiling effects (see this review for more details around models of ageing[20]).

There are several different theories about ageing. One model, based on understanding demographic patterns, highlights the notion of redundancy as a key aspect of understanding ageing ('reliability theory').[38] In this model, systems and organisms with greater inherent redundancy are better able to tolerate damage and insult accumulation, thereby having longer life expectancy. This explains why, as redundancy is used up over the life course, one observes mortality convergence at later life so that death rates become similar at advanced ages for different populations of the same species. It is suggested that early life damage may explain sociodemographic and geographical differences in age-related mortality rates due to the impact on initial redundancy. Weinert and Timiras propose four other classes of models for ageing:[39] (1) evolutionary; (2) molecular; (3) cellular; and (4) system-based. The disposable soma and antagonistic pleiotropy models argue that we have evolved to maximize our chances to reproduce and hence pass on our genes to the next generation. After reproductive age, the soma becomes disposable or genes that are beneficial at younger ages may actually become deleterious at older ages. Hanson and Gluckman have taken these ideas in their formulation of the developmental origins hypothesis,[40] where they put forward the concept of a predictive adaptive response (PAR). This occurs in earlier life and maximizes the chances of survival and reproduction, but in the longer term may be maladaptive as it may result in chronic diseases or more rapid ageing. These models assume time-limited reproductive ability, which is less true for men in societies where wealth may ensure continued reproduction into older ages. Furthermore, though the period of fertility is limited in women by the menopause, kinship networks can play an important role in the health and well-being of children and grandchildren, so older women may be crucially important for the health and development of their grandchildren.

The molecular models assume that with ageing comes either somatic mutations with resulting disease, for example cancer or errors in the fidelity of gene expression with failure of maintenance and repairs pathways. This phenomenon may be truly random due to chance or stochastic damage, or precipitated by environmental insults, for example radiation exposure. Peto and Doll in their rather provocatively titled commentary: 'There is no such thing as aging; old age is associated with disease but does not cause it',[41] made the logical point that a multi-stage model of cancer (though it has been applied to other conditions such as motor neurone disease (MND)[42]) requires that the transformation of a normal epithelial stem cell into a growing cancer involves: 'several consecutive changes in the genetic material of that cell, with the rate of progression of a partially altered cell from one stage to another being largely unaffected by age'.

Cellular senescence theories argue that there is a finite limit to the number of cellular replicative cycles and this may be related to the length of telomeres (cellular clock), protective complexes found at the end of eukaryotic chromosomes.[43] Whilst studies are not always consistent, telomere shortening is associated with mortality and a variety of ageing-related diseases. However, genetic and environmental factors are both relevant for the maintenance of telomeres and it has been suggested that: 'because telomere length is affected by so many non-genetic factors, measures of telomere length maintenance may be a proxy for assessing the "exposome"—that is, all of the exposures promoting disease'.[43] This would capture an accumulation of adverse exposures, although it is also possible that exposures at certain developmental stages may have far greater impact on telomere length (sensitive period) than at other stages of the life course. Further studies are required to examine longitudinal changes in telomere length in relation to the timing of the same exposures. Other mechanisms for damage include free radical exposure and wear and tear mechanisms. Finally, a systems-based approach assumes that various physiological systems, such as neuroendocrine or immune function, decline with age, thus failing to maintain homeostasis or losing the ability to mount a specific response to external antigens. A lot of interest has centred around the hypothalamic-pituitary-adrenal axis and the stress hormone cortisol. Sapolsky argued that the cortisol response to external stressors was in the long term maladaptive due to its neurotoxicity, which in turn led to central damage to the negative feedback system. Thus, with ageing future stress responses were maintained for longer due to the lack of an appropriate negative feedback mechanism ('glucocorticoid cascade hypothesis').[44,45] Elegant animal studies provide supportive evidence for this hypothesis, but findings in humans are far less convincing.[46] Given the adaptive nature of this system it is also hard to interpret cross-sectional findings. So, for example, elevated levels of 24-hour cortisol or a raised cortisol awakening response, may actually be a positive adaptive response to a stressor in one period of time, but chronically may indicate a loss of dynamic alterations and reduced responsiveness. Finally, there may be a stage with reduced rather than elevated functioning analogous to insulin production in response to glucose, leading to diabetes.[46]

Given the dramatic lifestyle changes most populations have experienced over the last century, it might be assumed that this would manifest itself across generations in relation to ageing traits. Few studies have examined birth cohort effects on ageing phenotypes. A Danish comparison examined nonagenarians either born in 1905 or in 1915 and assessed them using the same instruments and with almost identical response rates. Unsurprisingly, the probability of survival to this age was higher in the 1915 cohort, but despite this reduced selection, subjects from the later cohort performed better on cognitive assessments and had better activities of daily living scores, although did not differ on physical performance tests such as grip strength, chair stand, or gait speed. These cognitive cohort advantages are even more evident and clinically relevant in relation to dementia prevalence. The Medical Research Council Cognitive Function and Ageing Study (MRC CFAS) was able to compare dementia prevalence in three areas using the same methodology over a 20-year period. CFAS-II, the later study, found an absolute decrease of 1.8% and an OR for CFAS II vs CFAS I of 0.7, 95% CI 0.6–0.9, p = 0.003). Again one might not have predicted this observation given the link between vascular disease and dementia and the reduction in cardiovascular disease case fatality over time with improved medical care.[47]

A more complex picture has emerged from a recent study using data from the Chinese Longitudinal Healthy Longevity study which compared three pairs of cohorts, aged 80–89, 90–99, and 100–105 born ten years apart.[48] Both mortality and disability were reduced in the later cohorts but in this case cognitive impairment increased, whilst physical performance decreased for the more contemporaneous cohorts. The authors argued that later cohorts had benefitted from progress in effective disease treatment, healthier lifestyles, and improved standards of living due to rapid socioeconomic development in China. These 'benefits of success' imply a delay in senescence and improved capacity. But the later cohort had more subjects who survived life-threatening conditions because of better medical care with reduced performance, which they termed the 'costs of success'. The contradictory findings for cognition as compared to the Danish cohort were explained by differences in educational opportunities. Surprisingly, the later Chinese cohorts had lower educational levels than the earlier cohorts, probably due to domestic wars and greater childhood poverty. This was in stark contrast to the Danish experience, where educational levels improved over time. These findings have important implications for predicting future trends of health and social care needs but also highlight the importance of potential different life course influences.

Life Course Influences on Neurodegenerative Diseases

Evidence from meta-analysis of observational studies suggest that there are seven potentially modifiable risk factors for AD: diabetes, midlife hypertension, midlife obesity, physical inactivity, depression, smoking, and low educational attainment. The association between depression and AD is more complex as it could be part of a pre-clinical AD phenotype and a similar association has also been seen with anxiety.[49] Assuming independent effects, it has been estimated that these combined factors account for around 50% of the population attributable risk, which reduced to around 30% after mutual adjustment.[50] A relative reduction of 10% per decade in the prevalence of each of the seven risk factors, assuming a causal relationship, could reduce the prevalence of AD in 2050 by 8.3% worldwide.

Some of these risk factors (obesity, diabetes, mid-life hypertension) have well-established life course influences from *in utero* to post-natal and young adulthood,[8,51] though cognitive function and socioeconomic status may also impact on these risk factors, as well as smoking and physical inactivity in a bi-directional fashion. Untangling the causal pathway between these risk factors and cognitive function on all-cause mortality is challenging.[52] Barnett et al.[53] have argued that dementia risk begins at birth, through breastfeeding and post-natal nutrition influencing cognitive and brain development. Other potential exposures include: infections, stress, chemicals, and pesticides.[54] The establishment of lifelong behavioural patterns in earlier life is important because such patterns are more likely to be maintained. However, benefits may be greater during teenage years. A cross-sectional study of around 9000 women found that whilst reporting being active at any of four time points was beneficial, being active in the teen years had stronger effects than at 30 and 50 years.[55]

Educational attainment is of interest given its potential role on life course cognitive trajectories and as a proxy for peak cognitive function. Stern was the first to propose an active concept of cognitive reserve whereby brain function rather than brain size or the number of neurons or synapses was protective from pathology.[56] Thus, unlike a simple life course structural reserve—assessed by peak attainment in young adulthood—the brain has variations within its cognitive-processing mechanisms that allow it to use compensatory mechanisms when adjusting to neuropathological challenges such as neurofibrillary tangles found in AD. A simple structural model is often cited in relation to peak attained bone mass and future risk of an osteoporotic fracture, though even then the density and strength of the bone may determine fracture risk as well as total mass. Clearly there may or may not be interactions between anatomical and functional reserves. Richards and Deary have argued that the reserve model should be applied across the life course to cognitive development as well as cognitive function in adulthood.[57]

A meta-analysis found that lower educational level was associated with pooled OR of between 2.61 and 1.88 for increased prevalence and incidence of dementia respectively.[58] A qualitative review of the evidence also found that higher education had no effect on the age of onset of dementia, showed accelerated cognitive decline after clinical onset, had no effect on the age of death, had a higher level of clinical performance on initial assessment and if anything was associated with greater brain pathology in post-mortem and imaging studies among those with dementia. The largest neuropathological study, the EClipSE collaboration, examined 872 brain donors, 56% of whom had dementia at death.[59] Greater educational years was associated with a reduced risk of dementia and greater brain weight, but had no protective effect on the accumulation of neurodegenerative pathologies. Education was seen to mitigate the effect of pathology so that at any given pathological burden, more education was associated with a lower risk of cognitive decline. Given the highly correlated associations between education and a wide variety of other risk factors,[60] interpreting the causal nature of such an association is problematic, but two further strands of evidence lend weight to the causal importance of education. Mendelian randomization (MR),[61,62] is a method that uses the unconfounded association between genetic instruments and a phenotype of interest as an indirect measure of the association with the relevant outcome. In this case, assuming the instrumental variable assumptions are valid, any association cannot be due to either reverse causation (as with the depression risk factor) and confounding as the instrument can be empirically shown to not be associated with known confounders and implicitly with unknown confounders. The major limitations of MR studies are: (1) they require large sample sizes as the genetic instruments are generally modest in effect and (2) it is hard to exclude pleiotropic effects so that any possible genetic effects may be mediated through other pathways than the exposure, though this is less likely with a large number of genetic instruments. A recent MR study of around 8000 participants from the Health and Retirement study cohort (HRS) using three single nucleotide polymorphisms (SNPs) as a genetic risk score for education found a modest (1.1%) reduction in dementia risk with per year of schooling, but the 95% CI was consistent with chance. This has now been extended by a much larger study using 74 SNPs with 17,008 AD cases and 37,154 controls. A standard deviation increase in school years (3.5 years) was associated with a reduced odds ratio of 0.63 (95% CI 0.48 to 0.83, $p<0.001$) of AD.[63] Furthermore, the HRS study cited above was able to test the causal effect of educational years by using the 'natural experiment' of variations in state-level school policies in the USA.[64] This found that for every year increase in school years there was a 9.5% decrease in dementia risk (95% CI -14.8 to -4.2%). Whilst educational attainment is completed between the adolescent and young adult years, we should not assume that any interventions are only of value in this critical time-period. Higher educational level may lead to extrinsic compensation through various adaptations. More educated people will usually have occupations that are more intellectually demanding or have greater resources to partake in intellectual social activities, resulting in greater cognitive stimulation and consistent with the 'use it or lose it' hypothesis. It is therefore possible that cognitive compensatory mechanisms start in early life but require maintenance over adulthood and could therefore be modified in a positive fashion over decades.

Conclusion

A life course approach highlights the variety of different aetiological models that may contribute to ageing and the aetiology of various clinical entities including neurodegenerative disorders. It also forces one to consider how exposures accumulate over time both in terms of the number of adverse experiences, their duration, but also the timing which may have a disproportionate influence on later life intermediaries or outcomes. Most importantly it highlights the need for primary and secondary prevention across the whole of the life course rather than merely focussing on mid or later life.

REFERENCES

1. Bloom DE, Chatterji S, Kowal P, Lloyd-Sherlock P, McKee M, Rechel B, et al. Macroeconomic implications of population ageing and selected policy responses. *Lancet.* 2015; 385(9968): 649–57.
2. Brookmeyer R, Gray S, Kawas C. Projections of Alzheimer's disease in the United States and the public health impact of delaying disease onset. *American Journal of Public Health.* 1998; 88–9: 1337–42.
3. Barnett K, Mercer SW, Norbury M, Watt G, Wyke S, Guthrie B. Epidemiology of multimorbidity and implications for health care, research, and medical education: a cross-sectional study. *Lancet.* 2012; 380(9836): 37–43.
4. Salisbury C. Multimorbidity: redesigning health care for people who use it. *Lancet.* 2012; 380(9836): 7–9.
5. Beard JR, Bloom DE. Towards a comprehensive public health response to population ageing. *Lancet.* 2015; 385(9968): 658–61.
6. Fries JF. Ageing, natural death, and the compression of morbidity. *N Engl J Med* 1980; 313: 407–28.
7. Chatterji S, Byles J, Cutler D, Seeman T, Verdes E. Health, functioning, and disability in older adults–present status and future implications. *Lancet.* 2015; 385(9967): 563–75.
8. Whalley LJ, Dick FD, McNeill G. A life-course approach to the aetiology of late-onset dementias. *Lancet Neurology.* 2006; 5(1): 87–96.
9. Wirdefeldt K, Adami HO, Cole P, Trichopoulos D, Mandel J. Epidemiology and etiology of Parkinson's disease: a review of the evidence. *European Journal of Epidemiology.* 2011; 26: S1–S58.
10. Ben-Shlomo Y, Kuh D. A life course approach to chronic disease epidemiology: conceptual models, empirical challenges and interdisciplinary perspectives. *Int J Epidemiol.* 2002; 31(2): 285–93.
11. Kuh D, Davey Smith G. The life course and adult chronic disease: an historical perspective with particular reference to coronary heart disease. In: Kuh D, Ben-Shlomo Y (eds). *A Life Course Approach to Chronic Disease Epidemiology* (2nd edition). Oxford: Oxford University Press, 2004. pp15–40.
12. Barker DJP. *Mothers, Babies, and Disease in Later Life.* London: BMJ Publishing Group, 1994.
13. Gluckman PD, Hanson MA, Cooper C, Thornburg KL. Effect of in utero and early-life conditions on adult health and disease. *N Engl J Med.* 2008; 359(1): 61–73.
14. Gluckman PD, Hanson MA, Beedle AS. Early life events and their consequences for later disease: a life history and evolutionary perspective. *Am J Hum Biol.* 2007; 19(1): 1–19.
15. Rose G. The Strategy of Preventive Medicine. London: OUP, 1992.
16. Strachan D, Rose G. Strategies of prevention revisited: effects of imprecise measurement of risk factors on the evaluation of 'high-risk' and 'population-biased' approaches to prevention of cardiovascular disease. *J Clin Epidemiol.* 1991; 44: 1187–96.
17. Strachan DP. Respiratory and allergic diseases. In: Kuh D (ed.). *A Life Course Approach to Chronic Disease Epidemiology.* Oxford: OUP, 1997. pp101–120.
18. Lange P, Celli B, Agusti A, Boje Jensen G, Divo M, Faner R, et al. Lung-function trajectories leading to chronic obstructive pulmonary disease. *N Engl J Med.* 2015; 373(2): 111–22.
19. Spycher BD, Henderson J, Granell R, Evans DM, Smith GD, Timpson NJ, et al. Genome-wide prediction of childhood asthma and related phenotypes in a longitudinal birth cohort. *The Journal of Allergy and Clinical Immunology.* 2012; 130(2): 503–509.e7.
20. Ben-Shlomo Y, Cooper R, Kuh D. The last two decades of life course epidemiology, and its relevance for research on ageing. *International Journal of Epidemiology.* 2016; 45(4): 973–88.
21. Fjell AM, Westlye LT, Grydeland H, Amlien I, Espeseth T, Reinvang I, et al. Alzheimer disease neuroimaging I. Critical ages in the life course of the adult brain: nonlinear subcortical aging. *Neurobiology of Aging* 2013; 34(10): 2239–47.
22. Lyon J. Alzheimer outlook far from bleak. *JAMA* 2017; 317(9): 896–8.
23. Hedden T, Gabrieli JDE. Insights into the ageing mind: a view from cognitive neuroscience. *Nature Reviews Neuroscience.* 2004; 5(2): 87–96.
24. Singh-Manoux A, Kivimaki M, Glymour MM, Elbaz A, Berr C, Ebmeier KP, et al. Timing of onset of cognitive decline: results from Whitehall II prospective cohort study. *BMJ (Clinical research ed).* 2012; 344: d7622.
25. Krieger N. Theories for social epidemiology in the 21st century: an ecosocial perspective. *International Journal of Epidemiology.* 2001; 30: 668–77.
26. Doll R, Peto R, Boreham J, Sutherland I. Mortality in relation to smoking: 50 years' observations on male British doctors. *BMJ (Clinical research ed).* 2004; 328(7455): 1519.
27. Ben-Shlomo Y, Davey S, Shipley MJ, Marmot MG. What determines mortality risk in male former cigarette smokers? *American Journal of Public Health.* 1994; 84: 1235–42.
28. Band PR, Le ND, Fang R, Deschamps M. Carcinogenic and endocrine disrupting effects of cigarette smoke and risk of breast cancer. *Lancet.* 2002; 360: 1044–9.
29. Kuh D, Ben-Shlomo Y, Lynch J, Hallqvist J, Power C. Life course epidemiology. *J Epidemiol Community Health.* 2003; 57(10): 778–83.
30. Martyn CN, Greenwald SE. Impaired synthesis of elastin in walls of aorta and large conduit arteries during early development as an initiating event in pathogenesis of systemic hypertension. *Lancet.* 1997; 350: 953–5.
31. Alwin DF. Words have consequences. *The Journals of Gerontology Series B, Psychological Sciences and Social Sciences.* 2012; 67(2): 232–4.
32. Thiruchelvam M, McCormack A, Richfield EK, Baggs RB, Tank AW, Di Monte DA, et al. Age-related irreversible progressive nigrostriatal dopaminergic neurotoxicity in the paraquat and maneb model of the Parkinson's disease phenotype. *European Journal of Neuroscience.* 2003; 18(3): 589–600.
33. World Health Organization. World Report on Ageing and Health. Geneva: World Health Organization, 2015. 1(233).
34. Kuh D, Richards M, Cooper R, Hardy R, Ben-Shlomo Y. Life course epidemiology, ageing research, and maturing cohort studies: a dynamic combination for understanding healthy ageing. In: Kuh D, Cooper R, Hardy R, Richards M, Ben-Shlomo Y (eds). *A Life Course Approach to Healthy Ageing* (1st edition). Oxford: Oxford University Press, 2014. pp1–282.
35. Martin-Ruiz C, von Zglinicki T. A life course approach to biomarkers of ageing. In: Kuh D, Cooper R, Hardy R, Richards M, Ben-Shlomo Y, eds. *A Life Course Approach to Healthy Ageing.* Oxford: Oxford University Press, 2014. pp177–86.
36. Horvath S. DNA methylation age of human tissues and cell types. *Genome Biology.* 2013; 14(10): R115.
37. Belsky DW, Caspi A, Houts R, Cohen HJ, Corcoran DL, Danese A, et al. Quantification of biological aging in young adults.

Proceedings of the National Academy of Sciences of the United States of America. 2015; 112(130): E4104–10.
38. Gavrilov LA, Gavrilova NS. The quest for a general theory of aging and longevity. *Sci Aging Knowledge Environ*. 2003; 2003–28: RE5.
39. Weinert BT, Timiras PS. Invited review: Theories of aging. *Journal of Applied Physiology (Bethesda, Md: 1985)* 2003; 95(4): 1706–16.
40. Hanson MA, Gluckman PD. Early developmental conditioning of later health and disease: physiology or pathophysiology? *Physiological Reviews*. 2014; 94(4): 1027–76.
41. Peto R, Doll R. There is no such thing as aging. *BMJ*. 1997; 315: 1030–2.
42. Al-Chalabi A, Calvo A, Chio A, Colville S, Ellis CM, Hardiman O, et al. Analysis of amyotrophic lateral sclerosis as a multistep process: a population-based modelling study. *Lancet Neurology*. 2014; 13(11): 1108–13.
43. Blackburn EH, Epel ES, Lin J. Human telomere biology: A contributory and interactive factor in aging, disease risks, and protection. *Science*. 2015; 350(6265): 1193–8.
44. Sapolsky RM. *Stress, the Aging Brain, and the Mechanisms of Neuron Death*. London: MIT Press, 1992.
45. Sapolsky RM, Krey LC, McEwen BS. The neuroendocrinology of stress and aging: The glucocorticoid cascade hypothesis. *Endocrine Reviews*. 1986; 7: 284–301.
46. Ben-Shlomo Y, Gardner M, Lightman S. A life course approach to neuroendocrine systems: the example of the HPA axis. In: Kuh D, Cooper R, Hardy R, Richards M, Ben-Shlomo Y (eds). *A Life Course Approach to Healthy Ageing*. Oxford: Oxford University Press, 2014. pp1–282.
47. Tunstall-Pedoe H, Vanuzzo D, Hobbs M, Mähönen M, Zygimantas C, Kuulasmaa K, et al. WHO MONICA Project. Estimation of contribution of changes in coronary care to improving survival, event rates, and coronary heart disease mortality across the WHO MONICA project populations. *Lancet*. 2000; 355: 688–700.
48. Zeng Y, Feng Q, Hesketh T, Christensen K, Vaupel JW. Survival, disabilities in activities of daily living, and physical and cognitive functioning among the oldest-old in China: a cohort study. *Lancet*. 2017; 389(10079): 1619–29.
49. Gallacher J, Bayer A, Fish M, Pickering J, Pedro S, Dunstan F, et al. Does anxiety affect risk of dementia? Findings from the Caerphilly Prospective Study. *Psychosomatic Medicine*. 2009; 71(6): 659–66.
50. Norton S, Matthews FE, Barnes DE, Yaffe K, Brayne C. Potential for primary prevention of Alzheimer's disease: an analysis of population-based data. *Lancet Neurology*. 2014; 13(8): 788–94.
51. Barker DJ. Fetal origins of cardiovascular disease. *Ann Med*. 1999; 31(Suppl 1): 3–6.
52. Gallacher J, Bayer A, Dunstan F, Yarnell J, Elwood P, Ben-Shlomo Y. Can we understand why cognitive function predicts mortality? Results from the Caerphilly Prospective Study (CaPS). *Intelligence*. 2009; 37(6): 535–44.
53. Barnett JH, Hachinski V, Blackwell AD. Cognitive health begins at conception: addressing dementia as a lifelong and preventable condition. *BMC Medicine*. 2013; 11: 246.
54. Miller DB, O'Callaghan JP. Do early-life insults contribute to the late-life development of Parkinson and Alzheimer diseases? *Metabolism: Clinical and Experimental*. 2008; 57(Suppl 2): S44–9.
55. Middleton LE, Barnes DE, Lui L-Y, Yaffe K. Physical activity over the life course and its association with cognitive performance and impairment in old age. *Journal of the American Geriatrics Society*. 2010; 58(7): 1322–6.
56. Stern Y. Cognitive reserve in ageing and Alzheimer's disease. *Lancet Neurology*. 2012; 11(11): 1006–12.
57. Richards M, Deary IJ. A life course approach to cognitive reserve: a model for cognitive aging and development? *Annals of Neurology*. 2005; 58(4): 617–22.
58. Meng X, D'Arcy C. Education and dementia in the context of the cognitive reserve hypothesis: a systematic review with meta-analyses and qualitative analyses. *PlOS one*. 2012; 7(6): e38268.
59. Members ECC, Brayne C, Ince PG, Keage HAD, McKeith IG, Matthews FE, et al. Education, the brain and dementia: neuroprotection or compensation? *Brain: a Journal of Neurology*. 2010; 133(Pt 8): 2210–16.
60. Davey Smith G, Lawlor DA, Harbord R, Timpson N, Day I, Ebrahim S. Clustered environments and randomized genes: a fundamental distinction between conventional and genetic epidemiology. *PLOS medicine*. 2007; 4(12): e352.
61. Ebrahim S, Davey SG. Mendelian randomization: can genetic epidemiology help redress the failures of observational epidemiology? *Hum Genet*. 2008; 123(1): 15–33.
62. Davey Smith G, Ebrahim S. 'Mendelian randomization': can genetic epidemiology contribute to understanding environmental determinants of disease? *Int J Epidemiol*. 2003; 32(1): 1–22.
63. Anderson EL, Wade KH, Hemant G, Bowden J, Korologou-Linden R, Davey Smith G, et al. The causal effect of educational attainment on Alzheimer's disease: a two-sample Mendelian randomization study. *bioRxiv*. 2017. doi: https://doi.org/10.1101/127993
64. Nguyen TT, Tchetgen Tchetgen EJ, Kawachi I, Gilman SE, Walter S, Liu SY, et al. Instrumental variable approaches to identifying the causal effect of educational attainment on dementia risk. *Annals of Epidemiology*. 2016; 26(1): 71–6, e1–3.

4

Examining trends in dementia incidence and prevalence using an age-period-cohort framework

Kenneth M Langa, Eileen M Crimmins, and Mark D Hayward

Background

Dementia, a decline in memory and other cognitive functions leading to disability in daily function, is a common and feared geriatric condition. Over the past decade, dementia has been the focus of increasing attention from researchers, clinicians, and policymakers due to the projected significant increase in the number of dementia cases—and the associated burdens to patients, families, and government support programmes—that is expected to result from the worldwide growth in the elderly population. However, a growing number of population-based studies have reported that the age-specific risk of dementia in HICs has declined over the past 25 years, suggesting that trends in some combination of demographic, behavioural, medical, and environmental factors have led to a decrease in dementia risk, and may therefore mitigate some of the large growth in dementia cases projected for future decades.

Given the growing evidence that late-life dementia risk likely results from the summation of risk and protective factors that individuals experience across the life course from birth (even pre-birth) through old age, an 'age-period-cohort' perspective which clarifies trends in dementia using each of these different lenses may help in identifying potential causal pathways that affect dementia risk. For instance, widespread changes in health behaviours (e.g. smoking) and medical treatments (e.g. more widespread and intensive treatment of hypertension and high cholesterol) in many HICs around the world represent *period effects* in that they affected nearly all adult age groups, and may have contributed to a decrease in dementia risk in recent decades among older adults.

Cohort effects are those factors that selectively have an impact on individuals who are born in the same year (i.e. belong to the same 'birth cohort'). In the context of determining late-life dementia risk, environmental or social factors experienced during early-life (including *in utero*) that are likely to affect brain development may represent especially important cohort effects. For example, the prevalence of early-life infections,[1] as well as the adequacy of typical diets and nutrition levels among children,[2] may have an important effect on life expectancy, 'brain health' throughout life, and ultimately the risk for late-life dementia. As discussed in more detail below, increasing access to formal schooling opportunities and subsequent increases in levels of educational attainment in children around the world may also be an important cohort effect that has affected trends in late-life dementia risk among recent birth cohorts, possibly through the building of 'cognitive reserve' that allows individuals to compensate for age-related brain pathologies, thereby delaying or preventing dementia onset.[3]

Age is typically considered the most important and consistent risk factor for cognitive decline and dementia. Age: 'reflects biological and social processes internal to individuals and represent developmental changes across the life course'.[4] The close link between dementia and older age increases the public health and public policy importance of the expected large growth over the next few decades of the older population around the world.

Diagnostic Criteria for Dementia

Diagnostic criteria for dementia have evolved and been updated over the last few decades. In 2011, the US National Institute on Aging and US Alzheimer's Association (NIA-AA) updated the 1984 NINCDS-ADRDA diagnostic criteria to incorporate more recent clinical and basic science research regarding the natural history and causes of cognitive decline in adults.[5] The NIA-AA criteria for dementia are summarized below:

(1) Impairment in at least two of: memory, reasoning, visuospatial abilities, language; or changes in personality/behaviour; and
(2) The impairments 'interfere with the ability to function at work or at usual activities', and represent a decline from previous levels of functioning; and
(3) The impairments are not explained by delirium or psychiatric disorder.

A major evolution in the conceptualization of cognitive decline and dementia over the last 25 years is the identification of a symptomatic 'pre-dementia' stage, often termed MCI.[6,7] MCI is characterized by subjective and objective declines in cognitive function that are not severe enough to cause disability in daily function.[6] The identification of MCI and potential shifts over time in the diagnostic 'border' between MCI and dementia have important implications for identifying and measuring trends in dementia incidence and prevalence,[8] since changes in diagnostic thresholds may lead to differences in measured incidence and prevalence rates over time, separate from any 'true' change in the presence of dementia in the population under study.

Selected Recent Studies of Trends in the Incidence and Prevalence of Dementia

A growing number of recent studies have suggested a declining risk for dementia incidence or prevalence in HICs, including the USA, England, Netherlands, Sweden, and Denmark.[9] Findings from the Rotterdam Study, an ongoing population-based prospective cohort study, suggested that improved cardiovascular risk factor control may be leading to healthier brains. Dementia incidence decreased in cohorts of older adults in Rotterdam between 1990 and 2010, and brain MRIs performed in more recent cohorts show significantly less brain atrophy and fewer vascular-related brain lesions compared to MRIs performed in the earlier cohorts.[10]

Recent findings from the UK Cognitive Function and Ageing Study (CFAS) provide additional support for a declining risk of dementia in older adults over the last 20 years.[11] CFAS studied adults aged 65 and older in Cambridgeshire, Newcastle, and Nottingham in the early 1990s, and then again around 2010. Importantly, the same standardized algorithmic diagnostic process was used for both time periods in order to avoid a 'diagnostic drift', as described above, and to maximize the validity of the prevalence comparisons across the two time periods. Between 1991 and 2011, the age- and sex-standardized dementia prevalence declined from 8.3% to 6.5% between 1991 and 2011 in these regions in England. In addition to a decline in dementia prevalence during this time period, a follow-up analysis of CFAS data found that the incidence of dementia also declined significantly; the overall dementia incidence was 20.0 (95% CI: 16.9–23.8) per 1000 person-years in the earlier period, and 17.7 (95% CI: 15.2–20.9) in the later period.[12] Interestingly, the decline in incidence found in CFAS was significantly greater among men than among women.

In the USA, the prevalence of dementia among adults aged 65+ in the Health and Retirement Study was found to have declined from 11.6% to 8.8% between 2000 and 2012.[13] An increase in educational attainment among older US adults during the time period of the study was associated with some of the decline in dementia prevalence, and there was also some evidence that more aggressive treatment of cardiovascular risk factors (e.g. diabetes and hypertension) was associated with some of the decline. As in England, there is also evidence that dementia incidence has declined in recent decades in the USA; among older participants in the Framingham Heart Study, dementia incidence declined by about 20% per decade between 1977 and 2008, and the decline in risk was seen only among those with at least a high school education.[14]

Wu and colleagues recently performed a comprehensive review of 14 dementia incidence and prevalence studies from across Western Europe, the USA, Japan, and Nigeria.[15] Overall, the review concluded that there has been a reduction over the past few decades in the risk of developing dementia in HICs, with somewhat stronger and more consistent evidence for a decline in dementia incidence compared to dementia prevalence (which also reflects survival with dementia). No single risk or protective factor was identified that fully explained the trends in incidence and prevalence, but rising levels of educational attainment and better control of cardiovascular risk factors and disease (e.g. smoking, hypertension, diabetes, obesity, hyperlipidaemia, stroke, and heart disease) accounted for some of the declining risk in a number of the studies included in the review.

Finally, two recent studies have used the age-period-cohort framework to explore changes in dementia prevalence in both and HICs and LICs. Wu and colleagues performed a meta-analysis of dementia prevalence studies from mainland China, Hong Kong, and Taiwan for the years 1980–2012.[16] There were two main findings from the analysis. First, while the unadjusted prevalence of dementia increased monotonically and significantly from 2.1% of the age 60+ population in the earliest period (prior to 1990) to 5.7% in the latest period (2005–2012), this increasing trend was no longer significant after adjusting for differences across the periods in the diagnostic criteria used to identify dementia. Second, using the method of 'median polish', the authors found evidence for a cohort effect on dementia prevalence, with a higher prevalence of dementia in more recent birth cohorts. They hypothesize that those born more recently in China may have been at higher risk for dementia due to significant national events such as the Great Famine (1958–1961) and the Cultural Revolution (1966–1976), both of which may have had an effect on cognitive development in younger birth cohorts through their impact on nutrition and access to schooling, respectively. In addition, recent economic growth in China has been associated with an increase in cardiovascular risk factors (including smoking, diabetes, and hypertension), which may also be leading to an increase in dementia risk among more recent birth cohorts.

Leggett and colleagues explored whether higher levels of educational attainment among more recent birth cohorts in the USA were associated with better cognitive function.[17] Using data from the Americans' Changing Lives Study on 3617 adults aged 25 and older followed from 1986 to 2011, the analysis found evidence for significantly better cognitive function (as measured by the Short Portable Mental Status Questionnaire) across adulthood for those born between 1947 and 1961, compared to those born before 1932. In latent growth curve models, this cohort effect was nearly entirely explained by the higher level of education in the more recent birth cohorts.

Potential Causes of Trends in the Incidence and Prevalence of Dementia

As noted above, changes in recent decades in the level of educational attainment among older adults, and in the prevalence and treatment of cardiovascular risk factors, have been hypothesized as potential drivers of changes in the incidence and prevalence of dementia in countries around the world. There has been a worldwide trend toward increases in educational attainment over the last 40 years in both LICs and HICs; for instance, the proportion of 30–34-year-olds with a college education increased in HICs from 12% in 1970 to 27% in 2010, and from 3% to 11% in LICs.[18] Education is thought to affect brain biology, building cognitive reserve through neural pathways that allow individuals to better compensate for age-related inflammatory and vascular brain lesions, thereby delaying or preventing incident dementia.[3,19,20] Recent population-based brain autopsy data support the cognitive reserve hypothesis; higher levels of educational attainment were not associated with a lower burden of neurodegenerative and vascular neuropathology, but were associated with a lower risk of dementia before death (Eclipse Collaborative Members 2010).[21]

While there has been a general trend toward increasing levels of education around the world, there are significant international differences in the timing and magnitude of those increases that will likely lead to differences in dementia trends across countries. For instance, while there has been a significant increase in the level of educational attainment among older adults in the USA over the past few decades, there is likely to be no further significant increase in the next few decades, since education levels among those aged 65–69 now are similar to the education levels of those aged 25–29.[22] However, educational attainment among China's older population, for example, will continue to increase in the decades ahead because the education level of those aged 25–29 now is significantly higher than those aged 65–69.[22] Tracking dementia trends across countries with differing time trends in educational attainment may provide opportunities for a better understanding of the causal pathways leading from early-life education to late-life dementia risk.

Improvements in the prevention and treatment of cardiovascular risk factors (CRFs) and disease in recent decades may also have had an important impact on dementia risk among older adults, given the growing evidence of the overlap and interaction of cardiovascular risk factors, AD, and dementia.[23] Population-based autopsy studies have shown that mixed dementia, the combination of AD pathology and vascular pathology in the brain, is extremely common among older adults who die with dementia.[24,25,26] Recent studies have shown that having more CRFs in midlife is not only associated with a greater risk of cognitive decline in later life,[27] but is also associated with higher levels of amyloid protein in the brain, suggesting that CRFs may directly influence the development of AD pathology,[28] in addition to vascular pathology. This potentially close link and overlap between CRFs and the development of AD and vascular pathology raises the possibility that better treatment and control of these risk factors will decrease lifetime dementia risk. However, there are still significant uncertainties regarding if and how treatments for hypertension, diabetes, and hyperlipidaemia affect dementia risk,[29] including whether tighter control of these CRFs in midlife vs late-life is most important, as well as what are the most appropriate treatment targets to prevent or delay cognitive decline.[30]

Worldwide changes in hypertension recognition and control may be especially relevant to trends in dementia risk, given the close link between hypertension and stroke. For instance, in the USA, antihypertensive use increased from 54% to 73% of hypertensive adults between 1988 and 2008, with an accompanying increase in the rate of adequate blood pressure control from 27% to 50%.[31] A recent review of population-based studies of hypertension from around the world found similar improvements in blood pressure control in other HICs, with average systolic blood pressures declining significantly in recent decades, but an opposite trend in LICs in Asia and Africa.[32] These divergent trends in hypertension control, as well as other cardiovascular risk factors such as smoking, obesity, and diabetes across HICs and LICs will be very important to consider in future research on international comparisons of trends in dementia incidence and prevalence.

Trends in Late-life Dementia Prevalence and Incidence by Age, Period, and Cohort in the USA, 2000-2012

In this section, we use data from the US Health and Retirement Study collected from 2000 to 2012 to provide a comprehensive picture of dementia prevalence and the processes that affect change in prevalence. This nationally representative study of US adults was noted above as the source of national estimates of the decline in dementia prevalence in the USA.[13] It has also been used to make estimates of the prevalence of cognitive impairment without dementia (CIND),[33] and incident dementia.[34] We begin with a more detailed assessment of recent change in dementia prevalence US adults aged 65+, by looking at the age-specific prevalence every two years from 2000 to 2012, in order to add information on the consistency of the trend over time. As shown in Fig. 4.1, the decline in prevalence appears to be fairly steady over the 12-year period, supporting earlier reports. This pattern is reinforced by the similar downward trend in CIND, as both levels of cognitive impairment are trending downward together.

We show prevalence change over the 12-year period for men and women by age in Fig. 4.2. We find a fairly consistent pattern of decline between 2000 and 2012 for men across the age range, and for women at ages above 70. These figures suggest some movement to the right of the age curve so that the prevalence of dementia observed in 2000 is reached at an age that is a year or two later in 2012.

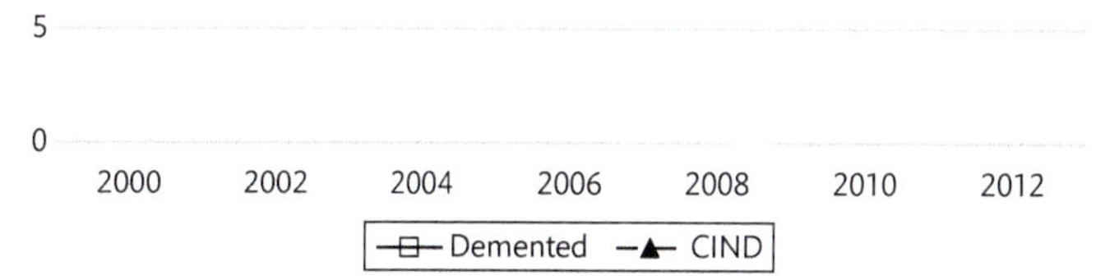

Fig. 4.1 Prevalence of dementia (per cent) and CIND, USA 65+ population: HRS 2000–2012.

Source: data from Langa, K. M., Larson, E., Crimmins, E. et al. A comparison of the prevalence of dementia in the United States in 2000 and 2012. *JAMA Internal Medicine*. 2017; 177(1): 51–58.

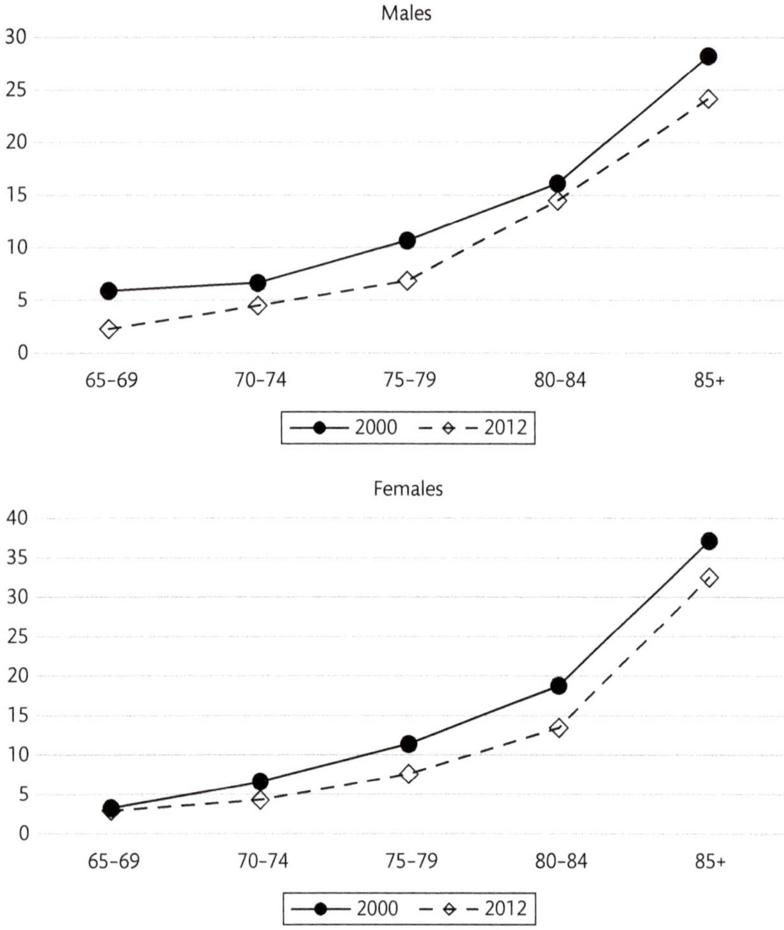

Fig. 4.2 Prevalence of dementia (per cent) by age and sex, USA 65+ population: HRS 2000–2012.

Switching to a cohort formulation of the data allows us to assess whether the reduction in dementia appears to characterize newer cohorts relative to earlier cohorts. Fig. 4.3 shows the percentage with dementia in birth cohorts ranging from 1923 to 1947. While there is not a lot of overlap in the age groups shown for these cohorts, generally most earlier points are above later points, indicating slight cohort improvement in later-born cohorts. Because the overlap across ages is limited, this may be shown more clearly in Fig. 4.4, which aligns the data for four age groups across either three or four cohorts. Most of these points indicate a trend toward

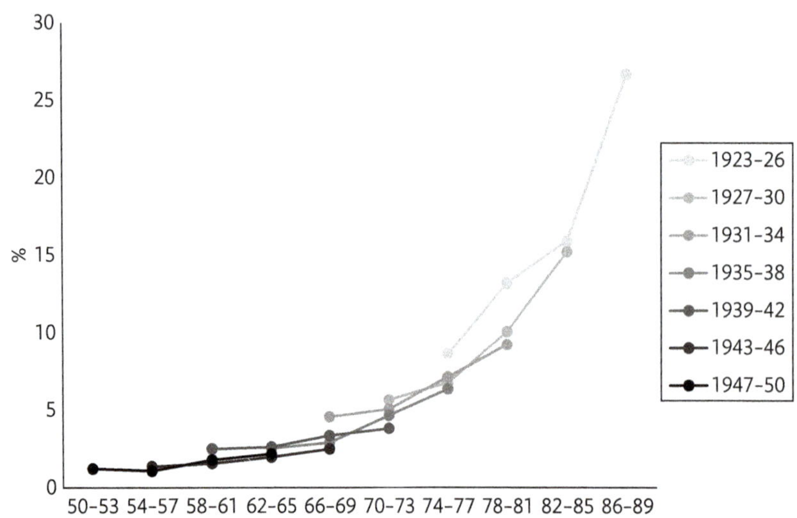

Fig. 4.3 Prevalence of dementia by birth cohort, USA: HRS 2000–2012.

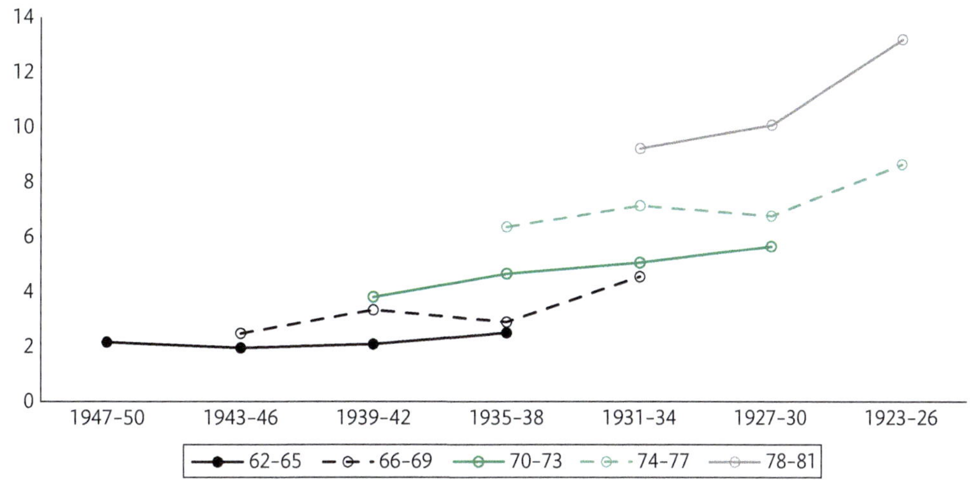

Fig. 4.4 Percentage with dementia at a given age for different birth cohorts, USA: HRS 2000–2012.

reduction in dementia prevalence in later cohorts at a given age. An exception is the last point, which shows an early baby boom cohort at the youngest age—62–65. The cohort declines are consistent and are relatively substantial. Table 4.1 shows that the cohort decline in dementia over 12 years at ages 62–65 is 13.5%, while those at older ages range from 26 to 45%. Thus later cohorts appear to have less dementia at a given age across the age range.

Prevalence actually tells us little about recent onset, as onset of dementia could have been at any time in a person's life when it is found at older ages. Recent incidence of dementia tells us more about current conditions. Incidence requires longitudinal data and a period of time in which to observe new cases. We can do this in the HRS by examining new cases among those who did not have dementia at either end of this 12-year time period. The availability of data allows us to look at four-year incidence over periods that are centred at 2002 and 2010—an eight-year span. Incidence curves by age are shown in Fig. 4.5. There is no suggestion of declining incidence over this period in the Health and Retirement Study (HRS) data. There is very little change in any age group, and only a hint of increase among the oldest women. If the odds of dementia onset in the four-year period is assessed using logistic regression models, the relative odds of dementia is the same in both periods (for men, 1.11 and 1.12 in the two periods and 1.12 and 1.13 for women in the two periods).

Another potential explanation for declining prevalence of dementia would be changing mortality among those who have dementia relative to those who do not. It is possible that mortality among those with dementia actually increased over time, leading to fewer survivors with dementia. However, we do not find evidence that this is the case; while mortality over our four-year observation window among HRS respondents with dementia is much higher than that among those without dementia (53% vs 16%), there is no difference in the four years after 2000 and the years after 2008.

Our investigation of the HRS data leads us to conclude that the evidence continues to point to declines in dementia prevalence among older US adults in recent decades, which correspond to regular improvement across cohorts that reflects lifetime experiences. This is in contrast to marked change in the processes that are currently affecting dementia prevalence such as the incidence rate and the rate of mortality, which appear relatively stable across this short period of investigation.

Table 4.1 Changes in dementia prevalence for birth cohorts at specified age in 2000 and 2012

	Difference, 2000-2012	% Decline	Birth cohort 2000	Birth cohort 2012
Ages 62-65	-0.34	13.5	1935-38	1947-50
Ages 66-69	-2.06	45.3	1931-34	1943-46
Ages 70-73	-1.84	32.4	1927-30	1939-42
Ages 74-77	-2.28	26.4	1923-26	1947-50

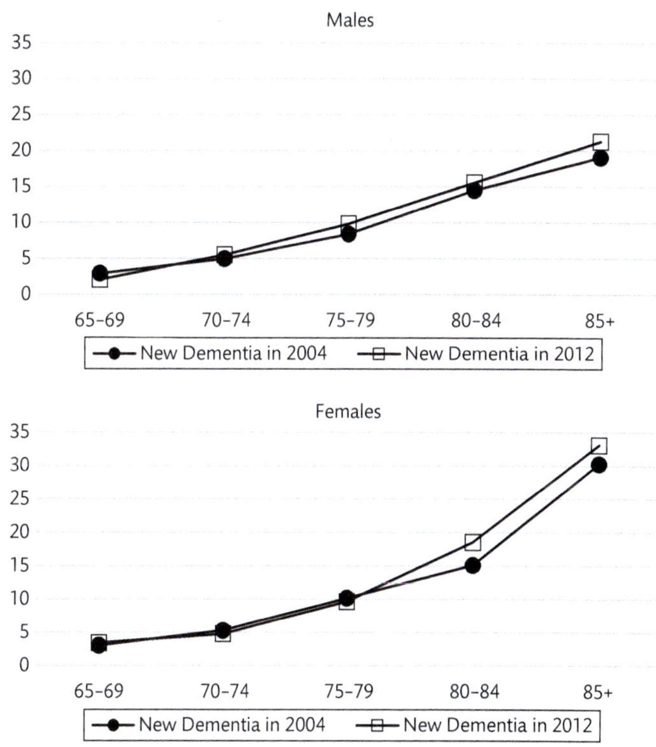

Fig. 4.5 Incidence of new dementia over four years among those without dementia in 2000 and 2008, USA: HRS 2000–2012.

Conclusion

The future large growth in the elderly population around the world makes a better understanding of the current and future incidence and prevalence of dementia especially important for patients, their families, and government support programmes. The individual risk for late-life dementia appears to be a function of diverse factors that span the entire life course, including the amount and quality of early-life education and social interactions, the total burden of midlife cardiovascular risk factors, and the extent of later-life physical and cognitive activity. The complexity of the interactions among social and medical factors across the life course, and how those factors ultimately affect later-life brain health and dementia risk, makes an age-period-cohort perspective on understanding trends in dementia incidence and prevalence especially valuable.

Recent evidence from population-based studies in countries around the world, including the new US data presented in this chapter, point to a declining incidence and prevalence of dementia in HICs, although the evidence is expectedly mixed, given the complexity of risk factors and their interactions across the life course as noted above. Current evidence suggests that the trends in LMICS may be different to those in HICs, perhaps due to different trends in key causal factors such as cardiovascular risk factors. Future population-based studies can use the cross-country variation in trends in education, cardiovascular risk factors, and health and social policies to better understand the causal factors that lead to late-life dementia risk, as well as better project the total societal burden of dementia as populations age around the world.

REFERENCES

1. Finch CE, Crimmins EM. Inflammatory exposure and historical changes in human life-spans. *Science*. 2004; 305(5691): 1736–9.
2. Zhang Z, Gu D, Hayward MD. Childhood nutritional deprivation and cognitive impairment among older Chinese people. *Soc Sci Med*. 2010; 71(5): 941–9.
3. Stern Y. Cognitive reserve in ageing and Alzheimer's disease. *Lancet Neurology*. 2012; 11(11): 1006–12.
4. Yang Y, Land KC. *Age-period-cohort Analysis: New Models, Methods, and Empirical Applications*. Boca Raton, FL: CRC Press, 2013. p1.
5. McKhann GM, Knopman DS, Chertkow H, Hyman BT, Jack CR, Kawas CH. et al. The diagnosis of dementia due to Alzheimer's disease: recommendations from the National Institute on Aging-Alzheimer's Association workgroups on diagnostic guidelines for Alzheimer's disease. *Alzheimer's & Dementia*. 2011; 7(3): 263–9.
6. Albert MS, DeKosky ST, Dickson D, Dubois B, Feldman HH, Fox NC, et al. The diagnosis of mild cognitive impairment due to Alzheimer's disease: recommendations from the National Institute on Aging-Alzheimer's Association workgroups on diagnostic guidelines for Alzheimer's disease. *Alzheimer's & Dementia*. 2011; 7(3): 270–9.
7. Langa KM, Levine D. The diagnosis and management of mild cognitive impairment: A clinical review. *JAMA*. 2014; 312(23): 2551–61.
8. Matthews FE, Stephan BC, Bond J, McKeith I, Brayne C; Medical Research Council Cognitive Function and Ageing Study. Operationalization of mild cognitive impairment: a graphical approach. *PLOS Med*. 2007; 4(10): 1615–19.
9. Larson E, Yaffe K, Langa KM. New insights into the dementia epidemic. *New England Journal of Medicine*. 2013; 369(24): 2275–7.
10. Schrijvers EM, Verhaaren BF, Koudstaal PJ, Hofman A, Ikram MA, Breteler MM. Is dementia incidence declining? Trends in dementia incidence since 1990 in the Rotterdam Study. Neurology. 2012; 78(19): 1456–63.
11. Matthews FE, Arthur A, Barnes LE, Bond J, Jagger C, Robinson L, et al. A two-decade comparison of prevalence of dementia in individuals aged 65 years and older from three geographical areas of England: results of the Cognitive Function and Ageing Study I and II. *Lancet*. 2013; 382(9902): 1405–12.
12. Matthews FE, Stephan B, Robinson L, Jagger C, Barnes L, Arthur A, et al. Cognitive Function and Ageing Studies (CFAS) Collaboration. A two-decade dementia incidence comparison from the Cognitive Function and Ageing Studies I and II. *Nature Communication*, 2016; 7: 11398.
13. Langa KM, Larson E, Crimmins E, Faul J, Levine D, Kabeto M, et al. A comparison of the prevalence of dementia in the United States in 2000 and 2012. *JAMA Internal Medicine*. 2017; 177(1): 51–8.
14. Satizabal CL, Beiser AS, Chouraki V, Chene G, Dufouil C, Seshadri S. Incidence of dementia over three decades in the Framingham Heart Study. *N Engl J Med*. 2016; 374(6): 523–32.
15. Wu YT, Beiser AS, Breteler MMB, Fratiglioni L, Helmer C, Hendrie HC, et al. The changing prevalence and incidence of dementia over time—current evidence. *Nat Rev Neurol*. 2017 (online ahead of print).
16. Wu YT, Lee HY, Norton S, Prina AM, Fleming J, Matthews FE, et al. Period, birth cohort and prevalence of dementia in mainland China, Hong Kong and Taiwan: a meta-analysis. *Int J Geriatr Psychiatry*. 2014; 29(12): 1212–20.
17. Leggett A, Clarke P, Zivin K, McCammon RJ, Elliott MR, Langa KM. Recent improvements in cognitive functioning among older US adults: How much does increasing educational attainment explain? *J Gerontol B Psychol Sci Soc Sci*. 2017 (online ahead of print).
18. Becker GS, Hubbard WHJ, Murphy KM. Explaining the worldwide boom in higher education of women. *J Human Capital*. 2010; 4(3): 203–41.
19. Meng X, D'Arcy C. Education and dementia in the context of the cognitive reserve hypothesis: a systematic review with meta-analyses and qualitative analyses. *PLOS One*. 2012; 7(6): e38268.
20. Valenzuela MJ, Sachdev P. Brain reserve and dementia: a systematic review. *Psychol Med*. 2005; 35: 1–14.
21. Eclipse Collaborative Members, 2010. Education, the brain and dementia: neuroprotection or compensation? *Brain*. 2010; 133: 2210–16.
22. Lutz W, Butz W, Samir KC. *World Population and Human Capital in the Twenty-First Century*. Oxford: Oxford University Press, 2014.
23. Snyder HM, Corriveau RA, Craft S, Faber JE, Greenberg SM, Knopman D, et al. Vascular contributions to cognitive impairment and dementia including Alzheimer's disease. *Alzheimers Dement*. 2015; 11(6): 710–17.
24. MRC CFAS (Neuropathology Group of the Medical Research Council Cognitive Function and Aging Study). Pathologic correlates of late onset dementia in a multicentre, community based population in England and Wales. *Lancet*. 2001; 357: 169–75.
25. Schneider JA, Arvanitakis Z, Bang W, Bennett DA. Mixed brain pathologies account for most dementia cases in community-dwelling older persons. *Neurology*. 2007; 69: 2197–204.

26. Sonnen JA, Larson EB, Crane PK, Haneuse S, Li G, Schellenberg GD, et al. Pathological correlates of dementia in a longitudinal, population-based sample of aging. *Ann Neurol.* 2007; 62: 406–13.
27. Gottesman RF, Schneider AL, Albert M, Alonso A, Bandeen-Roche K, Coker L, et al. Midlife hypertension and 20-year cognitive change: the atherosclerosis risk in communities neurocognitive study. *JAMA Neurol.* 2014; 71(10): 1218–27.
28. Gottesman RF, Schneider AL, Zhou Y, Coresh J, Green E, Gupta N, et al. Association between midlife vascular risk factors and estimated brain amyloid deposition. *JAMA.* 2017; 317(14): 1443–50.
29. Williamson JD, Launer LJ, Bryan RN, Coker LH, Lazar RM, Gerstein HC, et al. Action to control cardiovascular risk in diabetes memory in diabetes investigators. Cognitive function and brain structure in persons with type 2 diabetes mellitus after intensive lowering of blood pressure and lipid levels: a randomized clinical trial. *JAMA Intern Med.* 2014; 174(3): 324–33.
30. Dufouil C, Brayne C. The continuing challenge of turning promising observational evidence about risk for dementia to evidence supporting prevention. *JAMA Intern Med.* 2014; 174(3): 333–5.
31. Egan BM, Zhao Y, Axon RN. US trends in prevalence, awareness, treatment, and control of hypertension, 1988–2008. *JAMA.* 2010; 303(20): 2043–50.
32. NCD Risk Factor Collaboration (NCD-RisC). Worldwide trends in blood pressure from 1975 to 2015: a pooled analysis of 1479 population-based measurement studies with 19·1 million participants. *Lancet.* 2017; 389(10064): 37–55.
33. Plassman B, Langa KM, Fisher G, Heeringa SG, Weir DR, Ofstedal MB, et al. Prevalence of cognitive impairment without dementia in the United States. *Annals of Internal Medicine.* 2008; 148(6): 427–34.
34. Plassman B, Langa KM, McCammon R, Fisher GG, Potter GG, Burke JR, et al. Incidence of dementia and cognitive impairment, not dementia in the US. *Annals of Neurology.* 2011; 70(3): 418–26.

5

Overview of common designs, measures of effect, and biases in neuroepidemiological studies

Derrick A Bennett

Fundamentals of Epidemiological Study Design

Observational epidemiological studies can be subdivided into *descriptive* studies to describe the frequency and patterns of a given neurologic disorder in the population, and *analytic* studies to identify and test whether specific risk factors are associated with the neurological disorder of interest.[1] Experimental studies usually implement some kind of intervention in order to assess the effects on the neurological disorder. Fig. 5.1 shows a schematic of the major study designs that will be covered in this chapter.

Sampling

A fundamental approach to epidemiological research is to take a sample or subset of subjects from a larger defined population to study factors that are linked to the research question about the neurological disorder of interest (such as the onset of a disease, disease severity, or death from the disease). Statistical inference involves drawing conclusions about the population on the basis of a sample and differences may be observed to sampling variation (whereby even though samples may be random and the population does not change we would not expect each sample to give an identical result).[2] An example would be when investigators conduct studies in different settings and in different countries, there will always be differences in the results due to sampling variation. There are several different sampling schemes and these are outlined in Box 5.1.

Researchers are usually interested in determining whether the inferences that can be drawn from their study are correct for the individuals in the sample itself (*internal validity*) as well as whether the sample is a good representation of the 'source population' (*external validity*). In general, if a researcher wishes to conduct an epidemiological study of a neurological disorder, being able to collect data in a sample that is entirely representative of the source population would be almost impossible, and if it was possible, usually very expensive. In practice, many epidemiologic studies of neurological disorders (and many other chronic conditions) are conducted in non-representative populations where internal validity of the study can be achieved during the design and conduct. Generally, it is more important that a study is internally valid than externally valid (or generalizable) because if a study lacks internal validity the fact that it is representative of the source population is of little value.[1]

Person-time and rates

In order to draw reliable conclusions about the distributions of disease in a population, it is important to define the *numerator* and *denominator*. This includes knowing whether one or both numbers measures time. It should be defined whether the numerator is measuring *cases* or *events* and what population the denominator represents. Usually the denominator will represent the *person-time* (which is the multiple of the number of individuals over the time period of concern) and could be in years or months (i.e. person-years or person-months). *Rates* are used to measure of the frequency with which an event occurs in a defined population in a defined time (e.g. number of deaths per hundred thousand Britons in one year). A rate has a time dimension, whereas a proportion (e.g. number of Britons with AD divided by the total population) does not.

Descriptive epidemiological studies are particularly useful for assessing *prevalence* or *incidence* (see Box 5.2 for details). Even in a chronic disease, the manifestations are often intermittent, so as a consequence the point prevalence that is based on a single point in time tends to underestimate the neurological condition's total frequency. If repeated or continuous assessments of the same individuals with the neurological condition are possible, the period prevalence would provide a better estimate.

There are two different measures of incidence (cumulative incidence and the incidence rate (see Box 5.2 for details), and the choice between them depends on the study design. Incidence may be estimated from either a *fixed population* of subjects or a *dynamic population* (a group that is open to changes such as those due to births, deaths, or migrations). This changing denominator can be overcome by relating the

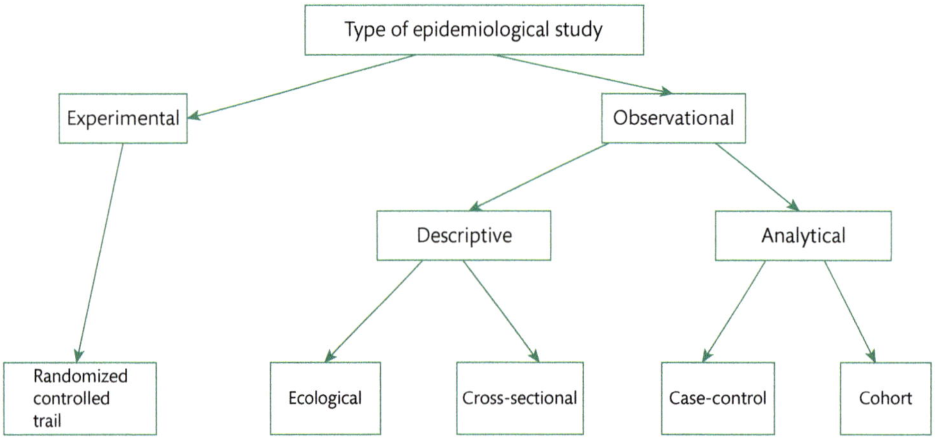

Fig. 5.1 A schematic of the major study designs.

numbers of new cases to the *person-time at risk*, calculated by adding together the periods during which each individual member of the population is at risk during the measurement period. The incidence rate and prevalence ratios are often expressed as the number with the neurological disorder per 100,000 population, for ease of presentation. Incidence rates and prevalence ratios for neurologic disorders will often vary according to personal characteristics such as gender, age, and race/ethnicity. Information on how disease incidence and prevalence vary according to these factors often provides the first clues about risk factors for a neurologic disorder.

Descriptive Epidemiological Studies

Investigative epidemiology begins with descriptive studies that aim to understand a neurologic disorder. The aim of such a study is to estimate how common or frequent the disorder is in the general population. Differences in disease frequency between subgroups of the population (such as those based on ethnicity or geographic location) may help identify risk factors for disease. The following subsections give a brief overview of the main types of descriptive epidemiological studies, with examples from the contemporary neurological literature.

Ecological studies

Ecological studies are designed to investigate associations between exposures and outcomes in populations (or groups) rather than in individuals.[3] Ecological studies tend to try and identify correlations between exposures and groups defined by geographical region (country, city), or by time (calendar period, birth cohort). Ecological studies may be useful for two reasons.[4] First, because it has been recognized that, even when studying individual level risk factors, population level studies can play an important role in identifying the most relevant public health problems to be tackled, and in hypothesis-generation of potential causes. Second, some risk factors for disease genuinely operate at the population level and under certain specific circumstances they may directly cause disease, but more realistically they may lead to disease because they are determinants of exposure to individual level risk factors.[5] For example, being poor in a rich country or neighbourhood may be more detrimental than having the same income level in a poor country or neighbourhood, and this is likely to be because of problems of social exclusion and lack of access to services and resources.[6] These types of studies suffer from a problem known as the *ecological fallacy* that occurs when associations seen in the groups under study are assumed to be also occurring at the individual level. An example of the ecological fallacy is that almost any chronic disease that is associated with affluence or

Box 5.1 Common types of sampling in epidemiology

Random sampling: this is where each person has the same chance of being selected for the study from the source population.

Stratified sampling: this is when the source population is divided into strata with the characteristics of interest such as age, sex, or ethnicity and individuals are then selected randomly from within each stratum.

Multi-stage sampling: this involves taking random samples at different levels from the source population.[56] The primary sampling unit could be city or province, the secondary sampling unit is a district or suburb, the tertiary sampling unit is street and the final sampling unit could be individuals within a household.

Cluster-sampling: this involves sampling groups of individuals such as schools, neighbourhoods, patients that attend a particular type of health practitioner, or cities, instead of sampling each individual separately.[57]

Box 5.2 Metrics used in descriptive epidemiology

Prevalence: is a count of existing number of people (usually as a percentage) with a disease of interest in a population.

Point prevalence: is the number of people with the disease of interest at a particular point in time.

Period prevalence: is the number of people with disease of interest during a specified time period (e.g. one year).

Incidence: this is a count of the new cases of the disease of interest in a defined population.

Cumulative incidence: is the proportion of people that develop the disease of interest during a specified time period, for example, within one month or one-year.

Incidence rate: is a measure of how quickly the disease of interest is occurring in the population. It is the ratio of the number of new cases to the total person-time at risk (where person-time is defined as the sum of time that each at risk individual contributes to the study).

Relationship between measures: incidence, prevalence, and duration of disease can provide a simple estimate of one measure from the other by the relationship: Prevalence = (incidence) × (average duration of disease).

Source: data from Hennekens, C.H., Buring, J.E. *Epidemiology in Medicine*. Lippincott Williams & Wilkins; 1987.

the adoption of a 'westernized lifestyle' has also been found to be associated, at the national level, with sales of television sets.[4] A recent published example of an ecological study in the neurological literature is the one by Lavados et al.[7] This study investigated whether regional differences in stroke mortality rates in Chile could be related to the variability in distribution of cardiovascular risk factors, the quality of medical care, or socioeconomic status. The authors found that risk of death from stroke in Chile was associated with age, sex, and being resident in four specific regions of the country.[7]

Cross-sectional studies

The aim of a *cross-sectional study* is to describe the health of a population and therefore these types of study need to be externally valid (i.e. they need to be representative sample of the source population). Cross-sectional studies measure both the exposure and disease in an individual at some specific point in time and provide information on the frequency of disease in a population at one point in time. Unfortunately, they do not provide direct evidence of the sequence of events and as a consequence only prevalence can be reliably estimated. For example, in the UK, the Health Survey for England (HSE) is a series of annual surveys about the health of people living in England. A structured interview containing key questions with each eligible person in the household is followed by a nurse visit for those who agree to take part. Each year, there is also a particular focus on a population group, disease, or condition.[8]

Box 5.3 Effect size metrics used in analytic epidemiology

The following measures are often used in cohort studies:

Relative risk or risk ratio: this ratio of the incidence of an event of interest in the exposed group to the incidence of the event of interest in the unexposed group.

Rate ratio: the ratio of incidence rate of the event of interest in the exposed group to the incidence rate of the event of interest in the unexposed group.

Risk difference: this is the difference between the risk of the event of interest in the exposed group and the risk of the event of interest in the unexposed group.

The following effect size metric is often used in a case-control study:

Odds ratio: this is the ratio of the odds of exposure in cases compared with the odds of the exposure in controls.

Measures of population impact used in case-control or cohort studies.

These measures assess the public health impact of an exposure assuming that the association between the exposure and disease is causal and are mainly used for cohort studies but can be used for case-control studies as well.

Population attributable risk (PAR): PAR is the difference in the rate or risk of disease for the population compared to the unexposed.

Population attributable risk fraction (PAF): PAF is the proportion of cases for an outcome of interest that can be attributed to a given risk factor among the entire population.

Source: data from Hennekens, C.H., Buring, J.E. *Epidemiology in Medicine*. Lippincott Williams & Wilkins; 1987; data from Jackson, R, Ameratunga, S., Broad, J. et al. (2006). The GATE frame: critical appraisal with pictures. *Evid Based Med*; 11: 35–38.

Analytical Epidemiological Studies

There are two major types of analytical epidemiological studies and each of them can be used to compare exposed and unexposed groups: cohort studies (or follow-up studies) and case-control studies. The main goal of analytic epidemiological studies of neurological disorders is to identify associations between putative risk factors and relevant neurologic outcomes. The risk factors and neurological outcomes are selected on the basis of the key research question. For example, many analytical epidemiological studies would collect information on several putative risk factors such as gender, age, lifestyle factors (e.g. smoking, alcohol, physical inactivity), environmental exposures, and molecular or genetic markers, in order to ascertain whether an association exists between these putative factors and a given neurological disorder. How this can be achieved through appropriate design of such studies will now be described.

Cohort studies

A classical prospective *cohort study* may be defined as a sample of the overall 'source population' to follow-up over a period of time. Exposures in the participants are measured at the outset of the study and their disease experience during follow-up is recorded. A *cohort study* is the best way to ascertain both the incidence and natural history of a disorder. All participants (both exposed and unexposed) in a cohort study must be at risk of developing the outcome or outcomes of interest. Box 5.3 describes some of the key metrics used in analytical epidemiology.

An example of a prospective cohort study is the Rotterdam Study that began in 1990 in the city of Rotterdam in the Netherlands. The study targets neurological disorders as well as several other chronic diseases of old age.[9] The Rotterdam Study included individuals living in a well-defined subgroup, (the Ommoord district) in the source population (the city of Rotterdam), in the Netherlands, and by 2008, the cohort included about 15,000 subjects aged 45 years or over. The participants in the Rotterdam Study were followed for a variety of neurological disorders such as stroke, Parkinson's disease, AD, and other dementias, as well as other chronic diseases of old age (such as macular degeneration, glaucoma, osteoporosis, and cancer).[10] The Rotterdam Study has contributed a large body of evidence to both neurological epidemiology and chronic disease epidemiology in general.[10] In terms of neurological research this study has identified that vascular risk factors are associated with poorer cognitive performance,[11] and has also ascertained that several lifestyle factors are associated with the risk of dementia and AD.[12,13] The Rotterdam Study has also contributed to large-scale collaborations that have identified novel genes underlying the risk of AD and stroke.[14,15]

Case-control studies

In very general terms a *case-control study* (aka retrospective study design) involves a group of subjects with the disease (the cases) and a second group without the disease (the controls). The frequency of past exposure to the putative risk factor is then determined in both groups (usually by asking the subjects to report their past exposure by the use of a standardized self-report questionnaire), and compared. If more cases are exposed than controls then this is an indication that the exposure may be a risk factor for the disease.[16]

The two key criteria that investigators should adhere to are: (1) there must be a clear and explicit definition of the criteria for diagnosis of a case and any eligibility criteria used for case selection; (2) controls should come from the same 'source population' as the cases, and their selection should be independent of the exposure or exposures of interest.[16] Generally, it is often preferred to use incident (new) cases rather than prevalent (existing) cases in a case-control study due to the fact that prevalent cases may have changed their behaviour or the disease itself may have altered the exposure of interest.[17] Case-control studies may seem simple, but choosing a control group can be more challenging than at first glance and a clear rationale for choice of control is required.[18,19] After clearly defining cases and controls, relevant data on exposures and other important variables has been collected, the investigator then aims to calculate a measure of effect for the case-control study of the neurological disorder. The OR and its associated CI is used as a measure of the strength of the association between an exposure and the neurological disorder (see Box 5.3). It is often stated in epidemiological textbooks that for rare diseases the OR calculated from a case-control study provides a good estimate of the relative risk (rate-ratio) as defined in a cohort study.[20] However, if the case-control is nested within a cohort study (i.e. cases and controls sampled from a well-defined 'source population') and the controls are selected longitudinally throughout the course of the study (often referred to as 'incidence density sampling') the resulting OR will approximate the rate-ratio for the 'source population'.[17,21]

A recent example of a well-designed case-control study of a neurological disorder is the one performed by Billioti de Gage and colleagues.[22] In this study the authors aimed to investigate the relationship between the risk of AD and exposure to benzodiazepines started at least five years before, considering both the dose-response relationship and an early symptom indicating the onset of a disease or illness (such as prodromal (anxiety, depression, insomnia)) possibly linked with treatment.[22] The authors report on a case-control study among older people (age >66) living in the community in the province of Quebec (Canada) and who were members of the public drug plan from 1 January 2000 to 31 December 2009. The source population included random samples of 38,741 people with a diagnosis or treatment (such as cholinesterase inhibitors or memantine) related to dementia for cases and 86,259 people without these conditions for controls, and the controls were selected by using an incidence density sampling strategy.[22]

Bias and Confounding in Epidemiological Study Designs

Bias

All types of epidemiological study can be prone to bias and biased studies produce results that differ systematically from the truth. The key biases in epidemiological studies are *selection bias* and *information bias*. Selection bias can arise from an absence of comparability between groups being studied or due to the people included in the study being non-representative of the source population due to non-response. Information bias can occur if the exposure data is collected in a non-standardized manner and it may differ between those with and those without the neurological disorder of interest. Table 5.1 summarizes the different types of selection and information biases, and steps to be taken to avoid these biases, when designing an epidemiological study.

Confounding

The major problem with all observational epidemiological studies is *confounding*. A *confounding factor* is one which is associated with the exposure of interest and is also associated with the neurological disorder of interest. In descriptive epidemiological studies death rates and disease rates are usually strongly related to age and often differ by sex. These rates therefore depend critically on the age-sex composition of the population of interest and thus it is very misleading to use overall crude rates when comparing two populations (unless they have identical age-sex structures). Standardization is a method used in descriptive epidemiology in order to produce comparable measures between populations or subgroups adjusted by major confounders such as differences in the age-sex structure of the populations or subgroups being compared.[23] Examples include comparing geographical regions (such as cities, counties, or countries) or certain groups (such as different occupations). There are two methods, known as direct and indirect standardization, and both methods use a 'standard population'. The choice of method is usually determined by the availability of the data and by their relative accuracy. Direct standardization is preferred when there are small numbers of events in any of the age-sex strata of the study populations as this method is more accurate. Indirect standardization is preferred if for some reason it is not possible to obtain national data on age-sex specific rates.

In analytical epidemiology, investigators should address confounding either at the design stage of the study or at the analysis stage using statistical techniques (such as stratification or multivariable regression analyses).[24] Matching controls to cases at the design stage of the study is one approach to minimizing the effects of confounding. Matching aims to minimize confounding by reducing systematic differences between those with the disease and those without the disease in terms of the confounding factors.[25] If the neurological condition of interest was multiple sclerosis (MS) gender is known to be associated with many risk factors for MS.[26] If the gender distribution of those with the disease is different from that of those without the disease, failure to take this confounder into account at the design or analysis stage can lead to spurious results. It is important at the analysis stage to assess whether the magnitude of the effect size (e.g. OR or rate ratio) could have been influenced by confounding by producing an adjusted effect size that takes into account potential confounding factors using multivariable regression models.[27] If the magnitude of the adjusted effect size is not substantially altered after adjustment for all known confounding factors then the investigator may then believe that their results are robust (although there may still be residual confounding due to unknown or unmeasured confounders).

Matching case-control studies are the most common design and the matching may be done for convenience or to improve precision.[28] The increase in efficiency occurs because it ensures similar numbers of cases and controls in each of the strata as defined by the confounder.[28] Matching should be used carefully as cases and controls should not be matched on variables that the investigator may be interested in assessing as having possible associations with the neurological disorder in the future.[29] Not only should exposure variables not be included, but neither should variables that are closely related to these variables. In addition, so-called *overmatching* should be avoided, as, if the controls are too similar to the cases, then the study may fail to detect a 'true association' between the exposure and the neurological disorder, even if one exists.[28–30]

Table 5.1 Bias in epidemiological study designs

Form of bias	Method to deal with this bias at the design stage
Selection bias	
What is selection bias? This type of bias occurs when the selection of the study participants for an epidemiological study is not representative of the entire 'source population' at risk.	A clear description of the 'source population' and how individuals with the neurological disorder and individuals without the neurological disorder were ascertained and classified.
Types of selection bias	
Extreme exposure status: This can occur in a cross-sectional survey if the subjects sampled were from either high or low-income status, neither of which would be representative of the overall. Differential diagnosis or referral of cases in a case-control study.	Strict inclusion and exclusion criteria can be applied in order to produce homogeneous groups.
Selection related to exposure: This can occur in a case-control or cohort study if the subjects selected for the study are somehow related to the exposure of interest.	An investigator may decide to utilize multiple control groups (such as group of community controls and a group of hospital controls) in order to ascertain whether their effect size is influenced by potential selection bias.
Non-response bias: A particular form of selection bias is non-response bias, where subjects that agree to participate in a study are different from those that decline or those that withdraw from a study are different to those that remain in the study.	Processes are in place that are used to re-contact non-responders to encourage these individuals to participate in the study. If possible the reasons for declining to participate should be documented
Information bias	
What is information bias? This occurs in an epidemiological study when the information that has been collected is incomplete or incorrect for some reason.	This can be circumvented by having well-designed questionnaires with in-built logical, validation and range checks.
Types of information bias	
Recall bias: This is a form of information bias that can occur in case-control studies when there is a difference between cases and controls in the accuracy and completeness of exposure information.	This can be circumvented by having several approaches to obtain exposure history details. Also the use of memory aids, such as photographs, diaries, and calendars can help participants remember exposures.[16]
Misclassification bias: This is a form of information bias that can occur where subjects are incorrectly assigned to one group when they should be in another.	For outcome status this can be avoided by having a clear definition of how someone will be classified as having the neurological disorder or not (e.g. ICD-10 code or CT/MRI scan). For exposures this can be by having objective questions and several approaches to obtain exposure history details (such as biomarkers of exposure).
Non-differential misclassification bias: This applies to the situation when the degree of misclassification in the groups is of the same magnitude and can lead to underestimation of the effect size metric of interest.	For outcome status this can be avoided by using accepted or 'gold-standard criteria' for the neurological disorder (if possible).
Differential-misclassification bias: This is more serious than non-differential misclassification bias as the degree of misclassification differs between the groups and can lead to either over- or under-estimation of the effect.	For outcome status this can be avoided by using accepted or 'gold-standard criteria' for the neurological disorder (if possible). For exposures a clear standard definition of exposed and unexposed can avoid this problem.
Measurement bias: This can occur when the methods of measurements are consistently dissimilar among groups of participants or if the presence of the outcome directly affects the measurement process.	Can be reduced by the use of a consistent approach to measurement for the groups being compared. Avoidance of measurement processes that are directly affected by the outcome of interest can also reduce this bias.
Interviewer bias: This can occur if interviewers are aware of the study hypothesis and subconsciously or consciously gather data selectively	One way to reduce this is to try to blind (or mask) to case-control status or the research hypothesis from the person who is collecting risk factor information or interviewing subjects.

Experimental Epidemiological Study Designs

The advantage of experimental studies in epidemiology are that they are less susceptible to confounding because the investigator determines who is exposed and who is unexposed. The main advantage is due to the fact that, if the exposure is allocated randomly to groups and the number of individuals *randomized* is sufficiently large then both measured and unmeasured confounding are more likely to be equally balanced between the groups. The most common design is the randomized controlled trial.

Randomized controlled trials

In the simplest parallel group RCT design to test the efficacy of a novel drug in the treatment of a specific disease, some patients with the disease are randomized to receive the new drug and some are randomized to be given the best existing drug. The two groups are then compared prospectively for incidence of disease and other important outcomes (also known as endpoints) of interest. Some of the key metrics that can be derived from an RCT are described in Box 5.4.

When conducting experimental studies it is usual have information reported in the protocol on research ethics committee approval (also known as institutional review boards) who will be concerned with informed consent (Do participants in the study fully understand the risks as well as the benefits of the study?), autonomy (Are participants physically and mentally capable of deciding what they will allow to be done to them?), and whether there is sufficient uncertainty to justify randomization.[31] In general, a high-quality RCT needs to utilize the following principles: (1) proper randomization; (2) have an appropriate comparison group and blinding (masking) of participants; (3) use intention-to-treat analyses; and (4) avoid conducting numerous unspecified data-driven subgroup analyses

Box 5.4 Metrics used in randomized controlled trials

Binary outcomes

	Event	No-event	Total
Treated	a	b	a + b
Control	c	d	c + d
Total	a + c	b + d	a + b +c +d

Relative risk or risk ratio (RR): the ratio of the risk of a given event in treated group of participants compared to the control group [a/(a + b) ÷ c/(c + d)].

Relative risk reduction (RRR): the proportion of the initial or baseline risk which was eliminated by a given treatment/intervention or by avoidance of exposure to a harmful factor.

The RRR is calculated as (1 − RR)*100%.

Odds ratio (OR): the ratio of the odds of a given event in the treated group of participants compared to the control group [a/b ÷ c/d].

Absolute risk reduction (ARR): the difference in risk of a given event, between two the treated and control groups [a/(a+b) - c/(c+d)].

Number needed to treat (NNT): the number of patients needed to be treated in order to prevent one additional event (and is the reciprocal of ARR, i.e. 1/ARR).

Continuous outcomes

	Mean	Sample size	Standard deviation	Standard error
Treated	M_t	N_t	SD_t	$SE_t = SD_t/\sqrt{N_t}$
Control	M_c	N_c	SD_c	$SE_c = SD_c/\sqrt{N_c}$

Mean difference: this is the difference in means between the treated and control group (e.g. $M_t – M_c$).

Standardized mean difference: this is the difference in means between the treated and control divided by the standard error of the mean difference (e.g. $(M_t – M_c) / \sqrt{(SE_t^2 + SE_c^2)}$).

to investigate effect modification.[32] More details and rationale for these key design issues in an RCT are outlined in Table 5.2.

An example of a large neurological trial is MRC CRASH RCT that aimed to assess the effect of corticosteroids on death and disability after head injury.[33] A group of 10,008 patients with head injury and a Glasgow Coma Scale score of 14 or less, within 8 hours of injury, were randomly allocated to a 48-hour infusion of corticosteroid (methylprednisolone) or placebo, with the primary outcome measures being death from any cause within two weeks of injury and death or disability at six months.[33]

Causality and Effect Modification

Well-designed epidemiological studies and RCTs play an important role in medical research. Analytical epidemiological studies can identify important hypotheses that can be tested in subsequent experimental studies. For both these designs the sample selection should be robust and the study size should be large enough to obtain an effect size estimate with a sufficiently narrow CI to be able to meaningfully answer the research question of interest (see Box 5.5 for more details).

Assessing causality

Observational epidemiology can only identify an association, but RCTs are considered to be the most robust study design for assessing *causality* in medical research due to their prospective nature and control of confounding factors.[34] Determining the cause of disease is a complex and inter-related process and it is rare to find a single exposure or factor that will directly cause one disease in epidemiology. Bradford-Hill[35] (Box 5.6) proposed some criteria for causality which have been used by epidemiologists as a guide in order to enhance the understanding of the disease process.

Table 5.2 Key properties of a good randomized controlled trial

Requirement for a good randomized controlled trial	Rationale for the requirement
1. Proper randomization (allocation to the particular drug is done by a probabilistic random process that ensures balance for known and unknown factors).	Specifically, the purpose of *randomization* is to assign patients to groups in a way that gives each patient an equal chance of falling into one or the other group; this should ensure that all factors are balanced between groups. Altman and Bland outline some common methods of randomization used in experimental studies.[48] Commonly accepted methods of administering the randomization include: centralized randomization by computer or telephone, randomization scheme controlled by pharmacy, numbered or coded containers administered sequentially to enrolled participants, on site computer system which can only be accessed after entering the characteristics of an enrolled participant.
2. Minimize bias (patients, clinicians and outcome evaluators should be unaware of the treatment allocation to the particular drug, and an adequate comparator group should be used).	*Blinding (or masking)* is necessary so that there is no risk of knowledge of the treatment received can influence the assessment of the patient. Altman and Schulz discuss practical ways to blind an RCT and other studies.[49,50] In a randomized controlled trial one of the treatments is included in the trial as a basis for comparison and it may be either an active treatment or a *placebo*. A true placebo is an inert or inactive treatment otherwise identical in appearance, taste, and mode of administration to the active treatment.[50]
3. Intention to treat analyses (the treatment efficacy is based treatment allocated rather than treatment received—that is the statistical analyses are performed according to the randomized groups regardless of adherence).	An *intention-to-treat analysis* is defined as: 'All patients randomly allocated to one of the treatments in a trial should be analysed together as representing that treatment, whether or not they completed, or indeed received that treatment.'[51] This is deemed to be the most robust and unbiased way to investigate the efficacy of a treatment. Despite this being the most robust form of analysis, in practice, these analyses have been found to be conducted and reported inconsistently.[52] Loss to follow-up can make intention-to-treat analyses more difficult and the researcher needs to make plausible assumptions about the outcome of those patients lost to follow-up otherwise the estimated treatment effect could be biased.[53]
4. Minimize the number of data-driven subgroup analyses.	Essentially *the more the data is divided up the more false-positive results are likely to be observed.* Analysing many subgroups can produce chance results, particularly if they have not been pre-specified beforehand. Rothwell suggests that if important subgroup effects are anticipated trials should be powered to detect them reliably.[54] Assman et al. stress the importance of statistical tests of interactions when analysing subgroups in an RCT.[55]

Box 5.5 Sample size

Sample size considerations for analytical epidemiological study designs and RCTs are extremely important because if a study is too small then it is unlikely that the investigators will be able to detect a modest, but clinically important, difference.[34]

Conversely, if a study is too large then time and resources will be wasted. Prior to the commencement of a study the investigators should therefore spend a reasonable length of time deciding on a feasible sample size required in order to meet the goals of the study.

The key components required for a sample size calculation for epidemiological studies are described in the references by Charan and Biswas[60] and Schlesselman[61] and for randomized trials by Schulz and Grimes.[62]

In order to ascertain whether an association between an exposure and a neurological disorder is causal, the investigator has to demonstrate that the association cannot be explained by chance, methodological flaws, bias, or by confounding. Doll[36] suggested that the essential criterion for causality is temporal sequence, as in some circumstances the strength of association may be so great (as with some occupational risk factors), and other evidence is lacking, that other criteria such as plausibility and consistency are irrelevant.

Effect modification

Effect modification occurs when the magnitude of the effect of the primary exposure on an outcome (i.e. the association) differs depending on the level of a third variable. In this situation, computing an overall estimate of association is misleading. One common way of dealing with *effect modification* is to examine the association separately for each level of the third variable. Effect modification (also called statistical interaction), is present when the association between exposure and disease is stronger in certain subgroups of the study subjects than in others. If effect modification is present, it may suggest new hypotheses to explain the interaction between the characteristic that defines the subgroups and association between exposure and disease. When effect modification is found in subgroups in either an observational or experimental study where it was not hypothesized, it should be evaluated in terms of the Bradford-Hill criteria (particularly the magnitude, probability, and biological plausibility), to determine whether it is real. Generally, large sample sizes are required to have sufficient statistical power to detect subgroup effects reliably in both observational and experimental epidemiology. However, information from both these types of design can make an important contribution to new knowledge.[37]

Box 5.6 Key criteria for assessing causality from epidemiological studies

The following criteria were proposed by Bradford-Hill.

Temporal sequence: this must be ascertained as an exposure cannot be deemed to be causal if it did not occur before the effect. The time period between the exposure and the disease must make biological sense and can only be determined via prospective studies.

Strength of association: this determines how important a specific exposure is in the disease process. The effect of the exposure can be quantified by computing some useful statistic which measures the strength of association.

Consistency of effect: observing similar associations in different populations and via different study designs can suggest that the findings are robust.

Biological plausibility: the association should make sense in terms of the biological mechanisms leading to the disease outcome of interest.

Dose-response: this informs the investigator that as the frequency or duration of the exposure increases, so the strength of the disease association also increases, therefore providing some evidence of the exposure being causal.

Specificity of effect: this means that if a specific exposure leads a specific disease, then this is good evidence of causality. A strong association with disease of a particular factor in the presence of other known risk factors is evidence of specificity (i.e. the association is independent of other known risk factors for the neurological disorder). The removal of an exposure or risk factor which leads to decreased risk of disease also provides evidence of specificity.

Source: data from Hill AB. The Environment and Disease: Association or Causation? *Proceedings of the Royal Society of Medicine*. 1965; 58(5):295–300.

Conclusion

Descriptive and analytical epidemiological methods can be used to assess trends and healthcare planning, such as those methods employed in the international Global Burden of Disease and Injuries (GBD) project that has aimed to assess trends in common neurological conditions such as stroke,[38,39] as well as rarer conditions.[40] The general aim of the GBD project has been to inform policymakers about the particular health challenges faced by their country and use this information to align health systems in order to better serve the host population.[41] The GBD has gone beyond estimating disease prevalence to incorporate risk factor prevalence and to quantify the impact in terms of disability adjusted life years (DALYs) and years of life lost due to the disease or risk factor, or healthy life expectancy.[42]

It should also be emphasized that not only do studies in neuroepidemiology need to be well designed and conducted, but also the findings need to be reported to a high standard. Good reporting strategies for neuroepidemiological studies facilitate the synthesis of the evidence (e.g. via systematic reviews), and are therefore of critical importance. Checklists and reporting standards are common for particular types of studies. For example, the Strengthening the Reporting of Observational studies in Epidemiology (STROBE) guidelines[43] are well known and widely used for analytical epidemiology (i.e. case-control studies, cohort studies, and cross-sectional studies). There are also reporting guidelines such as CONSORT for RCTs.[44] These types of reporting guidelines serve to help researchers design and undertake robust studies and can also assist reviewers and potential users of research outputs to assess validity and reliability. A neurological specific checklist, the Standards of Reporting of Neurological Disorders (STROND) that aims to facilitate more consistent, transparent, and contextualized reporting of descriptive and clinical studies in neuroepidemiology has been recently published[45,46] and examples of good reporting of the STROND items in the context of the MS literature has also been reported.[47] As there are now vast amounts of neurological research being published each year the ability to assimilate, critically appraise, and apply research findings has become essential and this chapter has endeavoured to make this difficult task somewhat easier for the early career researcher in neuroepidemiology.

REFERENCES

1. Grimes DA, Schulz KF. An overview of clinical research: the lay of the land. Lancet. 2002; 359(9300): 57–61. Epub 26 January 2002.
2. Altman DG, Bland JM. Uncertainty and sampling error. BMJ. 2014; 349.
3. Grimes DA, Schulz KF. Descriptive studies: what they can and cannot do. Lancet. 2002; 359(9301): 145–9. Epub 26 January 2002.
4. Pearce N. The ecological fallacy strikes back. Journal of Epidemiology and Community Health. 2000; 54(5): 326–7.
5. Susser M. The logic in ecological: I. The logic of analysis. American Journal of Public Health. 1994; 84(5): 825–9.
6. Yen IH, Kaplan GA. Neighborhood social environment and risk of death: multilevel evidence from the Alameda County Study. American Journal of Epidemiology. 1999; 149(10): 898–907.
7. Lavados PM, Díaz V, Jadue L, Olavarría VV, Cárcamo DA, Delgado I. Socioeconomic and cardiovascular variables explaining regional variations in stroke mortality in Chile: an ecological study. Neuroepidemiology. 2011; 37(1): 45–51.
8. England HSfE. Health Survey for England. Health and Social Care Information Centre: https://digital.nhs.uk/data-and-information/publications/statistical/health-survey-for-england/health-survey-for-england-2015.
9. Hofman A, Breteler MB, van Duijn C, Krestin G, Pols H, Stricker BC, et al. The Rotterdam Study: objectives and design update. European Journal of Epidemiology. 2007; 22(11): 819–29.
10. Hofman A, Brusselle GO, Murad S, van Duijn C, Franco O, Goedegebure A, et al. The Rotterdam Study: 2016 objectives and design update. European Journal of Epidemiology. 2015; 30(8): 661–708.
11. Breteler MMB, Claus JJ, Grobbee DE, Hofman A. Cardiovascular disease and distribution of cognitive function in elderly people: the Rotterdam study. BMJ. 1994; 308(6944): 1604–8.
12. Ott A, Slooter AJC, Hofman A, van Harskamp F, Witteman JCM, Van Broeckhoven C, et al. Smoking and risk of dementia and Alzheimer's disease in a population-based cohort study: the Rotterdam Study. Lancet. 1998; 351(9119): 1840–3.
13. Ruitenberg A, van Swieten JC, Witteman JCM, Mehta KM, van Duijn CM, Hofman A, et al. Alcohol consumption and risk of dementia: the Rotterdam Study. Lancet. 2002; 359(9303): 281–6.
14. Desikan RS, Schork AJ, Wang Y, Thompson WK, Dehghan A, Ridker PM, et al. Polygenic overlap between C-reactive protein, plasma lipids, and Alzheimer disease. Circulation. 2015; 131(23): 2061–9.
15. Ikram MA, Seshadri S, Bis JC, Fornage M, DeStefano AL, Aulchenko YS, et al. Genomewide Association Studies of Stroke. New England Journal of Medicine. 2009; 360(17): 1718–28.
16. Schulz KF, Grimes DA. Case-control studies: research in reverse. Lancet. 2002; 359(9304): 431–4. Epub 15 February 2002.
17. Pearce N. Classification of epidemiological study designs. International Journal of Epidemiology. 2012; 41(2): 393–7.
18. Grimes DA, Schulz KF. Compared to what? Finding controls for case-control studies. Lancet. 2005; 365(9468): 1429–33.
19. Wacholder S, McLaughlin JK, Silverman DT, Mandel JS. Selection of controls in case-control studies: I. Principles. American Journal of Epidemiology. 1992; 135(9): 1019–28.
20. Hennekens C, Buring J. Epidemiology in Medicine. Boston: Little, Brown and Co., 1987.
21. Pearce N. What does the odds ratio estimate in a case-control study? International Journal of Epidemiology. 1993; 22(6): 1189–92.
22. Billioti de Gage S, Moride Y, Ducruet T, Kurth T, Verdoux H, Tournier M, et al. Benzodiazepine use and risk of Alzheimer's disease: case-control study. BMJ. 2014; 349.
23. Naing NN. Easy way to learn standardization: direct and indirect methods. Malaysian Journal of Medical Sciences: MJMS. 2000; 7(1): 10–15.
24. McNamee R. Regression modelling and other methods to control confounding. Occupational and Environmental Medicine. 2005; 62(7): 500–506.
25. Sedgwick P. Why match in case-control studies? BMJ. 2012; 344.
26. Wolfson C, Granieri E, Lauer K. Case-control studies in multiple sclerosis. Neurology. 1997; 49(2 Suppl 2): S5–S14.
27. Kirkwood BR, Sterne JAC. Essential Medical Statistics. Oxford: Wiley-Blackwell, 2003.
28. Pearce N. Analysis of matched case-control studies. BMJ. 2016; 352.
29. Thomas SV, Suresh K, Suresh G. Design and data analysis case-controlled study in clinical research. Annals of Indian Academy of Neurology. 2013; 16(4): 483–7.
30. Marsh JL, Hutton JL, Binks K. Removal of radiation dose response effects: an example of over-matching. BMJ. 2002; 325(7359): 327–30.
31. Chan A-W, Tetzlaff JM, Gøtzsche PC, Altman DG, Mann H, Berlin JA, et al. SPIRIT 2013 explanation and elaboration: guidance for protocols of clinical trials. BMJ. 2013; 346.
32. C. Baigent, R. Peto, R. Gray, S. Parish, R. Collins. Large-scale randomized evidence: trials and meta-analyses of trials. Oxford: Oxford University Press, 2011.
33. CRASH, Collaborative, Group. Effect of intravenous corticosteroids on death within 14 days in 10,008 adults with clinically significant head injury (MRC CRASH trial): randomised placebo-controlled trial. Lancet. 2004; 364(9442): 1321–8.
34. Collins R, MacMahon S. Reliable assessment of the effects of treatment on mortality and major morbidity, I: clinical trials. Lancet. 2001; 357(9253): 373–80.
35. Bradford-Hill A. The environment and disease: association or causation? Proceedings of the Royal Society of Medicine. 1965; 58(5): 295–300.
36. Doll RS. Proof of causality: deduction from epidemiological observation. Perspectives in Biology and Medicine. 2002; 45(4): 499–515.
37. MacMahon S, Collins R. Reliable assessment of the effects of treatment on mortality and major morbidity, II: observational studies. Lancet. 2001; 357(9254): 455–62.
38. Krishnamurthi RV, Feigin VL, Forouzanfar MH, Mensah GA, Connor M, Bennett DA, et al. Global and regional burden of first-ever ischaemic and haemorrhagic stroke during 1990–2010: findings from the Global Burden of Disease Study 2010. Lancet Global Health. 2013; 1(5): e259–e81.
39. Feigin VL, Forouzanfar MH, Krishnamurthi R, Mensah GA, Connor M, Bennett DA, et al. Global and regional burden of stroke during 1990–2010: findings from the Global Burden of Disease Study 2010. Lancet. 383(9913): 245–55.
40. Whiteford HA, Ferrari AJ, Degenhardt L, Feigin V, Vos T. The Global Burden of Mental, neurological and substance use disorders: an analysis from the Global Burden of Disease Study 2010. PLOS One. 2015; 10(2): e0116820.

41. Murray CJL, Lopez AD. Measuring the Global Burden of Disease. New England Journal of Medicine. 2013; 369(5): 448–57.
42. Murray CJL, Barber RM, Foreman KJ, Ozgoren AA, Abd-Allah F, Abera SF, et al. Global, regional, and national disability-adjusted life years (DALYs) for 306 diseases and injuries and healthy life expectancy (HALE) for 188 countries, 1990–2013: quantifying the epidemiological transition. Lancet. 2015; 386(10009): 2145–91.
43. von Elm E, Altman DG, Egger M, Pocock SJ, Gotzsche PC, Vandenbroucke JP. The Strengthening the Reporting of Observational Studies in Epidemiology (STROBE) statement: guidelines for reporting observational studies. PLOS Medicine. 2007; 4(10): e296.
44. Schulz KF, Altman DG, Moher D. CONSORT 2010 statement: Updated guidelines for reporting parallel group randomised trials. Journal of Pharmacology & Pharmacotherapeutics. 2010; 1(2): 100–107.
45. Bennett DA, Brayne C, Feigin VL, Barker-Collo S, Brainin M, Davis D, et al. Development of the standards of reporting of neurological disorders (STROND) checklist: a guideline for the reporting of incidence and prevalence studies in neuroepidemiology. European Journal of Epidemiology. 2015; 30(7): 569–76.
46. Bennett DA, Brayne C, Feigin VL, Barker-Collo S, Brainin M, Davis D, et al. Explanation and elaboration of the standards of reporting of neurological disorders checklist: a guideline for the reporting of incidence and prevalence studies in neuroepidemiology. Neuroepidemiology. 2015; 45(2): 113–37.
47. Fiest KM, Marrie RA, Jette N, Bennett DA. The Standards of Reporting of Neurological Disorders (STROND) checklist: Application to multiple sclerosis. Multiple Sclerosis Journal. 2016; 23(1): 23–33.
48. Altman DG, Bland JM. How to randomise. BMJ. 1999; 319(7211): 703–4.
49. Altman DG, Schulz KF. Concealing treatment allocation in randomised trials. BMJ. 2001; 323(7310): 446–7.
50. Schulz KF, Grimes DA. Allocation concealment in randomised trials: defending against deciphering. Lancet. 2002; 359(9306): 614–18. Epub 28 February 2002.
51. Newell DJ. Intention-to-treat analysis: implications for quantitative and qualitative research. International Journal of Epidemiology. 1992; 21(5): 837–41.
52. Hollis S, Campbell F. What is meant by intention to treat analysis? Survey of published randomised controlled trials. BMJ. 1999; 319(7211): 670–4.
53. Akl EA, Briel M, You JJ, Sun X, Johnston BC, Busse JW, et al. Potential impact on estimated treatment effects of information lost to follow-up in randomised controlled trials (LOST-IT): systematic review. BMJ. 2012; 344.
54. Rothwell PM. Subgroup analysis in randomised controlled trials: importance, indications, and interpretation. Lancet. 365(9454): 176–86.
55. Assmann SF, Pocock SJ, Enos LE, Kasten LE. Subgroup analysis and other (mis)uses of baseline data in clinical trials. Lancet. 2000; 355(9209): 1064–9.
56. Sedgwick P. Units of sampling, observation, and analysis. BMJ. 2015; 351.
57. Sedgwick P. Cluster sampling. BMJ. 2014; 348.
58. Bennett DA, Feigin VL. Fundamental statistical and epidemiological concepts. In: Bennett DA, Feigin VL (eds). Handbook of Clinical Neuroepidemiology. New York: Nova Science Publishers, 2007. p690.
59. Pocock SJ, McMurray JJV, Collier TJ. Making sense of statistics in clinical trial reports: Part 1 of a 4-part series on statistics for clinical trials. Journal of the American College of Cardiology. 2015; 66(22): 2536–49.
60. Charan J, Biswas T. How to calculate sample size for different study designs in medical research? Indian Journal of Psychological Medicine. 2013; 35(2): 121–6.
61. Schlesselman JJ. Sample size requirements in cohort and case-control studies of disease. Am J Epidemiol. 1974; 99(6): 381–4. Epub 1 June 1974.
62. Schulz KF, Grimes DA. Sample size calculations in randomised trials: mandatory and mystical. Lancet. 2005; 365(9467): 1348–53.

6

Conducting research in low- and middle-income settings

Maëlenn Guerchet, Rosie Mayston, and A Matthew Prina

Introduction

Patel and Kim[1] described the vast research gap in publishing between HICs and LMICs in 2007, when only 3.7% of published research in psychiatry was reported to originate from LMICs. There are no up-to-date figures for this phenomenon, which has been labelled as the 10:90 divide,[2] but we imagine that even though some progress has been made, there is still an enormous gap between research published in HICs and LMICs. This gap is driven by a number of factors, including: (1) higher rejections rates of submitted manuscripts from LMICs;[1] (2) editorial attitudes (we recommend you read the letter from Peter Tyrer in International Psychiatry);[3] (3) and lack of psychiatric and neurological journals based in LMIC (in 2009 this was only 5.5% in LMICs, but all were based in MICs).[4]

This research gap in psychiatry, however, is not only the result of publishing processes, but it can also be linked to lower levels of research in LMIC settings. Increasing the volume of high quality research in LMICs is vital. Whilst understanding the applicability of results to a specific local context is important, synthesized evidence is vital to scientists and decision makers alike. Currently, most of systematic reviews and meta-analyses published in the neuropsychiatric literature are comprised largely of studies carried out in HIC settings. Given sociocultural, health system, and geopolitical differences between the LMICs and HICs, results from studies carried out in high resource countries are clearly not generalizable to a truly global context. This needs to change. It is clear that there is an increased appetite for research in global mental health, as demonstrated by the increased number of funding options that are currently available.[5]

It is important to note that this chapter has been written from a specific perspective: namely that of researchers based in the UK with experience of collaborative partnerships with colleagues living and working in LMIC settings. Most of the information given in this chapter is relevant to neuropsychiatric research, but could also be generalized to research in any health domain. However, as they are not based on biological markers of pathology like in other medical disciplines, psychiatric concepts (at the core of any measurement process in epidemiology) are strongly influenced by cultural factors.[6] Cultural issues are therefore highly relevant in psychiatric research, especially regarding measurement and epidemiological research. With care, sensitivity, and commitment, we believe partnerships between researchers in HICs and LMICs can be both productive and enjoyable for those involved. However, this work is not without its challenges: differences in perspectives should not be ignored. In particular, it is essential that researchers from HICs recognize the privilege, relative wealth, and opportunities their country of origin affords. Accordingly, in this chapter we focus on how a delicate balance may be achieved, wherein HIC researchers may offer their skills, knowledge, and labour in such a way that this contributes to the development of capacity, evidence, and understanding, whilst recognizing that these contributions should be complementary and considered supplementary to those of local service users, researchers, and clinicians. There remains an undeniable need for the development of research capacity in many LMICs. In addition, the vast majority of research funding comes from HICs. Researchers from HICs are well resourced and arguably have more time to focus upon research skills and career development, compared to LMIC colleagues who typically squeeze research activities into busy clinical jobs embedded in under-resourced and overstretched health systems. For these and many other reasons, we believe that researchers from HICs have an important role to play in global mental health research. We hope that by reading this more people will be encouraged to explore opportunities for collaborative research with colleagues in LMIC to address emerging and neglected neuropsychiatric priorities.

This chapter aims to highlight challenges and opportunities of carrying out collaborative research in LMICs, based on our experience of working with many partners across diverse settings.[7–10] However, we must highlight the diversity of low and middle-income settings. The World Bank classification, based on country income using gross national income (GNI) per capita, might not be relevant to experiences of health and illness, treatment, and services. Pace of health service development is highly heterogeneous within LMIC, such that carrying out research in well-resourced Chinese clinics might not be so different from working in a HIC hospital. Our experience is mainly based in low-income settings, although some of the ideas covered here are more generalizable across LMICs or rural areas of HICs. Based on this experience we have divided this chapter into three sections: (1) foundations for research; (2) data collection; and (3) impact and sustainability, as these phases of research present specific issues that need to be addressed. The approach that we have described in this chapter is the result of our direct experience, and we cannot guarantee that it will work for everyone and in every setting.

Foundations for Research

Community engagement/partnerships

Arguably, a degree of community engagement is essential to the implementation of health research. It is an ethical imperative that research is designed to benefit the population groups from which participants are recruited. In the absence of interactions with local stakeholders, it is impossible to ascertain the relevance of research to local needs. Community-based participatory research provides a framework which integrates community concerns and priorities, aiming to ensure that the voices of stakeholders are heard and ultimately promoting 'mutual credibility and trust' between research teams and the communities in which they work.[11] Although there is some evidence that community involvement in the development of mental and neurological services may have diffuse beneficial effects for healthcare workers, service users, and their families,[12] the extent to which different levels of participation result in genuine transformation and empowerment is uncertain. Nonetheless, efforts towards stakeholder involvement and building genuine collaborations with local partners in LMIC are to be welcomed. Impact of any kind is unlikely to be achieved without strong local partnerships. Expectations of 'impact' from international donor agencies and a commitment to funding-related activities means that there is an additional imperative for HIC researchers to think more carefully about their engagement.

Partnerships between universities can be an excellent starting point for broader community engagement. However, in settings where a combination of civil society, non-governmental organizations, and government agencies are central to health and development, it is important to step outside the confines of academic circles. It is important that engagement occurs at each stage of the research. Early substantive involvement, at the time of conception of the research idea, with policymakers, researchers, providers, and service users will strengthen the proposed research and provide a solid foundation for the development of productive relationships. Theory of change workshops, a participatory method for mapping the goals and process of change, are one possible mechanism for structuring this early inter-sectoral engagement and indeed can be used to shape future research activities.[13] It is important to create space for ongoing dialogue with partners. Depending on feasibility, this might take the form of face-to-face meetings, capacity building workshops, regular newsletters, or webinars/Skype conference calls. Involvement of partners in dissemination activities can be used as a mechanism for expressing appreciation for their participation throughout the lifetime of the project and is an excellent way of ensuring that research findings reach the attention of decision makers and other stakeholders. Although there are some excellent examples related to health systems and policy development,[14] in general, service user involvement in research has been woefully neglected in LMIC settings. Structural barriers exist to user involvement, including societal stigma of neuropsychiatric conditions which can inhibit participation in research,[15] but it is important that efforts are made to build capacity in this area.

Ethics

Although many of the ethical considerations that apply to working with vulnerable populations globally are equally relevant in LMIC settings, working in settings where people living with neuropsychiatric conditions may be particularly disempowered and underserved by health systems incurs its own challenges. Local partnerships are a good way to identify local institutional review boards that can be used to obtain local ethical approvals for research. Local partners are also often the first source of information for HIC researchers, regarding sensitivity to ethical concerns for specific service user groups, populations, and communities. The discrepancy in power which is common of encounters between researchers and research participants is often exaggerated in LIC settings, particularly if the researcher is a cultural outsider from a former colonizer nation. In clinical research settings, this can be particularly problematic as it is easy for potential research participants to elide their participation in research with their use of healthcare.[16] The consent process can often inadvertently support therapeutic misconception: the challenge of differentiating individual benefits from potential for collective good is a significant challenge and is usually delegated to local fieldworkers and seldom scrutinized.[17] Ensuring that participants' expectations of research are realistic is essential to avoiding later resentment at not deriving direct benefits from participation. Clear language and careful training and supervision of fieldworkers is essential to avoiding misconceptions and ensuring potential participants understand that research activities are independent from the care they do or do not receive. Specific considerations should be given to the consent process and communication about research participation with individuals who may lack capacity. Other important considerations include understanding and practice related to confidentiality and data protection. There can often be significant discrepancy between internationalized ethical frameworks and localized practice in this area. Conceptions of privacy and confidentiality vary cross-culturally. Although often insisted upon by ethics committees, the cultural acceptability of interviewing vulnerable individuals alone, without the presence of family members is questionable in many settings. Equally, the expectation of obtaining research-dedicated confidential space in busy clinical settings is not always reasonable. Comprehensive contextual knowledge can aid research teams in navigating these and other ethical challenges associated with carrying out neuropsychiatric research in LMIC settings.

An additional challenge might arise when the research involves blood samples and genetic analyses. Acceptance of blood withdrawal for clinical or research purposes might be less common among the target population or groups participating in the research than would commonly be the case among the general population in HIC settings. Barriers include religious or traditional beliefs, which may mean that research participants perceive the gift of blood for research purposes to be both more risky and more extraordinary than would their counterparts in HIC. In order to allay concerns, it is important that the precise purpose of blood collection as well as detailed information about process are described to potential participants: how much blood will be taken, what will happen to it, what are the specific benefits of this component of participation. If the research team are able to deliver timely, intelligible results which will be of use to participants in terms of supporting self-management, the inclusion of health checks, such as blood pressure measurement or glucose levels should be considered. Providing there are sufficient available clinical resources to support interpretation and health services are available to enable further assessment, health checks can provide an ethical incentive that is both health promoting and often commonly welcomed by participants who would otherwise need to pay for a similar service. Having said this, it is also important to maintain clarity regarding the difference between non-essential benefits offered as compensation for participation in research and clinical services which will be offered in the same way regardless of participation, non-participation, or indeed withdrawal from research activities. Nonetheless, as would be the case in HIC settings, a significant level of refusals of this component of research is to be expected. Consequently, in the context of large epidemiological population-based surveys, if not linked to the main outcome, consenting to blood withdrawal may not be a mandatory condition to enter the study. Given legitimate cultural concerns and historical abuse of human samples by HIC researchers, it can be expected that blood sample protocols will be subjected to particularly stringent scrutiny by local ethics committees. When local resources hinder the execution of certain biological and/or genetic analyses in a country, or when adequate storage preserving samples quality is not ensured locally (e.g. lack of reliable equipment or space, potential power cuts, etc.), shipping them to another location, often a HIC in case of a multi-partner project, might be an appealing option in terms of delivering high quality results. However, local storage and processing of biological samples remain a preferable option to feedback timely results to the research participants and can be an opportunity to develop local capacity. If shipping is required, national and international laws and regulations need to be checked to ensure that the export of such samples is permitted. A material transfer agreement (MTA), which is a contract governing the transfer of tangible research materials between collaborating institutions/organizations when the recipient intends to use it for his/her own research purposes, is often needed. It defines the rights of both partners, the provider and the recipient, but it can be a lengthy process to get this contract established and approved, and therefore needs to be anticipated.

Training

Once ethical approvals have been obtained, training research teams (project co-ordinators, supervisors, and research assistants) is a key step in preparation for implementation of research. It often involves several core considerations: profile of the researchers, content of the training, evaluation of the training and continuous support.

- The profile of interviewers to recruit for data collection and research interviews is likely to be dependent upon available resources and necessary skills required. Local researchers such as community health workers or high school graduates may be more knowledgeable of the community and culture of the participants. Therefore, acceptability and feasibility of the research might be enhanced but training in research methods and scientific principles might have to be reinforced. Recruiting university graduates or medical students who have a better scientific understanding could solve this last aspect, but they might be more socio-culturally distant from the participants, hence lack insight into the lives and understanding of the participants, especially when the research is to be carried out in rural areas. When clinical skills are not required, interviewers do not necessarily need to be healthcare workers. The main qualifications to consider are aptitude, honesty, willingness, diligence, and problem-solving skills. Specific features can impact on the recruitment if, for example, the research is to be conducted in a particular language environment or if specific cultural, gender-based, or social norms are likely to affect the environment in which the research is to be carried out. To summarize, the decision regarding who to recruit may be mainly dependent on available resources and the characteristics that are most likely to yield the best quality research according to the research methods, questions and topic.
- The content of the training has to be carefully designed according to the setting, the research project, and the profile of the staff to train. Whatever the profile of the team of interviewer is, it is recommended that the training starts with an introduction to the research in which they will be involved in, including the definition and description of symptoms of the neuropsychiatric condition studied. Specific training may be considered if the research involves a condition for which awareness within the population and/or research workers is low, to reduce stigmatizing beliefs among research team members, or to enable them to talk about sensitive topics with confidence. The rationale of the research and its potential impact will also have to be clearly presented, using global evidence and the relevance to the local context, as well as the aims of the research programme and the justification for the research methods (population, setting (clinical or population-based), outcomes, and other variables of interest). Using a combination of didactic and participatory approaches is important during training to check understanding and ensure knowledge is correctly applied. For example, beneficial aspects during the training would be: (1) an interactive, engaging, and friendly learning environment; (2) the opportunity to learn from a group of 'experts with real-life experience'; (3) the intensity of the training; and (4) the time given to absorb the material and consolidate new knowledge. In general, a training including more case studies and practical examples instead of too much theory can foster a better understanding, as well as team-building exercises and more visual and graphic elements in presentations.
- Special attention might have to be given where interviewers are doctors from local health services, as it might be tempting for doctors or other clinical health workers, who feel that they know a patient well, to miss out certain parts of a structured assessment and fill out answers from their own previous knowledge. In order to avoid any impact upon training, the trainer might also have to consider certain factors impeding even participation (i.e. gender, educational background, age).
- A favourable training environment can be ensured if sufficient resources are allocated to it, including using a dedicated room with appropriate equipment and scheduling sufficient breaks with refreshments.

- At the end of the training, a 'consolidation' time can be required. The last few days can be devoted to role play between trainees and the use of vignettes, before carrying out pre-test of the instruments and mock interviews using 'dummy' participants. Carried out under the supervision of a trainer, those tools can also be used as an evaluation of the level of the interviewer. The trainer should give detailed feedback on the performance of the trainee at the end of each session. If the performance of the trainee is not satisfying, going over more training and again carrying out interviews with 'dummy' participants until the performance is judged acceptable is recommended. If concerns about the performance of an interviewer are raised at the early stages of data collection, they may need retraining.[18] The consolidation time can also be an opportunity to confront the trainees with any potential difficulties they can encounter on the field (i.e. communication problems, fatigue, or poor cooperation of the participants).
- Finally, ongoing supervision and support to the local research teams are probably as important as the initial training and will ensure consistent quality over time. Supervision will be discussed in more detail in the data collection section. Continuous support can take several forms and should be discussed between investigators. Local investigators and HIC researchers can agree on regular Skype meetings or calls, and/or visits at critical stages of the implementation of the research, for example.

The training is also an opportunity to work collaboratively with local resources. 'Training of trainers' (ToT) models might be a more suitable and sustainable way of ensuring training of the research workers as well as local capacity, especially in the case of a multisite, nationwide project or longitudinal research project. However, time, institutional support, and adequate resources are likely to influence the success of a ToT in health partnerships.[19] Local researchers and service users are key people with an undeniable expertise on the context that can be used while planning the training and also when developing local adaptations. Different models of training, which will not be described here, exist for health research and intervention in LMICs.[20]

Study population

Issues related to selection of study population and sampling in LMIC settings can be broken down into two sets of challenges: those that are related to the definition of the population and those that relate to sampling and recruitment. It should be noted that in this section we focus more on the definition of the population rather than sampling methods and recruitment. Recognition and definition of cases of neuropsychiatric conditions might be cross-culturally different and need to be considered alongside (see Box 6.1 on Measurement challenges in LMICs).

In the context of low and middle-income settings, neuropsychiatric research might be first implemented in health services such as hospitals or primary care centres, before population-based studies are developed.

In some LMIC settings, a large proportion of people living with neuropsychiatric conditions never make it to a biomedical service: traditional and religious healers may be the first port of call, if people receive any treatment at all.[32] The role of these providers in the frontline of addressing neuropsychiatric conditions has emerged recently and studies have focused on the potential for integration of non-biomedical providers (traditional or faith healers) into

Box 6.1 Measurement challenges in LMIC

The extent to which the use of diagnostic categories and tools developed in HICs results in a measurement bias has been an ongoing topic of debate in cross-cultural psychiatry and global mental health.[21,22] Cross-cultural psychiatric research has traditionally been polarized between etic and emic approaches.[23] The etic approach comes from a position of universalism and assumes that experiences of mental illness are similar across different cultural settings. Therefore, HIC approaches to measurement are appropriate. The obvious critique of this approach is that it represents an imposition of HIC ideas, seeking to impose homogeneity when the reality is heterogeneous. The emic approach comes from a relativist perspective and assumes that experiences of distress can only be understood in the context of a particular cultural setting. The core critique of this approach is that it negates what is shared cross-culturally and does not facilitate any kind of cross-cultural comparative research and learning.

Today, most global mental health researchers would probably situate themselves somewhere in the middle of the etic-emic dichotomy.[24] There is consensus that there is conceptual overlap across different cultural settings, but that this varies according to both the disorder and the cultural settings being compared. The extent of the shared aspects of experience of phenomena might lead to either: cultural adaptation of an instrument originally designed for use in a different setting or alternatively, the development of an indigenous instrument, the performance of which might be compared with existing instruments designed to measure similar constructs.[25] Preparatory qualitative work is a useful way of understanding the extent to which concepts of illnesses of the spirit, for example, overlap with mental disorders. If there is little conceptual overlap, researchers might consider using the results of qualitative preparatory work to identify items to include in a new indigenous questionnaire. These might be combined with items from existing measures if qualitative work fails to identify concepts which are deemed to be important from expert opinion or clinical practice.[26] If there is a greater degree of conceptual overlap, researchers may wish to focus on ensuring a careful process of translation and back translation of the original instrument followed by necessary minor modifications.[27] In both cases, it is important to carry out pilot testing of the new or adapted instruments, followed by any further necessary revisions, before carrying out a full assessment of the psychometric properties of the instrument. Remember that developing an instrument from scratch is rarely advisable: this takes time and is expensive. It should be remembered that deficiencies of instruments are often over-estimated; adaptations can often be made in order to make them culturally appropriate.

An additional measurement challenge that can affect selection of diagnostic tool is the feasibility of neuro-diagnostic tests (like head CT, brain MRI, EEG, EMG, and CSF analysis).[28] These are largely dependent upon expensive high tech facilities, which are gradually becoming more accessible and reducing costs. Take the following example: until January 2015 there was no MRI in the Lao People's Democratic Republic. To date, there is still no neuro-imaging at all in Central African Republic. Unfortunately, if one is to carry out research in this context, the best that can be done is to strengthen the study protocol and identify the most reliable way to establish a diagnosis without these kinds of facilities. In the case of dementia research, it could be the use of further psychometric tests (such as the Free and Cued Selective Reminding Test)[29] allowing better characterization of cognitive impairments and even dementia subtypes. Additionally, a thorough assessment of disability and dependence, which are strongly associated with dementia, would enable a check on the validity of diagnosis. Outcomes might not be the only variables that are challenging to measure in low and middle-income settings. Methods for ascertaining demographic and socioeconomic status may need adaptation in order to be valid in some settings. For example, in countries for which birth registrations were not common for older generations, age may be reliably estimated using historical landmarks, such as a pandemic influenza in Nigeria or a solar eclipse in Benin.[30,31]

public health systems.[33] Neuropsychiatric 'cases' being most likely to be treated in the non-biomedical sector, researchers considering carrying out research in these facilities need to recognize that research participants are unlikely to be representative of those living with the condition residing in the area, let alone the country as a whole. In general, researchers can expect to encounter: more severe/chronic cases; people living with the condition who have families with sufficient resources and/or social capital to travel to the facility; and people living in the local urban area. Nonetheless, conducting research in tertiary institutions (i.e. large or university hospitals where specialists are practising) should not be dismissed: working in these settings often offers collaborative opportunities with experienced senior clinicians, more likely to have an orientation towards research, and based in a comparatively well-resourced environment. There are specific issues related to clinic-based research and selection of study location which are not dealt with here.[6,34–36]

In the case of population surveys, a common limitation encountered in low and middle-income settings is that it can be difficult to trace a reliable and/or up-to-date census or register (i.e. electoral lists, telephone directories) on which one can rely on for the sampling, as often happens in HIC. This might preclude the realization of any probabilistic sampling methods. Alternatives can be considered. One can be to implement a door-to-door survey in a geographically defined catchment area.[37,38] However, no urban or rural catchment area can hope to be representative of the aggregate characteristics of the city or country as a whole and the door-knocking will constitute an additional stage to the study protocol, as the area will need to be strictly defined and mapped where a house numbering system is not in place. This can therefore be a time and resource consuming process. Another alternative is to conduct a study within a health and demographic surveillance site (HDSS), in collaboration with the local institutions leading them and/or a global network coordinating them, such as the INDEPTH network.[39] Those DSS, located primarily in Africa, Asia, and Oceania, are effective and comprehensive data collection systems focusing on the populations of small, clearly delineated geographic areas. Initial and repeat censuses of the population are performed, registering each individual resident and recording their associated information, such as socioeconomic and behavioural data, health outcomes, and vital events.[40–42] Those sites are usually open and amenable to all types and forms of collaboration with external institutions that wish to engage in research with them. The INDEPTH network is now implementing a new generation of population surveillance operations, the Comprehensive Health and Epidemiological Surveillance System (CHESS), capable of timely delivery of high-quality data for disease-specific and pathogen-specific morbidity, together with data for overall and cause-specific mortality.[43] In both situations (door-knocking or HDSS), working in a defined and restricted geographical area might facilitate regular contacts, collaboration, and communication with the local authorities and the community as well as data collection.

Data Collection

Recruitment and minimizing loss to follow-up

As described in previous sections relating to building solid foundations for research, engagement with stakeholders from the conception of the study and throughout its duration is essential to achieving successful and impactful research. Good levels of community awareness and buy-in are crucial to attaining an acceptable recruitment rate, ultimately ensuring a sample that is representative of the base population. In addition to general engagement activities, it might be important to consider specific activities targeted at recruitment (e.g. community awareness meetings).[44] As ever, it is important to consult with local partners regarding the most appropriate content and structure of materials to support the achievement of recruitment goals (visual materials for populations with low or variable literacy rates, co-opting a local knowledge broker, often a community or religious leader, to facilitate or attend recruitment-related events).

Recruitment of participants in the research might be maximized with an efficient training of the interviewers and good knowledge of the community. Interviewers need to be well prepared to approach participants and understand the procedures for locating households and participants. A good coordination of the team will also ensure efficiency and security by:

- Contacting the right households and participants.
- Having a positive image amongst the community.
- Organizing cost-efficient and secure transportation for the interviewers (this might involve the cost of a dedicated vehicle and driver in rural areas for long distances with dispersed households).
- Ensuring that the interviewers are making contacts with the participants at appropriate time, particularly in rural areas (i.e. avoid arriving at households at peak harvest time when everyone is likely to be working long hours in the field). In some regions, seasonality, namely rainy seasons, can make transportation and interviews in rural areas particularly challenging.

Data collection

In HICs, ethics committees commonly emphasize that research interviews need to take place in a quiet, private environment with only the individual participant and the interviewer present (although there are exceptions to this). Researchers should be alert to tensions between the expectations of HIC ethics committees and the reality of carrying out research in LMICs. There are both practical and cultural reasons why conducting research interviews in LMICs can sometimes differ vastly from interviews with similar purpose and content carried out in HICs. Overstretched public clinics often lack private space for clinical encounters, let alone research activities. Understandings and prioritization of confidentiality and privacy vary cross-culturally: in some settings, other clinicians or family members being present for research interview might be either unavoidable or considered more acceptable than a one-to-one encounter between interviewer and interviewee.[26] In the case of a population survey, interviews are commonly performed in the participant's own home, unless the participant specifically requests to be assessed at a clinical centre (see Fig. 6.1). Two interviewers working together may provide better security if working in 'dangerous' areas or may reduce the amount of time spent in the household, thus minimizing disruption to the family's routine, if several people are to be interviewed in the same household.

For longitudinal studies, working in LMIC can sometimes provide additional challenges to minimizing loss to follow-up. Common methodologies used to maximize retention, such as regular newsletters or telephone contacts with participants present

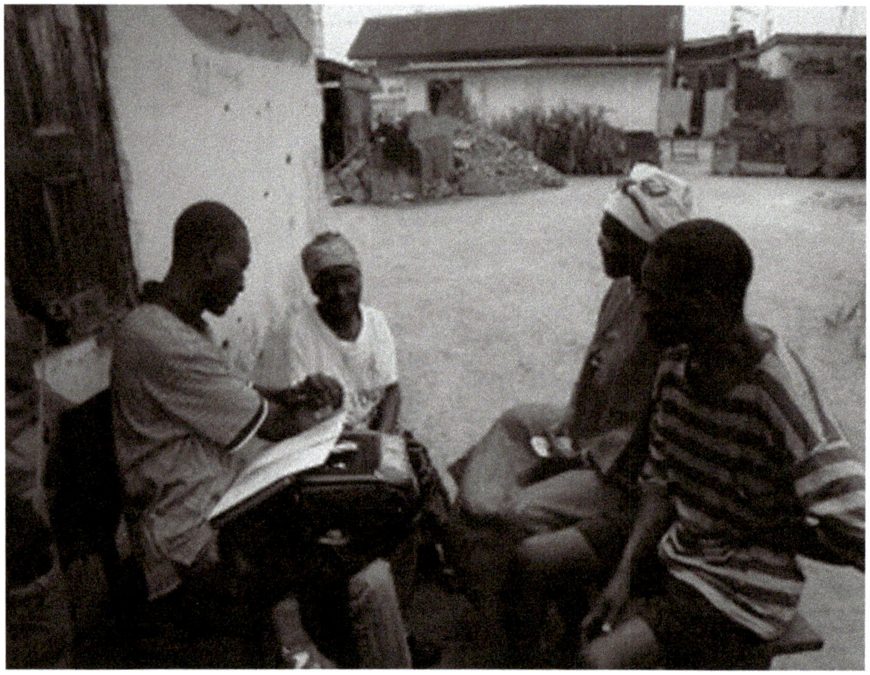

Fig. 6.1 Interview of an older adult, EDAC study, Congo, 2009.

might their own challenges. For example, email and postal services are unlikely to offer good coverage of study participants, especially in rural areas. Although mobile phone penetration has expanded rapidly in recent years, they cannot necessarily be considered a reliable mechanism for contacting participants. In many areas, mobile phones remain a collective resource, shared by members of the same household. This presents an ethical challenge, particularly if the nature of the research is sensitive. In addition, phones running out of credit or charge can mean they can be sometimes unused for long periods.[45]

Data management and quality control

As technologies are advancing, debates around the means of data collection are becoming more common. While coding or collecting data on paper sheets or questionnaires can provide a reassuring paper trail audit and minimize risks associated with power cuts and surges that may be damaging to electronic devices, collection on laptops or tablets is becoming a more feasible option in many settings. There are potential advantages and disadvantages associated with each approach. Although digital approaches offer the advantage of producing a relatively clean final dataset, extensive work is required to translate the paper questionnaire to the digital format, and test and amend this version to ensure usability. This process can be time consuming and should only really be considered if the relevant technological expertise to support this work is locally available. Computerized questionnaires can contain automatic checks and skips that facilitate the flow of the interview but potentially obscure any mistakes made by interviewers. Paper questionnaires necessitate double entry of data which can be a useful first step in quality assurance, offering the first opportunity for identification of mistakes, lack of clarity in recording of answers by interviewers, which can be addressed promptly by research supervisors. The final consideration is data security. A weatherproof, secure location that facilitates the storage of paper documents is essential. Even if data is primarily collected digitally, consent forms and other materials are usually on paper and need to be stored. A reliable power source without surges and long periods of lack of power is essential for digital devices in order to ensure data is not lost. The safety of both staff and devices should be considered.

Data quality can sometimes be at risk due to the challenges of carrying out research in LMICs. In some cases, researchers cannot expect to achieve the same level of accuracy as compared to studies carried out in highly calibrated research focused facilities in HICs (see Fig. 6.2). A pragmatic approach is key here: given the lack of evidence in some areas, a carefully designed population-based survey where all reasonable efforts have been made to maximize data quality, but where the margin of error is likely to be larger than that of similar findings conducted in HICs is a valuable contribution to the evidence base. The lack of precision of certain tools used to ascertain these neuropsychiatric disorders in some contexts is recognized and might impact current epidemiological data. However, important advances in psychiatric epidemiology have been made (especially in measurement equivalence across cultures), making the argument that many mental disorders are prevalent globally and are associated with high levels of distress and/or impairment.[46] A recent systematic review of qualitative literature on how depression is experienced around the world showed that diagnostic and associated features described in the DSM criteria are consistent with the most frequently mentioned symptoms of depression at both regional and global levels.[47] However, certain DSM non-diagnostic symptoms were also more prominent in some regions than some diagnostic features. These results support the need to continue investigating expressions of distress in order to adapt instruments for regional variations without dismissing entirely the use of standard instrument based on western models, as core

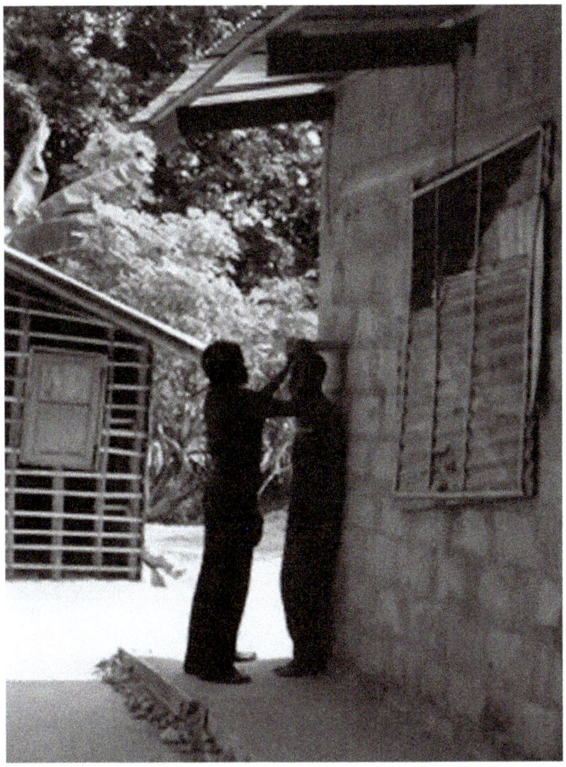

Fig. 6.2 Height measurement in a rural setting, Congo, 2012.

features were retrieved globally. Considering the large gaps in existing epidemiological data, this work is important in highlighting the global burden of mental disorders and informing the development of evidence-based local and global health and social policies, including national plans (e.g. Ethiopia) and mhGAP.[48,49]

These challenges notwithstanding, there are several important steps that may be taken to preserve data quality. Many of these are not dissimilar to challenges associated with managing research in HIC, although as indicated previously, particular attention should be paid to the skill sets, knowledge, and background of research staff which may be more diverse in LMIC settings. Capacity of staff to undertake consistent, high-quality work in line with study protocols is key: processes described regarding training and supervision are essential. Specific procedures include: review of completed research interview data by the research supervisor to identify issues related to completeness, unusual patterns of response, or high levels of missing data, which can then be addressed in supervision. Regular team meetings will allow the coordinator to discuss the issues encountered on the field as well as keeping the team motivated and interested in their work during the whole length of the study.[18] In addition to these, it may be important for a senior member of the research team to make ad hoc field visits to observe research team members in action. This may uncover additional issues related to acceptability of research activities, which interviewers may be reticent to report during supervision. Finally, usual procedures for evaluating data quality should be carried out by the data manager or study co-coordinator: for example range checks to check distributions and identify any outliers which require further elucidation.

Impact and Sustainability

Data analysis/dissemination

A crucial component of research comes after the data has been collected. Untapped data is sitting on many computers unanalysed. Equally, half-finished, or yet to be submitted manuscripts can also linger on our hard drives or desks for so long that we end up forgetting they even existed. This situation is common in both HICs and LMICs, but different issues are likely to underpin this phenomenon. In LMICs this is often the result of low research capacity and a lack of time specifically allocated to research activities.

Highly specialized data management, statistical analysis skills, and knowledge may be less common in LMIC settings, as also advanced training in epidemiological methods. Costs of some of the training, software, and equipment needed to carry out those analyses can be prohibitive. Although support from researchers in HICs can be sought, it is important that local capacity to carry out analyses in LMICs is developed. Some of the barriers to data analysis can be overcome by utilizing freely available open access software such as R,[50] a widely-used language and environment for statistical computing and graphics. Using this software can, however, be challenging for someone who has never used a statistical package before, compared to the more familiar (and costly) interface of SPSS, for example. Thus, training becomes a requirement. Although this is one of the biggest challenges, training using freely available online resources is slowly becoming feasible, particularly now that Internet access is increasingly ubiquitous.

Analysing the data is not the last hurdle, and unfortunately many papers never see the light of the day. Preparation of articles can be challenging, particularly if English is not the author's first language. Overseas collaborators may have an important role to play in editing and drafting articles, but it is important that efforts are made to address the disparity wherein a large proportion of papers originating from LMICs have a first author from a HIC.[1] International journals should also adopt more lenient policies, mostly relating to language and to the preparation of the manuscript following authors' guidelines, which can be complex, time-consuming, and culture-bound.

Dissemination of results using other means is also vital, and this can include policy briefs, public engagement workshops, reports, and use of social media among others. As part of the INDEP project,[9] for example, the Peruvian Principal Investigator of the study collaborated with the media school to produce a documentary of the research carried out, which is now freely available on the Internet.[51] Although this type of dissemination is not appropriate for every research project, it is important to engage in diverse dissemination activities which aim to reach a variety of audiences. Online repositories allowing the archive of manuscripts that have not yet been peer-reviewed or published are also starting to appear (i.e. BioRxiv).[52] This process can have some advantages, including speeding up the dissemination of results, before submission to a peer-reviewed journal. The Wellcome Trust is also encouraging this process.[53] In order to increase the reach of research, selecting the open access option should also be encouraged given that many journals waive or discount the open access publication fee for researchers based in LMICs.

Sustainability

Although arguably mental health has recently emerged as a bona fide field of global health, neuropsychiatric conditions have long been neglected by governments, international donors, and researchers. As a result, there remains a large disparity in the quantity, quality, and impact of neuropsychiatric research carried out in LMIC settings, relative to the burden of disease.[54] This is indicative of a lack of capacity and a lack of resources for research. It is essential that research teams think beyond the lifetime of the research project to build capacity for future research led by local teams. This will be crucial to ensuring the indigenization of research to address local priorities.[55] Although short-term, capacity-building programmes undoubtedly result in the advancement of knowledge and skills among some individuals, greater attention needs to be paid to issues such as developing regional collaborative networks and research culture if sustainable impacts are to be achieved. It may be helpful to carry out a needs assessment among stakeholders at the start of a project to guide the development of future capacity-building activities.[56] ToT models of capacity-building are currently underused in the context of mental health research in LMICs, despite evidence of effectiveness in other settings. In addition, it is important to consider possible mechanisms for evaluating the impact of capacity-building activities upon longer-term impacts, including, but not limited to, career advancements, publications with lead authors from LMIC, as well as successful grant applications from principal investigators.[56]

Conclusion

Collaborative and multicentre research programmes across different settings are contributing to strengthened partnerships between HIC and LMIC research, improved research capacity, and increased outputs from LMICs. Equity in those partnerships is key if the research is aiming at a real impact in policy and practice. However cross-cultural work is not always easy and calls for sensitivity and respect, including a recognition that scientific expertise and knowledge should be considered alongside more specific and local forms of knowledge and understandings. We have attempted to highlight specific examples where these differences might become challenges and made what we hope are pragmatic suggestions to address them. The current rise in funding opportunities in global health (starting from a very low base) should be seen as an opening to establish and maximize collaborations in order to perform high-quality research in LMIC and finally put neuropsychiatric research on global public health agendas.

REFERENCES

1. Patel V, Kim YR. Contribution of low- and middle-income countries to research published in leading general psychiatry journals, 2002–2004. Br J Psychiatry. 2007; 190: 77–8.
2. Saxena S, Paraje G, Sharan P, Karam G, Sadana R. The 10/90 divide in mental health research: trends over a 10-year period. Br J Psychiatry. 2006; 188: 81–2.
3. Tyrer P. The editor's dilemma: assessing papers of low-income countries. International Psychiatry. 2008; 5(79).
4. Kieling C, Herrman H, Patel V, Tyrer P, Mari JJ. A global perspective on the dissemination of mental health research. Lancet. 2009; 374(9700): 1500.
5. Global health funding reaches new high as funding priorities shift. (press release). Institute for Health Metrics and Evaluation (IHME) 2014.
6. Patel V. Cultural issues in measurement and research. Practical Psychiatric Epidemiology. Oxford: Oxford University Press, 2003. p414.
7. Guerchet M, Mbelesso P, Ndamba-Bandzouzi B, Pilleron S, Desormais I, Lacroix P, et al. Epidemiology of dementia in Central Africa (EPIDEMCA): protocol for a multicentre population-based study in rural and urban areas of the Central African Republic and the Republic of Congo. Springerplus. 2014; 3: 338.
8. Lund C, Alem A, Schneider M, Hanlon C, Ahrens J, Bandawe C, et al. Generating evidence to narrow the treatment gap for mental disorders in sub-Saharan Africa: rationale, overview and methods of AFFIRM. Epidemiol Psychiatr Sci. 2015; 24(3): 233–40.
9. Mayston R, Guerra M, Huang Y, Sosa AL, Uwakwe R, Acosta I, et al. Exploring the economic and social effects of care dependence in later life: protocol for the 10/66 research group INDEP study. Springerplus. 2014; 3: 379.
10. Prina AM, Acosta D, Acostas I, Guerra M, Huang Y, Jotheeswaran AT, et al. Cohort profile: the 10/66 study. Int J Epidemiol. 2016; 1–10.
11. Mosavel M, Simon C, van Stade D, Buchbinder M. Community-based participatory research (CBPR) in South Africa: engaging multiple constituents to shape the research question. Soc Sci Med. 2005; 61(12): 2577–87.
12. Petersen I, Baillie K, Bhana A, Mental H, Poverty Research Programme C. Understanding the benefits and challenges of community engagement in the development of community mental health services for common mental disorders: lessons from a case study in a rural South African subdistrict site. Transcult Psychiatry. 2012; 49(3-4): 418–37.
13. Breuer E, Lee L, De Silva M, Lund C. Using theory of change to design and evaluate public health interventions: a systematic review. Implement Sci. 2016; 11: 63.
14. Semrau M, Lempp H, Keynejad R, Evans-Lacko S, Mugisha J, Raja S, et al. Service user and caregiver involvement in mental health system strengthening in low- and middle-income countries: systematic review. BMC Health Serv Res. 2016; 16: 79.
15. Mayston R, Alem A, Habtamu A, Shibre T, Fekadu A, Hanlon C. Participatory planning of a primary care service for people with severe mental disorders in rural Ethiopia. Health Policy Plan. 2016; 31(3): 367–76.
16. Appelbaum PS, Roth LH, Lidz C. The therapeutic misconception—informed consent in psychiatric research. Int J Law Psychiat. 1982; 5(3-4): 319–29.
17. Reynolds L, Cousins T, Newell ML, Imrie J. The social dynamics of consent and refusal in HIV surveillance in rural South Africa. Social Science & Medicine. 2013; 77: 118–25.
18. 10/66 Dementia Research Group. Population-based Study Manual—version 3.0. King's College London, London: Institute of Psychiatry, 2004: 8–9.
19. Mormina M. A conceptual framework for ToT interventions in global health; executive summary. THET. https://www.thet.org/wp-content/uploads/2017/07/Executive-summary-final-161123.pdf.

20. Murray LK, Dorsey S, Bolton P, Jordans MJ, Rahman A, Bass J, et al. Building capacity in mental health interventions in low resource countries: an apprenticeship model for training local providers. Int J Ment Health Syst. 2011; 5(1): 30.
21. Summerfield D. Afterword: against 'global mental health'. Transcult Psychiatry. 2012; 49(3-4): 519–30.
22. Whitley R. Global Mental Health: concepts, conflicts and controversies. Epidemiol Psychiatr Sci. 2015; 24(4): 285–91.
23. Sartorius NK. Translation of health status instruments. In: Kuyken J (ed.). Quality of Life Assessment: International Perspectives. Berlin: Springer, 1994. pp3–18.
24. Patel V. Explanatory models of mental illness in sub-Saharan Africa. Soc Sci Med. 1995; 40(9): 1291–8.
25. Patel V, Simunyu E, Gwanzura F, Lewis G, Mann A. The Shona Symptom Questionnaire: the development of an indigenous measure of common mental disorders in Harare. Acta Psychiatr Scand. 1997; 95(6): 469–75.
26. Mayston R, Habtamu K, Medhin G, Alem A, Fekadu A, Habtamu A, et al. Developing a measure of mental health service satisfaction for use in low income countries: a mixed methods study. BMC Health Serv Res. 2017; 17(1): 183.
27. World Health Organization. Process of translation and adaptation of instruments Available from: http://www.who.int/substance_abuse/research_tools/translation/en/.
28. McLane HC, Berkowitz AL, Patenaude BN, McKenzie ED, Wolper E, Wahlster S, et al. Availability, accessibility, and affordability of neurodiagnostic tests in 37 countries. Neurology. 2015; 85(18): 1614–22.
29. Grober E, Buschke H, Crystal H, Bang S, Dresner R. Screening for dementia by memory testing. Neurology. 1988; 38(6): 900–903.
30. Ogunniyi A, Osuntokun BO. Determination of ages of elderly Nigerians through historical events: validation of Ajayi-Igun 1963 listing. West Afr J Med. 1993; 12(4): 189–90.
31. Paraiso MN, Houinato D, Guerchet M, Agueh V, Nubukpo P, Preux PM, et al. Validation of the use of historical events to estimate the age of subjects aged 65 years and over in Cotonou (Benin). Neuroepidemiology. 2010; 35(1): 12–16.
32. Demyttenaere K, Bruffaerts R, Posada-Villa J, Gasquet I, Kovess V, Lepine JP, et al. Prevalence, severity, and unmet need for treatment of mental disorders in the World Health Organization World Mental Health Surveys. JAMA. 2004; 291(21): 2581–90.
33. Gureje O, Nortje G, Makanjuola V, Oladeji B, Seedat S, Jenkins R. The role of global traditional and complementary systems of medicine in treating mental health problems. Lancet Psychiatry. 2015; 2(2): 168–77.
34. Thornicroft G, Patel V. Global Mental Health Trials. Oxford: Oxford University Press, 2014. p336.
35. Hartge P, Cahill J. Field methods in Epidemiology. In: RKJ, Greenland S, Lash TL (eds). Modern Epidemiology (3rd edition). Wolters Kluwer: Lippincott Williams & Wilkins, 2008.
36. Miller AL, Lopez L, Gonzalez JM, Dassori A, Bond G, Velligan D. Public-academic partnerships: research in community mental health settings: a practicum experience for researchers. Psychiatr Serv. 2008; 59(11): 1246–8.
37. Prince M, Ferri CP, Acosta D, Albanese E, Arizaga R, Dewey M, et al. The protocols for the 10/66 dementia research group population-based research programme. BMC Public Health. 2007; 7: 165.
38. Guerchet M, Houinato D, Paraiso MN, von Ahsen N, Nubukpo P, Otto M, et al. Cognitive impairment and dementia in elderly people living in rural Benin, west Africa. Dement Geriatr Cogn Disord. 2009; 27(1): 34–41.
39. INDEPTH Network. Better Health Information for Better Health Policy. Available from: http://www.indepth-network.org.
40. Garenne MDG, Pison G, Aaby P. Introduction. In: Press C (ed.). Prospective Community Studies in Developing Countries. Oxford: Oxford University Press, 1997. pp1–15.
41. INDEPTH Network. Population, Health, and Survival at INDEPTH Sites. Population and Health in Developing Countries. Ottawa, Canada: International Development Research Centre, 2002.
42. Tollman SM, Zwi AB. Health system reform and the role of field sites based upon demographic and health surveillance. Bull World Health Organ. 2000; 78(1): 125–34.
43. Sankoh O, Network I. CHESS: an innovative concept for a new generation of population surveillance. Lancet Glob Health. 2015; 3(12): e742.
44. Asher L, Fekadu A, Hanlon C, Mideksa G, Eaton J, Patel V, et al. Development of a Community-Based Rehabilitation Intervention for People with Schizophrenia in Ethiopia. PLOS One. 2015; 10(11): e0143572. countries: a mixed methods study. BMC Health Serv Res. 2017; 17(1): 183.
45. Davies T, Schneider M, Nyatsanza M, Lund C. 'The sun has set even though it is morning': Experiences and explanations of perinatal depression in an urban township, Cape Town. Transcult Psychiatry. 2016; 53(3): 286–312.
46. Gureje O, Stein DJ. Disorders, Diagnosis, and Classification. In: Patel V, Minas H, Cohen A, Prince M, editors. Global Mental Health: Principles and Practice. Oxford: Oxford University Press, 2013.
47. Haroz EE, Ritchey M, Bass JK, Kohrt BA, Augustinavicius J, Michalopoulos L, et al. How is depression experienced around the world? A systematic review of qualitative literature. Soc Sci Med. 2017; 183: 151–62.
48. World Health Organization. mhGAP intervention guide for mental, neurological and substance use disorders in non-specialized health settings: mental health Gap Action Programme (mhGAP)—version 2.0. Geneva: World Health Organization; 2016. Contract No.: ISBN 978 92 4 154979 0.
49. Ministry of Health, Federal Democratic Republic of Ethiopia. National Mental Health Strategy 2012/13—2015/16, 2012.
50. Olayinka OO, Mbuyi NN. Epidemiology of Dementia among the Elderly in Sub-Saharan Africa. International Journal of Alzheimer's Disease. 2014: 195750.
51. 10/66 Dementia Research Group. Caring for older people in Peru (Sobrellevando). Available from: https://www.youtube.com/watch?v=qNr5Vta17PQ.
52. Wang H, Gao T, Wimo A, Yu X. Caregiver time and cost of home care for Alzheimer's disease: a clinic-based observational study in Beijing, China. Ageing International. 2010; 35(2): 153–65.
53. Wellcome Trust. News—We now accept preprints in grant applications. Available from: https://wellcome.ac.uk/news/we-now-accept-preprints-grant-applications
54. Thornicroft G, Cooper S, Bortel TV, Kakuma R, Lund C. Capacity building in global mental health research. Harv Rev Psychiatry. 2012; 20(1): 13–24.
55. World Health Organization. Mental Health and Development. Geneva: World Health Organization; 2010.
56. Schneider M, Sorsdahl K, Mayston R, Ahrens J, Chibanda D, Fekadu A, et al. Developing mental health research in sub-Saharan Africa: capacity building in the AFFIRM project. Glob Ment Health. 2016; 3.

7

Trial designs, including observational to interventional

Edo Richard

Introduction

Observational epidemiology has taught us a lot about the development of neurological and neuropsychiatric disease over time. Longitudinal cohorts, followed for years or decades, have given valuable insights in risk factors for stroke, dementia, depression, and many other diseases.[1,2] In addition, they have revealed early symptoms, sometimes preceding clinical disease onset by many years, such as olfactory loss in PD and declining blood pressure in the years before onset of cognitive decline.[3,4] Treatment effects are often inferred based on the association between medication use and the occurrence or progression of symptoms or disease. But how do we translate this overwhelming amount of observational information into useful interventions that benefit our patients or persons at risk? This chapter will discuss the translation from observational data to interventional studies and the methodological considerations that are encountered.

From Observations to Interventions

Apart from understanding how factors throughout life influence the development of disease, results from observational cohort studies can also serve as the basis for the design of intervention studies. Due to the nature of observational cohort research, many resulting interventions will entail primary or secondary prevention, rather than treatment of manifest disease.

When is observational evidence sufficient?

To start with, observational evidence should be strong, consistent, and of a magnitude that is potentially clinically relevant, that is, individuals, groups of individuals, or society as a whole may benefit from an intervention. Systematic literature review with appropriate grading of potential sources of bias in design and reporting is essential before engaging in a clinical trial. The Cochrane risk of bias tool is a useful tool to assess potential sources of bias.[5] Preferably results from multiple cohorts are pooled in a quantitative meta-analysis and show a consistent association between a potential treatment target and the outcome of interest. When quantitative meta-analysis is not possible, for instance due to large heterogeneity in populations, interventions, outcomes, and follow-up duration of the different studies, a narrative approach can be used for a systematic review, which can yield specific patterns in results from different studies. Translation of findings from a single cohort study into an intervention trial is rarely advised, because reproducibility of the specific finding is unknown.

Even in the presence of overwhelming observational evidence of an association between a specific factor and a disease, treatment or elimination of the factor will not automatically lead to the prevention of the disease or prevention of decline in the case of chronic conditions. An illustrative example is the association between hyperhomocysteinaemia and dementia. In spite of a repeatedly reported association, interventions aiming to reduce the homocystein level in the blood probably do not lead to the reduction of dementia.[6,7]

Bias in observational research

Several sources of bias may influence the interpretation of the results from observational cohorts studies. A common source is spectrum bias, which refers to the population under study. The spectrum varies widely, from population-representative cohorts, to highly selected tertiary referral centre case series. Observational evidence across this spectrum can be valuable, as long as the external validity is kept in mind when translating the findings into an intervention study, which should target the same population. Even when the population under study is well described, bear in mind that there is always participation bias, that is, of those eligible to the study, persons deciding not to participate tend to be different from those who participate. This participation bias will also occur when performing an intervention study, but not necessarily leading to the same selection. Selective dropout is an important source of bias. If the outcome under study is dementia, but those with dementia tend to terminate their participation due to their condition, the interpretation of a longitudinal association of a risk factor with the outcome of interest is influenced.

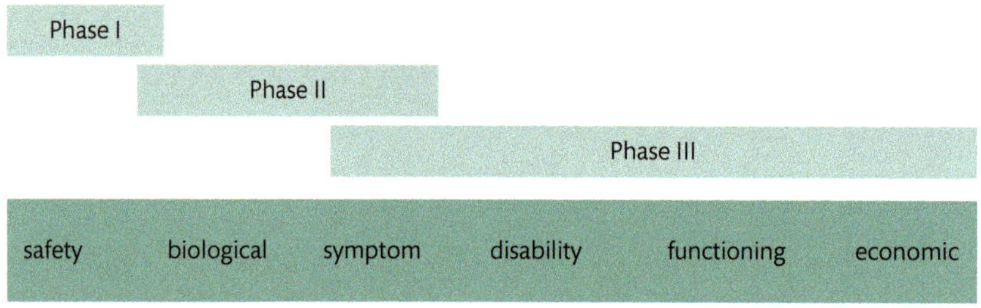

Fig. 7.1 Trial phase in relation to outcome. Phases of trial design with accompanying levels of outcome assessment. The different level of outcome assessment (in dark green) in relation to the phases of study (light green).

Phases in clinical trials

Four phases of clinical trials can be identified (Fig.7.1). A *phase I* study involves usually healthy volunteers and focuses on pharmacodynamics and pharmacokinetics. In this phase safety and tolerability are determined in a small sample size. *Phase II* studies can cover a wide range of designs. The main aim in phase II studies is to determine biological activity (or effect) of the drug under study. Whereas in phase I, often the maximally tolerated dosage is determined from a safety perspective, phase II studies can also focus on dose-finding. Multiple arms with different dosages are often used. Findings from phase II studies should inform the researchers on whether it is plausible that an effect of the drug can be detected in a *phase III* trial. It can also inform researchers on feasibility of recruitment of the target population and outcome assessment. Properly performed phase II trials can prevent expensive and lengthy phase III trials exposing large numbers of participants to ineffective drugs. The often-used term 'proof of concept study' usually also refers to a phase II study.

Phase III trials are designed to show effectiveness of an intervention. They typically have several hundreds to several thousands of participants, depending on the expected effect size of the intervention. Many neurological conditions have a long disease course, complicating the design of phase III trials. Although it is tempting to use intermediate (or surrogate) outcomes for such trials, proven clinically relevant benefit is required before regulatory approval is granted (see paragraph 'Choosing your outcomes' for discussion on outcomes). Since long-term effects and rare but serious side effects can often not be sufficiently determined in phase III trials, *phase IV* studies are often performed. This is also referred to as post-marketing surveillance.

Trial registration

The design and analysis plan of an RCT should be carefully prepared and published in a publicly accessible registry before the start of the trial. Details on target population, intervention, and primary and secondary outcomes should all be registered. This prevents the risk of undue adaptation of the study and analysis plan during the study and influence by the conduct and potential interim results of the trial. Registration can, for instance, be done at: www.clinicaltrials.gov or www.isrctn.org.

Research Question, Population and Outcomes

Defining your research question

It may seem obvious, but it is extremely relevant to define your main and secondary research questions. This determines all other aspects of the trial design. With advancing medical science, more and better treatments have become the standard of care. The research question will therefore often be whether a new intervention can have added value over existing treatments. Sometimes the question will be whether a new intervention can be equally effective, but with less side effects or a more patient-friendly intervention. This requires a different design and a different sample size calculation (see below).

Choosing your population

When designing an RCT based on findings from observational cohort studies, the definition of the RCT population should more or less match the population in which the original association was described. Observational cohorts can be population-representative cohorts (i.e. all people in a certain age range are included), population-based cohorts focusing on a specific subgroup in the population (e.g. women in a certain age range or all persons in a specific catchment area who are registered with their GP as having hypertension), or can contain those with a disease or a characteristic, but not necessarily representing all people with that condition (e.g. a tertiary memory clinic cohort of persons with mild cognitive impairment (MCI) or a primary care depression cohort). RCT populations in general are rarely population-representative, tend to be much more restrictive, and are usually limited by extensive inclusion and exclusion criteria. This is illustrated by an often dramatic difference in the number of participants screened and percentage actually recruited into an RCT. Recruiting a population into an RCT which is very different from the population in which the original association was found can result in a higher chance of a null-finding. In addition, too strict selection criteria also limit the generalizability of the findings, risking either broad implementation in a large group of people who were never represented in the RCT or a type II error, that is, concluding an intervention is not effective at large, whereas it might have been effective if the right population were studied.

Choosing your outcomes

Choosing the appropriate outcome for an intervention study is crucial. Several aspects have to be taken into account. Here, only the outcomes for phase III trials are discussed. Outcomes for phase II trials do not always need to be clinically relevant, although before designing a phase III trial, potential effect on clinically relevant parameters should be plausible. Outcome assessment can occur at different levels, including functioning, disability, disease-level, symptom level, biological parameter, and health-economics. (Fig. 7.1) The definition of the right primary outcome is very important. Determining the outcome beforehand reduces the chance of spurious findings and is essential.

Clinical outcomes

Before results of an RCT can lead to wide implementation, clinical relevance of a trial result has to be established. In primary or secondary prevention research, such as cardiovascular risk management to prevent (recurrent) stroke, efficacy is typically assessed based on incident disease (stroke) or mortality using a time-to-event analysis, such as for instance in the PROGRESS trial.[8] These are hard outcomes, which we generally agree are clinically relevant. Sometimes composite clinical outcomes including disease and mortality are used. In neuropsychiatric disease research, establishing efficacy is far less straightforward. Often outcome is assessed at the symptom level. For instance in dementia research the score on a neuropsychologial test battery is used, or in depression research the score on a depression assessment instrument such as the Hospital Anxiety and Depression Scale (HADS).[9] But when is an effect clinically relevant? A good example is the research on the efficacy of acetylcholinesterase inhibitors (AChEI) for mild to moderate dementia. In the original publications, on which the current wide prescription of these drugs in some countries is based, a 24-month difference of two points on the Alzheimer's Disease Assessment Scale-cognitive subscale, which ranges 0–70, was reported.[10] Although a statistically significant difference between intervention and control arms, the clinical relevance is questionable. Even more difficult to interpret are the commonly used composite standardized scores from a neuropsychological test battery. The effect size is usually expressed as a z-score, where $z = 1$ equates with one standard deviation (SD) difference. But how should we interpret a difference of 0.06 SD difference? Is that clinically relevant? Or will it translate into a clinically relevant difference in functioning or even dementia incidence on the long term? These questions are not answered, and urge us to interpret the effect on intermediate outcomes with great caution.

From a patient perspective, measuring functioning in daily life or quality of life are far more relevant. Generic handicap scales exist, such as the Academic Medical Centre Linear Disability Scale (ALDS).[11] Disease-specific scales such as, for instance, the Expanded Disability Status Scale (EDSS) for use in multiple sclerosis (MS) also exist.[12] Most of these disease-specific scales are ordinal, complicating analysis; often this is ignored and changes are analysed on a continuous scale. This complicates interpretation and often leads to interpretations that are not necessarily supported by the data.

Health-related quality of life (QoL) is difficult to assess. The most widely used instruments are the 36-item Short Form (SF-36) and the EQ-5D. These instruments assess different dimensions of QoL, including physical functioning, social functioning, psychological functioning, perception of overall QoL, and perception of health status. Some instruments, such as the EQ-5D can be used in health economic analyses, including cost-effectiveness analyses. They can be used to assess quality adjusted life years (QALY). The actual costs per gained life year in reasonable health can then be calculated. Whether the costs of an intervention per QALY justify large-scale implementation depends on many factors and differs per country.

Intermediate outcomes

For some conditions it is not practicable or reasonably feasible to use hard clinical outcomes, due to either low incidence rate or long time lag between intervention and occurrence of outcome of interest. A good example is the prevention of dementia. Interventions targeting risk factors for dementia could include midlife hypertension or obesity, based on consistent results from observational cohorts.[2] However, dementia incidence is extremely low in midlife. Therefore an unrealistically long follow-up, a staggering sample size, or both, would be required to detect an effect of an intervention targeting these midlife risk factors.[13] Intermediate outcomes accurately reflecting risk of dementia would be helpful. In cardiovascular risk management, such outcomes exist, for example the Framingham risk score or the SCORE.[14] But for most neurological and neuropsychiatric diseases such reliable risk estimators do not exist, and of those risk prediction tools that do exist, to date none has been validated for use as an outcome measure, that is, validated for evaluating change of risk.

Clinical intermediate outcomes can be based on risk factors, such as, for instance, the CAIDE dementia risk score, which estimates the risk of dementia 20 years later for those in midlife.[15] However, it is unknown whether a change in such a risk score will translate into an actual change in dementia risk. Another type of intermediate clinical outcome is a detailed assessment of a series of symptoms in a specific domain, such as results on a neuropsychological test battery for cognition, the Unified Parkinson's Disease Rating Scale (UPDRS) for parkinsonism or the Scale for the Assessment and Rating of Ataxia (SARA). Such scores aim to reflect functioning in a certain domain. Sometimes a so-called 'minimally clinically important difference' has been determined on this type of outcome, in an attempt to create a cut-off above which a clinically relevant treatment effect can be assumed. These cut-offs tend to change and are often a matter of debate. Also, it ignores the fact that neuropsychiatric diseases usually do not have a linear progression, and short-term (e.g. 6–12 months) effects will not necessarily sustain over time. Finally, a clinical intermediate outcome can be a single symptom or sign, for instance muscle strength.

Biological intermediate outcomes

These are often referred to as biomarkers, and can include, for instance, measures of cerebral atrophy on neuroimaging, protein levels in CSF or blood, changes on an EEG, or change in nerve conduction velocity on EMG. An important prerequisite for the use of these parameters is that there is reasonable evidence that changes on these parameters will translate into clinically detectable effects. Often this is not the case. In neuroimaging the correlation between severity of abnormalities on MRI and clinical symptoms is poor, particularly with advancing age. Whether a change on such a biological outcome measure as a result of an intervention will translate into a clinically detectable effect is usually unknown. Therefore biological and clinical intermediate outcomes are often combined in phase II trials to collect sufficient support both mechanistically and clinically before engaging into a phase III trial.

Adverse events

All serious expected and unexpected adverse events should be monitored. The tendency to detect any possible side effect using a long list of symptoms and signs that may occur in all participants in a trial usually results in the obligatory but uninformative paragraph that 80–90% of study participants suffered side effects (suggesting that there was no difference between placebo and control groups). Much more informative is a separate depiction of all serious adverse events (SAE). Phase III trials are not powered to detect a small but relevant difference in SAEs. Therefore, even small differences in SAEs which are not statistically significant, are reason for a phase IV study.

Study Design and Methodology

Choosing the right study design

To evaluate the effect of a new treatment, comparison to a control group is warranted. The most common type of study is the RCT. Randomization is considered the supreme way of allocating a treatment condition to research participants. It reduces the chance of many sources of bias, most notably allocation bias. In non-randomized studies there is always the risk of selective treatment allocation by clinicians, for instance based on the belief of a clinician in the effectiveness of a treatment or based on the prognosis of a patient. In addition to prevention of allocation bias, randomization will result in balanced groups, avoiding the need for adjustment for imbalances at baseline between groups. The most common types of RCT will be discussed here.

Parallel group RCT is the most straightforward and most commonly used type of RCT. Randomization is usually in a 1:1 manner, with individuals randomized to one group receiving the treatment under study or the other group receiving a control condition. This can be placebo, care as usual, or another drug or treatment. This type of RCT is most commonly used and is very suitable for drug trials.

Cluster-RCT is usually a parallel group design as well, but the main characteristic of this type of RCT is that a group of people is randomized to a specific condition. There can be several reasons to use a cluster-RCT design. Often this approach is used when delivery of an intervention is best achieved by targeting a group and there is a high chance of contamination (i.e. treatment of the intervention arm is (partly) delivered to the people in the control condition). For instance, in the Prevention of Dementia by Intensive Vascular care trial (preDIVA), nurse-led optimization of vascular risk factors in primary care to reduce the risk of dementia was delivered.[16] If individually randomized, different patients within one primary care practice would have to receive different treatments by the same practice nurse. This leads to a high risk of contamination, and therefore complete primary care practices were randomized to the intervention or control condition. This type of trial is also suitable for the evaluation of public health interventions, which can be delivered at the community level. Complete communities or municipalities can then be randomized. Outcome assessment is typically at the individual level. Because clustering of characteristics within communities and the effective number of units of randomization is smaller, this study design leads to a loss of statistical power and this has to be taken into account in the sample size calculation.

Factorial design RCT aims to test two interventions within one RCT. If properly applied the two treatments can be studied in one factorial design RCT with less participants than when investigated in two separate RCTs. The largest gain in sample size reduction can be achieved when the two interventions are very unlikely to interact with each other. With increasing interaction between the interventions, the sample size will have to be increased. The simplest and most common form is the 2 x 2 factorial design (Fig. 7.2). Only 25%

	Intervention X	control
Intervention Y	a	b
control	c	d

effect of intervention x: a + c vs. b + d
effect of intervention y: a + b vs. c + d

Fig. 7.2 Factorial design. Illustration of factorial design RCT.

of participants receive double placebo, 25% receive intervention x and placebo, 25% receive intervention y and placebo, and 25% receive intervention x and y. Recruitment and adherence to the interventions in this type of trial may be more challenging.

Non-inferiority trials are also referred to as equivalence trials. Sometimes the research question is not whether a new treatment is better than an existing treatment, but whether it is equally good. Obviously there must then be another good reason why the new treatment would be preferred over an existing treatment. This could be user friendliness (oral administration vs injection), costs, or fewer side effects. A good example is the evaluation of whether the much less intensive and cheaper behavioural activation therapy is non-inferior to intensive and expensive cognitive behavioural therapy for the treatment of depression.[17] This type of RCT is only appropriate if an effective therapy already exists. The non-inferiority margin has to be established in advance, that is, the margin within which the new treatment is considered 'not inferior'. This margin is often a matter of debate, but a commonly used margin is 20–40%, which means that a 20–40% smaller effect on the outcome of interest would still be considered non-inferior. The interpretation of the result of a non-inferiority trial is depicted in Fig. 7.3.

Cross-over design is where participants serve as their own controls. Participants are randomized to either first receive active treatment and then placebo or vice versa. A wash-out period may be necessary between the two treatment periods. This design has fairly limited applicability. Several assumptions are required. First of all it is only applicable for treatments with direct and short-lasting effects, such as pain relief or reduction of blood pressure and not for treatments influencing the disease course. One has to ensure that the effect wanes and no carry-over of the effect into the next treatment period will occur. Therapies with clear and recognizable side-effects will lead to de-blinding even more than in regular parallel group RCTs, since participants will have used both active treatment and placebo subsequently. It may sometimes be attractive to use this design when it is difficult to recruit large groups of people with the condition under study

Pragmatic trials and implementation research

Whereas results from most RCTs (sometimes referred to as *explanatory trials*) cannot easily be translated to the wider population with a specific condition in daily practice, healthcare policy and decision makers require information on effectiveness in a real-world setting. This requires different types of research, including *pragmatic trials* and other forms of *implementation research* designs.[18,19]

Pragmatic trials aim for high external validity by embedding a new intervention in daily practice as much as possible. Few or no exclusion criteria apply (as opposed to most RCTs focusing mainly on high internal validity and a homogeneous population fulfilling strict inclusion and exclusion criteria), specific treatment choices

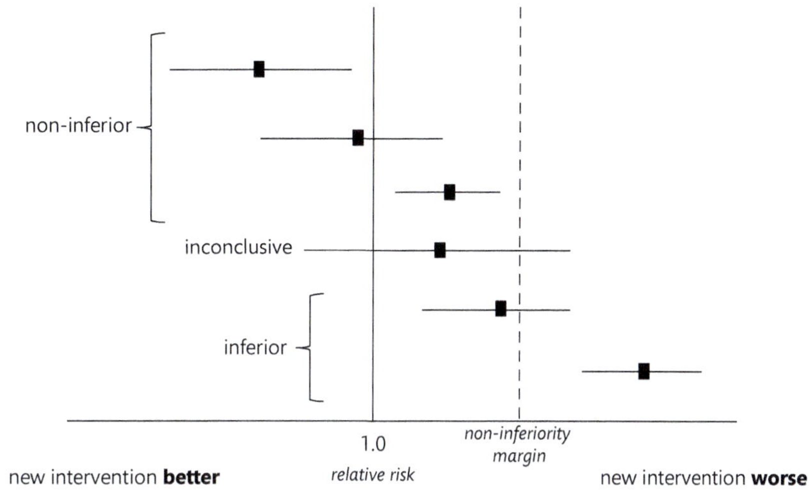

Fig. 7.3 Non-inferiority trial design. Interpretation of the results of a non-inferiority trial. Results of the upper three studies lead to the conclusion of non-inferiority; the upper one represents superiority.

are left to the discretion of the treating physician, and collect data on a range of clinically relevant outcomes using resources other than a case record form only, including, for instance, electronic medical records. Outcomes reflecting the intervention in a real-world setting include acceptability, adoption, appropriateness, feasibility, fidelity, cost, and sustainability.[19] These so-called *implementation outcomes* can be assessed in parallel with effectiveness outcomes. In reality, clinical trials do not have to be purely explanatory or purely pragmatic. One should always search for the appropriate balance between internal and external validity, based on the research question addressed.

Natural experiments

Particularly for studying the impact of public health interventions, a randomized design may not always be feasible. Evaluation of the effect of such an intervention can still take place, assessing it as a *natural experiment*.[20] A good example is the introduction of new legislation prohibiting smoking in public places. Such an approach in the UK led to a small but significant fall in hospital admissions for acute coronary syndrome.[21] Such an approach could be conceivable in the field of neuropsychiatry as well, for instance when implementing better access to primary mental healthcare facilities, using hospitalization for severe depression as an outcome. Interpretation of natural experiment data is obviously very prone to bias, so should be done with caution. Health policy changes and societal changes can easily confound the effect of the intervention under study. Nevertheless, for some interventions, particularly with a strong (biological) plausibility, this type of result may serve to support the implementation of certain public health interventions.

Other, *non-randomized types of trials* may be used on occasions in which randomization is not feasible or not practicable and a non-randomized controlled study can be performed. For instance the TRUTH study assesses whether intravenous alteplase for the treatment of acute stroke can safely and effectively be administered to those with a high initial blood pressure, which is then actively lowered using intravenous labetalol.[22] Severe hypertension was a contraindication in the original alteplase trials. Some centres started actively reducing blood pressure and then administered alteplase. Other centres consider hypertension a contraindication and don't administer alteplase. Randomization appeared impossible due to strong beliefs between different centres. Therefore a non-randomized design, comparing outcome in those patients between study centres was started. Unbalanced groups and selective recruitment leading to spectrum bias in some centres are important potential sources of bias of this approach.

In rare diseases it is also often not possible to perform an adequately powered RCT. Small series treated with a new treatment can then be compared to historical cohorts. Interpretation should be with great caution. Only major effects when compared to very comparable and preferably contemporary historical cohorts can be carefully interpreted as evidence for effectiveness of the intervention. An important source of bias when comparing historical cohorts is the improvement in medical care as a whole. For instance, the introduction of stroke units has improved outcome in patients with acute stroke.[23] If a new intervention was compared to a historical cohort identical in patient characteristics at hospital admission ten years earlier, who were never admitted to a stroke unit, the effect of stroke unit admission could be accidentally interpreted as a treatment effect of the new intervention.

Randomization

The main aim is to ensure that the two study groups are comparable and to avoid any allocation bias by researchers. The randomization process should be designed to avoid any form of selection bias, that is, it should be unpredictable for the researchers to which condition the next patient will be randomized. The most basic form of randomization is simple randomization. A computer algorithm can generate the treatment allocation. In studies with a small sample size this can lead to imbalance between groups due to chance. Commonly the ratio of treatment allocation is 1:1, but in principle the algorithm can generate any ratio. This approach can be appropriate for large RCTs where in individual centres large numbers of participants are recruited. At any point during the study, imbalance between the number of participants assigned to each group can occur due to chance.

An often-used variant is blocked randomization.[24] The main advantage is that treatment allocation is balanced throughout the study. Usually blocks of four are used. The order of treatment allocation within the blocks can vary and blocks with different order are randomly assigned. This ensures that in multicentre trials, all centres will always recruit both intervention and control participants, but the treatment allocation of the next participant is still unpredictable.

When concerned that imbalance for a specific factor may occur due to chance, randomization can be stratified. A computer algorithm can guard balancing, for instance across age groups, to avoid more participants with a high age allocated to a specific treatment arm due to chance. In a multicentre, or even multinational trial, large differences in study population may occur. In such cases stratification by centre may be appropriate.

Blinding

To avoid bias on the side of both participant and researcher, a double blind design is in general the preferred trial design. However, there are instances in which this is not feasible and other designs are acceptable.

A double-blind design is almost always possible for drug treatments and this is what should be aimed for. The treatment allocation code should only be broken in case of medical urgency. The placebo should be identical in appearance and a licensed pharmacy should be responsible for the preparation of the study drugs. In invasive treatments, including surgical interventions, it is usually not possible to blind the treating physician. Sometimes the patient can be blinded for surgical interventions, for instance when two surgical techniques are compared but the approach is comparable. When the healthcare workers delivering the intervention cannot be blinded (single-blind study), it is crucial that the person evaluating the outcome is blinded. When both the participant and those delivering the intervention cannot be truly blinded, for instance in the case of lifestyle interventions, the outcome assessor should always be blinded. This is referred to as a PROBE design (Prospective Open Label Blinded Endpoint).[25] Adequate blinding of participants can be evaluated by asking the participants which treatment arm they think they were assigned to.

Participant considerations

It is advisable to have representatives of the target population of an intervention involved in the study design phase. This is particularly relevant when evaluating complex interventions requiring motivated research participants, such as with lifestyle interventions or when using new ways of treatment delivery such as eHealth or telemedicine. This can help avoiding the design of an intervention that the target population will not be able or willing to adhere to when implemented on a large scale. Also during an intervention study, gaining insight in the experiences of the target population can be extremely valuable. Qualitative research methods, including in-depth interviews and focus groups, can yield important information required for successful implementation. Reasons for (non-)adherence and experiences with the intervention itself can only be properly evaluated using qualitative research with a purposive sample from the target population.

Sample Size

General considerations

Underpowered studies should be avoided at all times, because they constitute a waste of resources and raise serious ethical concerns.[26] Whereas in drug trials a rigorous process involving phase I and II trials usually precedes phase III trials, this will often not be the case in trials based on observations from cohort studies, since treatments will often involve existing drugs with known safety profiles and/or non-medical interventions, sometimes for new indications. In general, potential treatment effects tend to be grossly overestimated based on observational data. Since the magnitude of an association or treatment effect tends to decline after a first report, it is crucial to take all reports of sufficient quality into account when calculating the sample size. A poor sample size calculation can result in a trial which is clear beforehand will not be able to answer a research question. In addition to the waste of financial and personnel resources, it leads to futile exposure of research participants, which is an ethical concern. At the same time, although far less likely to happen, overpowered studies should be avoided for partly the same reasons as underpowered studies. In this case the excess number of research participants exposed to the burden of trial participation raises ethical concerns as well.

Sample size calculation

Actual sample size calculations are beyond the scope of this textbook. Here we describe some general considerations when planning an RCT.

Dropout is rarely overestimated by those who design trials and a realistic estimate of dropout should be made, for which oversampling is required. Dropout is highly dependent on the primary outcome. For a pragmatic outcome, such as, for instance, all-cause dementia, dropout can be extremely low, even in very long trials, since the participant does not have to be assessed in person.[16] On the other hand, for primary outcomes requiring serious time and effort of the participants, such as extensive neuropsychological testing, dropout can be high (and selective, severely affecting interpretation). Non-adherence is not dropout. In principle, all RCTs should be analysed using the intention to treat principle, to ensure external validity of the trial results. A pre-specified sensitivity analysis on those who are adherent to the intervention can be performed, but cannot be considered as conclusive for treatment effect and the sample size calculation should not be based on this analysis.

Sample size is dependent on the study design and the type of primary analysis. For a repeated measures analysis, for instance, a smaller sample size or shorter study duration may be sufficient. The previously mentioned non-inferiority design has impact on the sample size, generally leading to a larger sample size required to determine non-inferiority. In a cluster-randomized trial, subjects within a cluster tend to be more similar to each other than to subjects outside the cluster. For instance socioeconomic status tends to cluster within postcodes, so when randomizing municipalities, the effective sample size is reduced due to a lack of contrast between the subjects within a cluster. The magnitude of the resulting intra-cluster correlation coefficient (rho) determines the required increase in sample size. Failure to adapt the sample size accordingly will lead to an underpowered study and an increased risk of a type

II error. A thorough sample size calculation can have major influence on the study design and may also lead to the conclusion that a study is not feasible.

Ethical Issues

Main principles

The general principles of ethical conduct in medical research have been extensively discussed.[27] The seven essential criteria for ethical conduct of clinical research are value, scientific validity, fair selection of participants, favourable benefit/risk balance, independent review, informed consent, and respect for participants.[28]

Foremost, a clinically relevant question needs to be addressed, with relevance for a clearly defined group, which can range from a specific population with a specific condition to the complete population from a public health perspective. Particularly when designing a prevention trial based on population-representative observational data, it is essential that the impact of a positive trial at the population level is taken into account. A health-economic evaluation is essential, before results from such an RCT can be translated into a large-scale prevention strategy.

Informed consent

The principles are no different from participating in observational studies. Informed consent is the voluntary agreement to participate in research. It has a moral, legal, and instrumental role. From a moral perspective, it acknowledges participants' autonomy and self-governance and ensures participation is voluntarily. From a legal perspective, a signed informed consent is required for participation in an RCT, and it ensures the participant is adequately informed not only about the purpose of the study, but also about the procedures and potential benefits and harms. It is instrumental, because it supports a trusting relationship between researchers and participants. As such it enhances the quality of the study due to increased commitment and reduced dropout from a study.

Control condition

An RCT should be conducted when there is equipoise concerning the effect of an intervention. This implies that clinicians recruiting participants truly doubt whether the intervention under study will be effective. This justifies the randomization process and the administration of a control or placebo condition. Control conditions can be either care as usual, or a control intervention, which can be a placebo drug, a sham therapy, or a control therapy not expected to be effective (but neither potentially harmful).

Reporting of Results

Results from clinical trials should be reported in accordance with the Consolidated Standards for Reporting of Trials (CONSORT) statement.[29] Reporting of results should not depend on the outcome of the study. Not reporting trials with neutral (or even negative) findings seriously jeopardizes the interpretation of treatment effects as a whole. Selective reporting of positive trial results is likely, as funnel plots created in the context of meta-analyses often indicate potential publication bias towards small positive trials. This is another reason for registration of clinical trials before starting them.

REFERENCES

1. Cole MG, Dendukuri N. Risk factors for depression among elderly community subjects: a systematic review and meta-analysis. Am J Psychiatry. 2003; 160(6): 1147–56.
2. Ligthart SA, Moll van Charante EP, Van Gool WA, Richard E. Treatment of cardiovascular risk factors to prevent cognitive decline and dementia: a systematic review. Vasc Health Risk Manag. 2010; 6:775–85.
3. Postuma RB, Berg D. Advances in markers of prodromal Parkinson disease. Nat Rev Neurol. 2016; 12(11): 622–34.
4. Skoog I, Lernfelt B, Landahl S, Palmertz B, Andreasson LA, Nilsson L, et al. 15-year longitudinal study of blood pressure and dementia. Lancet. 1996; 347(9009): 1141–5.
5. Cochrane Group. Cochrane Handbook for Systematic Reviews of Interventions. Accessed 2/12/2019: http://training.cochrane.org/handbook.
6. Ford AH, Almeida OP. Effect of homocysteine lowering treatment on cognitive function: a systematic review and meta-analysis of randomized controlled trials. J Alzheimer's Dis. 2012; 29(1): 133–49.
7. Wald DS, Kasturiratne A, Simmonds M. Serum homocysteine and dementia: meta-analysis of eight cohort studies including 8669 participants. Alzheimer's Dement. 2011; 7(4): 412–7.
8. Group PC. Randomised trial of a perindopril-based blood-pressure-lowering regimen among 6105 individuals with previous stroke or transient ischaemic attack. Lancet. 2001; 358(9287): 1033–41.
9. Zigmond AS, Snaith RP. The hospital anxiety and depression scale. Acta Psychiatr Scand. 1983; 67(6): 361–70.
10. Rosler M, Anand R, Cicin-Sain A, Gauthier S, Agid Y, Dal-Bianco P, et al. Efficacy and safety of rivastigmine in patients with Alzheimer's disease: international randomised controlled trial. BMJ. 1999; 318(7184): 633–8.
11. Holman R, Lindeboom R, Vermeulen M, de Haan RJ. The AMC Linear Disability Score project in a population requiring residential care: psychometric properties. Health Qual Life Outcomes. 2004; 2: 42.
12. Kurtzke JF. Rating neurologic impairment in multiple sclerosis: an expanded disability status scale (EDSS). Neurology. 1983; 33(11): 1444–52.
13. Richard E, Andrieu S, Solomon A, Mangialasche F, Ahtiluoto S, Moll van Charante EP, et al. Methodological challenges in designing dementia prevention trials—the European Dementia Prevention Initiative (EDPI). J Neurol Sci. 2012; 322(1–2): 64–70.
14. Prochaska JJ, Velicer WF, Nigg CR, Prochaska JO. Methods of quantifying change in multiple risk factor interventions. Prev Med. 2008; 46(3): 260–5.
15. Kivipelto M, Ngandu T, Laatikainen T, Winblad B, Soininen H, Tuomilehto J. Risk score for the prediction of dementia risk in 20 years among middle aged people: a longitudinal, population-based study. Lancet Neurology. 2006; 5(9): 735–41.
16. Moll van Charante EP, Richard E, Eurelings LS, van Dalen JW, Ligthart SA, van Bussel EF, et al. Effectiveness of a 6-year multidomain vascular care intervention to prevent dementia (preDIVA): a cluster-randomised controlled trial. Lancet. 2016; 388(10046): 797–805.

17. Richards DA, Ekers D, McMillan D, Taylor RS, Byford S, Warren FC, et al. Cost and Outcome of Behavioural Activation versus cognitive behavioural therapy for depression (COBRA): a randomised, controlled, non-inferiority trial. Lancet. 2016; 388(10047): 871–80.
18. Tunis SR, Stryer DB, Clancy CM. Practical clinical trials: increasing the value of clinical research for decision making in clinical and health policy. JAMA. 2003; 290(12): 1624–32.
19. Peters DH, Adam T, Alonge O, Agyepong IA, Tran N. Implementation research: what it is and how to do it. BMJ. 2013; 347: f6753.
20. Craig P, Cooper C, Gunnell D, Haw S, Lawson K, Macintyre S, et al. Using natural experiments to evaluate population health interventions: new Medical Research Council guidance. J Epidemiol Community Health. 2012; 66(12): 1182–6.
21. Pell JP, Haw S, Cobbe S, Newby DE, Pell AC, Fischbacher C, et al. Smoke-free legislation and hospitalizations for acute coronary syndrome. N Engl J Med. 2008; 359(5): 482–91.
22. Zonneveld TP, Algra A, Dippel DW, Kappelle LJ, van Oostenbrugge RJ, Roos YB, et al. The ThRombolysis in UnconTrolled Hypertension (TRUTH) protocol: an observational study on treatment strategy of elevated blood pressure in stroke patients eligible for IVT. BMC Neurol. 2015; 15: 241.
23. Kalra L, Evans A, Perez I, Knapp M, Donaldson N, Swift CG. Alternative strategies for stroke care: a prospective randomised controlled trial. Lancet. 2000; 356(9233): 894–9.
24. Matts JP, Lachin JM. Properties of permuted-block randomization in clinical trials. Control Clin Trials. 1988; 9(4): 327–44.
25. Hansson L, Hedner T, Dahlof B. Prospective randomized open blinded end-point (PROBE) study. A novel design for intervention trials. Prospective Randomized Open Blinded End-Point. Blood Press. 1992; 1(2): 113–9.
26. Berge E, Salman RA, van der Worp HB, Stapf C, Sandercock P, Sprigg N, et al. Increasing value and reducing waste in stroke research. Lancet Neurology. 2017; 16(5): 399–408.
27. Beauchamp TCJ. Principles of Biomedical Ethics. Oxford: Oxford University Press, 2001.
28. Emanuel EJ, Wendler D, Grady C. What makes clinical research ethical? JAMA. 2000; 283(20): 2701–11.
29. Consort. Transparent Reporting of Trials. Accessed 2/12/ 2019: http://www.consort-statement.org.

8

Cardiometabolic morbidities and dementia

Chengxuan Qiu, Davide Liborio Vetrano, and Laura Fratiglioni

Introduction

Dementia has been recognized as a global public health priority owing to its huge societal and economic impacts.[1] Pooling data indicate that after 65 years of age, the prevalence of dementia doubles approximately every six years,[2] making dementia a condition typical of the older age. Indeed, up to 70% of dementia cases occur in people aged 75 years or older.[3,4] Recently, cumulative evidence has suggested that the incidence of dementia in Western Europe and North America might have declined in the past 3–4 decades,[5,6] partly due to improvement in the management of major cardiovascular risk factors and cardiovascular morbidities among young, middle-aged, and elderly people since the late 1970s. Given the accelerated increase in the worldwide ageing population, however, the global impact of dementia is projected to continuously increase in the coming decades.

Together with dementia, a number of other chronic health conditions (e.g. hypertension, diabetes, heart disease, and cerebrovascular disease) are fairly common among older people, with three out of four people aged 65 years or older being affected by two or more chronic diseases, a condition referred to as multimorbidity.[7] Thus, these chronic diseases, including dementia and cardiovascular morbidities, and ageing can be considered closely related processes, stemming from the progressive and lifelong accumulation of biological deficits and organ dysfunction that contribute to the progressive loss of resilience in older adults.[8]

The pathophysiological pathways leading to AD and other dementias can be influenced by numerous risk factors and morbid conditions experienced over the life course that do not necessarily involve only the central nervous system.[8] Scientific literature corroborates the idea of a body-mind connection in ageing: somatic and mental disorders coexist, interact, and influence each other, leading to complex phenotypes and boosting the occurrence of negative health events.[9] Shading light on the mechanisms that link somatic diseases and cognitive deterioration in ageing may help pave the way to new preventive and therapeutic intervention strategies that could delay the onset and progression of cognitive impairment and dementia.

In this chapter, we focus on epidemiological studies that investigate the relationship between cardiometabolic morbidity and dementia from a life-course perspective. Specifically, we seek to summarize the epidemiological literature concerning: (1) mixed dementia owing to cerebrovascular and neurodegenerative pathologies as the most common form of dementia in old age; (2) subclinical and clinical cardiovascular disease in relation to cognitive decline and dementia, as well as the potential pathophysiological mechanisms; and (3) cardiovascular comorbidities in dementia and their impact on care and prognosis of patients with dementia.

Cognitive Decline Does Not Always Lead to Alzheimer's Dementia

As people age, some domains of cognitive function start to decline from as early as 30 years of age.[10] The age-related cognitive decline may lead to cognitive impairment, from the lighter form such as cognitive impairment no dementia (CIND) and MCI to overt dementia of different types. CIND or MCI represents a stage of cognitive impairment in ageing where cognitive changes are serious enough to be noticed by individuals themselves or other persons, but the changes are not severe enough to interfere with daily life or functional independence.[11,12] Several studies have shown that people with CIND or MCI are at much higher risk of developing AD or other dementias than people with normal cognition. However, MCI (even subtype MCI) or CIND is a heterogeneous and complex clinical condition, and does not necessarily progress to dementia. Indeed, population-based follow-up studies of people with MCI or CIND suggested that around one-third of individuals with MCI or CIND remained stable or reverted to normal cognition over the next three to ten years, whereas only one-third of cases progressed to clinical dementia.[12–14]

People who receive a clinical diagnosis of AD do not always exhibit typical Alzheimer's pathology in their brain at post-mortem assessment, with ~20% being misclassified. On the other hand, many older people who fulfilled neuropathological criteria for AD at autopsy did not meet the clinical criteria for dementia before they died.[4] Traditionally, the two most common forms of dementia, AD and vascular dementia, have been studied as separate clinical entities, as they may show different neuropsychological profiles, especially in the initial phases. In the past two decades, however, clinical and population-based epidemiological studies have shown a considerable overlap in symptomatology and risk factors between AD and vascular dementia: ~50% of patients with clinically diagnosed AD could be reclassified as having AD with a vascular component (e.g. cerebrovascular disease, heart disease, diabetes, and hypertension).[4,15] This suggests that in most cases, vascular and neurodegenerative mechanisms may contribute to the expression of the dementia syndrome among the elderly. In addition, post-mortem and neuroimaging studies have revealed a substantial overlap in pathophysiological process and neuropathologies, such that most cases of clinically diagnosed dementia, and even AD in older people living in the community, show mixed vascular and neurodegenerative pathologies in the brain,[4,16] which confirms the findings from clinical studies. Indeed, cerebral macrovascular (e.g. atherosclerosis and infarcts), microvascular (e.g. lacunar infarcts, white matter lesions, and microbleeds), and neurodegenerative pathologies might co-occur and interact during the ageing process causing cumulative brain damages, which in turn could accelerate cognitive decline and promote clinical expression of MCI and dementia.[16,17] These findings have important implications for the treatment and preventive intervention aimed to delay dementia onset as most lifestyle and vascular risk factors are modifiable.

Of note, vascular cognitive impairment (VCI) has been proposed to represent a global diagnostic category for a heterogeneous group of cognitive disorders that are presumed to have a vascular cause.[18] Specifically, VCI includes the entire spectrum of cognitive disorders associated with all forms of vascular brain injury, ranging from MCI of vascular origin that does not meet the diagnostic criteria for dementia, to clinically overt dementia that is due to cerebrovascular disease (pure vascular dementia, e.g. post-stroke dementia and multi-infarct dementia), and mixed cerebrovascular and neurodegenerative disease (mixed dementia).

The Heart-brain Connection in Ageing and Dementia

Subclinical atherosclerosis and dementia

Atherosclerosis is a systemic disorder that progresses with age and ageing. Atherosclerosis involves simultaneously large and medium arteries of organs such as heart, brain, and the lower extremity. It has been well established that markers of subclinical atherosclerosis at various organs are predictive of future cardiovascular events. In the past two decades, numerous epidemiological studies have linked various markers of subclinical atherosclerosis with cognitive impairment and dementia in middle-aged and elderly populations.

Peripheral atherosclerosis

A low ankle-brachial index (ABI) (e.g. ABI <0.9) is a clinical marker of lower extremity peripheral atherosclerosis. Several population-based cohort studies have shown that a low ABI is associated with an increased risk of dementia and cognitive impairment,[4,16] and their association is supported by a systematic review.[19] In addition, a low ABI was associated with poor performance in verbal memory test, which could be attenuated when magnetic resonance imaging (MRI) markers of vascular brain lesions were taken into account.[20] These studies indicate that peripheral atherosclerosis may be involved in the development of cognitive disorders in old age through its link with brain lesions.

Carotid atherosclerosis

The Rotterdam Study reported a cross-sectional association between various markers of severe carotid atherosclerosis (e.g. carotid plaques and carotid intima-media thickness) and an increased likelihood of dementia and AD.[21] Furthermore, several population-based studies showed that carotid atherosclerosis, even clinically silent, was associated with cognitive decline, cognitive impairment, and dementia among middle-aged and older populations.[16,22] Systematic reviews concluded that asymptomatic carotid stenosis was associated with cognitive impairment.[23] In addition, the Framingham Heart Study suggested that internal carotid stenosis and increased internal carotid artery intima-media thickness were associated with imaging markers of brain lesions such as silent cerebral infarcts, white matter hyperintensities (WMHs), and grey matter atrophy. This suggests that the association of carotid atherosclerosis with cognitive disorders in old age may be mediated through those vascular brain lesions.[24]

Arterial stiffness

Arterial stiffness assessed with increased carotid femoral pulse wave velocity (PWV) is a marker for subclinical cardiovascular disease. Population-based studies have demonstrated a cross-sectional association between the increased severity of arterial stiffness and poor cognitive performance. For instance, the Icelandic Age, Gene/Environment Susceptibility (AGES)-Reykjavik Study showed that PWV parameters were associated with lower brain volumes, imaging markers of cerebral small vessel disease (SVD), and lower scores on tests of various cognitive domains.[25] Systematic review supports the cross-sectional association of measures of greater arterial stiffness with various markers of cerebral SVD, the major brain pathology underlying cognitive impairment and dementia in old age.[26] However, reports on a longitudinal association of increased PWV with cognitive decline and cognitive impairment has been less consistent across studies. The follow-up data from the Rotterdam Study showed no evidence for the association of PWV with subsequent cognitive decline or risk of dementia,[27] whereas the Baltimore Longitudinal Study of Aging showed an association of a higher carotid-femoral PWV with a faster decline in executive function and a screening measure of cognitive function weighted for memory and concentration.[28] The Health, Aging, and Body Composition Study supported an association of a higher PWV with a faster cognitive decline and a greater likelihood of cognitive impairment among community-dwelling older adults.[29] Furthermore, central arterial stiffness, measured with increased aortic PWV, is associated with reduced white matter volume and grey matter integrity, as well as with a faster cognitive decline and an increased risk of MCI and dementia among older adults.[30,31] Systematic reviews found rather consistent evidence supporting an association between arterial stiffness and clinical phenotypes of cognitive ageing.[32]

Coronary artery calcium

Coronary artery calcium score is a reliable measure of cumulative burden of coronary artery plaques. Several well-established cohort studies have assessed the associations of coronary artery calcification with brain lesions and phenotypes of cognitive ageing. The AGES-Reykjavik Study suggested that coronary artery calcification was associated with an increased likelihood of dementia.[33] In the Rotterdam Study, the larger volume of coronary artery calcification was associated with lower motor and processing speed, as well as with smaller grey matter volume and reduced white-matter microstructural integrity.[34] Furthermore, the Cardiovascular Health Study showed that coronary artery calcium score was associated with an increased risk of cognitive impairment and dementia, even among very old people (e.g. age ≥80 years), and that the association appeared to be largely mediated through vascular brain lesions (e.g. infarcts and WMHs).[16,35] The longitudinal data from the Multi-Ethnic Study of Atherosclerosis suggested that among middle-aged and elderly people (age 45–84 years), a higher coronary artery calcium score was associated with an increased risk of dementia in a dose-response manner.[36] Even among middle-aged adults (43–55 years of age), a greater volume of subclinical coronary artery calcium was found to be correlated with worse performance in memory and psychomotor speed tests.[37] These studies support the notion that coronary atherosclerosis is associated with cognitive impairment and dementia in middle-aged and older adults, and that vascular brain lesions may play a part in their association.

Cardiovascular disease and dementia

Coronary heart disease

In the past two decades, findings from epidemiological studies that explored the association of coronary heart disease (CHD) with dementia have been inconsistent. Two population-based studies in Finland and the USA failed to demonstrate an association between midlife CHD and an increased risk of dementia in late life.[38,39] On the contrary, several other population and registry-based studies supported an association of angina pectoris and myocardial infarction with the risk of dementia.[16] In the Cardiovascular Health Study, a 30% increased risk of dementia was reported for people suffering from myocardial infarction or angina pectoris, and such an association was attenuated when markers of brain lesions such as WMHs and ventricular enlargement were taken into consideration.[40] Similarly, the Women's Health Initiative Memory Study and the Swedish Twin Registry found a two-fold increased risk of dementia associated with a history of myocardial infarction, and a 45% increased risk related to angina pectoris.[41,42] The follow-up data from the Rotterdam Study cohort suggested that unrecognized myocardial infarction defined by electrocardiogram and interview, but not recognized myocardial infarction, was associated with an increased risk of dementia in men, not in women.[43] Systematic reviews support the view that CHD is prospectively associated with an increased risk of global cognitive deficits and dementia.[16,44,45] Finally, population-based studies have shown that a higher level of plasma high-sensitivity cardiac troponin T, a biomarker of myocardial injury, was associated with worse cognitive performance, accelerated cognitive decline, and an increased risk of dementia.[46,47] This suggests that even subclinical myocardial injury might contribute to the development of cognitive impairment and dementia.

Atrial fibrillation

Atrial fibrillation (AF) could contribute to up to five-fold increased risk of stroke, a major risk factor for cognitive decline, cognitive deficits, and dementia. Indeed, a link of AF with cognitive decline and dementia has been reported by numerus population-based studies, and has been supported by systematic reviews and meta-analyses. For instance, in the Cardiovascular Health Study cohort, data showed that elderly individuals with AF exhibited a steeper global cognitive decline and worse performance in processing speed, especially in the presence of stroke.[48] In a Finnish cohort of middle-aged people, AF occurring in late life, but not in midlife, was associated with an over two-fold increased risk of dementia.[39] In a meta-analysis of 21 cross-sectional and cohort studies, AF was associated with an approximately 40% increased risk of cognitive impairment in the general population, whereas in people with a history of clinical stroke, AF was associated with a 2.7-fold increased risk for cognitive impairment.[49] More recently, the Whitehall II cohort study of middle-aged adults (age 45–69 years) showed that AF was associated with an accelerated cognitive decline and a higher risk of dementia, and that the association was partly explained by the development of incident stroke and cardiovascular disease in people with AF.[50] With regard to specific cognitive domains, cross-sectional data from the AGES-Reykjavik Study suggested that AF was associated with impairment in memory, but not in processing speed and executive function.[51] Finally, the post-hoc analyses of data from two randomized controlled trials of patients with vascular disease or at high risk of diabetes showed that AF was associated with a 30% higher risk of cognitive decline and dementia.[52,53] However, whether optimal treatment of AF (e.g. anticoagulants) may decrease the risk of cognitive decline and dementia in people with AF remains to be clarified.

Heart failure

Heart failure and poor cognitive function frequently coexist in older people. In the Kungsholmen Project in central Stockholm, heart failure was associated with an over 80% increased risk of dementia and AD among very old people (age ≥75 years), and the increased risk could be partially counteracted by use of antihypertensive drugs.[54] The Cardiovascular Health Study showed that heart failure was associated with an approximately 50% increased risk of developing dementia.[55] Similarly, the Finnish study of a middle-aged cohort revealed an association of heart failure in late life, but not in midlife, with an increased risk of dementia.[39] A systematic review found evidence suggesting that heart failure was associated with an elevated risk of dementia and AD as well as with worse performance in global cognitive function, memory, attention, and mental flexibility, possibly through its impact on diminished cardiac function, cerebral hypoperfusion, and emboli.[44] In addition, the systematic review of cohort studies showed that the association between heart failure and a rapid cognitive decline could be partly buffered by the use of cardiovascular medications,[56] indicating that the risk of cognitive decline appears to be modifiable with cardiac treatment.

Cardiovascular comorbidities in dementia

Comorbidity in dementia is referred to as any additional co-existing ailment in a patient with dementia. Comorbid medical conditions, especially cardiovascular comorbidities, are highly prevalent in patients with dementia. For instance, the large-scale health insurance claims data in Germany showed that the prevalence of cardiovascular comorbidities among patients with dementia was 46.3% for cardiac insufficiency, 39.8% for coronary artery disease, and 32.4% for stroke.[57] In the Swedish Dementia Registry of over 30,000 patients with dementia in the primary care settings, the prevalence of cardiovascular comorbidities was 23% for ischaemic heart disease, 20% for cerebrovascular disease, 19% for atrial fibrillation, and 15% for heart failure, with cardiovascular medications being used in ~70% of patients with vascular and mixed dementia.[58] A Spanish study showed that in the primary care settings, hypertension (38–45%) and diabetes (15–21%) were the two most frequent comorbidities of dementia both for men and women.[59] In addition, a large-scale population-based study of patients with dementia in the long-stay (≥60 days) home care settings in Canada showed that chronic multimorbidity was present in nearly 90% of patients with dementia.[60] Indeed, literature reviews have suggested that comorbidities are more prevalent in people with dementia than those demographically matched controls.[9,61,62] In addition, the Baltimore Longitudinal Study of Aging study showed that the accumulation of chronic diseases was associated with an accelerated decline in specific cognitive domains such as verbal fluency and executive function.[63] A systematic review also found an association between a higher burden of comorbidities and a faster progression of dementia and AD.[61] This suggests that accelerated deterioration of physical health is associated with an accelerated decline in mental health in ageing. Taken together, these studies suggest that somatic disorders, especially cardiovascular comorbidities, significantly contribute to the progressive decline in cognitive and physical functioning in ageing and in patients with dementia, and thus result in functional dependency, poor quality of life, and a shorter survival.

In people with dementia, the presence of cardiovascular comorbidity not only contributes to poor outcomes but also often creates complex challenges for patient care. Literature review has suggested that the presence of comorbid chronic conditions in dementia has a strong impact on the management and care of patients, and poses an additional burden to caregivers.[9] First, the diagnosis and management of comorbid conditions in people with dementia may be undermined because dementia often dominates clinical encounters and shifts attention away from comorbidities.[64] In practice, people with dementia are subject to an increased risk of substantial delays in the recognition of additional comorbid health conditions, and dementia also imposes limitations in the management of comorbidities as well as in compliance. Furthermore, comorbidity *per se* and management of comorbid health conditions in dementia significantly increase the burden of health and social care agencies and caregivers. Indeed, a large population-based retrospective cohort study based on electronic health records in the UK suggested that the higher number of comorbidities in people with dementia not only led to a poorer survival but also considerably increased the use of healthcare service (e.g. primary care consultations, medical prescriptions, and hospital admissions).[65] These findings imply that comorbidity should be taken into consideration when allocating resources and planning care for people with dementia. Taken together, early recognition and proper management of treatable comorbidities (e.g. cardiovascular comorbidities) in dementia may help health and social care providers maximize the well-being of people with dementia.

Atherosclerosis Cascade over the Life Course and Dementia

Current evidence supports a strong association of cardiovascular disorders with an accelerated cognitive decline and an increased risk of MCI and dementia (Table 8.1).[4,16,66] They share not only common vascular risk factors (e.g. smoking, high blood pressure, and diabetes) but also pathophysiological pathways (e.g. inflammation, oxidative stress, and vascular damages) underlying such an association. From a life-course perspective, cardiovascular risk factors occurring in young adulthood onward and the subsequent development of subclinical atherosclerosis and arteriosclerosis in midlife, as well as clinical cardiovascular and cerebrovascular diseases in midlife and old ages, contribute to an accelerated cognitive decline and an increased risk of MCI and dementia later in life through various biological and neuropathological pathways. Indeed, in the past two decades, numerous population-based post-mortem and neuroimaging studies have revealed that cognitive phenotypes in ageing, including the rate of cognitive decline and clinical expression of cognitive impairment and dementia syndrome, are largely due to the overall burden of mixed cerebral macro- and microvascular disease and neurodegenerative pathology.[4,16,67] The vascular and neuropathological pathways leading to accelerated cognitive decline and dementia are briefly summarized in Fig. 8.1.

First, cerebral SVD (e.g. lacunar infarcts, WMHs, microbleeds, and microinfarcts) and disruption of the blood-brain barrier (BBB) and brain network connectivity, resulting from long-term exposures

Table 8.1 Different levels of connection between the cardiovascular system and the brain: from risk factors to comorbidities

Cardiovascular risk factors and related disorders associated with dementia				Cardiovascular Comorbidities in dementia
Cardiovascular risk factors	Subclinical atherosclerosis	Cardiovascular disease	Vascular brain lesions	
Smoking Hypertension Diabetes Obesity Hyperlipidaemia Physical inactivity Diet (fats, sodium)	Peripheral artery disease Carotid atherosclerosis Arterial stiffness or aortic stiffness Coronary artery calcification	Coronary heart disease Angina pectoris Myocardial infarction Atrial fibrillation Heart failure	Clinical stroke Small vessel disease: subcortical infarcts, lacunes, white matter lesions, microbleeds, enlarged perivascular spaces, amyloid angiopathy	Hypertension Diabetes Coronary heart disease Myocardial infarction Atrial fibrillation Heart failure

Source: data from Winblad B., Amouyel P., Andrieu S., et al. Defeating Alzheimer's disease and other dementias: a priority for European science and society. *Lancet Neurol.* 2016;15(5):455-532; data from Qiu C., Fratiglioni L. A major role for cardiovascular burden in age-related cognitive decline. *Nat Rev Cardiol.* 2015;12(5):267-277; data from Fratiglioni L., Qiu C. Epidemiology of dementia. In Dening T, Thomas A, (eds). *The Oxford Textbook of Old Age Psychiatry.* 2nd Ed. Oxford, UK: Oxford University Press 2013, pp. 389-413.

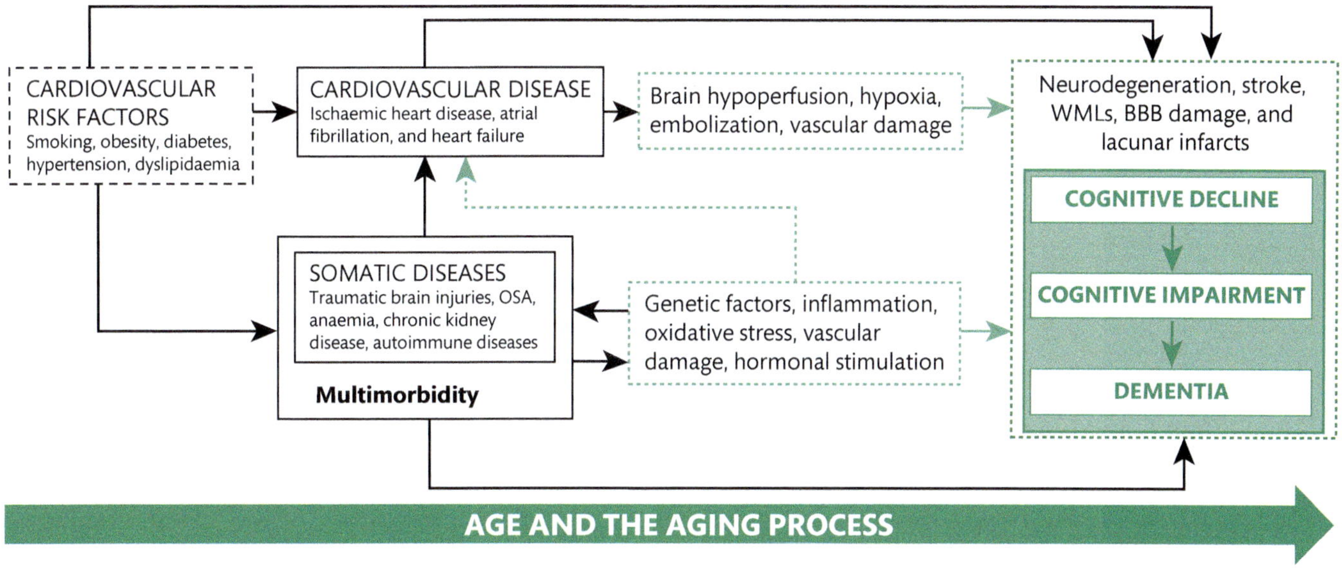

Fig. 8.1 Cardiovascular risk factors, cardiovascular morbidities, brain lesions, and cognitive phenotypes in ageing over the life course.
OSA = obstructive sleep apnea; WMLs = white matter lesions; BBB = blood-brain barrier.

to cardiovascular risk factors from early life onward, have emerged as important mechanisms leading to cognitive decline and dementia later in life.[68–70] In addition, arterial stiffness or atherosclerosis, as a marker for clinical cardiovascular disease, may be linked to cognitive decline and dementia through its impact on cerebral macro- and microvascular lesions. The neuropathological data from the UK Medical Research Council Cognitive Function and Ageing Study suggested an association between systemic cardiovascular health (e.g. ischaemic heart disease) and cerebral microinfarcts,[71] supporting the view that cardiovascular lesions and cerebral SVD may be interrelated in the ageing process.

Second, post-mortem and neuroimaging studies have also linked midlife vascular risk factors (e.g. smoking and hypertension) to brain neurodegenerative pathologies (e.g. amyloid-β, neuritic plaques, and global and regional brain atrophy).[72–74] In addition, the structural brain MRI studies and the Pittsburgh compound B (PiB)-positron emission tomography studies have revealed the associations of the Framingham Cardiovascular Risk Score not only with grey matter atrophy and reduced white matter microstructural integrity, but also with the burden of cerebral amyloid-β as quantified with a Global PiB index, suggesting that aggregated cardiovascular risk factors may be also amyloidogenic.[75–77] Furthermore, emerging evidence has supported the associations of cerebral hypoxia and cardiovascular disease (e.g. coronary heart disease and atrial fibrillation) with neurofibrillary tangles and neuritic plaques, the hallmarks of Alzheimer pathology.[78–80] This suggests that cardiovascular disease may contribute to the burden of brain neurodegenerative pathologies.

Third, cerebral atherosclerosis or arteriosclerosis and neurodegeneration share common biological and pathophysiological mechanisms, such as inflammation, oxidative stress, and toxic amyloid-β peptide deposition, and both conditions frequently coexist in people with dementia or cognitive impairment. However, evidence supporting their direct association has been mixed.[16,81] This implies that although common aetiological or reciprocally synergistic pathophysiological mechanisms may promote both atherosclerotic and neurodegenerative lesions in the brain, they may represent coinciding processes in the ageing process that converge to cause additive brain damage, thus leading to accelerated cognitive decline, cognitive impairment, and clinical manifestation of the dementia syndrome.[17,82]

Finally, artery stiffness and increased central pulse pressure may cause haemodynamic stress in the heart and the brain, which in turn may result in structural brain changes, insufficient cerebral blood perfusion, and cerebral hypoxia.[16,25] In addition, reduced cardiac output, cerebral hypoperfusion, or cerebral embolic events, owing to haemodynamic effects of CHD, AF, and heart failure, might predispose older people to accelerated cognitive decline and an increased risk of dementia.[49] Also, AF and heart failure can be linked to cognitive impairment, cognitive decline, and dementia, by causing silent vascular brain lesions such as lacunar infarcts, WMHs, and microbleeds.[16,83]

Summary

From a life course perspective, long-term exposures to cardiovascular risk factors from early life onward, together with advancing age, could cause subclinical atherosclerosis and clinical cardiovascular disease, and such a pathophysiological process also significantly contributes to the accelerated cognitive decline and increased risk of dementia in later life. As a result, the accelerated cognitive decline in ageing, when progressing to overt dementia, often ends with mixed dementia due to cerebrovascular and neurodegenerative pathologies in the brain. The body-mind (or heart-brain) connection in ageing and dementia or the lifespan atherosclerosis cascade in dementia has significant implications for the development of preventive and therapeutic interventions to delay the onset of cognitive impairment and dementia as many cardiovascular risk factors are modifiable and cardiovascular diseases are amenable to effective treatment. Furthermore, chronic comorbid conditions, especially cardiometabolic and cardiovascular comorbidities, are highly prevalent among people with dementia. The presence of comorbid conditions in dementia contributes to poor outcomes (e.g. hospital admission, functional dependency, and poor survival), creates complex challenges for patient care, and substantially increases the burden of health and social care agencies and caregivers. In this regard, early recognition and management of treatable cardiovascular comorbidities in dementia may help health and social care providers maximize the well-being of people with dementia.

REFERENCES

1. World Health Organization (WHO) and Alzheimer's Disease International (ADI). Dementia: a public health priority. Geneva: World Health Organization, 2012.
2. Prince M, Bryce R, Albanese E, Wimo A, Ribeiro W, Ferri CP. The global prevalence of dementia: a systematic review and metaanalysis. Alzheimer's Dement. 2013; 9(1): 63–75. e2.
3. Fratiglioni L, Qiu C. Prevention of cognitive decline in ageing: dementia as the target, delayed onset as the goal. Lancet Neurology. 2011; 10(9): 778–9.
4. Winblad B, Amouyel P, Andrieu S, et al. Defeating Alzheimer's disease and other dementias: a priority for European science and society. Lancet Neurology. 2016; 15(5): 455–532.
5. Wu YT, Fratiglioni L, Matthews FE, Lobo A, Breteler MM, Skoog I, Brayne C. Dementia in western Europe: epidemiological evidence and implications for policy making. Lancet Neurology. 2016; 15(1): 116–24.
6. Wu YT, Beiser AS, Breteler MMB, et al. The changing prevalence and incidence of dementia over time—current evidence. Nat Rev Neurol. 2017; 13(6): 327–39.
7. Calderón-Larrañaga A, Vetrano DL, Onder G, et al. Assessing and measuring chronic multimorbidity in the older population: A proposal for its operationalization. J Gerontol A Biol Sci Med Sci. 2017; 72(10): 1417–23.
8. Whalley LJ, Dick FD, McNeill G. A life-course approach to the aetiology of late-onset dementias. Lancet Neurology. 2006; 5(1): 87–96.
9. Bunn F, Burn AM, Goodman C, et al. Comorbidity and dementia: a scoping review of the literature. BMC Med. 2014; 12: 192.
10. Salthouse TA. When does age-related cognitive decline begin? Neurobiol Aging. 2009; 30(4): 507–14.
11. Winblad B, Palmer K, Kivipelto M, et al. Mild cognitive impairment—beyond controversies, towards a consensus: report of the International Working Group on Mild Cognitive Impairment. J Intern Med. 2004; 256(3): 240–6.
12. Livingston G, Sommerlad A, Orgeta V, et al. Dementia prevention, intervention, and care. Lancet. 2017; 390(10113): 2673–734.
13. Palmer K, Wang HX, Bäckman L, Winblad B, Fratiglioni L. Differential evolution of cognitive impairment in nondemented older persons: results from the Kungsholmen Project. Am J Psychiatry. 2002; 159(3): 436–42.
14. Palmer K, Bäckman L, Winblad B, Fratiglioni L. Mild cognitive impairment in the general population: occurrence and progression to Alzheimer disease. Am J Geriatr Psychiatry. 2008; 16(7): 603–11.
15. Agüero-Torres H, Kivipelto M, von Strauss E. Rethinking the dementia diagnoses in a population-based study: what is Alzheimer's disease and what is vascular dementia? A study from the Kungsholmen Project. Dement Geriatr Cogn Disord. 2006; 22(3): 244–9.
16. Qiu C, Fratiglioni L. A major role for cardiovascular burden in age-related cognitive decline. Nat Rev Cardiol. 2015; 12(5): 267–77.
17. Casserly I, Topol E. Convergence of atherosclerosis and Alzheimer's disease: inflammation, cholesterol, and misfolded proteins. Lancet. 2004; 363(9415): 1139–46.
18. Gorelick PB, Scuteri A, Black SE, et al. Vascular contributions to cognitive impairment and dementia: a statement for healthcare professionals from the American Heart Association/American Stroke Association. Stroke. 2011; 42(9): 2672–713.
19. Guerchet M, Aboyans V, Nubukpo P, Lacroix P, Clément JP, Preux PM. Ankle-brachial index as a marker of cognitive impairment and dementia in general population: a systematic review. Atherosclerosis. 2011; 216(2): 251–7.
20. Shaik MA, Venketasubramanian N, Cheng CY, Wong TY, Vrooman H, Ikram MK, et al. Ankle brachial index, MRI markers and cognition: The Epidemiology of Dementia in Singapore study. Atherosclerosis. 2017; 263: 272–7.
21. Hofman A, Ott A, Breteler MM, et al. Atherosclerosis, apolipoprotein E, and prevalence of dementia and Alzheimer's disease in the Rotterdam Study. Lancet. 1997; 349(9046): 151–4.
22. Yan Z, Liang Y, Shi J, et al. Carotid stenosis and cognitive impairment amongst older Chinese adults living in a rural area: a population-based study. Eur J Neurol. 2016; 23(1): 201–4.
23. Chang XL, Zhou HQ, Lei CY, et al. Association between asymptomatic carotid stenosis and cognitive function: a systematic review. Neurosci Biobeha Rev. 2013; 37(8): 493–9.
24. Romero JR, Beiser A, Seshadri S, et al. Carotid artery atherosclerosis, MRI indices of brain ischemia, aging, and cognitive impairment: the Framingham study. Stroke. 2009; 40(5): 1590–6.
25. Mitchell GF, van Buchem MA, Sigurdsson S, et al. Arterial stiffness, pressure and flow pulsatility and brain structure and function: the Age, Gene/Environment Susceptibility-Reykjavik study. Brain. 2011; 134(Pt 11): 3398–407.
26. van Sloten TT, Protogerou AD, Henry RM, Schram MT, Launer LJ, Stehouwer CD. Association between arterial stiffness, cerebral small vessel disease and cognitive impairment: A systematic review and meta-analysis. Neurosci Biobehav Rev. 2015; 53: 121–30.
27. Poels MM, van Oijen M, Mattace-Raso FU, et al. Arterial stiffness, cognitive decline, and risk of dementia: the Rotterdam study. Stroke. 2007; 38(3): 888–92.
28. Waldstein SR, Rice SC, Thayer JF, Najjar SS, Scuteri A, Zonderman AB. Pulse pressure and pulse wave velocity are related to cognitive decline in the Baltimore Longitudinal Study of Aging. Hypertension. 2008; 51(1): 99–104.
29. Zeki Al Hazzouri A, Newman AB, Simonsick E, et al. Pulse wave velocity and cognitive decline in elders: the Health, Aging, and Body Composition study. Stroke. 2013; 44(2): 388–93.
30. Pase MP, Beiser A, Himali JJ, et al. Aortic stiffness and the risk of incident mild cognitive impairment and dementia. Stroke. 2016; 47(9): 2256–61.
31. Maillard P, Mitchell GF, Himali JJ, et al. Effects of arterial stiffness on brain integrity in young adults from the Framingham Heart Study. Stroke. 2016; 47(4): 1030–6.
32. Singer J, Trollor JN, Baune BT, Sachdev PS, Smith E. Arterial stiffness, the brain and cognition: a systematic review. Ageing Res Rev. 2014; 15: 16–27.
33. Vidal JS, Sigurdsson S, Jonsdottir MK, et al. Coronary artery calcium, brain function and structure: the AGES-Reykjavik Study. Stroke. 2010; 41(5): 891–7.
34. Bos D, Vernooij MW, Elias-Smale SE, et al. Atherosclerotic calcification relates to cognitive function and to brain changes on magnetic resonance imaging. Alzheimer's Dement. 2012; 8(5 Suppl): S104–S111.

35. Kuller LH, Lopez OL, Mackey RH, et al. Subclinical cardiovascular disease and death, dementia, and coronary heart disease in patients 80+ years. J Am Coll Cardiol. 2016; 67(9): 1013–22.
36. Fujiyoshi A, Jacobs DR Jr, Fitzpatrick AL, et al. Coronary artery calcium and risk of dementia in MESA (Multi-Ethnic Study of Atherosclerosis). Circ Cardiovasc Imaging. 2017; 10(5): pii. e005349.
37. Reis JP, Launer LJ, Terry JG, et al. Subclinical atherosclerotic calcification and cognitive functioning in middle-aged adults: the CARDIA study. Atherosclerosis. 2013; 231(1): 72–7.
38. Bursi F, Rocca WA, Killian JM, et al. Heart disease and dementia: a population-based study. Am J Epidemiol. 2006; 163(2): 135–41.
39. Rusanen M, Kivipelto M, Levälahti E, et al. Heart diseases and long-term risk of dementia and Alzheimer's disease: a population-based CAIDE study. J Alzheimer's Dis. 2014; 42(1): 183–91.
40. Rosano C, Newman AB. Cardiovascular disease and risk of Alzheimer's disease. Neurol Res. 2006; 28(6): 612–20.
41. Eriksson UK, Bennet AM, Gatz M, Dickman PW, Pedersen NL. Nonstroke cardiovascular disease and risk of Alzheimer disease and dementia. Alzheimer Dis Assoc Disord. 2010; 24(3): 213–19.
42. Haring B, Leng X, Robinson J, et al. Cardiovascular disease and cognitive decline in postmenopausal women: results from the Women's Health Initiative Memory Study. J Am Heart Assoc. 2013; 2(6): e000369.
43. Ikram MA, van Oijen M, de Jong FJ, et al. Unrecognized myocardial infarction in relation to risk of dementia and cerebral small vessel disease. Stroke. 2008; 39(5): 1421–1426.
44. de Bruijn RF, Ikram MA. Cardiovascular risk factors and future risk of Alzheimer's disease. BMC Med. 2014; 12: 130.
45. Deckers K, Schievink SHJ, Rodriquez MMF, et al. Coronary heart disease and risk for cognitive impairment or dementia: Systematic review and meta-analysis. PLOS One. 2017; 12(9): e0184244.
46. Schneider AL, Rawlings AM, Sharrett AR, et al. High-sensitivity cardiac troponin T and cognitive function and dementia risk: the atherosclerosis risk in communities study. Eur Heart J. 2014; 35(27): 1817–24.
47. Wijsman LW, de Craen AJ, Trompet S, et al. High-sensitivity cardiac troponin T is associated with cognitive decline in older adults at high cardiovascular risk. Eur J Prev Cardiol. 2016; 23(13): 1383–92.
48. Thacker EL, McKnight B, Psaty BM, et al. Atrial fibrillation and cognitive decline: a longitudinal cohort study. Neurology. 2013; 81(2): 119–25.
49. Kalantarian S, Stern TA, Mansour M, Ruskin JN. Cognitive impairment associated with atrial fibrillation: a meta-analysis. Ann Intern Med. 2013; 158(5 Pt 1): 338–46.
50. Singh-Manoux A, Fayosse A, Sabia S, et al. Atrial fibrillation as a risk factor for cognitive decline and dementia. Eur Heart J. 2017; 38(34): 2612–18.
51. Stefansdottir H, Arnar DO, Aspelund T, et al. Atrial fibrillation is associated with reduced brain volume and cognitive function independent of cerebral infarcts. Stroke. 2013; 44(4): 1020–5.
52. ONTARGET Investigators, Yusuf S, Teo KK, Pogue J, et al. Telmisartan, ramipril, or both in patients at high risk for vascular events. N Engl J Med. 2008; 358(15): 1547–59.
53. TRANSCEND Investigators, Yusuf S, Teo K, Anderson C, et al. Effects of the angiotensin-receptor blocker telmisartan on cardiovascular events in high-risk patients intolerant to angiotensin-converting enzyme inhibitors: a randomised controlled trial. Lancet. 2008; 372(9644): 1174–83.
54. Qiu C, Winblad B, Marengoni A, Klarin I, Fastbom J, Fratiglioni L. Heart failure and risk of dementia and Alzheimer disease: a population-based cohort study. Arch Intern Med. 2006; 166(9): 1003–8.
55. Gure TR, Blaum CS, Giordani B, et al. Prevalence of cognitive impairment in older adults with heart failure. J Am Geriatr Soc. 2012; 60(9): 1724–9.
56. Hajduk AM, Kiefe CI, Person SD, Gore JG, Saczynski JS. Cognitive change in heart failure: a systematic review. Circ Cardiovasc Qual Outcomes. 2013; 6(4): 451–60.
57. Bauer K, Schwarzkopf L, Graessel E, Holle R. A claims data-based comparison of comorbidity in individuals with and without dementia. BMC Geriatr. 2014; 14: 10.
58. Cermakova P, Johnell K, Fastbom J, et al. Cardiovascular diseases in ~30,000 patients in the Swedish Dementia Registry. J Alzheimer's Dis. 2015; 48(4): 949–58.
59. Poblador-Plou B, Calderón-Larrañaga A, Marta-Moreno J, et al. Comorbidity of dementia: a cross-sectional study of primary care older patients. BMC Psychiatry. 2014; 14: 84.
60. Mondor L, Maxwell CJ, Hogan DB, et al. Multimorbidity and healthcare utilization among home care clients with dementia in Ontario, Canada: A retrospective analysis of a population-based cohort. PLOS Med. 2017; 14(3): e1002249.
61. Haaksma ML, Vilela LR, Marengoni A, et al. Comorbidity and progression of late onset Alzheimer's disease: A systematic review. PLOS One. 2017; 12(5): e0177044.
62. Snowden MB, Steinman LE, Bryant LL, et al. Dementia and co-occurring chronic conditions: a systematic literature review to identify what is known and where are the gaps in the evidence? Int J Geriatr Psychiatry. 2017; 32(4): 357–71.
63. Fabbri E, An Y, Zoli M, et al. Association between accelerated multimorbidity and age-related cognitive decline in older Baltimore Longitudinal Study of Aging participants without dementia. J Am Geriatr Soc. 2016; 64(5): 965–72.
64. Fox C, Smith T, Maidment I, et al. The importance of detecting and managing comorbidities in people with dementia? Age Ageing. 2014; 43(6): 741–3.
65. Browne J, Edwards DA, Rhodes KM, Brimicombe DJ, Payne RA. Association of comorbidity and health service usage among patients with dementia in the UK: a population-based study. BMJ Open. 2017; 7(3): e012546.
66. Fratiglioni L, Qiu C. Epidemiology of dementia. In: Dening T, Thomas A (eds). The Oxford Textbook of Old Age Psychiatry (2nd edition). Oxford: Oxford University Press, 2013, pp389–413.
67. Gold G, Giannakopoulos P, Herrmann FR, Bouras C, Kövari E. Identification of Alzheimer and vascular lesion thresholds for mixed dementia. Brain. 2007; 130(Pt 11): 2830–6.
68. Kalaria RN. Cerebrovascular disease and mechanisms of cognitive impairment: evidence from clinicopathological studies in humans. Stroke. 2012; 43(9): 2526–34.
69. Qiu C, Sigurdsson S, Zhang Q, et al. Diabetes, markers of brain pathology and cognitive function: the Age, Gene/Environment Susceptibility-Reykjavik Study. Ann Neurol. 2014; 75(1): 138–46.
70. Wang R, Fratiglioni L, Kalpouzos G, et al. Mixed brain lesions mediate the association between cardiovascular risk burden and cognitive decline in old age: A population-based study. Alzheimer's Dement. 2017; 13(3): 247–56.
71. Richardson K, Stephan BC, Ince PG, Brayne C, Matthews FE, Esiri MM. The neuropathology of vascular disease in the

Medical Research Council Cognitive Function and Ageing Study (MRC CFAS). Curr Alzheimer Res. 2012; 9: 687–96.

72. Knopman DS, Penman AD, Catellier DJ, et al. Vascular risk factors and longitudinal changes on brain MRI: the ARIC study. Neurology. 2011; 76(22): 1879–85.
73. Shah NS, Vidal JS, Masaki K, et al. Midlife blood pressure, plasma β-amyloid, and the risk for Alzheimer disease: the Honolulu Asia Aging Study. Hypertension. 2012; 59(4): 780–6.
74. Rodrigue KM, Rieck JR, Kennedy KM, Devous MDSr, Diaz-Arrastia R, Park DC. Risk factors for β-amyloid deposition in healthy aging: vascular and genetic effects. JAMA Neurol. 2013; 70(5): 600–6.
75. Reed BR, Marchant NL, Jagust WJ, DeCarli CC, Mack W, Chui HC. Coronary risk correlates with cerebral amyloid deposition. Neurobiol Aging. 2012; 33(9): 1979–87.
76. Villeneuve S, Reed BR, Madison CM, et al. Vascular risk and Aβ interact to reduce cortical thickness in AD vulnerable brain regions. Neurology. 2014; 83(1): 40–7.
77. Wang R, Fratiglioni L, Laukka EJ, et al. Effects of vascular risk factors and APOE ε4 on white matter integrity and cognitive decline. Neurology. 2015; 84(11): 1128–35.
78. Salminen A, Kauppinen A, Kaarniranta K. Hypoxia/ischemia activate processing of Amyloid Precursor Protein: impact of vascular dysfunction in the pathogenesis of Alzheimer's disease. J Neurochem. 2017; 140(4): 536–49.
79. Honjo K, Black SE, Verhoeff NP. Alzheimer's disease, cerebrovascular disease, and the β-amyloid cascade. Can J Neurol Sci. 2012; 39(6): 712–28.
80. Dublin S, Anderson ML, Heckbert SR, et al. Neuropathologic changes associated with atrial fibrillation in a population-based autopsy cohort. J Gerontol A Biol Sci Med Sci. 2014; 69(5): 609–15.
81. Yarchoan M, Xie SX, Kling MA, et al. Cerebrovascular atherosclerosis correlates with Alzheimer pathology in neurodegenerative dementias. Brain. 2012; 135(Pt 12): 3749–56.
82. Strozyk D, Dickson DW, Lipton RB, et al. Contribution of vascular pathology to the clinical expression of dementia. Neurobiol Aging. 2010; 31(10): 1710–20.
83. Chen LY, Lopez FL, Gottesman RF, et al. Atrial fibrillation and cognitive decline-the role of subclinical cerebral infarcts: the Atherosclerosis Risk in Communities study. Stroke. 2014; 45(9): 2568–74.

SECTION 2
Neurodegenerative disorders

9

Early onset Alzheimer's disease

Ratnavalli Ellajosyula

Introduction

Early onset Alzheimer's disease (EOAD) refers to AD presenting before 65 years.[1] This is considered an arbitrary construct based on employment and retirement age. However, the term is commonly used in clinical practice and has replaced 'presenile dementia'. The case of Auguste D, a 51-year-old woman described by Alzheimer was the earliest case of EOAD.[2] It shares common features with late onset AD (LOAD), including amnestic clinical presentation,[1] pathology,[3] hippocampal atrophy on magnetic resonance imaging scan (MRI) of the brain,[4] cerebrospinal fluid biomarkers,[5–7] and extent and distribution of amyloid on Pittsburgh Compound B (PiB) positron emission tomography (PET).[8] Though the similarities outweigh the differences, there are certain clinical, genetic, and biological distinctions.[9] Up to 5% of the EOAD is familial (EOFAD).[10,11] and 50% of EOFAD is due to highly penetrant mutations in three genes, presenilin 1 (*PSEN1*), presenilin 2 (*PSEN2*), and amyloid precursor protein (APP).[12–16] The discovery of these mutations in EOFAD has contributed immensely to our understanding, and confirmed a central role for amyloid in the pathogenesis of AD.

EOAD is uncommon and constitutes 2–10% of AD,[17] but due to the fact that it affects younger patients, who are employed or productive, there are more personal, psychological, familial, and social consequences. This chapter will review the epidemiology of EOAD.

Epidemiology

Prevalence

Estimating prevalence is important to measure disease burden and plan health services in the community. Studies on the epidemiology of EOAD are few, in contrast to LOAD, because of the formidable challenges and expense of conducting a large population study investigating an uncommon condition, with the likelihood of only an unreliable frequency estimate. A summary of the major studies with methodology and the prevalence rates are shown in Tables 9.1 and 9.2. Studies which have been done primarily in the elderly, and which happen to contain prevalence rates for the overlapping group in the 60–64-year range have been omitted.

Six studies[18–23] have specifically investigated prevalence of early onset dementia (EOD) and three of these were on AD (one also looked at frontotemporal dementia).[18,21,23] Other studies focused on the elderly, but also provided data for the younger age groups.[24–29]

The quoted prevalence estimates of EOAD in the various studies ranged from 15 to 200 per 100,000 of the population. Two studies from the UK, with similar case ascertainment of contacting all health providers and reviewing hospital records, reported nearly the same prevalence (15 and 17/100,000) for the 45–65-year population.[19,20] Campion et al., from Rouen, France,[21] determined the prevalence of EOAD as 41.2 in the 41–60-year range population. Ikejima and others from Japan used a postal questionnaire for case ascertainment in Ibaraki prefecture near Tokyo.[22] They found a prevalence of 22.3 but vascular dementia was commonest (42.5%), and AD accounted for 25.6% of cases. Similar estimates (25.5) have been observed in a cross-sectional registry study from Brescia County, Italy, more recently.[23] A total of 175 cases of EOD, 81 AD, were seen in a population of 317,107, using primarily the consolidated electronic database among the network of participating centres. A study from Pitea River Valley, Sweden, recruited cases prospectively over two years and found a prevalence of 28/100,000 in the 40–64-year age group.[29] An older cross-sectional registry study from the northern region, UK, exclusively on AD,[18] identified the highest number of patients with EOAD (227). The prevalence estimate for the age range 45–64 years was 34.6/100,000. This study also reported incidence rates and survival. Using a centralized medical record linkage system from Mayo clinic, Rochester, USA, which included general practice records and nursing homes, Kokmen et al.[27] found three cases of EOAD in a population of 9431, giving a prevalence rate of 31/100,000 for the 45–64-year age group. A study from Finland in the 1980s[24] using hospital data and community agencies reported a prevalence estimate of 46.7 for the 45–64-year age group/100,000 population. The population surveys have identified fewer cases of AD. The Rotterdam study identified four cases in a population of 2613 giving a rate of 200/100,000 for the 55–64-year age group.[28] In a rural population from Cache County, Utah, USA, all the households and institutions were screened using interviews and neurological examination to detect severe dementia but yielded only one case of AD in a population of 5489.[25] Another study from Finland, found only two cases of AD in 6120 people in the 30–64-year range population, giving a prevalence of 32.7.[26]

Table 9.1 Summary of methodology of various prevalence studies in early onset Alzheimer's disease ordered from most recent to older

Study	Location	Age range of study population (years)	Study design	Case ascertainment	Type of dementia	Diagnostic criteria	Methods
Borroni et al. 2011[23]	Italy: Brescia County	41–60	Cross-sectional/registry	Postal enquiry to all clinics Electronic data base and dementia register	AD and FTD	NINCDS-ADRDA	Neuropsychology, MRI
Ikejima et al. 2009[22]	Japan: Ibaraki	20–64	Cross-sectional/registry	2 step postal survey Health and care service providers	All	DSM III-R for dementia DSM IV	Neuroimaging in 50%
Harvey et al. 2003[20]	UK: London	30–64	Cross-sectional/registry	Health service providers, Hospital information systems, case registers	All	NINCDS-ADRDA	50%-CDR, behavioural pathology in AD rating scale, CAMDEX, cognitive assessment 83% neuroimaging
Ratnavalli et al. 2002[19]	UK: Cambridgeshire	45–64	Cross-sectional/registry	Special clinic databases—memory clinic, EOD Inpatient records, Health care services	All	DSM-III-R NINCDS-ADRDA	ACE, neuroimaging, neuropsychology, neuropsychiatry
Campion et al. 1999[21]	France: Rouen	41–60	Cross-sectional/registry	All referrals to neurology department	AD	NINCDS-ADRDA	Neuropsychology, CT scan
Andreasen et al. 1999[29]	Sweden: Pitea River Valley	40–90+	Registry Prospective	Attending clinic	All	NINCDS-ADRDA	Neuropsychology, CT scan
Ott et al. 1995[28]	Netherlands: Rotterdam	55–90+	Population	All residents 3 stage evaluation	All	DSM –III-R NINCDS-ADRDA	Screening –MMSE, GMS-A, CAMDEX, clinical examination, MRI, neuropsychology
Newens et al. 1993[18]	UK: Northern Health Region	45–64	Registry Retrospective	Computerized records of all hospitals. Supplementary sources -health providers	AD	DSM-III-R	Variable clinical, imaging and neuropsychology. Clinical algorithm for AD diagnosis
Kokmen et al. 1989[27]	USA: Rochester, Minnesota	46–106	Cross-sectional/registry	Computerized medical records of Mayo clinic and others	All	DSM-III NINCDS-ADRDA	Clinical evaluation, neuropathology in some
Sulkava et al. 1985[26]	Finland	30–85+	Population—40 study areas throughout country	2 stage Health exam—screening and clinical phase	All (severe only)	DSM III	Cognitive tests for memory Imaging in some
Schoenberg et al. 1985[25]	USA: Mississippi, Copiah County	40+	Population—all residents	2 stage- enumeration and screening interview Neurological examination	All (severe only)	Clinical	Examination, neuropathology in few
Molsa et al. 1982[24]	Finland: Turku	40+	Cross-sectional/registry	Hospitals, health service providers	All	Clinical	Some neuropsychological tests, neurological examination, interview

AD, Alzheimer's disease; FTD, Frontotemporal dementia; MMSE, Minimental Status examination; ACE, Addenbrooke's clinical examination; CDR, clinical dementia rating scale; MRI, magnetic resonance imaging; CT, computerized tomography; GMS-A, Geriatric mental state schedule; CAMDEX, Cambridge examination for mental disorders of the elderly; DSM, Diagnostic and Statistical manual of mental disorders, R-revised; NINCDS-ADRDA, National Institute of Neurological disorders and communicative disorders-Alzheimer's disease and related disorders association; EOD, Early onset dementia.

Table 9.2 Prevalence studies in early onset Alzheimer's disease ordered from most recent to older

					Prevalence/100,000 (95% Confidence Intervals)			
Reference	Population at risk	Early onset dementia cases	Alzheimer's disease cases n (%)	Age range (years)	Early onset dementia	Alzheimer's Disease	Men	Women
Borroni et al. 2011[23]	317,107	175	81 (46.3%)	45–64	55.2 (47.0–63.4)	25.5 (20.0-31.1)	24.9 (17.2-32.7)	26.11 (18.1-34.2)
Ikejima et al. 2009[22]	852,889	710	190 (26.8%)	45–64	83.3 (77.4–89.6)	22.3 (19.3-25.7)		
Harvey et al. 2003[20]	117,236	115	41 (35.7%)	45–64 30–64	98.1 (81.1–118)	17.4 (12.6-23.6) 35 (25.1-47.4)		
Ratnavalli et al. 2002[19]	72,815	60	11 (18.3%)	45–64	81 (62.8–104.5)	15.1 (8.4-27.0)	10.9 (4.2-28.1)	19.3 (9.4-39.9)
Campion et al. 1999[21]	94,593	–	39	41–60	–	41.2	23.9	57.7
Andreasen et al. 1999[29]	18,918	8	6 (75%)	40–64	38	28		
Ott et al. 1995[28]	2613	11	4 (36.4%)	55–64	421	200	200	100
Newens et al. 1993[18]	655,800	–	227	45–64		34.6 (30.3-39.5)	30.6 (24.8-37.3)	38.5 (32.3-45.9)
Kokmen et al. 1989[27]	9431	10	3 (30%)	45–64 55–59 60–64	81	31.8 (6.6-92.9) *	0 0	152 91
Sulkava et al. 1985[26]	6120	16	2 (12.5%)	30–64	260	32.7 (3.9-118.0)*	0	60
Molsa et al. 1982[24]	36,409	34	17	45–64	93.38	46.7 (27.2-74.7)*	38.3	53.1
Schoenberg et al. 1985[25]	5489		1	40–64		18.2 (0.5-101.4)*		

* CI calculated by Newens et al.[18]

From India, two studies reporting on dementia in the elderly population, also give estimates of prevalence for EOAD as 29 (55–64 years) from rural north India,[30] and 23.6/100,000 (50–64 years) from urban Mumbai.[31] The Maracaibo aging study (MAS) from Venezuela, where 42% of the evaluated population was 55–64 years old, reported prevalence for AD as 56/100,000 person-years for this age range.[32] A population survey using cross-sectional multistage cluster sampling technique in four regions of China yielded a rate of 204/100,000 for the 55–64-year age group.[33]

Incidence

Incidence rates are important for estimating risk in different age groups. The longitudinal cohorts based on incident cases are, methodologically, the best instrument to evaluate survival for EOD. Incidence studies are particularly difficult because they require either a repeated measurement of prevalence or the longitudinal observation of population to detect new cases. This is particularly so for an uncommon disease like EOAD and thus there are even fewer studies on the incidence (Table 9.3). Incidence rate from Cambridgeshire, UK, for age range 45–64 years was 4.2/100,000.[34] A recent registry study from Girona, Spain found an incidence rate of 5.7/100,000 in 30–64-year age range.[35] A study from Mayo Clinic reported a low rate of 4.4 for the 30–59-year age range,[36] while a Sweden study estimate was 13 for the 40–64-year age range.[29] Annual incidence rate was 2.4/100,000 in the Jewish population aged 40–60 years,[37] based on a retrospective review of cases entering institutions using age at symptom onset. The incidence rates were slightly more in women but not significant. Two studies from the UK in the 1990s, using health service and hospital case record review reported different figures. The study from Scotland[38] reported an incidence of 22.6 for the 40–64-year age group, while the figures were much lower from the Northern Health region, 7.2/100,000.[18]

Methodological Issues

There is considerable disparity between the prevalence and incidence estimates because of several methodological issues, including age range of the population studied, the setting, heterogeneity in study design, and sampling methods, which makes comparisons across studies difficult. Most studies have identified only a few cases of EOAD, with a few exceptions.[18,22]

The majority of the prevalence and incidence studies are from Europe. The findings from more economically developed countries may not be applicable to developing nations. The methods of sampling are also different. The Finnish study used a two-stage stratified cluster sampling method.[26] Ott et al. surveyed the population of Netherlands as a whole.[28] A door-to-door survey of household population was carried out in Copiah County, USA, but also ascertained cases from institutions for AD.[25] Many of the available studies have used a cross-sectional design, contacting all health services and providers in a defined catchment area to identify the early onset dementia cases.[18–24] In addition to reviewing hospital records in the area, secondary sources like community resource teams, general practitioners, social services, and nursing homes have also been tapped for case identification.[18–20,22,24] An assumption by the registry studies is that when dementia occurs in young age, the patient would come to the attention of health services. While this is highly likely, low education, socioeconomic, and immigration status may be barriers for seeking access to healthcare services. Registry studies have reported lower prevalence rates than the population studies.[19,20,22,23] It is quite possible that some of the cases are still not coming to the attention of healthcare services in the registry studies.

The population studies have used a brief screening tool or questionnaire to detect cases, which was followed by more extensive evaluation for the screen positive individuals.[25,26,28] The sensitivity of the screening instrument may not be 100%. AD was diagnosed

Table 9.3 Incidence studies in early onset Alzheimer's disease ordered from most recent to older

Reference	Study location	Study type	Age range (years)	Incidence/100,000 (95% Confidence intervals)			
				Early onset dementia	Alzheimer's disease	Men	Women
Garre-Olmo et al. 2010[35]	Spain: Girona	Registry -7 hospitals	30-64 45-64	13.4 (11.3-15.8) 11.9	5.7 (4.3-7.3)		
Mercy et al. 2008[34]	UK: Cambridgeshire	Registry	45-64	11.5 (8.6-15.0)	4.2 (2.5-6.6)		
Andreasen et al. 1999[29]	Sweden: Pitea River Valley	Prospective- Registry	40-64		13		
McGonigal et al.[38]	Scotland	Registry	40-64		22.6		
Newens et al. 1993[18]	UK: Northern Health Region	Health service and Case note review	45-64	94	7.2 (5.8-8.8)	6.5	7.8
Schoenberg et al.[36] 1987	USA: Minnesota, Rochester	Health records of Mayo clinic	30-59	19.2 (10.2-32.8)	4.4 (0.9-12.8)	3.1 (0.1-17.3)	5.6 (0.7-20.2)
Treves et al. 1986[37]	Israel	National neurologic disease Registry, hospital records	40-60		2.4 (1.9-3.0)		
Molsa et al. 1982[24]	Finland: Turku	Health registry	45-64		11.1 (6.3-17.8)		

using various editions of the diagnostic and statistical manual of mental disorders (DSM criteria[39,40])[18,22,26] or the National Institute of Neurological disorders and communicative disorders-Alzheimer's disease and related disorders association (NINCDS-ADRDA[41]) criteria.[19–21,23,27–29] A few have used a clinical algorithm.[24,25] The Finnish study used the label 'degenerative dementia' to indicate AD.[26] Pathology or genetic results when available were used to confirm diagnosis.[20,21,27] Memory impairment is no longer essential to make a clinical diagnosis of AD according to the recent criteria of the National Institute on Aging-Alzheimer's association (NIA-AA)[42] and the IWG.[43] Patients presenting at younger age may have atypical presentations, like logopenic aphasia, posterior cortical atrophy, and frontal dysexecutive syndrome and behavioural symptoms and may not necessarily have memory impairment.[44–46] Likelihood of an atypical presentation can be seen in one of every three EOAD patients.[9,47] All the reported studies diagnosed AD only when memory impairment was present. Patients seen at specialist clinics are usually more extensively evaluated and have detailed neuropsychology and neuroimaging. Neuroimaging, which is necessary to rule out a mixed dementia (as cerebrovascular pathology may coexist with AD), has not been done in all studies.[24,25]

Most studies have defined the symptom onset to include patients younger than 65 years, while Newens et al.[18] used age at diagnosis. The former approach may increase the prevalence estimates. On the other hand, prevalence as estimated by age at diagnosis may underestimate and affect comparisons of age specific rates across various studies. Insidious onset in AD makes the symptom onset difficult to define, while a delay in diagnosis may reduce the age specific prevalence rates. EOAD is sometimes particularly difficult to diagnose because of the atypical presentation.[9,44–47] Certain studies have included only severe dementia, but the criteria to define severity was different.[25,26]

Studies specifically looking at EOD used a cut-off of 65 years, but the age range studied varied. Some have included even younger age groups, in the 20s[22] and 30s,[20,26] while others studied the 45–64-age range.[18,19] Studies which include a broader age range have quoted lower prevalence because of the effect of including younger age groups. As the prevalence increases with age, looking at only the upper end of early onset age range would yield higher prevalence rates, as in the Rotterdam study.[28] This also makes comparisons across studies difficult.

Risk Factors

Age

Similar to LOAD, where age is the biggest risk factor, two studies have indicated that the prevalence[18,20,22] and incidence rates[18] in EOAD approximately doubled with each five-year increase in age (Fig. 9.1).

Gender

Women have an increased risk of AD, but this is inconclusive in EOAD. Incidence was significantly higher for women in the study from Scotland (28.2 vs 16.5/100,000 for 40–64 year age range).[38] Campion et al. found the prevalence to be higher in women.[21] A few studies do not comment on gender differences in EOAD,[20,29] while others found slightly higher age adjusted prevalence rates for women, which were not significant.[18,23,26] In a few studies, all cases were women, but this was not considered significant as the numbers were too small.[27]

Race

Race as a risk factor in EOAD is poorly studied. Age and sex adjusted incidence rates were higher (2.9/100,000) for those born in Europe or America compared to those born in Africa or Asia (1.4) in the study from Israel.[37] There is no other epidemiological study which provides this information. Using a C-Path online data repository (CODR), with information on 3000 patients registered for AD clinical trials, a study found that a significantly higher proportion of EOAD patients were Native Americans and Hispanics, but this could reflect an enrolment bias.[48]

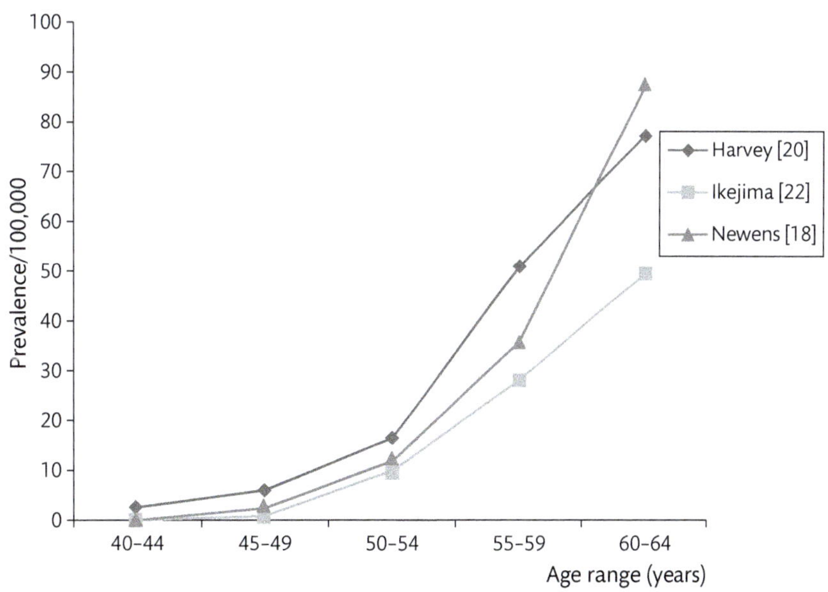

Fig. 9.1 Age specific prevalence rates in early onset Alzheimer's disease.

Other risk factors

There is no information on role of other risk factors in EOAD. In the analysis of CODR data, vascular risk factors were significantly less in the EOAD group as compared to LOAD.[48] Well-designed prospective cohort studies and multicentre case-control studies in EOAD are needed to evaluate risk factors in more detail.

Genetics

Family history of dementia was more common in the registry study from Spain in EOAD compared to LOAD (42.6% vs 30.6%).[35] In the only population based genetic study, Campion et al. determined prevalence of autosomal dominant form of early onset AD (ADEOAD, with onset before 61 years) in Rouen, France as 5.3 people/100,000 at risk for ages 41–60 years.[21] They defined autosomal dominant EOAD (ADEOAD) as occurrence of at least three EOAD cases in three generations. They screened 34 ADEOAD families and found *PSEN1* mutations in 56% and APP mutations in 15%. None had *PSEN2* mutations.

Apolipoprotein ε4 genotype

The apolipoprotein Eε4 (APOEε4) allele is the most important genetic risk factor for sporadic AD.[49] Around 50–65% AD patients are ε4 carriers, while only 20–25% of the general population are positive for one or more of the ε4 allele.[9] Instead of increasing the lifetime risk of developing AD, age at onset is decreased in heterozygous ε4 allele carriers.[50,51] Homozygous carriers develop AD up to ten years earlier than people who do not have this allele.[50] In a Dutch population study in Rotterdam and four northern provinces of Netherlands on the association of APOE and risk of EOAD, APOE4 genotyping was done in 175 (89%) patients.[52] The frequency of ApoEε4 allele was 2.3 times higher among patients when compared to controls and 1.6 times more common in those with family history compared to those without. This study reported an increased risk of EOAD for subjects homozygous for APOEε4 irrespective of family history, but increased risk was seen in heterozygotes, only when there was positive family history.

Patients with EOAD who are APOEε4 negative are more likely to have non-amnestic presentations,[7,53,54] more rapid progression,[55] and more cortical atrophy[56,57] and hypometabolism in the posterior regions.[58] Thus, there appear to be more undiscovered factors interacting with genes modulating the clinical phenotype.

Survival

Data from a handful of studies suggests that the average survival in EOAD patients is less than age and gender matched controls. The median survival was similar in three studies, 8.1 years from Israel,[37] 7.4 years in the Northern Health region, UK,[18] and 7.6 years from Scotland.[38] Age at onset and gender did not affect the survival in the studies from UK but survival was longer if onset occurred before age 55 years in the Israeli study. Younger people (EOAD) are expected to survive longer than older adults (LOAD) because of better general health and fewer comorbidities. To account for the effect of age, longevity quotient (LQ) (which is the proportion of expected survivors who actually survived, expressed as a percentage) has been used by Newens et al.[18] The five-year survival following diagnosis for incident cases was 64% and LQ was 69%. This study did not find any evidence of a more malignant course in EOAD as compared to LOAD. Numerous variables affect survival, like the nature and source of the sample, sex ratios, ratio of mild to severe cases, diagnostic criteria, comorbid conditions, and the point from which survival is estimated (onset, diagnosis, or prevalence date).

Studies from memory clinics using Cox proportional hazards suggest that the mortality risk in EOAD is significantly higher compared to LOAD.[59,60]

Time trends

There is hardly any literature on time trends in incidence in EOAD. In the only available paper, incidence of AD was stable over a decade (1975–1984) and remained equal for men and women.[61] This included the 50–64 age group. There was no birth cohort effect for AD.

Conclusion

EOAD is uncommon but understanding the biology and pathogenesis is crucial, as illustrated by the discovery of mutations in the ADEOAD, which shed light on the role of amyloid cascade in the pathogenesis of AD. Estimating the burden of disease in the population is difficult as epidemiological data are sparse. There is marked variation in the prevalence and incidence rates and in the methodology of the studies. Most of the studies are also from developed nations. There may be true differences across regions and countries due to different risk or protective factors but this remains to be evaluated. Cross-cultural and national studies with standardized methodology are necessary to understand both the burden of the disease and to direct and develop therapy and carry out clinical trials.

REFERENCES

1. Rossor MN, Fox NC, Mummery CJ, Schott JM, Warren JD. The diagnosis of young-onset dementia. Lancet Neurology. 2010; 9(8): 793–806.
2. Maurer K, Volk S, Gerbaldo H. Auguste D and Alzheimer's disease. Lancet. 1997; 349: 1546–9.
3. Blessed G, Tomlinson BE, Roth M. The association between quantitative measures of dementia and of senile change in the cerebral grey matter of elderly subjects. Brit J Psychiatry. 1968; 114(512): 797–81.
4. van de Pol LA, Hensel A, Barkhof F, Gertz HJ, Scheltens P,van der Flier WM. Hippocampal atrophy in Alzheimer disease: age matters. Neurology. 2006; 66: 236–8.
5. Bouwman FH, Schoonenboom NS, Verwey NA, et al. CSF biomarker levels in early and late onset Alzheimer's disease. Neurobiol Aging. 2009; 30: 1895–901.
6. Dickerson BC, Wolk DA. Dysexecutive versus amnesic phenotypes of very mild Alzheimer's disease are associated with distinct clinical, genetic and cortical thinning characteristics. J Neurol Neurosurg Psychiatry. 2011; 82: 45–51.
7. van der Flier WM, Schoonenboom SN, Pijnenburg YA, Fox NC, Scheltens P. The effect of APOE genotype on clinical phenotype in Alzheimer disease. Neurology. 2006; 67: 526–7.

8. Rabinovici GD, Furst AJ, Alkalay A, et al. Increased metabolic vulnerability in early-onset Alzheimer's disease is not related to amyloid burden. Brain. 2010; 133: 512–28.
9. van der Flier W, Pijnenburg YA, Fox NC and Scheltens P. Early-onset versus late-onset Alzheimer's disease: the case of the missing APOE ε4 allele. Lancet Neurology. 2011; 10: 280–8.
10. Wu L, Rosa-Neto P, Hsiung GY, et al. Early-onset familial Alzheimer's disease (EOFAD). Can J Neurol Sci. 2012; 39: 436–45.
11. Lleo A, Blesa R, Queralt R, et al. Frequency of mutations in the presenilin and amyloid precursor protein genes in early-onset Alzheimer disease in Spain. Arch Neurol. 2002; 59: 1759–63.
12. Goate A, Chartier-Harlin MC, Mullan M, et al. Segregation of a missense mutation in the amyloid precursor protein gene with familial Alzheimer's disease. Nature. 1991; 349: 704–6.
13. Levy-Lahad E, Wasco W, Poorkaj P, et al. Candidate gene for the chromosome 1 familial Alzheimer's disease locus. Science. 1995; 269: 973–7.
14. Levy E, Carman MD, Fernandez-Madrid IJ, et al. Mutation of the Alzheimer's disease amyloid gene in hereditary cerebral hemorrhage, Dutch type. Science. 1990; 248: 1124–6.
15. Rogaev EI, Sherrington R, Rogaeva EA, et al. Familial Alzheimer's disease in kindreds with missense mutations in a gene on chromosome 1 related to the Alzheimer's disease type 3 gene. Nature. 1995; 376: 775–8.
16. Sherrington R, Rogaev EI, Liang Y, et al. Cloning of a gene bearing missense mutations in early-onset familial Alzheimer's disease. Nature. 1995; 375: 754–60.
17. Cauwenberghe CV, Broeckhoven CV, Sleegers K. The genetic landscape of Alzheimer's disease: clinical implications and perspectives. Genetics in Medicine. 2016; 8: 421–30.
18. Newens AJ, Forster DP, Kay DW, Kirkup W, Bates D, Edwardson J. Clinically diagnosed presenile dementia of the Alzheimer type in the Northern Health Region: ascertainment, prevalence, incidence and survival. Psychol Med. 1993; 23: 631–44.
19. Ratnavalli E, Brayne C, Dawson K, Hodges JR. The prevalence of frontotemporal dementia. Neurology. 2002; 58: 1615–21.
20. Harvey RJ, Skelton-Robinson M, Rossor MN. The prevalence and causes of dementia in people under the age of 65 years. J Neurol Neurosurg Psychiatry. 2003; 74: 1206–9.
21. Campion D, Dumanchin C, Hannequin D, et al. Early onset autosomal dominant Alzheimer disease: prevalence, genetic heterogeneity, and mutation spectrum. Am J Hum Genet. 1999; 65: 664–70.
22. Ikejima C, Yasuno F, Mizukami K, Sasaki M, Tanimukai S, Asada T. Prevalence and causes of early-onset dementia in Japan: a population-based study. Stroke 2009; 40: 2709–14.
23. Borroni B, Alberici A, Grassi M, et al. Prevalence and demographic features of early-onset neurodegenerative dementia in Brescia County, Italy. Alzheimer Dis Assoc Disord. 2011; 25: 341–4.
24. Molsa P, Marttila RJ, Rinne UK. Epidemiology of dementia in a Finnish population. Acta Neurol Scand. 1982; 65: 541–52.
25. Schoenberg BS, Anderson DW, Haerer AF. Severe dementia: prevalence and clinical features in a biracial US population. Arch Neurol. 1985; 42: 740–3.
26. Sulkava R, Wikstrom J, Aromaa A, et al. Prevalence of severe dementia in Finland. Neurology. 1985; 35: 1025–9.
27. Kokmen E, Beard CM, Offord KP, Kurland LT. Prevalence of medically diagnosed dementia in a defined United States population: Rochester, Minnesota, January 1, 1975. Neurology. 1989; 39: 773–6.
28. Ott A, Breteler MM, van Harskamp F, et al. Prevalence of Alzheimer's disease and vascular dementia: association with education. The Rotterdam study. BMJ. 1995; 310: 970–3.
29. Andreasen N, Blennow K, Sjodin C, Winblad B, Svardsudd K. Prevalence and incidence of clinically diagnosed memory impairments in a geographically defined general population in Sweden. The Pitea Dementia Project. Neuroepidemiology. 1999; 18: 144–55.
30. Chandra V, Ganguli M, Pandav R, Johnston J, Belle S, DeKosky ST. Prevalence of Alzheimer's disease and other dementias in rural India: The Indo-US study. Neurology. 1998; 51: 1000–8.
31. Vas CJ, Pinto C, Panikker D, Noronha S, Deshpande N, Kulkarni L, et al. Prevalence of dementia in an urban Indian population. Int Psychogeriatr. 2001; 13: 439–50.
32. Molero AE, Pino-Ramirez G, Maestre GE. High prevalence of dementia in a Caribbean population. Neuroepidemiology. 2007; 29: 107–12.
33. Zhang ZX, Zahner GE, Roman GC, et al. Dementia subtypes in China: prevalence in Beijing, Xian, Shanghai, and Chengdu. Arch Neurol. 2005; 62: 447–53.
34. Mercy L, Hodges JR, Dawson K, Barker RA, Brayne C. Incidence of early-onset dementias in Cambridgeshire, United Kingdom. Neurology. 2008; 71: 1496–9.
35. Garre-Olmo J, Genis batlle D, del Mar Fernandez M, et al. Incidence and subtypes of early-onset dementia in a geographically defined general population. Neurology. 2010; 75: 1249–55.
36. Schoenberg BS, Kokmen E, Okazaki H. Alzheimer's disease and other dementing illnesses in a defined United States population: incidence rates and clinical features. Ann Neurol. 1987; 22: 724–9.
37. Treves T, Korczyn ADK, Zilber N, et al. Presenile dementia in Israel. Arch Neurol. 1986; 43: 26–9.
38. McGonigal G, Thomas B, Mcquade C, Starr JM, Maclennan WJ, Whalley LJ. Epidemiological of Alzheimer's presenile dementia in Scotland, 1974–1988. BMJ. 1993; 306: 680–3.
39. American Psychiatric Association. Diagnostic and statistical manual of mental disorders (3rd edition revised). Washington, DC: American Psychiatric Association, 1987.
40. American Psychiatric Association. Diagnostic and Statistical Manual of Mental Disorders (4th edition). American Psychiatric Association, Washington, DC, 1993.
41. McKhann G, Drachman D, Foilstein M, Katzman R, Price D, Stadlan E. Clinical diagnosis of Alzheimer's disease: report of the NINCDS-ADRDA Work group. Neurology. 1984; 34: 939–44.
42. McKhann, GM, Knopman, DS, Chertkow, H et al. The diagnosis of dementia due to Alzheimer's disease: recommendations from the National Institute on Aging-Alzheimer's Association workgroups on diagnostic guidelines for Alzheimer's disease. Alzheimer's Dement. 2011; 7: 263–9.
43. Dubois, B, Feldman, HH, Jacova, C et al. Revising the definition of Alzheimer's disease: a new lexicon. Lancet Neurology. 2010; 9: 1118–27.
44. Gorno-Tempini, ML, Hillis, AE, Weintraub, S et al. Classification of primary progressive aphasia and its variants. Neurology. 2011; 76: 1006–14.
45. Crutch, SJ, Schott, JM, Rabinovici, GD et al. Shining a light on posterior cortical atrophy. Alzheimer's Dement. 2013; 9: 463–5.
46. Ossenkoppele, R, Pijnenburg, YA, Perry, DC et al. The behavioural/dysexecutive variant of Alzheimer's disease: clinical, neuroimaging and pathological features. Brain. 2015; 138: 2732–49.

47. Koedam, EL, Lauffer, V, van der Vlies, AE, van der Flier, WM, Scheltens, P, Pijnenburg, YA. Early-versus late-onset Alzheimer's disease: more than age alone. J Alzheimer's Dis. 2010; 19: 1401–8.
48. Panegyres PK, Chen HY and the Coalition against Major Diseases (CAMD). Early-onset Alzheimer's disease: a global cross-sectional Analysis. Eur J Neurol. 2014; 21: 1149–54.
49. Strittmatter WJ, Roses AD. Apolipoprotein E and Alzheimer disease. Proc Natl Acad Sci USA. 1995; 92: 4725–7.
50. Blacker D, Haines JL, Rodes L, et al. ApoE-4 and age at onset of Alzheimer's disease: the NIMH genetics initiative. Neurology. 1997; 48: 139–47.
51. Meyer MR, Tschanz JT, Norton MC, et al. APOE genotype predicts when–not whether–one is predisposed to develop Alzheimer disease. Nat Genet. 1998; 19: 321–2.
52. Van Duijn Cm, de Knijff P, Cruts M, Wehnert A, Havekes LM, Hofman A, et al. Apolipoprotein E4 allele in a population-based study of early-onset Alzheimer's disease. Nat Genet. 1994; 1: 74–8.
53. Snowden JS, Stopford CL, Julien CL, et al. Cognitive phenotypes in Alzheimer's disease and genetic risk. Cortex. 2007; 43: 835–45.
54. Schott JM, Ridha BH, Crutch SJ, et al. Apolipoprotein E genotype modifies the phenotype of Alzheimer disease Arch Neurol. 2006; 63: 155–6.
55. van der Vlies AE, Koedam EL, Pijnenburg YA, Twisk JW, Scheltens P, van der Flier WM. Most rapid cognitive decline in APOE ε4 negative Alzheimer's disease with early onset. Psychol Med. 2009; 39: 1907–11.
56. Pievani M, Rasser PE, Galluzzi S, et al. Mapping the effect of APOEε4 on gray matter loss in Alzheimer's disease in vivo. Neuroimage. 2009; 45: 1090–8.
57. Gutierrez-Galve L, Lehmann M, Hobbs NZ, et al. Patterns of cortical thickness according to APOE genotype in Alzheimer's disease. Dement Geriatr Cogn Disord. 2009; 28: 476–85.
58. Hirono N, Hashimoto M, Yasuda M, et al. The effect of APOE ε4 allele on cerebral glucose metabolism in AD is a function of age at onset. Neurology. 2002; 58: 743–50.
59. Koedam EL, Pijnenburg YA, Deeg DJ, Baak MM, van der Vlies AE, Scheltens P, van der Flier WM. Early onset dementia is associated with higher mortality. Dement Geriatr Cogn Disord. 2008; 26: 147–52.
60. Chang JK, Hong CH, Lee Ks et al. Mortality risk after diagnosis of early-onset Alzheimer's disease versus late onset Alzheimer's disease: A propensity score matching analysis. J Alz Disease. 2017; 56: 1341–8.
61. Rocca WA, Bonaiuto S, Lippi A, et al. Prevalence of clinically diagnosed Alzheimer's disease and other dementing disorders: a door-to-door survey in Appignano, Macerata Province, Italy. Neurology. 1990; 40: 626–31.

10

Huntington's disease

Juliana R Dutra, Tanya P Garcia, and Karen Marder

Introduction

Huntington's disease (HD) is a progressive neurodegenerative disorder, inherited in an autosomal dominant fashion with typical onset during adult life. It is caused by an expansion in the cytosine adenine guanine (CAG) trinucleotide repeat in exon 1 of the huntingtin (HTT) gene on chromosome 4p16.3, which encodes the huntingtin protein. CAG repeat length is inversely correlated with age of onset of HD, which is defined clinically by extrapyramidal signs. Individuals with 40 or more repeats will develop HD if they live a normal life span. Individuals with 36 to 39 CAG repeats have reduced penetrance and generally late onset. The onset is gradual over many years, beginning with a pre-manifest phase during which a triad of symptoms begin to emerge: extrapyramidal movements, cognitive impairment, and behavioural changes. The clinical diagnosis of manifest HD occurs when the emergence of specific extrapyramidal signs occurs.

Among the neurodegenerative disorders, HD is unique in that the genetic cause is primarily a single gene disorder, it is autosomal dominant and fully penetrant, and the age at onset can be predicted. These unique features of HD have facilitated the design of longitudinal observational studies. The multicentre studies have analysed individuals at risk (known mutation in first-degree relative), and individuals with pre-manifest and manifest HD. Clinical data is based on the Unified Huntington's Disease Rating Scale (UHDRS) and biological data (DNA, blood and cerebrospinal fluid analysis, and neuroimaging). The results of these observational studies are leading to better understanding of the natural history of the disease, identifying potential biomarkers, and facilitating the design of new clinical trials with possible disease modifying agents.

Definition

Evaluation of disease onset

HD is associated with motor signs, including chorea, dystonia, bradykinaesia, and oculomotor impairments. The specificity of the extrapyramidal signs has led to the current definition of motor diagnosis: the time when a rater believes with ≥99% confidence that a subject's extrapyramidal signs are unequivocally associated with HD.[1] The confidence in the clinical diagnosis is expressed through the diagnostic confidence level (DCL) on the UHDRS. The DCL is a five-category ordinal rating scale from 0 to 4 where 0 denotes no motor abnormalities and 4 denotes unequivocal >99% confidence of diagnosis of HD.

For the past 20 years, the UHDRS exam and DCL scoring have been the primary measures for assessing HD onset. However, recent work has emerged promoting re-evaluations of the assessment criteria. The primary reason for this re-evaluation stems from the fact that the DCL score focuses solely on the motor aspect of HD, whereas the disease also encompasses cognitive and psychiatric impairments.

One potential refinement of the HD onset criteria is based on a pure cognitive assessment.[2] Cognitive impairments are known to emerge 10–15 years before a motor diagnosis[3] and cognitive decline has been a marker of disease progression. In a three-year longitudinal study of cognitive variables based on the PREDICT-HD study, Paulsen and Long[2] showed that the rate of change for the Trail Making Test and Symbol Digit Modalities Test differed significantly between carriers of expanded CAG repeats and controls, all of whom showed no detectable signs of motor abnormalities. The worsening cognitive performance of these cases over time suggests that cognitive onset may precede motor onset. A purely cognitive definition for HD onset could provide an earlier time point for intervention.

A diagnosis based solely on motor or solely on cognitive impairment, however, still does not capture the multi-level complexities of HD. A more holistic criterion is, for example, the multidimensional definition proposed by Biglan et al.:[4] clinicians evaluate HD diagnosis using motor as well as cognitive, behavioural, and functional components. Comparing the multidimensional criteria for HD diagnosis with the previous standard led to a larger proportion of patients receiving an earlier diagnosis.

Reilmann et al.[5] also favour a more holistic approach for HD diagnosis. They suggest that clinicians assess HD diagnoses using multiple aspects of the UHDRS—motor, cognitive, behavioural and functional exams—and all available medical history including whether or not the subject is genetically confirmed (i.e. subject has ≥36 CAG repeats). These 'natural history criteria' for diagnosis proposed by Reilman et al. better account for a patient's individual experience with HD (e.g. symptoms, genetic, and family history), and thus has the power to detect disease progression earlier.

Results from recent longitudinal studies further support the push towards a multidimensional assessment for HD diagnosis. Using 12 years of data from over a thousand subjects in PREDICT-HD, Long et al.[6] showed that including 34 variables from motor, imaging, cognitive, functional, psychiatric, and demographic measures increased the ability to predict age at onset better than a model that predicts age at onset using only CAG repeats and age. The results imply that a better understanding of a subject's disease progression can be learned from simultaneously accounting for the multiple impairments, not just one-dimensional aspects. Similar results have been seen in HD imaging studies[7] that simultaneously analyse multiple brain regions compared to individual assessments. Garcia and Müller showed that analysis of multiple brain regions can more accurately identify those regions that influence age of motor onset than univariate analysis because the former better captures the data complexity (e.g. correlations between brain regions).[7]

Practical issues in assessing HD onset

Despite evidence that supports multilevel criteria for evaluating HD diagnosis, there are three key practical limitations. First, assessments of the multiple HD impairments (motor, cognitive, behavioural, functional) should, in theory, be evaluated by the same rater at each visit to minimize rater variability. For example, Biglan et al.[4] showed that if the same rater assessed subjects using two different criteria (e.g. multidimensional motor diagnosis and standard motor-based diagnosis), then the rater would generally (89.8%) report the same age at diagnosis under both criteria. If different raters used the two different criteria, then each rater would generally report a different age at diagnosis under each criterion. Therefore, to minimize discrepancies when different raters are used, uniformity in rater training is essential, which is achieved through annual training modules (e.g. European HD Network).

A second practical limitation is collecting variables that demand large resources (e.g. imaging which requires MRI and quantitative motor testing that requires instrumentation). Not all clinical studies can feasibly and/or economically collect such data, although imaging data and quantitative motor testing have been shown to improve predictions of age at motor onset.

A third limitation is the limited frequency of patient assessments (observational studies tend to have fewer visits than clinical trials). More frequent visits would allow raters to detect impairments sooner, but increasing the number of visits incurs economical and time burdens on patients and their families.[8] Instead, the modern development of sensors, microelectronics, and telecommunications now provide inexpensive, wearable systems to track HD impairments more frequently, even at the convenience of a patient's home setting[8,9] and the possibility of having all assessments by the same rater(s). Wearable systems have allowed tracking gait,[8] UHDRS motor exam components except for rigidity and balance,[9] and cognition via the Montreal Cognitive Assessment,[10] which consists of visual and verbal assessments to detect MCI. While these studies have demonstrated the feasibility of wearable systems and telemedicine in detecting HD impairments, more studies are needed with larger patient cohorts (studies mentioned had sample sizes under 20) and longer study duration to more accurately determine the reliability and validity of these virtual assessments. In addition, these virtual assessments of patients do require adequate technology (e.g. reasonable Internet connection speed, sound, and lighting) for accurate assessment.

Disease Progression

The UHDRS is a clinical rating scale that assesses four different domains: motor performance, cognitive function, behavioural abnormalities, and functional capacity.[1] It is largely used in longitudinal observational studies as a way to define disease onset and to measure disease progression.

Motor

The motor component of the UHDRS consists of 31 questions, rated from 0 to 4 points, with 4 indicating the most severe impairment. The motor items are distributed among oculomotor function, chorea, dystonia, bradykinesia, and rigidity. The sum of all 31 items is referred as to total motor score (TMS), which is an important measure in many HD studies.

Observational studies have shown increasing motor impairments as HD progresses. In COHORT[11] and TRACK-HD[12] individuals with manifest HD had a significant motor performance decline when compared to controls over 36 months, and an annual increase in the TMS of approximately 3.0 points per year. Chorea and dystonia also tend to increase over time; however, the rate of increase of chorea substantially slows in individuals with advanced HD.[11]

Cognitive

The cognitive assessment of the UHDRS is composed of three tests: verbal fluency, Symbol Digit Modalities Test, and Stroop test.[1]

Like motor impairments, cognitive impairments also increase as HD progresses, with cognitive impairments tending to appear before motor impairments.[3] In the COHORT study, Dorsey et al.[11] analysed 333 clinically diagnosed HD individuals and 142 controls. The mean Mini Mental State Examination (MMSE) scores, and the mean verbal fluency scores, decreased by 0.7 point per year (SE = 0.07 and 0.16 respectively). The mean Symbol Digit Modality test scores decreased by 1.5 points per year (SE = 0.13). Colour naming scores, on the Stroop test decreased by 1.8 points per year (SE = 0.19), word reading scores declined by 3.1 points per year (SE = 0.25), and interference scores declined by 1.3 points per year (SE = 0.16). All these changes were significantly greater than the changes observed among controls ($P < 0.001$). In addition, 58 individuals with early HD who reported no functional impairment (Total Functional Capacity score of 13 (range 0–13)) scored an average 1 point worse on the MMSE, and 10–20% worse on the verbal fluency, Symbol Digit and Stroop test when compared to 142 controls. Similarly, in the TRACK-HD study,[12] cognitive measures showed a decline over a 36-month analysis in HD participants.

Behaviour

The behavioural component of the UHDRS consists of 28 items assessing frequency and severity of mood, anxiety, aggression, psychosis, and other behavioural abnormalities.[1] The behavioural impairment may not worsen as uniformly as motor and cognitive impairments. The progression of behavioural changes is more challenging to assess. Participants with less severe behavioural symptoms tend to participate in longitudinal observational studies, which might create a selection bias. As a result, a modest worsening[11] and no significant difference[12] in behaviour measures between HD and controls over 36 months are reported. Most importantly behavioural data such as depression may be self-limited, or may respond to treatment.

Functional capacity

The functional section of the UHDRS has three sub-items. One of them is the Total Functional Capacity Scale (TFC), which is a 14-unit scale (0–13) with higher scores indicating higher function. The annual rate of decline in TFC is an important outcome measure in HD clinical trials, and it ranges between 0.4 to 1.4 points among different studies.[1,11–18] The higher TFC decline of 1.4 was found in an HD study conducted in Venezuela[18] and it might be explained by the younger age of this population, relative inaccessibility to healthcare, and comorbid disorders.[11] The TFC was designed to capture early disability in people with HD, and individuals with longer disease duration or those who have a lower TFC at baseline, present less rapid annual rate of TFC decline, probably reflecting a floor effect.[15] Functional scales are being developed for people with pre-manifest HD, to capture subtle changes in their instrumental activities of daily life.

Pre-manifest HD

Understanding that changes in HD begin many years prior to the conventional definition of disease onset (DCL = 4), makes the pre-manifest phase a target for early intervention in future clinical trials. To understand changes in the pre-manifest stage, well-designed, longitudinal observational studies have been conducted, including PREDICT-HD,[19] TRACK-HD,[20] and PHAROS.[21]

The PREDICT-HD study examined 1013 pre-manifest HD and 301 controls between 2001 and 2012, and observed significant differences on motor, cognitive, psychiatric, and functional domains.[22] The participants were separated into three groups, based on an estimation of disease burden and the probability of motor onset. Individuals with less disease burden, and >12.78 years from estimated diagnosis did not show significant changes in TMS and TFC compared to controls. However, they demonstrated lower scores on four cognitive measures (Symbol Digit Modality Test, Stroop-word, University of Pennsylvania Smell Identification Test, and Trail Making Test) and one psychiatric measure (Frontal System Behavioral Scale) over time. Participants with higher disease burden, and who were <7.59 years from estimated diagnosis had significant changes in TMS, all cognitive measures, TFC, and eight of nine psychiatric variables. The result suggests that progression is faster in individuals closer to disease onset. The discrepancy in profile between individuals with different estimated HD onset was also reported in participants in TRACK-HD.[12] The results from TRACK-HD showed a progressive worsening on motor and cognitive measures, and increased apathy over 36 months in individuals who were fewer than 10.8 years from predicted HD onset, when compared to controls. This contrasted with little evidence of decline in individuals who were at least 10.8 years or more from predicted disease onset.

The presence of MCI was reported in participants with pre-manifest HD from PREDICT-HD study.[23] MCI is defined as at least one cognitive domain fall 1.5 or more standard deviations below the comparison group. Analysing 575 pre-HD individuals and 160 controls, Duff et al. found that almost 40% of pre-HD participants met the criteria for MCI. The majority (18.4%) presented as non-amnestic MCI. Within both amnestic and non-amnestic subtypes, single-domain MCI was more common than multiple-domain (26% and 13.9% respectively). Within all pre-manifest HD participants, the most common impairment was in processing speed followed by episodic memory and visuospatial processing.

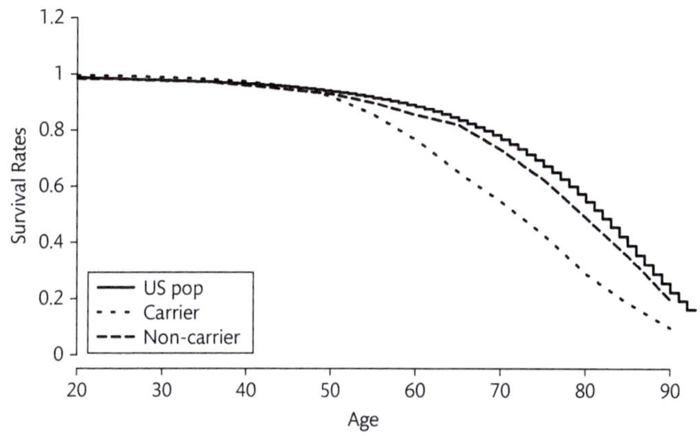

Fig. 10.1 Probability of survival for carriers and noncarriers of the Huntington disease gene mutation. Survival probabilities are compared with the general US Population.

Mortality

The progressive decline from disease onset to death is typically 15–25 years.[24,25] A higher risk of death was associated with increased CAG length (HR 1.09 for 1-point triplet repeat, p = 0.002) and age of onset (HR 1.05 for 1-point year increase, p = 0.022) in a retrospective HD study composed of 135 Italian individuals with manifest HD. The relationship between older age of onset and shorter disease duration may be partially explained by a shorter life expectancy in older individuals.[25] Pneumonia and heart failure are the most frequent causes of death.[24,25]

Fig. 10.1 displays the probability of survival as a function of age for individuals that are carriers of the gene mutation and those who are not (non-carriers). Observe that the probability of survival for non-carriers closely approximates the survival probabilities for the general US population, whereas the probability of survival for carriers of the gene mutation decreases faster after age 40.

Genetics

The Venezuelan kindred constituted a remarkable effort, that started in 1979, to document clinical and genetic data based on the world's largest genetically related HD community. It involved ten generations and 18,149 individuals, with 956 participants presenting fully penetrant HD.[26] Data analysis from this study was responsible for localizing the HD gene on chromosome 4 (4p16.3).[27] Ten years after the HD gene was mapped, haplotype analysis of linkage disequilibrium was performed on a segment of the short arm of chromosome 4, with the discovery of an expanded, unstable CAG trinucleotide repeat.[28]

CAG repeat length

A CAG repeat length of ≤26 is normal. Repeats between 27 and 35 are considered intermediate allele (IA), representing 1.5–5.8% of cases in the general population and HD families.[29] The presence of 36–39 repeats confers reduced penetrance, and a later disease onset.[30] In a population-based study composed of 7315 participants from the USA, British Columbia, and Scotland, 15 individuals presented a CAG repeat length in the reduced penetrance range, representing a frequency of 0.205% individuals.[31] The estimation of disease penetrance is 63.9% (55.5–73.2%) for age 65 and 74.2% (64.2–84.2%) for age 75 based on analyses of 176 individuals with CAG length between 36 and 39 (95% confidence interval).[32] Individuals with ≥40 CAG repeats will invariably develop HD (fully penetrant range) if they live a normal lifespan.

Carriers of intermediate allele (IA) (CAG repeat size between 27 and 35 repeats) may be subject to meiotic instability leading to expansion of the CAG repeat into the disease range in the next generation.[33–35] Studies have found a 'new' mutation rate of 10% or greater, more common than initially thought.[36,37] New mutation cases tend to occur during paternal IA transmission, and although its mechanisms are still unclear, the increased number of cell divisions in male gametogenesis may play a role. However, a new mutation following maternal transmission of an IA has also been reported.[34] What remains unclear is whether carrying an IA is associated with phenotypic changes in later life. A study based on data from an observational study of individuals at risk for HD (PHAROS) showed that individuals with IA presented more behavioural symptoms, especially apathy and suicidal ideation, when compared to controls at baseline and after four years of follow-up.[33] However, another longitudinal observational study,[35] did not find an association between IA and behavioural changes. They reported that mild chorea was more common in older individuals with IA when compared to older controls. However, age was the most important factor contributing to motor change. In addition to the clinical manifestations, there is also a report of functional imaging abnormalities[38] and neuropathological evidence of HD within the IA range.[39]

CAG repeat length and disease onset

Age of onset is inversely correlated with the CAG repeat length. The greater the CAG repeat length, the younger the age of onset. The usual age of onset is between 21 and 50 years old, with a mean CAG repeat of 45.72. Late onset occurs after 50 years old, with a mean repeat length of 41.85.[26] CAG repeat length determines approximately 60% of the variation in age at onset with other genetic and environmental factors accounting for the remaining variance.[26]

A juvenile form of HD is defined by age at onset ≤20 years old, and a mean CAG repeat length of 60.15.[26] This form is more commonly inherited through the paternal lineage, which is more prone to expansion of the CAG repeat size, leading to anticipation in the next generation.[40] It is characterized by the presence of tremor, bradykinesia, and dystonia, rather than chorea, which is commonly seen in non-juvenile HD. In addition, cerebellar signs, epilepsy, myoclonus, and spasticity can also occur. Juvenile HD is rare, with an incidence of 0.70 per million patient-year, and a prevalence of 6.77/million according to a population-based study performed in the UK from 1999 to 2010.[41]

CAG repeat length and disease progression

In studying the effect of CAG repeat length on HD progression, early studies either did not detect an association[42,43] or revealed a modest one.[44,45] More recent findings show some contradictory findings regarding the effect of CAG expansion on HD progression, but some contradictions have been remedied after the statistical analysis has been corrected. The contradictions and corrections are discussed next.

In regards to neurodegeneration, CAG repeat length has been shown to be significantly correlated with changes in the basal ganglia,[46] striatal atrophy rate, and volume,[47] but not with cortical and subcortical cross-sectional areas.[48] In a one-year longitudinal study of regional grey matter loss, Ruocco et al.[48] found that patients with at least 55 CAG repeats had faster rates of atrophy, particularly in the frontal and cerebellar areas. While these findings have implications in monitoring disease-modifying therapies, more longitudinal prospective studies are needed.

In regards to clinical progression, several studies have evaluated the impact of CAG repeat length on clinical measures assessed with the UHDRS. Overall, CAG repeat length accounts for at most 6% of the variability in clinical progression, although it does have statistically significant impact on several motor, cognitive, and functional measures, but not behavioural.[14]

No significant association has been found with functional capacity either measured via TFC scale[17,49] or activities of daily living.[45] A significant correlation between CAG repeats and functional capacity exists, however, under the inclusion of two extreme cases: individuals with over 90 CAG repeats who had onset before ten years.[49] In this case, having the number of CAG repeats at the upper edge of the pathological range naturally led to an aggressive form of HD which had a sharp impact on functional capacity.

In a prospective study on over 20 years of clinical data, Rosenblatt et al.[45] demonstrated that CAG repeat length has a statistically significant, but small effect on the progression rates of neurological signs, motor impairment (except chorea), cognition, and daily function. Effect sizes of CAG repeats on these progression rates was at most 0.25. The prospective, 30-month clinical treatment study by Ravina et al.[14] found similar significant associations, but the effect was stronger after controlling for age at the time of assessment (a confounding factor). In fact, in a re-analysis of similar data that adjusted for the confounding factor of age at onset, Rosenblatt et al.[50] found that the correlation between CAG repeat length and progression of UHDRS clinical variables at least doubled.

These results suggest that modest or undetectable associations between CAG repeat length and disease progression may be from methodological differences in testing for associations. Particularly, adjusting for confounding factors such as age at assessment[14] or age at onset[50] can meaningfully impact study conclusions. Some studies have adjusted for disease duration[44,45,48] to meaningfully capture the effect of CAG repeat length on HD progression, but disease duration is an estimated quantity that depends on a subject reporting the symptoms and thus leads to high variability. Therefore, future studies assessing the effects of CAG repeat length on HD progression should be careful to adjust for confounding factors.

Predicting HD motor onset using family history data

In some clinical studies of HD, the genetic mutation status of an individual is not known because of high costs or practical limitations (e.g. a family member is deceased). Instead, family history information collected through so-called kin-cohort studies can still help to inform HD onset.

Kin-cohort studies involve a sample of (usually diseased) subjects referred to as probands that are genotyped. Disease history and age at onset in the probands' first-degree relatives are obtained through validated interviews.[51] The relatives' genotype information, however, is not collected because of practical considerations (e.g. high costs). Instead, the probability that the relative has the genetic mutation is computed under the assumption of Mendelian transmission using information about the relative's relationship to the proband and the proband's mutation status.[52] The relatives' ages at onset and probability of having the genetic mutation are used to estimate the likeliness of onset occurring via survival models. Information from the probands can also be utilized, but this may lead to ascertainment bias: when the mutation carrier probands are not a representative sample of the population of HD mutation carriers. Ascertainment bias is difficult to adjust,[53] and easily avoided by excluding the probands from the analysis.

One area of kin-cohort research is estimating the probability of onset by a certain age without making any assumptions about the exact probability form. In the statistics literature, this type of estimator is known as 'non-parametric' and it allows flexibility and avoids errors from misspecifying the model.

Wang et al.,[54] Qin et al.,[55] and Ma and Wang[56] developed a family of flexible non-parametric estimators for kin-cohort data that provide clinically meaningful estimates of the cumulative risk of onset. Within the family of estimators, the so-called weighted least squares estimator[56] is easiest to compute and has the smallest variability (i.e. confidence bands of the estimated probability of onset are narrowest). The developed models for cumulative risk of onset have key benefits to clinical studies of HD. The models serve as time-dependent positive and negative predictive values of the HD mutation test[57] and provide a numerical summary of cumulative risk by a certain age associated with a positive mutation test. These modeling aspects are particularly helpful for predicting the risk of developing HD in the next k-years (i.e. five years) given the subject's current age.

A current limitation of the non-parametric models is that they do not directly include patient covariate information. Chen et al.[58] and Ma and Wang[59] remedied this by the well-used Langbehn et al. model[60] for predicting age of motor onset for kin-cohort data. Both models incorporate the CAG repeat information from the family members into the subject specific information by assuming that a relative inherits the same CAG repeat length as his/her proband, if the proband has the gene mutation. Although such an assumption oversimplifies the gamete transmission process, the models can be adapted to a more realistic process such as modelling that transmission from fathers may result in an increased CAG repeat length compared to transmission from mothers.

Under this simplified assumption of inherited CAG repeat length, Chen et al.[58] and Ma and Wang[59] predict age of motor onset using information from first-degree relatives. Both models lead to lower estimates of penetrance than when using probands alone. A potential reason for this difference is that the proband data may consist of a biased clinical sample of pre-manifest expanded CAG repeat or diagnosed subjects. Probands with more severe disease or with earlier age at onset may be more likely to participate. Pre-manifest probands might be undersampled and therefore may not be a fair representative sample of the entire HD population, especially under-representing subjects at risk. The family data may also be a better representative of the population since the family members are included in the analysis only through the inclusion of the probands, not their own HD disease status.

Descriptive Epidemiology

Incidence

The incidence of HD appears to be higher in Europe, North America, and Australia than in Asia. It has not been examined in Africa. A meta-analysis evaluated the incidence of HD in eight studies based on retrospective records in different geographic regions from 1985 to 2010, including two studies from North America, two from Asia, one from Australia, and three from Europe.[61] The mean incidence was 0.38 per 100,000 per year (95% CI: 0.16–0.94; $p < 0.0001$). The incidence of HD in Asia ranged from 0.046 to 0.16 per 100,000 per year. In contrast, the incidence was higher in Europe, North America, and Australia, ranging from 0.11 to 0.8 per 100,000 per year. The incidence did not change over time, based on one study from Taiwan[62] and one from Australia.[63]

Prevalence

Prevalence estimations of HD suggest more than a ten-fold difference among regions. A low prevalence of 0.40 per 100,000 is reported in Asia (Hong Kong, Japan, South Korea, and Taiwan). This contrasts with a prevalence of 7.33 per 100,000 in North America, 6.68 per 100,000 in the UK, 3.60 per 100,000 in Western Europe, and 5.63 per 100,000 in Australia.[64] Interestingly, the lower prevalence in Asians compared to Caucasians is also seen among UK migrants from the Indian subcontinent (1.35, 95% CI 0.79–2.16 per 100,000) when compared to the UK population.[65]

In South Africa, similar prevalence was reported for Caucasians (2.22 per 100,000) and mixed race subpopulations (2.17 per 100,000), although a lower prevalence was estimated for the black African subpopulation (0.01 per 100,000).[66] The low prevalence of HD among black Africans from South Africa differs from a higher prevalence among blacks from North America (6.37 per 100,000), which may be partially explained by mixed race ancestry among African Americans.[67]

Trend

Rawlins et al.[64] reported a trend of 15–20% increase per decade in HD prevalence in Australia (between 1954 and 1996), North America (between 1950 and 2012), UK (between 1950 and 2010), and Western Europe (between 1930 and 2007). There was no evidence of a significant increase in prevalence in Asia or Central and Eastern Europe. The availability of genetic testing and increased awareness of HD by physicians might have led to an increase in diagnosis. In addition, the overall increase in life expectancy and the availability of symptomatic medications for HD may have resulted in an increase in survival. It could also represent an increase in mutation rates, and consequently an increase in incidence. However, a study performed in the UK suggests that the incidence did not change between 1990 and 2010.[68]

Biological explanations

There are some possible explanations for the difference in prevalence between populations. The HD mutation is believed to have originated in Western Europe and then spread to other regions, primarily North America and Australia, with emigration.[69]

The CAG repeat length on the normal chromosome in individuals of European descent has a mean size of 18.4 ± 3.7, while

African, Chinese, and Japanese populations have a significantly smaller repeat size (16.2 ± 2.5, 16.4 ± 1.5, and 16.6 ± 1.3, respectively). This suggests that the normal chromosome in Europeans is more likely to be unstable, for example generating an IA, which is an allele with 27–35 repeats, that can eventually expand into the size range that causes HD.[69]

The presence of different haplogroups within the HTT might be responsible for instability.[70] Three haplogroups were identified in the HTT region, A, B, and C. In individuals of European descent, HD chromosomes are almost exclusively (95%) haplogroup A. In contrast, haplogroup A accounts for only 53% of chromosomes in individuals carrying a CAG repeat length <27. Haplogroup C was also common on normal chromosomes (41%) and completely absent in HD chromosomes. In the general population (<27 CAG), 62% of individuals with high normal CAG repeats (mean CAG = 19.8 ± 2.7) have a tendency to carry the haplogroup A, whereas 43% of individuals with low normal range (mean CAG = 17.3 ± 2.1) carry haplogroup A. Analysing variants of haplogroup A, it was found that A1 and A2 variants confer the highest risk of expanded CAG repeat, while A4 and A5 are protective. Chinese and Japanese general populations lack variants A1 and A2 and have a high frequency of A5, and up to 20% of European population have A1 and A2 variants.[70]

The CCG polymorphic region adjacent to the CAG repeat in HTT might also be related to the difference observed between the prevalence of HD in Asian and non-Asian populations. Individuals with HD of Caucasian descent have a strong association between the expanded CAG allele and the adjacent CCG size of seven, being present in 67.8% of wild-type (WT) HTT and 94.4% of mutant-type (MT). However, in individuals of Chinese and Japanese descent there is an increased frequency of CCG allele with ten repeats on the affected chromosome, and no significant association between CAG and CCG length.[69] This suggests that HD mutations in Asian versus Caucasians may have arisen from different ancestral lineages.[61]

Disease Modifiers

Genetic modifiers of age at onset

Although the CAG repeat length is the major factor associated with disease onset, there is still variability between individuals within the same family and even among individuals with the same number of repeats.[26] Supporting this idea, reports of identical twins with the HD mutation show a discordance in age at disease onset.[71,72] Previous studies analysed potential genetic modifiers that could account for this discrepancy. The length of the normal CAG repeats in heterozygotes did not show association with 'residual age of onset'. In addition, being homozygous for the HD mutation, had no significant effect. Common genetic variation at the HTT haplotype also did not modify the disease onset.[73]

A genome-wide association (GWA) analysis composed of 2131 subjects with 40–53 CAG repeats, and European ancestry, identified potential loci on chromosome 15, that could accelerate or delay the onset of the disease by 6.1 years and 1.4 years, respectively; and on chromosome 8 that could accelerate disease onset by 1.6 years.[73] This suggests that by including large numbers of participants, variants that modify age at onset may be discovered.

Environmental modifiers of age at onset

The variability in age of onset not explained by CAG repeat length, or other genetic factors, is attributed to unidentified environmental factors.[26] The contribution of lifestyle factors as potential modulators of neurodegeneration in HD still requires further investigation, leading to formal recommendations to delay age of onset in pre-symptomatic individuals.[74]

Cognitive stimulation

Analysing retrospectively the role of cognitive stimulation in a European cohort of HD patients (n = 891), López-Sendón et al.[75] reported that more years of education was associated with an earlier age at HD onset. However, the authors suggested that this finding might be related to increased awareness of symptoms among more educated HD individuals, which may anticipate their diagnosis. A smaller study with a more extensive analysis of intellectual scores, based on leisure activities, formal education, occupation, and domestic duties did not show any association between cognitive stimulation and age of onset.[76] Based on the PHAROS cohort of individuals followed prospectively, there was no association between reported cognitive enrichment and age at onset.[77]

Physical activity

Increase in levels of physical activity was not associated with phenoconversion in 154 HD individuals. However, the presence of a passive lifestyle (i.e. activities that require little or no initiative, or lacking in physical or intellectual challenge) was associated with earlier age of onset.[76] In the PHAROS study, there was no correlation between physical activity and age at onset.[77]

Diet

Dietary intake was evaluated by Marder et al. based on PHAROS participants.[78,79] In pre-symptomatic individuals (CAG ≥ 37) a higher caloric intake, but not body mass index (BMI), was associated with a higher repeat length and a higher probability of HD onset occurring in the next five years. It was suggested that an increased caloric intake may be necessary to maintain BMI in pre-symptomatic individuals, given the increased energy expenditure due to subtle motor changes or a hypermetabolic state.[78] The same group reported that a diet with high levels of dairy products was associated with a two-fold increased risk of phenoconversion. This finding could be secondary to a lower urate levels, which is associated with a faster progression in manifest HD.[79] Lifestyle factors were analysed in 737 participants from PHAROS. A greater exposure to caffeinated soda, but no other caffeinated beverages, was significantly associated with phenoconversion. Exposure to tobacco, alcohol, non-steroidal anti-inflammatory drugs, corticosteroids, oestrogens (in women), and head injury were not associated with development of HD.[77] The intake of caffeine was also reported in a retrospective French study composed of 80 HD participants. They found that an increased intake of caffeine (greater than 190 mg/day) was associated with an earlier age at onset of up to four years, after controlling for CAG repeat length, gender, and smoking.[80]

Future Directions

Understanding the overall progression of HD is critical to the timing of therapeutic interventions and design of effective clinical trials. Progress in understanding HD development has exploded in the analysis of motor decline,[81,82] cognitive decline,[2,83] and neurodegeneration.[12] These analyses have provided important but one-dimensional views of HD progression. A more holistic approach that considers multiple facets of the disease has the potential to provide a more comprehensive framework to more effectively understand the disease and ultimately identify biomarkers important for disease tracking.[84] In addition, such a holistic framework can better account for data nuances, thus allowing for more precise and less variable parameter estimates (i.e. smaller standard errors). This translates to higher power and smaller sample sizes when designing clinical trials. As statistical methodologies progress in better analysing HD data, it also becomes imperative that such methods become available to scientific researchers in user-friendly formats. A particular need, for example, is a point-and-click software that allows researchers to input a patient's information and compute his/her individual risk for HD motor diagnosis based on estimated trajectories of clinical decline and neurodegeneration. Such a tool would not only be beneficial to HD but can also serve as a starting point for evaluating the risk and pattern of progression for AD and PD which share features with HD.[85]

REFERENCES

1. Unified Huntington's Disease Rating Scale: reliability and consistency. Huntington Study Group. Movement Disorders. 1996; 11(2): 136–42.
2. Paulsen JS, Long JD. Onset of Huntington's disease: Can it be purely cognitive? Movement Disorders. 2014; 29(11): 1342–50.
3. Stout JC, Paulsen JS, Queller S, Solomon AC, Whitlock KB, Campbell JC, et al. Neurocognitive signs in prodromal Huntington disease. Neuropsychology. 2011; 25(1): 1–14.
4. Biglan KM, Zhang Y, Long JD, Geschwind M, Kang GA, Killoran A, et al. Refining the diagnosis of Huntington disease: the PREDICT-HD study. Frontiers in Aging Neuroscience. 2013; 5: 12.
5. Reilmann R, Leavitt BR, Ross CA. Diagnostic criteria for Huntington's disease based on natural history. Movement Disorders. 2014; 29(11): 1335–41.
6. Long JD, Paulsen JS, Investigators P-H, Coordinators of the Huntington Study G. Multivariate prediction of motor diagnosis in Huntington's disease: 12 years of PREDICT-HD. Movement Disorders. 2015; 30(12): 1664–72.
7. Garcia TP, Muller S. Cox regression with exclusion frequency-based weights to identify neuroimaging markers relevant to Huntington's disease onset. Annals of Applied Statistics. 2016.
8. Andrzejewski KL, Dowling AV, Stamler D, Felong TJ, Harris DA, Wong C, et al. Wearable sensors in Huntington disease: a pilot study. Journal of Huntington's Disease. 2016; 5(2): 199–206.
9. Bull MT, Darwin K, Venkataraman V, Wagner J, Beck CA, Dorsey ER, et al. A pilot study of virtual visits in Huntington disease. Journal of Huntington's Disease. 2014; 3(2): 189–95.
10. Abdolahi A, Bull MT, Darwin KC, Venkataraman V, Grana MJ, Dorsey ER, et al. A feasibility study of conducting the Montreal Cognitive Assessment remotely in individuals with movement disorders. Health Informatics Journal. 2016; 22(2): 304–11.
11. Dorsey ER, Beck CA, Darwin K, Nichols P, Brocht AF, Biglan KM, et al. Natural history of Huntington disease. JAMA Neurology. 2013; 70(12): 1520–30.
12. Tabrizi SJ, Scahill RI, Owen G, Durr A, Leavitt BR, Roos RA, et al. Predictors of phenotypic progression and disease onset in premanifest and early-stage Huntington's disease in the TRACK-HD study: analysis of 36-month observational data. Lancet Neurology. 2013; 12(7): 637–49.
13. Meyer C, Landwehrmeyer B, Schwenke C, Doble A, Orth M, Ludolph AC, et al. Rate of change in early Huntington's disease: A clinicometric analysis. Movement Disorders. 2012; 27(1): 118–24.
14. Ravina B, Romer M, Constantinescu R, Biglan K, Brocht A, Kieburtz K, et al. The relationship between CAG repeat length and clinical progression in Huntington's disease. Movement Disorders. 2008; 23(9): 1223–7.
15. Marder K, Zhao H, Myers RH, Cudkowicz M, Kayson E, Kieburtz K, et al. Rate of functional decline in Huntington's disease. Neurology. 2000; 54(2): 452.
16. Bamford KA, Caine ED, Kido DK, Cox C, Shoulson I. A prospective evaluation of cognitive decline in early Huntington's disease: functional and radiographic correlates. Neurology. 1995; 45(10): 1867–73.
17. Feigin A, Kieburtz K, Bordwell K, Como P, Steinberg K, Sotack J, et al. Functional decline in Huntington's disease. Movement Disorders. 1995; 10(2): 211–4.
18. Penney JB, Young AB, Shoulson I, Starosta-Rubenstein S, Snodgrass SR, Sanchez-Ramos J, et al. Huntington's disease in Venezuela: 7 years of follow-up on symptomatic and asymptomatic individuals. Movement Disorders. 1990; 5(2): 93–9.
19. Paulsen JS, Hayden M, Stout JC, et al. Preparing for preventive clinical trials: The PREDICT-HD study. Archives of Neurology. 2006; 63(6): 883–90.
20. Tabrizi SJ, Langbehn DR, Leavitt BR, Roos RAC, Durr A, Craufurd D, et al. Biological and clinical manifestations of Huntington's disease in the longitudinal TRACK-HD study: cross-sectional analysis of baseline data. Lancet Neurology. 2009; 8(9): 791–801.
21. The Huntington Study Group PI. At risk for Huntington disease: The PHAROS (prospective Huntington at risk observational study) cohort enrolled. Archives of Neurology. 2006; 63(7): 991–6.
22. Paulsen JS, Long JD, Johnson HJ, Aylward EH, Ross CA, Williams JK, et al. Clinical and biomarker changes in premanifest Huntington disease show trial feasibility: a decade of the PREDICT-HD Study. Frontiers in Aging Neuroscience. 2014; 6: 78.
23. Duff K, Paulsen J, Mills J, Beglinger LJ, Moser DJ, Smith MM, et al. Mild cognitive impairment in prediagnosed Huntington disease. Neurology. 2010; 75(6): 500–7.
24. Heemskerk AW, Roos RA. Aspiration pneumonia and death in Huntington's disease. PLOS Curr. 2012; 4: RRN1293.
25. Rinaldi C, Salvatore E, Giordano I, De Matteis S, Tucci T, Cinzia VR, et al. Predictors of survival in a Huntington's disease population from Southern Italy. Canadian Journal of Neurological Sciences. 2014; 39(01): 48–51.
26. Wexler NS, Lorimer J, Porter J, Gomez F, Moskowitz C, Shackell E, et al. Venezuelan kindreds reveal that genetic and environmental factors modulate Huntington's disease age of onset.

Proceedings of the National Academy of Sciences of the United States of America. 2004; 101(10): 3498–503.
27. Gusella JF, Wexler NS, Conneally PM, Naylor SL, Anderson MA, Tanzi RE, et al. A polymorphic DNA marker genetically linked to Huntington's disease. Nature. 1983; 306(5940): 234–8.
28. MacDonald ME, Ambrose CM, Duyao MP, Myers RH, Lin C, Srinidhi L, et al. A novel gene containing a trinucleotide repeat that is expanded and unstable on Huntington's disease chromosomes. Cell. 1993; 72(6): 971–83.
29. Semaka A, Kay C, Doty CN, Collins JA, Tam N, Hayden MR. High frequency of intermediate alleles on Huntington disease-associated haplotypes in British Columbia's general population. American Journal of Medical Genetics Part B, Neuropsychiatric Genetics: the official publication of the International Society of Psychiatric Genetics. 2013; 162B(8): 864–71.
30. Panegyres PK, Shu CC, Chen HY, Paulsen JS. Factors influencing the clinical expression of intermediate CAG repeat length mutations of the Huntington's disease gene. Journal of Neurology. 2015; 262(2): 277–84.
31. Kay C, Collins JA, Miedzybrodzka Z, Madore SJ, Gordon ES, Gerry N, et al. Huntington disease reduced penetrance alleles occur at high frequency in the general population. Neurology. 2016; 87(3): 282–8.
32. Quarrell OW, Rigby AS, Barron L, Crow Y, Dalton A, Dennis N, et al. Reduced penetrance alleles for Huntington's disease: a multi-centre direct observational study. Journal of Medical Genetics. 2007; 44(3): e68.
33. Killoran A, Biglan KM, Jankovic J, Eberly S, Kayson E, Oakes D, et al. Characterization of the Huntington intermediate CAG repeat expansion phenotype in PHAROS. Neurology. 2013; 80(22): 2022–7.
34. Semaka A, Kay C, Belfroid RD, Bijlsma EK, Losekoot M, van Langen IM, et al. A new mutation for Huntington disease following maternal transmission of an intermediate allele. European Journal of Medical Genetics. 2015; 58(1): 28–30.
35. Cubo E, Ramos-Arroyo MA, Martinez-Horta S, Martinez-Descalls A, Calvo S, Gil-Polo C, et al. Clinical manifestations of intermediate allele carriers in Huntington disease. Neurology. 2016; 87(6): 571–8.
36. Falush D, Almqvist EW, Brinkmann RR, Iwasa Y, Hayden MR. Measurement of mutational flow implies both a high new-mutation rate for Huntington disease and substantial underascertainment of late-onset cases. American Journal of Human Genetics. 2001; 68(2): 373–85.
37. Almqvist EW, Elterman DS, MacLeod PM, Hayden MR. High incidence rate and absent family histories in one quarter of patients newly diagnosed with Huntington disease in British Columbia. Clinical Genetics. 2001; 60(3): 198–205.
38. Squitieri F, Esmaeilzadeh M, Ciarmiello A, Jankovic J. Caudate glucose hypometabolism in a subject carrying an unstable allele of intermediate CAG33 repeat length in the Huntington's disease gene. Movement Disorders. 2011; 26(5): 925–7.
39. Kenney C, Powell S, Jankovic J. Autopsy-proven Huntington's disease with 29 trinucleotide repeats. Movement Disorders. 2007; 22(1): 127–30.
40. Sun Y-M, Zhang Y-B, Wu Z-Y. Huntington's Disease: Relationship Between Phenotype and Genotype. Molecular Neurobiology. 2016: 1–7.
41. Douglas I, Evans S, Rawlins MD, Smeeth L, Tabrizi SJ, Wexler NS. Juvenile Huntington's disease: a population-based study using the General Practice Research Database. BMJ Open. 2013; 3(4).
42. Ashizawa T, Wong LJ, Richards CS, Caskey CT, Jankovic J. CAG repeat size and clinical presentation in Huntington's disease. Neurology. 1994; 44(6): 1137–43.
43. Claes S, Van Zand K, Legius E, et al. Correlations between triplet repeat expansion and clinical features in Huntington's disease. Archives of Neurology. 1995; 52(8): 749–53.
44. Brandt J, Bylsma FW, Gross R, Stine OC, Ranen N, Ross CA. Trinucleotide repeat length and clinical progression in Huntington's disease. Neurology. 1996; 46(2): 527–31.
45. Rosenblatt A, Liang K-Y, Zhou H, Abbott MH, Gourley LM, Margolis RL, et al. The association of CAG repeat length with clinical progression in Huntington disease. Neurology. 2006; 66(7): 1016–20.
46. Aylward EH, Li Q, Stine OC, Ranen N, Sherr M, Barta PE, et al. Longitudinal change in basal ganglia volume in patients with Huntington's disease. Neurology. 1997; 48(2): 394–9.
47. Henley SMD, Wild EJ, Hobbs NZ, Scahill RI, Ridgway GR, MacManus DG, et al. Relationship between CAG repeat length and brain volume in premanifest and early Huntington's disease. Journal of Neurology. 2009; 256(2): 203–12.
48. Ruocco HH, Bonilha L, Li LM, Lopes-Cendes I, Cendes F. Longitudinal analysis of regional grey matter loss in Huntington disease: effects of the length of the expanded CAG repeat. Journal of Neurology, Neurosurgery & Psychiatry. 2008; 79(2): 130–5.
49. Squitieri F, Cannella M, Simonelli M. CAG mutation effect on rate of progression in Huntington's disease. Neurological Sciences. 2002; 23(2): s107–s8.
50. Rosenblatt A, Kumar BV, Mo A, Welsh CS, Margolis RL, Ross CA. Age, CAG repeat length, and clinical progression in Huntington's disease. Movement Disorders. 2012; 27(2): 272–6.
51. Marder K, Levy G, Louis ED, Mejia–Santana H, Cote L, Andrews H, et al. Accuracy of family history data on Parkinson's disease. Neurology. 2003; 61(1): 18–23.
52. Khoury MJ, Beaty TH, Cohen BH. Fundamentals of genetic epidemiology. New York: Oxford University Press, 1993.
53. Begg CB. On the use of familial aggregation in population-based case probands for calculating penetrance. Journal of the National Cancer Institute. 2002; 94(16): 1221–6.
54. Wang Y, Garcia TP, Ma Y. Nonparametric estimation for censored mixture data with application to the Cooperative Huntington's Observational Research Trial. J Am Stat Assoc. 2012; 107(500): 1324–38.
55. Qin J, Garcia TP, Ma Y, Tang MX, Marder K, Wang Y. Combining isotonic regression and EM algorithm to predict genetic risk under monotonicity constraint. Ann Appl Stat. 2014; 8(2): 1182–208.
56. Ma Y, Wang Y. Estimating disease onset distribution functions in mutation carriers with censored mixture data. Journal of the Royal Statistical Society. 2014: 63(1): 1–23.
57. Heagerty PJ, Zheng Y. Survival Model Predictive Accuracy and ROC Curves. Biometrics. 2005; 61(1): 92–105.
58. Chen T, Wang Y, Ma Y, Marder K, Langbehn DR. Predicting disease onset from mutation status using proband and relative data with applications to Huntington's disease. Journal of Probability and Statistics. 2012; 375935.
59. Ma Y, Wang Y. Nonparametric modeling and analysis of association between Huntington's disease onset and CAG repeats. Stat Med. 2014; 33(8): 1369–82.
60. Langbehn DR, Brinkman RR, Falush D, Paulsen JS, Hayden MR, on behalf of an International Huntington's Disease Collaborative G. A new model for prediction of the age of onset

and penetrance for Huntington's disease based on CAG length. Clinical Genetics. 2004; 65(4): 267–77.

61. Pringsheim T, Wiltshire K, Day L, Dykeman J, Steeves T, Jette N. The incidence and prevalence of Huntington's disease: a systematic review and meta-analysis. Movement Disorders. 2012; 27(9): 1083–91.
62. Chen YY, Lai CH. Nationwide population-based epidemiologic study of Huntington's disease in Taiwan. Neuroepidemiology. 2010; 35(4): 250–4.
63. McCusker EA, Casse RF, Graham SJ, Williams DB, Lazarus R. Prevalence of Huntington disease in New South Wales in 1996. Med J Aust. 2000; 173(4): 187–90.
64. Rawlins MD, Wexler NS, Wexler AR, Tabrizi SJ, Douglas I, Evans SJ, et al. The prevalence of Huntington's disease. Neuroepidemiology. 2016; 46(2): 144–53.
65. Shiwach RS, Lindenbaum RH. Prevalence of Huntington's disease among UK immigrants from the Indian subcontinent. British Journal of Psychiatry. 1990; 157(4): 598–99.
66. Hayden MR, MacGregor JM, Beighton PH. The prevalence of Huntington's chorea in South Africa. S Afr Med J. 1980; 58(5): 193–6.
67. Folstein SE, Chase GA, Wahl WE, McDonnell AM, Folstein MF. Huntington disease in Maryland: clinical aspects of racial variation. American Journal of Human Genetics. 1987; 41(2): 168–79.
68. Wexler NS, Collett L, Wexler AR, Rawlins MD, Tabrizi SJ, Douglas I, et al. Incidence of adult Huntington's disease in the UK: a UK-based primary care study and a systematic review. BMJ Open. 2016; 6(2).
69. Squitieri F, Andrew SE, Goldberg YP, Kremer B, Spence N, Zelsler J, et al. DNA haplotype analysis of Huntington disease reveals clues to the origins and mechanisms of CAG expansion and reasons for geographic variations of prevalence. Human Molecular Genetics. 1994; 3(12): 2103–14.
70. Warby SC, Montpetit A, Hayden AR, Carroll JB, Butland SL, Visscher H, et al. CAG expansion in the Huntington disease gene is associated with a specific and targetable predisposing haplogroup. American Journal of Human Genetics. 2009; 84(3): 351–66.
71. Friedman JH, Trieschmann ME, Myers RH, Fernandez HH. Monozygotic twins discordant for Huntington disease after 7 years. Archives of Neurology. 2005; 62(6): 995–7.
72. Panas M, Karadima G, Markianos M, Kalfakis N, Vassilopoulos D. Phenotypic discordance in a pair of monozygotic twins with Huntington's disease. Clinical Genetics. 2008; 74(3): 291–2.
73. Lee J-M, Wheeler Vanessa C, Chao Michael J, Vonsattel Jean Paul G, Pinto Ricardo M, Lucente D, et al. Identification of genetic factors that modify clinical onset of Huntington's disease. Cell. 2015; 162(3): 516–26.
74. Mo C, Hannan AJ, Renoir T. Environmental factors as modulators of neurodegeneration: insights from gene-environment interactions in Huntington's disease. Neuroscience and Biobehavioral Reviews. 2015; 52: 178–92.
75. López-Sendón JL, Royuela A, Trigo P, Orth M, Lange H, Reilmann R, et al. What is the impact of education on Huntington's disease? Movement Disorders. 2011; 26(8): 1489–95.
76. Trembath MK, Horton ZA, Tippett L, Hogg V, Collins VR, Churchyard A, et al. A retrospective study of the impact of lifestyle on age at onset of Huntington disease. Movement Disorders. 2010; 25(10): 1444–50.
77. Tanner C, Marder K, Eberly S, Biglan K, Oakes D, Shoulson I. Selected health and life style factors and time to phenoconversion in Huntington's disease (S47.003). Neurology. 2014; 82(10 Supplement).
78. Marder K, Zhao H, Eberly S, Tanner CM, Oakes D, Shoulson I, et al. Dietary intake in adults at risk for Huntington disease: Analysis of PHAROS Research Participants. Neurology. 2009; 73(5): 385–92.
79. Marder K, Gu Y, Eberly S, Tanner CM, Scarmeas N, Oakes D, et al. Relationship of Mediterranean diet and caloric intake to phenoconversion in Huntington disease. JAMA Neurology. 2013; 70(11): 1382–88.
80. Simonin C, Duru C, Salleron J, Hincker P, Charles P, Delval A, et al. Association between caffeine intake and age at onset in Huntington's disease. Neurobiology of Disease. 2013; 58: 179–82.
81. Long JD, Paulsen JS, Marder K, Zhang Y, Kim J-I, Mills JA, et al. Tracking motor impairments in the progression of Huntington's disease. Movement Disorders. 2014; 29(3): 311–19.
82. Liu D, Long JD, Zhang Y, Raymond LA, Marder K, Rosser A, et al. Motor onset and diagnosis in Huntington disease using the diagnostic confidence level. Journal of Neurology. 2015; 262(12): 2691–8.
83. Paulsen JS, Smith MM, Long JD, investigators tPH, Group cotHS. Cognitive decline in prodromal Huntington disease: implications for clinical trials. Journal of Neurology, Neurosurgery & Psychiatry. 2013; 84(11): 1233–9.
84. Fan J, Han X, Gu W. Estimating false discovery proportion under arbitrary covariance dependence. J Am Stat Assoc. 2012; 107(499): 1019–35.
85. Ross CA, Tabrizi SJ. Huntington's disease: from molecular pathogenesis to clinical treatment. Lancet Neurology. 2011; 10(1): 83–98.

11

Idiopathic Parkinson's disease and classification of parkinsonisms

Valentina Gallo, Honglei Chen, and Neil Pearce

Introduction

Two hundred years after its first description by Dr James Parkinson, Parkinson's disease (PD) diagnosis still heavily relies on clinical symptoms, the same symptoms originally described as comprising the clinical picture of *paralisis agitans* in Parkinson's 'Essay on the Shaking Palsy':

> 'Involuntary tremulous motion, with lessened muscular power, in parts not in action and even when supported; with a propensity to bend the trunk forwards, and to pass from a walking to a running pace: the senses and intellects being uninjured'
>
> (J. Parkinson, 'An Essay on the Shaking Palsy', 1817).

The term 'shaking palsy' emphasized the presence of a tremor that was distinct from those caused by epilepsy, alcoholism, or stroke. Parkinson also noted that the disease came on gradually, beginning in the hands and arms before moving through the rest of the body, and noted the weariness, inconvenience, and anguish it provoked in its victims.[1] Late 19th-century histological studies had linked the disease with changes in the *substantia nigra* of the midbrain, and the aftermath of the encephalitis lethargica epidemics of the 1910s and 1920s confirmed this view.[1] During the early 1960s, researchers began experiments administering small doses of levodopa in patients with post-encephalitic parkinsonism, and in *Awakenings*, published in 1973,[2] Oliver Sacks described the 'unlocking' of such patients at the Beth Abraham Hospital in New York, with larger doses of the drug.

Since 1817, major scientific improvements have enabled better descriptions of the neuropathology and pathophysiology of this condition. However, considerably less success has been achieved in terms of understanding the causes, preventing the disease, or developing curative treatments.

Cardinal Signs

PD is primarily characterized by motor symptoms; these include bradykinesia with rigidity and/or rest tremor, according to the latest diagnostic criteria.[3] Bradykinesia is defined as slowness of movement together with a decrement in amplitude or speed (or progressive hesitations/halts) as movements are continued.[3] Rigidity is assessed on 'slow passive movement of major joints with the patient in a relaxed position and the examiner manipulating the limbs and neck'.[3] Tremor is typically 4–6 Hz amplitude, at rest, but is suppressed during movement initiation.[3]

Nowadays, an increasingly more prominent role is being given to non-motor symptoms of PD; efforts are accordingly being made to produce a re-classification of clinical subtypes.

Neuropathology

The pathological hallmark of PD is the loss of dopaminergic neurons in the substantia nigra pars compacta of the midbrain, accompanied by cytoplasmic and axonal accumulations of α-synuclein, called Lewy bodies.[4,5] However, some heterogeneity (e.g. in some PINK1, Parkins, and LRRK2 mutation carriers nigral neuronal loss is not accompanied by Lewy bodies), suggests that more than one pathway leads to loss of dopaminergic signalling.[6] Moreover, this typical pathology in the basal ganglia is always accompanied by α-synuclein deposits in other areas of the central nervous system, and it is not the first area to show these changes. The Braak hypothesis, based on a cross-sectional study of post-mortem neuropathological examinations, proposes that brain pathology begins in the olfactory nucleus, the medulla oblongata, or even the enteric nervous system (stage 1), and then extends with a caudal-rostral spread through the brain stem (stage 2), and midbrain, including the substantia nigra (stage 3), to the cerebral cortex (stages 4–6).[5,7] Gut-to-brain spread would follow mainly the vagus nerve, and the observation that vagotomy may decrease the risk of PD reinforces this hypothesis.[8,9] This may explain the occurrence of additional clinical signs and symptoms in PD, such as psychiatric disorders (e.g. anxiety, depression, and cognitive impairment), and autonomic dysfunction (e.g. hypotension, urinary and erectile dysfunctions). Moreover, this theory is also coherent with the observation of non-motor symptoms, usually manifesting several years before disease onset, such as gastrointestinal (e.g. constipation,) and olfactory dysfunction.[10]

Diagnosis and Classification of Parkinsonism

Parkinsonism is principally divided into primary and secondary types. While potential causes of secondary parkinsonism should always be investigated and—when possible—treated,[11] primary parkinsonism embraces a number of neurodegenerative disorders of multifactorial origin. The most common type of primary parkinsonism is PD. The group of degenerative disorders commonly labelled as atypical parkinsonism are listed in Box 11.1. The designation 'atypical' mainly refers to the poor levodopa response and the early manifestation of additional clinical features such as ophthalmoparesis, dysautonomia, apraxia, or dementia.[12] Finally, the differential diagnosis of parkinsonism also encompasses a wide range of rare hereditary degenerative disorders that should be taken into account if the clinical presentation is not typical.

The gold standard for the diagnosis of PD is given by the post-mortem examination of the brain. In the last few decades, numerous efforts have been undertaken in order to identify the ideal combination of clinical criteria able to best predict *in vivo* the neuropathological features. To date, the most universally recognized criteria for the diagnosis of PD are from the Parkinson's Disease Society Brain Bank (PDSBB).[13] This is based on the presence of two cardinal symptoms (bradykinesia and at least another one among rigidity, resting tremor, and postural instability), and some exclusion (e.g. treatment with neuroleptic drug) and supportive criteria (e.g. unilateral onset).[14]

Box 11.1 Classification of parkinsonism

Primary parkinsonism

Parkinson's disease

Atypical parkinsonisms

Progressive supranuclear palsy (PSP)
Multiple system atrophy (MSA)
Cortico-basal degeneration
ALS-parkinsonism-dementia (Guam complex)

Secondary parkinsonism

Drugs-induced (antipsychotics, antiemetics, and dopamine-depleting drugs)
Infectious (post-encephalitic)
Toxins (i.e. MTPT)
Vascular
Trauma (i.e. pugilistic encephalopathy)
Brain tumours
Hydrocephalus
Hypoxia
Metabolic

Familial neurodegenerative diseases causing parkinsonism

Huntington chorea
Wilson's disease
Hellevorden-Spatz disease
Familial basal ganglia calcification
Familial parkinsonism with peripheral neuropathy
Neuroacanthocytosis

Source data from Bohlhalter S, Kaegi G. Parkinsonism: heterogeneity of a common neurological syndrome. *Swiss Med Wkly*. 2011; 141: w13293.

The Movement Disorder Society (MDS) Clinical Diagnostic criteria proposed a similar classification as the PDSBB (bradykinesia, rigidity, and/or rest tremor) but excluding postural instability.[3] According to this criteria, after confirmation of parkinsonism, a clinical diagnosis of PD is based on: absolute exclusion criteria (which rule out the disease), red flags (which must be counterbalanced by supportive criteria), and positive supportive criteria. These are combined to determine diagnostic certainty as clinically probable PD, or clinically established PD.[3] Recently, these criteria have been validated in a cohort of PD cases assessed with the PDSBB criteria confirming that over 90% of cases diagnosed according to the PDSBB criteria also fulfilled the MDS criteria.[15]

However, clinico-pathological studies demonstrate that even under optimal conditions, where consensus among neurologists expert in movement disorders is used to reach diagnoses, only 82% of the cases showed nigral degeneration with Lewy body accumulation.[14] This has not improved over the last 25 years, and it is only marginally improved by expertise of the doctors making the diagnosis, being slightly higher when an expert in movement disorder was involved.[16,17] In particular, diagnosis accuracy is problematic in the early phases of the disease, as clinical hallmark of other parkinsonisms may not have emerged.[16] The most frequent misdiagnoses in clinic-based studies reviewed recently were MSA and PSP, while essential tremor was the most frequent in community-based studies.[16] With the increasingly ageing of populations, a possible further challenge for PD diagnosis is the late onset of the disease, as it is when this might manifest as part of mixed neuropathology featuring the co-occurence of more than one neurodegenerative proteinopathy.[16]

None of these sophisticated clinical criteria can be easily applied in epidemiological studies. There is no unanimous consensus on which definition should be used in population-based studies. Depending on the specific study questions and design, sensitivity or specificity of the diagnosis of PD—in particular with regards to other atypical parkinsonisms—is favoured. Ideally, both methods co-exist in the same ascertainment procedure to both maximize power and enable sensitivity analyses.[18] Wherever it is not possible to rely on expert diagnoses, assessing single signs and symptoms might represent the best way to bridge accuracy of assessment and clinical relevance of the nosological classification, also increasing reproducibility.[19]

In Table 11.1, the currently available cohort studies investigating PD in prospective settings are listed alongside their main characteristics. The methods to define PD in these population-based epidemiological investigations varied across studies. In the Rotterdam study, out of 132 subjects with incident parkinsonism identified through intense case ascertainment, only 67 (51%) had PD.[20] In the NeuroEPIC4PD study, out of 881 PD cases identified, a total of 474 (54%) were labelled as definite or very likely according to a matrix combining the amount and quality of data available from the clinical records, and the degree of certainty of the neurologist performing the case ascertainment.[18] According to a record-linkage incidence study in Olmsted County, Minnesota, less than half (154, 42%) of the 364 parkinsonism cases identified in the 15-year period 1976–1990 could be defined as PD using the stricter criteria, 215 using the intermediate criteria (59% of all parkinsonism), and 266

Table 11.1 Cohort studies which have investigated the association between risk factors for Parkinson's disease

Study, place	Age at baseline	Sample size	Incident cases	Case ascertainment	Longest Follow-up	Active update of exposure information	Notes
Atherosclerosis Risk in Communities (ARIC) Study, USA [23–25]	45–64 years	15,792 participants (55% women; 27% African Americans)	106 (73 probable and 33 possible [25])	• Self-reported drug use • Self-reported diagnosis • Hospital records • Death certificates	1987–2010 (23 years)	Yes	Blood samples collected at all clinical visits
Cancer Prevention Study (CPS) –II Nutrition, USA [26–34]	50–79 years	184,190 participants (53% women)	605	• Self-reported • Medical records	1992–2005 (13 years)	Yes (for a portion of participants)	
The Agricultural Health Study (AHS), USA [35–42]	12–92 years	84,739 participants (28% women)	~400	• Self-reported diagnosis • In-person visit using National Institute of Neurological Disorders and Stroke/UK Brain Bank criteria[43]	1993–2015 (22 years)	Yes	Farming and movement evaluation (FAME) designed as a nested case-control study
Finnish cohort study, Finland[44]	25–74 years	51,552 participants (51% women)	633	• Drug registry	1972–2002 (30 years)	No	
Finnish Mobile Clinic Health Examination Survey (FMC), Finland[45–47]	30–59 years	10,962 participants (48% women)	101	• Drug registry • Validation of a subsample through clinical record review	1966–1994 (28 years)	No	Age-restricted subsamples used for individual analyses
Health Professional Follow-up Study (HPFS), USA	40–75 years	51,500 men	438	• Self-reported • Medical records review	1986–2006 (20 years)	Yes	
Honolulu-Asia Aging Study (HAAS), USA	45–68 years	8006 men	128	Before 1991: • Hospital and outpatient clinical record review • Death certificate review 1991–1993: • Active screening through semi-structured interview, technician evaluation • Neurologist confirmed diagnosis[48]	1965–1993 (28 years)	No	
NeuroEPIC4PD, Europe (UK, Italy, Greece, Netherlands, Germany, Sweden, Spain)[18]	35–70 years	220,494 participants (62% women)	881 (199 definite; 275 very likely; 146 probable; 261 possible)	• Self-reported • Drug registries • Hospital records • General practitioner records • All data available reviewed by a neurologist	1992–2006 (14 years)	No	Blood samples collected at recruitment
Nurses' Health Study (NHS),[49] USA	30–55 years	121,700 women	508	• Self-reported • Medical records	1976–2008 (32 years)	Yes	
Rotterdam Study,[50] Netherlands	55+ years	7983 participants (59% women)	88	• In person clinical diagnosis by a neurologist	1990–2004 (14 years)	Yes	
Physician Health Study (PHS),[51] USA	40–84 years	22,071 men participating in a trial on aspirin and β carotene for the prevention of cancer	616	• Self-reported	1982–2008 (26 years)	No	Diagnosis was validated via medical records review by a physician in a subsample of 73

(continued)

Table 11.1 Continued

Study, place	Age at baseline	Sample size	Incident cases	Case ascertainment	Longest Follow-up	Active update of exposure information	Notes
National Institutes of Health-American Association of Retired Persons Diet and Health Study (NIH-AARP),[52] USA	50–71 years	318,261 (41% women) (53)	2432	• Self-reported • A subsample validated through medical record review	1995–2006 (11 years)	No	Saliva collected for genetic analysis
Shanghai Women Health Study (SWHS),[54] China	40–70 years	74,941 women	95, of whom 76 with medically confirmed diagnosis	• Self-reported • Confirmed either with clinical examination or record review	1996–2011 (15 years)	Yes	Urine, blood and saliva collected at baseline
Singapore Chinese Health Study (SCHS)[55,56]	45–74 years	63,257 (55% women)	157	• Self-reported • Hospital records • Parkinson's disease registries	1993–2005 (17 years)	No	

Adapted with permission from Ascherio A., and Schwarzschild M. A. The epidemiology of Parkinson's disease: risk factors and prevention. *Lancet Neurology*, 15(12):1257–72. DOI:https://doi.org/10.1016/S1474-4422(16)30230-7

using the broad criteria (73% of all parkinsonism).[21] General practice records have been shown to be relatively accurate, the diagnosis of probable PD was confirmed in 83% of the cases by expert consensus, including 2% in whom atypical features were found but were insufficient to invalidate the diagnosis of PD.[17] Overall, the specificity and sensitivity of the diagnosis of PD and parkinsonism in population-based studies is of great relevance, especially when older populations are included. The prevalence of parkinsonian symptoms in the general population increases with age, reaching about 15% among people 65–74 years of age, 30% among those 75–84, and 52% among those 85 and older.[19] Similarly, the incidence of parkinsonism per 1000 person-years increases with age and has been estimated to be 36.0 for adults <75 years of age, 94.8 for those 75–84, and 160.5 for those 85 years or older.[22]

Burden of Disease

In 2016, an estimated 6.1 million (95% uncertainty interval (UI) 5.0–7.3) had PD, accounting for of 3·2 million (95% UI 2.6–4.0) DALYs, and 211,296 deaths (95% UI 167,771–265,160), globally. PD has a median age-standardized incidence rate in HIC of 14 per 100,000 people/year in the total population, and 160 per 100,000 people aged 65 years or older (57); the corresponding lifetime risk in the USA is 2% for men and 1.3% for women aged ≥40 years.[58] Age-adjusted PD prevalence appears to be lower in Africa than in Europe and the Americas,[59–61] most likely due to shorter survival. Incidence in Asia is similar to that in Europe and the Americas.[62,63] To what extent these differences could be genetically or environmentally driven is not clear. Data on ethnic-specific incidence of PD (mainly from the USA) are not consistent,[64–66] and in general it is unusual for ethnic differences to be genetically determined.[67] A recent ecological study suggested that concentrations of selenium, strontium, and manganese in soil could contribute to geographic variations in USA. However, this evidence is relatively weak.

The incidence of PD is low before age 50 and increases with age in both sexes.[58,68] It is not clear if the decrease in incidence observed after age 80 is real or due to artefacts such as underdiagnoses in older ages, comorbidity (frailty), or increased prevalence of cognitive impairment which is an exclusion criterion for the diagnosis of PD.[58,68,69] Men are more affected than women, with a M:F ratio around 1.5,[70] ranging from 1.3 to 2.0 in most studies.[69] However, in some European studies the incidence in men and women was similar;[71,72] and the M:F ratio was 0.95 in studies involving Asian populations (specifically Chinese and Japanese)[73] and was also similar among Asian living in the USA.[65] It is not clear whether the increased risks in men are due to greater susceptibility, increased exposures to causal agent(s), or both.[70,74]

Time trends

A recent analysis of the Global Burden of Disease Study 2016 has reported a more than doubling prevalence of PD from 1990 (2.5 million (95% UI 2.0–3.0)) to 2016 (6.1 million (95% UI 5.0–7.3)), globally.[75] This increase cannot be attributed solely to ageing populations, as the age-standardized prevalence rates have also risen in the same period. In 2016, PD was responsible of 3.2 million (95% UI 2.6–4.0) DALYs and 211,296 deaths (95% UI 167,771–265,160), globally. From 1990 to 2016, the age-standardized prevalence of PD increased in all regions except for Southern Latin America, Eastern Europe, and Oceania.[75] Incidence rates of both PD and parkinsonism were found to remain stable in some studies,[76,77] but to have increased from 1976 to 2005 in Minnesota (USA), although this increase was mainly driven by the incidence among people over 70 years.[78] In Europe, different trends were observed: a 6% yearly decline of PD incidence between 1999 and 2009 was reported in UK; however, this was probably explained by improved diagnosis given that in the same period an increase of parkinsonism incidence was also observed.[79] Similarly, a decline in incidence of PD and parkinsonism was observed in the Rotterdam study between 1990s and 2010s.[80]

Clinical Subtypes

Many attempts have been made to classify PD cases, principally in order to predict response to treatment, and survival, specifically with regards to comorbidities. Initial classifications were based on clinical observation and on motor symptoms. One of the first classifications distinguished cases by age of onset, where young age of onset (YOPD) cases were those with symptoms beginning before age 40[81] (but also 55 years in some other studies).[82] The older the age of onset, the more severe the postural instability, bradykinesia, autonomic dysfunction, global cognitive impairment, and hyposmia.[83] Older patients also had worse motor symptoms and a greater dopaminergic deficit.[83] On the contrary, younger age of onset is associated with a slower rate of disease progression, better preserved cognitive function, and better prognosis, overall.[82,84] However, patients with earlier age of onset typically develop more motor fluctuations and dyskinesias.[85]

The initial classification of PD based on motor symptoms divided patients into postural instability/gait difficulty (PIGD) and tremor-dominant (TD) subtypes.[86–88] Other classifications reflect similar broad categories with and without tremor; for example the akinetic/rigid form was defined to describe tremor-free patients with significant axial rigidity, which largely overlaps with the formerly known PIGD-dominant subtype.[89] Overall, patients presenting predominantly with resting tremor at onset tend to have a slower progression,[90] while the PIGD-dominant phenotype involves a faster cognitive decline.[91,92] Nonetheless, this classification has been criticized as PIGD and akinetic/rigid features may only be markers of older age, disease progression, and concomitant comorbidities.[93,94] A further advancement in classification involves incorporating non-motor symptoms:[95] patients with REM-behaviour disorder (RBD) have been reported to have a higher prevalence of cognitive impairment and more autonomic dysfunction,[96–98] and in some studies also a faster motor progression and a higher proportion of akinetic-rigid subtype.[99,100] Similarly, orthostatic hypotension has been associated with a higher risk of dementia.[96,99] Dementia has also been shown to be associated with more rapid disease progression.[101,102]

Currently, an increasing amount of clinical epidemiological research involves data-driven classifications, where cluster analysis is used to define categories according to a large number of clinical, demographic, and genetic factors, without an *a priori* ranking of the importance of these.[94] To date, the results are not conclusive, as they depend on the amount and quality of data used to generate them: samples are often selected on strict clinical criteria, with limited data on non-motor symptoms, and lack of longitudinal follow-up providing reliable information on prognosis.[94] For a complete review of the state of the art of the subtypes classification in PD, see the work of Fereshtehnejad and Postuma.[94] Current efforts to improve classification involve the incorporation of genetic and biomarker information into the classification in order to identify potential pathophysiological mechanisms underlying PD subtypes.[94,103]

Genetic Risk Factors

PD aggregates in families,[104] and approximately 5–10% of all cases are monogenic forms caused by highly penetrant but rare genetic mutations. The remaining cases are likely due to complex gene-environment interactions involving more common single nucleotide polymorphisms (SNPs) with weaker effect sizes.[6] Therefore, the genetic factors contributing to PD range from rare mutations with large effects (fully or highly penetrant), to more common genetic variants with modest effects on disease risk. Interestingly, co-occurrence of rare causative mutations and risk-increasing variants in the same genes (i.e. *SNCA*, and *LRRK2*) have been described.[6] Below, only the main confirmed monogenic forms (autosomal dominant and recessive) are described: comprehensive overviews, including the SNPs modulating PD risk in more complex gene-environment interactions, can be found in recent reviews.[6,105]

Three genes have been implicated in the autosomal-dominant transmission of the disease. The first to be identified was the *SNCA* gene on chromosome 4q22.1, encoding for α-synuclein which aggregates in Lewy bodies. A number of pathogenic missense mutations were identified over time.[106–110] Interestingly, structural aberrations of the chromosomal region containing the wild-type *SNCA* sequence, such as duplications[111,112] and triplications[113] were also identified in relation to PD. Subjects with *SNCA* missense mutations or multiplications often show dementia and may also present with atypical characteristics such as pyramidal signs, myoclonus, or seizures.[6] The exact toxic mechanisms exerted by α-synuclein are not clear yet; hypotheses include the possibility that it is the soluble form that exerts a toxic effect and it is therefore stored in the Lewy bodies as a mechanism of defence, or that Lewy body themselves lead to neuronal death.[114] Nor it is clear how α-synuclein proteins or aggregates generated in one neuron spread to other neighbouring neurons: a 'prion-protein-like' mechanism responsible for the spread has been postulated.[115,116]

Mutations in *LRRK2* (leucine-rich repeat kinase 2), inherited in an autosomal-dominant manner, are the most frequent in PD.117,118 At least six highly penetrant, pathogenic mutations have been described in *LRRK2*.[119,120] Interestingly, the *LRRK2* mutations have an estimated high-carrier frequency even among so-called 'sporadic' cases, that is, without family history, in particular among North African Arabs and Ashkenazi Jews (10–39%), while this is very low among Asians (0.1%).[119]

The latest autosomal dominant PD gene, *VPS35*, encoding a vacuolar protein sorting 35 retromer complex component, was identified by whole-exome next-generation sequencing.[121,122] At least one mutation on this gene has been confirmed to be causative. The VPS35 protein is involved in the retrograde transport of proteins and thus supports the hypothesis that altered vesicle formation and trafficking is one of the mechanisms underlying PD.[6]

Three genes have been identified as responsible for autosomal recessive homozygous or heterozygous loss-of-function mutations in PD: *PARK2* (known as Parkin),[123] *PINK1*,[124] and *PARK7* (known as DJ-1).[125] While mutations in these genes are relatively rare among PD cases in general, they appear to be responsible for a substantial proportion of early-onset PD.[6] Parkin is the most commonly mutated autosomal recessive gene, and accounts for 8.6% of the early-onset (<50 years) cases, followed by PINK1 (3.7%) and DJ-1 (0.4%).[6]

A large number of different mutations have been described for these genes; for further details; see the review by Lill.[6] The clinical characteristics of *Parkin*, *PINK1*, and *DJ-1* mutation carriers are comparable, with typical signs and symptoms of classical PD responsive to levodopa. In subjects with *Parkin* mutations, additional dystonic features have also been reported, while psychiatric signs and symptoms have repeatedly been described in those carrying *PINK1* mutations.[6] Dysfunctions ascribed to the proteins encoded by these genes have all been linked to mitochondrial dysfunction, accumulation of abnormal and misfolded proteins, impaired protein clearance and oxidative stress.[126] The evidence suggests the presence of a common pathway of neuroprotective signalling cascade, in which each of them plays a role.[126]

An additional autosomal recessive mutation in *DNAJC6* (encoding a member of heat shock protein family, Auxilin) has also been described in a handful of cases as a cause of early-onset PD, predominately with atypical signs and symptoms.[6] Auxilin is a clathrin-associated protein expressed predominately in neurons and enriched in nerve terminals, suggesting again that vesicle trafficking is an important feature in PD pathogenesis.[6]

While mutations in the *DNAJC6* are responsible for both PD cases and forms of atypical parkinsonism, other genes have been shown to be associated predominantly to atypical parkinsonism. A number of additional genes may also cause monogenic PD, but these are awaiting replication.[6]

The increasing recognition that PD has a high molecular and phenotypic heterogeneity supports the role of gene-environment interactions, and/or epigenetic changes resulting from environmental exposures.[10,12,127,128] This would partly explain the incomplete concordance between monozygotic and dizygotic twins for PD.[129] Some epigenetic mechanisms have recently been implicated in PD pathogenesis;[130] in particular, α-synuclein can link with histones and inhibit their acetylation,[131] which is largely attributable to its effect on Sirt2, a particular histone deacetylase. For a review on mechanisms, please refer to Urdinguio et al.[130]

Environmental Risk and Protective Factors

Smoking

There is strong and consistent epidemiological evidence that cigarette smoking reduces the risk of PD. An initial meta-analysis including 44 case-control studies and 4 cohort studies, estimated a pooled relative risk of PD of 0.59 (95% CI 0.54–0.63) for ever vs never smokers, and a relative risk of 0.39 (95% CI 0.32–0.47) for current smokers compared to never smokers.[132] Twelve years later, an updated meta-analysis, including 61 case-control and eight cohort studies, estimated a very similar association.[133] This association appears to be consistent in men and women and is not confounded or modified by educational level. Comparable inverse associations found for cigarette smoking were also observed for pipe and cigar smoking in men.[134] Dose-response relationships of decreased risk of PD have consistently been found, with increasing smoking duration and intensity and decreasing time since last smoking.[30,53,134,135] One large cohort study reported that duration and recentness of smoking were more important than smoking intensity in reducing PD risk.[53,136]

Non-causal explanations that have been proposed include: information bias—if PD diagnosis is less frequently reported on death certificates and clinical records of smokers; competing risks—due to higher mortality of younger smokers due to causes other than PD; confounding—if smoking and PD share some common genetic or environmental cause, that is, a low-risk-taking personality; or reverse causality. Information bias can be minimized in properly conducted prospective studies, which in turn give estimates of the association between smoking and PD slightly stronger than those from case-control studies.[132,135,137] Publication bias has been addressed and evaluated in meta-analyses and deemed to be negligible.[132,137] The problem of competing risks can be partly (but not completely) overcome by taking age into account appropriately in analyses of longitudinal studies.[135] Confounding and reverse causality are more difficult to rule out given that PD has a long prodromal period whose definition is still matter of debate. The implication of dopamine in the brain reward circuit and observation that treatment with levodopa could in some cases trigger pathological gambling behaviour in PD,[138] led to the hypothesis that people who will develop the disease may have a low risk-taking personality, less prone to addiction. This personality trait could be genetically determined or be a very early consequence of subtle dopamine shortage in the brain. However, a recent study exploring causal pathways of the inverse association between smoking and PD ruled out all the alternative explanations, concluding that the evidence supports a causal effect.[135]

Genetic factors may affect the propensity to initiate smoking,[139] and smoking is highly concordant among twins;[140] however, within twin pairs, PD is inversely associated with the dose (in packs/years) of smoking.[140] Furthermore, evidence from twin studies argues against a prominent role of genetic factors in this association as it is only slightly attenuated in dizygotic twins when compared to monozygotic twins.[140]

More difficult is the assessment of reverse causality. A recent analysis of the Danish registries suggests that quitting smoking before disease onset was easier for PD cases than for controls, and cases were less likely to use nicotine substitutes.[136] However, this potential reverse causality has been further explored using parental smoking as an instrumental variable associated with smoking in the offspring (the index subjects).[141] The negative association between parental smoking and PD is evidence against reverse causality; although we cannot rule out confounding due to an infectious/toxic agent in a family affecting both parental smoking and the future PD risk in offspring.[141] Finally, an inverse association between passive smoking and PD has been detected in some case-control studies,[142] although not always at significant level,[143] but not in others.[144] Recently, this association has been confirmed in a prospective setting.[135]

Coffee and tea

Drinking coffee has been inversely associated with risk of PD (RR 0.75, 95% CI 0.68–0.82) in a meta-analysis of 26 epidemiological studies.[145] A dose-response meta-analysis based on 13 studies estimated an overall inverse association between the highest coffee intake vs the lowest, with a RR of 0.65 (95% CI 0.56–0.74), which was only slightly attenuated after adjusting for smoking (RR 0.68, 95% CI 0.58–0.79).[146] A non-linear relationship with a significant reduced risk of PD for coffee intake up to three cups/day, and a plateau effect further increasing the number of cups/day was shown. In turn, a significant linear dose-response relationship of reduced PD risk increasing the amount of caffeine consumption was observed with a decreased risk of 17% (RR 0.83, 95% CI 0.76–0.92) for every 200 mg/day of caffeine consumed.[146]

The association between coffee consumption and PD has been investigated among non-smokers in two separate analyses in the Cancer Prevention Study II finding in both cases a significant and stronger inverse association in men but not in women.[26,33] However, this may be in part due to postmenopausal oestrogen use: coffee consumption was significantly associated with reduced risk of PD in never oestrogen user, while it was not associated in ever users.[33] These results, consistent with others,[147–149] support the hypothesis that postmenopausal oestrogen modifies the effect of caffeine on risk of PD, being a competitive inhibitor of its metabolism.[150]

Some exposure misclassification is also likely in epidemiological studies of coffee consumption, as types of coffee, brewing methods, and caffeine content may vary considerably from country to country and across continents. In general, stronger associations are found in Europe—where coffee is known to have an higher density of caffeine—compared to America;[146] consistent with a possible role of caffeine, a meta-analysis of the association between decaffeinated coffee and PD found little or no evidence of a protective effect (RR 0.94, 95% CI 0.78–1.12).[146]

A Genome-Wide Association and Interaction Study (GWAIS) tested each SNP's main effect and its interaction with coffee drinking, adjusting for sex and age, and detected as significant the rs4998386 and its neighbouring SNP in *GRIN2A* which encodes for a NMDA-glutamate-receptor subunit and regulates excitatory neurotransmission in the brain.[151] Compared to light coffee drinkers with the wild-type genotype (rs4998386_CC), the risk of PD was decreased by 18% in heavy coffee drinker with the same genotype, and by 59% in heavy coffee drinkers with the SNP (rs4998386_TC). These SNPs were also reported to be associated with the methylation pattern of the *GRIN2A* gene.[152] These results were replicated in a Swedish population,[153] but not in a pooled analysis including four independent European and US studies.[154] Other studies investigating gene-environment interaction in coffee drinking and PD did not find strong associations.[155]

Drinking tea has also been associated with a reduced risk of PD: a meta-analysis including eight original papers estimated a RR 0.63 (95% CI 0.49–0.81) for tea drinking, and a RR 0.61 (95% CI 0.50–0.74) after adjustment for cigarette smoking.[146] A decreased risk of 26% for every two cups/day increment for tea consumption was found.[146] A study in Singapore replicated the inverse association with PD for black tea, but not for green tea after adjustment for smoking and caffeine intake.[55] A case-control study in Argentina observed a similar inverse association for coffee, tea, and yerba mate intake.[156]

Brain injury

Traumatic brain injury has been hypothesized as a causative factor for PD on the basis of several different possible pathogenetic associations. Traumatic brain injury is known to cause a breakdown of the brain blood barrier (BBB) and to induce an inflammatory reaction in the brain that can be long-lasting;[157–159] mitochondrial function is disrupted after head injury, and glutamate release due to traumatic head injury further increases energy demands;[160,161] and head injury leads to accumulation of synuclein.[162–164] Nevertheless, epidemiological evidence is not consistent.

Case-control studies of head injury and PD are often difficult to interpret, mainly because of the potential for reverse causality. A large nationwide record-linkage study in Denmark including more than 13,000 PD cases found a significant association between traumatic brain injury and PD (OR 1.5, 95% CI 1.4–1.7), but the analysis of temporal patterns showed a maximum risk 0–3 months before PD diagnosis.[165] A population-based case-control study of PD in Canada, including 403 cases and 405 controls, showed a significant association between PD and injuries involving concussion (OR: 2.1, 95% CI 1.3–3.3) and unconsciousness (OR: 2.6, 95% CI 1.4–5.0); these effects remained for injuries that occurred long before diagnosis.[166] An analysis of 93 twin pairs discordant for PD found a statistically significant association between head injury and PD (OR 3.8, 95% CI 1.3–11). The association was similar when only head traumas occurring ten years before diagnosis were included (OR 3.2, 95% CI 1.1–11).[167]

Case-control studies in Germany[168] and Finland[169] did not find associations between PD and mild traumatic brain injury. A population-based record-linkage study in the USA, including 196 PD cases found no association with concussion with amnesia but without loss of consciousness (OR 1.0, 95% CI 0.1–7.1).[170] Some older studies found statistically significant associations between head traumas and PD,[168,171–173] while some others did not.[174–179] Some of this evidence has been recently reviewed as part of the International Collaboration on Mild Traumatic Brain Injury Prognosis.[180] Two recent population based studies reported that the association might depend on age at head injury, suggesting higher risk associated with head injuries occurred at younger age.[181,182]

A study of causes of death among retired sportsmen of the American Football League found a non-statistically significantly increased risk of PD compared to the general population.[183] Another recent study found a more than three-fold increased risk of PD among people with post-traumatic stress disorders.[184]

Diet, including dairy products and uric acid

No compelling evidence has been produced on the association between dietary intake of vitamins,[185,186] total fat or different fatty acids,[69] or flavonoids[185] intake and PD risk. Iron has been proposed as a risk factor for PD given that it accumulates in the substantia nigra;[187] however, total iron intake was not found to be associated with PD risk,[188] nor the number of blood donations, which is in turn associated with iron and ferritin body levels.[189] Conversely, in some studies, iron deficient anaemia has been associated with an increased risk of PD,[190] in one study, irrespective of iron supplementation use.[191] Epidemiological studies investigating the role of single nutrients in this context are hampered not only by well-known limitations (e.g. errors in exposure assessment, correlation among food items), but also by the association between pesticide contamination and PD, which might alter analyses of specific food items (i.e. berries) in relation to PD. In a large cohort study, analysis of dietary patterns has indicated that a diet characterized by high intakes of fruit, vegetables, and fish, was associated with a reduced risk of PD (RR 0.78 (95% CI 0.56–1.07) for the highest vs lowest quintile).[192]

High milk consumption has been associated with an increased risk of PD.[69] These findings are consistent across studies in both the USA[31,193,194] and Europe.[195,196] A recent meta-analysis calculated an increased risk of PD for dairy product intake (highest vs lowest level OR 1.40 (95% CI 1.20–1.63)), which was much stronger for men than for women.[197] The resulting association was found to be driven by consumption of milk and cheese, and not present for yogurt and butter, and the authors estimated that the risk of PD increased by

17% (95% CI 6%–30%) for every 200 g/day increment in milk intake.[197] The possible mechanisms underlying this association are not clear. One of the hypotheses is that milk could be contaminated with toxic substances responsible for the biological effect: for example in the Honolulu Asia Aging Study, the association of milk consumption with lower neuronal density in the substantia nigra and higher risk for PD may be explained by heptachlor contamination which occurred decades ago.[194,198] Another hypothesis postulates that the effect of milk could be mediated by its properties of reducing uric acid levels because of the uricosuric effect of its proteins.[199]

Uric acid is the end product in the metabolism of purines and has potent antioxidant properties. Epidemiological studies have consistently shown an inverse association between uric acid and PD in prospective studies. An initial meta-analysis of three large prospective studies estimated a combined RR of 0.80 (95% CI 0.71–0.90) for each standard deviation (1.3 mg/dL) increase in blood urate concentration,[200] which was subsequently confirmed by other evidence, in particular among men.[23,201–203] Some,[204,205] but not all,[206] genetic studies also suggest an association between specific SNPs in the SLC2A9, an urate transporter strongly associated with blood urate levels, and reduced risk of PD. Similar genetic studies, including a study using a Mendelian randomization (MR) approach found that SNPs associated with lower circulating uric acid levels were also associated with a faster clinical progression of the disease.[69,207]

Occupational and environmental exposures, including pesticides

Associations between a range of occupational and environmental exposures and PD have been observed, including organochlorines, certain metals (manganese and iron), and organic solvents.[74,208–214]

A recent meta-analysis[215] assessed the risk of PD in relation to welding, reporting a weighted RR of 0.85 (95% CI 0.82–0.89). Conversely, the same authors found no association between exposure to metals in other forms.[216–220]

A meta-analysis of the association between electromagnetic fields and PD, including two case-control[221,222] and eight prospective studies,[223–230] calculated an overall RR of 1.07 (95% CI 0.97–1.19). However, this was probably due to recall bias, as repeating the analysis in the prospective studies only, the estimate of the association was null.[215] Consistently, another meta-analysis on very-low electromagnetic fields and PD came to the same conclusion of no association.[231] Anecdotal evidence suggests an association between exposure to some solvents and risk of PD,[232–235] but this was not confirmed in larger studies.[236]

Perhaps the strongest evidence of occupational causes of PD relates to agricultural work and pesticide exposure. Farmers and agricultural workers have been shown to be at increased risk of PD in several key studies,[237–239] consistent with the hypothesis that exposure to pesticides could increase the risk of PD.[74] In fact, a role of pesticides was first hypothesized following the observation that people injecting drugs containing 1-methyl-4phnyl-1,2,3,6-tetrahydropyridine (MPTP) (a neurotoxin structurally similar to the herbicide paraquat) developed an acute parkinsonian syndrome.[240] MPTP is metabolized by the monoamine oxidase B becoming a substrate of the dopamine transporter, which inhibits the mitochondrial complex I leading to the degeneration of dopaminergic neurons. MPTP-induced animal models are currently used for investigating *in vivo* mechanisms of PD.[241] A recent meta-analysis, including 39 case-control, 4 cohort, and 3 cross-sectional studies, estimated an overall increased risk of PD among the exposed of 1.6 (95% CI 1.4–1.9) compared to unexposed, with strong associations for herbicides (OR = 1.4, 95% CI 1.1–1.8), and insecticides (OR = 1.5, 95% CI 1.1–2.1), but not for fungicides (OR 1.0, 95% CI 0.7–1.4).[242] The high heterogeneity between studies (I^2 = 63.5%, p = 0.001) was mainly explained by differences in exposure assessment, with higher estimates coming from more objective assessments using job titles rather than self-report. Difficulty in assessing exposure to different compounds remains an open challenge; evidence on single chemicals is still limited. The associations with paraquat and rotenone (another herbicide inhibitor of the mitochondrial complex I) are among the most established.[41] Among insecticides, some studies support an association with organochlorines,[47,243–245] particularly dieldrin. A stronger dose-response relationship with intensity of exposure compared to duration[246] for tremor-dominant PD[246] and for late-onset PD compared to early-onset,[243] were observed in relation to pesticide exposure. On the basis of current evidence, PD has been recognized as an occupational disease in agriculture professionals in France under specific conditions.[247] Few gene-environment interactions have been proposed to play a role in the association between pesticides and PD,[248–251] but to date none of them have been replicated.

Additional investigations on occupational risk factors and PD indicate that being in an occupation with night shifts,[252] working in transport or communication,[253] having a processing occupation,[253] or having been exposed to whole body vibrations[254] are all inversely associated with the condition. Conversely, being a physician,[219] a biological scientist,[227] or a teacher,[227] working in agriculture or horticulture,[239] or in churches[227] have all been associated with an increased risk of PD. In addition, exposure to cats and cattle was also associated with an increased risk.[255] A higher educational level is positively associated with the risk of PD,[219] and, consistently, occupational complexity, a refined way to measure intellectual engagement at work with data, people, but not with things, was also associated with an increased risk of PD, particularly in men.[256] However, overall, it is difficult to interpret these findings, and it is therefore likely that many of them are chance findings.

Drugs, including NSAIDs, calcium channel blockers, statins

A meta-analysis including prospective studies investigating the association between non-steroidal anti-inflammatory drug (NSAID) use and incidence of a total of 2779 PD cases, estimated a pooled RR of 0.73 (95% CI 0.63–0.85) for ibuprofen use and 1.12 (95% CI 1.01–1.23) for aspirin use. Use of other NSAIDs or acetaminophen was not associated with PD risk.[257] To date, the overall epidemiological evidence indicates no association between NSAIDs and PD, apart from ibuprofen. Despite initial theories of a generic anti-inflammatory role contrasting the microglia response to neurodegeneration, this prompted the search for potential preventive mechanisms specific to ibuprofen, the most prominent of which is activation of PPARγ, a proposed therapeutic target for PD.[69,258–260]

Following the proposed neuroprotective effect of some anti-hypertensive drugs, the use of dihydropyridine calcium channel blockers was investigated in relation to PD, and it was found to be associated with a reduced risk in some studies,[261–264] although not in all of them.[265,266] These drugs inhibit oxidative stress in mitochondria (as shown by some animal studies), and are therefore currently being investigated as disease modifying agents in a clinical trial in PD cases.[69]

Several studies have investigated the association between statin use and risk of PD, but the evidence is not clear-cut. A meta-analysis of eight studies (including about 15,000 cases) showed an overall significant inverse association (RR 0.77, 95% CI 0.64–0.92); however, larger studies showed consistently weaker and non-significant associations, making publication bias difficult to rule out.[267] Moreover, subsequent studies showed contrasting results.[25,268] Further, most of the available studies did not account for potential confounding by indication. In a recent longitudinal study that controlled for plasma cholesterols, statin use was associated with a higher risk for PD.[25] However, this analysis was based on a small number of exposed cases. Biologically, statins have been shown to have potent anti-inflammatory effects, but they also decrease plasma concentration of coenzyme Q10, a component of the mitochondrial respiratory chain, which has been hypothesized to confer protection against neurodegeneration in PD.[269] The effect of simvastatin in PD is currently being investigated in clinical trials.[69]

Oher lifestyle factors

The relationship between socioeconomic status and PD is unclear, with both positive[270] and inverse[77] relationships being observed, with additional studies finding no association.[271]

Overall, no association between BMI and PD was observed in epidemiological studies. A meta-analysis including ten prospective studies found no increased risk of PD per 5 kg/m^2 of BMI (RR 1.00, 95% CI 0.89–1.12).[272] However, a significant increased risk of PD was observed with increasing the midlife triceps skinfold thickness in the Honolulu Heart Programme,[273] with increasing the waist circumference and waist-to-hip ratio in never smokers,[274] and with increasing the BMI in Finnish men.[275] This suggests that neither BMI nor fat mass per se, but fat distribution and metabolic syndrome may be more relevant in modulating PD risk.[69]

A meta-analysis of almost 1000 PD cases showed a modest inverse association with alcohol intake, consistent among case-control and cohort studies (RR 0.86, 95% CI 0.75–1.0), with a linear dose-response relationship.[276] Moreover, in a very large Swedish study, alcohol misuse (defined as hospital admission with a diagnosis of alcohol use disorder) has been associated with an increased PD risk (RR 1.4, 95% CI 1.3–1.5),[277] suggesting non-linearity at very high doses.

The higher incidence of PD in men than in women, suggests that hormonal/reproductive factors may play a role in the disease. However, to date, no convincing evidence exists on the role of reproductive factors such as age at menarche, use of oral contraceptives, pregnancy, or menopause history.[278–281] Only post-menopausal hormone replacement was associated with an increased risk of PD in some studies,[33,280] but not all.[278–280] Collectively, these results suggest counterintuitively that post-menopausal hormone replacement may be associated, if anything, with an increased risk of PD.[69] One of the hypotheses that may explain these findings is that this association may be modified by caffeine:[26,149,282] risks of PD in women drinking higher amounts of coffee would be decreased among those using hormone replacement therapy, and increased among those not using the therapy.[33]

Physical activity is inversely associated with the risk of PD: a meta-analysis of five studies estimated a RR of 0.66 (95% CI 0.57–0.78).[283] The possibility of reverse causality, given the potential very long prodromal phase of the disease, is weakened by the observation that the negative association was present in high school, college, and in early adulthood;[284,285] nevertheless, it cannot be completely ruled out. Physical activity could exert a neuroprotective effect mainly through neuroplasticity.[286]

Comorbidities

Cancer

A growing body of evidence suggests that people with PD have a decreased risk of almost all cancers. The risk of cancer in people affected by PD is estimated to be decreased by 27% compared to those not affected (RR 0.73, 95% CI 0.63–0.83).[287] This association is probably partially, but not completely, driven by the inverse association with smoking: the risk reduction was 40% for smoking-related cancer (RR 0.60, 95% CI 0.55–0.67), but only 18% for non-smoking-related cancers (RR 0.82, 95% CI 0.70–0.95).[287]

On the other hand, the risk of PD has been shown to be more than doubled in subjects who suffered from melanoma (OR 2.11, 95% CI 1.26–3.54);[288] this association is stronger in men than women. The risk of melanoma among people living with PD is somewhat weaker (OR 1.44, 95% CI 1.06–1.96).[288] Timing of comorbidity is important given that it has been hypothesized that melanoma could be associated with PD treatment. In fact, the synthesis of both dopamine (used in the treatment of PD) and melanin share biochemical pathways: levodopa, the precursor of the neurotransmitter dopamine, is also a substrate for the formation of melanins.[289] However, data collected from early PD cases in clinical trials (not treated with levodopa) indicated that the increased risk of melamona in PD precedes the treatment with levodopa.[290–292] The presence of a common genetic factor among these diseases has been suggested by the observation that PD risk increased with decreasing darkness of hair colour.[293] However, gene variants known to be associated with melanoma were not confirmed in large PD case series,[294] nor were gene variants associated with PD associated with melanoma risk.[295] Nonetheless, a recent study of rare variants identified TYR—encoding for tyrosinase, an enzyme for the production of neuromelanin, a pathogenic allele for recessive albinism—to be more common in PD cases than controls.[296] A recent meta-analysis estimated an overall increased risk of PD for red compared to black hair of 1.68 (95% CI 1.07–2.64) and a for the MC1R (the melanocortin-1 receptor gene, strongly tied to red hair/fair skin) p.R151C SNP of 1.1 (95% CI 1.00-1.21).[297]

Diabetes

Research on the comorbidity between PD and diabetes is not consistent, with some studies reporting a positive association,[44,298–301] but others no association.[28,302] A meta-analysis of case-control studies shows that the risk of PD in diabetic people is reduced (OR 0.75, 95% CI 0.58–0.98).[303] This is consistent with the observation in Finland of a 50% lower PD risk (RR 0.5, 95% CI 0.30–0.83) in people with metabolic syndrome; association mostly driven by elevated fasting plasma glucose (0.52, 95% CI

0.3–0.89).[304] A possible explanation for these inconsistent results is the presence of a complex interaction between PD and insulin resistance, which is possibly mediated by factors such as increased levels of uric acid, which is negatively associated with PD, but is a risk factor for diabetes.[305] Furthermore, PD risk among people with diabetes could be reduced by use of antidiabetic drugs such as metformin.[69,306]

Hypercholesterolaemia

The association between hypercholesterolaemia and PD has been extensively investigated, mostly with inconsistent results. In some studies, hypercholesterolaemia has been associated with a significant decreased risk of PD,[282,307] in others with a significant increased risk.[302,308] An underlying confounder or effect modifier is probably the explanation for this inconsistency.[69]

Non-motor Symptoms

> 'The disease is of long duration: to connect, therefore, the symptoms which occur in its later stages with those which mark its commencement, requires a continuance of observation of the same case, or at least a correct history of its symptoms, even for several years'
>
> (Reproduced from Parkinson J. *An Essay on the Shaking Palsy*. London. Neely and Jones. 1817).

In addition to cardinal motor signs, PD patients also suffer from a wide range of non-motor symptoms, ranging from hyposmia and depression early on, to dementia and hallucinations that often occur at later stages of the disease. These symptoms are prevalent among PD patients and adversely affect their quality of life.[309] More importantly, accumulating evidence suggests that some non-motor symptoms may develop years prior to the clinical diagnosis of PD. These include olfactory impairment,[310] depression,[311–314] anxiety,[311–313,315] RBD,[316–319] excessive daytime sleepiness,[320,321] autonomic dysfunction such as constipation,[322–324] and lower heart rate variability.[325] As discussed earlier, these propdromal symptoms may potentially be explained by the sequential extranigral pathologies as implicated by the Braak hypothesis.[5] These prodromal pathologies of PD may take decades to develop.[326] A later extension of this hypothesis further posits that the synucleinopathy may even start in the periphery, for example in the enteric nerves in the gut and later spread retrogradely to brainstem via the vagus nerve.[327,328] Although the Braak hypothesis itself is still somewhat controversial,[329,330] it presents an intriguing possibility that the extra-nigra, nondopaminergic pathologies are intrinsic to early PD pathogenesis and prodromal non-specific symptoms of PD could well be part of the disease's natural history.[326]

Clinical studies and epidemiological surveys have clearly shown that these non-motor symptoms are common among PD patients. A recent meta-analysis reported the prevalence of selected non-motor symptoms among PD patients:[331] hyposmia was the most prevalent, affecting 75.5% of the patients, followed by constipation (50%), anxiety (39.9%), RBD (37.0%), depression (36.6%), and excessive daytime sleepiness (33.9%). Data on the prevalence of these symptoms in the prodromal stage of PD are scarce; but again, hyposmia was the most prevalent (35.5%), followed by depression (23.0%), constipation (20.0%), anxiety (18.8%), and RBD (17.9%). However, interpretation of these data on symptom prevalence is subject to a number of limitations. First, individual studies vary substantially in assessment methods, symptom definition, and patient characteristics. Many of the available studies used self-report checklists to identify non-motor symptoms;[332] whilst convenient in large surveys they may not objectively capture symptoms. Further, most symptoms may have a spectrum of severity, which may be progressive and more heterogeneous at early stages. In addition, dichotomization of continuous symptoms will result in misclassifications, particularly for less severe symptoms. For example, there may be more measurement errors in the evaluation of hyposmia than anosmia, even with an objective sense of smell identification test.[333]

Relationships of prodromal non-motor symptoms to Parkinson's disease

The evidence in support of prodromal symptoms of PD comes primarily from large prospective population-based cohorts that were initially established for research on cancer and cardiovascular diseases,[310,324,325] retrospective examination of archived medical records,[323] and clinical follow-up of individuals with specific symptoms such as RBD.[318,334] The number of prospective studies is limited; however, the evidence to date has been fairly consistent.[331,335] Clinical studies suggest that up to 80% of polysomnography-confirmed RBD patients will eventually develop PD or a related synucleinopathy.[334] Other symptoms are less specific to PD but are generally associated with 2–5 times higher risk of developing PD.[336]

Importance of studying prodromal non-motor symptoms in Parkinson's disease

The mounting evidence for prodromal symptoms of PD, coupled with the Braak hypothesis, has generated substantial interest in evaluating whether these symptoms, alone or with other markers, can predict future development of PD.[336,337] Such research will lead to more targeted research for risk characterization or even early disease identification and intervention. For example, polysomnograph-confirmed RBD patients may represent a target population for potential neuroprotection clinical trials.[334] Although much less specific than RBD, several studies have identified olfactory impairment as the most important symptom in predicting PD or differentiating PD patients from controls.[338–340] In addition, if the presence of various non-motor symptoms in the same individual indeed represents common or similar underlying pathogeneses that may eventually lead to PD, the presence of multiple symptoms may be much more predictive for PD than individual symptoms.[331]

Equally important, research on prodromal symptoms of PD may offer an unprecedented opportunity to understand PD aetiology.[327,328,341] A major challenge in the aetiological research of PD is that during the decades-long prodromal stage of neurodegeneration, many factors may come into play at various time points by initiating relevant pathology or modifying its progression. Neither current animal models nor epidemiological studies with clinically diagnosed disease outcome have been able to mimic or reconstruct this complex decades-long process. As a consequence, even the most robust epidemiological findings on PD (e.g. smoking and PD) are subject to alternative explanations such as reverse causation and unmeasured confounding.[342]

A better characterization of these non-motor symptoms in the prodromal development of PD may bring a higher resolution to this process by identifying factors that contribute to prodromal symptoms and factors that modify their progression to clinical PD.[336] More importantly, we expect this will enable us to examine novel aetiological hypotheses of PD. Examples include the 'two-hit' hypothesis,[328,341] the microbiome hypothesis,[343] and the prion-like hypothesis.[344]

In summary, although the epidemiological research on prodromal symptoms of PD is still in its infancy, such research holds great promise that may eventually shift the paradigm of PD aetiological research to target its origin(s) and may lead to early disease identification and intervention.[336]

Treatment

The mainstay of PD management is symptomatic treatment with drugs that increase dopamine concentrations or directly stimulate dopamine receptors.[345,346] However, therapy is initiated after the clinical motor onset of disease when more than 50% of dopaminergic neurons have typically already been lost.[347] Starting treatment in the pre-clinical (motor) phase could possibly attenuate or even reverse the neurodegenerative process. Reasons for the current absence of such preventive or disease-modifying treatment options are the inability to diagnose PD at pre-clinical stages and, related to this, only an incomplete understanding of the pathogenic mechanisms leading to neuronal dysfunction and neurodegeneration in PD in the first place.[348] Moreover, management strategies for many of the disabling features that occur in late stages of the disease, such as motor symptoms that do not respond to dopaminergic therapies or develop as complications of long-term dopaminergic drug use, as well as an array of non-motor symptoms, are poor.[345] These symptoms lead to major impairments in the patients' quality of life and present a large burden for family members and caregivers.[349]

Natural History and Prognosis

Disease progression is characterized by worsening of motor features, which initially can be managed with symptomatic therapies. However, as the disease advances, complications emerge related to long-term symptomatic treatment, including motor and non-motor fluctuations, dyskinesia, and psychosis.[350,351] In late-stage PD, treatment-resistant motor and non-motor features are prominent, including axial motor symptoms such as postural instability, freezing of gait, falls, dysphagia, and speech dysfunction. After about 17 years post-diagnosis, up to 80% of patients with PD have freezing of gait and falls, and up to 50% of patients report choking.[350,351] Autonomic symptoms, such as urinary incontinence, constipation with the need for daily laxatives, and symptomatic postural hypotension, are common non-motor features in these late stages of PD.[350–352] Dementia occurs in 83% of patients with PD of at least 20 years' disease duration.[352] These levodopa-resistant symptoms of late-stage PD contribute substantially to disability and are strong predictors of a need for admission to an institution and/or mortality.[353]

According to data from the population-based CamPaIGN cohort,[354] ten years after diagnosis 55% of the people with PD have died, 68% have developed postural instability, 46% have developed dementia, and only 23% have a 'good outcome'. At the time of diagnosis, those with a good outcome were younger, had a tremor-dominant disease, better cognitive function, and lower depression scores and comorbidities.[354] In Table 11.2, results from the main studies reporting prognosis of PD cohorts are summarized.

Mortality rates vary from 20% in 11 years[355] to 55% in 10 years,[354] probably reflecting sample selection and study design. In the CamPaIGN study, mortality is not different from the general UK

Table 11.2 Main population and hospital-based studies assessing Parkinson's disease progression and prognosis

	Length of follow-up	Mortality rate	Causes of death	Postural instability (or HY* stage 3)	Dementia	Good outcome
Sydney Multicentre study, 1999,[350] Australia	10 years	38% in 10 years SMR 1.58, 95% CI 1.21–2.02	Pneumonia (30%) and cardiovascular diseases (21%)	48% at 10 years	N/A	10% at 10 years
Sydney Multicentre study, 2008,[352] Australia	20 years	74% in 20 years SMR (between 3 and 20 years) 2.5, 95% CI 2.0–3.0	Pneumonia (25%)	92% at 20 years	83% at 20 years	7.4 ‰ at 20 years
Hospital-based incident cohort, 2012,[356] China	11 years	29% in 11 years SMR 1.1, 95% CI 0.8–1.5	Pneumonia (64%) and cancer (18%)	63% at 11 years	49% at 11 years	N/A
CamPaIGN study, 2013,[354] UK	10 years	55% in 10 years SMR 1.29, 95% CI 0.97-1.61	Pneumonia (33%) and cancer (19%)	68% at 10 years	46% at 10 years	23% at 10 years
PROPARK, 2014,[357] Netherlands	5 years	N/A	N/A	N/A	26.1% at 2.56 years	N/A
Singapore study, 2015, [355] Singapore	11 years	20% in 11 years	Infections/ sepsis (54%) cardiovascular disease (17%) cancer (10%)	N/A	N/A	N/A

* Hoehn-Yahr scale: SMR = Standardised Mortality Ratios; PG = Postural instability and gait difficulty (or PIGD); TD = Tremor dominant.

population (SMR 1.29, 95% CI 0.97–1.61), although the study was only 61% powered to detect as significant SMRs of 1.3 at 5% level. The most common causes of death among people with PD were pneumonia (33% of cases) and cancer (19%).[354] Pneumonia was the most frequent cause of death reported by all studies,[350,352,354–357] followed by cancer[355,356] and cardiovascular diseases.[350,355] Interestingly, in 40% of the cases identified by the CamPaIGN study, PD was considered to be neither the underlying nor the contributing cause of death. In the study, median time from diagnosis to death was 10.3 years, and baseline predictors of death were older age of onset, and history of smoking.[354]

About two-thirds of the subjects in the CamPaIGN study living with PD develop postural instability over approximately ten years.[350,354,356] Those who developed postural instability, did so in a median time of 4.7 years; older age and non-tremor dominant form of the disease were the baseline predictors for developing postural instability.[354]

Almost half of the people living with PD develop a cognitive decline during the first ten years of disease progression. [354,356] In the CamPaIGN study the incidence of dementia in people with PD was estimated to be 2.6 times higher than the incidence among people 65 or older in the Cambridge population (estimated from the MRC-CFA study).[358] Older age, cognitive problems at diagnosis, and the MAPT H1/H1 genotype were the only predictors of dementia onset in people with PD.[354] An analysis of extensive data coming from 3200 people with PD in North America and Europe produced a prediction algorithm for the development of cognitive impairment in people with PD. The algorithm included age at onset, baseline mini-mental examination state (MMSE), years of education, motor exam score, sex, depression, and β-glucocerebrosidase (GBA) mutation. This cognitive risk score predicted cognitive impairment within ten years of disease onset with an area under the curve (AUC) greater than 0.85. Subjects scoring in the highest quartile had a relative risk for global cognitive impairment compared with those in the lowest quartile of 18.4, (95% CI 9.4–36.1).[359]

The impact of disease subtype on prognosis is controversial. The analysis of non-dopaminergic symptoms and motor-complications in patients presenting with the PIGD or the tremor dominant form of the disease showed that the former had worse scores of cognitive function, depression, autonomic dysfunction, psychotic symptoms, motor complications, and faster cognitive deterioration, compared to TD patients.[360] This suggests that PIGD is a valuable proxy for disease advancement, rather than a specific phenotype. It should therefore be used as an indicator of prognosis.[360]

Future Directions and Conclusions

To date, strategies for PD treatment have not been successful, mainly due to the fact that at the time of the diagnosis the neurodegeneration process in the central nervous system is well under way. Ideally, the efficacy of some of the studied compounds should be tested at earlier stages of neurodegeneration. The study of non-motor symptoms at population level yields an important promise of being able to identify people who will develop the motor symptoms of PD, at earlier stages with a good probability. Once this predictive model is established, it will be possible to test potential disease-modifying molecules at earlier stages of neural degeneration. This will also have a tremendous impact on their potential success, and therefore on both people living with PD and their families.

REFERENCES

1. Barnett R. Parkinson's disease. *Lancet*. 2016; 387(10015): 217.
2. Sacks O. *Awakenings*. New York: 1st Vintage Books, 1973.
3. Postuma RB, Berg D, Stern M, Poewe W, Olanow CW, Oertel W, et al. MDS clinical diagnostic criteria for Parkinson's disease. *Mov Disord*. 2015; 30(12): 1591–601.
4. Spillantini MG, Schmidt ML, Lee VM, Trojanowski JQ, Jakes R, Goedert M. Alpha-synuclein in Lewy bodies. *Nature*. 1997; 388(6645): 839–40.
5. Braak H, Del Tredici K, Rub U, de Vos RA, Jansen Steur EN, Braak E. Staging of brain pathology related to sporadic Parkinson's disease. *Neurobiol Aging*. 2003; 24(2): 197–211.
6. Lill CM. Genetics of Parkinson's disease. *Mol Cell Probes*. 2016; 30(6): 386–96.
7. Braak H, Del Tredici K. Invited Article: Nervous system pathology in sporadic Parkinson disease. *Neurology*. 2008; 70(20): 1916–25.
8. Svensson E, Horvath-Puho E, Thomsen RW, Djurhuus JC, Pedersen L, Borghammer P, et al. Vagotomy and subsequent risk of Parkinson's disease. *Ann Neurol*. 2015; 78(4): 522–9.
9. Liu B, Fang F, Pedersen NL, Tillander A, Ludvigsson JF, Ekbom A, et al. Vagotomy and Parkinson disease: A Swedish register-based matched-cohort study. *Neurology*. 2017; 88(21): 1996–2002.
10. Schrag A, Horsfall L, Walters K, Noyce A, Petersen I. Prediagnostic presentations of Parkinson's disease in primary care: a case-control study. *Lancet Neurology*. 2015; 14(1): 57–64.
11. Esper CD, Factor SA. Failure of recognition of drug-induced parkinsonism in the elderly. *Mov Disord*. 2008; 23(3): 401–4.
12. Bohlhalter S, Kaegi G. Parkinsonism: heterogeneity of a common neurological syndrome. *Swiss Med Wkly*. 2011; 141: w13293.
13. Gibb WR, Lees AJ. The relevance of the Lewy body to the pathogenesis of idiopathic Parkinson's disease. *J Neurol Neurosurg Psychiatry*. 1988; 51(6): 745–52.
14. Hughes AJ, Daniel SE, Kilford L, Lees AJ. Accuracy of clinical diagnosis of idiopathic Parkinson's disease: a clinico-pathological study of 100 cases. *J Neurol Neurosurg Psychiatry*. 1992; 55(3): 181–4.
15. Malek N, Lawton MA, Grosset KA, Bajaj N, Barker RA, Ben-Shlomo Y, et al. Utility of the new Movement Disorder Society clinical diagnostic criteria for Parkinson's disease applied retrospectively in a large cohort study of recent onset cases. *Parkinsonism Relat Disord*. 2017; 40: 40–6.
16. Rizzo G, Copetti M, Arcuti S, Martino D, Fontana A, Logroscino G. Accuracy of clinical diagnosis of Parkinson disease: A systematic review and meta-analysis. *Neurology*. 2016; 86(6): 566–76.
17. Schrag A, Ben-Shlomo Y, Quinn N. How valid is the clinical diagnosis of Parkinson's disease in the community? *J Neurol Neurosurg Psychiatry*. 2002; 73(5): 529–34.
18. Gallo V, Brayne C, Forsgren L, Barker RA, Petersson J, Hansson O, et al. Parkinson's disease case ascertainment in the EPIC cohort: the NeuroEPIC4PD Study. *Neurodegener Dis*. 2015; 15(6): 331–8.
19. Bennett DA, Beckett LA, Murray AM, Shannon KM, Goetz CG, Pilgrim DM, et al. Prevalence of parkinsonian signs and associated mortality in a community population of older people. *N Engl J Med*. 1996; 334(2): 71–6.

20. de Lau LM, Giesbergen PC, de Rijk MC, Hofman A, Koudstaal PJ, Breteler MM. Incidence of parkinsonism and Parkinson disease in a general population: the Rotterdam Study. *Neurology*. 2004; 63(7): 1240–4.
21. Bower JH, Maraganore DM, McDonnell SK, Rocca WA. Influence of strict, intermediate, and broad diagnostic criteria on the age- and sex-specific incidence of Parkinson's disease. *Mov Disord*. 2000; 15(5): 819–25.
22. Buchman AS, Leurgans SE, Yu L, Wilson RS, Lim AS, James BD, et al. Incident parkinsonism in older adults without Parkinson disease. *Neurology*. 2016; 87(10): 1036–44.
23. Chen H, Mosley TH, Alonso A, Huang X. Plasma urate and Parkinson's disease in the Atherosclerosis Risk in Communities (ARIC) study. *Am J Epidemiol*. 2009; 169(9): 1064–9.
24. The Atherosclerosis Risk in Communities (ARIC) study: design and objectives. The ARIC investigators. *Am J Epidemiol*. 1989; 129(4): 687–702.
25. Huang X, Alonso A, Guo X, Umbach DM, Lichtenstein ML, Ballantyne CM, et al. Statins, plasma cholesterol, and risk of Parkinson's disease: a prospective study. *Mov Disord*. 2015; 30(4): 552–9.
26. Palacios N, Gao X, McCullough ML, Schwarzschild MA, Shah R, Gapstur S, et al. Caffeine and risk of Parkinson's disease in a large cohort of men and women. *Mov Disord*. 2012; 27(10): 1276–82.
27. Palacios N, Gao X, O'Reilly E, Schwarzschild M, McCullough ML, Mayo T, et al. Alcohol and risk of Parkinson's disease in a large, prospective cohort of men and women. *Mov Disord*. 2012; 27(8): 980–7.
28. Palacios N, Gao X, McCullough ML, Jacobs EJ, Patel AV, Mayo T, et al. Obesity, diabetes, and risk of Parkinson's disease. *Mov Disord*. 2011; 26(12): 2253–9.
29. Thacker EL, Chen H, Patel AV, McCullough ML, Calle EE, Thun MJ, et al. Recreational physical activity and risk of Parkinson's disease. *Mov Disord*. 2008; 23(1): 69–74.
30. Thacker EL, O'Reilly EJ, Weisskopf MG, Chen H, Schwarzschild MA, McCullough ML, et al. Temporal relationship between cigarette smoking and risk of Parkinson disease. *Neurology*. 2007; 68(10): 764–8.
31. Chen H, O'Reilly E, McCullough ML, Rodriguez C, Schwarzschild MA, Calle EE, et al. Consumption of dairy products and risk of Parkinson's disease. *Am J Epidemiol*. 2007; 165(9): 998–1006.
32. Ascherio A, Chen H, Weisskopf MG, O'Reilly E, McCullough ML, Calle EE, et al. Pesticide exposure and risk for Parkinson's disease. *Ann Neurol*. 2006; 60(2): 197–203.
33. Ascherio A, Weisskopf MG, O'Reilly EJ, McCullough ML, Calle EE, Rodriguez C, et al. Coffee consumption, gender, and Parkinson's disease mortality in the cancer prevention study II cohort: the modifying effects of estrogen. *Am J Epidemiol*. 2004; 160(10): 977–84.
34. Chen H, Jacobs E, Schwarzschild MA, McCullough ML, Calle EE, Thun MJ, et al. Nonsteroidal anti inflammatory drug use and the risk for Parkinson's disease. *Ann Neurol*. 2005; 58(6): 963–7.
35. Alavanja MC, Sandler DP, McMaster SB, Zahm SH, McDonnell CJ, Lynch CF, et al. The Agricultural Health Study. *Environ Health Perspect*. 1996; 104(4): 362–9.
36. Furlong M, Tanner CM, Goldman SM, Bhudhikanok GS, Blair A, Chade A, et al. Protective glove use and hygiene habits modify the associations of specific pesticides with Parkinson's disease. *Environ Int*. 2015; 75: 144–50.
37. Goldman SM, Kamel F, Ross GW, Jewell SA, Bhudhikanok GS, Umbach D, et al. Head injury, alpha-synuclein Rep1, and Parkinson's disease. *Ann Neurol*. 2012; 71(1): 40–8.
38. Kamel F, Goldman SM, Umbach DM, Chen H, Richardson G, Barber MR, et al. Dietary fat intake, pesticide use, and Parkinson's disease. *Parkinsonism Relat Disord*. 2014; 20(1): 82–7.
39. Shrestha S, Kamel F, Umbach DM, Beane Freeman LE, Koutros S, Alavanja M, et al. Nonmotor symptoms and Parkinson disease in United States farmers and spouses. *PLOS One*. 2017; 12(9): e0185510.
40. Kirrane EF, Bowman C, Davis JA, Hoppin JA, Blair A, Chen H, et al. Associations of ozone and PM2.5 concentrations with Parkinson's disease among participants in the Agricultural Health Study. *J Occup Environ Med*. 2015; 57(5): 509–17.
41. Tanner CM, Kamel F, Ross GW, Hoppin JA, Goldman SM, Korell M, et al. Rotenone, paraquat, and Parkinson's disease. *Environ Health Perspect*. 2011; 119(6): 866–72.
42. Kamel F, Tanner C, Umbach D, Hoppin J, Alavanja M, Blair A, et al. Pesticide exposure and self-reported Parkinson's disease in the agricultural health study. *Am J Epidemiol*. 2007; 165(4): 364–74.
43. Gelb DJ, Oliver E, Gilman S. Diagnostic criteria for Parkinson disease. *Arch Neurol*. 1999; 56(1): 33–9.
44. Hu G, Jousilahti P, Bidel S, Antikainen R, Tuomilehto J. Type 2 diabetes and the risk of Parkinson's disease. *Diabetes Care*. 2007; 30(4): 842–7.
45. Saaksjarvi K, Knekt P, Mannisto S, Lyytinen J, Jaaskelainen T, Kanerva N, et al. Reduced risk of Parkinson's disease associated with lower body mass index and heavy leisure-time physical activity. *Eur J Epidemiol*. 2014; 29(4): 285–92.
46. Weisskopf MG, Knekt P, O'Reilly EJ, Lyytinen J, Reunanen A, Laden F, et al. Polychlorinated biphenyls in prospectively collected serum and Parkinson's disease risk. *Mov Disord*. 2012; 27(13): 1659–65.
47. Weisskopf MG, Knekt P, O'Reilly EJ, Lyytinen J, Reunanen A, Laden F, et al. Persistent organochlorine pesticides in serum and risk of Parkinson disease. *Neurology*. 2010; 74(13): 1055–61.
48. Ward CD, Gibb WR. Research diagnostic criteria for Parkinson's disease. *Adv Neurol*. 1990; 53: 245–9.
49. Palacios N, Fitzgerald KC, Hart JE, Weisskopf MG, Schwarzschild MA, Ascherio A, et al. Particulate matter and risk of Parkinson disease in a large prospective study of women. *Environ Health*. 2014; 13: 80.
50. Bornebroek M, de Lau LM, Haag MD, Koudstaal PJ, Hofman A, Stricker BH, et al. Nonsteroidal anti-inflammatory drugs and the risk of Parkinson disease. *Neuroepidemiology*. 2007; 28(4): 193–6.
51. Driver JA, Logroscino G, Lu L, Gaziano JM, Kurth T. Use of non-steroidal anti-inflammatory drugs and risk of Parkinson's disease: nested case-control study. *BMJ*. 2011; 342: d198.
52. Dong J, Beard JD, Umbach DM, Park Y, Huang X, Blair A, et al. Dietary fat intake and risk for Parkinson's disease. *Mov Disord*. 2014; 29(13): 1623–30.
53. Chen H, Huang X, Guo X, Mailman RB, Park Y, Kamel F, et al. Smoking duration, intensity, and risk of Parkinson disease. *Neurology*. 2010; 74(11): 878–84.
54. Chen H, Ding D, Wang J, Zhao Q, Meng H, Li H, et al. Parkinson's disease research in a prospective cohort in China. *Parkinsonism Relat Disord*. 2015; 21(10): 1200–04.
55. Tan LC, Koh WP, Yuan JM, Wang R, Au WL, Tan JH, et al. Differential effects of black versus green tea on risk of

Parkinson's disease in the Singapore Chinese Health Study. *Am J Epidemiol.* 2008; 167(5): 553–60.

56. Tan LC, Methawasin K, Tan EK, Tan JH, Au WL, Yuan JM, et al. Dietary cholesterol, fats and risk of Parkinson's disease in the Singapore Chinese Health Study. *J Neurol Neurosurg Psychiatry.* 2016; 87(1): 86–92.
57. Hirtz D, Thurman DJ, Gwinn-Hardy K, Mohamed M, Chaudhuri AR, Zalutsky R. How common are the 'common' neurologic disorders? *Neurology.* 2007; 68(5): 326–37.
58. Elbaz A, Bower JH, Maraganore DM, McDonnell SK, Peterson BJ, Ahlskog JE, et al. Risk tables for parkinsonism and Parkinson's disease. *J Clin Epidemiol.* 2002; 55(1): 25–31.
59. Winkler AS, Tutuncu E, Trendafilova A, Meindl M, Kaaya J, Schmutzhard E, et al. Parkinsonism in a population of northern Tanzania: a community-based door-to-door study in combination with a prospective hospital-based evaluation. *J Neurol.* 2010; 257(5): 799–805.
60. Dotchin C, Msuya O, Kissima J, Massawe J, Mhina A, Moshy A, et al. The prevalence of Parkinson's disease in rural Tanzania. *Mov Disord.* 2008; 23(11): 1567–672.
61. Okubadejo NU, Bower JH, Rocca WA, Maraganore DM. Parkinson's disease in Africa: A systematic review of epidemiologic and genetic studies. *Mov Disord.* 2006; 21(12): 2150–6.
62. Zhang ZX, Roman GC, Hong Z, Wu CB, Qu QM, Huang JB, et al. Parkinson's disease in China: prevalence in Beijing, Xian, and Shanghai. *Lancet.* 2005; 365(9459): 595–7.
63. Tan LC, Venketasubramanian N, Jamora RD, Heng D. Incidence of Parkinson's disease in Singapore. *Parkinsonism Relat Disord.* 2007; 13(1): 40–3.
64. Mayeux R, Marder K, Cote LJ, Denaro J, Hemenegildo N, Mejia H, et al. The frequency of idiopathic Parkinson's disease by age, ethnic group, and sex in northern Manhattan, 1988–1993. *Am J Epidemiol.* 1995; 142(8): 820–7.
65. Van Den Eeden SK, Tanner CM, Bernstein AL, Fross RD, Leimpeter A, Bloch DA, et al. Incidence of Parkinson's disease: variation by age, gender, and race/ethnicity. *Am J Epidemiol.* 2003; 157(11): 1015–22.
66. Wright Willis A, Evanoff BA, Lian M, Criswell SR, Racette BA. Geographic and ethnic variation in Parkinson disease: a population-based study of US Medicare beneficiaries. *Neuroepidemiology.* 2010; 34(3): 143–51.
67. Pearce N, Foliaki S, Sporle A, Cunningham C. Genetics, race, ethnicity, and health. *BMJ.* 2004; 328(7447): 1070–72.
68. Bower JH, Maraganore DM, McDonnell SK, Rocca WA. Incidence and distribution of parkinsonism in Olmsted County, Minnesota, 1976–1990. *Neurology.* 1999; 52(6): 1214–20.
69. Ascherio A, Schwarzschild MA. The epidemiology of Parkinson's disease: risk factors and prevention. *Lancet Neurology.* 2016; 15(12): 1257–72.
70. Wooten GF, Currie LJ, Bovbjerg VE, Lee JK, Patrie J. Are men at greater risk for Parkinson's disease than women? *J Neurol Neurosurg Psychiatry.* 2004; 75(4): 637–9.
71. Granieri E, Carreras M, Casetta I, Govoni V, Tola MR, Paolino E, et al. Parkinson's disease in Ferrara, Italy, 1967 through 1987. *Arch Neurol.* 1991; 48(8): 854–7.
72. de Rijk MC, Launer LJ, Berger K, Breteler MM, Dartigues JF, Baldereschi M, et al. Prevalence of Parkinson's disease in Europe: A collaborative study of population-based cohorts. Neurologic Diseases in the Elderly Research Group. *Neurology.* 2000; 54(11 Suppl 5): S21–23.
73. Taylor KS, Cook JA, Counsell CE. Heterogeneity in male to female risk for Parkinson's disease. *J Neurol Neurosurg Psychiatry.* 2007; 78(8): 905–6.
74. Bronstein J, Carvey P, Chen H, Cory-Slechta D, DiMonte D, Duda J, et al. Meeting report: consensus statement-Parkinson's disease and the environment: collaborative on health and the environment and Parkinson's Action Network (CHE PAN) conference 26–28 June 2007. *Environ Health Perspect.* 2009; 117(1): 117–21.
75. Collaborators GBDPsD. Global, regional, and national burden of Parkinson's disease, 1990-2016: a systematic analysis for the Global Burden of Disease Study 2016. *Lancet Neurology.* 2018; 17(11): 939–53.
76. Akushevich I, Kravchenko J, Ukraintseva S, Arbeev K, Yashin AI. Time trends of incidence of age-associated diseases in the US elderly population: Medicare-based analysis. *Age Ageing.* 2013; 42(4): 494–500.
77. Lix LM, Hobson DE, Azimaee M, Leslie WD, Burchill C, Hobson S. Socioeconomic variations in the prevalence and incidence of Parkinson's disease: a population-based analysis. *J Epidemiol Community Health.* 2010; 64(4): 335–40.
78. Savica R, Grossardt BR, Bower JH, Ahlskog JE, Rocca WA. Time trends in the incidence of Parkinson disease. *JAMA Neurol.* 2016; 73(8): 981–9.
79. Horsfall L, Petersen I, Walters K, Schrag A. Time trends in incidence of Parkinson's disease diagnosis in UK primary care. *J Neurol.* 2013; 260(5): 1351–7.
80. Darweesh SK, Koudstaal PJ, Stricker BH, Hofman A, Ikram MA. Trends in the Incidence of Parkinson disease in the general population: the Rotterdam Study. *Am J Epidemiol.* 2016; 183(11): 1018–26.
81. Quinn N, Critchley P, Marsden CD. Young onset Parkinson's disease. *Mov Disord.* 1987; 2(2): 73–91.
82. Schrag A, Schott JM. Epidemiological, clinical, and genetic characteristics of early-onset parkinsonism. *Lancet Neurology.* 2006; 5(4): 355–63.
83. Pagano G, Ferrara N, Brooks DJ, Pavese N. Age at onset and Parkinson disease phenotype. *Neurology.* 2016; 86(15): 1400–7.
84. Hely MA, Morris JG, Reid WG, O'Sullivan DJ, Williamson PM, Broe GA, et al. Age at onset: the major determinant of outcome in Parkinson's disease. *Acta Neurol Scand.* 1995; 92(6): 455–63.
85. Salawu FK. Patient considerations in early management of Parkinson's disease: focus on extended-release pramipexole. *Patient Prefer Adherence.* 2012; 6: 49–54.
86. Jankovic J, McDermott M, Carter J, Gauthier S, Goetz C, Golbe L, et al. Variable expression of Parkinson's disease: a base-line analysis of the DATATOP cohort. The Parkinson Study Group. *Neurology.* 1990; 40(10): 1529–34.
87. Hurt CS, Alkufri F, Brown RG, Burn DJ, Hindle JV, Landau S, et al. Motor phenotypes, medication and mood: further associations with impulsive behaviours in Parkinson's disease. *J Parkinsons Dis.* 2014; 4(2): 245–54.
88. Lewis SJ, Foltynie T, Blackwell AD, Robbins TW, Owen AM, Barker RA. Heterogeneity of Parkinson's disease in the early clinical stages using a data driven approach. *J Neurol Neurosurg Psychiatry.* 2005; 76(3): 343–8.
89. Rajput AH, Voll A, Rajput ML, Robinson CA, Rajput A. Course in Parkinson disease subtypes: A 39-year clinicopathologic study. *Neurology.* 2009; 73(3): 206–12.
90. Jankovic J, Kapadia AS. Functional decline in Parkinson disease. *Arch Neurol.* 2001; 58(10): 1611–15.

91. Alves G, Larsen JP, Emre M, Wentzel-Larsen T, Aarsland D. Changes in motor subtype and risk for incident dementia in Parkinson's disease. *Mov Disord*. 2006; 21(8): 1123–30.
92. Burn DJ, Rowan EN, Minett T, Sanders J, Myint P, Richardson J, et al. Extrapyramidal features in Parkinson's disease with and without dementia and dementia with Lewy bodies: A cross-sectional comparative study. *Mov Disord*. 2003; 18(8): 884–9.
93. Kotagal V. Is PIGD a legitimate motor subtype in Parkinson disease? *Ann Clin Transl Neurol*. 2016; 3(6): 473–7.
94. Fereshtehnejad SM, Postuma RB. Subtypes of Parkinson's Disease: What Do They Tell Us About Disease Progression? *Curr Neurol Neurosci Rep*. 2017; 17(4): 34.
95. Marras C. Subtypes of Parkinson's disease: state of the field and future directions. *Curr Opin Neurol*. 2015; 28(4): 382–6.
96. Anang JB, Gagnon JF, Bertrand JA, Romenets SR, Latreille V, Panisset M, et al. Predictors of dementia in Parkinson disease: a prospective cohort study. *Neurology*. 2014; 83(14): 1253–60.
97. Postuma RB, Bertrand JA, Montplaisir J, Desjardins C, Vendette M, Rios Romenets S, et al. Rapid eye movement sleep behavior disorder and risk of dementia in Parkinson's disease: a prospective study. *Mov Disord*. 2012; 27(6): 720–6.
98. Sixel-Doring F, Trautmann E, Mollenhauer B, Trenkwalder C. Associated factors for REM sleep behavior disorder in Parkinson disease. *Neurology*. 2011; 77(11): 1048–54.
99. Lee JE, Kim KS, Shin HW, Sohn YH. Factors related to clinically probable REM sleep behavior disorder in Parkinson disease. *Parkinsonism Relat Disord*. 2010; 16(2): 105–8.
100. Kumru H, Santamaria J, Tolosa E, Iranzo A. Relation between subtype of Parkinson's disease and REM sleep behavior disorder. *Sleep Med*. 2007; 8(7–8): 779–83.
101. Riedel O, Klotsche J, Spottke A, Deuschl G, Forstl H, Henn F, et al. Cognitive impairment in 873 patients with idiopathic Parkinson's disease. Results from the German Study on Epidemiology of Parkinson's Disease with Dementia (GEPAD). *J Neurol*. 2008; 255(2): 255–64.
102. Rolinski M, Szewczyk-Krolikowski K, Tomlinson PR, Nithi K, Talbot K, Ben-Shlomo Y, et al. REM sleep behaviour disorder is associated with worse quality of life and other non-motor features in early Parkinson's disease. *J Neurol Neurosurg Psychiatry*. 2014; 85(5): 560–6.
103. Thenganatt MA, Jankovic J. Parkinson disease subtypes. *JAMA Neurol*. 2014; 71(4): 499–504.
104. Bonifati V, Fabrizio E, Vanacore N, De Mari M, Meco G. Familial Parkinson's disease: a clinical genetic analysis. *Can J Neurol Sci*. 1995; 22(4): 272–9.
105. Klein C, Westenberger A. Genetics of Parkinson's disease. *Cold Spring Harb Perspect Med*. 2012; 2(1): a008888.
106. Polymeropoulos MH, Lavedan C, Leroy E, Ide SE, Dehejia A, Dutra A, et al. Mutation in the alpha-synuclein gene identified in families with Parkinson's disease. *Science*. 1997; 276(5321): 2045–7.
107. Kruger R, Kuhn W, Muller T, Woitalla D, Graeber M, Kosel S, et al. Ala30Pro mutation in the gene encoding alpha-synuclein in Parkinson's disease. *Nat Genet*. 1998; 18(2): 106–8.
108. Zarranz JJ, Alegre J, Gomez-Esteban JC, Lezcano E, Ros R, Ampuero I, et al. The new mutation, E46K, of alpha-synuclein causes Parkinson and Lewy body dementia. *Ann Neurol*. 2004; 55(2): 164–73.
109. Lesage S, Anheim M, Letournel F, Bousset L, Honore A, Rozas N, et al. G51D alpha-synuclein mutation causes a novel parkinsonian-pyramidal syndrome. *Ann Neurol*. 2013; 73(4): 459–71.
110. Kiely AP, Asi YT, Kara E, Limousin P, Ling H, Lewis P, et al. Alpha-synucleinopathy associated with G51D SNCA mutation: a link between Parkinson's disease and multiple system atrophy? *Acta Neuropathol*. 2013; 125(5): 753–69.
111. Chartier-Harlin MC, Kachergus J, Roumier C, Mouroux V, Douay X, Lincoln S, et al. Alpha-synuclein locus duplication as a cause of familial Parkinson's disease. *Lancet*. 2004; 364(9440): 1167–9.
112. Ibanez P, Bonnet AM, Debarges B, Lohmann E, Tison F, Pollak P, et al. Causal relation between alpha-synuclein gene duplication and familial Parkinson's disease. *Lancet*. 2004; 364(9440): 1169–71.
113. Singleton AB, Farrer M, Johnson J, Singleton A, Hague S, Kachergus J, et al. alpha-Synuclein locus triplication causes Parkinson's disease. *Science*. 2003; 302(5646): 841.
114. Lill CM, Bertram L. Towards unveiling the genetics of neurodegenerative diseases. *Semin Neurol*. 2011; 31(5): 531–41.
115. Brettschneider J, Del Tredici K, Lee VM, Trojanowski JQ. Spreading of pathology in neurodegenerative diseases: a focus on human studies. *Nat Rev Neurosci*. 2015; 16(2): 109–20.
116. Walsh DM, Selkoe DJ. A critical appraisal of the pathogenic protein spread hypothesis of neurodegeneration. *Nat Rev Neurosci*. 2016; 17(4): 251–60.
117. Zimprich A, Biskup S, Leitner P, Lichtner P, Farrer M, Lincoln S, et al. Mutations in LRRK2 cause autosomal-dominant parkinsonism with pleomorphic pathology. *Neuron*. 2004; 44(4): 601–7.
118. Paisan-Ruiz C, Jain S, Evans EW, Gilks WP, Simon J, van der Brug M, et al. Cloning of the gene containing mutations that cause PARK8-linked Parkinson's disease. *Neuron*. 2004; 44(4): 595–600.
119. Healy DG, Falchi M, O'Sullivan SS, Bonifati V, Durr A, Bressman S, et al. Phenotype, genotype, and worldwide genetic penetrance of LRRK2-associated Parkinson's disease: a case-control study. *Lancet Neurology*. 2008; 7(7): 583–90.
120. Ross OA, Soto-Ortolaza AI, Heckman MG, Aasly JO, Abahuni N, Annesi G, et al. Association of LRRK2 exonic variants with susceptibility to Parkinson's disease: a case-control study. *Lancet Neurology*. 2011; 10(10): 898–908.
121. Zimprich A, Benet-Pages A, Struhal W, Graf E, Eck SH, Offman MN, et al. A mutation in VPS35, encoding a subunit of the retromer complex, causes late-onset Parkinson disease. *Am J Hum Genet*. 2011; 89(1): 168–75.
122. Vilarino-Guell C, Wider C, Ross OA, Dachsel JC, Kachergus JM, Lincoln SJ, et al. VPS35 mutations in Parkinson disease. *Am J Hum Genet*. 2011; 89(1): 162–7.
123. Kitada T, Asakawa S, Hattori N, Matsumine H, Yamamura Y, Minoshima S, et al. Mutations in the parkin gene cause autosomal recessive juvenile parkinsonism. *Nature*. 1998; 392(6676): 605–8.
124. Valente EM, Abou-Sleiman PM, Caputo V, Muqit MM, Harvey K, Gispert S, et al. Hereditary early-onset Parkinson's disease caused by mutations in PINK1. *Science*. 2004; 304(5674): 1158–60.
125. Bonifati V, Rizzu P, van Baren MJ, Schaap O, Breedveld GJ, Krieger E, et al. Mutations in the DJ-1 gene associated with autosomal recessive early-onset parkinsonism. *Science*. 2003; 299(5604): 256–9.
126. Fitzgerald JC, Plun-Favreau H. Emerging pathways in genetic Parkinson's disease: autosomal-recessive genes in Parkinson's disease—a common pathway? FEBS J. 2008; 275(23): 5758–66.

127. Burbulla LF, Kruger R. Converging environmental and genetic pathways in the pathogenesis of Parkinson's disease. *J Neurol Sci*. 2011; 306(1–2): 1–8.
128. Ali SF, Binienda ZK, Imam SZ. Molecular aspects of dopaminergic neurodegeneration: gene-environment interaction in parkin dysfunction. *Int J Environ Res Public Health*. 2011; 8(12): 4702–13.
129. Wirdefeldt K, Gatz M, Reynolds CA, Prescott CA, Pedersen NL. Heritability of Parkinson disease in Swedish twins: a longitudinal study. *Neurobiol Aging*. 2011; 32(10): 1923 e1–8.
130. Urdinguio RG, Sanchez-Mut JV, Esteller M. Epigenetic mechanisms in neurological diseases: genes, syndromes, and therapies. *Lancet Neurology*. 2009; 8(11): 1056–72.
131. Kontopoulos E, Parvin JD, Feany MB. Alpha-synuclein acts in the nucleus to inhibit histone acetylation and promote neurotoxicity. *Hum Mol Genet*. 2006; 15(20): 3012–23.
132. Hernan MA, Takkouche B, Caamano-Isorna F, Gestal-Otero JJ. A meta-analysis of coffee drinking, cigarette smoking, and the risk of Parkinson's disease. *Ann Neurol*. 2002; 52(3): 276–84.
133. Li X, Li W, Liu G, Shen X, Tang Y. Association between cigarette smoking and Parkinson's disease: A meta-analysis. *Arch Gerontol Geriatr*. 2015; 61(3): 510–16.
134. Ritz B, Ascherio A, Checkoway H, Marder KS, Nelson LM, Rocca WA, et al. Pooled analysis of tobacco use and risk of Parkinson disease. *Arch Neurol*. 2007; 64(7): 990–97.
135. Gallo V, Vineis P, Cancellieri M, Chiodini P, Barker RA, Brayne C, et al. Exploring causality of the association between smoking and Parkinson's disease. *Int J Epidemiol*. 2019; 48(3): 912–25.
136. Ritz B, Lee PC, Lassen CF, Arah OA. Parkinson disease and smoking revisited: ease of quitting is an early sign of the disease. *Neurology*. 2014; 83(16): 1396–402.
137. Breckenridge CB, Berry C, Chang ET, Sielken RL, Jr, Mandel JS. Association between Parkinson's disease and cigarette smoking, rural living, well-water consumption, farming and pesticide use: systematic review and meta-analysis. *PLOS One*. 2016; 11(4): e0151841.
138. Crockford D, Quickfall J, Currie S, Furtado S, Suchowersky O, El-Guebaly N. Prevalence of problem and pathological gambling in Parkinson's disease. *Journal of GAMBLING STUDIES/ co-sponsored by the National Council on Problem Gambling and Institute for the Study of Gambling and Commercial Gaming*. 2008; 24(4): 411–22.
139. Madden PA, Heath AC, Pedersen NL, Kaprio J, Koskenvuo MJ, Martin NG. The genetics of smoking persistence in men and women: a multicultural study. *Behavior Genetics*. 1999; 29(6): 423–31.
140. Tanner CM, Goldman SM, Aston DA, Ottman R, Ellenberg J, Mayeux R, et al. Smoking and Parkinson's disease in twins. *Neurology*. 2002; 58(4): 581–8.
141. O'Reilly EJ, Chen H, Gardener H, Gao X, Schwarzschild MA, Ascherio A. Smoking and Parkinson's disease: using parental smoking as a proxy to explore causality. *Am J Epidemiol*. 2009; 169(6): 678–82.
142. Searles Nielsen S, Gallagher LG, Lundin JI, Longstreth WT, Jr., Smith-Weller T, Franklin GM, et al. Environmental tobacco smoke and Parkinson's disease. *Mov Disord*. 2012; 27(2): 293–6.
143. Mellick GD, Gartner CE, Silburn PA, Battistutta D. Passive smoking and Parkinson disease. *Neurology*. 2006; 67(1): 179–80.
144. Tanaka K, Miyake Y, Fukushima W, Sasaki S, Kiyohara C, Tsuboi Y, et al. Active and passive smoking and risk of Parkinson's disease. *Acta Neurol Scand*. 2010; 122(6): 377–82.
145. Costa J, Lunet N, Santos C, Santos J, Vaz-Carneiro A. Caffeine exposure and the risk of Parkinson's disease: a systematic review and meta-analysis of observational studies. *J Alzheimers Dis*. 2010; 20(Suppl 1): S221–38.
146. Qi H, Li S. Dose-response meta-analysis on coffee, tea and caffeine consumption with risk of Parkinson's disease. *Geriatr Gerontol Int*. 2014; 14(2): 430–9.
147. Ascherio A, Zhang SM, Hernan MA, Kawachi I, Colditz GA, Speizer FE, et al. Prospective study of caffeine consumption and risk of Parkinson's disease in men and women. *Ann Neurol*. 2001; 50(1): 56–63.
148. Ross GW, Abbott RD, Petrovitch H, Morens DM, Grandinetti A, Tung KH, et al. Association of coffee and caffeine intake with the risk of Parkinson disease. *JAMA*. 2000; 283(20): 2674–9.
149. Ascherio A, Chen H, Schwarzschild MA, Zhang SM, Colditz GA, Speizer FE. Caffeine, postmenopausal estrogen, and risk of Parkinson's disease. *Neurology*. 2003; 60(5): 790–5.
150. Pollock BG, Wylie M, Stack JA, Sorisio DA, Thompson DS, Kirshner MA, et al. Inhibition of caffeine metabolism by estrogen replacement therapy in postmenopausal women. *Journal of Clinical Pharmacology*. 1999; 39(9): 936–40.
151. Hamza TH, Chen H, Hill-Burns EM, Rhodes SL, Montimurro J, Kay DM, et al. Genome-wide gene-environment study identifies glutamate receptor gene GRIN2A as a Parkinson's disease modifier gene via interaction with coffee. *PLOS Genetics*. 2011; 7(8): e1002237.
152. Hamza TH, Hill-Burns EM, Scott WK, Vance JM, Factor SA, Zabetian CP, et al. Glutamate receptor gene GRIN2A, coffee, and Parkinson disease. *PLOS Genetics*. 2014; 10(11): e1004774.
153. Yamada-Fowler N, Fredrikson M, Soderkvist P. Caffeine interaction with glutamate receptor gene GRIN2A: Parkinson's disease in Swedish population. *PLOS One*. 2014; 9(6): e99294.
154. Ahmed I, Lee PC, Lill CM, Searles Nielsen S, Artaud F, Gallagher LG, et al. Lack of replication of the GRIN2A-by-coffee interaction in Parkinson disease. *PLOS Genetics*. 2014; 10(11): e1004788.
155. Yamada-Fowler N, Soderkvist P. Coffee, genetic variants, and Parkinson's disease: gene-environment interactions. *Journal of Caffeine Research*. 2015; 5(1): 3–10.
156. Gatto EM, Melcon C, Parisi VL, Bartoloni L, Gonzalez CD. Inverse association between yerba mate consumption and idiopathic Parkinson's disease. A case-control study. *J Neurol Sci*. 2015; 356(1–2): 163–7.
157. Gentleman SM, Leclercq PD, Moyes L, Graham DI, Smith C, Griffin WS, et al. Long-term intracerebral inflammatory response after traumatic brain injury. *Forensic Sci Int*. 2004; 146(2–3): 97–104.
158. Lenzlinger PM, Morganti-Kossmann MC, Laurer HL, McIntosh TK. The duality of the inflammatory response to traumatic brain injury. *Mol Neurobiol*. 2001; 24(1–3): 169–81.
159. Schmidt OI, Heyde CE, Ertel W, Stahel PF. Closed head injury—an inflammatory disease? *Brain Res Brain Res Rev*. 2005; 48(2): 388–99.
160. Arundine M, Tymianski M. Molecular mechanisms of glutamate-dependent neurodegeneration in ischemia and traumatic brain injury. *Cell Mol Life Sci*. 2004; 61(6): 657–68.
161. Liu PK, Robertson CS, Valadka A. The association between neuronal nitric oxide synthase and neuronal sensitivity in the brain after brain injury. *Ann N Y Acad Sci*. 2002; 962: 226–41.
162. Newell KL, Boyer P, Gomez-Tortosa E, Hobbs W, Hedley-Whyte ET, Vonsattel JP, et al. Alpha-synuclein immunoreactivity is present in axonal swellings in neuroaxonal

dystrophy and acute traumatic brain injury. *J Neuropathol Exp Neurol*. 1999; 58(12): 1263–8.
163. Smith DH, Uryu K, Saatman KE, Trojanowski JQ, McIntosh TK. Protein accumulation in traumatic brain injury. *Neuromolecular Med*. 2003; 4(1–2): 59–72.
164. Uryu K, Giasson BI, Longhi L, Martinez D, Murray I, Conte V, et al. Age-dependent synuclein pathology following traumatic brain injury in mice. *Exp Neurol*. 2003; 184(1): 214–24.
165. Rugbjerg K, Ritz B, Korbo L, Martinussen N, Olsen JH. Risk of Parkinson's disease after hospital contact for head injury: population based case-control study. *BMJ*. 2008; 337: a2494.
166. Harris MA, Shen H, Marion SA, Tsui JK, Teschke K. Head injuries and Parkinson's disease in a case-control study. *Occup Environ Med*. 2013; 70(12): 839–44.
167. Goldman SM, Tanner CM, Oakes D, Bhudhikanok GS, Gupta A, Langston JW. Head injury and Parkinson's disease risk in twins. *Ann Neurol*. 2006; 60(1): 65–72.
168. Seidler A, Hellenbrand W, Robra BP, Vieregge P, Nischan P, Joerg J, et al. Possible environmental, occupational, and other etiologic factors for Parkinson's disease: a case-control study in Germany. *Neurology*. 1996; 46(5): 1275–84.
169. Kuopio AM, Marttila RJ, Helenius H, Rinne UK. Environmental risk factors in Parkinson's disease. *Mov Disord*. 1999; 14(6): 928–39.
170. Bower JH, Maraganore DM, Peterson BJ, McDonnell SK, Ahlskog JE, Rocca WA. Head trauma preceding PD: a case-control study. *Neurology*. 2003; 60(10): 1610–15.
171. Semchuk KM, Love EJ, Lee RG. Parkinson's disease: a test of the multifactorial etiologic hypothesis. *Neurology*. 1993; 43(6): 1173–80.
172. De Michele G, Filla A, Volpe G, De Marco V, Gogliettino A, Ambrosio G, et al. Environmental and genetic risk factors in Parkinson's disease: a case-control study in southern Italy. *Mov Disord*. 1996; 11(1): 17–23.
173. Taylor CA, Saint-Hilaire MH, Cupples LA, Thomas CA, Burchard AE, Feldman RG, et al. Environmental, medical, and family history risk factors for Parkinson's disease: a New England-based case control study. *Am J Med Genet*. 1999; 88(6): 742–9.
174. Bharucha NE, Stokes L, Schoenberg BS, Ward C, Ince S, Nutt JG, et al. A case-control study of twin pairs discordant for Parkinson's disease: a search for environmental risk factors. *Neurology*. 1986; 36(2): 284–8.
175. Williams DB, Annegers JF, Kokmen E, O'Brien PC, Kurland LT. Brain injury and neurologic sequelae: a cohort study of dementia, parkinsonism, and amyotrophic lateral sclerosis. *Neurology*. 1991; 41(10): 1554–7.
176. Morano A, Jimenez-Jimenez FJ, Molina JA, Antolin MA. Risk-factors for Parkinson's disease: case-control study in the province of Caceres, Spain. *Acta Neurol Scand*. 1994; 89(3): 164–70.
177. Martyn CN, Osmond C. Parkinson's disease and the environment in early life. *J Neurol Sci*. 1995; 132(2): 201–6.
178. Werneck AL, Alvarenga H. Genetics, drugs and environmental factors in Parkinson's disease. A case-control study. *Arq Neuropsiquiatr*. 1999; 57(2B): 347–55.
179. McCann SJ, LeCouteur DG, Green AC, Brayne C, Johnson AG, Chan D, et al. The epidemiology of Parkinson's disease in an Australian population. *Neuroepidemiology*. 1998; 17(6): 310–17.
180. Marras C, Hincapie CA, Kristman VL, Cancelliere C, Soklaridis S, Li A, et al. Systematic review of the risk of Parkinson's disease after mild traumatic brain injury: results of the International Collaboration on Mild Traumatic Brain Injury Prognosis. *Archives of Physical Medicine and Rehabilitation*. 2014; 95(3 Suppl): S238–44.
181. Gao J, Liu R, Zhao E, Huang X, Nalls MA, Singleton AB, et al. Head injury, potential interaction with genes, and risk for Parkinson's disease. *Parkinsonism Relat Disord*. 2015; 21(3): 292–6.
182. Taylor KM, Saint-Hilaire MH, Sudarsky L, Simon DK, Hersh B, Sparrow D, et al. Head injury at early ages is associated with risk of Parkinson's disease. *Parkinsonism Relat Disord*. 2016; 23: 57–61.
183. Lehman EJ, Hein MJ, Baron SL, Gersic CM. Neurodegenerative causes of death among retired National Football League players. *Neurology*. 2012; 79(19): 1970–4.
184. Chan YE, Bai YM, Hsu JW, Huang KL, Su TP, Li CT, et al. Post-traumatic stress disorder and risk of Parkinson disease: a nationwide longitudinal study. *Am J Geriatr Psychiatry*. 2017; 25(8): 917–23
185. Agim ZS, Cannon JR. Dietary factors in the etiology of Parkinson's disease. *Biomed Res Int*. 2015; 2015: 672838.
186. Takeda A, Nyssen OP, Syed A, Jansen E, Bueno-de-Mesquita B, Gallo V. Vitamin A and carotenoids and the risk of Parkinson's disease: a systematic review and meta-analysis. *Neuroepidemiology*. 2014; 42(1): 25–38.
187. Dexter DT, Wells FR, Lees AJ, Agid F, Agid Y, Jenner P, et al. Increased nigral iron content and alterations in other metal ions occurring in brain in Parkinson's disease. *J Neurochem*. 1989; 52(6): 1830–6.
188. Logroscino G, Gao X, Chen H, Wing A, Ascherio A. Dietary iron intake and risk of Parkinson's disease. *Am J Epidemiol*. 2008; 168(12): 1381–8.
189. Logroscino G, Chen H, Wing A, Ascherio A. Blood donations, iron stores, and risk of Parkinson's disease. *Mov Disord*. 2006; 21(6): 835–8.
190. Savica R, Grossardt BR, Carlin JM, Icen M, Bower JH, Ahlskog JE, et al. Anemia or low hemoglobin levels preceding Parkinson disease: a case-control study. *Neurology*. 2009; 73(17): 1381–7.
191. Hong CT, Huang YH, Liu HY, Chiou HY, Chan L, Chien LN. Newly diagnosed anemia increases risk of Parkinson's disease: a population-based cohort study. *Sci Rep*. 2016; 6: 29651.
192. Gao X, Chen H, Fung TT, Logroscino G, Schwarzschild MA, Hu FB, et al. Prospective study of dietary pattern and risk of Parkinson disease. *Am J Clin Nutr*. 2007; 86(5): 1486–94.
193. Chen H, Zhang SM, Hernan MA, Willett WC, Ascherio A. Diet and Parkinson's disease: a potential role of dairy products in men. *Ann Neurol*. 2002; 52(6): 793–801.
194. Park M, Ross GW, Petrovitch H, White LR, Masaki KH, Nelson JS, et al. Consumption of milk and calcium in mid-life and the future risk of Parkinson disease. *Neurology*. 2005; 64(6): 1047–51.
195. Saaksjarvi K, Knekt P, Lundqvist A, Mannisto S, Heliovaara M, Rissanen H, et al. A cohort study on diet and the risk of Parkinson's disease: the role of food groups and diet quality. *Br J Nutr*. 2013; 109(2): 329–37.
196. Kyrozis A, Ghika A, Stathopoulos P, Vassilopoulos D, Trichopoulos D, Trichopoulou A. Dietary and lifestyle variables in relation to incidence of Parkinson's disease in Greece. *Eur J Epidemiol*. 2013; 28(1): 67–77.
197. Jiang W, Ju C, Jiang H, Zhang D. Dairy foods intake and risk of Parkinson's disease: a dose-response meta-analysis of prospective cohort studies. *Eur J Epidemiol*. 2014; 29(9): 613–19.
198. Abbott RD, Ross GW, Petrovitch H, Masaki KH, Launer LJ, Nelson JS, et al. Midlife milk consumption and substantia nigra neuron density at death. *Neurology*. 2016; 86(6): 512–19.

199. Choi HK, Atkinson K, Karlson EW, Willett W, Curhan G. Purine-rich foods, dairy and protein intake, and the risk of gout in men. *N Engl J Med.* 2004; 350(11): 1093–1103.
200. Weisskopf MG, O'Reilly E, Chen H, Schwarzschild MA, Ascherio A. Plasma urate and risk of Parkinson's disease. *Am J Epidemiol.* 2007; 166(5): 561–7.
201. O'Reilly EJ, Gao X, Weisskopf MG, Chen H, Schwarzschild MA, Spiegelman D, et al. Plasma urate and Parkinson's disease in women. *Am J Epidemiol.* 2010; 172(6): 666–70.
202. Jain S, Ton TG, Boudreau RM, Yang M, Thacker EL, Studenski S, et al. The risk of Parkinson disease associated with urate in a community-based cohort of older adults. *Neuroepidemiology.* 2011; 36(4): 223–9.
203. Gao X, O'Reilly EJ, Schwarzschild MA, Ascherio A. Prospective study of plasma urate and risk of Parkinson disease in men and women. *Neurology.* 2016; 86(6): 520–6.
204. Facheris MF, Hicks AA, Minelli C, Hagenah JM, Kostic V, Campbell S, et al. Variation in the uric acid transporter gene SLC2A9 and its association with AAO of Parkinson's disease. *J Mol Neurosci.* 2011; 43(3): 246–50.
205. Gonzalez-Aramburu I, Sanchez-Juan P, Jesus S, Gorostidi A, Fernandez-Juan E, Carrillo F, et al. Genetic variability related to serum uric acid concentration and risk of Parkinson's disease. *Mov Disord.* 2013; 28(12): 1737–40.
206. Gao J, Xu H, Huang X, Chen H. Short communication: genetic variations of SLC2A9 in relation to Parkinson's disease. *Transl Neurodegener.* 2013; 2(1): 5.
207. Simon KC, Eberly S, Gao X, Oakes D, Tanner CM, Shoulson I, et al. Mendelian randomization of serum urate and Parkinson disease progression. *Ann Neurol.* 2014; 76(6): 862–8.
208. Di Monte DA. The environment and Parkinson's disease: is the nigrostriatal system preferentially targeted by neurotoxins? Lancet Neurology. 2003; 2(9): 531–8.
209. Cannon JR, Greenamyre JT. The role of environmental exposures in neurodegeneration and neurodegenerative diseases. *Toxicol Sci.* 2011; 124(2): 225–50.
210. Gao HM, Hong JS. Gene-environment interactions: key to unraveling the mystery of Parkinson's disease. *Prog Neurobiol.* 2011; 94(1): 1–19.
211. Ross CA, Smith WW. Gene-environment interactions in Parkinson's disease. *Parkinsonism Relat Disord.* 2007; 13 (Suppl 3): S309–315.
212. Cannon JR, Greenamyre JT. Gene-environment interactions in Parkinson's disease: specific evidence in humans and mammalian models. *Neurobiol Dis.* 2013; 57: 38–46.
213. Dick FD, De Palma G, Ahmadi A, Scott NW, Prescott GJ, Bennett J, et al. Environmental risk factors for Parkinson's disease and parkinsonism: the Geoparkinson study. *Occup Environ Med.* 2007; 64(10): 666–72.
214. Caudle WM, Guillot TS, Lazo CR, Miller GW. Industrial toxicants and Parkinson's disease. *Neurotoxicology.* 2012; 33(2): 178–88.
215. Gunnarsson LG, Bodin L. Parkinson's disease and occupational exposures: a systematic literature review and meta-analyses. *Scand J Work Environ Health.* 2017; 43(3): 197–209.
216. Coon S, Stark A, Peterson E, Gloi A, Kortsha G, Pounds J, et al. Whole-body lifetime occupational lead exposure and risk of Parkinson's disease. *Environ Health Perspect.* 2006; 114(12): 1872–6.
217. Feldman AL, Johansson AL, Nise G, Gatz M, Pedersen NL, Wirdefeldt K. Occupational exposure in parkinsonian disorders: a 43-year prospective cohort study in men. *Parkinsonism Relat Disord.* 2011; 17(9): 677–82.
218. Firestone JA, Lundin JI, Powers KM, Smith-Weller T, Franklin GM, Swanson PD, et al. Occupational factors and risk of Parkinson's disease: a population-based case-control study. *Am J Ind Med.* 2010; 53(3): 217–23.
219. Frigerio R, Elbaz A, Sanft KR, Peterson BJ, Bower JH, Ahlskog JE, et al. Education and occupations preceding Parkinson disease: a population-based case-control study. *Neurology.* 2005; 65(10): 1575–83.
220. Gorell JM, Johnson CC, Rybicki BA, Peterson EL, Kortsha GX, Brown GG, et al. Occupational exposures to metals as risk factors for Parkinson's disease. *Neurology.* 1997; 48(3): 650–8.
221. Noonan CW, Reif JS, Yost M, Touchstone J. Occupational exposure to magnetic fields in case-referent studies of neurodegenerative diseases. *Scand J Work Environ Health.* 2002; 28(1): 42–8.
222. Savitz DA, Checkoway H, Loomis DP. Magnetic field exposure and neurodegenerative disease mortality among electric utility workers. *Epidemiology.* 1998; 9(4): 398–404.
223. Feychting M, Jonsson F, Pedersen NL, Ahlbom A. Occupational magnetic field exposure and neurodegenerative disease. *Epidemiology.* 2003; 14(4): 413–19; discussion 27–8.
224. Hakansson N, Gustavsson P, Johansen C, Floderus B. Neurodegenerative diseases in welders and other workers exposed to high levels of magnetic fields. *Epidemiology.* 2003; 14(4): 420–6; discussion 7–8.
225. Johansen C, Olsen JH. Mortality from amyotrophic lateral sclerosis, other chronic disorders, and electric shocks among utility workers. *Am J Epidemiol.* 1998; 148(4): 362–8.
226. Johansen C. Exposure to electromagnetic fields and risk of central nervous system disease in utility workers. *Epidemiology.* 2000; 11(5): 539–43.
227. Park RM, Schulte PA, Bowman JD, Walker JT, Bondy SC, Yost MG, et al. Potential occupational risks for neurodegenerative diseases. *Am J Ind Med.* 2005; 48(1): 63–77.
228. Roosli M, Lortscher M, Egger M, Pfluger D, Schreier N, Lortscher E, et al. Mortality from neurodegenerative disease and exposure to extremely low-frequency magnetic fields: 31 years of observations on Swiss railway employees. *Neuroepidemiology.* 2007; 28(4): 197–206.
229. Savitz DA, Loomis DP, Tse CK. Electrical occupations and neurodegenerative disease: analysis of US mortality data. *Arch Environ Health.* 1998; 53(1): 71–4.
230. Tanner CM, Ross GW, Jewell SA, Hauser RA, Jankovic J, Factor SA, et al. Occupation and risk of parkinsonism: a multicenter case-control study. *Arch Neurol.* 2009; 66(9): 1106–13.
231. Huss A, Koeman T, Kromhout H, Vermeulen R. Extremely low frequency magnetic field exposure and Parkinson's disease—a systematic review and meta-analysis of the data. *Int J Environ Res Public Health.* 2015; 12(7): 7348–56.
232. Reis J, Benbrick E, Bonneterre V, Spencer PS. Parkinson's disease and solvents: is there a causal link? *Rev Neurol* (Paris). 2016; 172(12): 761–5.
233. Hageman G, van der Hoek J, van Hout M, van der Laan G, Steur EJ, de Bruin W, et al. Parkinsonism, pyramidal signs, polyneuropathy, and cognitive decline after long-term occupational solvent exposure. *J Neurol.* 1999; 246(3): 198–206.
234. Ohlson CG, Hogstedt C. Parkinson's disease and occupational exposure to organic solvents, agricultural chemicals and mercury—a case-referent study. *Scand J Work Environ Health.* 1981; 7(4): 252–6.
235. Petersen MS, Halling J, Bech S, Wermuth L, Weihe P, Nielsen F, et al. Impact of dietary exposure to food contaminants

on the risk of Parkinson's disease. *Neurotoxicology*. 2008; 29(4): 584–90.

236. Brouwer M, Koeman T, van den Brandt PA, Kromhout H, Schouten LJ, Peters S, et al. Occupational exposures and Parkinson's disease mortality in a prospective Dutch cohort. *Occup Environ Med*. 2015; 72(6): 448–55.
237. Hertzman C, Wiens M, Snow B, Kelly S, Calne D. A case-control study of Parkinson's disease in a horticultural region of British Columbia. *Mov Disord*. 1994; 9(1): 69–75.
238. Gorell JM, Johnson CC, Rybicki BA, Peterson EL, Richardson RJ. The risk of Parkinson's disease with exposure to pesticides, farming, well water, and rural living. *Neurology*. 1998; 50(5): 1346–50.
239. Tuchsen F, Jensen AA. Agricultural work and the risk of Parkinson's disease in Denmark, 1981–1993. *Scand J Work Environ Health*. 2000; 26(4): 359–62.
240. Langston JW, Ballard P, Tetrud JW, Irwin I. Chronic Parkinsonism in humans due to a product of meperidine-analog synthesis. *Science*. 1983; 219(4587): 979–80.
241. Ritz BR, Paul KC, Bronstein JM. Of pesticides and men: a California story of genes and environment in Parkinson's disease. *Current Environmental Health Reports*. 2016; 3(1): 40–52.
242. van der Mark M, Brouwer M, Kromhout H, Nijssen P, Huss A, Vermeulen R. Is pesticide use related to Parkinson disease? Some clues to heterogeneity in study results. *Environmental Health Perspectives*. 2012; 120(3): 340–7.
243. Elbaz A, Clavel J, Rathouz PJ, Moisan F, Galanaud JP, Delemotte B, et al. Professional exposure to pesticides and Parkinson disease. *Annals of Neurology*. 2009; 66(4): 494–504.
244. Hancock DB, Martin ER, Mayhew GM, Stajich JM, Jewett R, Stacy MA, et al. Pesticide exposure and risk of Parkinson's disease: a family-based case-control study. *BMC Neurology*. 2008; 8:6.
245. Richardson JR, Roy A, Shalat SL, Buckley B, Winnik B, Gearing M, et al. beta-Hexachlorocyclohexane levels in serum and risk of Parkinson's disease. *Neurotoxicology*. 2011; 32(5): 640–5.
246. Moisan F, Spinosi J, Delabre L, Gourlet V, Mazurie JL, Benatru I, et al. Association of Parkinson's disease and its subtypes with agricultural pesticide exposures in men: a case-control study in France. *Environmental Health Perspectives*. 2015; 123(11): 1123–9.
247. Elbaz A, Moisan F. The scientific bases to consider Parkinson's disease an occupational disease in agriculture professionals exposed to pesticides in France. *J Epidemiol Community Health*. 2016; 70(4): 319–21.
248. Elbaz A, Levecque C, Clavel J, Vidal JS, Richard F, Amouyel P, et al. CYP2D6 polymorphism, pesticide exposure, and Parkinson's disease. *Annals of Neurology*. 2004; 55(3): 430–4.
249. Dutheil F, Beaune P, Tzourio C, Loriot MA, Elbaz A. Interaction between ABCB1 and professional exposure to organochlorine insecticides in Parkinson disease. *Archives of Neurology*. 2010; 67(6): 739–45.
250. Lee PC, Rhodes SL, Sinsheimer JS, Bronstein J, Ritz B. Functional paraoxonase 1 variants modify the risk of Parkinson's disease due to organophosphate exposure. *Environment International*. 2013; 56: 42–7.
251. Fitzmaurice AG, Rhodes SL, Cockburn M, Ritz B, Bronstein JM. Aldehyde dehydrogenase variation enhances effect of pesticides associated with Parkinson disease. *Neurology*. 2014; 82(5): 419–26.
252. Chen H, Schernhammer E, Schwarzschild MA, Ascherio A. A prospective study of night shift work, sleep duration, and risk of Parkinson's disease. *Am J Epidemiol*. 2006; 163(8): 726–30.
253. Dick S, Semple S, Dick F, Seaton A. Occupational titles as risk factors for Parkinson's disease. *Occup Med* (Lond). 2007; 57(1): 50–56.
254. Harris MA, Marion SA, Spinelli JJ, Tsui JK, Teschke K. Occupational exposure to whole-body vibration and Parkinson's disease: results from a population-based case-control study. *Am J Epidemiol*. 2012; 176(4): 299–307.
255. Harris MA, Tsui JK, Marion SA, Shen H, Teschke K. Association of Parkinson's disease with infections and occupational exposure to possible vectors. *Mov Disord*. 2012; 27(9): 1111–7.
256. Valdes EG, Andel R, Sieurin J, Feldman AL, Edwards JD, Langstrom N, et al. Occupational complexity and risk of Parkinson's disease. *PLOS One*. 2014; 9(9): e106676.
257. Gao X, Chen H, Schwarzschild MA, Ascherio A. Use of ibuprofen and risk of Parkinson disease. *Neurology*. 2011; 76(10): 863–9.
258. Asanuma M, Miyazaki I. Nonsteroidal anti-inflammatory drugs in experimental parkinsonian models and Parkinson's disease. *Curr Pharm Des*. 2008; 14(14): 1428–34.
259. Asanuma M, Miyazaki I. Common anti-inflammatory drugs are potentially therapeutic for Parkinson's disease? *Exp Neurol*. 2007; 206(2): 172–8.
260. Tsuji T, Asanuma M, Miyazaki I, Miyoshi K, Ogawa N. Reduction of nuclear peroxisome proliferator-activated receptor gamma expression in methamphetamine-induced neurotoxicity and neuroprotective effects of ibuprofen. *Neurochem Res*. 2009; 34(4): 764–74.
261. Becker C, Jick SS, Meier CR. Use of antihypertensives and the risk of Parkinson disease. *Neurology*. 2008; 70(16 Pt 2): 1438–44.
262. Ritz B, Rhodes SL, Qian L, Schernhammer E, Olsen JH, Friis S. L-type calcium channel blockers and Parkinson disease in Denmark. *Ann Neurol*. 2010; 67(5): 600–6.
263. Pasternak B, Svanstrom H, Nielsen NM, Fugger L, Melbye M, Hviid A. Use of calcium channel blockers and Parkinson's disease. *Am J Epidemiol*. 2012; 175(7): 627–35.
264. Lee YC, Lin CH, Wu RM, Lin JW, Chang CH, Lai MS. Antihypertensive agents and risk of Parkinson's disease: a nationwide cohort study. *PLOS One*. 2014; 9(6): e98961.
265. Simon KC, Gao X, Chen H, Schwarzschild MA, Ascherio A. Calcium channel blocker use and risk of Parkinson's disease. *Mov Disord*. 2010; 25(12): 1818–22.
266. Ton TG, Heckbert SR, Longstreth WT, Jr, Rossing MA, Kukull WA, Franklin GM, et al. Calcium channel blockers and beta-blockers in relation to Parkinson's disease. *Parkinsonism Relat Disord*. 2007; 13(3): 165–9.
267. Undela K, Gudala K, Malla S, Bansal D. Statin use and risk of Parkinson's disease: a meta-analysis of observational studies. *J Neurol*. 2013; 260(1): 158–65.
268. Lin KD, Yang CY, Lee MY, Ho SC, Liu CK, Shin SJ. Statin therapy prevents the onset of Parkinson disease in patients with diabetes. *Ann Neurol*. 2016; 80(4): 532–40.
269. Shults CW, Oakes D, Kieburtz K, Beal MF, Haas R, Plumb S, et al. Effects of coenzyme Q10 in early Parkinson disease: evidence of slowing of the functional decline. *Arch Neurol*. 2002; 59(10): 1541–50.
270. Li X, Sundquist J, Sundquist K. Socioeconomic and occupational groups and Parkinson's disease: a nationwide study based on hospitalizations in Sweden. *Int Arch Occup Environ Health*. 2009; 82(2): 235–41.

271. Caslake R, Taylor K, Scott N, Gordon J, Harris C, Wilde K, et al. Age-, gender-, and socioeconomic status-specific incidence of Parkinson's disease and parkinsonism in northeast Scotland: the PINE study. *Parkinsonism Relat Disord.* 2013; 19(5): 515–21.
272. Wang YL, Wang YT, Li JF, Zhang YZ, Yin HL, Han B. Body mass index and risk of Parkinson's disease: a dose-response meta-analysis of prospective studies. *PLOS One.* 2015; 10(6): e0131778.
273. Abbott RD, Ross GW, White LR, Nelson JS, Masaki KH, Tanner CM, et al. Midlife adiposity and the future risk of Parkinson's disease. *Neurology.* 2002; 59(7): 1051–7.
274. Chen H, Zhang SM, Schwarzschild MA, Hernan MA, Willett WC, Ascherio A. Obesity and the risk of Parkinson's disease. *Am J Epidemiol.* 2004; 159(6): 547–55.
275. Hu G, Jousilahti P, Nissinen A, Antikainen R, Kivipelto M, Tuomilehto J. Body mass index and the risk of Parkinson disease. *Neurology.* 2006; 67(11): 1955–9.
276. Zhang D, Jiang H, Xie J. Alcohol intake and risk of Parkinson's disease: a meta-analysis of observational studies. *Mov Disord.* 2014; 29(6): 819–22.
277. Eriksson AK, Lofving S, Callaghan RC, Allebeck P. Alcohol use disorders and risk of Parkinson's disease: findings from a Swedish national cohort study 1972–2008. *BMC Neurol.* 2013; 13: 190.
278. Simon KC, Chen H, Gao X, Schwarzschild MA, Ascherio A. Reproductive factors, exogenous estrogen use, and risk of Parkinson's disease. *Mov Disord.* 2009; 24(9): 1359–65.
279. Rugbjerg K, Christensen J, Tjonneland A, Olsen JH. Exposure to estrogen and women's risk for Parkinson's disease: a prospective cohort study in Denmark. *Parkinsonism Relat Disord.* 2013; 19(4): 457–60.
280. Liu R, Baird D, Park Y, Freedman ND, Huang X, Hollenbeck A, et al. Female reproductive factors, menopausal hormone use, and Parkinson's disease. *Mov Disord.* 2014; 29(7): 889–96.
281. Rocca WA, Bower JH, Maraganore DM, Ahlskog JE, Grossardt BR, de Andrade M, et al. Increased risk of parkinsonism in women who underwent oophorectomy before menopause. *Neurology.* 2008; 70(3): 200–9.
282. Huang X, Abbott RD, Petrovitch H, Mailman RB, Ross GW. Low LDL cholesterol and increased risk of Parkinson's disease: prospective results from Honolulu-Asia Aging Study. *Mov Disord.* 2008; 23(7): 1013–18.
283. Yang F, Trolle Lagerros Y, Bellocco R, Adami HO, Fang F, Pedersen NL, et al. Physical activity and risk of Parkinson's disease in the Swedish National March Cohort. *Brain: Journal of Neurology.* 2015; 138(Pt 2): 269–75.
284. Chen H, Zhang SM, Schwarzschild MA, Hernan MA, Ascherio A. Physical activity and the risk of Parkinson disease. *Neurology.* 2005; 64(4): 664–9.
285. Xu Q, Park Y, Huang X, Hollenbeck A, Blair A, Schatzkin A, et al. Physical activities and future risk of Parkinson disease. *Neurology.* 2010; 75(4): 341–8.
286. Hirsch MA, Iyer SS, Sanjak M. Exercise-induced neuroplasticity in human Parkinson's disease: What is the evidence telling us? *Parkinsonism Relat Disord.* 2016; 22(Suppl 1): S78–81.
287. Bajaj A, Driver JA, Schernhammer ES. Parkinson's disease and cancer risk: a systematic review and meta-analysis. *Cancer Causes Control.* 2010; 21(5): 697–707.
288. Liu R, Gao X, Lu Y, Chen H. Meta-analysis of the relationship between Parkinson disease and melanoma. *Neurology.* 2011; 76(23): 2002–9.
289. Fiala KH, Whetteckey J, Manyam BV. Malignant melanoma and levodopa in Parkinson's disease: causality or coincidence? *Parkinsonism Relat Disord.* 2003; 9(6): 321–7.
290. Constantinescu R, Romer M, Kieburtz K, Group DIotPS. Malignant melanoma in early Parkinson's disease: the DATATOP trial. *Mov Disord.* 2007; 22(5): 720–2.
291. Schwid SR, Bausch J, Oakes D, Schuchter L, Tanner C, Forrest M, et al. Cancer incidence in a trial of an antiapoptotic agent for Parkinson's disease. *Mov Disord.* 2010; 25(12): 1801–8.
292. Constantinescu R, Elm J, Auinger P, Sharma S, Augustine EF, Khadim L, et al. Malignant melanoma in early-treated Parkinson's disease: the NET-PD trial. *Mov Disord.* 2014; 29(2): 263–5.
293. Gao X, Simon KC, Han J, Schwarzschild MA, Ascherio A. Genetic determinants of hair color and Parkinson's disease risk. *Ann Neurol.* 2009; 65(1): 76–82.
294. Lubbe SJ, Escott-Price V, Brice A, Gasser T, Hardy J, Heutink P, et al. Is the MC1R variant p.R160W associated with Parkinson's? *Ann Neurol.* 2016; 79(1): 159–61.
295. Meng S, Song F, Chen H, Gao X, Amos CI, Lee JE, et al. No association between Parkinson disease alleles and the risk of melanoma. *Cancer Epidemiol Biomarkers Prev.* 2012; 21(1): 243–5.
296. Lubbe SJ, Escott-Price V, Gibbs JR, Nalls MA, Bras J, Price TR, et al. Additional rare variant analysis in Parkinson's disease cases with and without known pathogenic mutations: evidence for oligogenic inheritance. *Hum Mol Genet.* 2016; 25(24): 5483–9.
297. Chen X, Feng D, Schwarzschild MA, Gao X. Red hair, MC1R variants, and risk for Parkinson's disease—a meta-analysis. *Ann Clin Transl Neurol.* 2017; 4(3): 212–16.
298. Schernhammer E, Hansen J, Rugbjerg K, Wermuth L, Ritz B. Diabetes and the risk of developing Parkinson's disease in Denmark. *Diabetes Care.* 2011; 34(5): 1102–8.
299. Sun Y, Chang YH, Chen HF, Su YH, Su HF, Li CY. Risk of Parkinson disease onset in patients with diabetes: a 9-year population-based cohort study with age and sex stratifications. *Diabetes Care.* 2012; 35(5): 1047–49.
300. Driver JA, Smith A, Buring JE, Gaziano JM, Kurth T, Logroscino G. Prospective cohort study of type 2 diabetes and the risk of Parkinson's disease. *Diabetes Care.* 2008; 31(10): 2003–5.
301. Xu Q, Park Y, Huang X, Hollenbeck A, Blair A, Schatzkin A, et al. Diabetes and risk of Parkinson's disease. *Diabetes Care.* 2011; 34(4): 910–15.
302. Simon KC, Chen H, Schwarzschild M, Ascherio A. Hypertension, hypercholesterolemia, diabetes, and risk of Parkinson disease. *Neurology.* 2007; 69(17): 1688–95.
303. Lu L, Fu DL, Li HQ, Liu AJ, Li JH, Zheng GQ. Diabetes and risk of Parkinson's disease: an updated meta-analysis of case-control studies. *PLOS One.* 2014; 9(1): e85781.
304. Saaksjarvi K, Knekt P, Mannisto S, Lyytinen J, Heliovaara M. Prospective study on the components of metabolic syndrome and the incidence of Parkinson's disease. *Parkinsonism Relat Disord.* 2015; 21(10): 1148–55.
305. Kim SC, Liu J, Solomon DH. Risk of incident diabetes in patients with gout: a cohort study. *Arthritis Rheumatol.* 2015; 67(1): 273–80.
306. Wahlqvist ML, Lee MS, Hsu CC, Chuang SY, Lee JT, Tsai HN. Metformin-inclusive sulfonylurea therapy reduces the risk of Parkinson's disease occurring with Type 2 diabetes in a Taiwanese population cohort. *Parkinsonism Relat Disord.* 2012; 18(6): 753–58.

307. de Lau LM, Koudstaal PJ, Hofman A, Breteler MM. Serum cholesterol levels and the risk of Parkinson's disease. *Am J Epidemiol.* 2006; 164(10): 998–1002.
308. Hu G, Antikainen R, Jousilahti P, Kivipelto M, Tuomilehto J. Total cholesterol and the risk of Parkinson disease. *Neurology.* 2008; 70(21): 1972–9.
309. Soh SE, Morris ME, McGinley JL. Determinants of health-related quality of life in Parkinson's disease: a systematic review. *Parkinsonism & Related Disorders.* 2011; 17(1): 1–9.
310. Ross GW, Petrovitch H, Abbott RD, Tanner CM, Popper J, Masaki K, et al. Association of olfactory dysfunction with risk for future Parkinson's disease. *Ann Neurol.* 2008; 63(2): 167–73.
311. Ishihara-Paul L, Wainwright NW, Khaw KT, Luben RN, Welch AA, Day NE, et al. Prospective association between emotional health and clinical evidence of Parkinson's disease. *European Journal of Neurology.* 2008; 15(11): 1148–54.
312. Shiba M, Bower JH, Maraganore DM, McDonnell SK, Peterson BJ, Ahlskog JE, et al. Anxiety disorders and depressive disorders preceding Parkinson's disease: a case-control study. *Movement Disorders.* 2000; 15(4): 669–77.
313. Bower JH, Grossardt BR, Maraganore DM, Ahlskog JE, Colligan RC, Geda YE, et al. Anxious personality predicts an increased risk of Parkinson's disease. *Movement Disorders.* 2010; 25(13): 2105–13.
314. Fang F, Xu Q, Park Y, Huang X, Hollenbeck A, Blair A, et al. Depression and the subsequent risk of Parkinson's disease in the NIH-AARP Diet and Health Study. *Movement Disorders.* 2010; 25(9): 1157–62.
315. Weisskopf MG, Chen H, Schwarzschild MA, Kawachi I, Ascherio A. Prospective study of phobic anxiety and risk of Parkinson's disease. *Movement Disorders.* 2003; 18(6): 646–51.
316. Claassen DO, Josephs KA, Ahlskog JE, Silber MH, Tippmann-Peikert M, Boeve BF. REM sleep behavior disorder preceding other aspects of synucleinopathies by up to half a century. *Neurology.* 2010; 75(6): 494–9.
317. Iranzo A, Molinuevo JL, Santamaria J, Serradell M, Marti MJ, Valldeoriola F, et al. Rapid-eye-movement sleep behaviour disorder as an early marker for a neurodegenerative disorder: a descriptive study. *Lancet Neurology.* 2006; 5(7): 572–7.
318. Schenck CH, Bundlie SR, Mahowald MW. Delayed emergence of a parkinsonian disorder in 38% of 29 older men initially diagnosed with idiopathic rapid eye movement sleep behaviour disorder. *Neurology.* 1996; 46(2): 388–93.
319. Postuma RB, Gagnon JF, Vendette M, Fantini ML, Massicotte-Marquez J, Montplaisir J. Quantifying the risk of neurodegenerative disease in idiopathic REM sleep behavior disorder. *Neurology.* 2009; 72(15): 1296–1300.
320. Abbott RD, Ross GW, White LR, Tanner CM, Masaki KH, Nelson JS, et al. Excessive daytime sleepiness and subsequent development of Parkinson disease. *Neurology.* 2005; 65(9): 1442–6.
321. Gao J, Huang X, Park Y, Hollenbeck A, Blair A, Schatzkin A, et al. Daytime napping, nighttime sleeping, and Parkinson disease. *American Journal of Epidemiology.* 2011; 173(9): 1032–8.
322. Abbott RD, Ross GW, Petrovitch H, Tanner CM, Davis DG, Masaki KH, et al. Bowel movement frequency in late-life and incidental Lewy bodies. *Movement Disorders.* 2007; 22(11): 1581–6.
323. Savica R, Carlin JM, Grossardt BR, Bower JH, Ahlskog JE, Maraganore DM, et al. Medical records documentation of constipation preceding Parkinson disease: a case-control study. *Neurology.* 2009; 73(21): 1752–8.
324. Gao X, Chen H, Schwarzschild MA, Ascherio A. A prospective study of bowel movement frequency and risk of Parkinson's disease. *American Journal of Epidemiology.* 2011; 174(5): 546–51.
325. Alonso A, Huang X, Mosley TH, Heiss G, Chen H. Heart rate variability and the risk of Parkinson disease: the Atherosclerosis Risk in Communities study. *Annals of Neurology.* 2015; 77(5): 877–83.
326. Hawkes CH, Del Tredici K, Braak H. A timeline for Parkinson's disease. *Parkinsonism & Related Disorders.* 2010; 16(2): 79–84.
327. Hawkes CH, Del Tredici K, Braak H. Parkinson's disease: a dual-hit hypothesis. *Neuropathology and Applied Neurobiology.* 2007; 33(6): 599–614.
328. Hawkes CH, Del Tredici K, Braak H. Parkinson's disease: the dual hit theory revisited. *Ann N Y Acad Sci.* 2009; 1170: 615–22.
329. Dickson DW, Uchikado H, Fujishiro H, Tsuboi Y. Evidence in favor of Braak staging of Parkinson's disease. *Movement Disorders.* 2010; 25(Suppl 1): S78–82.
330. Burke RE, Dauer WT, Vonsattel JP. A critical evaluation of the Braak staging scheme for Parkinson's disease. *Annals of Neurology.* 2008; 64(5): 485–91.
331. Chen H, Zhao EJ, Zhang W, Lu Y, Liu R, Huang X, et al. Meta-analyses on prevalence of selected Parkinson's nonmotor symptoms before and after diagnosis. *Transl Neurodegener.* 2015; 4(1): 1.
332. Chaudhuri KR, Martinez-Martin P, Brown RG, Sethi K, Stocchi F, Odin P, et al. The metric properties of a novel non-motor symptoms scale for Parkinson's disease: results from an international pilot study. *Movement Disorders.* 2007; 22(13): 1901–11.
333. Hummel T, Konnerth CG, Rosenheim K, Kobal G. Screening of olfactory function with a four-minute odor identification test: reliability, normative data, and investigations in patients with olfactory loss. *Annals of Otology, Rhinology, and Laryngology.* 2001; 110(10): 976–81.
334. Postuma RB, Gagnon JF, Bertrand JA, Genier Marchand D, Montplaisir JY. Parkinson risk in idiopathic REM sleep behavior disorder: preparing for neuroprotective trials. *Neurology.* 2015; 84(11): 1104–13.
335. Noyce AJ, Bestwick JP, Silveira-Moriyama L, Hawkes CH, Giovannoni G, Lees AJ, et al. Meta-analysis of early nonmotor features and risk factors for Parkinson disease. *Ann Neurol.* 2012; 72(6): 893–901.
336. Chen H, Burton EA, Ross GW, Huang X, Savica R, Abbott RD, et al. Research on the premotor symptoms of Parkinson's disease: clinical and etiological implications. *Environ Health Perspect.* 2013; 121(11–12): 1245–52.
337. Berg D, Marek K, Ross GW, Poewe W. Defining at-risk populations for Parkinson's disease: lessons from ongoing studies. *Movement Disorders.* 2012; 27(5): 656–65.
338. Berg D, Postuma RB, Adler CH, Bloem BR, Chan P, Dubois B, et al. MDS research criteria for prodromal Parkinson's disease. *Movement Disorders.* 2015; 30(12): 1600–11.
339. Nalls MA, McLean CY, Rick J, Eberly S, Hutten SJ, Gwinn K, et al. Diagnosis of Parkinson's disease on the basis of clinical and genetic classification: a population-based modelling study. *Lancet Neurology.* 2015; 14(10): 1002–9.
340. Liu R, Umbach DM, Peddada SD, Xu Z, Troster AI, Huang X, et al. Potential sex differences in nonmotor symptoms in early drug-naive Parkinson disease. *Neurology.* 2015; 84(21): 2107–15.
341. Reichmann H. View point: etiology in Parkinson's disease. Dual hit or spreading intoxication. *J Neurol Sci.* 2011; 310(1–2): 9–11.

342. Ritz B, Rhodes SL. After half a century of research on smoking and PD, where do we go now? *Neurology.* 2010; 74(11): 870–1.
343. Felice VD, Quigley EM, Sullivan AM, O'Keeffe GW, O'Mahony SM. Microbiota-gut-brain signalling in Parkinson's disease: Implications for non-motor symptoms. *Parkinsonism Relat Disord.* 2016; 27:1–8.
344. Stopschinski BE, Diamond MI. The prion model for progression and diversity of neurodegenerative diseases. *Lancet Neurology.* 2017; 16(4): 323–32.
345. Kalia LV, Lang AE. Parkinson's disease. *Lancet.* 2015; 386(9996): 896–912.
346. Goetz CG, Pal G. Initial management of Parkinson's disease. *BMJ.* 2014; 349: g6258.
347. Cheng HC, Ulane CM, Burke RE. Clinical progression in Parkinson disease and the neurobiology of axons. *Ann Neurol.* 2010; 67(6): 715–25.
348. AlDakheel A, Kalia LV, Lang AE. Pathogenesis-targeted, disease-modifying therapies in Parkinson disease. *Neurotherapeutics.* 2014; 11(1): 6–23.
349. Saarni SI, Harkanen T, Sintonen H, Suvisaari J, Koskinen S, Aromaa A, et al. The impact of 29 chronic conditions on health-related quality of life: a general population survey in Finland using 15D and EQ-5D. *Qual Life Res.* 2006; 15(8): 1403–14.
350. Hely MA, Morris JG, Traficante R, Reid WG, O'Sullivan DJ, Williamson PM. The Sydney multicentre study of Parkinson's disease: progression and mortality at 10 years. *J Neurol Neurosurg Psychiatry.* 1999; 67(3): 300–307.
351. Hely MA, Morris JG, Reid WG, Trafficante R. Sydney multicenter study of Parkinson's disease: non-L-dopa-responsive problems dominate at 15 years. *Movement Disorders.* 2005; 20(2): 190–9.
352. Hely MA, Reid WG, Adena MA, Halliday GM, Morris JG. The Sydney multicenter study of Parkinson's disease: the inevitability of dementia at 20 years. Mov Disord. 2008; 23(6): 837–44.
353. Coelho M, Ferreira JJ. Late-stage Parkinson disease. *Nat Rev Neurol.* 2012; 8(8): 435–42.
354. Williams-Gray CH, Mason SL, Evans JR, Foltynie T, Brayne C, Robbins TW, et al. The CamPaIGN study of Parkinson's disease: 10-year outlook in an incident population-based cohort. *J Neurol Neurosurg Psychiatry.* 2013; 84(11): 1258–64.
355. Oosterveld LP, Allen JC, Jr., Reinoso G, Seah SH, Tay KY, Au WL, et al. Prognostic factors for early mortality in Parkinson's disease. *Parkinsonism Relat Disord.* 2015; 21(3): 226–30.
356. Auyeung M, Tsoi TH, Mok V, Cheung CM, Lee CN, Li R, et al. Ten year survival and outcomes in a prospective cohort of new onset Chinese Parkinson's disease patients. *J Neurol Neurosurg Psychiatry.* 2012; 83(6): 607–11.
357. Zhu K, van Hilten JJ, Marinus J. Predictors of dementia in Parkinson's disease; findings from a 5-year prospective study using the SCOPA-COG. *Parkinsonism Relat Disord.* 2014; 20(9): 980–5.
358. Matthews F, Brayne C, Medical Research Council Cognitive F, Ageing Study I. The incidence of dementia in England and Wales: findings from the five identical sites of the MRC CFA Study. *PLOS Med.* 2005; 2(8): e193.
359. Liu G, Locascio JJ, Corvol JC, Boot B, Liao Z, Page K, et al. Prediction of cognition in Parkinson's disease with a clinical-genetic score: a longitudinal analysis of nine cohorts. *Lancet Neurology.* 2017; 16(8): 620–9.
360. van der Heeden JF, Marinus J, Martinez-Martin P, Rodriguez-Blazquez C, Geraedts VJ, van Hilten JJ. Postural instability and gait are associated with severity and prognosis of Parkinson disease. *Neurology.* 2016; 86(24): 2243–50.

12

Dementia and Parkinson's disease

Rodolfo Savica and Pierpaolo Turcano

Introduction

Parkinson's disease (PD) and cognitive decline have been extensively associated throughout numerous studies. In the first description of PD by James Parkinson in 1817 there was already hinted the presence of cognitive decline during the later stage of disease.[1] AD, the most common form of neurodegenerative disorder, can also present with signs and symptoms that may be attributable to parkinsonism and related disorders.

PD and dementing syndromes can be considered as a continuum of the same spectrum of the degeneration. In fact, pathologically the diffuse deposit of abnormal proteins beyond the basal ganglia can lead to a dementing disease.[2] Indeed, the ascending hypothesis of neurodegeneration reported by Braak, highlights how synuclein deposits causing Lewy bodies (LBs) can progressively involve the entire cortex in stages IV and V of the disease, whereas it is limited to the basal ganglia in stage III.[3] Thus, in the later stages of disease the cortical involvement would cause a dementing disorder due to the spreading of LBs beyond the basal ganglia. Nevertheless, the ascending hypothesis is only one of the different patterns of neurodegeneration associated with PD; thus, cognitive decline does not always occur at the later stages of PD.[4]

PD and AD, for example, share a number of common characteristics that should be considered, such as increasing incidence and prevalence with age, and relative rarity of genetic dominant causes of disease.[5]

However, the most relevant common feature that has important epidemiologic implications is the multiplicity of the clinical phenotypes that can contribute to the unique challenges in the diagnosis and identification of such disorders.

Using a simplistic approach, it is possible to differentiate between two different kinds of cognitive decline associated with PD: cognitive impairment/dementia that occurs before or at the immediate onset of the diagnosis of PD and cognitive impairment/dementia occurring in the later stages of the disease. In addition, there are also the parkinsonian symptoms that are present in patients with long-standing dementing illnesses, non-primarily defined as motor disorders (AD, fronto-temporal dementia (FTD), etc.).

It is extremely important to consider and weight these differences in studying the epidemiologic association of PD and other forms of dementias.

Generally the presence of cognitive decline/dementia within the clinical phenotype of PD defines two conditions: dementia with Lewy bodies (DLB) and Parkinson's disease dementia (PDD). The difference between DLB and PDD is based on the temporal onset of the memory decline: when occurring within one year from the onset of parkinsonism (or two years in the clinical setting) it is defined as DLB; when present after one year (or two in clinical settings) it is defined as PDD.[6]

From a clinical standpoint it may be difficult to differentiate between these two entities since they may share the same clinical features such as hallucinations, cognitive fluctuations, and RBD. Moreover, the underlying pathological hallmark is the same for PD, DLB, and PDD:[7] these three diseases all present the deposit of LBs as the main pathology protein aggregates; however, the presence of beta-amyloid, tau aggregates, and other less frequent pathological hallmarks can be observed.[8] In addition to the accumulation of pathological proteins within the brain tissues, other factors may lead to the same phenotypic expression, such as the presence of cerebrovascular disease, that may contribute to the cognitive impairments of these patients and to the extrapyramidal signs.[9,10] Moreover, recent studies pointed out the importance of neuroinflammation in PD; neuroinflammatory mechanisms may in fact play a pivotal role in the progression of neurodegeneration seen in these patients, contributing to the phenotypic expression of the parkinsonian symptoms.[11]

As mentioned above, there is a strong coexistence of AD pathology in patients with DLB[12] (~87%[13]). Furthermore, AD pathology can also be present in PD in about 40% of PD patients.[14] However, the accumulation of LBs is not always sufficient for the development of dementia in all the cases of PD; in fact, there are cases of PD with high burden of LBs that may not have dementia.[15] Although the presence of β-amyloid plaques and LBs on brain autopsy may be associated with a higher cognitive impairment[16] and it may be a better predictor of dementia compared with the accumulation of LBs or β-amyloid alone.[15]

Age is absolutely crucial in these disorders; in fact, the presence of dementia or cognitive decline is a common feature of elderly parkinsonian patients. Epidemiological data show that the akinetic-rigid form of PD featuring axial involvement with minimal tremor seems to be affecting the more elderly population;[17,18] additionally, DLB and PDD seem to be more common later in life compared to PD without dementia.

Prevalence, Incidence, and Survival of Parkinson's Disease and Dementia

The prevalence of a disease refers to the number of events, in a given population at a designated point in time. The incidence of the disease is defined as the number of new cases of a given disease during a defined period of time in a specified population.[19]

DLB is the second most common type of degenerative dementia and the second most common parkinsonism in older people, accounting for about 10–15% of cases on autopsy.[20]

When the studies explore individuals who are older than 65 years the prevalence of DLB ranged from 0.1%[21] to 2.0% of the population;[22] whereas the prevealence of DLB in all dementias varied between between 2.8%[23] to 30.5%.[22] Notably, the higher prevalence has been reported in studies conducted in Europe: namely 30.5% in North London,[22] and 21.9% in Finland.[24]

Incidence studies have been relatively limited to this date. The Cache County Study, in Utah (USA), estimated an incidence rate of 0.1% of DLB cases a year in the general population of people older than 65 years of age, which corresponds to a 3.2% rate of incident case of DLB of the cases of dementia.[25]

A pivotal study on the projects of prevalence of dementias for 2030 and 2050 reported that the prevalence of DLB in 2050 will increase by 131% in the USA.[26]

In Olmsted County, Minnesota, the incidence of DLB was 3.5 per 100,000 person years and as expected it increases with age (especially after 60 years of age); it was higher in men than in women.[27] The incidence of PDD was 2.5 per 100,000 person years overall and was increasing with age, but was similar in men and women (2.3 vs 2.7).

A recent study reported on how the presence of cognitive decline may have a relevant role in shortening the survival of patients with PD when compared with controls.

In Olmsted county, Minnesota, we observed that patients with incident diagnosis of PD had a moderate increased risk of mortality as compared to PDD and DLB. This study further highlights the relevance of cognitive decline as a crucial phenotypical characteristic dictating the disease progression and prognosis.[28] The burden of neurofibrillary tangles (NFT) within the brain tissues of PDD and DLB patients inversely correlates with the interval between the onset of motor symptoms and the onset of dementia; moreover, the accumulation of NFT has been shown to negatively impact the overall survival of these patients.[29] Similar results have been found in the same study when the burden of cerebral neuritic plaques has been assessed. The presence of AD-type pathology might therefore not only be related to a physiologic ageing process, but it may actually be pivotal for both the pathogenesis and the disease progression of synucleinopathies, influencing the onset of dementia and the overall survival of the patients.

Classification of Motor and Cognitive Phenotypes of Parkinsonism

The presence of cognitive impairments and the relationship with the different forms of parkinsonism is very much influenced by the adherence to different clinical criteria adopted.[30] The clinical criteria, indeed, may shift the epidemiological results depending on whether more or less lenient criteria are considered.

This relevant relationship between criteria and cognition of parkinsonism is able to significantly modify the results of epidemiological data. For example, the data of the Rochester Epidemiological Project (REP) in the Olmsted County in Minnesota are clearly affected by this phenomenon. Adding cognitive impairment translated to broaden the criteria and completely change the incidence curves of parkinsonism. The presence of dementia led to an increase of the curve rising even after age 80 for both sexes. Whereas this was very different in the cases without dementia; when broader clinical criteria, including demented patients, were adopted, the incidence rate of PD was higher in men than women, and this sex difference is more striking at older ages.

Epidemiological data show concordantly that the phenotype of parkinsonism shifts with ageing from a pure form of motor diseases to a motor plus cognitive phenotype. This is true for DLB and PDD. In fact, the presence of parkinsonism along with dementia is probably a common feature of subjects who develop parkinsonism after a certain age. The motor phenotype in older ages is more likely an axial parkinsonism characterized by postural instability, masked face, and no tremor.[17] DLB and the DLB prodromal stages are probably the most common clinical form of parkinsonism after 80 years of age.[31]

Clinical phenotypes of Parkinson's disease with dementia

The clinical criteria for DLB proposed in the Consensus conference havecognitive disorder and parkinsonism the main features.[6,32]

Parkinsonism as one of the main features of DLB may help differentiate DLB from pure AD.[33] However, the parkinsonism associated with DLB seems to have clinical characteristics that are different from the PD cases; indeed, resting tremor does not seem to be consistently associated with DLB. However, early observation pointed out that resting tremor was the most common motor symptom of DLB.[34] A number of other symptoms can be more strongly associated with DLB, such as myoclonus, psychiatric symptoms, dysautonomia, and sleep and wakeful disturbances. Some of these features can be present early on in the course of the disease such as, complex visual hallucinations[35] and dream enactment behaviour disorders.[36] Nonetheless, DLB is still a challenging diagnosis to make even for a movement disorders specialist; a recent meta-analysis showed that about 20% of DLB diagnoses are incorrect.[37] The presence of cognitive symptoms shared by other disorders such as PDD and AD, the overlap of some pathological features among different diseases, and the co-occurrence of vascular pathology, especially in the oldest population that may mimic some of the discussed symptoms, may in fact lead to a frequent clinical misdiagnosis of this disease.

Environmental factors and methodological challenge

Environmental risk factors play a crucial role in the development and physiopathology of all neurodegenerative disorders. Numerous studies have been associated with PD, but limited information is available for PD with dementia of all type. No studies have explored the risk or protective factors for PD with dementia or DLB. The relatively low prevalence and the difficulties in the diagnosis make traditional population-based epidemiological investigations very challenging; the phenotypic heterogeneity adds to the complexity. Case-control studies that use prevalent cases from tertiary centres (memory or movement disorder clinics) are likely to be subject to various biases that make conclusions uncertain. Despite this, we strongly advocate for the importance of such studies, It will be some time before studies on risk factors for DLB from unbiased studies will be available.

On the other hand, there is some available evidence on incidental LB disease. Interestingly, the risk factors that have a significant association with PD have also been reported to have the same association with incidental LBD. Caffeine intake, occupation, years of education, head injury, and number of children seem to be risk factors not only for PD but also for incidental LBD.[38] Unfortunately the data was limited and warrants caution in the interpretation, but it is very likely that the patients with incidental LBD may have the same environmental risk factors of PD, but a different individual/environmental predisposition can lead to a different phenotype of degeneration.

Future of Epidemiology of PD, PDD, and DLB

The number of cases of all the neurodegenerative diseases will increase in the near future. The oldest old are the population segment with the fastest rate of expansion and will become five times bigger by 2050. The major consequence of these changes will be the substantial increase of the number of cases with dementia or with cognitive involvement and the decline of subjects with primarily motor diseases. According to these changes because LBD is the dementia of the oldest old, prevalence and incidence of LBD will strongly increase.

In addition, there will be a better clinical recognition of the clinical diagnosis of DLB.[39] Thus, the increased awareness of the diagnosis will further increase the recognition and the number of cases affected by PD with dementia; however, the diagnosis is possible only after a long period of time and many specialist visits.[40] Overlapping of symptoms of AD with LBD is another additional important factor. Lastly, DLB seems to recognize more comorbidities than AD, with more vascular burden and psychiatric diseases.[41]

Frailty is a complex condition characterized by reduced response to acute and chronic conditions of stress, making the single individual more vulnerable.[42] Many of the characteristics associated with frailty are also impaired in PD, PDD, and DLB. Moreover, the addition of co-pathologies in PD is responsible both for the total amount of frailty at baseline and the rapidity of progression.[43]

REFERENCES

1. Parkinson J, Whittingham C. *An Essay on the Shaking Palsy.* London: Whittingham and Rowland for Sherwood, Neely, and Jones, 1817. p66.
2. Tamo W, Imaizumi T, Tanji K, Yoshida H, Mori F, Yoshimoto M, et al. Expression of alpha-synuclein, the precursor of non-amyloid beta component of Alzheimer's disease amyloid, in human cerebral blood vessels. *Neurosci Lett.* 2002; 326(1): 5–8.
3. Braak H, Del Tredici K, Rub U, de Vos RA, Jansen Steur EN, Braak E. Staging of brain pathology related to sporadic Parkinson's disease. *Neurobiol Aging.* 2003; 24(2): 197–211.
4. Savica R, Knopman DS. *Dementia with Lewy Bodies, in Neurodegeneration* (eds) A Schapira, Z Wszolek, TM Dawson, N Wood. Oxford: Wiley, 2017. pp83–92.
5. Logroscino G. *Imaging IN Neurodegenerative Disorders*, ed. L Saba. Oxford: Oxford University Press, 2014. p592.
6. McKeith IG, Boeve BF, Dickson DW, Halliday G, Taylor JP, Weintraub D, et al. Diagnosis and management of dementia with Lewy bodies: Fourth consensus report of the DLB Consortium. *Neurology.* 2017; **89**(1): 88–100.
7. Dickson DW, Braak H, Duda JE, Duyckaerts C, Gasser T, Halliday GM, et al. Neuropathological assessment of Parkinson's disease: refining the diagnostic criteria. Lancet Neurology. 2009; 8(12): 1150–7.
8. Halliday GM, Holton JL, Revesz T, Dickson DW. Neuropathology underlying clinical variability in patients with synucleinopathies. Acta Neuropathol. 2011; 122(2): 187–204.
9. Toledo JB, Arnold SE, Raible K, Brettschneider J, Xie SX, Grossman M, et al. Contribution of cerebrovascular disease in autopsy confirmed neurodegenerative disease cases in the National Alzheimer's Coordinating Centre. Brain. 2013; 136(Pt 9): 2697–706.
10. Hatate J, Miwa K, Matsumoto M, Sasaki T, Yagita Y, Sakaguchi M, et al. Association between cerebral small vessel diseases and mild parkinsonian signs in the elderly with vascular risk factors. Parkinsonism Relat Disord. 2016; 26: 29–34.
11. Hirsch EC, Hunot S. Neuroinflammation in Parkinson's disease: a target for neuroprotection? Lancet Neurology. 2009; 8(4): 382–97.
12. McKeith IG, Galasko D, Kosaka K, Perry EK, Dickson DW, Hansen LA, et al. Consensus guidelines for the clinical and pathologic diagnosis of dementia with Lewy bodies (DLB): report of the consortium on DLB international workshop. Neurology. 1996; 47(5): 1113–24.
13. McKeith IG, Ballard CG, Perry RH, Ince PG, O'Brien JT, Neill D, et al. Prospective validation of consensus criteria for the diagnosis of dementia with Lewy bodies. Neurology. 2000; 54(5): 1050–8.
14. Jellinger KA, Seppi K, Wenning GK, Poewe W. Impact of coexistent Alzheimer pathology on the natural history of Parkinson's disease. J Neural Transm (Vienna). 2002; 109(3): 329–39.
15. Hepp DH, Vergoossen DL, Huisman E, Lemstra AW, Berendse HW, Rozemuller AJ. Distribution and load of amyloid-beta pathology in Parkinson disease and dementia with Lewy bodies. J Neuropathol Exp Neurol. 2016; 75(10): 936–45.
16. Sarro L, Senjem ML, Lundt ES, Przybelski SA, Lesnick TG, Graff-Radford J, et al. Amyloid-beta deposition and regional grey matter atrophy rates in dementia with Lewy bodies. Brain. 2016; 139(Pt 10): 2740–50.
17. McKeith I. Dementia in Parkinson's disease: common and treatable. Lancet Neurology. 2004; 3(8): 456.
18. Levy G, Tang MX, Cote LJ, Louis ED, Alfaro B, Mejia H, et al. Motor impairment in PD: relationship to incident dementia and age. Neurology. 2000; 55(4): 539–44.
19. Last JM and International Epidemiological Association. *A Dictionary of Epidemiology* (4th edition). New York: Oxford University Press, 2001. xx, p196.
20. McKeith I, Mintzer J, Aarsland D, Burn D, Chiu H, Cohen-Mansfield J, et al. Dementia with Lewy bodies. Lancet Neurology. 2004; 3(1): 19–28.
21. de Silva HA, Gunatilake SB, Smith AD. Prevalence of dementia in a semi-urban population in Sri Lanka: report from a regional survey. Int J Geriatr Psychiatry. 2003; 18(8): 711–15.

22. Stevens T, Livingston G, Kitchen G, Manela M, Walker Z, Katona C. Islington study of dementia subtypes in the community. Br J Psychiatry. 2002; 180: 270–6.
23. Yamada T, Hattori H, Miura A, Tanabe M, Yamori Y. Prevalence of Alzheimer's disease, vascular dementia and dementia with Lewy bodies in a Japanese population. Psychiatry Clin Neurosci, 2001; 55(1): 21–5.
24. Rahkonen T, Eloniemi-Sulkava U, Rissanen S, Vatanen A, Viramo P, Sulkava R. Dementia with Lewy bodies according to the consensus criteria in a general population aged 75 years or older. J Neurol Neurosurg Psychiatry. 2003; 74(6): 720–24.
25. Miech RA, Breitner JC, Zandi PP, Khachaturian AS, Anthony JC, Mayer L. Incidence of AD may decline in the early 90s for men, later for women: the Cache County study. Neurology. 2002; 58(2): 209–18.
26. Bach JP, Ziegler U, Deuschl G, Dodel R, Doblhammer-Reiter G. *Projected numbers of people with movement disorders in the years 2030 and 2050.* Mov Disord. 2011; 26(12): 2286–90.
27. Savica R, Grossardt BR, Bower JH, Boeve BF, Ahlskog JE, Rocca WA. Incidence of dementia with Lewy bodies and Parkinson disease dementia. JAMA Neurol. 2013; 70(11): 1396–402.
28. Savica R, Grossardt BR, Bower JH, Ahlskog JE, Boeve BF, Graff-Radford J, et al. Survival and causes of death among people with clinically diagnosed synucleinopathies with parkinsonism: a population-based study. JAMA Neurol. 2017; 74(7): 839–46.
29. Irwin DJ, Grossman M, Weintraub D, Hurtig HI, Duda JE, Xie SX, et al. Neuropathological and genetic correlates of survival and dementia onset in synucleinopathies: a retrospective analysis. Lancet Neurology. 2017; 16(1): 55–65.
30. Bower JH, Maraganore DM, McDonnell SK, Rocca WA. Influence of strict, intermediate, and broad diagnostic criteria on the age- and sex-specific incidence of Parkinson's disease. Movement Disorders. 2000; 15(5): 819–25.
31. Savica R, Grossardt BR, Bower JH, Ahlskog JE, Rocca WA. Incidence and pathology of synucleinopathies and tauopathies related to parkinsonism. JAMA Neurology. 2013; 1–7.
32. McKeith IG. Consensus guidelines for the clinical and pathologic diagnosis of dementia with Lewy bodies (DLB): report of the Consortium on DLB International Workshop. J Alzheimers Dis. 2006; 9(3 Suppl): 417–23.
33. Ferman TJ, Smith GE, Boeve BF, Ivnik RJ, Petersen RC, Knopman D, et al. DLB fluctuations: specific features that reliably differentiate DLB from AD and normal aging. Neurology. 2004; 62(2): 181–7.
34. Crystal HA, Dickson DW, Lizardi JE, Davies P, Wolfson LI. Antemortem diagnosis of diffuse Lewy body disease. Neurology. 1990; 40(10): 1523–8.
35. Manford M, Andermann F. Complex visual hallucinations. Clinical and neurobiological insights. Brain. 1998; 121(Pt 10): 1819–40.
36. Claassen DO, Josephs KA, Ahlskog JE, Silber MH, Tippmann-Peikert M, Boeve BF. REM sleep behavior disorder preceding other aspects of synucleinopathies by up to half a century. Neurology. 2010; 75(6): 494–9.
37. Rizzo G, Arcuti S, Copetti M, Alessandria M, Savica R, Fontana A, et al. Accuracy of clinical diagnosis of dementia with Lewy bodies: a systematic review and meta-analysis. J Neurol Neurosurg Psychiatry. 2018; 89(4): 358–66.
38. Frigerio R, Fujishiro H, Maraganore DM, Klos KJ, DelleDonne A, Heckman MG, et al. Comparison of risk factor profiles in incidental Lewy body disease and Parkinson disease. Arch Neurol. 2009; 66(9): 1114–9.
39. Litvan I, MacIntyre A, Goetz CG, Wenning GK, Jellinger K, Verny M, et al. Accuracy of the clinical diagnoses of Lewy body disease, Parkinson disease, and dementia with Lewy bodies: a clinicopathologic study. Arch Neurol. 1998; 55(7): 969–78.
40. Galvin JE, Duda JE, Kaufer DI, Lippa CF, Taylor A, Zarit SH. Lewy body dementia: the caregiver experience of clinical care. Parkinsonism Relat Disord. 2010; 16(6): 388–92.
41. Fereshtehnejad, SM, Damangir S, Cermakova P, Aarsland D, Eriksdotter M, Religa D. Comorbidity profile in dementia with Lewy bodies versus Alzheimer's disease: a linkage study between the Swedish Dementia Registry and the Swedish National Patient Registry. Alzheimers Res Ther. 2014; 6(5–8): 65.
42. Erekson EA, Fried TR, Martin DK, Rutherford TJ, Strohbehn K, Bynum JP. Frailty, cognitive impairment, and functional disability in older women with female pelvic floor dysfunction. Int Urogynecol J. 2015; 26(6): 823–30.
43. Buchman AS, Yu L, Wilson RS, Schneider JA, Bennett DA. Association of brain pathology with the progression of frailty in older adults. Neurology. 2013; 80(22): 2055–61.

13

Amyotrophic lateral sclerosis (ALS) and fronto-temporal dementia (FTD)

Giancarlo Logroscino and Adriano Chiò

Introduction

Amyotrophic lateral sclerosis (ALS) is characterized by the presence of neurodegeneration of both upper and lower motor neurons and for a long time has been thought of as a pure motor disease. Clinical heterogeneity of ALS is based on the differential involvement of both upper and motor neurons but also on the involvement of other neuronal systems beyond motor neurons, especially cognition. This has been recognized particularly after the discovery of C9ORF72, a gene responsible for an important part of cases both of sporadic and familial ALS and frontotemporal dementia (FTD) as well.[1,2]

In this new approach, based on integration of observations with different methodology, FTD and ALS are considered to be part of a unique spectrum of overlapping genetic, neuropathological, and clinical diseases. Therefore we decided to describe the epidemiology of these two diseases in two sections of this chapter.

Amyotrophic Lateral Sclerosis

Descriptive epidemiology methods: the ALS registries

ALS is a progressive neurodegenerative disorder involving primarily the motor system, but affecting also other systems; the extent and the order of regions involved varies across individuals and populations.[3] The difficulties of case classification have increased after the recognition of non-motor symptoms as part of the main clinical features of ALS. Part of the challenge in early case identification and proper classification stems from mixing issues related to the diagnosis with issues related to different phenotypes at onset.[4] The change of diagnosis from simple motor phenotype to more complex phenotypes is going to strongly affect the recruitment in future epidemiologic studies. This is relevant also considering that the use of El Escorial criteria as the main criteria for diagnosis, based primarily on motor symptoms and signs, has determined an improvement in the quality and the consistency of the results across epidemiological studies.[5] The El Escorial Criteria are, however, strongly influenced by the idea of ALS as almost exclusively a disease of motor neurons.

Over the past 20 years, the design of ALS epidemiological studies has progressed, at least in Europe, therefore to focus on a prospective, population-based methodology, employing the El Escorial criteria, multiple and heterogeneous sources of data to ensure complete case ascertainment. The first study to use this approach was the Scottish ALS register in the early 1980s.[6] In the following years in Italy (in three regions: Piedmont,[7] Lombardy,[8] and Puglia[9]), in Ireland,[10] and then more recently in Holland,[11] the UK,[12] and in Catalonia, Spain,[13] a series of population-based registries have been implemented.

Registries as an organized collection of data, primarily clinical, have been built up mainly for cancer. A registry has been defined as: 'the file of data concerning all cases of a particular disease or other health relevant conditions in a defined population such that cases can be related to a population-base'.[14]

The registry is technically different from a simple clinical data base because the collection of data is systematic.[15] The two key concepts in a registry are: (1) the definition of a population at risk over time; (2) the geographic boundaries of the area of interest where the population is localized. This organization requires the knowledge of the size of the base-population and the count of the ALS cases that over time appear in the population at risk. The first ALS registry with the key described characteristics was organized in Scotland in the late 1980s.[16] For rare diseases like ALS this requires the survey of a network of clinical centres in a geographic area with a big base population (at least one million). This network should include all the diagnostic facilities to which a subject for whom ALS is suspected would go to have a diagnostic evaluation. The number of links in the network depends on the organization of the system and this can vary across different countries. In Ireland almost all cases go to the Motor Neuron disease centre in Dublin, similarly in the Netherlands, Dutch patients go to Utrecht and in Piedmont, Italy, there are two main ALS centres in Turin and in Novara. However, in Puglia, Italy, there are three main centres for ALS diagnosis (Tricase, Bari, San Giovanni Rotondo), but there are another ten facilities quite active and independent in the diagnosis and care of ALS patients even if with low numbers per year. In Milan, Lombardy, there are five ALS facilities and in the remining part of Lombardy at least other fifteen. The organization of SLALOM, the registry in Lombardy[17] and of SLAP in

Puglia[9] is therefore more complex, requiring a difficult collection from many sources, very challenging to keep over long time period.

However, if the collection of data is kept over a time period of several years it is possible to collect data on natural history of ALS, prognosis, and time trends. It is then possible to have estimates useful for causal research as well for public health planning and care delivery.

ALS incidence and prevalence around the world

Most of studies on incidence and prevalence have been conducted in Europe. A recent meta-analyses, examining all the published literature, showed that ALS incidence in the world was 1.75/100,000, 2.43 in men and 1.45 in women. The data were based on the pooling together of studies where more than 13,000 cases and 825 millions of person-years-follow-up were analysed.[18]

The incidence in Europe was quite homogeneous, ranging from 1.9 in Northern Europe, 2.2 in Southern Europe, and 2.3 in Western Europe.

The crude incidence of the studies on populations of European ancestry (Europe, North America, and New Zealand) was about 2/100,000. The highest incidence in Europe was reported in the Faroe Islands (3.6/100,000),[19] while the lowest was in Serbia 0.5/100,000. These data on average are consistent with the EURALS study, the first collaborative study of European registries in Europe, where the incidence was 2.7/10,000 and the age of onset was 65 years (see Table 13.1).[20] In this data set the interval first symptom-diagnosis was one year and the age-incidence curve showed a peak in the mid-seventies, mostly due to spinal cases in men.[17] The shape of the incidence curve is characterized by an earlier peak in men and a flatter curve in women (Figs. 13.1 and 13.2).

Confirming the importance of diagnostic criteria for quality of data, one of the sources of heterogenity in the meta-analyses[18] was the contrast between studies with diagnosis based on clinical judgement (1.29/100,000) and studies with diagnosis based on El Escorial criteria (1.9/100,000) characterized by higher incidence.

In recent years, studies have increasingly used capture-recapture methodology to measure the number of cases that were not identified within the registry. Based on this method in the Netherlands the incidence was 2.77 per 100,000 person-years (95% CI 2.63–2.91),[11] while it was 3.2 in Limousin, France (95% CI 2.81–3.56),[21] the highest measured in population-based studies.

The ALS prevalence has been analysed in few studies compared to incidence. The overall prevalence recently assessed in a systematic review was 5.40 or 39,863 prevalent cases in Europe.[15] The prevalence was very low in former Yugoslavia (Slovenia, Croatia, Serbia, Montenegro, Bosnia-Herzegovina, Kosovo, and Macedonia), but relatively high in the Netherlands and Italy (around 8/100,000). The highest prevalence has been estimated with the capture-recapture method in the Netherlands: 10.32 per 100,000 individuals (95% CI 9.78–10.86). Similar to incidence studies, prospective prevalence studies, based on ongoing collection of data over time, show higher estimates compared to retrospective prevalence studies.

In a systematic effort to determine an ALS registry in the USA, the collection of almost 30,000 cases in 2012 and 2013 showed a prevalence of 4.7 cases per 100,000 in the US population.[22] Overall, ALS was more common in the USA among whites, males, and persons aged 60–69 years. The differences in prevalence are much larger than in incidence. This is due to the differences in the ALS care systems, but also to the demanding task of collecting proper data for prevalence studies, especially when using administrative data.

Ancestry and ALS

The importance of ethnicity as a possible determinant of ALS incidence has been described in a review based on 61 studies.[23] A lower standardized incidence was observed in Asian populations. The recent systematic meta-analyses showed that ancestry can be a driver of variation of incidence.[18] In this perspective, data from mixed population are particularly useful. In a population-based study in Cuba, ALS mortality rate, a valid surrogate of incidence rate, was almost half in the mixed population (0.55/100,000) compared to white and and black people (about 0.9 in both ethnic groups).[24] Confirming the importance of ethnicity, in an area of high incidence (North America) in an ethnic non-Caucasian group, in American Indian and Alaska natives, the ALS incidence was particularly low (0.63/100,000).[25] The highest crude incidence has been described so far in the Faroe Islands.[19] This is a closed population in small islands, representing probably a genetic isolate. And as has been reported, the most recent studies in Caucasian population show an incidence over 3/100,000, especially if using the capture-recapture methodology.

Clinical measures in ALS population-based studies

The median age of ALS onset was about 65 years in Europe, while it is 59 in America and East Asia and lower in Libya and Israel.[3] The diagnostic delay was about 12 months in Europe, 10 in New Zealand, and much longer in the USA, about 17 months.[21] The sex ratio (males: females) was recently around 1:2 both in Europe and in the USA, while it is much higher in Iran and Uruguay (around

Table 13.1 Data from the EURALS five registries including the ALS incidence

	Follow-up (1998-1999)					ALS Registers details	
Registry	Denominator (py)	Cases	Crude incidence rate (per 100,000 py)	Days to diagnosis (median IQR)	Age at diagnosis (mean ± SD)	Year case ascertainment commenced	Reference population size
Ireland	7,455,000	154	2.06	280 (180–495)	63.2 ± 15.3	1993	3,917,203 (2002 census)
Lancashire, UK	3,246,334	54	1.66	389 (267–584)	65.4 ± 10.6	1986	1,623,667 (2001 census)
Lombardy, IT	9,895,108	194	1.96	255 (159–372)	61.9 ± 12.6	1998	4,947,554 (2001 census)
Piemonte, IT	8,815,564	265	3.00	240 (150–390)	65.9 ± 10.8	1995	4,341,733 (2006 est.)
Puglia, IT	7,959,576	130	1.63	271 (180–540)	62.5 ± 11.5	1998	4,086,613 (2001 census)
Scotland	10,124,022	231	2.28	270 (180–390)	66.5 ± 11.7	1989	5,062,011 (2001 census)

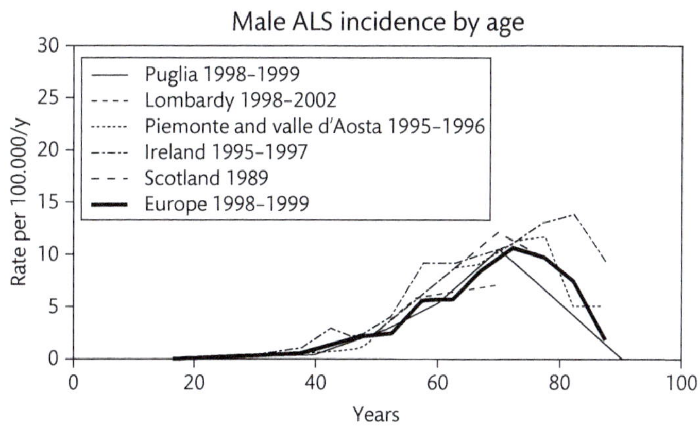

Fig. 13.1 ALS age–incidence curve for males.

2:2). The male-female ratio was much higher in older studies, probably suggesting a changing exposure for females in recent decades. Survival time was under 30 months in most of the studies conducted in Western, Central and South Europe; in the USA survival was between 30 and 40 months, while the longer published survivorship was described in Iran (40 months).

The bulbar onset was overall one-third of the total number of cases. Several reports indicated, however, a higher percentage in Northern Europe (more than 40%) compared to Southern Europe (34%).[3,20]

The number of familiar cases on average was about 4–5% but there are still uncertainties in the definition of a familial case.[26]

These data clearly show that the phenotypic heterogeneity of ALS is very important. Most of this variability is based on geographic location of the sample (living on a subcontinent explaining a large part of the variability: 80%).[3] A subcontinent inhabited by a specific population identified for ethnicity can be considered a surrogate of ethnic group and or ancestry.

Time trends

The absolute load of cases due to neurodegenerative diseases is increasing over time. Most of the increase is due to the ageing of the general population. In the Global Burden of Disease (GBD) study, ALS shows an increase of absolute numbers of about 22% of ALS, but a decrease in the age-standardized rates of 1.5% in the last ten years (comparing 2015 to 2005) both in count percentage and in change in years lived with disability. This is consistent with the

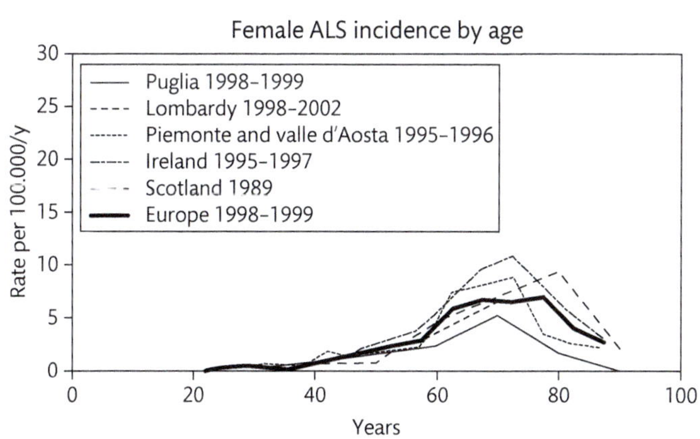

Fig. 13.2 ALS age–incidence curve for females.

similar change of neurological diseases that decrease by about 1.5 as age-standardized rates of years lived with disability, but increase by about 15% as absolute numbers.[27]

Time trend studies have been mainly based on studies on mortality. Recent data have been increasingly using resources from national database, especially in Scandinavian countries. These data suggest that both the incidence and mortality of ALS are increasing. Denmark data show an increase in risk of about 1% per year examining the period from 1970 to 2009.[28]

A recent study conducted in Norway,[29] using the Norwegian Cause of Death Registry, has described how ALS mortality increased throughout the whole period from 1951 to 2014 ($p < 0.001$), with a mean annual increase of 1.14%. The mortality increase was present only among those older than 60 years, but the rates fell significantly amongst the oldest old. The authors explain this trend by improvement in case ascertainment or in change over a long period of time of exposures that can be causal in ALS.

In contrast, a recent study conducted in the Irish Registry consistently with an age-period-cohort analysis shows no cohort effect but the initial signs of a period effect; with increasing incidence of ALS only in the most recently diagnosed group.[30]

In the future it is likely that the change in ALS clinical assessment, with an increased focus for atypical or non-motor phenotypes, will lead to an ALS incidence increase. ALS patient ascertainment[31] will modify time trends, with numbers consequently going up because of non-restriction to the classical motor phenotype. The evaluation of time trends through European registries are therefore important because of the high quality of the clinical assessment in evaluating in the future the time trends to compare similar entities. In recent data based on EC criteria, there was no significant time trend both in the Piedmont and Ireland registries, those with longer time of follow up.[32,33]

Environmental, behavioural, social, and medical factors in ALS

Several lines of evidences strengthen the idea that environmental risk factors are important in ALS but the data are so far quite elusive. The study of environmental risk factors for ALS is really challenging because most of the studies are case-control studies, characterized by small sample size, poor study design, including misclassification of exposure and recall, and selection bias. The assessment of environmental exposure is per se a challenge because of changes of exposure over time and difficulties in exposure assessment procedures.

The few prospective cohort studies are weak because of limited power and long time interval between the investigated exposures and disease onset. Another challenge is the different distribution of exposure prevalence in different populations, a factor that has often not been completely evaluated.

Education and SES Educational level is consistently inversely associated with the ALS risk in several studies in Europe. This has been recently confirmed in the EUROMOTOR, a multinational study based on population-based registries where the cases had a lower education compared to controls.[34] On the contrary in the USA, higher educational status and higher SES are associated with higher risk.[35] In a study conducted in New Jersey, the risk was particularly high in subjects within the best stratum of SES level (earning more than $120,000) (1.37, 95% CI: 1.02, 1.82).[36] The education has a different meaning socially in different countries and can be linked to different risk factors in the causal chain depending on the area of the study.

Physical activity Physical activity has always been a major focus of ALS aetiological research because of the clinical observation of ALS cases often being slim and reports of ALS as pathology in famous sport players.[37] In a case control study based in a tertiary US centre, where the risk was significantly increased for subjects who had always had a lean body shape and had been varsity athletes.[38]

In a cohort of 7325 male professional football players engaged by a football team from the Italian First and Second Divisions in a 30-year period (1970–2001) the risk of ALS was 6.5 measured as standardized mortality ratio (SMR), as compared to the risk in the general population.[39] The risk was significantly higher in younger subjects and the clinical onset was predominantly bulbar, in contrast with the general population, where bulbar onset is more common among older subjects. Interestingly, the longest duration of professional football activity was associated with the highest risk, showing the presence of a linear dose response. Highest risk of death due to ALS was also found in a cohort of professional American football players in the USA (RR = 4.3): the risk was particularly high in players in speed positions compared to non-speed positions (RR = 3.3).[40]

Most of the studies in the general population have not shown a significant increased risk for physical activity. Physical activity has been shown as protective in a big case-control study from the EURALS consortium[41] in which overall, sport-related and work-related physical activity were inversely associated with ALS risk. In the only prospective study conducted in the multinational study[42] in the European Prospective Investigation into Cancer and Nutrition (EPIC), a borderline protective effect of physical activity on the risk of dying of ALS was shown (RR = 0.67; CI 0.5–1.06).

In a case control study conducted in Italy by the EURALS group on the association between trauma ALS, the ORs were 3.07 (95% CI 1.86–5.05) for patients reporting 3+ traumatic events and 2.44 (95% CI 1.36–4.40) for severe traumatic events. The sensitivity analyses excluding recent events before disease onset confirmed the results.[41] An increased borderline risk was confirmed in data from the Danish National Register Patient (OR = 1.09, 95% CI: 0.99, 1.19). The risk was particularly elevated when it was at earlier ages (OR = 1.22, 95% CI: 1.08, 1.37).[43] A previous preliminary study with EURALS data was negative.[44]

Military service Two major papers indicated an increased risk among veterans of the Gulf War.[45,46] The only study assessing the association between military service and ALS in the general population was the Cancer Prevention Study 2 that found an increased ALS risk among subjects who served in the military independently from the period they served.[47]

These findings were recently confirmed in a study conducted among the Scottish Veterans Health Study[48] among 57,000 UK veterans and 173,000 civilians (HR 1.49, 95% C1.01–2.21, p = 0.046). The increased risk was, however, associated with a history of trauma or traffic accidents both in veterans and non-veterans.

In the National Longitudinal Mortality Study, following a cohort of about one million subjects, there were 471 ALS deaths. There was a slight increase of ALS risk in males who had served (RR: 1.23; 95% CI 0.98–1.53). The risk was particularly high for males who served in World War II (1.47; 95% CI 1.13–1.91). Similar results were present for females, but with larger confidence intervals.[49] All these results confirm that military service is a risk factor for ALS.

Smoking Smoking is the only risk factor that has been shown to be consistently associated with increased ALS risk in several studies. In the first formal meta-analyses (15 case control studies and 5 cohort studies), the pooled ALS RR (95% CI) was 1.28 (0.97–1.68) for current versus never smokers When stratifying for sex, the ALS risk was high only in women 1.66 (1.31–2.10).[50]

In the Epic cohort current smokers at recruitment had an almost two-fold increased risk of dying from ALS compared to subjects who never smoked (HR = 1.89, 95% CI 1.14–3.14).[51] In this study there was a clear dose effect because the number of years smoking linearly increased the ALS risk. In this study there was also an association between years since quitting smoking and reduction of risk.

In a collaborative analyses of five major US prospective cohorts, with follow-up ranging from 7 to 28 years[52] (the Nurses' Health Study, the Health Professionals Follow-up Study, the Cancer Prevention Study II Nutrition Cohort, the Multiethnic Cohort, and the National Institutes of Health-AARP, formerly known as the American Association of Retired Persons Diet and Health Study) with a base population of more than one million subjects and 832 ALS cases, smokers had a higher risk of ALS than never smokers (age- and sex-adjusted relative risks of 1.44 95% CI 1.23–1.68). Interestingly there was no dose-response, but the association was influenced by the age when smoking started.

In a large population-based study conducted in the Netherlands[53] with 494 patients with incident ALS and 1599 controls an increased risk was shown only in incident cases and for current smokers. Smoking was also associated with a worse prognosis (death hazard ratio = 1.51, 95% CI 1.07, 2.15).

In conclusion, the data consistently indicate that in ALS smoking is a risk factor. More data are needed to understand if the age of smoking initiation is more important than dose in determining the increase in risk.

Metals Among metals, lead has the most consistent reports of an association with ALS. Exposure to lead and heavy metal has been initially reported in clinical cases.[54,55] Acute exposure to a high dose of lead determines a well-known peripheral neuropathy.[56] A dose response relationship between lead dose and ALS risk has been reported.[57] Lead can be measured in the blood, CSF, and in the bone. Several studies show that patients with ALS have higher lead concentration compared to controls, but others studies do not;[58] the difficulty is that lead exposure measured in fluids does not reflect long-term exposure.

In a recent meta-analyses based on nine studies, the risk of developing ALS among individuals with exposure to lead was doubled (OR, 1.81; 95% CI 1.39–2.36).[59] In this study the attributable risk in sporadic cases was about 5%.

In a case-control study[60] from two major ALS centres in the USA, both metals (OR = 3.65; 95% CI 1.15, 11.60) and pesticides (OR = 6.50; 95% CI 1.78, 23.77)[61] have significantly increased the risk.

Fertilizers and pesticides Fertilizers and pesticides are used worldwide, especially in agriculture, and have been described as risk factors for all major neurodegenerative disease, particularly PD. The association with ALS has been described in several studies. A recent meta-analyses of 21 studies concluded that the risk of ALS was significantly increased with pesticide exposure (OR, 1.44; 95% CI 1.22–1.70) and with farmers (OR, 1.42; 95% CI 1.17–1.73), but was not significant with rural residence (OR, 1.25; 95% CI 0.84–1.87). The risk was particularly high for men and after expert judgement of pesticides exposure (RR = 2.07).[62]

The two cohort studies that used death certificate and self-report for exposure assessment were negative,[63,64] but the only cohort study that used expert judgement for exposure was positive.[61] Substantial evidence therefore links pesticide exposure to ALS risk.

Cardiovascular disease, metabolic diseases, and hormones An increasing interest has developed in the role of diabetes and glucose metabolism in ALS.[65] In Denmark, using a national administrative database on six million Danish residents, with a period of observation of about 30 years, a hospital admission for diabetes was associated with a reduction of ALS risk in the older age groups after age 61. In contrast, an increased ALS risk was associated with an admission before age 51. These results are consistent with the results of a Swedish study showing 50% of reduction in ALS risk for subjects over 70 with non-insulin dependent diabetes.[66] These results are opposed to the results of an Asian study where an increased risk of ALS was associated with diabetes only among the oldest. The study was conducted using an administrative database in Taiwan.[67]

The 'metabolic syndrome profile' has been hypothesized to be associated with a protective effect on ALS risk and with a better prognosis as well, in studies conducted in European populations. The role of altered lipid and glucose metabolism may counteract the increased energy requirement of ALS in Caucasian populations in the presence of a specific genotype.[68] On the other hand, diabetes as well as other vascular risk factors, including blood lipid levels and hypertension, may produce vascular damage or other less known mechanisms and this may increase the risk in some older groups of some populations.

In a case-control study conducted in Holland, data on medical conditions and use of medication were explored using a structured questionnaire. Hypercholesterolaemia (OR 0.76, 95% CI 0.63–0.92, P = 0.006), the use of statins (OR 0.45, 95% CI 0.35–0.59, P = 1.86 × 10(-9)), or immunosuppressive drugs (OR 0.26, 95% CI 0.08–0.86, P = 0.03) were associated with a decreased risk of ALS.[69]

In a study using the Oxford Record Linkage system, those without records of cardiovascular disease were at slight increased risk of ALS (RR: 1.14; 95% CI 1.05–1.22).[70] These results were not supported in similar studies conducted in the Netherlands, where vascular risk factors, measured clinically and biochemically, were not associated with ALS risk. Instead, ALS patients reported less use of cholesterol-lowering medication and had a lower premorbid BMI and lipid profile favourable on cardiovascular risk. These findings again may confirm the role of pathways linked to energy metabolism and consumption in the ALS pathogenesis.[71]

In Denmark in a case-control study with 3182 ALS residents and sex- and age-matched controls (100 per patient), CVD admission at least three years prior to the date of the ALS diagnosis was associated with cardiovascular risk profile (OR = 1.15; 95% CI 1.04–1.27) and with atherosclerosis (OR = 1.36; 95% CI 1.02–1.80).[72]

The data on medical conditions are still confusing for cardiovascular risk factors, but data on diabetes, lipids, and statins consistently indicate a protective role of low metabolism or high energy stores in ALS.

Frontolobar Degeneration and Frontotemporal Dementia

FTD descriptive/analytic

Frontolobar degeneration causes complex clinical syndromes: frontotemporal dementia (FTD) behavioural type with mostly behavioural symptoms and sparse cognitive symptoms, two forms with primary language involvement (the semantic variant and non-fluent aphasia), others involving mainly motor symptoms (progressive supranuclear palsy and cortico-basal degeneration). Furthermore the association of FTD of the behavioural type with motor neuron disease has been described as an additional phenotype. In the past there have been few epidemiological studies limited to a specific phenotype (mostly FTD behavioural type) or to specific age groups, generally under age 65, because these clinical syndromes are the more common causes of young onset dementias after AD.

The prevalence of FTD and other neurodegenerative early onset dementias (EOD) was measured in the city of Cambridge or East or South Cambridgeshire in a population of 325,000 in the age range 45–64. In this age range the prevalence was 81 (95% CI 62.8–104.5) per 100,000 in the 45- to 64-year age group for all dementias, while it was 15 per 100,000 (8.4 to 27.0) for FTD, with a surprising high prevalence among males (14:3).[73]

In contrast, in Japan the estimated prevalence of EOD in the target population was 42.3 per 100,000 (95% CI 39.4–45.4), while vascular dementia was the most frequent (42.5%) followed by AD (25.6%). FTD was only 2.6% of the total EOD.[74] In Italy, a study focusing on prevalence of EOD between age 45 and 65 found 55.1 per 100,000 inhabitants (95% CI 47.0–63.4) with about the same share respectively between AD and FTD: 25.5 and 29.6 per 100,000 inhabitants.[75]

In a study conducted in Holland the prevalence in all Holland was 1.1/100000 (95% CI 1.1–1.8) while in the Zuid Holland it was 2.5 (95% CI 2.1–3.5) with a peak at ages 60–69 of 9.1. The most likely explanation for this gap, considering also the characteristics of the Holland healthcare, is under-ascertainment outside the area of Zuid in the remaining part of the Dutch territory. The peak of prevalence measured as 4 in the age group of 45–65 was considerably lower than in UK where it was 15 in the same age group.[73]

Thus, the distribution of prevalence of FTD is strongly determined by the area of the study. Characteristics of the subtypes of dementias can explain the difference between Asian countries like Japan and European countries (particularly low prevalence of FTD in Asia), while difference in quality of case ascertainment may explain at least part of the difference within European countries.

The most recent and comprehensive study on the epidemiology of FTD has been conducted in two counties in the UK (Cambridgeshire and Norfolk) with a population of 1.7 million inhabitants.[76] There were no age limits and the study was designed to identify cases of FTD, corticobasal syndrome (CBS), progressive supranuclear palsy (PSP) including subjects with FTD, and motor neuron disease. Moreover, similarly to what has been done for ALS in EURALS, the ALS European collaborative study,[20] this study used multiple sources of case ascertainment. The prevalence of FTD, PSP, and CBS was 10.8/100,000. The incidence and mortality rates were very similar, at 1.61/100,000 and 1.56/100,000 person-years. The peak of age at diagnosis was around aged 70, with earliest age for FTD behavioural and oldest for PSP and non-fluent FTD. In this series only 23% underwent genetic screening and 15% were positive for some relevant known mutation. Also relevant was the particularly long interval between first symptom and diagnosis (about four years), underlying the difficulties of an early diagnosis.

Three other incidence FTD studies have been published so far. The only incidence study in the USA was conducted in Rochester (MN) using data from REP, the Rochester Epidemiologic Project were 2.2 for ages 40–49, 3.3 for ages 50–59, and 8.9 for ages 60–69.[77] For comparison, the corresponding rates for AD were 0.0, 3.3, and 88.9 in the same area. The number of cases in the numerator were extremely low due to the small size of the reference population (50,000 people).

In the UK, the incidence for all cases of primary dementia for the age range 45–64 years was estimated to be 11.5 cases per 100,000 person-years (95% CI 8.6–15.0). The incidence of FTD for the age range 45–64 years was estimated to be 3.5 cases per 100,000 person-years (95% CI 2.0–5.7); while AD was around 4.2.[78]

Using data from the Registry of Dementia of Girona (ReDeGi), a region in Spain with a reference population of subjects under age 65, the incidence of EOD for the age range 30–64 was 13.4 cases per 100,000 persons-year. Ten per cent were FTD and 42% AD.[79]

The most likely peak of incidence at onset is before age 70, while the peak of incidence based on diagnosis is later, between age 70 and 75, similarly to ALS (Fig. 13.3).

About one-third of FTD cases have a positive family history.[80] Very few studies have been published on environmental risk factor for FTD. With FTD in a case control study conducted in Holland with 80 patients and 124 controls, the only relevant risk factor was head trauma (RR: 3.3; CI 1.3–8.1). A non-significant association

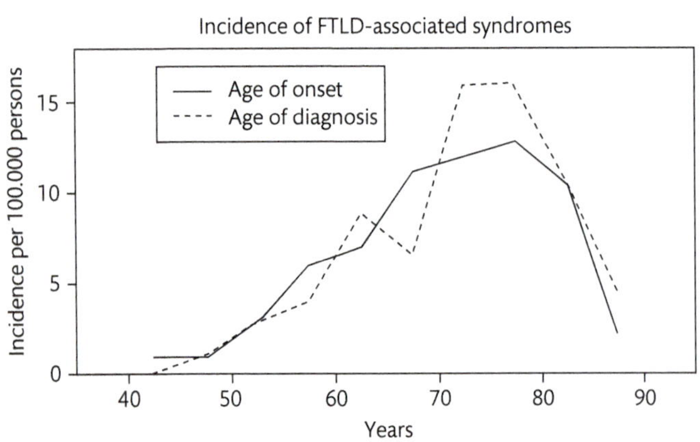

Fig. 13.3 FTD age incidence curve at onset and at diagnosis.

was described for thyroid diseases. The frontal lobe may be particularly sensitive to head trauma, including mild head trauma as the animal models show.[81]

In conclusion, the FTD epidemiology is based so far mainly on descriptive and genetic data.

As in other rare neurological diseases, the model should be the same for ALS, with multinational collaboration of population-based studies with prospective design, multisource for case ascertainment, and the same diagnostic criteria. The additional challenge is the difficulties of diagnosis, especially for the behavioural-type FTD. Many cases of FTD are labelled with psychiatric diagnosis or never diagnosed, especially at onset of disease and in the milder forms. The diagnosis is very late and the data from the Cambridgeshire and Norfolk register show a four-year interval that is much more than in other neurodegenerative diseases.

Genetic Epidemiology of ALS and FTD (Genetic Risk Factors)

In the last two decades, the understanding of ALS and FTD genetics has grown at an increasingly rapid pace.[82] Currently, more than 30 causative genes have been correlated to ALS and FTD. A large number of these genes may cause either ALS or FTD or both, and few of them seem to be exclusively related to one of the two diseases. These observations seem to mirror the pathology of the two disorders: TDP-43 cytoplasmic ubiquitinated aggregates are found, in fact, in about 95–97% of ALS cases and 40% of FTD cases, and *FUS* inclusions in 1% of ALS cases and 9% of FTD cases. SOD1 pathology seems to be exclusive of a small proportion of ALS patients (2%), while at least 50% of FTD patients have a tauopathy, which is the pathological hallmark of progranulin (PRGN) and microtubule-associated protein tau (MAPT) mutations.[83]

A growing body of information is accumulating concerning the ethnic differences in the distribution both of major ALS genes mutations and of minor genes influencing ALS age at onset and clinical course. However, very few systematic population-based studies have been performed, and most of them are related to the four more common genes (*SOD1*, *TARDBP*, *FUS*, and *C9orf72*). Moreover, all these studies have been performed in populations of European ancestry. The data from these studies are summarized in Table 13.1.

Large differences emerge from these studies. *SOD1* mutations are quite frequent in Scotland[84] and, to a less extent, in Piedmont,[85] while it is virtually absent in Ireland and the Netherlands.[86,87] The large number of *SOD1* cases in Scotland is, however, explained by the presence of a founder variant (p.I114T) (18 of the 21 identified cases).[84] The frequency of TARDBP is relatively similar in all populations, ranging from 0.5% in Ireland to 1.5% in Piedmont, with the notable exception of Sardinia, where about a quarter of ALS patients carry two different missense mutations of this gene (p.A382T and p.G295S), again representing two founder variants.[88] In this population, contrary to patients with different ancestry carrying the same mutation, *TARDBP* mutations are also characterized by a high frequency of comorbid FTD.[88] Finally, *C9orf72* has a rather different distribution in the examined populations, with a peak around 10% of ALS patients in Northern Europe and lower figures in Southern Europe (7% in Piedmont,

Italy).[84,85] Again, a higher frequency (13.6%) has been found in Sardinia, implying a founder effect in this isolated population.[88] A similar founder effect has been reported for the Finnish population for *SOD1* p.D90A missense mutation and for *C9orf72* GGGGCC expansion.[89]

Data on non-European populations are sparse and virtually no population-based studies have been published. Studies based on referral centres indicate that *C9orf72* expansions are rarer in patients of Japanese or Chinese ancestry compared to Europeans, while *SOD1*, *TARDBP*, and *FUS* mutations have a similar frequency.[90] Some genetic mutations are characterized by a particular elevated occurrence in restricted geographical areas. For example, mutations of *VAPB* gene are quite frequent in Brazil and very rarely described elsewhere, while recessively inherited mutations of the *Alsin* gene (ALS2) are almost exclusively identified in populations of Arab/Maghreb ancestry.[82]

The co-morbidity of ALS and FTD has been explored in one epidemiological study performed in Piedmont, Italy: 17 out of 32 (53.1%) of ALS patients carrying *C9orf72* expansion had bvFTD, more commonly those with a positive family history for ALS or FTD (66.7% of fALS and 12.5% of sALS).[85] Similarly, a genetic study performed on the patients of the Irish ALS register showed that of the 17 patients with C9orf72 expansion, 5 (29.4%) had bvFTD and 5 (29.4%) a milder cognitive impairment.[86] Concerning the other main ALS genes, the population-based study performed in Piedmont found that three out of seven patients (42.9%) with *TARDBP* missense mutations had bvFTD, while none of the ten patients with *SOD1* missense mutation had cognitive impairment.[91]

Systematic studies of the genetic determinants of FTD on population-based cohorts are lacking. In a clinical-based study, the hereditability of FTD has been estimated to be 41.8%, although a clear dominant transmission was found in only 10.2% of cases.[92] The most common gene identified in FTD patients is *C9orf72*, accounting for 25% of cases, followed by *MAPT* and *GRN*.[93]

In conclusion, genetic epidemiology of ALS and FTD is still in its beginnings. Future research is needed to better understand the population-specific genetic characteristics of ALS and to improve genetic counselling.

Prognostic Factors of ALS

Prognosis of ALS has been widely studied in the last decades, with several aims: first, to determine the outcome of the disease in the single patient/group of patients and second, to improve the design of clinical trials. Prognostic studies have been performed in different setting of patients: (1) subjects referring to ALS tertiary centres; (2) subjects enrolled in clinical trials; (3) epidemiological-based series of patients. Moreover, each study can be defined as prospective or retrospective, according to the type of observation over time. All these approaches have advantages and disadvantages. Studies based on referral centre series are generally quite large and characterized by a good quality of data collection, but suffer a strong referral bias inherent in the selection of patients attending tertiary centres (which are younger and have a better prognosis than non-attending ones).[94]

Studies based on patients enrolled in pharmacological trials have the advantages of the prospective collection and the good standardization of data, a high level of diagnostic accuracy, and the enrolment of a relatively homogenous population. Recently, a large database, the Pooled Resource Open-Access ALS Clinical Trials Database (PRO-ACT) (https://nctu.partners.org/ProACT/) has been created, containing records from over 10,700 ALS patients who participated in 23 phase II/III clinical trials.[95] The aim of this open resource is to generate models of ALS progression and to facilitate further clinical trials in ALS.[95] However, patients included in clinical trials represent a highly selected population, due to the strict enrolment criteria of pharmacological trials. In a population-based study, it has been shown that patients enrolled in clinical trials compared to the general ALS population were younger (56.2 years, SD 10.2, vs 65.1 years, SD 11.1), were less likely to have a bulbar onset (15.2% vs 32.7%), and to be female (37.2% vs 46.7%) and had a significantly longer survival (3.9 years vs 2.6 years).[96] This is partly due to the enrolment in clinical trials of prevalent patients instead of incident ones, and the exclusion of fast progressors and subjects with comorbid condition such as renal or liver failure.

Prognostic studies based on epidemiological populations are considered the best available methodological design for the study of rare disorders.[94] They have the advantage of allowing the application of uniform and definite diagnostic criteria and permit the assessment of prognostic factors in a standardized manner. Most importantly, the completeness of case ascertainment permits the analysis of the full clinical spectrum of the ALS population, in particular the old or very old cases, as demonstrated by the older mean age of onset observed in the registry cohorts compared to that of both retrospective epidemiological series and referral series. The drawbacks of epidemiological registries are long-term costs of a prospective follow-up and the complexity in organization and coordination. In this chapter we will therefore focus on prognostic factors as they have emerged from population-based studies, with some reference to other studies as comparison.

Overall survival Overall survival of ALS as reported in epidemiological studies ranges around 30 months from the onset of motor symptoms, at least one year shorter than that reported in clinical-based studies.[94] There are no clear indications that median survival increased in the last decade, despite the improvement of patients' care, the increased use of support therapies such as enteral nutrition (EN) and non-invasive ventilation (NIV), and the larger number of patients attending tertiary ALS centres.[33,97] In a study from Scotland a reduction of survival was found in the 1989–1998 period.[98]

Demographic factors Age is consistently considered the strongest prognostic factor in ALS, with a clear dose-effect relationship, that is, survival time decreases with increasing age of symptom onset. Conversely, the effect of gender is less clear, with some population-based studies indicating a shorter survival among women even after correction for age and bulbar onset,[97,99,100] and others showing a similar outcome in the two genders.[101–103] Race/ethnicity has been rarely studied in population-based surveys: in a study performed in New Jersey, Afro-Americans appeared to have a better prognosis (41 months) than Europeans (20 months) and Asians (30 months).[104]

Clinical features Bulbar or generalized onset appears to be a negative prognostic factors in almost all population-based studies.[97,98,100,102,103,105,106] In an extensive evaluation of ALS phenotypes, the best outcomes were observed in prevalent upper motor neuron ALS (76 months) and flail arm phenotypes (48 months), and the worst in respiratory (17 months) and bulbar phenotypes (24 months).[107] The large survival difference determined by clinical phenotypes has profound implications in the design of clinical trials and patient stratification. According to two population-based studies, comorbid FTD and executive/non-executive impairment are associated with a worse outcome,[108,109] partially related to a reduced efficacy of life-prolonging therapies (EN and NIV) in this population of patients.[91]

Diagnostic delay is an established prognostic factor in ALS: the longer the better the prognosis.[97,106,110] The finding of a worse prognosis in patients with a short time delay between onset and diagnosis is likely to indicate a more aggressive disease, which leads the patient to seek medical attention more rapidly and to be more readily diagnosed.[94]

The rate of disease progression, usually measured as the decline of ALSFRS-R scale over a given period of time, is related to the outcome of ALS, likely indicating that the pace of the loss of motor neurons is an intrinsic feature of each patient,[101,111,112] although ALSFRS-R decline is not linear over time.[111]

Nutritional status is also considered a prognostic factor in ALS. In a clinic-based study a body mass index (BMI) value ≤18.5 has been found to be an independent prognostic factor for death both in univariate and in multivariable analysis.[113] Recently, a retrospective study performed in the Limousin region, France, showed that weight loss >10% at diagnosis is an independent prognostic factor with an HR of 2.29 (95% CI 1.65–3.17).[112] Similarly, also respiratory status at diagnosis is strongly related to ALS prognosis.[107]

Lastly, there is no consensus that the El Escorial classification is related to ALS prognosis. A population-based study performed in Ireland did not show any effect,[114] while three studies performed in Italy and France and a recent study from Ireland showed that definite ALS at diagnosis was related to a worse prognosis than any other El Escorial diagnostic level.[101–103,115]

ALS genes Genetics has a strong influence on ALS phenotype and also modifies its outcome. In a population-based study comparing the four more common genes in the Caucasian population, it has been found that *FUS* has the worse prognosis, often with a survival under 12 months from onset even in presence of a young age at onset, followed by *C9orf72* GGGGCC expansion. TARDBP mutations seem to be the more benign.[85] The prognostic effect of *SOD1* depends on the specific mutation, with p.A4V probably carrying the worst prognosis and p.D90A the best, of the mutation spectrum. Among the large number of risk genes, the only one that has been studied in a population-based study is *ATXN2*: the presence of an intermediate-length (CAG) expansion (encoding 27–33 glutamines, polyQ) is not only a risk factor of ALS,[116] but is also related to a poorer prognosis, as demonstrated in the Piedmont and Valle d'Aosta ALS register (HR 2.79, 95% CI 1.67–4.64).[117]

Treatments Attending an ALS multidisciplinary clinic has been reported to increase survival in several population-based studies,[115,118,119] but not all.[120] The positive effect of ALS centres seems to be independent of all other considered prognostic factors (namely age, site of onset, enteral nutrition, and NIPPV), and has been therefore explained as a consequence of a comprehensive care of patients. However, these results should be considered cautiously, since they were not controlled and were based on a post-hoc analyses.

Riluzole remains the only drug which has been demonstrated to be effective in increasing ALS survival in a RCT.[121] Its positive effect on ALS outcome has been confirmed in several European population-based studies.[101,106,115,118,120]

There is no consensus on the effect on survival of EN in ALS patients, although in some epidemiological studies it emerged as a positive prognostic factor.[97,101] Conversely, non-invasive ventilation emerged as a positive prognostic factor in a RCT,[122] but not in epidemiological studies.[85,97] However, not surprisingly, the survival time of NIV has been found to be shorter in population-based studies than in studies based on referral centres.[96]

Other factors Cigarette smoking is a possible risk factor for ALS. In two population-based studies performed in Piedmont, Italy, and the Netherlands it has also been shown that current and former smokers have a shorter survival than never smokers, with a dose-response gradient;[53,123] the effect of smoking is not related to patients' respiratory status at time of diagnosis or to the co-occurrence of chronic obstructive pulmonary disease (COPD), a well-known complication of smoking.[123] In the same paper, COPD resulted as a strong independent negative prognostic factor of ALS (HR 1.46, 95% CI 1.06–2.01).[123] Conversely, alcohol consumption was not associated with survival in a Dutch population-based study.[53] In a population-based, case-control study performed in the Netherlands no significant association between nutrient intake and survival was found with multivariate Cox regression analysis.[124] Similarly, two studies on the same population did not find any association between survival and premorbid medical conditions or premorbid use of medication,[69] or with lifetime physical activity.[124]

FTD Prognosis

There are few studies examining survivorship in FTD, all in clinical settings of tertiary centres. Some studies have provided neuropathological confirmation of the clinical diagnosis. The first large series with neuropathology including both behavioural and language variants have described FTD as an aggressive disease with a median survivorship after diagnosis of about three years.[125] In this series there has also been a selection of subjects with the motor phenotype (FTD plus motor neuron disease and corticobasal degeneration (CBD)). In the FTD motor neuron disease group the median survivorship was only one year, while the subjects with tau deposition had better prognosis. The series with neuropathology select the cases with worst prognosis.

In a large clinical series, FTD had a shorter survivorship than AD from disease clinical onset (8.7 vs 11.8 years), but longer than the previous series. The survival in FTD was very similar to CBD/PSP that were considered as components of the FTD spectrum but analysed separately.[126]

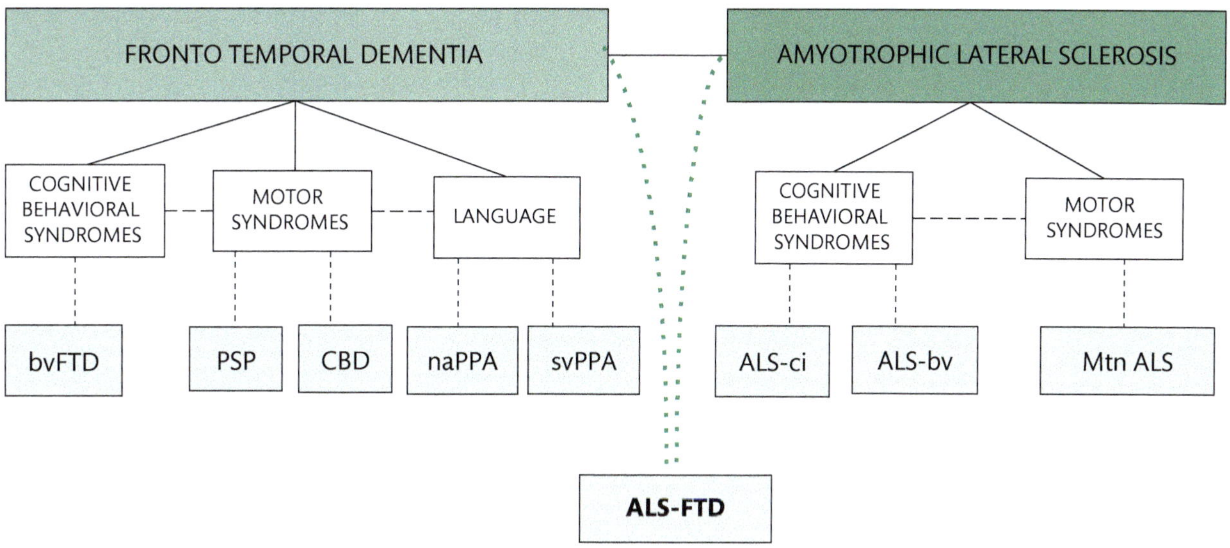

Fig. 13.4 ALS FTD spectrum: the clinical syndromes.

Interestingly, tests of frontal disfunction like reverse digit span and letter fluency predicted poor survival. In a more recent study, the presence of memory dysfunction was a marker of rapid progression, in association with family history for neurodegenerative diseases, stereotypic and compulsive behaviour, and deterioration of test of global cognition like MMSE and ACE (Addenbrooke Cognitive Examination).[127] In a recent clinical series the presence of language disorders was the only predictor of survival.[128] A recent meta-analysis showed a longer median survivorship.[129] In this paper the median survivorship was better in FTD and PFA (8 years) than in FTD with ALS (2.5 years), which had the worst prognosis. PSP and CBD, the other two forms with motor involvement, had a negative prognosis as well, while SD had a better prognosis (12 years).

It is important to mention that the behavioural variant has a non-progressive form that would be very important to identify at diagnosis.[130] These non-progressive cases are possibly phenocopies and not FTD with specific neuropathology.

The only study with a wide referral of FTD and PSP (national referral in Holland involving both memory clinics and nursing homes) has shown similar results with a survivorship of ten years in FTD and eight years in PSP. In this study patients with FTD with ALS were excluded.[131]

In conclusion, we have several prognostic indicators like motor and memory impairment, identified in studies in tertiary centres. However, longitudinal epidemiological studies are missing. Therefore the prognostic variables identified in clinical studies should be tested in the proper population settings.

Conclusions

FTD and ALS offer an interesting model for precision medicine: two distinct phenotypes at the extreme of the spectrum with intermediate phenotypes in the middle (Fig. 13.4). Many cases share a genetic risk factor (C9ORF72). There is also probably a neuropathological continuum with deposition of TDP 43 in both diseases.[132] There are several challenges: missing diagnosis of behavioural variants, uncertainties in disease classification, identification of early stages. Data on FTD risk factors are poor. The presence of a prospective, population-based registry in a specific geographic area including both ALS and the whole FTD spectrum is probably the best instrument to answer to all these questions.

REFERENCES

1. DeJesus-Hernandez M, Mackenzie IR, Boeve BF, Boxer AL, Baker M, Rutherford NJ, et al. Expanded GGGGCC hexanucleotide repeat in noncoding region of C9ORF72 causes chromosome 9p-linked FTD and ALS. Neuron. 2011; 72(2): 245–56.
2. Renton AE, Majounie E, Waite A, Simon-Sanchez J, Rollinson S, Gibbs JR, et al. A hexanucleotide repeat expansion in C9ORF72 is the cause of chromosome 9p21-linked ALS-FTD. Neuron. 2011; 72(2): 257–68.
3. Marin B, Logroscino G, Boumediene F, Labrunie A, Couratier P, Babron MC, et al. Clinical and demographic factors and outcome of amyotrophic lateral sclerosis in relation to population ancestral origin. Eur J Epidemiol. 2016; 31(3): 229–45.
4. Al-Chalabi A, Hardiman O, Kiernan MC, Chio A, Rix-Brooks B, van den Berg LH. Amyotrophic lateral sclerosis: moving towards a new classification system. Lancet Neurology. 2016; 15(11): 1182–94.
5. Logroscino G, Traynor BJ, Hardiman O, Chio A, Couratier P, Mitchell JD, et al. Descriptive epidemiology of amyotrophic lateral sclerosis: new evidence and unsolved issues. Journal of Neurology, Neurosurgery, and Psychiatry. 2008; 79(1): 6–11.
6. Forbes RB, Colville S, Parratt J, Swingler RJ. The incidence of motor neuron disease in Scotland. Journal of Neurology. 2007; 254(7): 866–9.
7. Incidence of ALS in Italy: evidence for a uniform frequency in Western countries. Neurology. 2001; 56(2): 239–44.
8. Beghi E, Millul A, Micheli A, Vitelli E, Logroscino G. Incidence of ALS in Lombardy, Italy. Neurology. 2007; 68(2): 141–5.

9. Logroscino G, Beghi E, Zoccolella S, Palagano R, Fraddosio A, Simone IL, et al. Incidence of amyotrophic lateral sclerosis in southern Italy: a population based study. Journal of Neurology, Neurosurgery, and Psychiatry. 2005; 76(8): 1094–8.
10. Traynor BJ, Codd MB, Corr B, Forde C, Frost E, Hardiman O. Incidence and prevalence of ALS in Ireland, 1995–1997: a population-based study. Neurology. 1999; 52(3): 504–9.
11. Huisman MH, de Jong SW, van Doormaal PT, Weinreich SS, Schelhaas HJ, van der Kooi AJ, et al. Population based epidemiology of amyotrophic lateral sclerosis using capture-recapture methodology. Journal of Neurology, Neurosurgery, and Psychiatry. 2011; 82(10): 1165–70.
12. Abhinav K, Stanton B, Johnston C, Hardstaff J, Orrell RW, Howard R, et al. Amyotrophic lateral sclerosis in South-East England: a population-based study. The South-East England register for amyotrophic lateral sclerosis (SEALS Registry). Neuroepidemiology. 2007; 29(1-2): 44–8.
13. Pradas J, Puig T, Rojas-Garcia R, Viguera ML, Gich I, Logroscino G. Amyotrophic lateral sclerosis in Catalonia: a population based study. Amyotrophic Lateral Sclerosis & Frontotemporal Degeneration. 2013; 14(4): 278–83.
14. Porta M. A Dictionary of Epidemiology (6h edition). Oxford: Oxford University Press, 2014. p243.
15. Chio A, Logroscino G, Traynor BJ, Collins J, Simeone JC, Goldstein LA, et al. Global epidemiology of amyotrophic lateral sclerosis: a systematic review of the published literature. Neuroepidemiology. 2013; 41(2): 118–30.
16. The Scottish Motor Neuron Disease Register: a prospective study of adult onset motor neuron disease in Scotland. Methodology, demography and clinical features of incident cases in 1989. Journal of Neurology, Neurosurgery, and Psychiatry. 1992; 55(7): 536–41.
17. Beghi E, Morrison KE. ALS and military service. Neurology. 2005; 64(1): 6–7.
18. Marin B, Boumediene F, Logroscino G, Couratier P, Babron MC, Leutenegger AL, et al. Variation in worldwide incidence of amyotrophic lateral sclerosis: a meta-analysis. International Journal of Epidemiology. 2017; 46(1): 57–74. doi: 10.1093/ije/dyw061. Review. PubMed PMID: 27185810; PubMed Central PMCID: PMC5407171.
19. Joensen P. Incidence of amyotrophic lateral sclerosis in the Faroe Islands. Acta Nneurologica Scandinavica. 2012; 126(1): 62–6.
20. Logroscino G, Traynor BJ, Hardiman O, Chio A, Mitchell D, Swingler RJ, et al. Incidence of amyotrophic lateral sclerosis in Europe. Journal of Neurology, Neurosurgery, and Psychiatry. 2010; 81(4): 385–90.
21. Marin B, Hamidou B, Couratier P, Nicol M, Delzor A, Raymondeau M, et al. Population-based epidemiology of amyotrophic lateral sclerosis (ALS) in an ageing Europe—the French register of ALS in Limousin (FRALim register). European Journal of Neurology: the official journal of the European Federation of Neurological Societies. 2014; 21(10): 1292–1300, e78–79.
22. Mehta P, Kaye W, Bryan L, Larson T, Copeland T, Wu J, et al. Prevalence of amyotrophic lateral sclerosis—United States, 2012–2013. Morbidity and Mortality weekly report Surveillance Summaries (Washington, DC). 2016; 65(8): 1–12.
23. Cronin S, Hardiman O, Traynor BJ. Ethnic variation in the incidence of ALS: a systematic review. Neurology. 2007; 68(13): 1002–7.
24. Zaldivar T, Gutierrez J, Lara G, Carbonara M, Logroscino G, Hardiman O. Reduced frequency of ALS in an ethnically mixed population: a population-based mortality study. Neurology. 2009; 72(19): 1640–5.
25. Gordon PH, Mehal JM, Holman RC, Rowland LP, Rowland AS, Cheek JE. Incidence of amyotrophic lateral sclerosis among American Indians and Alaska natives. JAMA Neurology. 2013; 70(4): 476–80.
26. Byrne S, Walsh C, Lynch C, Bede P, Elamin M, Kenna K, et al. Rate of familial amyotrophic lateral sclerosis: a systematic review and meta-analysis. Journal of Neurology, Neurosurgery, And Psychiatry. 2011; 82(6): 623–7.
27. GBD 2015 Disease and Injury Incidence and Prevalence Collaborators. Global, regional, and national incidence, prevalence, and years lived with disability for 310 diseases and injuries, 1990–2015: a systematic analysis for the Global Burden of Disease Study 2015. Lancet. 2016; 388(10053): 1545–602.
28. Seals RM, Hansen J, Gredal O, Weisskopf MG. Age-period-cohort analysis of trends in amyotrophic lateral sclerosis in Denmark, 1970–2009. American Journal of Epidemiology. 2013; 178(8): 1265–71.
29. Nakken O, Lindstrom JC, Tysnes OB, Holmoy T. Mortality trends of amyotrophic lateral sclerosis in Norway 1951–2014: an age-period-cohort study. Journal of Neurology. 2016; 263(12): 2378–85.
30. Tobin K, Gilthorpe MS, Rooney J, Heverin M, Vajda A, Staines A, et al. Age-period-cohort analysis of trends in amyotrophic lateral sclerosis incidence. Journal of Neurology. 2016; 263(10): 1919–26.
31. Hardiman O, Al Chalabi A, Brayne C, Glymour M, Beghi E, Van den Berg LH, et al. The changing picture of amyotrophic lateral sclerosis: lessons from European registers. J Neurol Neurosurg Psychiatry. 2017; 88(7): 557–63. doi: 10.1136/jnnp-2016-314495. Epub 11 March 2017. Review. PubMed PMID: 28285264.
32. Chio A, Mora G, Calvo A, Mazzini L, Bottacchi E, Mutani R. Epidemiology of ALS in Italy: a 10-year prospective population-based study. Neurology. 2009; 72(8): 725–31.
33. O'Toole O, Traynor BJ, Brennan P, Sheehan C, Frost E, Corr B, et al. Epidemiology and clinical features of amyotrophic lateral sclerosis in Ireland between 1995 and 2004. Journal of Neurology, Neurosurgery, and Psychiatry. 2008; 79(1): 30–32.
34. D'Ovidio F, Rooney J, Visser A, Vermeulen R, Veldink J, Van den Berg LH, et al. Critical issues in ALS case-control studies: the case of the Euro-MOTOR study. Amyotroph Lateral Scler Frontotemporal Degener. 2017; 18(5-6): 411–18. doi: 10.1080/21678421.2017.1285939. Epub 10 Feb 2017. PubMed PMID: 28594593.
35. Roberts AL, Johnson NJ, Chen JT, Cudkowicz ME, Weisskopf MG. Race/ethnicity, socioeconomic status, and ALS mortality in the United States. Neurology. 2016; 87(22): 2300–8.
36. Henry KA, Fagliano J, Jordan HM, Rechtman L, Kaye WE. Geographic variation of amyotrophic lateral sclerosis incidence in New Jersey, 2009–2011. American Journal of Epidemiology. 2015; 182(6): 512–19.
37. Kasarskis EJ, Winslow M. When did Lou Gehrig's personal illness begin? Neurology. 1989; 39(9): 1243–5.
38. Scarmeas N, Shih T, Stern Y, Ottman R, Rowland LP. Premorbid weight, body mass, and varsity athletics in ALS. Neurology. 2002; 59(5): 773–5.
39. Chio A, Benzi G, Dossena M, Mutani R, Mora G. Severely increased risk of amyotrophic lateral sclerosis among Italian professional football players. Brain. 2005; 128(Pt 3): 472–6.

40. Lehman EJ, Hein MJ, Baron SL, Gersic CM. Neurodegenerative causes of death among retired National Football League players. Neurology. 2012; 79(19): 1970–4.
41. Pupillo E, Messina P, Giussani G, Logroscino G, Zoccolella S, Chio A, et al. Physical activity and amyotrophic lateral sclerosis: a European population-based case-control study. Annals of Neurology. 2014; 75(5): 708–16.
42. Gallo V, Vanacore N, Bueno-de-Mesquita HB, Vermeulen R, Brayne C, Pearce N, et al. Physical activity and risk of amyotrophic lateral sclerosis in a prospective cohort study. Eur J Epidemiol. 2016; 31(3): 255–66.
43. Seals RM, Hansen J, Gredal O, Weisskopf MG. Physical trauma and amyotrophic lateral sclerosis: a population-based study using Danish National Registries. American Journal of Epidemiology. 2016; 183(4): 294–301.
44. Beghi E, Logroscino G, Chio A, Hardiman O, Millul A, Mitchell D, et al. Amyotrophic lateral sclerosis, physical exercise, trauma and sports: results of a population-based pilot case-control study. Amyotrophic Lateral Sclerosis: official publication of the World Federation of Neurology Research Group on Motor Neuron Diseases. 2010; 11(3): 289–92.
45. Horner RD, Kamins KG, Feussner JR, Grambow SC, Hoff-Lindquist J, Harati Y, et al. Occurrence of amyotrophic lateral sclerosis among Gulf War veterans. Neurology. 2003; 61(6): 742–9.
46. Haley RW. Excess incidence of ALS in young Gulf War veterans. Neurology. 2003; 61(6): 750–6.
47. Weisskopf MG, O'Reilly EJ, McCullough ML, Calle EE, Thun MJ, Cudkowicz M, et al. Prospective study of military service and mortality from ALS. Neurology. 2005; 64(1): 32–7.
48. Bergman BP, Mackay DF, Pell JP. Early adoption of screening and the changing pattern of cervical cancer in UK military women: evidence from the Scottish Veterans Health Study. Journal of the Royal Army Medical Corps. 2016; 162(5): 379–82.
49. Weisskopf MG, Cudkowicz ME, Johnson N. Military service and amyotrophic lateral sclerosis in a population-based cohort. Epidemiology (Cambridge, Mass). 2015; 26(6): 831–8.
50. Alonso A, Logroscino G, Hernan MA. Smoking and the risk of amyotrophic lateral sclerosis: a systematic review and meta-analysis. Journal of Neurology, Neurosurgery, and Psychiatry. 2010; 81(11): 1249–52.
51. Gallo V, Bueno-De-Mesquita HB, Vermeulen R, Andersen PM, Kyrozis A, Linseisen J, et al. Smoking and risk for amyotrophic lateral sclerosis: analysis of the EPIC cohort. Annals of Neurology. 2009; 65(4): 378–85.
52. Wang H, O'Reilly EJ, Weisskopf MG, Logroscino G, McCullough ML, Thun MJ, et al. Smoking and risk of amyotrophic lateral sclerosis: a pooled analysis of 5 prospective cohorts. Archives of Neurology. 2011; 68(2): 207–13.
53. de Jong SW, Huisman MH, Sutedja NA, van der Kooi AJ, de Visser M, Schelhaas HJ, et al. Smoking, alcohol consumption, and the risk of amyotrophic lateral sclerosis: a population-based study. American Journal of Epidemiology. 2012; 176(3): 233–9.
54. Livesley B, Sissons CE. Chronic lead intoxication mimicking motor neurone disease. BMJ. 1968; 4(5627): 387–8.
55. Campbell AM, Williams ER, Barltrop D. Motor neuron disease and exposure to lead. Journal of Neurology, Neurosurgery, and Psychiatry. 1970; 33(6): 877–85.
56. Thomson RM, Parry GJ. Neuropathies associated with excessive exposure to lead. Muscle & Nerve. 2006; 33(6): 732–41.
57. McGuire V, Longstreth WT, Jr, Nelson LM, Koepsell TD, Checkoway H, Morgan MS, et al. Occupational exposures and amyotrophic lateral sclerosis. A population-based case-control study. American Journal of Epidemiology. 1997; 145(12): 1076–88.
58. Kamel F, Umbach DM, Hu H, Munsat TL, Shefner JM, Taylor JA, et al. Lead exposure as a risk factor for amyotrophic lateral sclerosis. Neuro-degenerative Diseases. 2005; 2(3–4): 195–201.
59. Wang MD, Gomes J, Cashman NR, Little J, Krewski D. A meta-analysis of observational studies of the association between chronic occupational exposure to lead and amyotrophic lateral sclerosis. Journal of Occupational and Environmental Medicine. 2014; 56(12): 1235–42.
60. Malek AM, Barchowsky A, Bowser R, Heiman-Patterson T, Lacomis D, Rana S, et al. Environmental and occupational risk factors for amyotrophic lateral sclerosis: a case-control study. Neuro-degenerative Diseases. 2014; 14(1): 31–8.
61. Burns CJ, Beard KK, Cartmill JB. Mortality in chemical workers potentially exposed to 2,4-dichlorophenoxyacetic acid (2,4-D) 1945-94: an update. Occupational and Environmental Medicine. 2001; 58(1): 24–30.
62. Kang H, Cha ES, Choi GJ, Lee WJ. Amyotrophic lateral sclerosis and agricultural environments: a systematic review. Journal of Korean Medical Science. 2014; 29(12): 1610–7.
63. Weisskopf MG, Morozova N, O'Reilly EJ, McCullough ML, Calle EE, Thun MJ, et al. Prospective study of chemical exposures and amyotrophic lateral sclerosis. Journal of Neurology, Neurosurgery, and Psychiatry. 2009; 80(5): 558–61.
64. Kamel F, Umbach DM, Bedlack RS, Richards M, Watson M, Alavanja MC, et al. Pesticide exposure and amyotrophic lateral sclerosis. Neurotoxicology. 2012; 33(3): 457–62.
65. Kioumourtzoglou MA, Rotem RS, Seals RM, Gredal O, Hansen J, Weisskopf MG. Diabetes mellitus, obesity, and diagnosis of amyotrophic lateral sclerosis: a population-based study. JAMA Neurology. 2015; 72(8): 905–11.
66. Mariosa D, Kamel F, Bellocco R, Ye W, Fang F. Association between diabetes and amyotrophic lateral sclerosis in Sweden. European Journal of Neurology: the official journal of the European Federation of Neurological Societies. 2015; 22(11): 1436–42.
67. Sun Y, Lu CJ, Chen RC, Hou WH, Li CY. Risk of amyotrophic lateral sclerosis in patients with diabetes: a nationwide population-based cohort study. Journal of Epidemiology. 2015; 25(6): 445–51.
68. Dupuis L, Pradat PF, Ludolph AC, Loeffler JP. Energy metabolism in amyotrophic lateral sclerosis. Lancet Neurology. 2011; 10(1): 75–82.
69. Seelen M, van Doormaal PT, Visser AE, Huisman MH, Roozekrans MH, de Jong SW, et al. Prior medical conditions and the risk of amyotrophic lateral sclerosis. Journal of Neurology. 2014; 261(10): 1949–56.
70. Turner MR, Wotton C, Talbot K, Goldacre MJ. Cardiovascular fitness as a risk factor for amyotrophic lateral sclerosis: indirect evidence from record linkage study. Journal of Neurology, Neurosurgery, and Psychiatry. 2012; 83(4): 395–8.
71. Sutedja NA, van der Schouw YT, Fischer K, Sizoo EM, Huisman MH, Veldink JH, et al. Beneficial vascular risk profile is associated with amyotrophic lateral sclerosis. Journal of Neurology, Neurosurgery, and Psychiatry. 2011; 82(6): 638–42.
72. Kioumourtzoglou MA, Seals RM, Gredal O, Mittleman MA, Hansen J, Weisskopf MG. Cardiovascular disease and diagnosis of amyotrophic lateral sclerosis: A population based study. Amyotrophic Lateral Sclerosis & Frontotemporal Degeneration. 2016; 17(7–8): 548–54.

73. Ratnavalli E, Brayne C, Dawson K, Hodges JR. The prevalence of frontotemporal dementia. Neurology. 2002; 58(11): 1615–21.
74. Ikejima C, Yasuno F, Mizukami K, Sasaki M, Tanimukai S, Asada T. Prevalence and causes of early-onset dementia in Japan: a population-based study. Stroke; a Journal of Cerebral Circulation. 2009; 40(8): 2709–14.
75. Borroni B, Alberici A, Grassi M, Rozzini L, Turla M, Zanetti O, et al. Prevalence and demographic features of early-onset neurodegenerative dementia in Brescia County, Italy. Alzheimer Disease and Associated Disorders. 2011; 25(4): 341–4.
76. Coyle-Gilchrist IT, Dick KM, Patterson K, Vazquez Rodriquez P, Wehmann E, Wilcox A, et al. Prevalence, characteristics, and survival of frontotemporal lobar degeneration syndromes. Neurology. 2016; 86(18): 1736–43.
77. Knopman DS, Petersen RC, Edland SD, Cha RH, Rocca WA. The incidence of frontotemporal lobar degeneration in Rochester, Minnesota, 1990 through 1994. Neurology. 2004; 62(3): 506–8.
78. Mercy L, Hodges JR, Dawson K, Barker RA, Brayne C. Incidence of early-onset dementias in Cambridgeshire, United Kingdom. Neurology. 2008; 71(19):1496–9.
79. Garre-Olmo J, Genis Batlle D, del Mar Fernandez M, Marquez Daniel F, de Eugenio Huelamo R, Casadevall T, et al. Incidence and subtypes of early-onset dementia in a geographically defined general population. Neurology. 2010; 75(14): 1249–55.
80. Woollacott IO, Rohrer JD. The clinical spectrum of sporadic and familial forms of frontotemporal dementia. Journal of Neurochemistry. 2016; 138(Suppl 1): 6–31.
81. Rosso SM, Landweer EJ, Houterman M, Donker Kaat L, van Duijn CM, van Swieten JC. Medical and environmental risk factors for sporadic frontotemporal dementia: a retrospective case-control study. Journal of Neurology, Neurosurgery, and Psychiatry. 2003; 74(11): 1574–6.
82. Renton AE, Chio A, Traynor BJ. State of play in amyotrophic lateral sclerosis genetics. Nature Neuroscience. 2014; 17(1): 17–23.
83. Hardy J, Rogaeva E. Motor neuron disease and frontotemporal dementia: sometimes related, sometimes not. Experimental Neurology. 2014; 262 Pt B: 75–83.
84. Black HA, Leighton DJ, Cleary EM, Rose E, Stephenson L, Colville S, et al. Genetic epidemiology of motor neuron disease-associated variants in the population. Neurobiol Aging. 2017; (51): 178. e11–e20.
85. Chio A, Calvo A, Mazzini L, Cantello R, Mora G, Moglia C, et al. Extensive genetics of ALS: a population-based study in Italy. Neurology. 2012; 79(19): 1983–9.
86. Kenna KP, McLaughlin RL, Byrne S, Elamin M, Heverin M, Kenny EM, et al. Delineating the genetic heterogeneity of ALS using targeted high-throughput sequencing. Journal of Medical Genetics. 2013; 50(11): 776–83.
87. van Blitterswijk M, van Es MA, Hennekam EA, Dooijes D, van Rheenen W, Medic J, et al. Evidence for an oligogenic basis of amyotrophic lateral sclerosis. Human Molecular Genetics. 2012; 21(17): 3776–84.
88. Borghero G, Pugliatti M, Marrosu F, Marrosu MG, Murru MR, Floris G, et al. Genetic architecture of ALS in Sardinia. Neurobiol Aging. 2014; 35(12): 2882. e7–12.
89. Majounie E, Renton AE, Mok K, Dopper EG, Waite A, Rollinson S, et al. Frequency of the C9orf72 hexanucleotide repeat expansion in patients with amyotrophic lateral sclerosis and frontotemporal dementia: a cross-sectional study. Lancet Neurology. 2012; 11(4): 323–30.
90. Zou ZY, Zhou ZR, Che CH, Liu CY, He RL, Huang HP. Genetic epidemiology of amyotrophic lateral sclerosis: a systematic review and meta-analysis. Journal of Neurology, Neurosurgery, and Psychiatry. 2017; 88(7): 540–9. doi: 10.1136/jnnp-2016-315018. Epub 5 Jan 2017. Review. PubMed PMID: 28057713.
91. Chio A, Calvo A, Moglia C, Gamna F, Mattei A, Mazzini L, et al. Non-invasive ventilation in amyotrophic lateral sclerosis: a 10 year population based study. Journal of Neurology, Neurosurgery, and Psychiatry. 2012; 83(4): 377–81.
92. Rohrer JD, Guerreiro R, Vandrovcova J, Uphill J, Reiman D, Beck J, et al. The heritability and genetics of frontotemporal lobar degeneration. Neurology. 2009; 73(18): 1451–6.
93. Bang J, Spina S, Miller BL. Frontotemporal dementia. Lancet. 2015; 386(10004): 1672–82.
94. Chio A, Logroscino G, Hardiman O, Swingler R, Mitchell D, Beghi E, et al. Prognostic factors in ALS: A critical review. Amyotrophic Lateral Sclerosis: official publication of the World Federation of Neurology Research Group on Motor Neuron Diseases. 2009; 10(5–6): 310–23.
95. Zach N, Ennist DL, Taylor AA, Alon H, Sherman A, Kueffner R, et al. Being PRO-ACTive: What can a clinical trial database reveal about ALS? Neurotherapeutics: the Journal of the American Society for Experimental NeuroTherapeutics. 2015; 12(2): 417–23.
96. Chio A, Canosa A, Gallo S, Cammarosano S, Moglia C, Fuda G, et al. ALS clinical trials: do enrolled patients accurately represent the ALS population? Neurology. 2011; 77(15): 1432–7.
97. Rooney J, Byrne S, Heverin M, Corr B, Elamin M, Staines A, et al. Survival analysis of Irish amyotrophic lateral sclerosis patients diagnosed from 1995–2010. PLOS One. 2013; 8(9): e74733.
98. Forbes RB, Colville S, Cran GW, Swingler RJ. Unexpected decline in survival from amyotrophic lateral sclerosis/motor neuron disease. Journal of Neurology, Neurosurgery, and Psychiatry. 2004; 75(12): 1753–5.
99. Chancellor AM, Slattery JM, Fraser H, Swingler RJ, Holloway SM, Warlow CP. The prognosis of adult-onset motor neuron disease: a prospective study based on the Scottish Motor Neuron Disease Register. Journal of Neurology. 1993; 240(6): 339–46.
100. del Aguila MA, Longstreth WT Jr, McGuire V, Koepsell TD, van Belle G. Prognosis in amyotrophic lateral sclerosis: a population-based study. Neurology. 2003; 60(5): 813–19.
101. Chio A, Mora G, Leone M, Mazzini L, Cocito D, Giordana MT, et al. Early symptom progression rate is related to ALS outcome: a prospective population-based study. Neurology. 2002; 59(1): 99–103.
102. Pupillo E, Messina P, Logroscino G, Beghi E. Long-term survival in amyotrophic lateral sclerosis: a population-based study. Annals of Neurology. 2014; 75(2): 287–97.
103. Marin B, Couratier P, Arcuti S, Copetti M, Fontana A, Nicol M, et al. Stratification of ALS patients' survival: a population-based study. Journal of Neurology. 2016; 263(1): 100–111.
104. Jordan H, Fagliano J, Rechtman L, Lefkowitz D, Kaye W. Effects of demographic factors on survival time after a diagnosis of amyotrophic lateral sclerosis. Neuroepidemiology. 2015; 44(2): 114–20.
105. Zoccolella S, Beghi E, Palagano G, Fraddosio A, Guerra V, Samarelli V, et al. Analysis of survival and prognostic factors in amyotrophic lateral sclerosis: a population based study. Journal of Neurology, Neurosurgery, and Psychiatry. 2008; 79(1): 33–7.

106. Scotton WJ, Scott KM, Moore DH, Almedom L, Wijesekera LC, Janssen A, et al. Prognostic categories for amyotrophic lateral sclerosis. Amyotrophic Lateral Sclerosis: official publication of the World Federation of Neurology Research Group on Motor Neuron Diseases. 2012; 13(6): 502–8.
107. Chio A, Calvo A, Moglia C, Mazzini L, Mora G. Phenotypic heterogeneity of amyotrophic lateral sclerosis: a population based study. Journal of Neurology, Neurosurgery, and Psychiatry. 2011; 82(7): 740–6.
108. Phukan J, Elamin M, Bede P, Jordan N, Gallagher L, Byrne S, et al. The syndrome of cognitive impairment in amyotrophic lateral sclerosis: a population-based study. Journal of Neurology, Neurosurgery, and Psychiatry. 2012; 83(1): 102–8.
109. Montuschi A, Iazzolino B, Calvo A, Moglia C, Lopiano L, Restagno G, et al. Cognitive correlates in amyotrophic lateral sclerosis: a population-based study in Italy. Journal of Neurology, Neurosurgery, and Psychiatry. 2015; 86(2): 168–73.
110. Mateen FJ, Carone M, Sorenson EJ. Patients who survive 5 years or more with ALS in Olmsted County, 1925–2004. Journal of Neurology, Neurosurgery, and Psychiatry. 2010; 81(10): 1144–6.
111. Mandrioli J, Biguzzi S, Guidi C, Sette E, Terlizzi E, Ravasio A, et al. Heterogeneity in ALSFRS-R decline and survival: a population-based study in Italy. Neurological Sciences: official journal of the Italian Neurological Society and of the Italian Society of Clinical Neurophysiology. 2015; 36(12): 2243–52.
112. Marin B, Arcuti S, Jesus P, Logroscino G, Copetti M, Fontana A, et al. Population-based evidence that survival in amyotrophic lateral sclerosis is related to weight loss at diagnosis. Neuro-degenerative Diseases. 2016; 16(3–4): 225–34.
113. Desport JC, Preux PM, Truong TC, Vallat JM, Sautereau D, Couratier P. Nutritional status is a prognostic factor for survival in ALS patients. Neurology. 1999; 53(5): 1059–63.
114. Traynor BJ, Codd MB, Corr B, Forde C, Frost E, Hardiman OM. Clinical features of amyotrophic lateral sclerosis according to the El Escorial and Airlie House diagnostic criteria: a population-based study. Archives of Neurology. 2000; 57(8): 1171–6.
115. Rooney J, Heverin M, Vajda A, Burke T, Galvin M, Tobin K, et al. Survival analysis of geospatial factors in the Irish ALS cohort. Amyotrophic Lateral Sclerosis & Frontotemporal Degeneration. 2016; 17(7–8): 555–60.
116. Elden AC, Kim HJ, Hart MP, Chen-Plotkin AS, Johnson BS, Fang X, et al. Ataxin-2 intermediate-length polyglutamine expansions are associated with increased risk for ALS. Nature. 2010; 466(7310): 1069–75.
117. Chio A, Calvo A, Moglia C, Canosa A, Brunetti M, Barberis M, et al. ATXN2 polyQ intermediate repeats are a modifier of ALS survival. Neurology. 2015; 84(3): 251–8.
118. Traynor BJ, Alexander M, Corr B, Frost E, Hardiman O. Effect of a multidisciplinary amyotrophic lateral sclerosis (ALS) clinic on ALS survival: a population based study, 1996–2000. Journal of Neurology, Neurosurgery, and Psychiatry. 2003; 74(9): 1258–61.
119. Chio A, Bottacchi E, Buffa C, Mutani R, Mora G. Positive effects of tertiary centres for amyotrophic lateral sclerosis on outcome and use of hospital facilities. Journal of Neurology, Neurosurgery, and Psychiatry. 2006; 77(8): 948–50.
120. Zoccolella S, Beghi E, Palagano G, Fraddosio A, Guerra V, Lepore V, et al. ALS multidisciplinary clinic and survival. Results from a population-based study in Southern Italy. Journal of Neurology. 2007; 254(8): 1107–12.
121. Lacomblez L, Bensimon G, Leigh PN, Guillet P, Meininger V. Dose-ranging study of riluzole in amyotrophic lateral sclerosis. Amyotrophic Lateral Sclerosis/Riluzole Study Group II. Lancet. 1996; 347(9013): 1425–31.
122. Bourke SC, Tomlinson M, Williams TL, Bullock RE, Shaw PJ, Gibson GJ. Effects of non-invasive ventilation on survival and quality of life in patients with amyotrophic lateral sclerosis: a randomised controlled trial. Lancet Neurology. 2006; 5(2): 140–7.
123. Calvo A, Canosa A, Bertuzzo D, Cugnasco P, Solero L, Clerico M, et al. Influence of cigarette smoking on ALS outcome: a population-based study. Journal of Neurology, Neurosurgery, and Psychiatry. 2016; 87(11): 1229–33.
124. Huisman MH, Seelen M, van Doormaal PT, de Jong SW, de Vries JH, van der Kooi AJ, et al. Effect of presymptomatic body mass index and consumption of fat and alcohol on amyotrophic lateral sclerosis. JAMA Neurology. 2015; 72(10): 1155–62.
125. Hodges JR, Davies R, Xuereb J, Kril J, Halliday G. Survival in frontotemporal dementia. Neurology. 2003; 61(3): 349–54.
126. Roberson ED, Hesse JH, Rose KD, Slama H, Johnson JK, Yaffe K, et al. Frontotemporal dementia progresses to death faster than Alzheimer disease. Neurology. 2005; 65(5): 719–25.
127. Devenney E, Bartley L, Hoon C, O'Callaghan C, Kumfor F, Hornberger M, et al. Progression in behavioral variant frontotemporal dementia: a longitudinal study. JAMA Neurology. 2015; 72(12): 1501–9.
128. Garcin B, Lillo P, Hornberger M, Piguet O, Dawson K, Nestor PJ, et al. Determinants of survival in behavioral variant frontotemporal dementia. Neurology. 2009; 73(20): 1656–61.
129. Kansal K, Mareddy M, Sloane KL, Minc AA, Rabins PV, McGready JB, et al. Survival in frontotemporal dementia phenotypes: a meta-analysis. Dementia and Geriatric Cognitive Disorders. 2016; 41(1–2): 109–22.
130. Hornberger M, Shelley BP, Kipps CM, Piguet O, Hodges JR. Can progressive and non-progressive behavioural variant frontotemporal dementia be distinguished at presentation? Journal of Neurology, Neurosurgery, and Psychiatry. 2009; 80(6): 591–3.
131. Chiu WZ, Kaat LD, Seelaar H, Rosso SM, Boon AJ, Kamphorst W, et al. Survival in progressive supranuclear palsy and frontotemporal dementia. Journal of Neurology, Neurosurgery, and Psychiatry. 2010; 81(4): 441–5.
132. Neumann M, Sampathu DM, Kwong LK, Truax AC, Micsenyi MC, Chou TT, et al. Ubiquitinated TDP-43 in frontotemporal lobar degeneration and amyotrophic lateral sclerosis. Science (New York, NY). 2006; 314(5796): 130–3.

14

Rare neurodegenerative parkinsonism (PSP, MSA, CBD)

James B Rowe and Ian TS Coyle-Gilchrist

Introduction

There are many neurological disorders that are individually rare, but which between them constitute a substantial burden of disease, in social, health, and economic terms. Here, we focus on a group of rare neurodegenerative disorders that include progressive supranuclear palsy (PSP), corticobasal syndrome (CBS), and multiple system atrophy (MSA).

These disorders differ in many aspects of their pathology and clinical features, but historically they have often been considered together, in research, teaching and healthcare services. In this chapter, we discuss the evolving nomenclature that must be understood in order to appreciate the epidemiological evidence and its limitations. We then consider the features of these disorders that make epidemiological research especially difficult, including substantially overlapping features of disease and marked under-diagnosis. Finally, we consider the currently available data on prevalence and incidence, and suggest ways to improve the future evidence base so as to inform clinicians, policymakers, healthcare providers, and trialists.

The name of the rose

In reviewing the historical evidence, drawn from the last 50 years, one must set the data in the context of the understanding of these diseases as it was at the time. The interpretation of terms, and diagnostic labels, has not been constant. We will highlight the impact of these changes on the epidemiology.

PSP, CBS, and MSA are often lumped together under the collective term of 'Parkinson-plus' syndromes, or 'atypical parkinsonism'. These terms are widely used but nonetheless misleading. For example, typical PSP is not atypical, although it is distinct from other conditions. As an analogy, consider a camel—it is not an atypical horse, but a typical camel.

These three disorders are also pathologically and clinically quite different from idiopathic PD, and the term Parkinson-plus might lead the novice to understand that PSP, CBS, and MSA are forms of PD, which they are not. The term 'parkinsonism' refers to akinetic-rigidity, which is a core clinical feature of the classical presentations of these disorders. However, we shall see that even this supposedly core feature is no longer considered a universal feature of the syndromes which result from the pathological entities associated with PSP, CBS, and MSA. PSP may present without akinesia or motor rigidity, while MSA may present as ataxia without parkinsonism.

Progressive supranuclear palsy was described in 1964 by Steele et al.,[1] as a syndrome of axial akinetic-rigidity, supranuclear gaze palsy, bulbar dysfunction, and postural instability, with mild frontal cognitive impairment. They described characteristic neuropathology of neuronal loss, gliosis, and NFT affecting brainstem and subcortical nuclei. This pathology was subsequently shown to be a primary tauopathy with aggregates of hyperphosphorylated tau. Since 1996, this syndrome has generally been diagnosed according to the MDS criteria,[2] and the clinic-pathological correlation of this syndrome to tau pathology exceeds 90%.[3,4]

More recently, this syndrome has been called Richardson's syndrome, PSP-Richardson's syndrome, or PSP-RS. This is to distinguish it from other clinical syndromes that came to be recognized as having the same underlying pathology. For example, Williams et al.,[5] reported that half of cases in a large movement disorder brain bank series with PSP did not have Richardson's syndrome, but instead looked more like idiopathic PD, which they therefore termed PSP-parkinsonism, or PSP-P. Later, Respondek et al.,[6] examined the presenting clinical syndrome in a separate large series of cases with the pathology of PSP. The classical PSP-RS was shown to be a minority of the clinical presentations. PSP-P was as common, but so, too, were cases of abnormal behaviour, personality, speech, and language. The relative proportions of these clinical syndromes in relation to PSP pathology and PSP-mimics is summarised in Fig. 14.1B.

In 2016, the diagnostic criteria for PSP were radically re-written, to include multiple clinical syndromes, varying in clinical features (termed PSP-RS, PSP-P, PSP-F for frontal, PSP-CBS, and so on) and varying in the strength of clinic-pathological correlation.[7,8] So, when considering the data for prevalence or incidence of PSP, one must consider whether a study refers to PSP-RS clinical syndrome,

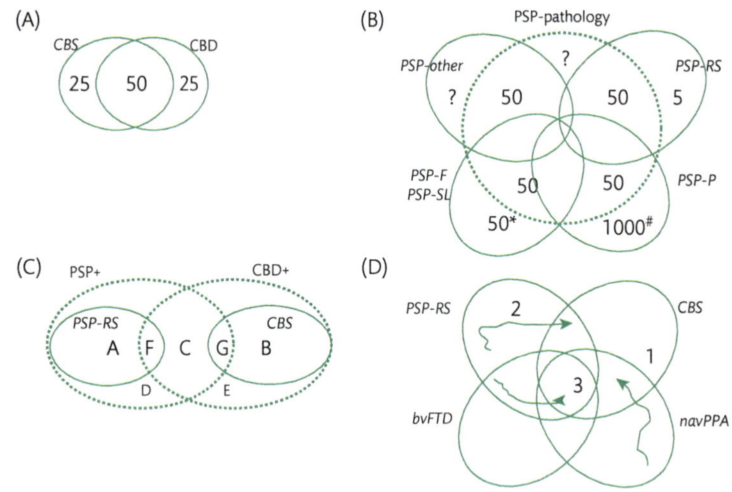

Fig. 14.1 Illustration of the challenges in diagnosis and clinic-pathological correlation which affect epidemiological studies. A. Corticobasal syndrome (CBS) and corticobasal degeneration (CBD, the pathology) overlap to a limited degree. The figures represent approximate percentages arising from post-mortem validation studies. B. Progressive supranuclear palsy (PSP) pathology has many phenotypic expressions, including Richardson's syndrome (PSP-RS), and PSP-parkinsonism (PSP-P), and presentations with changes in behaviour (PSP-F), speech and language (PSP-SL). The figures represent approximate proportions, as indicated by post-mortem studies. These syndromic variants have causes other than PSP pathology, rarely in the case of PSP-RS but very commonly in the case of PSP-P. C. Illustration of the problems arising from pooling prevalence estimates from studies which have focused on one or other syndrome. See text for details. D. Illustration of the challenge to epidemiology caused by the evolution of clinical syndromes over time, in three different cases. The accumulation of deficits leads to overlap or de-differentiation of cases. See text for descriptions of cases 1, 2, and 3.

or instead refers to any of the clinical syndromes that are now associated with the PSP pathology.

CBS has a similarly complex nosological history. First described as corticodentatonigral degeneration with neuronal achromasia,[9] and later corticobasoganglionic degeneration,[10] the disease became better known as corticobasal degeneration.[11] At first, the syndrome of asymmetric motor dysfunction, akinetic-rigidity, dystonia, myoclonus, apraxia, and alien limb, was strongly associated with a distinctive neuroglial pathology, with ballooned achromatic neurons in the cortex and tau inclusions in astrocytes and oligodendrocytes.[12] However, it became clear that clinicopathological correlations were poor, made worse by the proliferation of diagnostic criteria of varying sensitivity and specificity,[10,13,14,15,16] which were either lacking in pathological validation, or were biased towards cohorts with cognitive or motor syndromes, or were poorly operationalized for clinical application. New international consensus diagnostic criteria were developed in 2013,[16] which confirmed the convention of using CBS to refer to the clinical syndrome and CBD to refer to the pathology of corticobasal degeneration. The clinicopathological correlation remains limited at with around two-thirds of CBD cases displaying CBS, and two-thirds of CBS cases being cases by CBD (summarized in Fig. 14.1A).[17] So, when considering the data for prevalence or incidence of CBS/CBD, one must consider whether a study refers to CBS clinical syndrome, or to any of the clinical syndromes that are associated with the CBD-pathology.

Multiple system atrophy has two principal syndromic variants, currently known as MSA-C (cerebellar, referring to the ataxia), and MSA-P (parkinsonism, referring to akinetic rigidity). Both forms are associated with autonomic dysfunction, and relative preservation of cognition. The neuropathology of MSA includes glial cytoplasmic inclusions and degenerative changes to the basal ganglia, brainstem nuclei, cerebellum, intermediolateral columns, and Onuf's nucleus in the spinal cord. The inclusions are distinct from PSP and CBD, in that they contain a-synuclein but not tau. These current terms MSA-P and MSA-C[18,19] replaced striatonigral degeneration, sporadic olivopontocerebellar atrophy, and Shy Drager Syndrome. In centres of excellence, these criteria have good accuracy, around 85%,[20] but the accuracy in primary care cohorts or of early stage disease is likely to be much lower. In contrast to PSP and CBS/CBD, the criteria and nosology pertaining to MSA has been more stable during the period in which much of the epidemiological evidence was obtained.

Lumping, splitting, and double dipping

As the diagnostic criteria for PSP and CBS/CBD have been revised, it is increasingly apparent that there is an overlap between them. This is most evident in the mirror terms CBS-PSP[16] and PSP-CBS.[7] This is not battle for diagnostic territory, but reflects a maturing understanding of the spectral nature of these disorders. Indeed, some have proposed that PSP and CBS are merely phenotypic variants of a single disease.[21] Should the epidemiology 'lump' them together as a single pathological entity, or should the prevalence and incidence estimates recognize the phenotypic heterogeneity and 'split' cases into syndromic variants?

Whether epidemiological studies focus on one illness, say PSP, or another, say CBS, or consider them jointly will have a considerable impact on the estimated prevalence and incidence. Consider the situation illustrated in Fig. 14.1C. A study of PSP-RS alone, identifies cases A + F, and a separate study of CBS alone identifies cases B + G. There are additional cases D and C with PSP pathology but not the classical syndrome PSP-RS. Of these, cases C have some features of CBS, enough to exclude them from diagnosis of PSP-RS but not enough to include them as CBS under the criteria before.[16] There are cases E with CBD pathology but not CBS. There are also cases F with CBD-pathology but which mimic PSP-RS and cases G of PSP-pathology that cause CBS.

Depending on the study design, the estimated prevalence of PSP and CBS/CBD would vary widely. For example, a minimal study of PSP-RS might include only PSP cases A + F, while a second minimal study of CBS would include only cases G + B. If pooling across these studies, the combined prevalence estimate of PSP and CBS would be A + F + G + B, failing to include cases C who quite clearly have features of both PSP and CBS. In contrast, an inclusive study of clinical disorders caused by PSP pathology would include A + C + D + F + G, while the inclusive study of disorders caused by CBD would include B + C + E + F + G. If pooling across these two inclusive studies, the combined prevalence would be A + B + 2C + D + E + 2F + 2G, inadvertently 'double-dipping' and twice counting cases in classes C, F, and G. This risk is real, made more so with the strongly overlapping criteria for CBS-PSP[16] and PSP-CBS,[7] even allowing that the two criteria are not quite identical.

It is not for this chapter to assert whether it is better to be maximally specific (and therefore insensitive) in case ascertainment, or to be more inclusive (with lower specificity). However, we do highlight the risk of combining historical epidemiological studies, as the pooled estimates will be very inaccurate. As there are perhaps more cases of PSP pathology without PSP-RS than with it,[6] the risk of wildly inaccurate estimates is high if one is to pool across studies which have examined the syndromes separately.

Symptoms, diagnosis, uncertainty, and evolution

There are many challenges to accurate epidemiology of neurological disorders, but PSP, CBS/CBD, and MSA present some exceptional difficulties. A reader new to the topic might assume that whether a person has a disease is clear, even if there may be difficulties in identifying them within a population. One might acknowledge a finite mis-diagnosis rate and biases in case ascertainment, but still hold to an underlying assumption that one either does, or does not, have the illness. This assumption is not well founded. In contrast with discrete events such as stroke or hip fractures, PSP, CBS, and MSA progress gradually from asymptomatic pathology through to fulminant disease.

The diagnosis is usually established clinically in terms of probable PSP, CBS/CBD, or MSA, with a 'full house' of relevant symptoms and signs under the clinical diagnostic criteria and appropriate investigations. Some cases may be identified at an earlier stage, when the diagnosis is 'probable', in terms of consistent symptoms and signs and lack of exclusionary criteria, but with limited certainty or specificity. However, even before this stage, patients may have several years of symptoms, which in hindsight indicate the onset of their disease but which prospectively fall far short of enabling a diagnosis. Such an oligosymptomatic state may last for several years. For example, it typically takes three years from first symptoms onset to the diagnosis of PSP-RS.[22,23]. In an illness with mean duration of six years,[22,23] this period of undiagnosed but symptomatic disease represents approximately half of prevalent cases, were they to be diagnosed.

Furthermore, it is increasingly clear that a state of progressive pathology without symptoms can last for years or even decades. This evidence comes in part from post-mortem studies, in which PSP, MSA, and CBD pathology is identified in people without evident symptoms. In addition, even though PSP, CBD, and MSA are essentially sporadic diseases, they have much in common with other neurodegenerative disorders including frontotemporal lobar degeneration (FTLD) arising from tau mutations, PD from autosomal PARK mutations, HD from Huntingtin mutations, and progressive ataxias from SCA mutations.[24,25,26] In these genetic disorders, cognitive, brain imaging, and fluidic biomarkers have consistently shown 1–2 decades or asymptomatic prodromal neuropathology.[27,28,29] It is likely, therefore, that sporadic PSP, CBD, and MSA also have several years of asymptomatic pathology. To complicate diagnosis further, early symptoms may be insidious and not recognized as features of the illness, such as subtle affective and personality changes in the prodromal phase of PSP.[30] Alternatively, symptoms of the underlying pathology may be transiently elicited by acute illness or medication (e.g. neuroleptics), recovering on withdrawal, and re-emerging several years later.

A third problem is that many patients may evolve from one syndrome to another,[5,31] or gain clinical features that accumulate criteria for more than one syndrome.[23] Again, the sum of former prevalence estimates of single disorders would not accurately reflect the prevalence of the syndromes when considered together. This is illustrated in Fig. 14.1D, for three cases. Case one represents an individual whose initial syndrome is of non-fluent agrammatic primary progressive aphasia (formerly called progressive non-fluent aphasia). Many such patients develop a motor disorder with apraxia and dystonia that comes to resemble CBS. Case two represents a patient presenting with PSP-RS, but who again develops apraxia and dystonia, resembling CBS. Case three represents the evolution of a poorly differentiated tauopathy within the FTLD spectrum, accumulating clinical features of PSP-RS, bvFTD, and CBS, and lacking features to support a single classification. Such intermediate, progressive, and poorly differentiated cases are common.[23]

So how should an epidemiological study approach asymptomatic disease, prodromal stages, and the period of diagnostic uncertainty? The answer is with clarity of the precise research question, and awareness of the 'soft' transitions between states. With these caveats in mind, we now turn to the published evidence to support estimated prevalences and incidence of PSP, CBS/CBD, and MSA, individually.

Prevalence and Incidence of PSP

To date four studies have specifically attempted to determine the prevalence of PSP in Europe and the USA,[23,32,33,34] with two in Japan.[35,36] Golbe et al.[32] surveyed neurologists and chronic care facilities in a US district (population = 799,022). Suspected cases were reassessed by the study team, confirming 50 cases of symptomatic probable and possible PSP, corresponding largely to PSP-RS. This provides an estimated prevalence = 1.39/100,000.[32]

Schrag et al.[33] took a different approach in the UK, screening 15 urban general practice records (population = 121,608). Over 200 cases of possible Parkinsonian disease were declared, of whom 84% were assessed by a movement disorders specialist, leading to five cases of probable PSP and one of possible PSP. Interestingly, none of these six had been previously diagnosed with PSP, indicating a severe problem in under-diagnosis that may affect other studies. The crude and age-adjusted prevalence was of 4.9/100,000 and 6.4/

100,000 respectively. With the inclusion of additional patients with unclassifiable parkinsonism, which we speculate to include a high proportion of intermediate and overlap cases such as CBS-PSP or PSP-CBS (see Fig. 14.1C), one reaches an upper age-adjusted prevalence estimate 11.1/100,000.[33]

Nath et al.[34] used a similar methods across 35 general practices in the UK (population = 259,998). They confirmed 17 cases of probable or possible PSP, leading to crude and age adjusted prevalence 6.5/100,000 and 5/100,000 respectively. Ten additional cases of unclassified or atypical parkinsonism were found. In parallel, they received reports of 577 diagnoses of PSP across the UK (population = 59,236,500) and 80 cases in their region (population = 2,589,240). These alternate methods give an estimated age-adjusted prevalence of 1/100,000 nationally or 2.4/100,000 regionally.[34]

The fourth study included PSP within a broader study of all syndromes associated with frontotemporal lobar degeneration.[23] This PiPPIN study is notable for the inclusiveness of PSP-CBS and CBS-PSP, and the overlap between PSP and frontotemporal dementia. Patients were assigned to a single diagnostic class. Forty-eight prevalent cases of PSP were identified and a further 38 cases of CBS in a population of 1.69 million, allowing age and sex standardized point prevalence estimates of 2.9/100,000 and 2.3/100,000 respectively to be calculated.

In Japan, primary and secondary care case reporting after an awareness campaign revealed 12 cases of PSP (population = 66,465), giving an adjusted prevalence of 10/100,000.[37] A separate survey estimated Japanese PSP prevalence at 5.82/100,000.[38] A decade later, a follow-up study identified more cases, with adjusted prevalence 17.9/100,000.[35] However, the new study included a broader spectrum of syndromes associated with PSP pathology, including a probable sixteen cases of PSP-RS, four with possible PSP-RS, three with PSP-P, and two with PSP-PAGF.

Only limited data are available on the incidence of PSP. In the USA, one study reported an incidence of 0.3/100,000,[32] which was similar to the rate of 0.14/100,000 reported in a Russian cohort of incident cases of parkinsonism.[39] In the UK, the PiPPIN study, an epidemiological study of FTLD syndromes (PSP, CBS, and FTD), identified 19 incident cases of PSP (and nine additional cases of CBS) amongst a population of 1.69 million over two years. While standardized rates for the incidence of individual syndromes within the spectrum of FTLD are not reported, standardized incidence of FTLD as a whole was calculated at 1.61/100,000 person-years with PSP accounting for approximately one-third of incident cases. Mortality rates in this study were strikingly similar to incidence, serving as a further surrogate of incidence (assuming a steady state of disease).[23]

These studies all relied on patients having previously been assessed and diagnosed as having a Parkinsonian syndrome or PSP. It remains unclear is how common PSP is as a pathological process, rather than as a syndrome; how many patients with PSP pathology evade a formal diagnosis of PSP or other Parkinsonian syndrome during life; and how common the pathological findings are in the absence of any Parkinsonian syndrome.

A different methodology is required to try to resolve these issues. The Medical Research Council (CFAS),[40] and the Cambridge City Over 75 Cohort study (CC75C)[41] are long-term phenotyping studies of people aged over 64 (CFAS) or over 75 years (CC75C), and include a neuropathological arm. In 1991 CFAS recruited a representative sample of 13,004 people in the UK at five centres, plus 5222 at one centre in 1990. Subgroups were approached for potential brain donation, in the absence of an affective disorder of lack of insight (e.g. due to dementia), although invitation to donation was biased towards including participants with cognitive impairment.[42,43] Semiquantitative analysis of specific lesions and prediction of clinicopathological preliminary diagnosis were recorded by assessors blind to the subjects' previous clinical state or interview data using the protocol of the Consortium to Establish a Registry of Alzheimer's Disease,[44] with minor modifications.[42] Neuropathology in 695 participants revealed 4 people with PSP pathology. None had a diagnosis of PSP in their lifetime.

The proportion of CFAS participants with PSP pathology was therefore at least 0.016% or 16/100,000, whilst for CC75C cohort proportion was at least 0.046% or 46/100,000. The true number of participants who died with PSP pathology is likely to be even higher than this, since only 695/20,392 (3.4%) underwent post-mortem neuropathological examination, although recruitment is likely to have been biased towards those developing neuropathology. These results are not equivalent to prevalence estimates, of PSP reported by other studies, but nonetheless reveal three interesting issues.

First, presence of PSP pathology is much higher than one might immediately expect from the earlier population prevalence data. This may be due to the relatively short period of symptomatic disease relative to lengthy asymptomatic and prodromal stages. Second, the prevalence of a pathology would be greater than its associated syndrome as it does not depend upon the added requirements for identification and diagnosis during life. Third, the pathological diagnosis would include those patients with syndromic heterogeneity, and *forme fruste* cases. Neither cohort had an upper age limit, but cases below 65 would have been excluded, and these may be up to half of symptomatic cases.[23] Interestingly, one patient died aged 93, much older than the cases identified by Nath et al.,[34] but adding pathological support to the identification of prevalent cases of PSP and CBS in patients in their the ninth decade.[23] This illustrates that PSP may be present but under-diagnosed in the very elderly.

Corticobasal Degeneration

There are limited data on the epidemiology of CBS/CBD. From 534 incident cases of parkinsonism, Winter et al.[39] identified one case of CBS. Schrag et al.[33] identified no cases amongst their population of 121,628. In rural Japan, a study to investigate the prevalence of PD and atypical Parkinsonian syndromes found six cases from population = 66,465, giving an age-adjust prevalence of CBS of 6/100,000,[38] based on case notification from primary and secondary care organizations and case note reviews. An earlier study set in tertiary care in Japan identified 151 cases of probable CBD, 121 of whom had a classical syndrome, supporting a prevalence estimate of 1.7/100,000.[45] In the UK, the CAMPAIGN study of incident parkinsonism identified two cases of CBS from 309 incidence cases of parkinsonism in a single county (population ~700,000), but did not seek to identify prevalent cases.[46]

However, ascertainment limitations may affect CBD prevalence estimates in studies focused mainly on PD. For example, the PICNICS study of incident PD in the UK (county population ~700,000) identified 211 incident cases of parkinsonism in 28 months, including 172 cases of PD but no cases of CBS,[47] even though their study population was half of that of the earlier CAMPAIGN study and later PiPPIN study, which ten years later identified 38 prevalent cases and 9 incident cases of CBS using different ascertainment methods.[23] This suggests that a study of the incidence of PD is not necessarily a reliable means to estimate the prevalence or incidence of CBS. Moreover, an emphasis on motor CBS syndromes in earlier studies may have underestimated the prevalence of CBS presenting with cognitive, behavioural, speech, or language dysfunction. Moreover, CBS and CBD studies have drawn on multiple different sets of criteria, disabling comparisons across studies and territories.[10,13,16,48]

Multiple System Atrophy

There are more extensive data on the prevalence of MSA, in a wider range of countries than for PSP and CBS/CBD. Whilst issues of diagnostic accuracy remain, there has been a longer period of stability in clinical diagnostic criteria. The heterogeneity and insidious onset of MSA also mean that prevalence estimates are likely to be underestimates, being driven by classical presentations at later stages of disease when the diagnostic criteria are more specific. About two-thirds of patients with probable and possible MSA have MSA-P, while one-third have MSA-C,[49,50] although these two syndromic variants carry a similar prognosis that is contingent on the degree of autonomic dysfunction.[51]

In Scotland, in a multisource case 36-month prospective ascertainment in a primary care population of 311,357, the 17 incident cases of MSA-P comprised 1.4/100,000,[52] slightly lower than 20 cases of PSP-RS. This lies within the range of estimates of MSA-P in the studies from Moscow (0.11/100,000),[39] the USA (0.6/100,000),[53] Sweden (2.1/100,000),[54] and Iceland (0.7/100,000),[55] with MSA-P again more common than MSA-C.

In Iceland, a secondary care survey of cases of ten years identified nineteen cases, ten of whom were alive on the prevalence day, equating to prevalence 3.4/100 000.[55] This is similar to a concurrent UK-based primary case setting assessment, which estimated age-adjusted prevalence of at MSA 4.4/100,000 (two probable and two possible cases identified);[33] higher than the crude prevalence estimate in France in the late 1990s of 1.94/100,000,[56] but substantially lower than a Japanese estimate from a service-based case ascertainment study a decade later which identified 11 cases from a population of 66,465, giving an age-adjusted prevalence 13/100,000.[37] Of the nine men and two women, seven had probable MSA and four possible MSA: six with MSA-C and five with MSA-P. Using a very different approach, with door-to-door surveying of a population of nearly 1000 adults over 65 years old, a surprising 0.3% were found to carry a diagnosis of MSA, almost half that of PD.[57] This study is the exception, as other studies have placed the prevalence of MSA at less than one-tenth that of PD. From the other studies outlined above, the ratio of estimated prevalence to estimated incidence is reassuringly compatible with the life expectancy data in longitudinal studies, typically of 5–7 years.

However, prodromal symptoms in the form of REM-behaviour disorder (RBD) suggest that the population with possible or probable MSA underestimates the total symptomatic prevalence of MSA pathology. For example, 9/10 patients have RBD, in half of whom the sleep symptoms predated other clinical features.[58] Conversely, of 172 adults with RBD and neuropathology, half had developed sleep symptoms before other motor or cognitive deficits, including 19 with subsequent onset of MSA.[59] This suggests that a significant proportion of symptomatic MSA cases have RBD but not (yet) the classical syndromes of MSA-P or MSA-C. In other words, the symptoms of RBD can indicate an oligosymptomatic or *forme fruste* manifestation of MSA pathology, for several years before the other clinical features enable a definitive diagnosis.

Future Directions

The sporadic nature of PSP, CBS/CBD, and MSA mean that the identification of pre-manifest or prodromal symptoms has relied on serendipity, either clinically or within large-scale research studies such as the UK BioBANK, in whom it is likely that PSP, CBS, and MSA will emerge during follow up of 500,000 initially healthy adults. Such pre-manifest data would be invaluable in tracking the earliest symptoms related to sporadic disease, and ascertaining the true prevalence of symptomatic neuropathology. The advent of a diagnostic biomarker for presymptomatic disease as part of a population screening process would facilitate this, but such a biomarker has yet to be validated. The identification of premanifest disease would also offer the greatest prospect of impact on the long-term cost and burden of these diseases, with the advent of disease modifying therapies.

Until then, we face a difficult trade-off between sensitivity and specificity of clinical diagnostic criteria. Changing attitudes to postmortem examination, across time and cultures, also make it difficult to interpret regional and temporal differences in the incidence and prevalence of PSP, CBD, and MSA, without the gold standard of neuropathology. Changes in diagnostic criteria have the advantage of progress towards better accuracy, but reduce compatibility between studies.

It may therefore be that although the classical syndromes of PSP-R, CBS, and MSA are rare, the lifetime risk of symptoms arising from their corresponding neuropathologies is much higher than previously recognized. Coyle-Gilchrist estimated the lifetime risk of frontotemporal lobar degeneration (PSP, CBD plus frontotemporal dementia but excluding MSA) was as high as 1 in 742.[23] This is in line with the high rate of undiagnosed PSP pathology in the CFAS and CC75 population-based post-mortem studies.

In this review of the epidemiology of the 'rare' neurodegenerative disorders associated with parkinsonism, we have seen that each disease has clinical heterogeneity, indistinct nosological boundaries, and a long prodromal state. Understanding this heterogeneity in phenotypic expression will facilitate both progress in understanding the pathogenesis, but also improvements in stratified, mechanism-based treatment strategies to prevent or arrest the course of PSP, CBS, and MSA.

Conclusion

Considered individually PSP, CBS, and MSA are rare conditions but there is increasing evidence to suggest that they are commonly under-diagnosed. The criteria used in clinical diagnosis continue to evolve, partly in an effort to strengthen clinico-pathological correlations, seeking to predict underlying pathological mechanisms (and hence support further research towards disease modifying treatment), but also to provide a common framework to facilitate description of early clinical phenotypes and guide symptomatic therapies. While most epidemiological estimates of the prevalence and incidence of PSP, CBS, and MSA are based on clinically diagnosed cases the true prevalence of these diseases as pathological processes is likely to be much higher. This is not just because some cases may go unrecognized. Rather, many cases may be unrecognizable under the current criteria, either because they exist in pre- or oligo-symptomatic form or because the clinical syndrome they produce falls between the boundaries of currently recognized clinical syndromes. The transitions between syndromes over time, or loss of differentiation between them, adds further to the challenges of epidemiology, diagnosis, and treatment. However, progress in the epidemiological evaluation has been synergistic, with advances in understanding the pathogenesis of PSP, CBS/CBD and MSA, reflecting a radical revision of clinic-pathological correlations and insights into the heterogeneous phenotypic expression of each disease.

REFERENCES

1. Steele JC, Richardson JC, Olszewski J. Progressive supranuclear palsy. A heterogeneous degeneration involving the brain stem, basal ganglia and cerebellum with vertical gaze and pseudobulbar palsy, nuchal dystonia and dementia. *Archives of Neurology*. 1964; 10(April): 333–59.
2. Litvan I, Agid Y, Calne D, Campbell G, Dubois B, Duvoisin RC, et al. Clinical research criteria for the diagnosis of progressive supranuclear palsy (Steele-Richardson-Olszewski Syndrome): Report of the NINDS-SPSP International Workshop. *Neurology.* 1996; 47(1): 1–9.
3. Bensimon G, Ludolph A, Agid Y, Vidailhet M, Payan C, Leigh PN. Riluzole treatment, survival and diagnostic criteria in Parkinson plus disorders: the NNIPPS Study. *Brain.* 2009 132(1): 156–71. doi:10.1093/brain/awn291.
4. Litvan I, Bhatia KP, Burn DJ, Goetz CG, Lang AE, McKeith I, et al. SIC task force appraisal of clinical diagnostic criteria for Parkinsonian disorders. *Movement Disorders.* 2003; 18(5): 467–86. doi:10.1002/mds.10459.
5. Williams DR, Lees AJ. Progressive supranuclear palsy: clinicopathological concepts and diagnostic challenges. *Lancet Neurology.* 2009; 8(3): 270–9. doi:10.1016/S1474-4422(09)70042-0.
6. Respondek G, Stamelou M, Kurz C, Ferguson LW, Rajput A, Chiu WZ, et al. The phenotypic spectrum of progressive supranuclear palsy: a retrospective multicenter study of 100 definite cases. *Movement Disorders: official journal of the Movement Disorder Society.* 2014; 29(14): 1758–66. doi:10.1002/mds.26054.
7. Höglinger GU, Respondek G, Stamelou M, Kurz C, Josephs KA, Lang AE, et al. Clinical diagnosis of progressive supranuclear palsy: the Movement Disorder Society Criteria. *Movement Disorders: official journal of the Movement Disorder Society*. 2017. May. doi:10.1002/mds.26987.
8. Respondek G, Kurz C, Arzberger T, Compta Y, Englund E, Ferguson LW, et al. Which ante mortem clinical features predict progressive supranuclear palsy pathology? *Movement Disorders: official journal of the Movement Disorder Society*. May, 2007. doi:10.1002/mds.27034.
9. Rebeiz JJ, Kolodny EH, Richardson EP. Corticodentatonigral degeneration with neuronal achromasia. *Archives of Neurology.* 1968; 18(1): 20–33.
10. Lang AE, Riley DE, Bergeron C. Cortical-basal ganglionic degeneration. In: Calne DB (ed.) *Neurodegenerative Diseases.* Philadelphia: WB Saunders, 1994. pp877–94.
11. Gibb WR, Luthert PJ, Marsden CD. Corticobasal degeneration. *Brain: a Journal of Neurology.* 1989; 112(Pt 5)(October): 1171–92.
12. Forman MS, Zhukareva V, Bergeron C, Chin S, Grossman M, Clark C, et al. Signature tau neuropathology in gray and white matter of corticobasal degeneration. *American Journal of Pathology.* 2002; 160(6): 2045–53.
13. Kumar R, Bergeron C, Pollanen M, Lang AE. Cortical-basal ganglionic degeneration. In: Jankovic J, Tolosa E (eds) *Parkinson's Disease and Movement Disorders,* Baltimore: Williams and Wilkins, 1998. pp 297–316.
14. Boeve BF, Lang AE, Litvan I. Corticobasal degeneration and its relationship to progressive supranuclear palsy and frontotemporal dementia. *Annals of Neurology* 2003; 54(S5): S15–S19. doi:10.1002/ana.10570.
15. Bak TH, Hodges JR. Corticobasal degeneration: clinical aspects. *Handbook of Clinical Neurology.* 2008; 89: 509–21. doi:10.1016/S0072-9752(07)01247-X.
16. Armstrong MJ, Litvan I, Lang AE, Bak TH, Bhatia KP, Borroni B, et al. Criteria for the diagnosis of corticobasal degeneration. *Neurology.* 2013; 80(5): 496–503. doi:10.1212/WNL.0b013e31827f0fd1.
17. Alexander SK, Rittman T, Xuereb JH, Bak TH, Hodges JR, Rowe JB. Validation of the new consensus criteria for the diagnosis of corticobasal degeneration. *Journal of Neurology, Neurosurgery and Psychiatry.* 2014; February, jnnp-2013-307035. doi:10.1136/jnnp-2013-307035.
18. Gilman S, Low P, Quinn N, Albanese A, Ben-Shlomo Y, Fowler C, et al. Consensus statement on the diagnosis of multiple system atrophy. American Autonomic Society and American Academy of Neurology. *Clinical Autonomic Research: official journal of the Clinical Autonomic Research Society.* 1998; 8(6): 359–62.
19. Gilman S, Wenning GK, Low PA, Brooks DJ, Mathias CJ, Trojanowski JQ, et al. Second consensus statement on the diagnosis of multiple system atrophy. *Neurology.* 2008; 71(9): 670–6. doi:10.1212/01.wnl.0000324625.00404.15.
20. Osaki Y, Ben-Shlomo Y, Lees AJ, Daniel SE, Colosimo C, Wenning G, et al. Accuracy of clinical diagnosis of progressive supranuclear palsy. *Movement Disorders: official journal of the Movement Disorder Society.* 2004; 19(2): 181–9. doi:10.1002/mds.10680.
21. Scaravilli T, Tolosa E, Ferrer I. Progressive supranuclear palsy and corticobasal degeneration: lumping versus splitting. *Movement Disorders: official journal of the Movement Disorder Society.* 2005; 20 (Suppl 12) (August): S21–28. doi:10.1002/mds.20536.
22. O'Sullivan SS, Massey LA, Williams DR, Silveira-Moriyama L, Kempster PA, Holton JL, et al. Clinical outcomes of progressive supranuclear palsy and multiple system atrophy. *Brain: A Journal of Neurology.* 2008; 131(Pt 5): 1362–72. doi:10.1093/brain/awn065.
23. Coyle-Gilchrist IT, Dick KM, Patterson K, Vázquez Rodríquez P, Wehmann E, Wilcox A, et al. Prevalence, characteristics, and survival of frontotemporal lobar degeneration syndromes. *Neurology.* 2016; 86(18): 1736–43. doi:10.1212/WNL.0000000000002638.

24. Siuda J, Fujioka S, Wszolek ZK. Parkinsonian syndrome in familial frontotemporal dementia. *Parkinsonism and Related Disorders.* 2014; 20(9): 957–64. doi:10.1016/j.parkreldis.2014.06.004.
25. Sánchez MP, Gonzalo I, Avila J, De Yébenes JG. Progressive supranuclear palsy and tau hyperphosphorylation in a patient with a C212Y Parkin mutation. *Journal of Alzheimer's Disease.* 2002; 4(5): 399–404.
26. Lin, I-S, Wu RM, Lee-Chen G-J, Shan D-E, Gwinn-Hardy K. The SCA17 phenotype can include features of MSA-C, PSP and cognitive impairment. *Parkinsonism and Related Disorders.* 2007; 13(4): 246–9. doi:10.1016/j.parkreldis.2006.04.009.
27. Rohrer JD, Nicholas JM, Cash DM, van Swieten J, Dopper E, Jiskoot L, et al. Presymptomatic cognitive and neuroanatomical changes in genetic frontotemporal dementia in the Genetic Frontotemporal Dementia Initiative (GENFI) Study: a cross-sectional analysis. *Lancet Neurology.* 2015; 14(3): 253–62. doi:10.1016/S1474-4422(14)70324-2.
28. Bateman RJ, Xiong C, Benzinger TLS, Fagan AM, Goate A, Fox NC, et al. Clinical and biomarker changes in dominantly inherited Alzheimer's Disease. *New England Journal of Medicine.* 2012; 367(9): 795–804. doi:10.1056/NEJMoa1202753.
29. Tabrizi SJ, Scahill RI, Owen G, Durr A, Leavitt BR, Roos RA, et al. predictors of phenotypic progression and disease onset in premanifest and early-stage Huntington's disease in the TRACK-HD study: analysis of 36-Month observational data. *Lancet Neurology.* 2013; 12(7): 637–49. doi:10.1016/S1474-4422(13)70088-7.
30. Burrell JR, Hodges JR, Rowe JB. Cognition in corticobasal syndrome and progressive supranuclear palsy: a review. *Movement Disorders: official journal of the Movement Disorder Society.* 2014; 29(5): 684–93. doi:10.1002/mds.25872.
31. Kertesz A, McMonagle P, Blair M, Davidson W, Munoz DG. The evolution and pathology of frontotemporal dementia. *Brain: A Journal of Neurology.* 2005; 128(Pt 9): 1996–2005. doi:10.1093/brain/awh598.
32. Golbe LI, Davis PH, Schoenberg BS, Duvoisin RC. Prevalence and natural history of progressive supranuclear palsy. *Neurology.* 1988; 38(7): 1031–4.
33. Schrag A, Ben-Shlomo Y, Quinn NP. Prevalence of progressive supranuclear palsy and multiple system atrophy: a cross-sectional study. *Lancet.* 1999; 354(9192): 1771–5. doi:10.1016/S0140-6736(99)04137-9.
34. Nath U, Ben-Shlomo Y, Thomson RG, Morris HR, Wood NW, Lees AJ, et al. The prevalence of progressive supranuclear palsy (Steele–Richardson–Olszewski Syndrome) in the UK. *Brain.* 2001; 124(7): 1438–49. doi:10.1093/brain/124.7.1438.
35. Takigawa H, Kitayama M, Wada-Isoe K, Kowa H, Nakashima K. Prevalence of progressive supranuclear palsy in Yonago: change throughout a decade. *Brain and Behavior.* 2016; 6(12): e00557. doi:10.1002/brb3.557.
36. Kawashima M, Miyake M, Kusumi M, Adachi Y, Nakashima K. Prevalence of progressive supranuclear palsy in Yonago, Japan. *Movement Disorders: official journal of the Movement Disorder Society.* 2004; 19(10): 1239–40. doi:10.1002/mds.20149.
37. Osaki Y, Morita Y, Kuwahara T, Miyano I, Doi Y. Prevalence of Parkinson's disease and atypical Parkinsonian syndromes in a rural Japanese district. *Acta Neurologica Scandinavica.* 2011; 124(3): 182–7. doi:10.1111/j.1600-0404.2010.01442.x.
38. Kawashima M, Miyake M, Kusumi M, Adachi Y, Nakashima K. Prevalence of progressive supranuclear palsy in Yonago, Japan. Mov Disord. 2004; 19(10): 1239–40.
39. Winter Y, Bezdolnyy Y, Katunina E, Avakjan G, Reese JP, Klotsche J, et al. Incidence of Parkinson's disease and atypical parkinsonism: Russian population-based study. *Movement Disorders: official journal of the Movement Disorder Society.* 2010; 25(3): 349–56. doi:10.1002/mds.22966.
40. Brayne C, McCracken C, Matthews FE. Cohort Profile: The Medical Research Council Cognitive Function and Ageing Study (CFAS). *International Journal of Epidemiology.* 2006; 35 (5): 1140–45. doi:10.1093/ije/dyl199.
41. Fleming J, Zhao E, O'Connor DW, Pollitt PA, Brayne C. Cohort Profile: The Cambridge City over-75s Cohort (CC75C). *International Journal of Epidemiology.* 2007; 36(1): 40–6. doi:10.1093/ije/dyl293.
42. Xuereb JH, Brayne C, Dufouil C, Gertz H, Wischik C, Harrington C, et al. Neuropathological findings in the very old. results from the first 101 brains of a population-based longitudinal study of dementing disorders. *Annals of the New York Academy of Sciences.* 2000; 903(April): 490–6.
43. Brayne C, Nickson J, McCracken C, Gill C, Johnson AL, and Analysis Group of the MRC CFA Study. Cognitive function and dementia in six areas of England and Wales: the distribution of MMSE and prevalence of GMS organicity level in the MRC CFA study. The Medical Research Council Cognitive Function and Ageing Study (MRC CFAS). *Psychological Medicine.* 1998; 28(2): 319–35.
44. Mirra SS, Heyman A, McKeel D, Sumi SM, Crain BJ, Brownlee LM, et al. The Consortium to Establish a Registry for Alzheimer's Disease (CERAD). Part II. Standardization of the neuropathologic assessment of Alzheimer's disease. *Neurology.* 1991; 41(4): 479–86.
45. Morimatsu M, Negoro K. Provisional diagnostic criteria of corticobasal degeneration (CBD) and the survey of patients with CBD in Japan. *Rinshō Shinkeigaku = Clinical Neurology.* 2002; 42(11): 1150–3.
46. Foltynie T, Brayne C, Robbins TW, Barker RA. The cognitive ability of an incident cohort of Parkinson's patients in the UK. The CamPaIGN Study. *Brain.* 2004; 127(3): 550–60. doi:10.1093/brain/awh067.
47. Evans JR, Cummins G, Breen DP, Foltynie T, Mason SL, Brayne C, et al. Comparative epidemiology of incident Parkinson's disease in Cambridgeshire, UK. *Journal of Neurology, Neurosurgery, and Psychiatry.* 2016; 87(9): 1034–6. doi:10.1136/jnnp-2015-312581.
48. Boeve BF, Maraganore DM, Parisi JE, Ahlskog JE, Graff-Radford N, Caselli RJ, et al. Pathologic heterogeneity in clinically diagnosed corticobasal degeneration. *Neurology.* 1999; 53(4): 795–800.
49. Wenning GK, Geser F, Krismer F, Seppi K, Duerr S, Boesch S, et al. The natural history of multiple system atrophy: a prospective European cohort study. *Lancet Neurology.* 2013; 12(3): 264–74. doi:10.1016/S1474-4422(12)70327-7.
50. Coon EA, Sletten DM, Suarez MD, Mandrekar JN, Ahlskog JE, Bower JH, et al. Clinical features and autonomic testing predict survival in multiple system atrophy. *Brain: a Journal of Neurology.* 2015; 138 (Pt 12): 3623–31. doi:10.1093/brain/awv274.
51. Low PA, Reich SG, Jankovic J, Shults CW, Stern MB, Novak P, et al. Natural history of multiple system atrophy in the USA: a prospective cohort study. *Lancet. Neurology.* 2015; 14(7): 710–19. doi:10.1016/S1474-4422(15)00058-7.
52. Caslake R, Taylor K, Scott N, Harris C, Gordon J, Wilde K, et al. Age and gender-specific incidence of vascular parkinsonism,

progressive supranuclear palsy, and Parkinsonian-type multiple system atrophy in North East Scotland: the PINE Study. *Parkinsonism and Related Disorders.* 2014; 20(8): 834–9. doi:10.1016/j.parkreldis.2014.04.013.

53. Bower JH, Maraganore DM, McDonnell SK, Rocca WA. Incidence of progressive supranuclear palsy and multiple system atrophy in Olmsted County, Minnesota, 1976–1990. *Neurology.* 1997; 49(5): 1284–8.
54. Linder J, Stenlund H, Forsgren L. Incidence of Parkinson's disease and parkinsonism in Northern Sweden: a population-based study. *Movement Disorders: official journal of the Movement Disorder Society.* 2010; 25 (3): 341–8. doi:10.1002/mds.22987.
55. Bjornsdottir A, Gudmundsson G, Blondal H, Olafsson E. Incidence and prevalence of multiple system atrophy: a nationwide study in Iceland. *Journal of Neurology, Neurosurgery, and Psychiatry.* 2103; 84(2): 136–40. doi:10.1136/jnnp-2012-302500.
56. Chrysostome V, Tison F, Yekhlef F, Sourgen C, Baldi I, Dartigues JF. Epidemiology of multiple system atrophy: a prevalence and pilot risk factor study in Aquitaine, France. *Neuroepidemiology.* 2004; 23 (4): 201–8. doi:10.1159/000078506.
57. Trenkwalder C, Schwarz J, Gebhard J, Ruland D, Trenkwalder P, Hense HW, et al. Starnberg trial on epidemiology of parkinsonism and hypertension in the elderly. prevalence of Parkinson's disease and related disorders assessed by a door-to-door survey of inhabitants older than 65 years. *Archives of Neurology.* 1995: 52(10): 1017–22.
58. Palma J-A, Fernandez-Cordon C, Coon EA, Low PA, Miglis MG, Jaradeh S, et al. Prevalence of REM sleep behavior disorder in multiple system atrophy: a multicenter study and meta-analysis. *Clinical Autonomic Research: official journal of the Clinical Autonomic Research Society.* 2015; 25(1): 69–75. doi:10.1007/s10286-015-0279-9.
59. Boeve BF, Silber MH, Ferman TJ, Lin SC, Benarroch EE, Schmeichel AM, et al. Clinicopathologic correlations in 172 cases of rapid eye movement sleep behavior disorder with or without a coexisting neurologic disorder. *Sleep Medicine.* 2013; 14(8): 754–62. doi:10.1016/j.sleep.2012.10.015.

15

Posterior cortical atrophy

Keir XX Yong, SJ Crutch, and JM Schott

Nosology

Posterior cortical atrophy (PCA) was a term first introduced by Benson et al.,[1] although previous reports had existed of patients with progressive and relatively selective visual impairment despite having normal acuity.[2,3,4] Benson et al.[1] reported five patients who exhibited deficits in higher visual function and signs of Balint's and Gerstmann's syndrome, yet showed abnormal but relatively spared memory until later in the course of their disease. Subsequent neuropathological evaluation found that patients with clinical presentations consistent with PCA had hallmarks of AD in the form of NFTs and senile plaques.[5,6] While the majority of PCA cases are associated with AD pathology, likely contributing to the use of terms such as 'the visual variant of AD' or 'biparietal AD' to describe PCA,[7,8,9] some cases of PCA have been attributable to corticobasal degeneration (CBD), dementia with Lewy bodies (DLB), or prion disease.[10,11,12,13]

Clinical Presentation

The core behavioural phenotype of PCA involves prominent visuospatial and visuoperceptual impairment, features of Balint's (simultanagnosia, oculomotor apraxia, optic ataxia), and Gerstmann's syndrome (acalculia, agraphia, left-right disorientation, finger agnosia), and alexia and apraxia.[14,15] McMonagle et al.[14] reported that some of the most common symptoms of PCA were alexia, agraphia, simultanagnosia, acalculia, and optic ataxia. Longitudinal investigations indicate that the relative preservation of memory, language, and executive function observed in early stages of PCA tend to give way to more global cognitive impairment (see Fig. 15.1).[7,14] Observations of visual hallucinations, noted in up to 25% of PCA patients,[16] and dystonia might implicate underlying DLB or CBD.[15] Cases have been made for the classification of PCA as its own distinct nosological entity based on the uniformity of its clinical profile,[17] while others have argued that PCA exists on a continuum of phenotypic variation in AD and does not represent a discrete disease.[18]

Case study of a PCA patient

A 56-year-old lady presented with a three-year history of visual problems. Initial symptoms were difficulties telling the time when reading a clock face. This was followed by difficulties with reading, losing her place on the page particularly when moving from line to line. She gave up driving after two minor accidents. She subsequently reported more difficulties with numbers, decline in spelling, and problems both in writing and typing. Neither she nor her husband reported episodic memory to be a major problem. There was no relevant past medical or family history, and repeated ocular examinations were normal. On examination she gave a detailed history, but scored 19/30 on the mini-mental state examination. Bedside and formal neuropsychometry testing confirmed significant problems with tasks sensitive to parietal function, including calculation, spelling, praxis, dot counting, interpreting fragmented stimuli (Fig. 15.2), and she showed evidence of visual disorientation. The neurological examination was normal. An MRI scan revealed posterior cortical atrophy with relatively preserved hippocampi (Fig. 15.3). A CSF examination revealed elevated levels of tau and depressed levels of Aβ1-42 in keeping with AD. Amyloid PET scanning done on a research basis confirmed the presence of widespread cortical fibrillar amyloid deposition. She was diagnosed with PCA due to underlying AD, was commenced on donepezil, and was referred for post-diagnostic counselling and to the posterior cortical atrophy support group (http://www.raredementiasupport.org/pca/).

Pathology

Findings from pathological studies suggest the majority of PCA patients have underlying AD.[5,6,9,10,11] However, some cases of PCA have been associated with Lewy body pathology,[10,13] CBD,[6,10,11] subcortical gliosis, and prion disease.[10] Reporting pathological data for 21 PCA patients, Renner et al.[10] found Fourteen had AD pathology, including one with coexisting Parkinson disease had AD pathology, two had AD-Lewy body variant, one had DLB with coexisting subcortical gliosis, and two had prion-associated disease (CJD and fatal familial insomnia). A separate investigation found seven of seven PCA patients had AD pathology.[19]

In PCA patients with AD pathology, differences have been noted in the distribution of NFTs[6] or NFTs and senile plaques,[7,8] relative to typical Alzheimer's disease (tAD) patients. In PCA patients, differences have been localized,? particularly within occipital regions which are relatively unaffected in tAD, with pathological distribution increasing in densities from the primary visual cortex to the

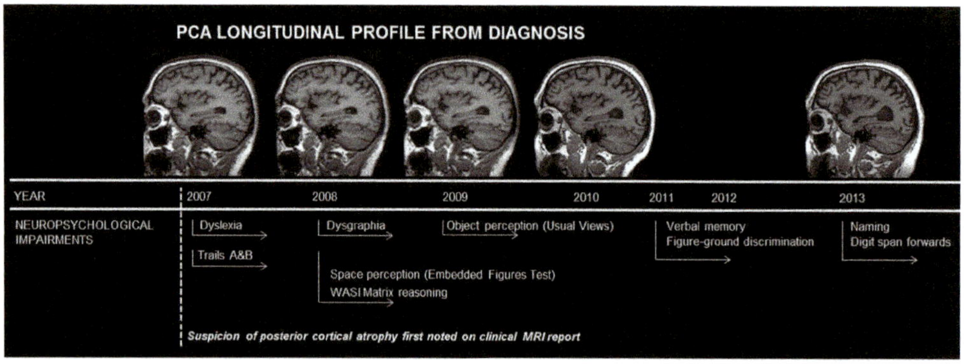

Fig. 15.1 Longitudinal investigation of an individual with PCA outlining neuroimaging, clinical, and neuropsychological data. Serial MR images are shown in sagittal view of the patient's right hemisphere. This individual was initially seen as a healthy control participant who subsequently developed PCA.

For a more detailed case description, see: Kennedy J, Lehmann M, Sokolska M, et al. Visualizing the emergence of posterior cortical atrophy. *Neurocase*. 2012; 18(3): 248–57. Adapted from Crutch, S. J., Schott, J. M., Rabinovici, G. D. et al. Consensus classification of posterior cortical atrophy. *Alzheimer's & Dementia*, 13(8): 870-884.

visual association areas[5,20,21] and lower densities reported in frontal regions.[7,21] However, while Tang-Wai et al.[6] found lower concentrations of senile plaques in hippocampal regions of PCA relative to tAD patients, similar plaque densities were found in other cortical areas; furthermore, Renner et al.[10] did not find evidence of differences in parietal burden of senile plaques or NFTs.

Pathological observations in PCA have been interpreted to reflect the particular involvement of cortical pathways between the striate, posterior parietal, and cingulate cortices. A disproportionate loss of Meynert cells in the striate cortex has been noted in PCA; such cells have long projections to area MT and the superior colliculus.[5,20] High densities of NFTs found in layer III of Brodmann areas 17, 18, and 19 suggests involvement of projections from areas 17 to 18 and feedforward projections from areas 18 and 19 to visual association areas. In addition, feedback projections are likely affected given high densities of NFTs in layers V and VI of area 18.[22] Such findings not only inform the understanding of AD pathogenesis; the selective vulnerability of certain cells to AD might help explain patterns of cognitive deficits.

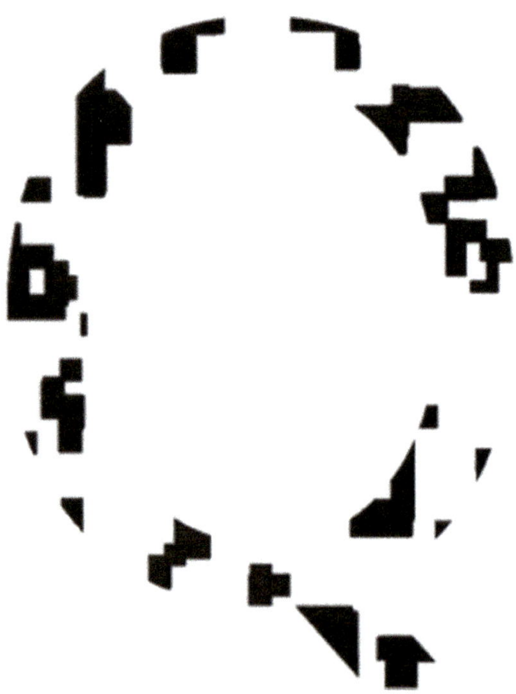

Fig. 15.2 Example of a fragmented letter, used to assess visuoperceptual function.

Biomarkers

Structural imaging

Consistent with the terminology of PCA, imaging techniques have identified atrophy particularly in posterior brain regions. Using voxel-based morphometry (VBM), cross-sectional studies have found reductions in grey matter volume in occipital, posterior parietal, and posterior temporal regions in PCA relative to healthy controls.[23,24,25,26] Comparisons of PCA and tAD patients have found lower grey matter volume in occipital and bilateral posterior parietal regions of the PCA group;[23,24] Lehmann et al.[23] also identified lower cortical thickness in the right superior parietal lobule of the PCA group and in the left entorhinal cortex in the tAD group. A comparison of hippocampi between PCA and tAD has identified increased hippocampal volume and differences in shape, particularly in the left superior hippocampus.[27] Factors related to the localization and degree of atrophy in PCA may include apolipoprotein (APOE) status and age at onset.[28] Longitudinal VBM analysis has revealed global patterns of grey matter loss in both PCA and tAD,[29] while cross-sectional grey matter volume and multivariate cortical thickness analysis comparing PCA, logopenic progressive aphasia (LPA), and early-onset tAD has indicated overlap in neuroimaging characteristics of the precuneus, posterior cingulate cortex, and left temporoparietal and medial temporal regions, possibly suggestive of different clinical syndromes representing points within an AD phenotypic spectrum.[25,30] It is worth noting that not all PCA patients show clear posterior atrophy;[14] the inconsistency of prominent atrophy noted at autopsy by Renner et al.[10] led them to suggest the use of posterior cortical dysfunction rather than PCA.

Diffusion tensor imaging (DTI) studies have identified white matter changes in posterior brain networks,[26] with one case study

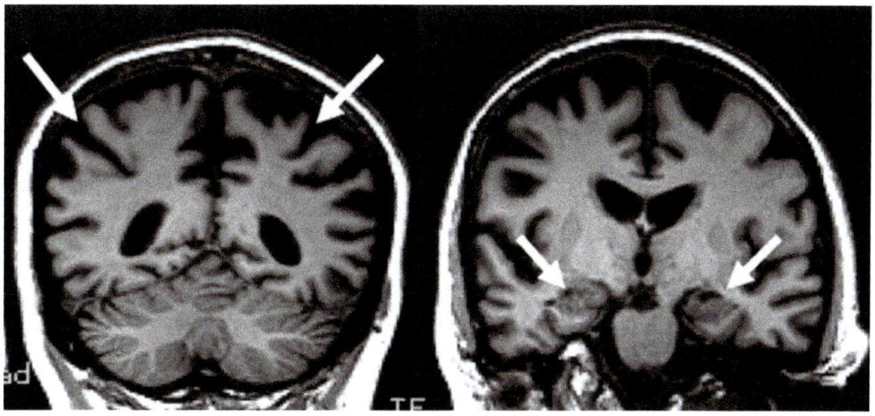

Fig. 15.3 Parietal volume loss (left panel), with preserved hippocampal volumes (right panel) in a patient with PCA.

suggesting particularly early involvement of the occipital lobe.[31] A recent investigation by Madhavan et al.[32] found changes in white matter tracts in the parietal and occipital lobes relative to patients with tAD and LPA.

Functional imaging

Functional imaging studies of PCA patients using single photon emission computed tomography (SPECT) and fluorodeoxyglucose-(FDG) PET point to hypometabolism in posterior cerebral hemispheres and hypoperfusion in occipital, parietal, and temporal cortices relative to healthy controls.[33–35] PCA and DLB have been shown to have overlapping regions of hypometabolism, with DLB patients showing a greater degree of hypometabolism in medial occipital, frontal, and temporal areas, and PCA patients showing greater asymmetry.[36] Some of these studies have also identified bilateral hypometabolism in the frontal eye fields compared to tAD patients;[33,34] such imaging findings may relate to oculomotor apraxia in PCA.[15]

Molecular imaging

Other imaging techniques include using PET ligands which bind to fibrillary forms of β-amyloid, including Pittsburgh compound-B (PiB) and florbetapir (18 F) PET. Such techniques have identified amyloid deposition distributed broadly across the cortex, in contrast to atrophy, hypometabolism, and reduced cerebral blood flow showing a more anterior-posterior gradient,[37,38] and have variously suggested increased amyloid-β deposits in occipital and parietal regions of PCA patients relative to tAD patients[37,39] or that no differences exist in amyloid plaque burden.[35,40] PCA patients with beta-amyloid deposition have been found to have a lesser degree of hypometabolism in medial occipital, frontal, anterior temporal, and caudate regions than DLB patients, but more asymmetric patterns of hypometabolism.[36] More recently, the development of tau PET tracers offer a means to assess regional tau aggregation.[41]

Cerebrospinal fluid

Analysis of cerebrospinal fluid (CSF) enables assessment of different biological processes implicated in AD. Established analyses include amyloid beta 1-42 (Aβ1-42), phosphorylated tau (P-tau) and 'total' tau (T-tau). Levels of Aβ1-42 are inversely correlated with amyloid load,[42] P-tau is correlated with neurofibrillary tangle burden,[43] and T-tau has been interpreted as a measure of the degree of neurodegeneration.[44] A CSF analysis by Seguin et al.[11] found that 17 of 22 PCA patients fulfilled biological criteria for tAD; of the remaining five patients, two exhibited a normal CSF profile but showed a PCA corticobasal syndrome (CBS). Whilst the CSF profile therefore principally reflect the presence/absence of AD pathology, there may be some subtle differences in PCA compared to tAD. Thus a recent study has identified that, relative to patients with both typical and atypical AD, PCA patients had lower levels of T-tau/P-tau and the lowest AβX-40/ AβX-42 ratios.[45]

Neuropsychology

Detailed neuropsychological assessment plays a significant role in the diagnosis and characterization of PCA. Standardized neuropsychological measures provide a means of evaluating whether patients fulfil proposed diagnostic criteria for PCA, and have practical implications for how patients should be treated clinically.[46] Future neuropsychological investigation may yield insights into the relationship between PCA and tAD, clarify whether discrete subtypes of PCA exist, offer ways to discriminate between different aetiologies underlying PCA, and provide suggestions of biological mechanisms underlying PCA through longitudinal assessment. The following sections are of relevance when considering how to administer and interpret cognitive assessments in PCA, given how measures intended to assess memory, language, and executive function may be susceptible to various deficits in visual domains. An area where such potential confounds have major implications is in clinical trial design, where outcome measures perceived to be appropriate for some patients (such as those with a primarily amnesic presentation of AD) may need to be carefully considered, particularly if involving a prominent visual component.

Visual processing abnormalities

Visuospatial impairment

Prominent deficits in visuospatial ability are some of the most frequent and striking characteristics of PCA. While visual disorientation emphasizes a deficit in the ability to localize a single object, higher-order visuospatial impairment is particularly associated with deficits in representing the spatial relationships between multiple objects and/or integrating spatial information across modalities (e.g. visuomotor tasks). Deficits in visuospatial ability can lead to poor performance on tasks such as position discrimination, dot counting, matching orientation, cancellation, or search tasks. Impaired performance on such tasks has been noted in a range of studies of PCA.[1,8,23,39,47–49]

Poor performance on measures of visuospatial ability may reflect visual neglect in some PCA patients; various studies have noted neglect,[4,26] with one recent group study identifying signs of neglect in 16 of 24 PCA patients,[50] which contrasts with earlier studies which reported much lower rates (15–20);[6,14] this discrepancy may be due to these investigations employing clinical examination, rather than neuropsychological measures. However, the line bisection and Bells test[51] used by Andrade et al.[50] are not 'pure' measures of neglect in PCA; they may be confounded by more general deficits in visuospatial and visuomotor ability, as well as the counterintuitive tendency of some PCA patients to misperceive large stimuli.

A diminished ability to recognize large rather than small pictures, words, and letters presented in isolation has been noted in PCA for some time.[48,52,53] This deficit has been referred to as the 'inverse size' effect,[54] and likely contributes to problems in scene perception in PCA[55] and clinical complaints of patients who report having particular difficulty in reading large font, such as newspaper headlines.[53] An inverse size effect on single word recognition in PCA has been associated with reduced grey matter volume in the superior posterior parietal lobule.[56] Such effects may reflect a reduced effective field of vision, associated with parietal and parieto-occipital damage.[57] Disproportionate deficits in perceiving stimuli presented in peripheral vision have been attributed to an inability to cope with high attentional demands,[57] although they may also relate to poor eye movement control, inefficient scanning strategies,[55] or visual field defects.[58,59]

Visuoperceptual impairment

Progressive and disproportionate deficits in object recognition were some of the earliest noted features of PCA.[1,4] Models of object recognition have specified that a deficit arising at the level of perceptual categorization subsequent to visual sensory processing presents as an apperceptive agnosia, while a deficit in semantic categorization presents as an associative agnosia.[60] The term apperceptive agnosia refers to patients with impaired object recognition; such patients demonstrate intact visual sensory functions and their impairment does not relate to a semantic deficit. Apperceptive agnosia has been linked to right parietal damage[61] and has been assessed using stimuli that degrade visual complexity, including everyday objects shown from different angles,[62] silhouette drawings of objects,[62] overlapping drawings,[63] incomplete line drawings,[64] or degraded letters.[61] Apperceptive agnosia has been noted in various case studies of PCA;[9,65] one group study observed that patients with apperceptive agnosias tended to have longer disease durations.[14] Two group studies have placed the incidence of visual agnosia at around 45–65% and have attributed these to deficits in apperception;[14,66] however, neither of these studies assessed performance on measures of early visual processing, such as shape detection or discrimination. All three PCA patients with visuoperceptual impairment from Sala et al.[67] had difficulties in form and line discrimination, emphasizing the likely contribution of early visual impairment towards higher-order visual deficits. In a study of 21 PCA patients, Lehmann et al.[23] found all 21 showed impaired performance on recognition tasks of fragmented letters and objects shown from unconventional angles; however, all patients also showed deficits on at least one measure of early visual processing.

Associative agnosia refers to patients who can construct a sufficient perceptual representation of an object, but the representation suffers from a loss of meaning.[68] Such patients often have bilateral temporal lesions,[69] although associative agnosia has been found in a patient with unilateral posterior temporal damage.[70] Selective associative agnosias tend to be rare in PCA, with group observations of visual agnosias in PCA not being attributed to semantic deficits.[14,66]

Another visuoperceptual deficit observed in PCA is prosopagnosia, which has been defined as a disproportionate impairment in recognizing faces relative to other objects. Prosopagnosia can result from damage to right occipito-temporal regions, although it is not a common consequence of such damage.[71] Problems identifying faces can be an early[65] and common (20–25%)[6,14,66] symptom of PCA, leading to suggestions of prosopagnosia as a supportive diagnostic feature for PCA.[6] However, disorders of face perception in PCA are rarely very selective; they have been accompanied by visual agnosias[14,65] and deficits in early visual processing.[67]

Early visual processing deficits

While deficits in higher-order visual domains, such as spatial or object perception, tend to be reported more frequently than disrupted early visual processing in PCA, it is likely that deficits in early visual processes at least contribute to higher-order visual problems.[72] Early visual dysfunction includes deficits in perceiving form, colour, motion, and single point localization and is associated with the occipital lobes.[60,73] Consistent with AD pathology in Brodmann areas 17–19 observed in PCA cases,[21] some investigations suggest widespread occipital lobe dysfunction in PCA, occurring as early as the primary visual area,[74] while colour after-effects in PCA have been interpreted as showing degeneration of excitatory neurons and relative preservation of inhibitory interneurons in V1.[53,75]

Visual localization relates to the inability to localize a single object and is often assessed using single point localization;[68] such localization deficits may constitute part of visuospatial impairment. Holmes and Horrax[76] gave the classic account of visual disorientation, reporting patients with difficulties in the localization, maintenance of fixation, and visual tracking of objects. The functional impact of visual disorientation is considerable, with many patients being unable to correctly reach for objects or walk across a room unaided.[68] Visual disorientation has been associated with damage to the occipital or occipitoparietal region[60] and forms one of the features of Balint's syndrome. Visual disorientation can be restricted to one half of the visual field;[77] in contrast, visuospatial disorders are mostly associated with right parietal damage and are not restricted to the contralateral visual field. Visual disorientation has been identified in PCA in a range of case studies,[9,39,53,75] a study of 21 PCA patients found 60% of them were impaired on a task of single point localization and 81% were impaired on dot counting.[23] Problems in visual localization may be variable, with visually-disorientated PCA patients sometimes being able to seemingly pinpoint small objects with surprising accuracy or better localize moving stimuli.[46,78]

Form perception is often assessed using tasks such as the Efron Squares test[79] or figure-ground detection, which are measures of shape discrimination or shape detection processes. Abnormalities in shape discrimination, shape detection, orientation discrimination, contour integration, form coherence, visual field detection, and colour perception have all been noted in PCA;[6,14,23,24,59,74,75] studies have identified how 65–80% of PCA patients showed impaired performance on a figure-ground detection task, while 67% showed deficits in shape discrimination.[23,55] Group studies have also suggested a varying incidence of hemianopia or quadrantanopia in PCA (5–78%);[14,24,59] this might reflect confounding visual phenomena such as the inverse size effect, neglect, or visual disorientation.

Acquired dyslexia

Acquired dyslexia often presents as an early[1,80] and common (80–95%)[14,66] symptom of PCA, and alexia is a proposed supportive feature of a diagnosis of PCA.[6,66] Various clinical reports exist of PCA patients having difficulty following text along a printed line or moving from one line to the next,[53] seeing lines of text in 'false order',[39] and losing their place on a page.[53] Empirical group investigations have identified that perceptual and spatial aspects of single word and text reading are the primary predictors of reading ability.[56,81,82] A combination of visual and oculomotor deficits likely contribute to text reading difficulties in PCA, including a restriction in the effective field of vision, neglect,[50] visual field defects,[59] abnormalities in fixation stability, and saccade generation (see Fig. 15.4)[83] and perceived motion of static stimuli.[53] A visual deficit that has been strongly implicated in limiting reading ability in PCA is excessive visual crowding, a form of inhibitory interaction where the identification of a target stimulus is undermined when presented among visual clutter. Normally a limiting factor on perception in healthy peripheral vision, PCA patients have demonstrated object recognition deficits in line with crowding, but with centrally-presented stimuli.[84,85] A better understanding of how particular deficits in aspects of visual processing and oculomotor characteristics in PCA relate to functional activities may inform strategies to better support patients.

Non-visual symptoms

Characteristic deficits of PCA are not restricted to visual domains; they include domains associated with dominant parietal function, including calculation, spelling and praxis),[14,34,49,65] consistent with clinical criteria considering elements of Gerstmann's syndrome core or supportive features of PCA.[6,66] Relative preservation of memory and semantics has been noted in PCA;[6,14,66] the majority of PCA patients do not show early episodic memory impairment as assessed clinically or through neuropsychological testing,[23,24] and demonstrate competent performance on semantic fluency and synonym discrimination tasks relative to both tAD patients[66] and healthy individuals.[23] Some studies have suggested that executive function is relatively preserved in PCA compared to tAD,[66] while others have found no evidence of differences between PCA and tAD patients.[86] An important caveat is that visual impairment can confound tasks with a visual component that intend to assess performance IQ or executive function, which likely accounts for PCA patients' performance IQ being lower than verbal IQ.[14]

Language disturbance

While verbal language has been considered relatively intact in PCA compared to visual domains,[14,66] there is evidence that some language skills are impaired in PCA. Benson et al.[1] noted how all five of the PCA patients he reported developed transcortical sensory aphasia, which included anomia and comprehension disorder. Subsequent studies have observed some prevalence of early language difficulties in PCA; out of 14 PCA patients, over a third presented with language complaints at disease onset,[25] 7 of 9 presented signs of anomia in spontaneous speech,[87] while another investigation found 24 of 27 PCA patients showed signs of anomia.[6] Studies comparing PCA with LPA patients have found overlapping deficits in phonemic fluency and word retrieval in response to verbal descriptions.[55,88] In the context of poor repetition of non-words and comprehension of longer sentences in the absence of syntactic deficits, it is possible that such performance could reflect weaknesses in phonological processing and short-term memory, particularly given the purported role of parietal systems in mediating the short-term phonological storage and retrieval of verbal information,[89] and/or damage to early stages of auditory processing.[90] Some phonological impairment has been noted in PCA, and there is an overlap in performance between PCA and LPA patients on tasks of non-word repetition, phonemic fluency, and prosody processing. Diminished aspects of auditory spatial processing have also been identified in PCA, including deficits in discriminating the position of stationary sounds relative to controls, and in discriminating moving versus stationary sounds relative to tAD patients.[91]

Dyspraxia

A common symptom in PCA is limb apraxia, which previous group studies have observed in around 95% of patients.[14,34] Previous reports exist of individuals presenting with progressive apraxia and symptoms suggestive of posterior cortical dysfunction but with

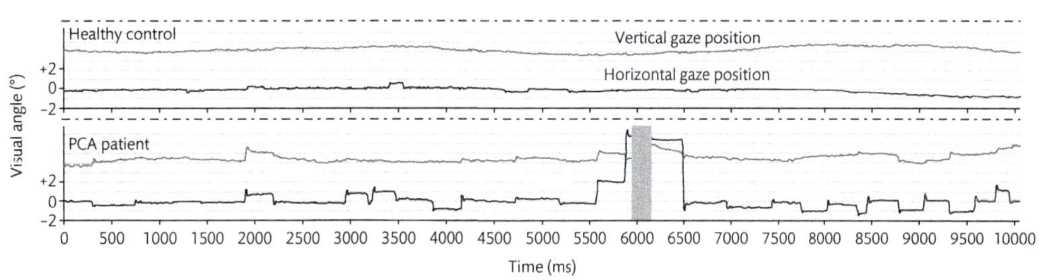

Fig. 15.4 Representative traces from a healthy control and a PCA patient in a single trial of the fixation task. The healthy control maintains steady fixation upon the target, whilst the PCA patient shows saccadic intrusions in the form of square-wave jerks and a large saccadic intrusion.

The upper plot (grey line) for each participant shows gaze position in the y (vertical) axis, the lower plot (black line) shows gaze position in the x (horizontal) axis. The location of the target stimulus is represented by lines behind the traces. The grey area in the plot for the PCA patient represents a blink, therefore x and y gaze coordinates are not available for this period.

Reproduced from Shakespeare TJ. Abnormalities of fixation, saccade and pursuit in posterior cortical atrophy. *Brain*, 138(7). 2015; 1976-1991.

relatively intact visual and memory function. Green et al.[92] identified how one AD patient whose recognition memory was within the normal range presented with prominent apraxia, along with difficulties performing mental arithmetic and hypoperfusion particularly within the posterior parietal cortex. Another case involves a patient who performed within the normal range on four tests of verbal and spatial memory and measures of early visual and visuoperceptual processing; the primary deficit was a progressive loss of manual praxis, with additional dyscalculia).[4] Regarding other motor features, Ryan et al.[93] found that 30% of 44 PCA patients had prominent limb rigidity; these patients showed an increased tendency to demonstrate more frequent and asymmetrical apraxia, and a cortical thickness analysis identified a greater degree of cortical thinning in the right hemisphere in these patients relative to PCA patients without limb rigidity. An apraxic presentation of PCA may reflect an overlap with CBD,[14] although it is worth noting that pathological data and CSF data for patients showing limb rigidity and apraxia have suggested underlying AD.[93]

Implications for classification

These detailed neuropsychological studies raise fundamental questions as to whether the term PCA should be restricted to those with early and prominent visual deficits, or might be extended to patients who present with progressive apraxia, acalculia, and/or spelling. Some investigations have been explicit in describing patients with apraxia as the leading symptom as having PCA,[65] with Aharon-Peretz et al. proposing that PCA represents two clinically-related behavioural phenotypes involving either predominant visuospatial impairment or apraxia. Suárez-González et al.[94] noted how patients presenting with prominent non-visual symptoms demonstrated visual processing impairments on formal neuropsychological assessment, despite not exhibiting clinically significant visual dysfunction. Whether the term PCA might be applicable to patients with progressive predominantly posterior dysfunction in the absence of prominent visual symptoms is one aspect of a broader discussion of the phenotypic spectrum of PCA. Based on findings from individual case reports, different subtypes of PCA have been proposed, including distinct parietal (dorsal), occipitotemporal (ventral), caudal forms (primary visual)[8,9] and a dominant parietal variant.[95] A group study of PCA noted deficits associated with occipital and temporal lobe damage, such as achromatopsia, hemianopia, visual agnosia, prosopagnosia, but found an overall pattern to be involving a disproportionate deficit in dorsal relative to ventral or primary visual processes;[14] future group longitudinal investigations involving comprehensive neuropsychological assessment might allow clarification of the considerable heterogeneity existing within the PCA syndrome.

Diagnostic/Research Criteria

The core clinical features of PCA include an insidious onset and gradual progression, presentation of visual impairment in the absence of significant ocular disease, an absence of stroke or tumour, relatively preserved episodic memory and the presence of any of the following symptoms: simultanagnosia, optic ataxia, oculomotor apraxia, dyspraxia, environmental disorientation or aspects of Gerstmann's syndrome. Supportive features include alexia, ideomotor apraxia, young age at onset and neuroimaging evidence of parieto-occipital atrophy or hypometabolism (see Table 15.1).[6,14,66,95] Such diagnostic criteria have reasonable agreement and have been mentioned in consensus criteria for atypical AD;[96] however, slight differences exist in definitions of PCA, which may result from variations of clinical experience at different centres and the fact that proposed criteria have not been validated in a wider population sample. Inconsistencies in terminology limit comparisons between studies, and likely contribute to inconsistencies in pathological or imaging literature.

Improving PCA terminology and promoting consistencies in the application of terminology has implications for studies investigating the epidemiology of PCA, and for considering the suitability of patients for future investigations, whether relating to disease characterization or therapeutic trials. There is a need for a consensus on a variety of issues: whether the term PCA should be applied to patients with a pure visual presentation, those with more global cognitive impairment but with visual deficits as the earliest presenting or most prominent feature, and those who present with apraxia, acalculia, or spelling difficulties, but do not show early or prominent visual impairment.[46] Original diagnostic criteria were composed before development of AD pathophysiological biomarkers. The availability of CSF, amyloid, and tau PET imaging, and post-mortem pathological data relates to questions of how best to label PCA at different levels. For example, PCA as a clinical syndrome versus PCA arising from specific underlying aetiologies (e.g. AD, DLB, CBD). Whether *in vivo* pathophysiological confirmation of underlying AD is available is of particular relevance, raising questions on the suitability of pharmacological interventions targeting amyloid or tau deposition in PCA patients, while syndromic classification might be sufficient for non-pharmacological, behavioural interventions. Even in patients who show low Aβ 1-42 and high total tau levels consistent with AD,[97] questions remain about the appropriateness of cognitive outcome measures intended to assess the efficacy of pharmacological interventions; examples of measures particularly susceptible to confounding include executive function tasks with a visuospatial component,[15] or visually mediated tasks testing episodic memory. In order to address some of these questions, the PCA Working Party, consisting of researchers representing 23 institutions in 9 countries, was set up to facilitate improvement and harmonization of the diagnostic criteria for PCA and promote better clinical and research practice.[72] Recent outcomes of the PCA Working Party include the largest investigation of genetic risk factors for PCA to date[98] and the first multicentre consensus classification criteria for PCA, comprising three classification levels for PCA defined at a syndromic (PCA) or disease level (e.g. PCA-AD, PCA-DLB).[95] Within Crutch and colleague's recent framework, classification levels correspond to the availability of clinical or pathophysiological biomarker evidence, while establishing terminology for cases where clinical features overlap with other neurodegenerative syndromes (PCA-plus).

Prevalence and Incidence

As the preceding sections demonstrate, there is considerable debate as to how PCA should be classified on neuropsychological grounds; whether PCA should be used as syndromic diagnosis encompassing any underlying pathology or should be restricted to those with AD; how existing diagnostic criteria should be applied; and even

Table 15.1 Clinical diagnostic criteria for PCA

Tang-Wai et al., 2004	Mendez et al., 2002	Crutch et al., 2017
Core features Insidious onset and gradual progression Presentation of visual complaints in the absence of significant primary ocular disease Relative preservation of anterograde memory and insight early in the disorder Disabling visual impairment throughout the disorder Absence of stroke or tumour Absence of early parkinsonism and hallucinations *Any of the following findings:* Simultanagnosia with or without optic ataxia or ocular apraxia Constructional dyspraxia Visual field defect Environmental disorientation Any of the elements of Gerstmann's syndrome **Supportive features** Alexia Presenile onset Ideomotor or dressing apraxia Prosopagnosia **Investigations** Neuropsychology: deficits referable to parietal and/or occipital regions Neuroimaging: focal or asymmetric atrophy in parietal and/or occipital regions on structural imaging Focal or asymmetric hypoperfusion/ hypometabolism in parietal and/or occipital regions on functional imaging	**Core diagnostic features (all must be present)** Insidious onset and gradual progression Presentation with visual complaints with intact primary visual functions Evidence of predominant complex visual disorder on examination Elements of Balint's syndrome Visual agnosia Dressing apraxia Environmental disorientation Proportionally less impaired deficits in memory and verbal fluency Relatively preserved insight with or without depression **Supportive diagnostic features** Presenile onset Alexia Elements of Gerstmann's syndrome Ideomotor apraxia Physical examination within normal limits **Investigations** Neuropsychology: predominantly impaired perceptual deficits Neuroimaging: predominantly occipitoparietal abnormality (especially on functional neuroimaging) with relative sparing of frontal and mesiotemporal regions	**Clinical features** Insidious onset Gradual progression Prominent early disturbance of visual ± other posterior cognitive functions Absence of tumour, significant vascular disease including stroke, afferent visual cause or identifiable cause (e.g. kidney failure) sufficient to explain symptoms **Cognitive features** Space perception deficit Simultanagnosia Object perception deficit Constructional dyspraxia Environmental agnosia Oculomotor apraxia Dressing apraxia Optic ataxia Alexia Left/right disorientation Acalculia Limb apraxia (not limb-kinetic) Apperceptive prosopagnosia Agraphia Homonymous visual field defect Finger agnosia Relatively spared anterograde memory, speech, nonvisual language, executive function and behaviour **Investigations** Neuropsychology: deficits predominantly within space and object perception domains Neuroimaging: predominant occipito-parietal or occipito-temporal atrophy/hypometabolism/ hypoperfusion on MRI/FDG-PET/SPECT

Source: data from Tang-Wai D.F. et al. Clinical, genetic, and neuropathologic characteristics of posterior cortical atrophy. *Neurology*. 2004; 12;63(7):1168-74; data from Mendez M.F. et al. Posterior cortical atrophy: clinical characteristics and differences compared to Alzheimer's disease. *Dement Geriatr Cogn Disord*. 2002;14(1):33-40; data from Crutch S.J. et al. Consensus classification of posterior cortical atrophy. *Alzheimer's & Dementia*. 2017;13(8):870-884.

whether PCA is a misnomer, given that there may not always be atrophy at least on structural MR imaging. Coupled with variable knowledge of PCA amongst different medical professionals, it follows that precise estimates of the prevalence and incidence of PCA are difficult to determine.

PCA is typically considered as a form of young-onset dementia (disease onset <65 years), with AD the most common aetiology. Prevalence rates of young-onset AD within the 45–64 year-old age group have been estimated to be between 15 to 35 cases per 100,000[99,100] and incidence rates estimated at 6–7 per 100,000.[99,101] To date, estimates of the prevalence of PCA or visual presentations of AD have been based on samples from secondary and/or tertiary services. Of 270 patients diagnosed with probable young-onset AD at a specialist centre, 13% were diagnosed with non-amnestic presentations, predominantly involving either visual or biparietal dysfunction characterized by visuospatial and praxic deficits.[102] Of 154 cases seen in a memory clinic, 4% had PCA,[103] while Snowden et al.[104] reported that out of 523 patients who attended a specialist centre for cognitive disorders, 5% had a visual presentation. Although Snowden et al.[104] specified that PCA related to patients with an initially visual presentation, in the context of whether different subtypes of PCA exist, it is possible that the diagnostic term might be applied to patients classified under other cognitive presentations, given how clinical classification of the 7% of patients with a language presentation included reading, writing, calculation, and spelling difficulties, and 3% of patients were defined as having an apraxic presentation.

In addition to issues surrounding classification of the PCA syndrome, the lack of population-based epidemiological studies likely relates to its relative rarity. Estimates of the incidence and prevalence of AD featuring predominant visual processing deficits may be informed through population-based studies comprising samples that are well-characterized in cognitive profile. A recent prospective population-based study of 5088 older adults identified incident late onset AD in 825 participants in whom cognitive data was available on memory, executive function, language, visuospatial ability, and attention; 14% demonstrated relatively pronounced impairment on scaled composite scores of visuospatial ability relative to other cognitive domains.[105] Participants within this subset almost exclusively did not fulfil criteria for PCA; however, such investigations may establish whether or not atypical AD subtypes represent extremities within a phenotypic disease spectrum, including whether certain risk factors predispose individuals to particular clinical presentations.

Consistent with the notion of PCA primarily presenting as a form of young-onset dementia, the largest, worldwide study published to date confirmed that of 302 cases fulfilling standard clinical criteria, the mean (SD) age was 58.9 (6.9) years;[98] and 83% had young-onset dementia. PCA patients with a wide range of ages have been reported (40–86 years:).[6] Some studies have reported that women are slightly over-represented (e.g. 59% of the sample reported by Schott et al.[99]), others have found no difference in gender distribution.[10,14,66]

Genetic and Environmental Risk Factors

To date, there has been no clear consensus as to the genetic basis of PCA. While a study of 40 PCA patients found 11 had a family history of dementia, none presented with a phenotype akin to PCA, and the incidence of family history in PCA does not significantly differ with that in tAD.[6,66] Mutations identified on the PS-1 gene[106] and the progranulin gene[107,108] have also been identified in patients with a PCA phenotype, but to all intents and purposes, PCA is a sporadic syndrome. It is possible that APOE ε4 status may differ between PCA and tAD patients; two studies have found around 20–30% of patients with a visual presentation of AD were ε4-positive, relative to over 80% of amnestic AD patients.[102,107] However, other studies have reported that around 45–55% of PCA patients were ε4-positive and suggested a lower prevalence of APOE ε4-positive tAD patients (55–75%).[6,25,87] The largest exploratory genome-wide association study of PCA to date involved analysis of 293 samples provided through efforts involving 11 international centres.[98] While a strong association was found at APOE, the risk associated with APOE was smaller than that observed for tAD. Three novel loci were nominated near CNTNAP5, FAM46A, and SEMA3C. These genes are implicated in intercellular communication processes within the central nervous system retinal signalling pathway abnormalities thought to be involved in the pathogenesis of retinitis pigmentosa and in the maturation of the visual system respectively; validation of these findings is currently underway.[96] Future investigations into the genotype of well-characterized PCA patients might shed light on the biological processes underlying PCA, and may offer insights into the possibility that reduced APOE ε4 allele load might confer some form of protection to medial temporal regions from AD pathogenesis.[110]

Factors such as smoking, nutrition, education, exercise, and traumatic brain injury are associated with the risk of early and late-onset AD in general[111–115] and there have been suggestions of neurodevelopmental differences in PCA manifesting in over-represented learning disability rates.[116] However, there is currently no compelling evidence for any specific risk for PCA. Consideration of risk factors for cerebrovascular disease has been recommended for clinical management of PCA.[111]

Supporting People with PCA

Pharmacological management of cognitive and behavioural symptoms in PCA

Symptomatic treatment for AD may be offered through pharmacological interventions; these include AChEIs (e.g. donepezil, galantamine, and rivastigmine) and an NMDA receptor antagonist (memantine). A NICE review has recommended AChEIs in the management of mild-to-moderate AD, while also recommending memantine for severe AD as well as patients with moderate AD who are unsuitable for or unable to tolerate AChEIs. In PCA, AChEIs have been noted to provide some clinical benefit,[118] although specific effects of AChEIs and memantine in PCA have yet to be thoroughly investigated. Recommending antidepressant drugs might be appropriate for PCA patients with persistent low mood, and treatments for parkinsonism (e.g. L-Dopa), myoclonus, or seizures may be appropriate in individual patients. As for other forms of AD (or other neurodegenerative diseases) there are currently no treatments proven to alter the progression or outcome of PCA.

Challenges to providing appropriate care for people with PCA

Patients with PCA may have particular care needs. The prominent visuospatial and visuoperceptual impairment occurring in PCA pose significant challenges to maintaining independent activities of daily living. At a relatively early point in the disease course, and often still at a working age, patients with PCA may be unable to drive due to diminished visuospatial ability, manage correspondence due to reading difficulties, dress independently due to apraxia, or leave the home unaccompanied due to topographical disorientation. Awareness of dependence on others may provoke feelings of guilt, frustration, or low mood, particularly when coupled with a relative sparing of insight until later in the disease.[28]

Sources of inappropriate care for individuals with PCA include the oversight of visual deficits in the context of dementia being perceived as a condition relating primarily, or solely, to memory function. Consequences of this may include group activities in day centres or residential care settings being visually mediated, without considering the barriers some PCA patients may face to engaging in such activities.[72] The relative preservation of memory, language, and insight in early stages of PCA does not preclude engagement in patient support group meetings, or psychological treatments. Disease-specific support group meetings, such as the PCA support group, promote the exchange of information and advice, both professional and personal, in addition to any social and emotional benefits of participation, and may fulfil an advocacy role in raising awareness about particular issues experienced by individuals with rarer forms of dementia.[28]

Future Directions

As previously outlined, various challenges limit the precision in estimating incidence and prevalence rates of PCA, with currently available information derived from samples recruited through single-centre clinical secondary and tertiary services. Prerequisites of population-based epidemiological studies of PCA include consistent application of terminology, development of consensus on diagnostic criteria, and acknowledgement of heterogeneity within the PCA spectrum. Furthermore, particular challenges to the implementation of population-based studies of PCA include its rarity and frequent misdiagnosis. The establishment of the international PCA Working party and subsequent formation of consensus classification criteria represent steps towards addressing these challenges and in facilitating multicentre investigations of PCA.[72,95] Given PCA's predominantly visual presentation and proposed subtypes, a representative sample may require identification of patients through a variety of specialist neurology, ophthalmology, neuro-ophthalmology, and psychiatric clinics and services. Particularly in light of limited prognostic information on PCA, future large-scale studies would ideally comprise longitudinal visits, with patients followed up to advanced disease stages. Findings from such investigations would promote better clinical management and care planning, clarify heterogeneity within the PCA syndrome, and enable exploration of factors relating to disease progression. Large-scale studies should seek to replicate recent genome-wide association findings implicating three novel genes in the development of PCA and estimating a smaller effect of APOE risk in PCA relative to tAD.[98] Questions on the appropriateness of cognitive outcome measures to assess efficacy of interventions are relevant to the inclusion of PCA-AD patients in AD-specific pharmacological trials, as well as the possibility of future pharmacological and non-pharmacological interventions specifically targeting PCA patients. Future population-based studies including both typical and atypical presentations of young onset AD, including PCA-AD, would not only help establish incidence and prevalence rates, but also may support the understanding of factors driving AD phenotypic heterogeneity.

REFERENCES

1. Benson DF, Davis RJ, Snyder BD. Posterior cortical atrophy. *Archives of Neurology*, 1988; 45(7): 789–93.
2. Morel F Les aires striée, parastriée et péristriée dans les troubles de la fonction visuelle au cours de la maladie d'Alzheimer. *Stereotactic and Functional Neurosurgery*. 1944; 6(5): 238–42.
3. Cogan DG. Visual disturbances with focal progressive dementing disease. *American Journal of Ophthalmology*. 1985; 100(1): 68–72.
4. De Renzi E. Slowly progressive visual agnosia or apraxia without dementia. *Cortex*. 1986; 22: 171–80.
5. Hof PR, Bouras C, Constantinidis J, Morrison JH. Selective disconnection of specific visual association pathways in cases of Alzheimer's-disease presenting with Balints syndrome. *Journal of Neuropathology and Experimental Neurology*. 2000; 49(2): 168–84. doi: 10.1097/00005072-199003000-00008.
6. Tang-Wai DF, Graff-Radford NR, Boeve BF, Dickson DW, Parisi JE, Crook R, et al. Clinical, genetic, and neuropathologic characteristics of posterior cortical atrophy. *Neurology*. 2004; 63(7): 1168–74.
7. Levine DN, Lee JM, Fisher CM. The visual variant of Alzheimer's disease: a clinicopathologic case study. *Neurology*. 1993; 43(2): 305–13.
8. Ross SK, Graham N, Stuart-Green L, Prins M, Xuereb J, Patterson K, et al. Progressive biparietal atrophy: an atypical presentation of Alzheimer's disease. *Journal of Neurology Neurosurgery and Psychiatry*. 1996; 61(4): 388–95.
9. Galton CJ, Patterson K, Xuereb JH, Hodges JR. Atypical and typical presentations of Alzheimer's disease: a clinical, neuropsychological, neuroimaging and pathological study of 13 cases. *Brain*. 2000; 123: 484–98. doi: 10.1093/brain/123.3.484.
10. Renner JA, Burns JM, Hou CE, McKeel DW, Storandt M, Morris JC. Progressive posterior cortical dysfunction—a clinicopathologic series. *Neurology*. 2004; 63(7): 1175–80.
11. Seguin J, Formaglio M, Perret-Liaudet A, Quadrio I, Tholance Y, Rouaud O, et al. CSF biomarkers in posterior cortical atrophy. *Neurology*. 2011; 76(21): 1782–8.
12. Mendez MF. Corticobasal ganglionic degeneration with Balint's syndrome. Journal of Neuropsychiatry and Clinical Neurosciences. 2000; 12(2): 273–5.
13. Tang-Wai DF, Josephs KA, Boeve BF, Dickson DW, Parisi JE, Petersen RC. Pathologically confirmed corticobasal degeneration presenting with visuospatial dysfunction. *Neurology*. 2003; 61(8): 1134–5.
14. McMonagle P, Deering F, Berliner Y, Kertesz A. The cognitive profile of posterior cortical atrophy. *Neurology*. 2006; 66(3): 331–8.
15. Crutch SJ, Lehmann M, Schott JM, Rabinovici GD, Rossor MN, Fox, NC. Posterior cortical atrophy. *Lancet Neurology*. 2012;11(2): 170–8.
16. Josephs KA, Whitwell JL, Boeve BF, Knopma, DS, Tang-Wai DF, Drubach DA, et al. Visual hallucinations in posterior cortical atrophy. *Archives of Neurology*. 2006; 63(10): 1427–32. doi: 10.1001/archneur.63.10.1427.
17. Tang-Wai D, Mapstone M. What are we seeing? Is posterior cortical atrophy just Alzheimer disease? *Neurology*. 2006; 66(3): 300–1. doi: 10.1212/01.wnl.0000202093.81603.d8.
18. Stopford CL, Snowden JS, Thompson JC, Neary D. Variability in cognitive presentation of Alzheimer's disease. *Cortex*. 2008; 44(2): 185–95. doi: 10.1016/j.cortex.2005.11.002.
19. Alladi S, Xuereb J, Bak T, Nestor P, Knibb J, Patterson K, et al. Focal cortical presentations of Alzheimer's disease. *Brain*. 2007; 130(Pt 10): 2636–45. doi: 130/10/2636 [pii]10.1093/brain/awm213.
20. Hof PR, Bouras C, Constantinidis J, Morrison JH. Balint's syndrome in Alzheimer's disease: specific disruption of the occipito-parietal visual pathway. *Brain Res*. 1989; 493(2): 368–75.
21. Hof PR, Vogt BA, Bouras C, Morrison JH. Atypical form of Alzheimer's disease with prominent posterior cortical atrophy: a review of lesion distribution and circuit disconnection in cortical visual pathways. *Vision Res*. 1997; 37(24): 3609–25. doi: S0042-6989(96)00240-4 [pii]10.1016/S0042-6989(96)00240-4.
22. von Gunten A, Bouras C, Kovari E, Giannakopoulos P, Hof PR Neural substrates of cognitive and behavioral deficits in atypical Alzheimer's disease. *Brain Res Rev*. 2006; 51(2): 176–211. doi: S0165-0173(05)00169-4 [pii]10.1016/j.brainresrev.2005.11.003.
23. Lehmann M, Crutch SJ, Ridgway GR, Ridha BH, Barnes J, Warrington EK, et al. Cortical thickness and voxel-based morphometry in posterior cortical atrophy and typical Alzheimer's disease. *Neurobiology of Aging*. 2011; 32(8): 1466–76. doi: 10.1016/j.neurobiolaging.2009.08.017.
24. Whitwell JL, Jack CR, Kantarci K, Weigand SD, Boeve BF, Knopman DS, et al. Imaging correlates of posterior cortical atrophy. *Neurobiology of Aging*. 2007; 28(7): 1051–61. doi: 10.1016/j.neurobiolaging.2006.05.026.
25. Migliaccio R, Agosta F, Rascovsky K, Karydas A, Bonasera S, Rabinovici GD et al. Clinical syndromes associated with posterior atrophy Early age at onset AD spectrum. *Neurology*. 2009; 73(19): 1571–8. doi: 10.1212/Wnl.0b013e3181c0d427.
26. Migliaccio R, Agosta F, Scola E, Magnani G, Cappa SF, Pagani E,et al. Ventral and dorsal visual streams in posterior cortical atrophy: A DT MRI study. *Neurobiology of Aging*. 2012; 33(11): 2572–84. doi: 10.1016/j.neurobiolaging.2011.12.025.
27. Manning EN, Macdonald KE, Leung KK, Young J, Pepple T, Lehmann M, et al. Differential hippocampal shapes in posterior

cortical atrophy patients: A comparison with control and typical AD subjects. *Human Brain Mapping.* 2015; 36(12), 5123–36.
28. Suárez-González A, Henley SM, Walton J, Crutch SJ. Posterior cortical atrophy: an atypical variant of Alzheimer disease. *Psychiatric Clinics of North America.* 2015; 38(2): 211–20.
29. Lehmann M, Barnes J, Ridgway GR, Ryan NS, Warrington EK, Crutch SJ, et al. Global gray matter changes in posterior cortical atrophy: a serial imaging study. Alzheimer's & Dementia. 2012; 8(6); 502–12.
30. Ridgway GR, Lehmann M, Barnes J, Rohrer JD, Warren JD, Crutch SJ, et al. Early-onset Alzheimer disease clinical variants multivariate analyses of cortical thickness. *Neurology.* 2012; 79(1): 80–4.
31. Duning T, Warnecke T, Mohammadi S, Lohmann H, Schiffbauer H, Kugel H, et al. Pattern and progression of white-matter changes in a case of posterior cortical atrophy using diffusion tensor imaging. *Journal of Neurology Neurosurgery and Psychiatry.* 2009; 80(4): 432–6. doi: 10.1136/jnnp.2008.153148.
32. Madhavan A, Schwarz CG, Duffy JR, Strand EA, Machulda MM, Drubach DA, et al. Characterizing white matter tract degeneration in syndromic variants of Alzheimer's disease: a diffusion tensor imaging study. *Journal of Alzheimer's Disease.* 2015; 49(3): 633–43.
33. Nestor PJ, Caine D, Fryer TD, Clarke J, Hodges JR. The topography of metabolic deficits in posterior cortical atrophy (the visual variant of Alzheimer's disease) with FDG-PET. *Journal of Neurology Neurosurgery and Psychiatry.* 2003; 74(11): 1521–9. doi: 10.1136/jnnp.74.11.1521.
34. Kas A, de Souza LC, Samri D, Bartolomeo P, Lacomblez L, Kalafat M, et al. Neural correlates of cognitive impairment in posterior cortical atrophy. *Brain.* 2011; 134: 1464–78. doi: 10.1093/Brain/Awr055.
35. Rosenbloom MH, Alkalay A, Agarwal N, Baker SL, ONeill JP, Janabi M, et al. Distinct clinical and metabolic deficits in Alzheimer's disease and posterior cortical atrophy are not related to amyloid distribution. *Neurology.* 2010; 74(9): A301.
36. Whitwell J, Graff-Radford J, Singh T, Drubach D, Senjem M, Spychalla A, et al. 18F-FDG PET in posterior cortical atrophy and dementia with Lewy bodies. *Journal of Nuclear Medicine.* 2016; jnumed-116.
37. Lehmann M, Ghosh PM, Madison C, Laforce R, Corbetta-Rastelli C, Weiner MW, et al. Diverging patterns of amyloid deposition and hypometabolism in clinical variants of probable Alzheimer's disease. *Brain.* 2013; 136: 844–58. doi: 10.1093/Brain/Aws327.
38. Lehmann M, Madison C, Ghosh PM, Miller ZA, Greicius MD, Kramer JH, et al. Loss of functional connectivity is greater outside the default mode network in nonfamilial early-onset Alzheimer's disease variants. *Neurobiology of Aging.* 2015; 36(10): 2678–86.
39. Tenuovuo O, Kemppainen N, Aalto S, Nagren K, Rinne JO. Posterior cortical atrophy: a rare form of dementia with in vivo evidence of amyloid-beta accumulation. *Journal of Alzheimer's Disease.* 2008; 15(3): 351–5.
40. de Souza LC, Corlier F, Habert MO, Uspenskaya O, Maroy R, Lamari F, et al. Similar amyloid-beta burden in posterior cortical atrophy and Alzheimer's disease. *Brain.* 2011; 134(Pt 7): 2036–43. doi: 10.1093/brain/awr130awr130 [pii].
41. Ossenkoppele R, Schonhaut DR, Baker SL, O'Neil J, Janabi M, Ghosh PM, et al. Tau, amyloid, and hypometabolism in a patient with posterior cortical atrophy. *Annals of Neurology.* 2015; 77(2): 338–42.
42. Strozyk D, Blennow K, White LR, Launer LJ. CSF Aβ 42 levels correlate with amyloid-neuropathology in a population-based autopsy study. *Neurology.* 2003; 60(4): 652–6.
43. Buerger K, Ewers M, Pirttilä T, Zinkowski R, Alafuzoff I, Teipel SJ, et al. CSF phosphorylated tau protein correlates with neocortical neurofibrillary pathology in Alzheimer's disease. *Brain.* 2006; 129(11): 3035–41.
44. Blennow K, Hampel H, Weiner M, Zetterberg H. Cerebrospinal fluid and plasma biomarkers in Alzheimer disease. *Nature Reviews Neurology.* 2010; 6(3): 131–44.
45. Paterson RW, Toombs J, Slattery CF, Nicholas JM, Andreasson U, Magdalinou NK et al. Dissecting IWG-2 typical and atypical Alzheimer's disease: insights from cerebrospinal fluid analysis. *Journal of Neurology.* 2015; 262(12): 2722–30.
46. Crutch SJ. Seeing why they cannot see: understanding the syndrome and causes of posterior cortical atrophy. *J Neuropsychol.* 2013; doi: 10.1111/jnp.12011.
47. Mizuno M, Sartori G, Liccione D, Battelli L, Campo R. Progressive visual agnosia with posterior cortical atrophy. Clinical Neurology and Neurosurgery. 1996; 98(2): 176–8.
48. Stark, ME, Grafman J, Fertig E. A restricted 'spotlight' of attention in visual object recognition. *Neuropsychologia.* 1997; 35(9): 1233–49. doi: 10.1016/S0028-3932(97)00049-3.
49. Delazer M, Karner E, Zamarian L, Donnemiller E, Benke T. Number processing in posterior cortical atrophy—a neuropsycholgical case study. Neuropsychologia. 2006; 44(1): 36–51. doi: S0028-3932(05)00173-9 (pii)10.1016/j.neuropsychologia.2005.04.013.
50. Andrade K, Samri D, Sarazin M, de Souza LC, Cohen L, Thiebaut de Schotten M, et al. Visual neglect in posterior cortical atrophy. *BMC Neurology.* 2010; 10. doi: Artn 68Doi 10.1186/1471-2377-10-68.
51. Gauthier L, Dehaut F, Joanette Y. The Bells test—a quantitative and qualitative test for visual neglect. *International Journal of Clinical Neuropsychology.* 1989; 11(2): 49–54.
52. Saffran EM, Fitzpatrick-DeSalme EJ, Coslett HB. Visual disturbances in dementia. *Modular Deficits in Alzheimer-type Dementia.* 1990; 44: 297–327.
53. Crutch SJ, Lehmann M, Gorgoraptis N, Kaski D, Ryan N, Husain M, et al. Abnormal visual phenomena in posterior cortical atrophy. *Neurocase.* 2011; 17(2): 160–77. doi: Pii 926575951Doi 10.1080/13554794.2010.504729.
54. Coslett HB, Stark M, Rajaram S, Saffran EM. Narrowing the spotlight: a visual attentional disorder in presumed Alzheimer's disease. Neurocase. 1995; 1(4): 305–18.
55. Shakespeare TJ, Yong KXX, Frost C, Kim LG, Warrington EK, Crutch SJ. Scene perception in posterior cortical atrophy: categorization, description and fixation patterns. *Frontiers in Human Neuroscience.* 2013; 7. doi: Artn 621Doi 10.3389/Fnhum.2013.00621.
56. Yong KX, Shakespeare TJ, Cash D, Henley SM, Warren JD, Crutch SJ. (Con)text-specific effects of visual dysfunction on reading in posterior cortical atrophy. *Cortex.* 2014; 57: 92–106.
57. Russell C, Malhotra P, Deidda C, Husain M. Dynamic attentional modulation of vision across space and time after right hemisphere stroke and in ageing. *Cortex.* 2013; 49(7): 1874–83. doi: 10.1016/j.cortex.2012.10.005 S0010-9452(12)00307-3 [pii].
58. Delaj L, D'Alessandro R, Stracciari A, Fonti C, Cretella L, Lodi R. Long-lasting hemianopia due to PCA. *Journal of Neurology.* 2010; 257(9): 1562–4.

59. Pelak VS, Smyth SF, Boyer PJ, Filley CM. Computerized visual field defects in posterior cortical atrophy. *Neurology*. 2011; 77(24): 2119–22. doi: 10.1212/Wnl.0b013e31823e9f2a.
60. Warrington EK. Visual deficits associated with occipital lobe lesions in man. *Experimental Brain Research Supplementum*. 1986; 11, 247–61.
61. Warrington EK, James M. Disorders of visual perception in patients with localised cerebral lesions. *Neuropsychologia*. 1967; 5(3): 253–66. doi: 10.1016/0028-3932(67)90040-1.
62. Warrington EK, James M. Visual apperceptive agnosia—a clinico-anatomical study of 3 cases. *Cortex*. 1998; 24(1): 13–32.
63. De Renzi E, Scotti G, Spinnler H. Perceptual and associative disorders of visual recognition. Neurology. 1969; 19(7): 634–42.
64. Gollin ES. Developmental studies of visual recognition of incomplete objects. *Perceptual and Motor Skills*. 1960; 11(3), 289–98.
65. Aharon-Peretz J, Israel O, Goldsher D, Peretz A. Posterior cortical atrophy variants of Alzheimer's disease. *Dement Geriatr Cogn Disord*. 1999; 10(6): 483–7. doi: 17194 [pii]17194.
66. Mendez MF, Ghajarania M, Perryman KM. Posterior cortical atrophy: clinical characteristics and differences compared to Alzheimer's disease. *Dementia and Geriatric Cognitive Disorders*. 2002; 14(1): 33–40.
67. Sala SD, Spinnler H, Trivelli C. Slowly progressive impairment of spatial exploration and visual perception. *Neurocase*. 1996; 2(4): 299–323.
68. McCarthy RA, Warrington EK. *Cognitive Neuropsychology: A Clinical Introduction*. Cambridge, MA: Academic Press, 1990.
69. Capitani E, Laiacona M, Mahon B, Caramazza A. What are the facts of semantic category-specific deficits? A critical review of the clinical evidence. *Cognitive Neuropsychology*. 2003; 20(3–6): 213–61. doi: 10.1080/02643290244000266.
70. McCarthy RA, Warrington EK. Visual associative agnosia: a clinico-anatomical study of a single case. *Journal of Neurology, Neurosurgery & Psychiatry*. 1986; 49(11): 1233–40.
71. De Renzi E, Perani D, Carlesimo GA, Silveri MC, Fazio F. Prosopagnosia can be associated with damage confined to the right hemisphere an MRI and PET study and a review of the literature. *Neuropsychologia*. 1994; 32(8): 893–902. doi: 0028-3932(94)90041-8 [pii].
72. Crutch SJ, Schott JM, Rabinovici GD, Boeve BF, Cappa SF, Dickerson BC, et al. Shining a light on posterior cortical atrophy. *Alzheimer's & Dementia*. 2012; 9(4): 463–5. doi: 10.1016/j.jalz.2012.11.004.
73. Farah MJ. The Cognitive Neuroscience of Vision. Oxford: Blackwell Publishing, 2000.
74. Metzler-Baddeley C, Baddeley RJ, Lovell PG, Laffan A, Jones RW. Visual impairments in dementia with Lewy bodies and posterior cortical atrophy. Neuropsychology, 2010; 24(1): 35.
75. Chan D, Crutch SJ, Warrington EK. A disorder of colour perception associated with abnormal colour after-images: a defect of the primary visual cortex. *J Neurol Neurosurg Psychiatry*. 2001; 71(4): 515–17.
76. Holmes G, Horrax G. Disturbances of spatial orientation and visual attention, with loss of stereoscopic vision. *Archives of Neurology and Psychiatry*. 1919; 1(4): 385.
77. Cole S, Warrington EK. Visual disorientation in homonymous half-fields. *Neurology*. 1962; 12: 257–63.
78. Midorikawa A, Nakamura K, Nagao T, Kawamura M. Residual perception of moving objects: dissociation of moving and static objects in a case or posterior cortical atrophy. *European Neurology*. 2008; 59(3–4): 152–8. doi: 10.1159/000114035.
79. 32.Efron R. What is perception?. In: *Proceedings of the Boston Colloquium for the Philosophy of Science 1966/1968*. Springer: Netherlands, 1969. pp137–73.
80. Berthier ML, Leiguarda R, Starkstein SE, Sevlever G, Taratuto AL. Alzheimer's-disease in a patient with posterior cortical atrophy. *Journal of Neurology Neurosurgery and Psychiatry*. 1991; 54(12): 1110–11. doi: 10.1136/jnnp.54.12.1110.
81. Mendez MF, Shapira JS, Clark DG. 'Apperceptive' alexia in posterior cortical atrophy. *Cortex*. 2007; 43(2): 264:70. doi: 10.1016/S0010-9452(08)70481-7.
82. Yong KX, Rajdev K, Shakespeare TJ, Leff AP, Crutch SJ. Facilitating text reading in posterior cortical atrophy. *Neurology*. 2015; 85(4): 339–48.
83. Shakespeare TJ, Kaski D, Yong KX, Paterson RW, Slattery CF, Ryan NS, et al. Abnormalities of fixation, saccade and pursuit in posterior cortical atrophy. Brain. 2015; 138(7): 1976–91.
84. Crutch SJ, Warrington EK. Foveal crowding in posterior cortical atrophy: a specific early-visual-processing deficit affecting word reading. *Cognitive Neuropsychology*. 2007; 24(8): 843–66. doi: 10.1080/02643290701754240.
85. Yong KX, Shakespeare TJ, Cash D, Henley SM, Nicholas J M, Ridgway GR et al. Prominent effects and neural correlates of visual crowding in a neurodegenerative disease population. Brain. 2014; 137(12): 3284–99.
86. Rosenbloom MH, Alkalay A, Agarwal N, Baker SL, O'Neil JP, Janabi M, et al. Distinct clinical and metabolic deficits in PCA and AD are not related to amyloid distribution. *Neurology*. 2011; 76(21): 1789–96.
87. Magnin E, Sylvestre G, Lenoir F, Dariel E, Bonnet L, Chopard G, et al. Logopenic syndrome in posterior cortical atrophy. *Journal of Neurology*. 2013; 260(2): 528–33. doi: 10.1007/s00415-012-6671-7.
88. Crutch SJ, Lehmann M, Warren JD, Rohrer JD. The language profile of posterior cortical atrophy. *Journal of Neurology Neurosurgery and Psychiatry*. 2013; 84(4): 460–66. doi: 10.1136/jnnp-2012-303309.
89. Jonides J, Schumacher EH, Smith EE, Koeppe RA, Awh E, Reuter-Lorenz PA, et al. The role of parietal cortex in verbal working memory. *Journal of Neuroscience*. 1998; 18(13): 5026–34.
90. Goll JC, Crutch SJ, Loo JHY, Rohrer JD, Frost C, Bamiou DE, et al. Non-verbal sound processing in the primary progressive aphasias. Brain. 2010; 133: 272–85. doi: 10.1093/Brain/Awp235.
91. Golden HL, Nicholas JM, Yong KX, Downey LE, Schott JM, Mummery CJ, et al. Auditory spatial processing in Alzheimer's disease. Brain. 2015; 138(1): 189–202.
92. Green RC, Goldstein FC, Mirra SS, Alazraki NP, Baxt JL, Bakay RA. Slowly progressive apraxia in Alzheimer's disease. Journal of Neurology, Neurosurgery & Psychiatry. 1995; 59(3): 312–5.
93. Ryan NS, Shakespeare TJ, Lehmann M, Keihaninejad S, Nicholas JM, Leung KK, et al. Motor features in posterior cortical atrophy and their imaging correlates. *Neurobiology of Aging*. 2014; 35(12): 2845–57.
94. Suárez-González A, Lehmann M, Shakespeare TJ, Yong KX, Paterson RW, Slattery CF, et al. Effect of age at onset on cortical thickness and cognition in posterior cortical atrophy. Neurobiology of Aging. 2016; 44: 108–13.
95. Crutch SJ, Schott J M, Rabinovici GD, Murray M, Snowden JS, van der Flier W, et al. Consensus classification of posterior cortical atrophy. *Alzheimer's & Dementia*. 2017; 13(8): 870–84.

96. Dubois B, Feldman HH, Jacova C, Hampel H, Molinuevo JL, Blennow K, et al. Advancing research diagnostic criteria for Alzheimer's disease: the IWG-2 criteria. *Lancet Neurology*. 2014; 13(6): 614–29.
97. Dubois B, Feldman HH, Jacova C, Dekosky ST, Barberger-Gateau P, Cummings J, et al. Research criteria for the diagnosis of Alzheimer's disease: revising the NINCDS-ADRDA criteria. *Lancet Neurology*. 2007; 6(8): 734–46. doi: 10.1016/S1474-4422(07)70178-3.
98. Schott JM, Crutch SJ, Carrasquillo MM, Uphill J, Shakespeare TJ, Ryan NS, et al. *Genetic risk factors for the posterior cortical atrophy variant of Alzheimer's disease*. Alzheimer's & Dementia. 2016; 12(8): 862–71.
99. Newens AJ, Forster DP, Kay DWK, Kirkup W, Bates D, Edwardson J. Clinically diagnosed presenile dementia of the Alzheimer type in the Northern Health Region: ascertainment, prevalence, incidence and survival. *Psychological Medicine*. 1993; 23(3): 631–44.
100. Renvoize E, Hanson M, Dale M. Prevalence and causes of young onset dementia in an English health district. *International Journal of Geriatric Psychiatry*. 2011; 26(1): 106–7.
101. Bickel H, Bürger K, Hampel H, Schreiber Y, Sonntag A, Wiegele B, et al. Presenile dementia in memory clinics—incidence rates and clinical features. *Der Nervenarzt*. 2006; 77(9): 1079–85.
102. Koedam EL, Lauffer V, van der Vlies AE, van der Flier WM, Scheltens P, Pijnenburg YA. Early-versus late-onset Alzheimer's disease: more than age alone. *Journal of Alzheimer's Disease*. 2010; 19(4): 1401–8.
103. Croisile DB. Benson's syndrome or Posterior Cortical Atrophy. *Orphanet Encyclopedia*. September 2004; 1–4.
104. Snowden JS, Stopford CL, Julien CL, Thompson JC, Davidson Y, Gibbons L, et al. Cognitive phenotypes in Alzheimer's disease and genetic risk. *Cortex*, 2007; 43(7): 835–45.
105. Crane PK, Trittschuh E, Mukherjee S, Saykin AJ, Sanders RE, Larson EB, et al. Incidence of cognitively defined late-onset Alzheimer's dementia subgroups from a prospective cohort study. *Alzheimer's & Dementia*. 2017; 13(12): 1307–16.
106. Sitek EJ, Narozanska E, Peplonska B, Filipek S, Barczak A, Styczynska M, et al. A patient with posterior cortical atrophy possesses a novel mutation in the Presenilin 1 gene. *PLOS One*. 2013; 8(4): doi: ARTN e61074DOI 10.1371/journal.pone.0061074.
107. Caroppo P, Belin C, Grabli D, Maillet D, De Septenville A, Migliaccio R, et al. Posterior cortical atrophy as an extreme phenotype of GRN mutations. JAMA Neurology. 2015; 72(2): 224–8.
108. Peng G, Liu P, He F, Luo B. Posterior cortical atrophy as a primary clinical phenotype of corticobasal syndrome with a progranulin gene rs5848 TT genotype. *Orphanet Journal of Rare Diseases*. 2016; 11(1): 1.
109. Schott JM, Ridha BH, Crutch SJ, Healy DG, Uphill J B, Warrington EK, et al. Apolipoprotein E genotype modifies the phenotype of Alzheimer disease. *Archives of Neurology*. 2006; 63(1): 155–6. doi: 10.1001/archneur.63.1.155.
110. Filippini N, Rao A, Wetten S, Gibson RA, Borrie M, Guzman D, et al. Anatomically-distinct genetic associations of APOE epsilon 4 allele load with regional cortical atrophy in Alzheimer's disease. *Neuroimage*. 2009; 44(3): 724–8. doi: 10.1016/j.neuroimage.2008.10.003.
111. Anstey KJ, von Sanden C, Salim A, O'Kearney R. Smoking as a risk factor for dementia and cognitive decline: a meta-analysis of prospective studies. *American Journal of Epidemiology*. 2007; 166(4): 367–78.
112. Peters R, Peters J, Warner J, Beckett N, Bulpitt C. Alcohol, dementia and cognitive decline in the elderly: a systematic review. *Age and Ageing*, 2008; 37(5), 505–12.
113. Morris MC. The role of nutrition in Alzheimer's disease: epidemiological evidence. *European Journal of Neurology*. 2009; 16(s1): 1–7.
114. Hamer M, Chida Y. Physical activity and risk of neurodegenerative disease: a systematic review of prospective evidence. *Psychological Medicine*. 2009; 39(1): 3–11.
115. Mendez MF, Paholpak P, Lin A, Zhang JY, Teng E. Prevalence of traumatic brain injury in early versus late-onset Alzheimer's disease. *Journal of Alzheimer's Disease*. 2015; 47(4): 985–93.
116. Miller ZA, Rosenberg LM, Stephens M, Mandelli ML, Rabinovici GD, Miller BL, et al. Learning disability status within the posterior cortical atrophy syndrome. *Alzheimer's & Dementia: the journal of the Alzheimer's Association*. 2015; 11(7): 245.
117. Shakespeare TJ, Crutch SJ, Fox NC. Posterior cortical atrophy: advice for diagnosis and implications for management. Neurodegenerative Disease Management, 2012; 2(6): 599–607.
118. Kim E, Lee Y, Lee J, Han SH. A case with cholinesterase inhibitor responsive asymmetric posterior cortical atrophy. *Clinical Neurology and Neurosurgery*. 2005; 108(1): 97–101.

16

Epidemiology of essential tremor

Elan D Louis

Introduction

Essential tremor (ET) is a chronic, progressive neurological disease. The motor feature that is the hallmark of the disease is a 4–12 Hz kinetic tremor that begins in the arms (Fig. 16.1) and may spread to additional body areas, particularly cranial regions (i.e. the neck, voice, jaw).[1–3] Additional motor features (gait ataxia)[4] as well as non-motor features (cognitive, psychiatric, sensory)[5] characterize the disease, although are not universal. ET is the most common tremor disorder and is also among the most prevalent neurological diseases.[6] The pathophysiology of ET is poorly understood, although it shares numerous key features with neurodegenerative disorders.[7–9] As with other progressive neurological diseases of later life (e.g. MND, PD), ET may represent a family of related diseases rather than a single disease entity.[10] The treatment options for ET are limited, with few available medications and limited efficacy of these.[11,12]

The epidemiology of ET is important for several reasons. First, it involves the study of the primary causes (i.e. aetiologies) of the disease, and this study will, it is hoped, lead to measures to prevent the disease. Second, the distribution of the disease within and across populations provides clues about underlying disease processes (i.e. pathophysiology). This chapter serves as a detailed review of the epidemiology of ET.

Case Definition and Additional Methodological Considerations

A primary issue that needs to be addressed when examining the epidemiology of a disorder is that of case definition. How does one define a case? Case definition in ET is problematic for a variety of reasons (Box 16.1). The first is that the clinical manifestations of the disease are relatively restricted. Despite the presence of a range of different types of tremor (rest, postural, kinetic, intentional),[1,2,13–15] additional motor features (gait ataxia, subclinical eye motion abnormalities),[4,16,17] and non-motor features,[5] kinetic tremor remains the predominant and hallmark feature.[13] This contrasts with PD, which is characterized by four hallmark features (tremor at rest, bradykinesia, rigidity, and postural and gait difficulty). Second, the hallmark clinical feature of ET, kinetic tremor, may be a feature of a myriad of disorders of both the central and peripheral nervous system;[1] thus, kinetic tremor is not specific to ET. Third, mild kinetic tremor of the arms is seen to some extent as a normal physical finding within the population and particularly in the elderly,[18,19] among whom ET is also the most prevalent.[6] Fourth, at present there remains no diagnostic test (serological, imaging, physiological, or pathological) to validate a clinical diagnosis of ET. Fifth, attempts at case definition in ET have been heavily influenced by the ascertainment of the cases. Thus, consensus definitions, while potentially useful because they reflect the opinions and experience of leaders in the field, have generally fallen short in ET because they have not been designed from an epidemiological perspective but rather from the perspective of the neurology clinic. While it is important to consider PD and dystonia in the exclusionary criteria, as one often does in clinic settings, from the population perspective, these are rare diseases and enhanced physiological tremor is far more common.[18,19] It is important for diagnostic criteria to attempt to exclude individuals with normal (enhanced physiological) tremor. This means that the criteria should specify in detail the extent of tremor that must be present to qualify for a diagnosis of ET. Present consensus criteria generally note that bilateral action tremor must be present, but do not specify the extent of tremor that must be present.[20,21] This is problematic for population-based studies because the prevalence of mild kinetic tremor is high in the normal population.

There are several additional methodological considerations that influence the study of the epidemiology of ET. First, tremor in ET may be mild, particularly when observed in cases which were ascertained from the population rather than from treatment settings. As a result, the prevalence of asymptomatic ET is high.[22] Because of this, screening questionnaires for ET generally lack sensitivity,[23] particularly among the many mild cases. Second, because the large majority of ET cases do not seek treatment,[24–26] clinic-based series of ET cases reflect a small proportion of ET cases whose selection is prone to bias resulting, for example, in increased ascertainment of both familial and young onset forms of the disease.[27,28] Therefore, one must carefully distinguish population-based from clinic-based studies of ET. Finally, cognitive deficits are more prevalent in ET cases than controls;[5] hence, the validity of self-reported information must take this into account.

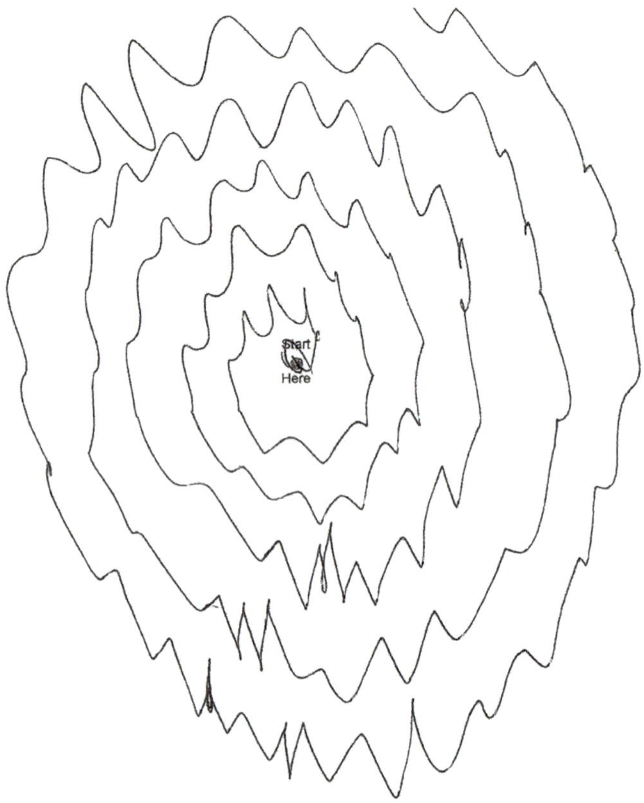

Fig. 16.1 The motor feature that is the hallmark of ET is kinetic tremor. This patient has attempted to draw an Archimedes spiral, and kinetic tremor is evident.

Descriptive Epidemiology

Incidence

There are only two published studies of the incidence of ET.[29,30] The first of these was a retrospective medical record review that utilized the records linkage system of the Rochester Epidemiology Project.[29] The records linkage system was designed to capture all health encounters of individuals living in Olmstead County, Minnesota. However, an entry into the medical record for ET-related tremor would have required, in all likelihood, that the issue be problematic enough to be recognized by the patient and then brought to medical attention, and further, be deemed important enough by the treating general medical doctor to necessitate a medical entry. Hence, individuals with mild tremor or individuals with other more pressing medical issues are not likely to have been entered, resulting in low estimates of disease prevalence and incidence. Indeed, the estimated prevalence of ET in that same study was very low (0.3%).[29] The authors reported an age-and sex-adjusted incidence of 23.7 per 100,000 US white population. This did not differ in men and women.

Box 16.1 Case definition in essential tremor: problematic areas

1. The clinical manifestations of ET are relatively restricted
2. The hallmark clinical feature of ET, kinetic tremor, may be a feature of a myriad of neurological disorders
3. Mild kinetic tremor of the arms is seen to some extent as a normal physical finding in the population
4. There remains no diagnostic test (serological, imaging, physiological, or pathological) to validate a clinical diagnosis of ET
5. Attempts at case definition in ET have been heavily influenced by the methods used to ascertain cases

In the second incidence study,[30] the authors estimated the incidence of ET among persons age 65 and older in three populations in central Spain. Eighty-three incident ET cases were identified among 3942 individuals assessed. The adjusted annual incidence rate was 616 per 100,000. Of interest is that 64 (77.1%) of 83 incident ET cases had not been diagnosed before the study assessment (i.e. they had not come to medical attention), thereby demonstrating the importance of population-based ascertainment of cases. The incidence of ET was considerably higher than that reported previously. The authors concluded that the incidence of ET was higher than previously recognized because a large proportion of patients with ET may not seek medical attention.

Prevalence

Precise estimates of disease prevalence are important because they form the numerical basis for planned public health initiatives, provide key data on the background occurrence of disease for family studies, and offer clues about the existence of underlying biological factors of possible mechanistic importance. The most recent review of disease prevalence indicated that there were 28 population-based prevalence studies of ET.[6] These twenty-eight studies were from nineteen countries and five continents (ten in Asia, eight in Europe, five in North America, four in Africa, and one in South America). Crude prevalence estimates had a broad range, from 0.01 to 20.5%, representing a 2050-fold difference between the lowest and highest estimates.[6]

A number of factors may account for the large difference in prevalence estimates. The age structure of the population is important, as the prevalence of ET increases with age.[6] For example, in a prevalence study in Saudi Arabia,[31] the vast bulk (90.5%) of enrollees were ≤40 years old (vs only 1.5% of enrollees who were over age 60) and similarly, in New Guinea,[32] 66.9% were under age 30 (vs only 3.9% who were over age 60). Likewise, in Nigeria,[33] 71.5% were ≤30 years old, whereas only 6.0% were age ≥60 years. As a result, the crude prevalence (including all ages) in these countries was low, ranging from 0.01 to 0.4%.[6] By contrast, a prevalence study conducted in Italy[34] had an older age structure (15.1% were age ≥60), as did a study among the Parsi community of India (44% were age ≥50),[35] yielding crude prevalence estimates (among all ages) of 0.4 and 1.6% (median = 1.0%).[6]

Another issue is whether each study participant was examined or whether they were screened first and then examined based on a positive response to a screening questionnaire. As noted above, screening questionnaires for ET have only modest sensitivity (generally in the range of 60–70%),[23,30] particularly for previously-undiagnosed, population-dwelling cases with mild ET. While several prevalence studies screened participants, they also provided data on the sensitivity of the screening questionnaire,[6] thereby allowing the reader to calculate an estimated prevalence that approximated a situation in which all participants had been examined. Studies that either did this or that examined each participant, generally provided higher estimates of prevalence.[6] A related issue is that neurologists, especially those who specialize in movement disorders, are better at diagnosing ET and are therefore more likely to provide accurate estimates of the prevalence of ET than general practitioners or non-physicians. Indeed, the proper diagnosis of ET can be challenging, with studies showing that 30–50% of 'ET' cases do not have ET, but rather, have other diagnoses.[36,37]

A final issue that could account for large difference in prevalence estimates is that of case definition. A sizable number of prevalence studies did not define the entity that was being studied (i.e. ET),[6] and this could have resulted in disparities in prevalence estimates. Furthermore, the large majority of studies used definitions that either did not specify the nature of the neurological examination that was performed on participants or the minimum severity of tremor that was required for a participant to qualify for a diagnosis of ET, and this likely further added to disparities in prevalence estimates.[6]

As discussed in the most recent review of disease prevalence, if one restricts prevalence studies of ET to those that were population-based, that provided complete data on all age groups, and that either examined each participant or provided data on the sensitivity of their screening questionnaire, then the crude prevalence of ET (across all ages) = 0.4%, and the crude prevalence range among persons aged 60–65 and older = 2.3–14.3% (median value = 6.3%).[6] In the most recent review of disease prevalence,[6] a meta-analysis of the 28 population-based prevalence studies was performed, using data from 2067 ET cases among a total of 462,746 participants screened. In that analysis, the estimated prevalence of ET (all ages) was 0.9% and, in a meta-analysis restricted to studies that provided data on cases aged ≥65 years, the estimated prevalence in that age group was 4.6%.[6]

Aside from age, other factors could influence prevalence. More than one-third of the 28 population-based prevalence studies showed a gender difference, with most of these demonstrating a higher prevalence of ET among men.[6] However, over all, the crude male prevalence: crude female prevalence = 1.08:1, indicating that gender is not a strong predictor of prevalence.[6]

Ethnic differences in the prevalence of ET, if present, might reflect differences in the prevalence of susceptibility genotypes; however, such differences could also reflect differences in exposure to environmental factors that have been associated with ET.[38] Although there may be ethnic differences in the prevalence of ET, as discussed below, there is a need for more data. Several studies have made direct comparisons between racial and/or ethnic groups. A population-based study in New Guinea reported differences in the prevalence of ET among populations that were defined by different languages, with a high prevalence in villagers living in the Bena Bena and Kamano populations vs a complete absence of ET cases among the Gimi or Yagaria.[32] Tan and colleagues[39] estimated the prevalence of ET in a community-based study in Singapore, comparing three ethnic groups: Singaporean Chinese, Malays, and Indians. The prevalence of ET was marginally higher in Indians than Chinese, and no Malays with ET were identified. A study in Copiah County, Mississippi, reported a non-significant trend for ET to be higher among whites than African-Americans, although the study relied on an initial screening questionnaire, and this could have biased results toward lower prevalence among less educated participants.[6,40] In a similar fashion, an initial study in northern Manhattan, New York, reported a non-significant trend toward higher prevalence in whites than African-Americans; however, that study also relied on an initial screening questionnaire.[6,41] By contrast, a later study of a different sample derived from the same population, which did not rely on a screening questionnaire, reported a significant ethnic difference in the prevalence of ET, with the prevalence among whites being the lowest.[42] Clearly, more data are needed.

To investigate this issue further, one may also examine data from studies that sampled different ethnic groups in the same country. For example, a study in the Basque region of Spain[43] reported a prevalence estimate that was similar to that in Madrid.[44] By contrast, a study of the Parsi community in Bombay, India,[35] reported a higher prevalence than a study largely of Hindus in West Bengal.[45] A major problem with these types of cross-study comparisons is that differences in study design (e.g. differences in the screening tool used or disparities in the definition of ET) could easily could account for any observed differences.

One may also compare studies that sampled different populations and ethnic groups while using similar or identical study protocols. For example, population-based studies in Turkey, Arabs in Israel, and Basques in Spain did not rely on screening questionnaires and all used the same examination and a similar definition of ET. The crude prevalence of ET was 0.8% (age ≥65 in Arabs in Israel),[46] 6.3% (age ≥60 years in Turkey),[47] 6.5% (age ≥61 years in Turkey),[48] and 6.4% (age ≥65 Basques in Spain),[43] suggesting that there may be regional and possibly ethnic differences in the prevalence of ET.[6] Here, as well, more data are needed.

Risk Factors

General

Age is a clear risk factor for ET. In the incidence study in Rochester, Minnesota, there was a clear age-associated increase in the incidence of ET, with the most dramatic rise beginning to occur in those who were entering their 50s.[29] The population-based study of the incidence of ET in Spain enrolled study subjects who were aged 65 and older; hence, the age-distribution was narrower than that of the prior study in Minnesota. In Spain, the incidence of ET increased in each age stratum (i.e. 568/100,000 (65–69 years), 583/100,000 (70–74 years), 754/100,000 (75–79 years), 810/100,000 (80–84 years)), until the oldest old, in which the sample size dropped off.[30] Prevalence studies have consistently shown a similar rise in the prevalence of ET with advancing age.[6]

Besides age, ethnicity may be a risk factor for ET, as reviewed above, although the data are mixed and additional data are needed. Finally, a family history of ET is a risk factor for ET, as the disease is in many cases familial.[49] These data will be reviewed below.

Environmental risk factors

While a family history of ET is a risk factor for ET, the aetiology of ET is not entirely genetic. In fact, in most series, the majority (>50%) of ET cases have not reported affected relatives,[50] and despite the high prevalence of the disease, families that are informative for genetic linkage studies have been difficult to locate. The existence of intra-familial differences in age of onset and severity of tremor,[24,49] also suggests that environmental factors may serve as modifiers of an underlying susceptibility genotype. Therefore, the environmental epidemiology of ET is an important area of study.

In terms of possible toxic causes of ET, the β-carboline alkaloids have been investigated extensively.[38] These are a group of naturally occurring chemicals that include harmane, harmine, harmaline, and others.[38,51] They are structurally similar to the neurotoxin 1-methyl-4-phenyl-1,2,3,6-tetrahydropyridine (MPTP), which forms the basis for one of the main toxin-induced animal models for PD.[52] Similar to MPTP, β-carboline alkaloids are very neurotoxic and administration of β-carboline alkaloids to a wide variety of laboratory animals produces an action tremor resembling that seen in patients with ET.[38,53] Humans exposed to intravenously administered harmine also develop an acute, coarse tremor.[38] While β-carboline alkaloids are produced endogenously,[54] one study estimated that dietary sources were 50 times greater than endogenous sources,[38,55] Harmane (1-methyl-9H-pyrido[3,4-b]indole) is particularly abundant in the human diet. Harmane and other β-carboline alkaloids are found in particularly high nanogram/gram concentrations in muscle foods (beef, chicken) and cooking leads furthermore to increased concentrations.[38] Indeed, the formation of β-carboline alkaloids in cooked meat is a function of both cooking temperature and time.[38] In addition to their high concentration in meat, β-carboline alkaloids are also present in plant-derived foods/substances, including coffee, ethanol, and tobacco.[38] In 2002, Louis et al.[56] demonstrated that blood harmane concentration was elevated in 100 ET patients in New York compared to 100 matched control subjects (median blood harmane: 5.21 g^{-10}/ml in cases vs 2.28 g^{-10}/ml in controls, $p = 0.005$). A larger replicate sample of 150 ET cases and 135 matched controls was published in 2008; while overall concentrations were lower in the replicate sample, the case-control difference persisted (median blood harmane: 2.61 g^{-10}/ml in cases vs 1.82 g^{-10}/ml in controls, $p = 0.016$).[57] A study of ET cases in Spain in 2013 similarly demonstrated elevated blood harmane concentrations in ET cases compared to controls.[58] A study of brain levels in that same year demonstrated elevated harmane concentrations in ET cases, and particularly among those with familial ET.[59] The links between this toxin and ET are of growing interest. Now, additional studies are needed to demonstrate that the exposure precedes the disease.

Human beings may be exposed to both organic and inorganic forms of lead through occupational and non-occupational sources.[38] In both laboratory animals and human beings, lead exposure may produce an acute or chronic progressive disorder in which action tremor is a prominent feature.[38,60] There is preliminary evidence that there may be an association between lead exposure and ET. In an initial study at a tertiary referral centre in New York,[61] blood lead concentrations were measured in 100 ET cases and 143 matched controls. Although in absolute terms, blood lead concentrations were low, these concentrations were higher in ET than in controls (median: 2.7 vs 2.3 mg/dl; $p = 0.038$). Blood lead concentration was later evaluated in another study at a hospital in Turkey[62] and the median blood lead concentration was 2.7 mg/dl in 105 ET cases vs 1.5 mg/dl in 105 controls ($p < 0.001$). The possible association of lead exposure with ET is intriguing, yet it needs to be further explored with additional replicate samples, preferably from population-based studies.[38] Furthermore, bone lead concentration, which is a more valid measure of chronic lead exposure than blood lead concentration, needs to be assessed in ET cases and controls.[38]

Patients with ET may use ethanol to temporarily lessen the amplitude of their tremor.[38] The generally accepted causal pathway is that having ET could lead to increased consumption of ethanol. Ethanol is also a known cerebellar toxin, resulting in marked loss of Purkinje cells.[38] Given the emerging links between ET and cerebellar pathology (especially, Purkinje cell),[63] this raises the question as to whether ethanol consumption might be associated with increased risk of incident ET, earlier age of onset of incident ET, or more rapid rate of progression of prevalent ET. In one study, lifetime ethanol consumption was assessed in a prospective, population-based study in central Spain of 3285 elderly participants, 76 of whom developed incident ET by follow-up. In an adjusted model, the baseline number of drink-years was marginally associated with a higher risk of incident ET (relative risk, $RR = 1.003$, $p = 0.059$). In an adjusted Cox model, the highest baseline drink-year quartile doubled the risk of incident ET ($RR = 2.29$, $p = 0.018$), while other quartiles were associated with more modest elevations in risk (RR in 3rd quartile = 1.82, $p = 0.10$; RR in 2nd quartile = 1.75, $p = 0.10$; RR in 1st quartile = 1.43, $p = 0.34$ vs non-drinkers $RR = 1.00$). With each higher drink-year quartile, the risk of incident ET increased an average of 23% ($p = 0.01$, test for trend).[64]

Numerous studies have demonstrated an association between cigarette smoking and lower risk of PD.[38,65] Three studies have examined smoking habits in ET cases compared to controls.[38,66–68] In the first,[66] the proportion of ET patients and controls who smoked was similar, yet the number of cigarette pack years was marginally lower in cases. The second was a population-based study in Madrid.[67] Ever smokers were approximately one half as likely to have prevalent ET when compared with never smokers ($OR = 0.58$, $p = 0.004$).[67] In the same cohort, the association between baseline smoking and incident ET was also examined.[68] Baseline pack years were lower in incident ET cases than controls ($p = 0.002$). Those in the highest baseline pack year tertile were one-third as likely to develop incident ET when compared to non-smokers (adjusted $RR = 0.29$, $p = 0.03$). Additional prospective studies are needed to further explore the possible protective effects of smoking on risk of ET.

Higher adherence to the Mediterranean diet (MeDi) has been related to degenerative disease and, with that in mind, adherence to the MeDi was calculated from a food frequency questionnaire administered in a case-control study of environmental epidemiology of ET in the New York Tri-State area.[69] In a study, 148 ET cases adhered less to MeDi than 250 controls ($p = 0.03$) and higher adherence to MeDi was associated with lower odds for ET ($OR = 0.78$, $p = 0.042$). This association has yet to be reproduced and the mechanisms that underlie this putative association merit further study.[69]

Using a similar rationale, that non-steroidal anti-inflammatory drugs (NSAIDs) have been shown to be inversely related to PD and AD, both of which may share common mechanisms with ET, investigators compared 92 ET cases to 107 controls (~1:1 matching) in terms of self-reported NSAID (especially ibuprofen) and aspirin use.[70] The proportion of NSAID or aspirin users (current or past) was similar in ET cases and controls (for current user, $p = 0.66$; for past user, $p = 0.90$).[70] Among users, however, the total dosage of ibuprofen was higher in controls than ET cases ($p = 0.04$). ET cases and controls did not differ with respect to aspirin use in the previous year. The data raise the possibility that ibuprofen use could have a potential protective role in ET.[70]

Head trauma has been associated with neurodegenerative disorders and, for this reason, was assessed in ET. History of head trauma was assessed in 274 ET cases and 3201 controls in a population-based study in central Spain. Thirty-two (11.7%) of 274 ET cases vs 260 (8.1%) of 3201 controls reported a history of serious head trauma (p = 0.04). In an adjusted model, participants who reported serious head trauma were 52% more likely to have ET (OR 1.52, p = 0.04). The data suggest that serious head trauma is associated with increased odds of ET. Additional studies are needed to reproduce this novel finding.[71]

Genetic risk factors in population-based studies

Both genetic and environmental factors are likely contributors to the aetiology of ET. In terms of the former, many large kindreds demonstrate an autosomal dominant pattern of inheritance.[3] In a population-based familial aggregation study, first-degree relatives of ET cases were nearly five times more likely to develop ET than were members of the general population, and ten times more likely if the proband's tremor began at an early age.[49] The two twin studies revealed a concordance for ET of approximately 60% in monozygotic twins, which was in excess of that seen in dizygotic twins.[72,73] The search for ET genes is ongoing and intensive.[74] Most of this work was not conducted in population-based studies, although there are exceptions. Thus, a genome-wide single nucleotide polymorphism (SNP) association study of ET in an Icelandic population identified an association with a marker in the LINGO1 (Leucine rich repeat and Ig domain containing 1) gene.[75] Since the initial report, numerous studies have replicated the association in independent ET case-control samples worldwide. Collectively, the data suggest that the *LINGO1* SNP rs9652490 confers modest risk for ET, with ORs in the range of 1.2–1.7, across different studies, making this the most robust genetic finding in ET to date. The leucine-rich repeat protein family plays important roles in a number of cellular processes, including neurodevelopment (e.g. neuronal differentiation and growth)[76] and in brain homeostatic processes such as cell migration and regeneration and in the regulation of axon guidance and branching.[77–79] The latter is of particular interest because recent controlled post-mortem studies have catalogued an array of changes in the cerebellar cortex, primarily involving the Purkinje cell and surrounding neuronal populations (e.g. basket cells), in the majority of ET cases.[63,80,81] Many of these changes involve what are thought to be primary alterations in Purkinje cell axonal architecture (e.g. increased torpedo formation) as well as secondary remodelling of both the Purkinje cell axonal processes (e.g. increased recurrent collateral formation, axonal branching, and terminal axonal sprouting) and the basket cell axonal processes (i.e. hypertrophy of basket cell axonal processes, which form an abnormal 'pinceau' structure around the Purkinje cell axon initial segment).[63,80,82,83]

Prognosis and Mortality

Prognosis

ET is generally viewed as a progressive disorder; as such, the prognosis is that the tremor will worsen over time. Despite this, there are few longitudinal data in patients with ET. In a study of 45 ET patients who were followed by a physician at Mayo Clinic, Jacksonville, Florida, for at least five years, the Tremor Rating Scale total score increased an average of two points per year during the observed study period, which represented an approximate 12% annual change.[84] One important caveat is that the study was clinic-based. Patients who elect to return for follow-up clinical visits are a self-selected group who often have tremor that is progressively worsening; patients with stable tremor are less inclined to return. Hence the study was likely to have overestimated the rate of decline in ET. In another research study in New York, investigators collected prospective, longitudinal data on tremor severity in 83 ET cases.[85] Unlike the other study, cases were not self-selected for follow-up based on a need for clinical care, as ascertainment was part of a research study. In that study, the median annual increase in tremor scores from baseline was 1.8–2.0%.[85] In another study, 44 ET patients were followed prospectively over a four-year period.[86] Accelerometry and surface electromyography were used to measure hand tremor every two years. The tremor amplitude increased 29% over the four-year period (approximately 7% per year).[86] That study also was clinic-based, like the one in Jacksonville.

Aside from an increase in the severity of arm tremor in ET with time, there is a tendency for the complexity of tremor to increase over time, both in terms of the spread of tremor to also involve cranial structures (e.g. head),[87] in terms of the directionality of the tremor (e.g. head tremor tends to become more multi-rather than uni-axial),[88] and in terms of the tendency to develop multiple types of tremor (e.g. rest tremor, intention tremor).[15,89]

Additional prognostic information can be gleaned from other sources. In a cross-sectional, clinical-epidemiological study at Columbia-University Medical Center, 335 ET patients with disease durations rating from 1–81 years underwent a single evaluation that included self-reported measures of tremor-related disability, performance-based measures of function, and neurologist-assessments of tremor type, location, and severity.[90] These cross-sectional data were used to produce clinical snapshots of the disease at each ten-year duration interval (i.e. <10, 10–19, 20–29, 30–39, ≥40 years). A variety of metrics of tremor severity increased across the ten-year time intervals.[90] By ≥40 years duration, one-third of patients had tremor in at least two cranial locations (neck, voice, jaw), and the proportion with high-amplitude tremor reached 20.3% (while drawing spirals), 33.8% (while drinking), and 60.8% (while using a spoon). Yet even in the longest tremor duration group, very few (<10%) were incapacitated (i.e. completely unable to perform the above-mentioned tasks), and one-third continued to exhibit no cranial tremor.[90] The data in the study paint a picture of progressive decade-by-decade decline in ET. Despite this, patients with long disease duration did not relentlessly converge upon the same end-stage of severe, functionally incapacitating, diffuse tremor.[90]

Finally, an important prognostic item in ET is that the disease increases the risk of developing both PD and AD. Thus, in a prospective, population-based study in central Spain, a cohort of 3813 older people were followed for a median of 3.3 years. Six (3.0%) of 201 ET cases developed incident PD versus 24 (0.7%) of 3574 controls (adjusted RR = 4.27, p = 0.002).[91] Furthermore, in prospective, population-based studies in both New York and Spain, the risk of incident dementia was 1.5–2.0 times higher in ET cases than age-matched controls.[92,93]

Mortality

Although it is often stated that mortality in ET cases and age-matched control subjects is similar, the data to support this statement are weak and this is an area of research that requires additional attention.

Several early investigators proposed that ET promotes longevity. In the early 1900s,[94] Minor promoted the idea of 'status macrobioticus multiparus', which was characterized by tremor, longevity, and fecundity in individuals with tremor and their relatives. He observed a disproportionately large number of elder persons in tremor families as compared to the general population of France. One in every 14.5 of his ET cases was ≥80 years old, compared to one in every 116 people in the general population of France according to 1876 census data. Three (0.4%) of the 683 relatives of his ET cases were 100 years of age or older, while the total number of citizens of this age in France was only 150 out of 40 million (0.0004%). Jankovic et. al.[95] examined data on parents of ET cases. The parents who were reported to have had tremor lived a median of eight years longer than did parents who did not have tremor. While one interpretation is that tremor confers a longevity factor, a more likely explanation, acknowledged by the authors, is that the risk of ET increases markedly with age, and older relatives are more likely to manifest tremor than are younger relatives. In other words, living to an older age may increase the likelihood of developing ET, rather than the reverse.

Others have published data that suggests that ET does not alter life span. In a retrospective study in Rochester, Minnesota, 266 ET patients were selected and their medical records abstracted.[29] The authors used a group of historical control subjects for comparison (i.e. persons of similar age and sex from the West North Central region of the USA). They found that survival after diagnosis of ET was comparable to that of the historical controls. Aside from the use of a historical control group as well as the retrospective study design, the study was problematic for other reasons. For example, participants were quite young (mean age at inception was 58 years and the mean length of follow-up was 9.7 years), suggesting that some of the cases may not have been followed into advanced age, when risk of mortality is likely to be higher.

Given the observation that ET shares numerous features with neurodegenerative disorders and that it may be a neurodegenerative disease itself,[7–9] conceptually, one would think it could shorten life span. Two studies are relevant here. First, a prospective, longitudinal, population-based design was used to compare the risk of mortality in participants with ET vs controls in three communities in central Spain.[96] The mean baseline age was 73.5 years. There were 33 (16.4%) deaths among 201 ET cases and 465 (13.9%) among 3337 controls. In an unadjusted Cox model, risk of mortality was increased in ET (RR = 1.59, p = 0.01).[96] In a Cox model that adjusted for a number of potential confounding factors (baseline age, gender, educational category, current ethanol drinking, use of antidepressant medication, and community), the risk of mortality remained increased in ET (RR = 1.45, p = 0.04).[96] In a longitudinal study of ageing in Danish twins, spirals were obtained on small subsample of 276 participants; higher spiral score was an independent risk factor for mortality.[97] Spiral scores of 0–2 were used as the reference. Mortality was increased in those with a spiral score of 3 (hazard ratio, HR = 1.23, p <0.01), further increased in those with a spiral score of 4 (HR = 1.51, p <0.01), and even further increased in those with a spiral score of 5–7 (HR = 1.83, p <0.01).

The data to date suggest that ET is associated with a modest but significant increased risk of mortality. Clearly, further study is needed.

Future Directions

ET remains one of the most prevalent neurological diseases.[6] Despite this, the treatment options for ET remain limited, with few medications and limited efficacy of those that are used.[11,12] The identification of environmental risk factors for ET is important as this will lead the way to interventional steps that could modify the risk of developing ET. The identification of susceptibility genes, and particularly those that operate on a population-level, is an important step in terms of understanding the broad biological basis for ET. Indeed, this is the first step in developing therapies that target specific biological events. For these reasons, work in the areas of analytical epidemiology, environmental epidemiology, and genetic epidemiology is particularly important.

REFERENCES

1. Louis ED. Clinical practice. Essential tremor. N Engl J Med. 2001; 345(12): 887–91.
2. Critchley M. Observations of essential (heredofamilial) tremor. Brain. 1949; 72(2): 113–39.
3. Bain PG, Findley LJ, Thompson PD, Gresty MA, Rothwell JC, Harding AE, et al. A study of hereditary essential tremor. Brain. 1994; 117 (4): 805–24.
4. Louis ED, Rao AK. Functional aspects of gait in essential tremor: a comparison with age-matched Parkinson's disease cases, dystonia cases, and controls. Tremor Other Hyperkinet Mov (NY). 2015; 5. doi: 10.7916/D8B27T7J.
5. Louis ED. Non-motor symptoms in essential tremor: A review of the current data and state of the field. Parkinsonism Relat Disord. 2016; 22(Suppl 1): S115–8.
6. Louis ED, Ferreira JJ. How common is the most common adult movement disorder? Update on the worldwide prevalence of essential tremor. Mov Disord. 2010; 25(5): 534–41.
7. Louis ED. Essential tremor: a common disorder of Purkinje neurons? *Neuroscientist*. 2016; 22(2): 108–18.
8. Bonuccelli U. Essential tremor is a neurodegenerative disease. J Neural Transm. 2012; 119(11): 1383–7.
9. Benito-Leon J. Essential tremor: a neurodegenerative disease? Tremor Other Hyperkinet Mov (NY). 2014; 4: 252.
10. Louis ED. 'Essential tremor' or 'the essential tremors': is this one disease or a family of diseases? Neuroepidemiology. 2014; 42(2): 81–9.
11. Diaz NL, Louis ED. Survey of medication usage patterns among essential tremor patients: movement disorder specialists vs general neurologists. Parkinsonism Relat Disord. 2010; 16(9): 604–7.
12. Louis ED, Rios E, Henchcliffe C. How are we doing with the treatment of essential tremor (ET)?: Persistence of patients with ET on medication: data from 528 patients in three settings. Eur J Neurol. 2010; 17(6): 882–4.
13. Louis ED. The primary type of tremor in essential tremor is kinetic rather than postural: cross-sectional observation

of tremor phenomenology in 369 cases. Eur J Neurol. 2013; 20(4): 725–7.
14. Louis ED, Hernandez N, Michalec M. Prevalence and correlates of rest tremor in essential tremor: cross-sectional survey of 831 patients across four distinct cohorts. Eur J Neurol. 2015; 22(6): 927–32.
15. Louis ED, Frucht SJ, Rios E. Intention tremor in essential tremor: prevalence and association with disease duration. Mov Disord. 2009; 24(4): 626–7.
16. Gitchel GT, Wetzel PA, Baron MS. Slowed saccades and increased square wave jerks in essential tremor. Tremor Other Hyperkinet Mov (NY). 2013; 3.
17. Kronenbuerger M, Konczak J, Ziegler W, et al. Balance and motor speech impairment in essential tremor. Cerebellum. 2009; 8(3): 389–98.
18. Louis ED, Ford B, Pullman S, Baron K. How normal is 'normal'? Mild tremor in a multiethnic cohort of normal subjects. Arch Neurol. 1998; 55(2): 222–7.
19. Louis ED, Wendt KJ, Ford B. Senile tremor. What is the prevalence and severity of tremor in older adults? Gerontology. 2000; 46(1): 12–6.
20. Bain P, Brin M, Deuschl G, et al. Criteria for the diagnosis of essential tremor. Neurology. 2000; 54: S7.
21. Deuschl G, Bain P, Brin M. Consensus statement of the Movement Disorder Society on Tremor. Ad Hoc Scientific Committee. Mov Disord. 1998; 13(Suppl 3): 2–23.
22. Louis ED, Ford B, Pullman SL. Prevalence of asymptomatic tremor in relatives of patients with essential tremor. Arch Neurol. 1997; 54(2): 197–200.
23. Louis ED, Ford B, Lee H, Andrews H. Does a screening questionnaire for essential tremor agree with the physician's examination? Neurology. 1998; 50(5): 1351–7.
24. Larsson T, Sjogren T. Essential tremor: a clinical and genetic population study. Acta Psychiatr Scand Suppl. 1960; 36(144): 1–176.
25. Rautakorpi I, Takala J, Marttila RJ, Sievers K, Rinne UK. Essential tremor in a Finnish population. Acta Neurol Scand. 1982; 66(1): 58–67.
26. Louis ED, Ottman R, Ford B, et al. The Washington Heights-Inwood Genetic Study of Essential Tremor: methodologic issues in essential-tremor research. Neuroepidemiology. 1997; 16(3): 124–33.
27. Louis ED, Barnes LF, Ford B, Ottman R. Family history information on essential tremor: potential biases related to the source of the cases. Mov Disord. 2001; 16(2): 320–4.
28. Louis ED, Ford B, Wendt KJ, Cameron G. Clinical characteristics of essential tremor: data from a community-based study. Mov Disord. 1998; 13(5): 803–8.
29. Rajput AH, Offord KP, Beard CM, Kurland LT. Essential tremor in Rochester, Minnesota: a 45-year study. J Neurol Neurosurg Psychiatry. 1984; 47(5): 466–70.
30. Benito-Leon J, Bermejo-Pareja F, Louis ED. Incidence of essential tremor in three elderly populations of central Spain. Neurology. 2005; 64(10): 1721–5.
31. al Rajeh S, Bademosi O, Ismail H, et al. A community survey of neurological disorders in Saudi Arabia: the Thugbah study. Neuroepidemiology. 1993; 12(3): 164–78.
32. Hornabrook RW, Nagurney JT. Essential tremor in Papua, New Guinea. Brain. 1976; 99(4): 659–72.
33. Osuntokun BO, Adeuja AO, Schoenberg BS, et al. Neurological disorders in Nigerian Africans: a community-based study. Acta Neurol Scand. 1987; 75(1): 13–21.
34. Salemi G, Savettieri G, Rocca WA, et al. Prevalence of essential tremor: a door-to-door survey in Terrasini, Sicily. Sicilian Neuro-Epidemiologic Study Group. Neurology. 1994; 44(1): 61–4.
35. Bharucha NE, Bharucha EP, Bharucha AE, Bhise AV, Schoenberg BS. Prevalence of essential tremor in the Parsi community of Bombay, India. Arch Neurol. 1988; 45(8): 907–8.
36. Schrag A, Muenchau A, Bhatia KP, Quinn NP, Marsden CD. Overdiagnosis of essential tremor. Lancet. 1999; 353(9163): 1498–9.
37. Jain S, Lo SE, Louis ED. Common misdiagnosis of a common neurological disorder: how are we misdiagnosing essential tremor? Arch Neurol. 2006; 63(8): 1100–4.
38. Louis ED. Environmental epidemiology of essential tremor. Neuroepidemiology. 2008; 31(3): 139–49.
39. Tan LC, Venketasubramanian N, Ramasamy V, Gao W, Saw SM. Prevalence of essential tremor in Singapore: a study on three races in an Asian country. Parkinsonism Relat Disord. 2005; 11(4): 233–9.
40. Haerer AF, Anderson DW, Schoenberg BS. Prevalence of essential tremor. Results from the Copiah County study. Arch Neurol. 1982; 39(12): 750–1.
41. Louis ED, Marder K, Cote L, et al. Differences in the prevalence of essential tremor among elderly African Americans, whites, and Hispanics in northern Manhattan, NY. Arch Neurol. 1995; 52(12): 1201–5.
42. Louis ED, Thawani SP, Andrews HF. Prevalence of essential tremor in a multiethnic, community-based study in northern Manhattan, New York, NY. Neuroepidemiology. 2009; 32(3): 208–14.
43. Bergareche A, De La Puente E, Lopez De Munain A, et al. Prevalence of essential tremor: a door-to-door survey in bidasoa, spain. Neuroepidemiology. 2001; 20(2): 125–8.
44. Benito-Leon J, Bermejo-Pareja F, Morales JM, Vega S, Molina JA. Prevalence of essential tremor in three elderly populations of central Spain. Mov Disord. 2003; 18(4): 389–94.
45. Das SK, Biswas A, Roy J, et al. Prevalence of major neurological disorders among geriatric population in the metropolitan city of Kolkata. J Assoc Physicians India. 2008; 56: 175–81.
46. Glik A, Masarwa M, Abuful A, et al. Essential tremor might be less frequent than Parkinson's disease in North Israel Arab villages. Mov Disord. 2009; 24(1): 119–22.
47. Dogu O, Sevim S, Camdeviren H, et al. Prevalence of essential tremor: door-to-door neurologic exams in Mersin Province, Turkey. Neurology. 2003; 61(12): 1804–6.
48. Sur H, Ilhan S, Erdogan H, et al. Prevalence of essential tremor: A door-to-door survey in Sile, Istanbul, Turkey. Parkinsonism Relat Disord. 2009; 15(2): 101–4.
49. Louis ED, Ford B, Frucht S, et al. Risk of tremor and impairment from tremor in relatives of patients with essential tremor: a community-based family study. Ann Neurol. 2001; 49(6): 761–9.
50. Louis ED. Etiology of essential tremor: should we be searching for environmental causes? Mov Disord. 2001; 16(5): 822–9.
51. Zetler G, Singbartl G, Schlosser L. Cerebral pharmacokinetics of tremor-producing harmala and iboga alkaloids. Pharmacology. 1972; 7(4): 237–48.
52. Langston JW, Langston EB, Irwin I. MPTP-induced parkinsonism in human and non-human primates—clinical and experimental aspects. Acta Neurol Scand Suppl. 1984; 100: 49–54.
53. Du W, Aloyo VJ, Harvey JA. Harmaline competitively inhibits [3H]MK-801 binding to the NMDA receptor in rabbit brain. Brain Res. 1997; 770(1–2): 26-9.

54. Gearhart DA, Collins MA, Lee JM, Neafsey EJ. Increased beta-carboline 9N-methyltransferase activity in the frontal cortex in Parkinson's disease. Neurobiol Dis. 2000; 7(3): 201–11.
55. Pfau W, Skog K. Exposure to beta-carbolines norharman and harman. J Chromatogr B Analyt Technol Biomed Life Sci. 2004; 802(1): 115–26.
56. Louis ED, Zheng W, Jurewicz EC, et al. Elevation of blood beta-carboline alkaloids in essential tremor. Neurology. 2002; 59(12): 1940–4.
57. Louis ED, Jiang W, Pellegrino KM, et al. Elevated blood harmane (1-methyl-9H-pyrido[3,4-b]indole) concentrations in essential tremor. Neurotoxicology. 2008; 29(2): 294–300.
58. Louis ED, Benito-Leon J, Moreno-Garcia S, et al. Blood harmane (1-methyl-9H-pyrido[3,4-b]indole) concentration in essential tremor cases in Spain. Neurotoxicology. 2013; 34: 264–8.
59. Louis ED, Factor-Litvak P, Liu X, et al. Elevated brain harmane (1-methyl-9H-pyrido[3,4-b]indole) in essential tremor cases vs controls. Neurotoxicology. 2013; 38: 131–5.
60. Coulehan JL, Hirsch W, Brillman J, et al. Gasoline sniffing and lead toxicity in Navajo adolescents. Pediatrics. 1983; 71(1): 113–17.
61. Louis ED, Jurewicz EC, Applegate L, et al. Association between essential tremor and blood lead concentration. Environ Health Perspect. 2003; 111(14): 1707–11.
62. Dogu O, Louis ED, Tamer L, et al. Elevated blood lead concentrations in essential tremor: a case-control study in Mersin, Turkey. Environ Health Perspect. 2007; 115(11): 1564–8.
63. Babij R, Lee M, Cortes E, et al. Purkinje cell axonal anatomy: quantifying morphometric changes in essential tremor versus control brains. Brain. 2013; 136: 3051–61.
64. Louis ED, Benito-Leon J, Bermejo-Pareja F. Population-based study of baseline ethanol consumption and risk of incident essential tremor. J Neurol Neurosurg Psychiatry. 2009; 80(5): 494–7.
65. Ritz B, Ascherio A, Checkoway H, et al. Pooled analysis of tobacco use and risk of Parkinson disease. Arch Neurol. 2007; 64(7): 990–7.
66. Jiménez-Jiménez FJ dT-HM, Alonso-Navarro H, et al. Environmental risk factors for essential tremor. Eur Neurol. 2007; 58(2): 106–13.
67. Benito-Leon J, Louis ED, Bermejo-Pareja F. Population-based case-control study of cigarette smoking and essential tremor. Mov Disord. 2008; 23(2): 246–52.
68. Louis ED, Benito-Leon J, Bermejo-Pareja F. Population-based prospective study of cigarette smoking and risk of incident essential tremor. Neurology. 2008; 70(19): 1682–7.
69. Scarmeas N, Louis ED. Mediterranean diet and essential tremor. A case-control study. Neuroepidemiology. 2007; 29(3–4): 170–7.
70. Pan J, Michalec M, Louis ED. Non-steroidal anti-inflammatory drug use and essential tremor. Neuroepidemiology. 2014; 43(2): 145–9.
71. Benito-Leon J, Louis ED, Labiano-Fontcuberta A, Bermejo-Pareja F. Serious head trauma preceding essential tremor: A population-based study (NEDICES). J Neurol Sci. 2015; 353(1–2): 116–21.
72. Tanner CM, Goldman SM, Lyons KE, et al. Essential tremor in twins: an assessment of genetic vs environmental determinants of etiology. Neurology. 2001; 57(8): 1389–91.
73. Lorenz D, Frederiksen H, Moises H, et al. High concordance for essential tremor in monozygotic twins of old age. Neurology. 2004; 62(2): 208–11.
74. Clark LN, Louis ED. Challenges in essential tremor genetics. Rev Neurol (Paris). 2015; 171(6–7): 466–74.
75. Stefansson H, Steinberg S, Petursson H, et al. Variant in the sequence of the LINGO1 gene confers risk of essential tremor. Nat Genet. 2009; 41(3): 277–9.
76. Halegoua S, Armstrong RC, Kremer NE. Dissecting the mode of action of a neuronal growth factor. Curr Top Microbiol Immunol. 1991; 165: 119–70.
77. Bormann P, Roth LW, Andel D, Ackermann M, Reinhard E. zfNLRR, a novel leucine-rich repeat protein is preferentially expressed during regeneration in zebrafish. Mol Cell Neurosci. 1999; 13(3): 167–79.
78. Brose K, Tessier-Lavigne M. Slit proteins: key regulators of axon guidance, axonal branching, and cell migration. Curr Opin Neurobiol. 2000; 10(1): 95–102.
79. Nguyen-Ba-Charvet KT, Chedotal A. Role of Slit proteins in the vertebrate brain. J Physiol Paris. 2002; 96(1–2): 91–8.
80. Louis ED, Faust PL, Vonsattel JP, et al. Neuropathological changes in essential tremor: 33 cases compared with 21 controls. Brain. 2007; 130(12): 3297–307.
81. Louis ED. Essential tremor: from bedside to bench and back to bedside. Curr Opin Neurol. 2014; 27(4): 461–7.
82. Kuo SH, Tang G, Louis ED, et al. Lingo-1 expression is increased in essential tremor cerebellum and is present in the basket cell pinceau. Acta Neuropathol. 2013; 125(6): 879–89.
83. Erickson-Davis CR, Faust PL, Vonsattel JP, et al. 'Hairy baskets' associated with degenerative Purkinje cell changes in essential tremor. J Neuropathol Exp Neurol. 2010; 69(3): 262–71.
84. Putzke JD, Whaley NR, Baba Y, Wszolek ZK, Uitti RJ. Essential tremor: predictors of disease progression in a clinical cohort. J Neurol Neurosurg Psychiatry. 2006; 77(11): 1235–7.
85. Louis ED, Agnew A, Gillman A, Gerbin M, Viner AS. Estimating annual rate of decline: prospective, longitudinal data on arm tremor severity in two groups of essential tremor cases. J Neurol Neurosurg Psychiatry. 2011; 82(7): 761–5.
86. Elble RJ, Higgins C, Hughes L. Longitudinal study of essential tremor. Neurology. 1992; 42(2): 441–3.
87. Louis ED. When do essential tremor patients develop head tremor? Influences of age and duration and evidence of a biological clock. Neuroepidemiology. 2013; 41(2): 110–15.
88. Robakis D, Louis ED. Head tremor in essential tremor: 'Yes-yes', 'no-no', or 'round and round'? Parkinsonism Relat Disord. 2016; 22: 98–101.
89. Cohen O, Pullman S, Jurewicz E, Watner D, Louis ED. Rest tremor in patients with essential tremor: prevalence, clinical correlates, and electrophysiologic characteristics. Arch Neurol. 2003; 60(3): 405–10.
90. Louis ED, Gerbin M, Galecki M. Essential tremor 10, 20, 30, 40: clinical snapshots of the disease by decade of duration. Eur J Neurol. 2013; 20(6): 949–54.
91. Benito-Leon J, Louis ED, Bermejo-Pareja F. Risk of incident Parkinson's disease and parkinsonism in essential tremor: a population based study. J Neurol Neurosurg Psychiatry. 2009; 80(4): 423–5.
92. Bermejo-Pareja F, Louis ED, Benito-Leon J. Risk of incident dementia in essential tremor: A population-based study. Mov Disord. 2007; 22(11): 1573–80.
93. Thawani SP, Schupf N, Louis ED. Essential tremor is associated with dementia: prospective population-based study in New York. Neurology. 2009; 73(8): 621–5.

94. Minor L. Neue Beobachtungen uber das erbliche Zittern. Russk Klin. 1929; 12: 713–25.
95. Jankovic J, Beach J, Schwartz K, Contant C. Tremor and longevity in relatives of patients with Parkinson's disease, essential tremor, and control subjects. Neurology. 1995; 45(4): 645–8.
96. Louis ED, Benito-Leon J, Ottman R, Bermejo-Pareja F. A population-based study of mortality in essential tremor. Neurology. 2007; 69(21): 1982–9.
97. Deuschl G, Petersen I, Lorenz D, Christensen K. Tremor in the elderly: Essential and aging-related tremor. Mov Disord. 2015; 30(10): 1327–34.

SECTION 3
Dementia as final common outcome

17

Detecting dementia early in populations

Amy R Borenstein

Introduction

Dementia is a syndrome characterized by loss of critical cognitive functions. As it progresses, social and occupational activities are increasingly limited. AD is the major subtype of dementia, and it is the most common and important diagnosis for public health. The incidence of clinical dementia increases after age 65 in a logarithmic fashion, doubling every five years.[1] There are currently approximately 36 million people in the world with dementia, most of it driven pathologically by AD, and this number is projected to increase to 115 million by 2050. Along with this increase in the number of affected people comes an ever-growing burden of the disease for individuals, families, healthcare systems, and society (https://www.ohchr.org/Documents/Issues/OlderPersons/Dementia/GAADReport.pdf).

Although the clinical disease of dementia occurs mostly in older ages, growing evidence suggests that the pathologic processes associated with it begin early with genetic risk, and that exposures encountered over the life course act cumulatively and interactively to result in this outcome.[1] Therefore, the presentation of dementia symptoms in older age should be regarded as the *result* of lifelong pathology, rather than the *beginning* of the disease process.[1] By the time dementia is clinically diagnosable, the pathologic process is likely irreversible.

Factors influencing the presentation of dementia

Important factors that play a role in the clinical presentation of AD include the pathologic disease substrate and load, the capacity of the brain to maintain function in the presence of this pathology (brain and cognitive reserve), as well as individual and group environmental and genetic characteristics and susceptibilities.

The Case for Multiple Pathologies

The relative contribution to dementia of individual pathologies and reserve will vary from person to person, as will the interactions between genetic and environmental risk factors, which can affect both pathologies and reserve. One important finding is that multiple pathologies are likely to coexist in older people. For example, in the Religious Orders Study and the Rush Memory and Aging Project in Chicago, of 179 individuals who came to autopsy at an average age of 87 and had 'probable AD' by NINCDS-ADRDA criteria,[2] 88% had only pathologic AD and 46% had mixed pathologies. Vascular infarcts accompanied Alzheimer neurodegeneration in 30% of the subjects, while 11% had AD with neocortical Lewy body disease, and 5% had all three pathologies.[3]

Vascular lesions are the most common co-pathology with AD lesions in the brains of older persons. The main question related to these lesions is the extent to which they influence cognition relative to AD pathology: do they additively lower cognition (i.e. add a second hit), or do the AD and vascular lesions combined result in more cognitive impairment than the two lesions alone? The Nun Study[4] was the first to report that, when combined with vascular infarcts, AD pathology was associated with a lower Mini-Mental Examination Score (3/30) than AD alone (15/30). Since the report in 1997, there have been several community autopsy samples[5–8] which have shown that a range of vascular lesions in the brain occur separately or in combination with AD pathology and other neurodegenerative lesions, including Lewy body pathology. Further, it is likely the combination and load of comorbid lesions that contribute to cognitive impairment and dementia.[6] In the Nun Study, the presence of vascular infarcts in the absence of AD pathology had little effect on cognition, with results similar to those with neither vascular nor AD pathology.[4] Similar findings demonstrating an additive model were later reported by the Religious Orders Study,[7] the Memory and Aging Project,[8] and the Adult Changes in Thought Study.[9] As non-AD pathologies increase in frequency in the oldest age groups, AD is less likely to cause clinical dementia by itself in the very old. Prevention of the most common non-AD pathology, vascular disease, would likely lead to a considerable decrease in the incidence of clinical dementia among people who fulfil neuropathologic criteria for AD (Fig. 17.1).

Determinants of Dementia over the Life Course

Although some have proposed that the beginning of AD occurs when biomarker changes become evident some 20–25 years before symptom onset,[10] it is likely that critical pathologic events are occurring behind the scenes decades earlier. For example, the accumulation of insoluble amyloid-ß (Aß) deposits (neuritic

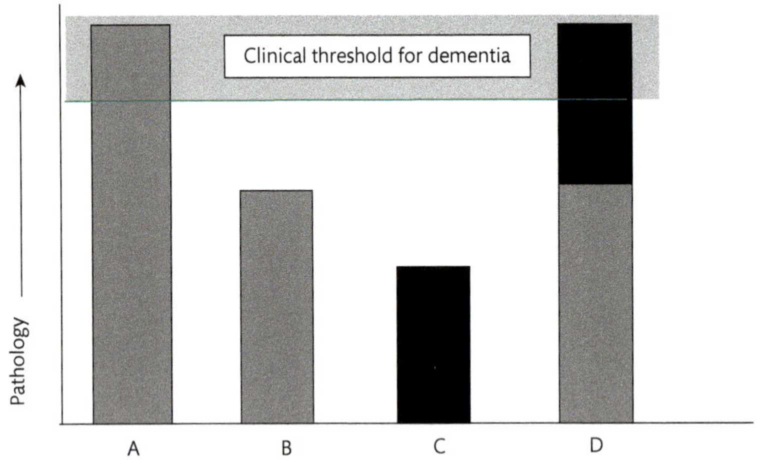

Fig. 17.1 Additive model for mixed neuropathologies in achieving the clinical threshold for dementia.

In Bar A, an individual has accumulated sufficient pathology to attain the clinical threshold for dementia and will therefore manifest symptoms. In Bar B, there is an accumulation of Alzheimer pathology or other pathology, but insufficient to meet the clinical threshold; thus, this individual will remain cognitively intact. In Bar C, there is some degree of vascular or other pathology, but again this individual will remain cognitively intact. In Bar D, the same amount of Alzheimer (or other) neuropathology is present as in Bar B, but there is mixed pathology, placing the individual over the clinical threshold for dementia.

plaques) and neurofibrillary tangles are seen as early as the second decade.[11] Other forms of beta amyloid, however, including soluble oligomers,[12,13] may be present over most of the life course and contribute to degeneration of synapses and neurons.[14]

The rate at which pathology accumulates in an individual is determined primarily by their genetic constitution. In less than 5% of AD cases, three major genetic variants cause a familial form of the disease (APP gene on chr 21) and PSEN genes (chr 1 and chr 14). The remainder are sporadic cases that are due to a complex set of genes, each contributing small effects. The exception is the apolipoprotein-ε4 allele, which raises the cumulative incidence of sporadic cases ranging from 18% to 38% at 70–75 years old, with estimates depending on the population, study setting (clinical vs community), and other methodologic factors such as differential loss of participants and definitions of exposure and outcome.[15]

Beside disease-modifying genes, age, sex, and race/ethnicity also influence the risk for developing dementia.[16] Additionally, exposures in gestation and early life, as well as environmental and socioeconomic conditions, predispositions to vascular diseases, depression and inflammation, diet, exercise, head injury, medications and other individual lifestyle activities, such as smoking and alcohol use, mental and social activities, play important roles in determining the onset of clinical disease.[1]

In addition, although there is a great deal of research ongoing on the concepts of brain[17,18] and cognitive reserve,[19] measures of reserve are rarely taken into account when determining risk for clinical onset of dementia/AD or how to detect the disease early. We know that pathology and reserve interact with one another, such that two individuals may have the same severity of pathology, but one may be demented, due to having exhausted a reserve capacity, while another with higher reserve capacity is able to substantially delay clinical onset of dementia, often remaining non-demented up to the time of their death.[1,20] This ability to mask signs of dementia is evident from studies of individuals who are positive for aggregated beta-amyloid on PET scans, yet retain apparent normal cognition, and from autopsy studies that show that approximately one-third of individuals with severe Alzheimer lesions remain non-demented during life.[1] The ability of such individuals to escape detection results in misclassification of the outcome and in the reduction of statistical power of longitudinal studies to identify risk factors for pathologies. Although education has commonly been used as a surrogate for reserve, it is but one component of this concept. Our ability to measure reserve accurately is critical to the success of both studies of risk factors for pathologies and clinical trials in which the amount of reserve can influence the power to assess agents aimed at modification of specific pathologies.

Genes and environmental exposures behave independently, cumulatively, and interactively to both increase or reduce pathology as well as to modify the brain's reserve capacity, and this trajectory is reflected in individual risk profiles across the life course (see Fig. 17.2).

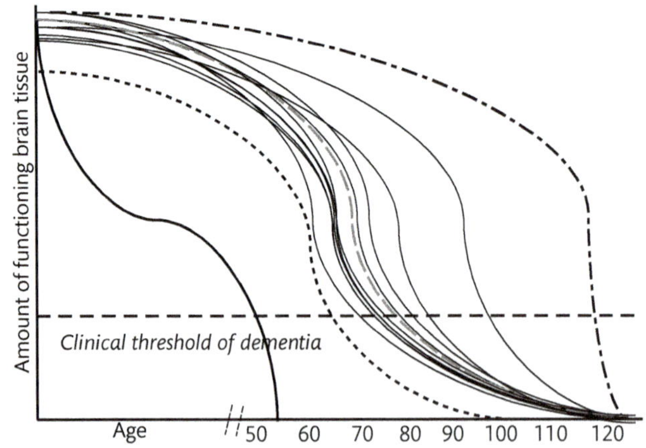

Fig. 17.2 Illustration of different trajectories toward cognitive impairment.

Legend. The solid bold line shows an individual with a familial mutation who will clinically express clinical dementia by age 50. Other curves show variable trajectories with different risk profiles, resulting in differences in clinical age of onset, The hatched line to the right shows an individual whose performance exceeds the threshold until very late in life and who can remain non-demented throughout their life span. Reproduced with permission from Borenstein A., and Mortimer J. *Alzheimer's Disease: Life Course Perspectives on Risk Reduction*. Academic Press; 2016. Copyright © 2016 Elsevier Inc. All rights reserved.

Phenotyping in clinical and epidemiologic research on dementia

The continuous trajectory of brain function has, for clinical purposes, been categorized into discrete stages. Over time, the stages have been increasingly refined to better reflect the continuum. Initially, the criteria for dementia and AD identified individuals after there was substantial loss in cognition and daily functioning. Most epidemiologic cohort studies that began in the 1990s or early 2000s have used dementia criteria developed by international guidelines in the Diagnostic and Statistical Manual[21–24] versions 3 and 4, or the International Classification of Diseases versions 9 and 10 (www.who.int/classifications/icd). Both of these guidelines emphasized memory loss and loss of independent ability to perform daily activities of living. In the newest version of this manual (DSM5), the term 'dementia' has been changed to 'Major Neurocognitive Disorder' (NCD), memory impairment has been de-emphasized, acknowledging that NCD may begin with a non-memory cognitive impairment. Guidelines give more focus on whether there has been a *decline* from a previous level in cognition that interferes with independence in everyday activities.

To diagnose probable or possible AD,[2] most epidemiologic cohort studies of dementia utilized the National Institute of Neurological and Communicative Disorders and Stroke (NINCDS) and the 1984 Alzheimer's Disease and Related Disorders Association (ADRDA) (NINCDS-ADRDA) criteria. Possible dementia was diagnosed if other co-existing morbidity was present that could explain some of the clinical presentation. The new criteria for AD, proposed in 2011,[25] take into account research showing that memory impairment may not be the primary cognitive deficit in all patients with AD, incorporate genetic information gained over the last three decades, and take the approach that the pathophysiology of AD does not differ by age or AD biomarkers. The three strata of AD defined by the new criteria are: (1) probable AD dementia; (2) possible AD dementia (as in the old criteria with modifications), and for research purposes only; (3) probable or possible AD dementia with evidence of the AD pathophysiological process (biomarkers of Aβ and neuronal injury), with no prioritization of one biomarker over another. The International Working Group-2 also proposed revision of AD diagnostic guidelines[26] that includes a clinical core of early and significant episodic memory loss, with supportive criteria including medial temporal lobe atrophy on structural MRI, abnormal CSF biomarkers, evidence of amyloid on PET or functional neuroimaging, or the presence of a proven autosomal dominant mutation in the immediate family. The use of biomarkers in the diagnosis of AD portends current proposals to move away from more clinical measures toward quantifiable biomarkers that can be measured in standardized ways.[27]

MCI was the first prodromal stage of AD dementia to be formally defined as a clinical entity. The original criteria defined a person without clinical dementia who had abnormal memory for their age, but normal (within 1.5 standard deviations) general cognitive function and no or very few impairments in activities of daily living.[28] In 2004, these criteria were broadened as it became apparent that subtypes of MCI could be defined (amnestic vs non-amnestic), and that these subtypes increased the risk for different dementia subtypes.[29]

In 2011, further refinements were also made to define symptoms in the phase prior to MCI, labelled the pre-clinical stage.[30] This first pre-clinical stage is biomarker evidence of β-amyloid accumulation on PET amyloid imaging or low A-β_{42} in cerebrospinal fluid (CSF) (amyloid positivity) with no detectable evidence of additional brain alterations that suggest neurodegeneration or subtle cognitive and/or behavioural symptoms. Stage 2 involves amyloid positivity *plus* evidence of synaptic dysfunction and/or early neurodegeneration (elevated CSF tau/phosphor-tau, hypometabolism as seen on FDG-PET, or cortical thinning or loss of grey matter in selected regions of interest, and/or hippocampal atrophy on volumetric MRI). Finally, stage 3 adds subtle cognitive decline to amyloid positivity and evidence of neurodegeneration.[1,31,32]

The use of these CSF and imaging biomarkers to diagnose AD will lead to more standardized, reproducible case definitions based on the presence of a pathology. However, currently, the move toward a more biomarker-based diagnosis raises important issues for epidemiologic studies. First, more methodologic work is needed before these biomarkers can be used for population-based research. The diagnostic characteristics of these proposed biologic and imaging biomarkers have not been evaluated as single or joint biomarkers in general clinical and community populations where there is a wide range of multiple brain pathologies and comorbid chronic disease. Additional methodologic work is needed in several core areas, including the extent to which pathologic levels of these biomarkers predict future functional impairments, the extent to which issues such as cognitive and brain reserve, as well as comorbidity, influence the biomarkers, and improved reliability and standardization of the measures. Further, it is not known how well the changes in these biomarkers reflect, or interact with, early changes in the continuum.

Since these measures can be costly and invasive, and need to be further validated if they are to be used in large population cohorts (as well as being used in clinical care and accepted by insurance companies), biomarker data are currently collected in subsets of cohorts, depending on the specific aim of the study. The 'representativeness' of these subsamples to the total cohort will depend on whether they differ in important ways related to the exposure and outcome.

Another issue concerning the use of CSF/imaging biomarkers is their transportability to places with poorly resourced medical care. This will lead to less information in places where this information is most needed (i.e. in rural areas or in LMICs, where AD is growing at a greater pace than in HICs.[33] This may result in a lack of standardization across studies of information depending on place, race/ethnicity, education, income, health status, access to healthcare, and a myriad of other variables that are related to the risk for AD. There are several research initiatives to identify blood-based biomarkers, which would enable a greater portion of the population to be tested.

Study Designs to Identify and Diagnose Cases in Large Studies

Given this background about the AD phenotype and related diagnostic schemas, we will next discuss different study designs to identify dementia and AD cases, in order of their utility and value.

Population-based cohorts

The gold standard for identifying and diagnosing cases is from populations that are well-characterized and studied prospectively over many years. In epidemiologic research, the need for standardized definitions of cases is critical to decreasing misclassification of outcomes. To standardize phenotyping, a protocol and standard operating procedure manual is needed, and accepted guidelines such as those described above should be followed for every participant in the study and over time. Typically, a population is carefully enumerated and screened with a global cognitive test, such as the Mini-Mental State Examination[34] or a similar screening instrument, such as the MOCA[35] or the 3MS.[36] Criteria are set for 'passing' or 'failing' based on pilot studies of the sensitivity and specificity of the cognitive screening instrument in the particular population being studied. If one is interested in enumeration of prevalence or incidence, it is important to work into the protocol an estimation of the false-negative rate of the test, to estimate the number of people who have dementia but are found to 'pass' the test.[1]

The success of the screening methodology depends on the cut-point set for test positivity. As there is a reciprocal relationship between sensitivity and specificity, if the goal of the study is finding all cases, one would set the sensitivity high and sacrifice specificity. This will result in working up more false-positive cases to find a true positive case, and can be a source of considerable expense for the study. However, if too low a cut-point is selected, it is possible that milder cases will be missed. This is less of an issue in longitudinal studies, which presumably will capture mild cases in the next exam, but may be an issue if the goal is to estimate the number of prevalent cases in the population.

One strategy to offset missing mild cases is to sample from different cognitive (and perhaps also age) strata. In this approach, the whole population is stratified by their cognitive screening test score and individuals are randomly sampled, usually in proportion to the expected number of cases within the strata, to undergo the clinical evaluation. For example, the low-performing stratum may be sampled at 100% and the high stratum at 10%.[37] Selected persons within these strata undergo the same clinical evaluation, and analyses of the data must take into account the sampling scheme. There is a wide range of protocols used to diagnose dementia and its subtypes: two or three-stage screening to increase the probability that the participant is likely a case that can be diagnosed with more and more detail, or one stage that includes all participants participating in all diagnostic activities. Data for diagnosis collected on the participants may include questionnaires, cognitive testing, a neurological and physical exam, a neuropsychological evaluation, a proxy interview about the participant's daily functioning, and measures of hearing, vision, and depression. The neuropsychological battery is typically administered by a psychometrist and interpreted by a neuropsychologist. Supporting data (blood and genetic tests, imaging, and biomarker studies) are built into the protocol. After all data have been collected on a participant, a consensus diagnosis is adjudicated at a meeting involving the study clinicians and neuropsychologists in which the diagnostic criteria are carefully completed and the final diagnosis is made by all clinical staff. The protocol may also have a built-in component for follow-up of incident cases, since some cases require further studies to meet all diagnostic criteria or to be able to subtype the dementia. Alternatively, algorithmic diagnoses may be determined. Typically, cohort studies are designed to see the participants every few years (usually 2–3 or every year if possible to avoid loss to follow-up and deaths). Participants are re-screened with the cognitive instrument and the diagnostic procedure is repeated to find incident cases. Having a complete ascertainment of incident cases is essential to a valid investigation. If the cohort is closed (no new participants are allowed in), most of the individuals who meet dementia criteria during the study will be discovered and enumerated. However, investigators must account for losses to follow-up, which, if excessive, can severely bias the findings. The most effective way to ensure identifying all cases is to set up mechanisms to review records from all sources in the community that see dementia patients, including nursing homes.

Health service-based cohorts

Population-based cohort studies are time and cost-consuming. Another design to identify cases is to use data based on records from health service organizations. This method is becoming more appealing in a world of big data, because the datasets already exist and are dynamically growing. Therefore, the sample sizes can be far greater than any single cohort. Such studies may use electronic data from country-wide registries such as those available in Scandinavian countries or HMO-type registries like that of Kaiser Permanente in California (https://healthy.kaiserpermanente. org/, Geisinger, in California, https://www.geisinger.org/, or the Clinical Practice Research Datalink https://www.cprd.com/Home/). Methods such as natural language processing and big data bioinformatics are rapidly becoming available to gain the optimal amount of insight into questions such as frequency of the disease in subpopulations, the effects of medications, or repeatedly measured levels of plasma-based diagnostics, or onset of new medical conditions. This design increases sample size, but at the cost of standardized measures of information.[38] However, very large samples of moderate to severe cases and the appropriate research questions can mitigate the effect this has on the measures of association if this misclassification is non-differential, that is, related only to either the exposure or the outcome of interest, but not to both. Another factor to account for is the lack of information on people who are at risk for, or have dementia, but who did not come to the attention of medical services. Although 'gate-keeping' can occur in population-based cohort studies as well, identification of the population using a census or similar method will allow the investigators to know several of the characteristics of individuals who are missing from their sample. Finally, these databases usually do not contain detailed and frequent measures related to the risk for, diagnosis of, and consequences of dementia, particularly in the early stages of the disease. This type of information would need to be obtained either from an already existing cohort with similar characteristics to the health service-based cohort, or a sub-study involving more intensive exams.

Other sources of data

Using only hospital discharge data to identify cases may only capture those cases that are advanced, have behavioural disturbances, or are admitted for another medical reason. If the aim of the study is to collect all cases that occur in the cohort, such discharge records should be reviewed. Similarly, death certificates do not typically report dementia as a primary cause of death, although it may be recorded as the secondary or contributing cause of death. This might change as the population ages and as the awareness of dementia increases in the medical community.

Conclusion

In populations, early detection and prevention need to begin early in life with genes and healthful lifestyles, respectively. Detecting dementia early relies not only on detecting pathologies in the brain, but also on being able to measure an individual's brain and cognitive reserve, since these interact to produce clinical disease. Today, we are able to detect dementia in research-based populations 20–25 years before clinical onset using biomarkers. However, use of biomarkers is expensive and invasive. When disease-modifying treatments become available, early detection of dementia in populations will become crucial. Since the expense of biomarker detection and treatment with biologically-modifying drugs among asymptomatic people will be out of reach for many global populations, we need to develop methods to detect dementia early using less expensive modalities, such as characterization by genetic risk. We also need to identify methods to measure brain and cognitive reserve and take these into account in identifying individuals at high risk for conversion from normal to impaired cognitive function.

REFERENCES

1. Borenstein AR, Mortimer JA. Alzheimer's Disease: Life Course Perspectives on Risk Reduction. San Diego, CA: Elsevier Academic Press, 2016.
2. McKhann G, Drachman D, Folstein M, Katzman R, Price D, Stadlan EM. Clinical diagnosis of Alzheimer's disease: report of the NINCDS-ADRDA Work Group under the auspices of Department of Health and Human Services Task Force on Alzheimer's Disease. Neurology. 1984; 34(7): 939–44.
3. Schneider JA, Arvanitakis Z, Leurgans SE, Bennett DA. The neuropathology of probable Alzheimer disease and mild cognitive impairment. Ann Neurol. 2009; 66(2): 200–8.
4. Snowdon DA, Greiner LH, Mortimer JA, Riley KP, Greiner PA, Markesbery WR. Brain infarction and the clinical expression of Alzheimer disease. The Nun Study. JAMA: the journal of the American Medical Association. 1997; 277(10): 813–7.
5. Gelber RP, Launer LJ, White LR. The Honolulu-Asia Aging Study: epidemiologic and neuropathologic research on cognitive impairment. Curr Alzheimer Res. 2012; 9(6): 664–72.
6. Flanagan M, Larson EB, Latimer CS, Cholerton B, Crane PK, Montine KS, et al. Clinical-pathologic correlations in vascular cognitive impairment and dementia. Biochimica et Biophysica Acta. 2016; 1862(5): 945–51.
7. Arvanitakis Z, Leurgans SE, Barnes LL, Bennett DA, Schneider JA. Microinfarct pathology, dementia, and cognitive systems. Stroke; a Journal of Cerebral Circulation. 2011; 42(3): 722–7.
8. Schneider JA, Arvanitakis Z, Bang W, Bennett DA. Mixed brain pathologies account for most dementia cases in community-dwelling older persons. Neurology. 2007; 69(24): 2197–204.
9. Montine TJ, Sonnen JA, Montine KS, Crane PK, Larson EB. Adult Changes in Thought study: dementia is an individually varying convergent syndrome with prevalent clinically silent diseases that may be modified by some commonly used therapeutics. Curr Alzheimer Res. 2012; 9(6): 718–23.
10. Jack CR, Jr, Holtzman DM. Biomarker modeling of Alzheimer's disease. Neuron. 2013; 80(6): 1347–58.
11. Braak H, Braak E. Frequency of stages of Alzheimer-related lesions in different age categories. Neurobiology of Aging. 1997; 18(4): 351–7.
12. Mucke L, Selkoe DJ. Neurotoxicity of amyloid beta-protein: synaptic and network dysfunction. Cold Spring Harbor Perspectives in Medicine. 2012; 2(7): a006338.
13. Lesne SE, Sherman MA, Grant M, Kuskowski M, Schneider JA, Bennett DA, et al. Brain amyloid-beta oligomers in ageing and Alzheimer's disease. Brain: a Journal of Neurology. 2013; 136(Pt 5): 1383–98.
14. Larson ME, Lesne SE. Soluble Abeta oligomer production and toxicity. Journal of Neurochemistry. 2012; 120(Suppl 1): 125–39.
15. Qian J, Wolters FJ, Beiser A, Haan M, Ikram MA, Karlawish J, et al. APOE-related risk of mild cognitive impairment and dementia for prevention trials: an analysis of four cohorts. PLOS Med. 2017; 14(3): e1002254.
16. Manly JJ. Critical issues in cultural neuropsychology: profit from diversity. Neuropsychology Review. 2008; 18(3): 179–83.
17. Mortimer JA. Important role of brain reserve in lowering the risk of Alzheimer's disease. Future Neurology. 2009; 4: 1–4.
18. Mortimer JA. The continuum hypothesis of Alzheimer's disease and normal aging: the role of brain reserve. Alzheimer Res. 1995; 1995(1): 67–70.
19. Stern Y. Cognitive reserve in ageing and Alzheimer's disease. Lancet Neurology. 2012; 11(11): 1006–12.
20. Stern Y. What is cognitive reserve? Theory and research application of the reserve concept. Journal of the International Neuropsychological Society. 2002; 8(3): 448–60.
21. Association AP. Diagnostic and Statistical Manual of Mental Disorders (3rd edition). Washington, DC: American Psychiatric Association, 1980.
22. Association AP. Diagnostic and Statistical Manual (3rd edition), revised. Washington, DC: American Psychiatric Association, 1987.
23. American Psychiatric Association. Diagnostic and Statistical Manual of Mental Disorders (4th edition), text revision. Washington, DC: American Psychiatric Association, 2000.
24. American Psychiatric Association. Diagnostic and Statistical Manual of Mental Disorders (5th edition). Arlington, V.: American Psychiatric Publishing, 2013.
25. McKhann GM, Knopman DS, Chertkow H, Hyman BT, Jack CR, Jr, Kawas CH, et al. The diagnosis of dementia due to Alzheimer's disease: recommendations from the National Institute on Aging-Alzheimer's Association workgroups on diagnostic guidelines for Alzheimer's disease. Alzheimer's & Dementia: the Journal of the Alzheimer's Association. 2011; 7(3): 263–9.
26. Dubois B, Feldman HH, Jacova C, Dekosky ST, Barberger-Gateau P, Cummings J, et al. Research criteria for the diagnosis of Alzheimer's disease: revising the NINCDS-ADRDA criteria. Lancet Neurology. 2007; 6(8): 734–46.
27. Karlawish J, Jack CR, Jr, Rocca WA, Snyder HM, Carrillo MC. Alzheimer's disease: The next frontier-Special Report 2017. Alzheimer's & Dementia: the Journal of the Alzheimer's Association. 2017; 13(4): 374–80.
28. Petersen RC, Smith, GE, Waring SC, Ivnik RJ, Tangalos EG, Kokmen E. Mild cognitive impairment: clinical characterization and outcome. Arch Neurol. 1999; 56: 303–8.
29. Lopez OL, Becker JT, Jagust WJ, Fitzpatrick A, Carlson MC, DeKosky ST, et al. Neuropsychological characteristics of mild cognitive impairment subgroups. J Neurol Neurosurg Psychiatry. 2006; 77(2): 159–65.

30. Sperling RA, Aisen PS, Beckett LA, Bennett DA, Craft S, Fagan AM, et al. Toward defining the preclinical stages of Alzheimer's disease: recommendations from the National Institute on Aging-Alzheimer's Association workgroups on diagnostic guidelines for Alzheimer's disease. Alzheimer's & Dementia: the Journal of the Alzheimer's Association. 2011; 7(3): 280–92.
31. Zwan MD, Villemagne VL, Dore V, et al. Subjective memory complaints in APOEe4 carriers are associated with high amyloid-beta burden. Journal of Alzheimer's Disease. 2016; 49(4): 1115–22.
32. Kryscio RJ, Abner EL, Jicha GA, Nelson PT, Smith CD, Van Eldik LJ, et al. Self-reported memory complaints: a comparison of demented and unimpaired outcomes. Journal of Prevention of Alzheimer's Disease. 2016; 3(1): 13–19.
33. Prince M, Ali GC, Guerchet M, Prina AM, Albanese E, Wu YT. Recent global trends in the prevalence and incidence of dementia, and survival with dementia. Alzheimer's Res Ther. 2016; 8(1): 23.
34. Folstein MF, Folstein SE, McHugh PR. 'Mini-mental state'. A practical method for grading the cognitive state of patients for the clinician. J Psychiatr Res. 1975; 12(3): 189–98.
35. Nasreddine ZS, Phillips NA, Bedirian V, Charbonneau S, Whitehead V, Collin I, et al. The Montreal Cognitive Assessment, MoCA: a brief screening tool for mild cognitive impairment. J Am Geriatr Soc. 2005; 53(4): 695–9.
36. Teng EL, Chui HC. The Modified Mini-Mental State (3MS) examination. Journal of Clinical Psychiatry. 1987; 48(8): 314–18.
37. Bienias JL, Beckett LA, Bennett DA, Wilson RS, Evans DA. Design of the Chicago Health and Aging Project (CHAP). Journal of Alzheimer's Disease. 2003; 5(5): 349–55.
38. Weiskopf NG, Weng C. Methods and dimensions of electronic health record data quality assessment: enabling reuse for clinical research. Journal of the American Medical Informatics Association. 2013; 20(1): 144–51.

18

The oldest-old and dementia at the end of life

María M Corrada and Claudia H Kawas

The Oldest-old

In 1997, Madame Jeanne-Louis Calment died in Arles, France, and established the world record for longest-lived human, having lived to more than 122 years of age. Although centenarians were previously a rarity, it is now estimated that more than half of all people who have been born in the developed world this century will reach their 100th birthday or even greater.[1] With these profound increases in life expectancy, the oldest-old, people aged 90 years and older, are the fastest growing segment of the population in most of the world. According to United Nations projections, in 2015 there were 16 million people aged 90 and older around the world (Table 18.1). By 2060, the 90+ population will be more than six times higher, reaching 113 million.[2] These individuals have the highest rates of dementia and disability and will present an enormous public health challenge.

The countries expected to have the largest number of 90+year-olds are in Asia, North and Latin America, and Europe. But by far the country with the largest number will be China, where the population of 90+year-olds will burgeon from 2.3 million to a stunning 28.6 million, eclipsing most of the other nations combined. The oldest-old population is not only growing in numbers but also as a percentage of the elderly population, people 65 and older. In 2015, 90+year-olds represented about 2.8% of the elderly world population but the number is expected to increase to 6% of the elderly population by 2060. In more developed regions (Europe, North America, Australia/New Zealand, and Japan), 90+year-olds will represent more than 10% of the elderly population.[2] Although poorly understood, many species show differences in longevity by sex, with females living longer on average than males. This differential longevity is also true for human men and women and is very consistent across all countries.[3] Thus, by age 90, there are three women alive for every man and the overwhelming majority of supercentenarians (people over 110 years) are women.[4]

Epidemiology of Dementia in the Oldest-old

For many years, scientists have known that prevalence and incidence of dementia is strongly associated with advancing age, making age by far the strongest risk factor for dementia. Essentially all studies have demonstrated a doubling of dementia risk with every five years of age, beginning at age 65 and extending to age 85.[5] For the oldest-old, however, it was not clear if this persistent doubling continued into the 10th decade and beyond because some studies suggested a levelling off, or even a reduction in dementia risk for oldest-old. Recent larger studies, however, have demonstrated that the risk of dementia continues to increase in the oldest-old.

Dementia prevalence

For studies with age-specific estimates above age 90, prevalence at age 90–95 ranges from 32%[6,7] to 48%[8] and at ages 95–99 from 41%[6] to 59%[9] (Fig. 18.1). Several centenarian studies have estimated dementia prevalence,[10] with estimates ranging from 42% in the Swedish Centenarian Study[11] to 76% in the New England Centenarian Study.[12] Most studies of nonagenarians and centenarians are consistent in showing higher dementia prevalence in women than men,[10,13] primarily a result of greater longevity in women, even in the presence of dementia.

Dementia incidence

Even more notable than the variability of prevalence rates is the striking variability in studies of dementia incidence rates in the oldest-old. Before age 85, incidence rates are fairly similar in most studies, with little variability (Fig. 18.1). In contrast, after age 90, estimates of incidence rates vary considerably. At age 90–95, rates range from 5% per year[35] to 19% per year,[36] a four-fold difference. At ages 95–99, incidence rates range from 7% per year[37] to 29% per year.[36] Moreover, although most studies show incidence rates increasing with age, some studies, such as the Rotterdam Study[35] and Rochester Epidemiology Project[37] do not appear to show increasing rates after age 90. In other studies, like the Cache County Study,[38] incidence rates appear to significantly decline after age 90. With larger studies, however, it is now clear that incidence of dementia continues to double with every five years of age after age 90, continuing the exponential increase demonstrated at younger ages.[5] In the 90+ Study,[39] one of the largest studies to date, rates doubled

Table 18.1 Projected oldest-old population (90+) 2015–2060: top ten countries (thousands)

Country	Year 2015	2060
China	2321	28,657
USA	2247	9247
India	1138	8511
Japan	1758	5800
Brazil	431	5315
Bangladesh	203	3066
Germany	694	2977
Mexico	328	2834
Italy	673	2676
Vietnam	378	2658
World	16,826	113,151

Note: Information extracted from United Nations Department of Economics and Social Affairs Population Division. World Population Prospects: the 2017 Revision.

Source: data from United Nations Department of Economics and Social Affairs Population Division. World Population Prospects: The 2017 Revision. https://population.un.org/wpp/Download/Standard/Population/ [Accessed: 15/07/19][2]

every 5.5 years after age 90, reaching a staggering 40% per year at ages 100+. In studies with enough men and women for adequate estimates, there were no clear differences in dementia incidence by sex.[10] In all likelihood, much of the variability in dementia estimates of published studies reflects differences in study population, dementia criteria, study size, follow-up length, and other methodological differences, rather than genuine differences in the dementia incidence of the different countries.[40,41]

Risk and protective factors for dementia

Risk and protective factors for dementia have primarily been studied in younger elderly with the assumption that these factors might also be relevant for the oldest-old. Age matters, however, and there is growing evidence that many factors identified as risk factors for AD and all-cause dementia in younger elderly do not apply to the oldest-old. For example, the e4 allele of the apolipoprotein E gene (APOEe4) is the strongest susceptibility gene for dementia and AD at younger ages and people with one or two copies of the e4 allele are at increased risk of dementia or AD.[42] But in the oldest-old, the APOEe4 allele is no longer associated with an increased risk of dementia.[43–45] The presence of the APOEe2 allele has been implicated as a protective factor for AD in younger elderly, but it is not related to dementia risk in the oldest-old.[44,45] The APOE2 allele, however, may account in part for the clinical-pathological discordance in people with high levels of AD pathology but who have no dementia.[46]

Hypertension is another risk factor that appears to have a different effect in very old age. During midlife, hypertension has been consistently found to be linked to a higher dementia risk,[47–50] but the association appears to change with age and is no longer a risk factor at older ages.[51,52] In fact, several studies have suggested that hypertension is associated with a lower risk of dementia in the very elderly.[53,54] Age of onset of hypertension may be a key variable here. In the 90+ Study, although people with a history of hypertension

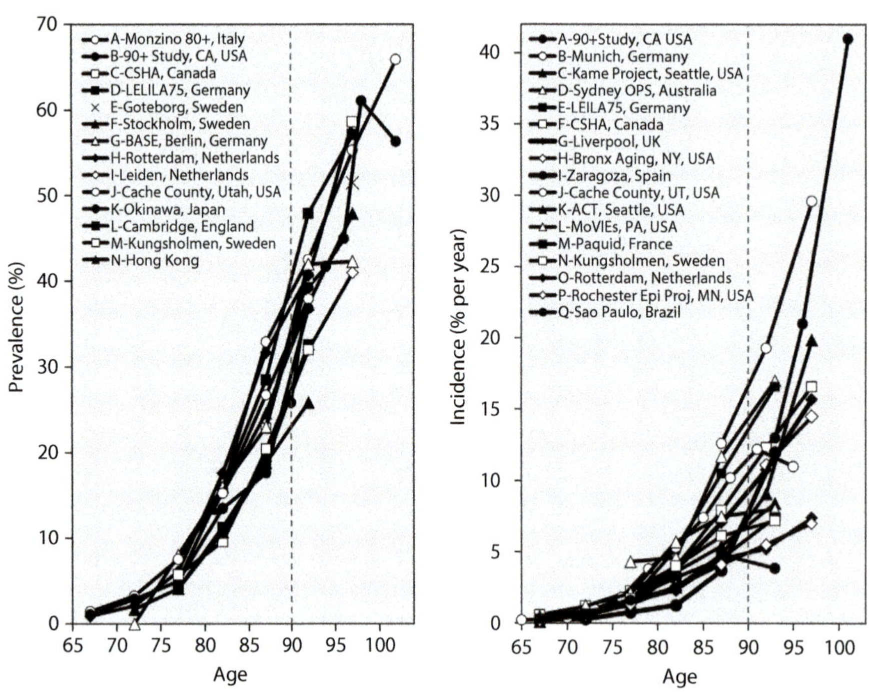

Fig. 18.1 Age-specific prevalence and incidence of dementia in studies with people aged 90+.

Note: prevalence studies: A-Monzino 80-plus, Italy;[14] B-90+ Study, California, USA;[13] C-CSHA, Canada;[9] D-LEILA75+, Germany;[8] E-Goteborg, Sweden;[15] F-Stockholm, Sweden;[16] G-BASE, Germany;[17] H-Rotterdam, Netherlands;[18] I-Leiden, Netherlands;[6] J-Cache County, Utah, US;[19] K-Okinawa, Japan;[20] L-Cambridge, England;[21] M-Kungsholmen, Sweden;[7] N-Hong Kong, China.[22]

Incidence studies: A-90+ Study, CA;[39] B-Munich, Germany;[36] C-Kame Project, Seattle;[23] D-Sydney OPS, Australia;[24] E-LEILA, Germany;[25] F-CSHA, Canada;[26] G-Liverpool, UK;[27] H-Bronx Aging, NY;[28] I-Zaragoza, Spain;[29] J-Cache County, UT;[38] K-ACT, Seattle WA;[30] L-MoVIEs, PA;[31] M-Paquid, France;[32] N-Kungsholmen, Sweden;[33] O-Rotterdam, Netherlands;[34] P-Rochester Epi Project, MN;[37] Q-Sao Paulo, Brazil.[35]

showed a lower risk of dementia, the effect was limited to people who developed hypertension later in life, in their 80s or 90s, compared with people who never developed hypertension.[54] High cholesterol also appears to have an association with dementia that changes with age,[55] being a risk factor in midlife and protective against dementia when present in the very elderly.[56,57]

Not all risk and protective factors behave differently in the oldest-old, however. For example, as in younger elderly, education continues to be associated with a lower risk of dementia[39] and better cognitive performance[58] among the oldest-old. Also, similar to younger ages, history of stroke or history of heart disease are associated with increased risk of dementia in the oldest-old.[54] Dementia in this age group is associated with a wide variety of neuropathologies (as discussed below) and risk and protective factors for each pathology are likely to differ. Thus, more research is necessary to better understand risk and protective factors in the oldest-old, especially in relation to different neuropathological processes.

Neuropathology

Delineating the causes of dementia and cognitive loss in extreme ageing has been a challenge. Although AD continues to be the most frequent dementia-associated pathology in the oldest-old, many other pathologic processes have been implicated and clinical pathologic studies have suggested a weakening in this age group of the association between dementia and AD as well as other neuropathologic changes. Moreover, several neuropathologic abnormalities infrequently detected in younger elderly become more common in the oldest-old and are strongly associated with dementia. Importantly, mixed pathologic processes become more frequent with advancing age, with about half of all 90+ individuals with dementia having two or more pathologic changes detected at autopsy.

Prevalence of neuropathologic changes and risk of dementia

AD pathology (neuritic amyloid plaques and neurofibrillary tangles) is the most prevalent dementia-related abnormality in the brains of the oldest-old. Approximately half of all individuals over age 90[59–62] have AD pathology consistent with intermediate or high likelihood of dementia due to AD defined by NIA-Reagan criteria.[63] Interestingly, despite the high prevalence of AD pathology in this age group, approximately 25% do not have amyloid deposition in the form of neuritic plaques, whereas virtually all have at least some neurofibrillary tangles in transentorhinal brain regions (Braak stage II or greater).[64–65] Compared with younger elderly, many non-AD pathologies are found more frequently in the oldest-old. These dementia-related pathologies include hippocampal sclerosis (HS) in 15–20% of all individuals,[62,66] microinfarcts in >50% with 15–20% having three or more,[62,67,68] moderate to severe amyloid angiopathy in 10–20%,[62,69] and severe white matter disease in 8–10%.[62] In contrast, Lewy bodies, large infarcts, frontotemporal degenerations, and PD are detected much less frequently, each occurring in only 1–4% of individuals in this age group.[70–73]

In the 90+ Study, the odds of dementia were much greater for many non-AD pathologies compared to AD.[62] Fig. 18.2 shows the odds of dementia associated with each type of pathologic abnormality, compared to not having that pathology. For AD, the OR for dementia was 2.2, whereas for some non-AD pathologies the ORs were greater than 10. It is also worth noting that two under-studied pathologies, microinfarcts and HS, occur most frequently in this age group and are highly associated with dementia. In three different cohorts, 3+ microinfarcts were shown to independently contribute to dementia, with a magnitude similar to high levels of neurofibrillary tangles (OR = 3–5).[69,74,75] In the 90+ Study, only microinfarcts in cortical regions other than occipital (mid-frontal, inferior parietal, and superior temporal) were related to dementia,

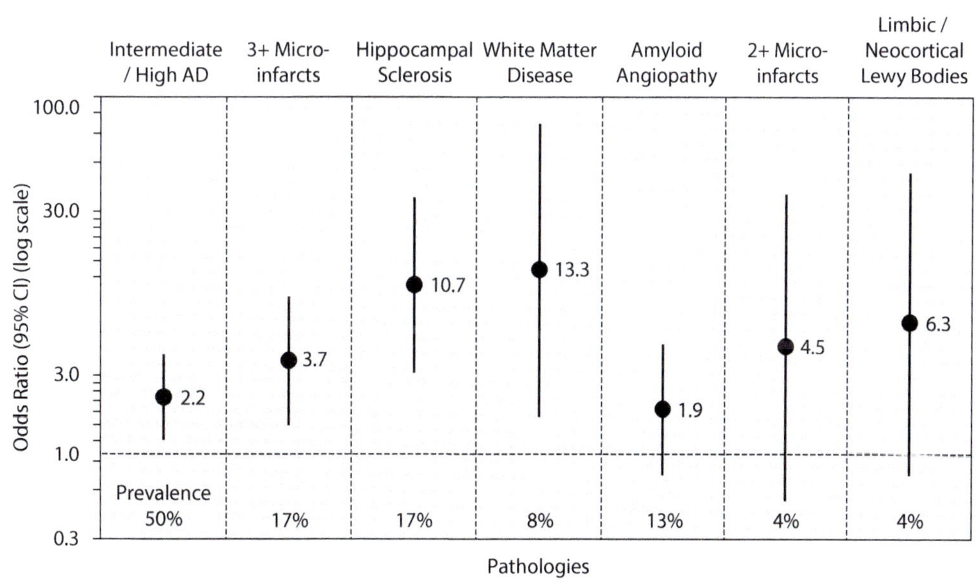

Fig. 18.2 Prevalence and odds of dementia for different pathologies: the 90+ study.

Note: AD = Alzheimer's disease. Odds of dementia and confidence intervals estimated from logistic regression adjusting for sex and age at death in 183 autopsied participants.

Source: Data from Kawas CH, Kim RC, Sonnen JA, et al. Multiple pathologies are common and related to dementia in the oldest-old: The 90+ Study. *Neurology*. 85(6): 535–42. Copyright © 2015, American Academy of Neurology. https://doi.org/10.1212/WNL.0000000000001831.

whereas microinfarcts in the occipital cortex or subcortical regions (basal ganglia and thalamus) were more frequent (>70% of all detected) but not related to dementia.[75] Even more striking is the very strong association of HS with dementia in this age group (OR = 10.7). HS accounts for as much as a third of all dementia in this age group and is rarely seen in individuals without dementia. We know little about these understudied pathologies, in part because neither microinfarcts nor HS is detectable with imaging or other diagnostic modalities, and they do not have validated clinical criteria for diagnosis during life. Because these pathologies can only be investigated in autopsied study participants, we also know little about risk or other factors that may be relevant to their clinical expression.

Single and mixed pathologies

The majority of oldest-old with dementia have two or more pathologic processes detected at autopsy.[60,66,76–78] Similar to younger elderly, the combination of AD and some form of vascular pathology is the most common co-occurrence, but all combinations exist.[60,62,79] Studies have shown that the number of pathologies is related to the likelihood and severity of dementia. In the 90+ Study, prevalence of dementia rose from 22% in people with 'no' pathologies to virtually all individuals (95%) that died with three or more pathologies. Among people with dementia, the severity of cognitive impairment increased from an average MMSE score of 17.7 (moderate dementia) in people with 'no' pathologies to an average MMSE score of 5.7 (severe dementia) in individuals with four or more pathologies, even with a similar duration of disease.[62] The Honolulu Asia Aging Study and the Nun Study demonstrated that total burden of comorbid neuropathologic abnormalities, rather than any single lesion type, was the most relevant determinant of cognitive impairment, often despite AD being the only clinical diagnosis assigned during life.[80] The authors noted that these findings present challenges to dementia and intervention research, as well as accurate clinical diagnosis.

When alone, non-AD pathologies appear more likely to result in dementia than intermediate/high AD pathology. In the 90+ Study, individuals with a single non-AD pathology (such as HS, severe white matter disease, or 3+ microinfarcts) were 12 times more likely to have dementia than individuals with no pathology, and the likelihood of dementia did not change with the addition of a second pathology. In contrast, individuals with intermediate/high AD pathology alone were only three times more likely to have dementia than individuals with no pathologies. However, when AD pathology was accompanied by a second pathology, the likelihood of dementia increased to the level of non-AD pathologies.[62] The ways in which pathologies may be additive or interact requires further study.

Clinical pathological discordance: dementia without pathology and pathology without dementia

Despite the high prevalence of pathologies at this age, investigators have also noted that the prevalence of dementia of unknown origin (i.e. dementia not clearly explained by the presence of any known pathological abnormality), increases in this age group, approaching 50%.[81] More recent studies suggest that consideration of other lesser studied pathologies such as microinfarcts and hippocampal sclerosis account for some of these cases of dementia. However, even with consideration of these pathologies, more than 20% of individuals in the tenth decade of life are noted to have dementia without obvious aetiology on autopsy.[82] Individuals with dementia but insufficient pathology to explain their cognitive losses do, in fact, generally have low levels of pathologic abnormalities, including very mild AD-type changes, amyloid angiopathy, or occasional microinfarcts. Additional research is necessary to determine whether combinations of these low levels of pathologic changes or other undetected pathologies contribute to dementia in these individuals.

The detection of cerebral pathologies in the brains of people without overt dementia is more prevalent in the oldest-old compared to any other age group. Approximately 30–40% of nonagenarians and centenarians without dementia during life have intermediate and high likelihood AD pathology at autopsy.[62,83] Although occurring less frequently, investigators have also noted the presence of other pathologic changes in non-demented individuals, including Lewy bodies, vascular disease, and HS.[62,83–85] We do not fully understand the implication of the presence of pathologies in people without dementia. One possibility is that at least some of these individuals are in preclinical stages of disease and would have developed dementia if they had lived longer. Alternatively, some oldest-old individuals may be 'resilient' to the deleterious effects of these pathologies through genetic, environmental, or other factors. A third possibility is that these individuals may appear resilient to AD pathology in part because they have not developed additional brain pathologic comorbidities such as microinfarcts. In the Honolulu Asian Aging Study and the Nun Study, no cognitive impairment in individuals with a high level of neurofibrillary tangles (Braak stage V) was strongly associated with minimal or no comorbid abnormalities, suggesting that the expression of dementia may be more related to the presence of other co-existing pathologies.[86]

Weakening of the association between AD pathology and dementia

Several investigators have noted a weakening of the relationship between AD pathology and dementia with advancing age.[65,87] This finding is likely related to the high prevalence of non-AD pathologies, the frequent occurrence of AD pathology in individuals without dementia in this age group, and, possibly, failure to detect known or unknown pathologic processes. In a large clinical pathological study from the Medical Research Council Cognitive Function and Ageing Study,[65] investigators noted a significant weakening of the association between neocortical neuritic plaques and dementia from an OR = 8.63 at 75 years of age to an OR = 2.48 at 95 years of age. In contrast, however, neocortical cerebral atrophy in this study maintained a relationship with age in persons with dementia at both 75 years of age (OR = 5.11) an 95 years of age (OR = 6.10) and thus distinguished the cohort with dementia from the cohort without dementia. Complementary findings were present in the Honolulu Asian Aging Study, where moderate or severe brain atrophy was independently associated with poor cognition, even after accounting for the influence of education and other dementia-related lesions.[79] We do not know the underlying pathophysiology of brain atrophy and it is hoped that future studies will elucidate underlying mechanisms or pathologic processes related to this important finding.

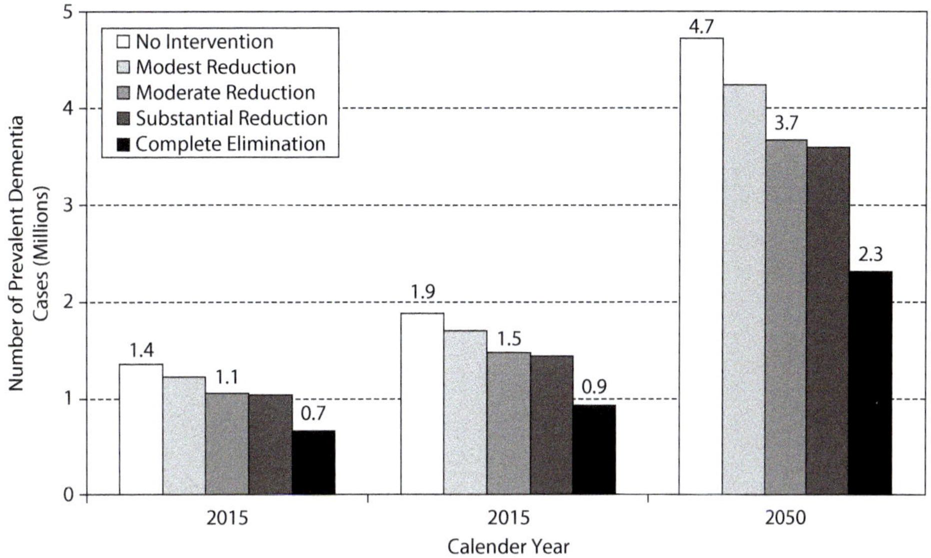

Fig. 18.3 US prevalence of dementia among persons aged 90 years and over in calendar years 2015, 2030, and 2050 with no intervention and four intervention scenarios to reduce Alzheimer's disease pathology.

Reproduced with permission from Brookmeyer R, Kawas CH, Abdallah N. Impact of interventions to reduce Alzheimer's disease pathology on the prevalence of dementia in the oldest-old. *Alzheimer's Dementia*. 12(3): 225–32. https://doi.org/10.1016/j.jalz.2016.01.004.

Dementia Projections and Potential Impact of AD-related Interventions

With the rapid growth of this segment of the population throughout much of the world, the number of people with dementia will present a staggering public health challenge. In the USA, the prevalence of dementia among the oldest-old will increase from 1.35 million in 2015 to 4.72 million in 2050, nearly the current number of dementia cases the USA currently has at all ages.[88,89] An area of intense research is the development of interventions targeting AD pathologic changes. Brookmeyer et al. estimated the impact on the prevalence of dementia in the oldest-old of different intervention scenarios to reduce or eliminate AD pathology (amyloid plaques and neurofibrillary tangles).[88] Moderate reductions in AD pathology would reduce dementia prevalence by approximately 22% and avert about one million dementia cases. If interventions were available that completely eliminated AD pathology, dementia prevalence in the oldest-old would be reduced by approximately 50%, averting nearly 2.4 million cases by 2050 (Fig. 18.3). Even in this scenario, however, at least half of dementia cases would remain, those cases attributed to pathological abnormalities other than AD. Although total elimination would significantly reduce the burden of dementia and have considerable public health impact, large numbers of dementia cases in the oldest-old would still remain.

Methodological Challenges in Studying Dementia in the Oldest-old

All studies present methodological challenges, but these are particularly apparent in studies of the oldest-old. Some of the challenges include very high mortality rates, a frail population with high rates of visual and hearing impairment, severe motor limitations, multiple comorbidities, and lack of normative cognitive data and validated diagnostic criteria. These challenges contribute to difficulty in enrolling and retaining participants for research, performing and interpreting cognitive assessments, and diagnosing dementia and its aetiology. In-depth reviews of issues related to diagnosing dementia and studying the oldest-old have been published previously.[90–92]

Experience in the 90+ Study

The 90+ Study is a study in Southern California, USA, established in 2003 to investigate dementia, disability, and frailty in the oldest-old. The study limited enrolment to people aged 90 and older so it could be designed specifically to fit the needs of the oldest-old and respond to some of the challenges of studying the oldest-old. Below we include a brief summary of how the 90+ Study addressed some of those challenges.

High mortality and consequently limited follow-up are a reality when studying the oldest-old. The 90+ Study sought to maximize the amount of longitudinal data collected by having frequent assessments at intervals of six months, shorter than the typical dementia study. A shorter interval allows for detection of shorter duration cases, detection of rapid change, and more data points for analyses of rates of decline in cognition or function. Another issue when studying very elderly participants who are often frail, have multiple chronic medical conditions and limited mobility, is that they are less likely to participate in research, leading to potential bias to our studies. The 90+ Study addressed some of these challenges by not limiting enrolment to people who could go to the research centre for evaluations. Instead, researchers visited participants at their homes, including nursing homes, assisted living, or wherever they resided. Although this approach is costly, it ensured the cohort reflected more accurately the full spectrum of cognitive and physical abilities of the oldest-old. To address the sensory impairments frequently present in oldest-old participants, assessment materials and stimuli were modified with larger and bolder print, and rather than presenting stimuli in one modality (either verbally or visually) stimuli was presented both verbally and in print. The magnitude of participant fatigue was a somewhat unexpected challenge and required shortening of all procedures. When available, short versions of tests were selected. In addition, the neuropsychological battery was kept short, and visits were divided into more than one encounter when needed. Because making decisions about function and cognition is challenging when physical limitations and other conditions are present, researchers relied heavily on information from informants who knew participants' cognition and function well. Informants were probed to determine the extent to which functional changes were the result of cognitive change, physical problems, or both.

Effect of methodology: follow-up interval and dementia incidence

As described above, incidence rates after age 90 show great variability between the different studies. Although real differences in incidence could exist in different studies, methodological factors are likely to account for much of the variability. Methodological reasons could include sample size, differences in assessment methods, and length of interval between evaluations. As noted previously, the 90+ Study selected a short follow-up interval of six months, shorter than the typical epidemiological study of dementia, to capture shorter duration cases and rapid changes in cognition. To demonstrate the effect that the length of follow-up intervals has on incidence rates, the 90+ Study calculated dementia incidence rates simulating different lengths of follow-ups. First, rates were calculated using the information for all available evaluations, which were every six months.[39] Then, rates were calculated by ignoring certain follow-up visits and only considering evaluations every 12 months or every 24 months. When the intervals between evaluations were longer, the resulting dementia incidence rates were lower than the original rates. Incidence rates were 28–34% lower for women and 35– 46% lower for men when using longer intervals (Fig. 18.4). It appears that people who develop dementia and die soon after are missed and not counted when longer follow-up intervals are used, resulting in underestimates of incidence rates. The underestimates seem to be particularly important for oldest-old men, most likely due to the shorter lifespan of men compared to women. Because most epidemiological studies of dementia have follow-up intervals much longer than six months, it is likely that these studies underestimate incidence rates of dementia in the oldest-old, explaining in part the variability in dementia rates observed worldwide.

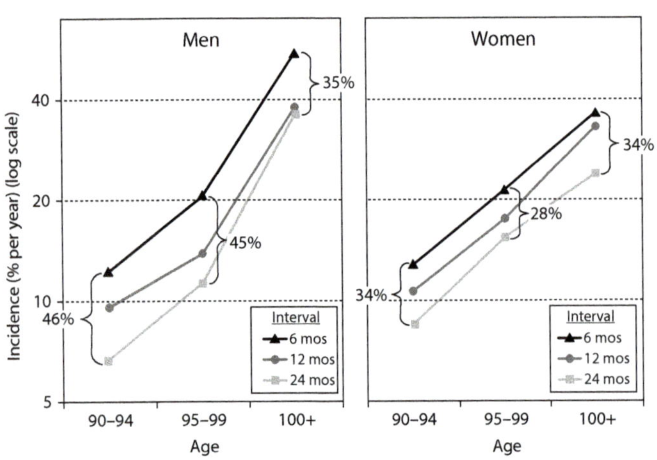

Fig. 18.4 Effect of length of follow-up interval on dementia incidence rates: the 90+ study.

Conclusion

The oldest-old are the fastest growing segment of the population, with the highest rates of dementia and disability. This population will quadruple in the coming decades and present an extraordinary public health challenge. Incidence rates for dementia top 40% per year in centenarians and dementia is related to multiple pathologic processes, including AD, which accounts for approximately half of all dementia at this age. Frequent non-AD pathologies in this age group, such as hippocampal sclerosis and microinfarcts, are poorly understood. Investigations of these pathologies are generally limited to autopsy studies because they cannot be reliably diagnosed during life, although there has been recent progress in developing MRI markers of microinfarcts.[93] Risk and protective factors for the various dementia-related pathologies are likely to differ, and require further investigation in order to facilitate the development of potential strategies to reduce the burden of dementia in this age group.

REFERENCES

1. Christensen K, Doblhammer G, Rau R, Vaupel JW. Ageing populations: the challenges ahead. Lancet. 2009; 374(9696): 1196–1208.
2. United Nations Department of Economics and Social Affairs Population Division. World population prospects: the 2017 revision. Data file. https://population.un.org/wpp/Download/Standard/Population/wpp2019_pop_f01_1_population_both_sexes.xlxs. Available from: htpps://esa.un.org/unpd/wpp.
3. Austad SN, Fischer KE. Sex differences in lifespan. Cell Metab. 2016; 23(6): 1022–33.
4. Supercentenarian Research Foundation. Gerontology Research Group World Supercentenarian Rankings List (Available from: http://supercentenarian-research-foundation.org/TableE.aspx).
5. Jorm AF, Jolley D. The incidence of dementia: a meta-analysis. Neurology. 1998; 51(3): 728–33.
6. Heeren TJ, Lagaay AM, Hijmans W, Rooymans HG. Prevalence of dementia in the 'oldest old' of a Dutch community. J Am Geriatr Soc. 1991; 39(8): 755–9.
7. Fratiglioni L, Grut M, Forsell Y, et al. Prevalence of Alzheimer's disease and other dementias in an elderly urban population: relationship with age, sex, and education. Neurology. 1991; 41: 1886–92.
8. Riedel-Heller SG, Busse A, Aurich C, Matschinger H, Angermeyer MC. Prevalence of dementia according to DSM-III-R and ICD-10: results of the Leipzig Longitudinal Study of the Aged (LEILA75+) Part 1. Br J Psychiatry. 2001; 179: 250–4.
9. Ebly EM, Parhad IM, Hogan DB, Fung TS. Prevalence and types of dementia in the very old: results from the Canadian Study of Health and Aging. Neurology. 1994; 44: 1593–600.
10. Yang Z, Slavin MJ, Sachdev PS. Dementia in the oldest old. Nat Rev Neurol. 2013; 9(7): 382–93.
11. Samuelsson SM, Alfredson BB, Hagberg B, et al. The Swedish Centenarian Study: A multidisciplinary study of five

consecutive cohorts at the age of 100. Int J Aging Hum Dev. 1997;45(3):223-53.
12. Silver MH, Newell K, Brady C, Hedley-White ET, Perls TT. Distinguishing between neurodegenerative disease and disease-free aging: correlating neuropsychological evaluations and neuropathological studies in centenarians. Psychosom Med. 2002; 64(3): 493–501.
13. Corrada MM, Brookmeyer R, Berlau D, Paganini-Hill A, Kawas CH. Prevalence of dementia after age 90: results from the 90+ Study. Neurology. 2008; 71(5): 337–43.
14. Lucca U, Tettamanti M, Logroscino G, et al. Prevalence of dementia in the oldest old: the Monzino 80-plus population based study. Alzheimer's Dement. 2015; 11(3): 258–70 e3.
15. Borjesson-Hanson A, Edin E, Gislason T, Skoog I. The prevalence of dementia in 95-year-olds. Neurology. 2004; 63(12): 2436–8.
16. von Strauss E, Viitanen M, De Ronchi D, Winblad B, Fratiglioni L. Aging and the occurrence of dementia: findings from a population-based cohort with a large sample of nonagenarians. Arch Neurol. 1999; 56(5): 587–92.
17. Wernicke TF, Reischies FM. Prevalence of dementia in old age: Clinical diagnoses in subjects aged 95 years and older. Neurology. 1994; 44: 250–3.
18. Ott A, Breteler MM, van Harskamp F, et al. Prevalence of Alzheimer's disease and vascular dementia: association with education. The Rotterdam study. BMJ. 1995; 310: 970–3.
19. Breitner JC, Wyse BW, Anthony JC, et al. APOE-epsilon4 count predicts age when prevalence of AD increases, then declines: the Cache County Study. Neurology. 1999; 53(2): 321–31.
20. Ogura C, Nakamoto H, Uema T, Yamamoto K, Yonemori T, Yoshimura T. Prevalence of senile dementia in Okinawa, Japan. COSEPO Group. Study Group of Epidemiology for Psychiatry in Okinawa. Int J Epidemiol. 1995; 24(2): 373–80.
21. O'Connor DW, Pollitt PA, Hyde JB, et al. The prevalence of dementia as measured by the Cambridge Mental Disorders of the Elderly Examination. Acta Psychiatr Scand. 1989; 79: 190–8.
22. Chiu HF, Lam LC, Chi I, et al. Prevalence of dementia in Chinese elderly in Hong Kong. Neurology. 1998; 50(4): 1002–9.
23. Borenstein AR, Wu Y, Bowen JD, et al. Incidence rates of dementia, Alzheimer disease, and vascular dementia in the Japanese American population in Seattle, WA: the Kame Project. Alzheimer Dis Assoc Disord. 2014; 28(1): 23–9.
24. Waite LM, Broe GA, Grayson DA, Creasey H. The incidence of dementia in an Australian community population: the Sydney Older Persons Study. Int J Geriatr Psychiatry. 2001; 16(7): 680–9.
25. Riedel-Heller SG, Busse A, Aurich C, Matschinger H, Angermeyer MC. Incidence of dementia according to DSM-III-R and ICD-10: results of the Leipzig Longitudinal Study of the Aged (LEILA75+), Part 2. Br J Psychiatry. 2001; 179: 255–60.
26. The Canadian Study of Health and Aging Working Group. The incidence of dementia in Canada. Neurology. 2000; 55(1): 66–73.
27. Copeland JR, McCracken CF, Dewey ME, et al. Undifferentiated dementia, Alzheimer's disease and vascular dementia: age- and gender-related incidence in Liverpool. The MRC-ALPHA Study. Br J Psychiatry. 1999; 175: 433–8.
28. Hall CB, Verghese J, Sliwinski M, et al. Dementia incidence may increase more slowly after age 90: results from the Bronx Aging Study. Neurology. 2005; 65(6): 882–6.
29. Lobo A, Lopez-Anton R, Santabarbara J, et al. Incidence and lifetime risk of dementia and Alzheimer's disease in a Southern European population. Acta Psychiatr Scand. 2011; 124(5): 372–83.
30. Kukull WA, Higdon R, Bowen JD, et al. Dementia and Alzheimer disease incidence: a prospective cohort study. Arch Neurol. 2002; 59: 1737–46.
31. Ganguli M, Dodge HH, Chen P, Belle S, DeKosky ST. Ten-year incidence of dementia in a rural elderly US community population: the MoVIES Project. Neurology. 2000; 54(5): 1109–16.
32. Letenneur L, Commenges D, Dartigues JF, Barberger-Gateau P. Incidence of dementia and Alzheimer's disease in elderly community residents of south-western France. Int J Epidemiol. 1994; 23(6): 1256–61.
33. Fratiglioni L, Viitanen M, von Strauss E, Tontodonati V, Herlitz A, Winblad B. Very old women at highest risk of dementia and Alzheimer's disease: incidence data from the Kungsholmen Project, Stockholm. Neurology. 1997; 48(1): 132–8.
34. Ruitenberg A, Ott A, van Swieten JC, Hofman A, Breteler MM. Incidence of dementia: does gender make a difference? Neurobiol Aging. 2001; 22(4): 575–80.
35. Nitrini R, Caramelli P, Herrera E, Jr, et al. Incidence of dementia in a community-dwelling Brazilian population. Alzheimer Dis Assoc Disord. 2004; 18(4): 241–6.
36. Fichter MM, Schroppel H, Meller I. Incidence of dementia in a Munich community sample of the oldest old. Eur Arch Psychiatry Clin Neurosci. 1996; 246(6): 320–8.
37. Edland SD, Rocca WA, Petersen RC, Cha RH, Kokmen E. Dementia and Alzheimer disease incidence rates do not vary by sex in Rochester, Minn. Arch Neurol. 2002; 59(10): 1589–93.
38. Miech RA, Breitner JC, Zandi PP, Khachaturian AS, Anthony JC, Mayer L. Incidence of AD may decline in the early 90s for men, later for women. The Cache County Study. Neurology. 2002; 58(2): 209–18.
39. Corrada MM, Brookmeyer R, Paganini-Hill A, Berlau D, Kawas CH. Dementia incidence continues to increase with age in the oldest-old: The 90+ Study. Ann Neurol. 2010; 67(1): 114–21.
40. Corrada M, Brookmeyer R, Kawas CH. Sources of variability in prevalence rates of Alzheimer's disease. Int J Epidemiol. 1995; 24(5): 1000–5.
41. Pioggiosi P, Forti P, Ravaglia G, Berardi D, Ferrari G, De Ronchi D. Different classification systems yield different dementia occurrence among nonagenarians and centenarians. Dement Geriatr Cogn Disord. 2004; 17(1–2): 35–41.
42. Farrer LA, Cupples LA, Haines JL, et al. Effects of age, sex, and ethnicity on the association between apolipoprotein E genotype and Alzheimer disease. A meta-analysis. APOE and Alzheimer Disease Meta Analysis Consortium. JAMA. 1997; 278(16): 1349–56.
43. Juva K, Verkkoniemi A, Viramo P, et al. APOE epsilon4 does not predict mortality, cognitive decline, or dementia in the oldest old. Neurology. 2000; 54(2): 412–5.
44. Qiu C, Kivipelto M, Aguero-Torres H, Winblad B, Fratiglioni L. Risk and protective effects of the APOE gene towards Alzheimer's disease in the Kungsholmen project: variation by age and sex. J Neurol Neurosurg Psychiatry. 2004; 75(6): 828–33.
45. Corrada MM, Paganini-Hill A, Berlau DJ, Kawas CH. Apolipoprotein E genotype, dementia, and mortality in the oldest old: The 90+ Study. Alzheimer's Dement. 2013; 9(1): 12–8.
46. Berlau DJ, Corrada MM, Head E, Kawas CH. APOE epsilon2 is associated with intact cognition but increased Alzheimer pathology in the oldest old. Neurology. 2009; 72(9): 829–34.

47. Launer LJ, Ross GW, Petrovitch H, et al. Midlife blood pressure and dementia: the Honolulu Asia Aging Study. Neurobiol Aging. 2000; 21(1): 49–55.
48. Kivipelto M, Helkala EL, Laakso MP, et al. Midlife vascular risk factors and Alzheimer's disease in later life: longitudinal, population based study. BMJ. 2001; 322(7300): 1447–51.
49. Yamada M, Kasagi F, Sasaki H, Masunari N, Mimori Y, Suzuki G. Association between dementia and midlife risk factors: the Radiation Effects Research Foundation Adult Health Study. J Am Geriatr Soc. 2003; 51(3): 410–14.
50. Whitmer RA, Sidney S, Selby J, Johnston SC, Yaffe K. Midlife cardiovascular risk factors and risk of dementia in late life. Neurology. 2005; 64(2): 277–81.
51. Li G, Rhew IC, Shofer JB, et al. Age-varying association between blood pressure and risk of dementia in those aged 65 and older: a community-based prospective cohort study. J Am Geriatr Soc. 2007; 55(8): 1161–7.
52. Ruitenberg A, Skoog I, Ott A, et al. Blood pressure and risk of dementia: results from the Rotterdam study and the Gothenburg H-70 Study. Dement Geriatr Cogn Disord. 2001; 12(1): 33–9.
53. Qiu C, Winblad B, Fratiglioni L. Low diastolic pressure and risk of dementia in very old people: a longitudinal study. Dement Geriatr Cogn Disord. 2009; 28(3): 213–19.
54. Corrada MM, Hayden KM, Paganini-Hill A, et al. Age of onset of hypertension and risk of dementia in the oldest-old: The 90+ Study. Alzheimer's Dement. 2017; 13(2): 103–10.
55. Mielke MM, Zandi PP, Shao H, et al. The 32-year relationship between cholesterol and dementia from midlife to late life. Neurology. 2010; 75(21): 1888–95.
56. Evans M, Kawas CH, Bullain SS, Corrada MM. Cholesterol, statins and the risk of dementia in the oldest-old: the 90+ Study. Neurology. 2014; 82(10 Supplement): S58.003.
57. Mielke MM, Zandi PP, Sjogren M, et al. High total cholesterol levels in late life associated with a reduced risk of dementia. Neurology. 2005; 64(10): 1689–95.
58. Skoog J, Backman K, Ribbe M, et al. A longitudinal study of the Mini-Mental State Examination in late nonagenarians and its relationship with dementia, mortality, and education. J Am Geriatr Soc. 2017; 65(6): 1296–300.
59. Schneider JA, Aggarwal NT, Barnes L, Boyle P, Bennett DA. The neuropathology of older persons with and without dementia from community versus clinic cohorts. J Alzheimer's Dis. 2009; 18(3): 691–701.
60. Jellinger KA, Attems J. Prevalence of dementia disorders in the oldest-old: an autopsy study. Acta Neuropathol. 2010; 119(4): 421–33.
61. Nelson PT, Head E, Schmitt FA, et al. Alzheimer's disease is not 'brain aging': neuropathological, genetic, and epidemiological human studies. Acta Neuropathol. 2011; 121(5): 571–87.
62. Kawas CH, Kim RC, Sonnen JA, Bullain SS, Trieu T, Corrada MM. Multiple pathologies are common and related to dementia in the oldest-old: the 90+ Study. Neurology. 2015; 85(6): 535–42.
63. Consensus recommendations for the postmortem diagnosis of Alzheimer's disease. The National Institute on Aging, and Reagan Institute Working Group on Diagnostic Criteria for the Neuropathological Assessment of Alzheimer's Disease. Neurobiol Aging. 1997; 18(4 Suppl): S1–12.
64. Braak H, Braak E. Frequency of stages of Alzheimer-related lesions in different age categories. Neurobiol Aging. 1997; 18(4): 351–7.
65. Savva GM, Wharton SB, Ince PG, Forster G, Matthews FE, Brayne C. Age, neuropathology, and dementia. N Engl J Med. 2009; 360(22): 2302–9.
66. Neltner JH, Abner EL, Jicha GA, et al. Brain pathologies in extreme old age. Neurobiol Aging. 2016; 37: 1–11.
67. Brayne C, Richardson K, Matthews FE, et al. Neuropathological correlates of dementia in over-80-year-old brain donors from the population-based Cambridge City over-75s cohort (CC75C) Study. J Alzheimer's Dis. 2009; 18(3): 645–58.
68. Smith EE, Schneider JA, Wardlaw JM, Greenberg SM. Cerebral microinfarcts: the invisible lesions. Lancet Neurology. 2012; 11(3): 272–82.
69. Sonnen JA, Larson EB, Crane PK, et al. Pathological correlates of dementia in a longitudinal, population-based sample of aging. Ann Neurol. 2007; 62(4): 406–13.
70. Imhof A, Kovari E, von Gunten A, et al. Morphological substrates of cognitive decline in nonagenarians and centenarians: a new paradigm? J Neurol Sci. 2007; 257(1–2): 72–9.
71. Sinka L, Kovari E, Gold G, et al. Small vascular and Alzheimer disease-related pathologic determinants of dementia in the oldest-old. J Neuropathol Exp Neurol. 2010; 69(12): 1247–55.
72. Ubhi K, Peng K, Lessig S, et al. Neuropathology of dementia with Lewy bodies in advanced age: a comparison with Alzheimer disease. Neurosci Lett. 2010; 485(3): 222–7.
73. Jellinger KA, Attems J. Prevalence and pathology of dementia with Lewy bodies in the oldest old: a comparison with other dementing disorders. Dement Geriatr Cogn Disord. 2011; 31(4): 309–16.
74. White L, Petrovitch H, Hardman J, et al. Cerebrovascular pathology and dementia in autopsied Honolulu-Asia Aging Study participants. Ann N Y Acad Sci. 2002; 977: 9–23.
75. Corrada MM, Sonnen JA, Kim RC, Kawas CH. Microinfarcts are common and strongly related to dementia in the oldest-old: the 90+ study. Alzheimer's Dement. 2016; 12(8): 900–8.
76. White L, Small BJ, Petrovitch H, et al. Recent clinical-pathologic research on the causes of dementia in late life: update from the Honolulu-Asia Aging Study. J Geriatr Psychiatry Neurol. 2005; 18(4): 224–7.
77. Schneider JA, Arvanitakis Z, Bang W, Bennett DA. Mixed brain pathologies account for most dementia cases in community-dwelling older persons. Neurology. 2007; 69(24): 2197–2204.
78. James BD, Bennett DA, Boyle PA, Leurgans S, Schneider JA. Dementia from Alzheimer disease and mixed pathologies in the oldest old. JAMA. 2012; 307(17): 1798–800.
79. Gelber RP, Launer LJ, White LR. The Honolulu-Asia Aging Study: epidemiologic and neuropathologic research on cognitive impairment. Curr Alzheimer Res. 2012; 9(6): 664–72.
80. White LR, Edland SD, Hemmy LS, et al. Neuropathologic comorbidity and cognitive impairment in the Nun and Honolulu-Asia Aging Studies. Neurology. 2016; 86(11): 1000–8.
81. Crystal HA, Dickson D, Davies P, Masur D, Grober E, Lipton RB. The relative frequency of 'dementia of unknown etiology' increases with age and is nearly 50% in nonagenarians. Arch Neurol. 2000; 57(5): 713–19.
82. Corrada MM, Berlau DJ, Kawas CH. A population-based clinicopathological study in the oldest-old: the 90+ Study. Curr Alzheimer Res. 2012; 9(6): 709–17.
83. Polvikoski T, Sulkava R, Myllykangas L, et al. Prevalence of Alzheimer's disease in very elderly people: a prospective neuropathological study. Neurology. 2001; 56(12): 1690–6.
84. Oinas M, Polvikoski T, Sulkava R, et al. Neuropathologic findings of dementia with Lewy bodies (DLB) in a population-based Vantaa 85+ study. J Alzheimer's Dis. 2009; 18(3): 677–89.

85. White L. Brain lesions at autopsy in older Japanese-American men as related to cognitive impairment and dementia in the final years of life: a summary report from the Honolulu-Asia aging study. J Alzheimer's Dis. 2009; 18(3): 713–25.
86. Latimer CS, Keene CD, Flanagan ME, et al. Resistance to Alzheimer disease neuropathologic changes and apparent cognitive resilience in the Nun and Honolulu-Asia Aging Studies. J Neuropathol Exp Neurol. 2017; 76(6): 458–66.
87. Haroutunian V, Schnaider-Beeri M, Schmeidler J, et al. Role of the neuropathology of Alzheimer disease in dementia in the oldest-old. Arch Neurol. 2008; 65(9): 1211–17.
88. Brookmeyer R, Kawas CH, Abdallah N, Paganini-Hill A, Kim RC, Corrada MM. Impact of interventions to reduce Alzheimer's disease pathology on the prevalence of dementia in the oldest-old. Alzheimer's Dement. 2016; 12(3): 225–32.
89. Alzheimer's Association. Alzheimer's disease facts and figures. Alzheimer's Dement. 2016; 12(4): 459–509.
90. Poon LW, Jazwinski M, Green RC, et al. Methodological considerations in studying centenarians: lessons learned from the Georgia Centenarian Studies. Annu Rev Gerontol Geriatr. 2007; 27(1): 231–64.
91. Brumback-Peltz C, Balasubramanian AB, Corrada MM, Kawas CH. Diagnosing dementia in the oldest-old. Maturitas. 2011; 70(2): 164–8.
92. Slavin MJ, Brodaty H, Sachdev PS. Challenges of diagnosing dementia in the oldest old population. J Gerontol A Biol Sci Med Sci. 2013; 68(9): 1103–11.
93. van Veluw SJ, Shih AY, Smith EE, et al. Detection, risk factors, and functional consequences of cerebral microinfarcts. Lancet Neurol. 2017; 16(9): 730–40.

SECTION 4
Vascular disorders

19

Global stroke burden and prevention strategies

Findings from GBD 2015

Rita Krishnamurthi and Valery L Feigin

Introduction

The global impact of stroke is high and increasing. Stroke is the second major cause of death and disability globally.[1,2] Approximately 20% of incident stroke results in death within the first month.[3] Of those who survive, approximately 30% will be left with permanent disabilities ranging from mild to moderate, and another 20–25% will experience another stroke,[4] although these figures vary depending on stroke subtype, and demographic factors such as age, sex, ethnicity, and geographic location.[5–7] The most common forms of disability after stroke include: one-sided paralysis, leading to difficulty in walking and self-care; speech impairment; visual impairment; cognitive impairment, including memory loss; and mood disturbances such as anxiety and depression.[8]

Quantifying the burden of stroke and temporal trends by regions and countries, as well as understanding the relative impact and contribution of risk factors to stroke burden is important for planning evidence-based stroke care, education, and prevention strategies, as well as directing the appropriate allocation of resources where they are needed. This chapter presents the findings of the most recent stroke burden over all and in terms of burden attributable to potentially modifiable risk factors from GBD 2015. The estimates are derived from (https://vizhub.healthdata.org/gbd-compare/) and http://ghdx.healthdata.org/gbd-results-tool.

Global Stroke Burden: GBD 2015

The GBD 2015 studies use a revised indicator of socioeconomic status, termed the sociodemographic index (SDI).[2] The SDI is derived from income per capita, average educational attainment in the population of those over 15, and total fertility rate. Fig. 19.1 shows the distribution of global SDI quintiles at national and some sub-national levels.[2] Most countries that are traditionally described as developed or HICs have the highest SDI, while those traditionally described as LICs have the lowest SDI. However, countries with high income, such as some Middle Eastern countries fall into a lower SDI quintile due to lower educational attainment and higher fertility rates.

Stroke Pathology, Subtypes and Ischaemic Stroke Subtypes

Stroke is a heterogeneous disease that occurs as a result of disruption of blood flow to the brain. The World Health Organization (WHO) defines stroke as 'rapidly developed clinical signs of local (or global) disturbance of cerebral function, lasting more than 24 hours or leading to death, with no apparent cause other than of vascular origin'.[9] The majority (approximately 80%) of strokes are ischaemic, resulting from the blockage of one or more blood vessels, while 20% of strokes are haemorrhagic, resulting from the rupture of blood vessels in the brain (intracerebral haemorrhage) or in the subarachnoid space surrounding the brain (subarachnoid haemorrhage). The symptoms, outcomes, and prognosis can vary depending on which pathological type of stroke has occurred. In addition, the causes and risk factors of stroke vary by subtype. For this reason, it is important to study stroke burden by its pathological type. At this stage of the GBD study development, intracerebral haemorrhage, and subarachnoid haemorrhage are combined into one category called haemorrhagic stroke. Stroke burden can be studied in terms of incidence (occurrence of first-ever-in-a-lifetime stroke), prevalence (the proportion of people living with stroke), mortality (death rates), and DALYs, derived from the sum of years of life lost (YLL) due to premature mortality and the years lost due to disability (YLD).[10]

Previous GBD studies have shown that the prevalence of stroke increased significantly between 1990 and 2010.[11] Most strokes occurred in developing countries, with prevalence of stroke increasing in developing countries between 1990 and 2010. While incidence, mortality, and DALY rates declined during this period, the absolute numbers of strokes, deaths, and DALYs increased significantly,

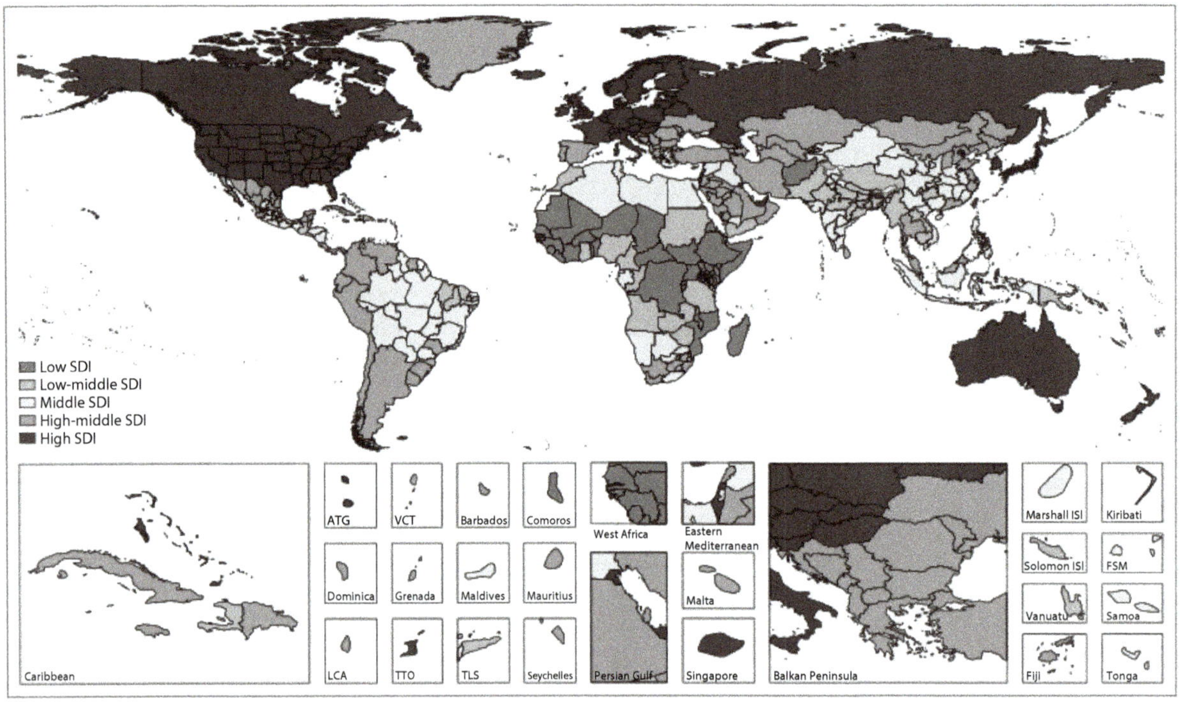

Fig. 19.1 Global distribution of SDI quintiles.

Reproduced from Wang HW, et al. Global, regional, and national life expectancy, all-cause mortality, and cause-specific mortality for 249 causes of death, 1980–2015: a systematic analysis for the Global Burden of Disease Study 2015. *The Lancet*, 388(10053): 1459–544. Copyright © 2016 The Author(s). Published by Elsevier Ltd. Distributed under the terms of the Creative Commons Attribution 4.0 International (CC BY 4.0). https://creativecommons.org/licenses/by/4.0/

particularly in those over 85 years of age. The incidence of haemorrhagic stroke had also increased significantly, with an 18.5% increase seen between 1990 and 2010.[12]

GBD 2015 Findings

The previous GBD findings have since been updated and are presented as GBD 2015 findings in the following sections.

Prevalence

In 2015 there were over 42 million prevalent strokes globally, compared to just over 26 million in 1990. Both the absolute numbers, and rates of prevalent stroke were highest in high SDI countries (over 9.5 million strokes, 741 per 100,000) compared to low SDI countries (2.1 million strokes, 391.5 per 100,000). The global prevalence of stroke varied by SDI region and country. Fig. 19.2 shows the global distribution of stroke prevalence per 100,000. Highest prevalence rates were seen in Russia, Ukraine, and surrounding countries to the east, followed by, Japan, Mongolia, Kazakhstan, China, and the UK, with the lowest in Mexico.

The prevalence of stroke in absolute numbers has increased globally since 1990. While numbers of prevalent strokes were lowest in low SDI regions, there was an approximate two-fold increase in numbers between 1990 and 2015. Middle SDI regions had the highest proportion of prevalent strokes.

Incidence

Globally there were over 8.9 million incident strokes in 2015. The highest number of incident strokes occurred in middle and high-middle SDI countries, and the lowest in low SDI countries. The global age-standardized incidence rates of stroke per 100,000 for 1990, and 2015 are shown in Table 19.1. The incidence rates of stroke were 2.5-fold higher in low SDI countries compared to high SDI countries in 2015, and this disparity had increased since 1990.

Ischaemic versus haemorrhagic stroke

The global age-standardized incidence rate of ischaemic stroke was 83.8 per 100,000 and for haemorrhagic stroke was 52.9 per 100,000 in 2015. Fig. 19.2 and 19.3 show temporal trends in incidence rates for the ischaemic and haemorrhagic stroke. Large disparities were seen, with incidence rates in low SDI being 5–6-fold higher than the highest SDI regions. The incidence of both subtypes of stroke has steadily reduced globally and in high SDI regions, but has remained high or even increased in low SDI regions since 1990. While the incidence rates of haemorrhagic strokes across all SDI quintiles was lower, the temporal and SDI patterns were similar to those for ischaemic stroke (Fig. 19.3).

Mortality

Globally there were over 6.3 million deaths due to stroke in 2015, with 53% of deaths due to haemorrhagic stroke. As shown in Fig. 19.4 age-standardized mortality rates were lowest in high SDI countries and declined sharply, particularly from 2000 to 2015. In contrast, low and low-middle SDI mortality rates were approximately 1.5-fold higher and did not decline as rapidly as high SDI regions. Globally, mortality rates for males and females were similar, but in high SDI, the rate in males was 26% higher than in females (Fig. 19.5).

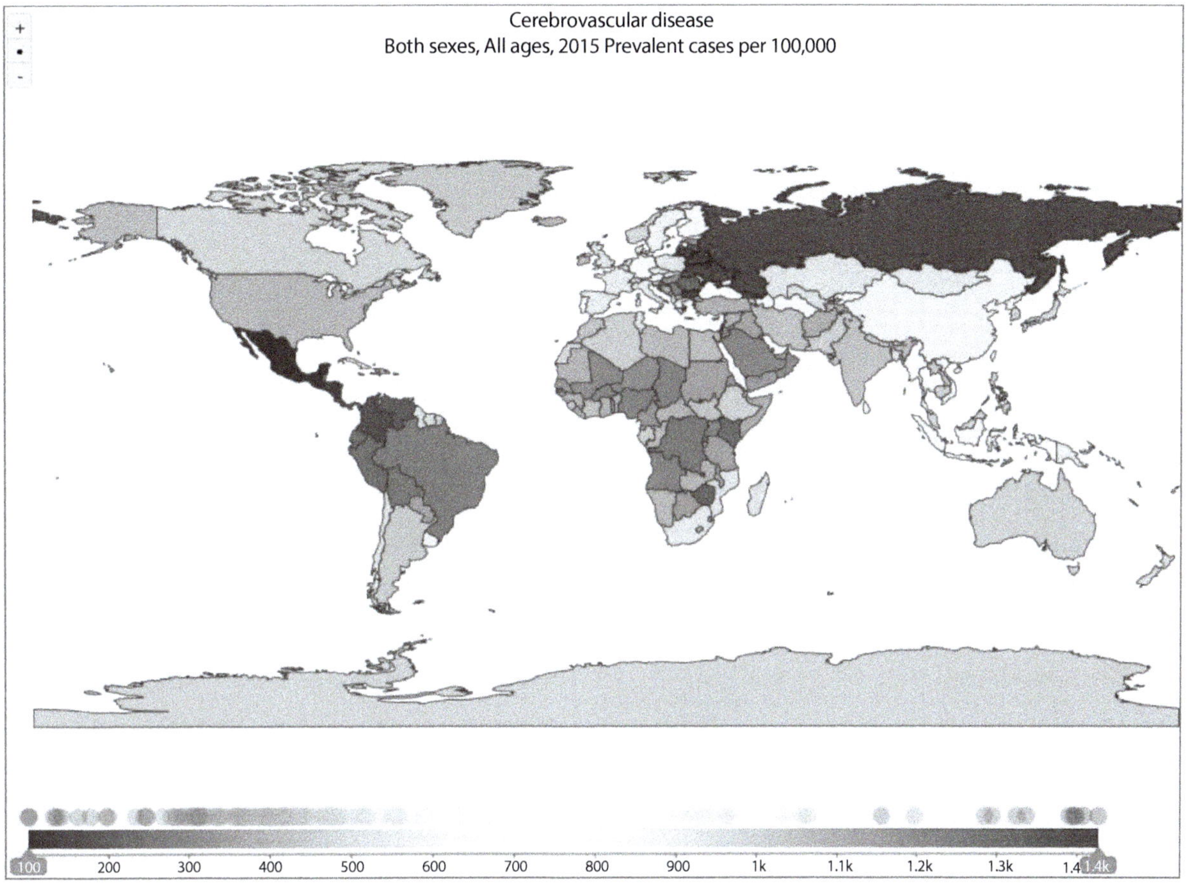

Fig. 19.2 Global stroke prevalence in 2015.

DALYs

There were over 118 million DALYs attributed to cerebrovascular disease in 2015, compared to just over 97 million in 1990. Absolute numbers of DALYs attributable to haemorrhagic stroke were 1.6-fold higher than that for ischaemic stroke globally and in low SDI countries, DALYs were 2.2-fold higher. In absolute numbers the highest proportion (35%) of DALYs associated with stroke were seen in middle SDI regions, and the lowest in low SDI regions (5.6%). In 2015, the highest DALY rates were seen in low SDI regions, and the lowest rates were in high SDI regions (Fig. 19.6). Both high and high-middle SDI regions have had a sharp decline in DALY rates since 1990, while the reductions in low and middle SDI regions were less prominent.

Prevalence of stroke risk factors

The GBD 2015 data also described the global distribution of DALYs attributable to 17 modifiable risk factors for stroke. Fig. 19.7 shows

Table 19.1 Temporal trends in stroke incidence rates, per 100,000

Year	Location	Incidence rates	95% CI
1990	Low SDI	206.27	218.6–193.1
1990	Global	173.98	182.2–165.7
1990	High SDI	126.13	132.2–120.6
2015	Global	136.83	143.5–130.1
2015	Low SDI	203.93	218.4–189.6
2015	High SDI	81.26	85.3–77.6

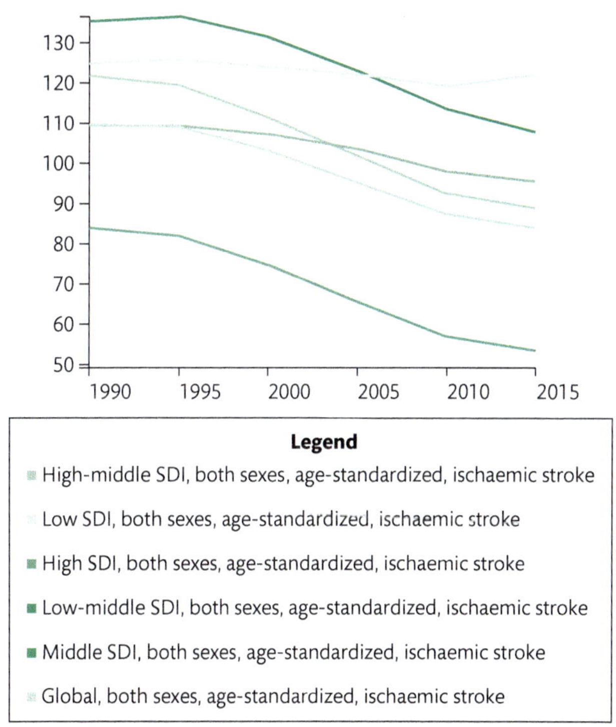

Fig. 19.3 Incidence rates of ischaemic stroke by SDI (per 100,000).

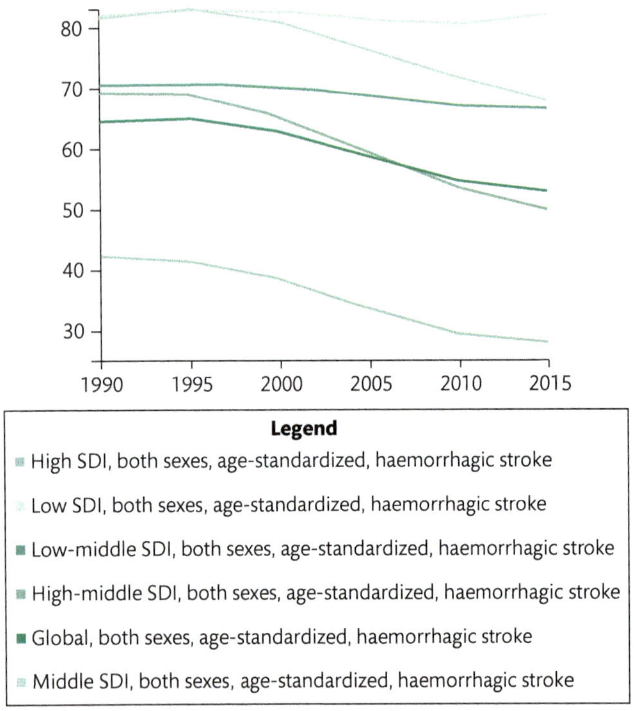

Fig. 19.4 Incidence rates of haemorrhagic stroke by SDI (per 100,000).

the DALYs attributed to risk factors in 21 regions in 2013.[13] The contribution of high blood pressure and smoking to increased DALY rates was greatest in Russia and other Eastern European countries, while air pollution contributed most to increased DALYs in Central, East, and West Africa and Asia. Fewer DALYs were attributed to a diet low in fruits, and this was prominent mainly on Russia, and South-East Asia.

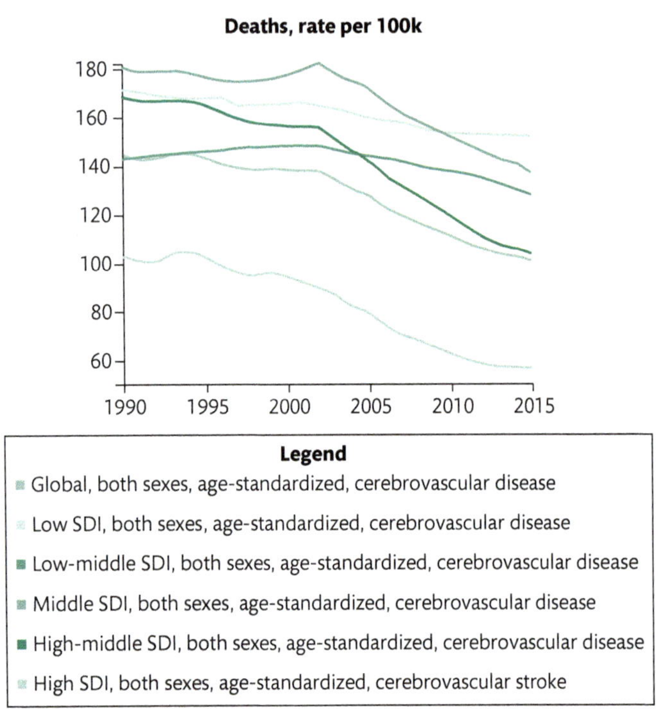

Fig. 19.5 Global stroke death rates by SDI regions (per 100,000).

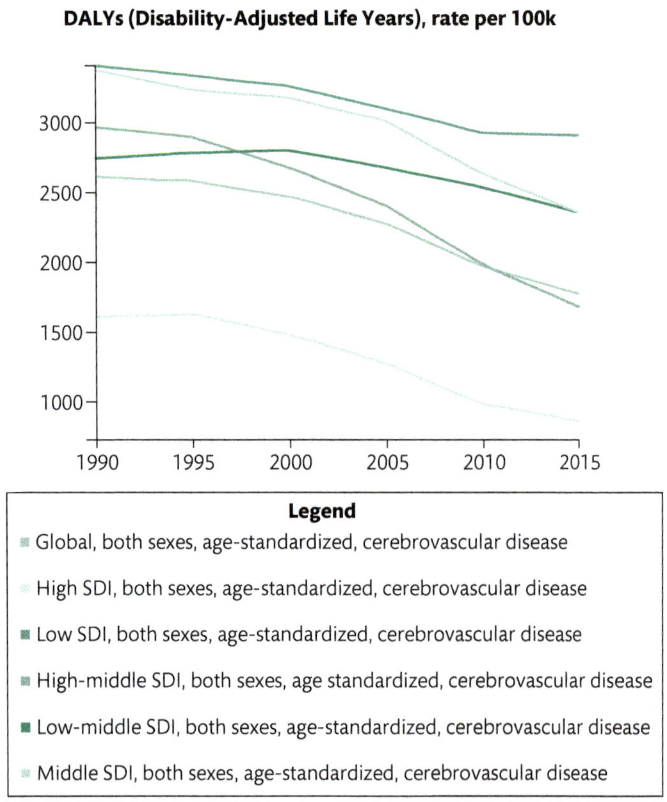

Fig. 19.6 DALY rates of stroke by SDI (per 100,000).

Fig. 19.8 shows the global trends in death rates attributed to major stroke risk factors. High blood pressure had the greatest impact on death rates, but a decline was seen from 1990 to 2015 in death rates due to high blood pressure. Other risk factors contributing to stroke deaths were air pollution, a diet high in sodium, a diet low in fruits, and tobacco smoking. The relative contribution of these risk factors to stroke deaths was approximately 2–3-fold lower than that of high blood pressure.

In 2013 (Fig. 19.7) globally, systolic blood pressure was consistently ranked the number 1 risk factor attributable to 64.1% of DALYs, followed by the diet low in fruits, high body mass index (BMI) (apart from Asia), and a diet high in sodium.[13,14] However, the study found significant geographical variation in the population attributable fraction of risk factors. In particular, air pollution had a significantly greater impact on stroke burden in eastern, western, and central sub-Saharan Africa, than in North America, Europe, Australasia, and high-income Asia Pacific countries.[13]

Sex differences in stroke burden

By GBD 2015 estimates, stroke incidence and mortality rates were higher in males than in females across all age groups, and overall (Table 19.2 and Table 19.3). Age-standardized incidence rates were significantly higher in males than in females. The same trend was seen separately for DALYs by stroke subtypes, with haemorrhagic stroke DALYs 1.4-fold higher and ischaemic stroke DALYs cases 1.2-fold higher in males than females. Similarly, mortality rates in males were significantly higher than in females across all age groups. The age-standardized mortality rate in males was 30% higher in males. Mortality rates in both males and females increased significantly with increasing age.

Rank: 1–5; 6–10; 11–15; >15

Risk factor	Global	High-income Asia pacific	Western Europe	Australasia	High-income North America	Central Europe	Southern Latin America	Eastern Europe	East Asia	Tropical Latin America	Central Latin America	South-East Asia	Central Asia	Andean Latin America	North Africa and Middle East	Caribbean	South Asia	Oceania	Southern sub-Saharan Africa	Eastern sub-Saharan Africa	Central sub-Saharan Africa	Western sub-Saharan Africa
High systolic blood pressure	1	1	1	1	1	1	1	1	1	1	1	1	1	1	1	1	1	1	1	1	1	1
Diet low in fruits	2	2	4	4	3	4	4	3	2	3	4	2	2	3	3	3	2	3	2	2	2	2
High body-mass index	3	6	2	2	2	2	2	2	6	2	2	6	3	2	2	2	8	2	3	5	5	4
Diet high in sodium	4	3	6	10	6	3	8	6	3	4	8	8	4	7	4	12	5	13	7	9	11	8
Smoking	5	4	5	5	5	6	5	5	4	6	6	4	6	6	8	5	7	5	5	8	10	12
Diet low in vegetables	6	5	3	3	4	5	3	4	11	5	3	3	5	4	5	4	4	4	4	4	4	5
Ambient particulate matter (2.5 μm) pollution	7	8	11	14	12	8	12	10	5	9	9	9	8	9	6	11	6	15	11	12	6	6
Household air pollution from solid fuels	8	..	..	..	..	..	15	..	7	14	12	5	12	11	14	7	3	6	8	3	3	3
Diet low in whole grains	9	7	9	8	9	7	6	7	8	7	5	7	7	5	7	6	10	7	10	10	7	9
High fasting plasma glucose	10	10	10	9	7	11	7	9	9	8	7	10	9	10	9	10	9	8	9	11	8	11
Low physical activity	11	9	8	6	8	10	11	11	13	11	13	11	13	12	10	8	12	9	13	14	12	10
Low glomerular filtration rate	12	12	7	7	13	9	10	12	14	10	10	14	10	8	11	9	11	12	6	7	9	7
Alcohol use	13	11	12	11	10	12	9	8	12	12	11	15	11	14	16	15	15	11	12	13	14	14
Lead exposure	14	14	14	13	15	14	16	15	10	15	16	12	14	15	13	13	13	14	14	6	13	13
High total Cholesterol	15	13	13	12	11	13	13	13	16	13	14	13	15	13	12	14	14	10	15	15	15	15
Second-hand smoke	16	15	15	15	16	15	14	14	15	16	17	16	16	17	15	17	16	16	16	16	16	16
Diet high in sugar-sweetened beverages	17	16	16	16	14	16	17	16	17	17	15	17	17	16	17	16	17	17	17	17	17	17

Fig. 19.7 DALYs attributable to risk factors in 21 regions, from GBD 2013.

Reproduced with permission from Feigin V.L. et al. Global burden of stroke and risk factors in 188 countries, during 1990–2013: a systematic analysis for the Global Burden of Disease Study 2013. *The Lancet*. 2016 Aug; 15(9): 913–924. DOI:https://doi.org/10.1016/S1474-4422(16)30073-4.

When comparing sex differences in stroke burden by SDI quintiles, differences between males and females in both burden and temporal trends emerge (Fig. 19.9). DALYs in females decreased with increasing SDI, while in males this drop was only seen in the high SDI group. Moreover, DALYs were lower in females than males, except in low SDI countries. The greatest differences were seen in middle and high-middle countries, where DALY rates in males were much higher (by 995 and 890 DALYs per 100,000 per annum respectively).

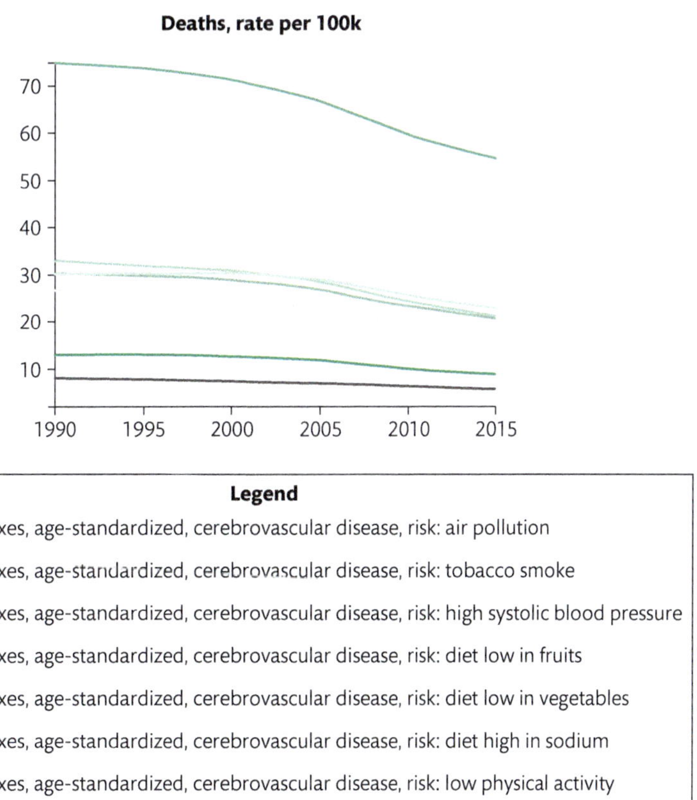

Fig. 19.8 Trends in stroke deaths attributed to risk factors (per 100,000).

Table 19.2 Global incidence rates in males and females, per 100,000

	Age group	Incidence rate	95% CI	
Females	15–49 years	23.34	25.62	21.2
Males	15–49 years	32.06	35.12	29.34
Females	50–69 years	226.42	244.59	208.23
Males	50–69 years	321.33	345.75	297.05
Females	70+ years	968.78	1035.67	903.84
Males	70+ years	1018.93	1089.69	949.43
Females	Age-standardized	123.03	129.25	116.92
Males	Age-standardized	151.3	158.54	143.87

Mortality rates follow a similar pattern, where mortality rates are higher in females in low SDI countries, while death rates in males are higher, particularly in middle and low-middle SDI countries. The difference in mortality rates between males and females was greatest in middle and high-middle SDI countries (Table 19.3).

Conversely, incidence rates decreased with increasing SDI quintiles, with the lowest incidence rates for both males and females seen in the high SDI countries. The incidence rate for females was again higher than for males in low SDI countries, but not in the other SDI quintiles. As with mortality and DALY rates the greatest difference in incidence rates was seen in middle and HMICs.

Table 19.3 Global mortality rates in males and females, per 100,000

	Age group	Mortality rate	95% CI	
Females	15–49 years	8.45	9.07	7.93
Males	15–49 years	14.26	15.03	13.48
Females	50–69 years	112.41	118.14	107.41
Males	50–69 years	177.96	185.36	170.8
Females	70+ years	974.59	1005.01	946.88
Males	70+ years	1077.21	1112.91	1047.24
Females	Age-standardized	88.28	91.32	85.62
Males	Age-standardized	115.61	119.54	112.15

Prevention Strategies

The risk factors for stroke are classed as modifiable and non-modifiable. The most important non-modifiable risk factor for stroke are age and sex, as increasing age and being a male significantly increase the risk of stroke.[15,16] Race or ethnicity is another non-modifiable risk factor for stroke, with Black Americans, Asians, and Pacific Islanders tending to have a higher risk of stroke than those of European or white ethnicity; non-white Hispanics have a lower risk of stroke compared to White Americans.[17]

Despite the contribution of non-modifiable risk factors, stroke is potentially highly preventable, with the control of contributing modifiable risk factors. The INTERSTROKE studies found that 90% of strokes are attributable to ten potentially modifiable risk factors: history of high blood pressure, low physical activity, apolipoprotein ratio, unhealthy diet, psychosocial factors, waist to hip ratio, current smoking, cardiac causes, alcohol consumption, and diabetes mellitus.[18,19] These factors contributed to stroke risk consistently across regions, sex, and age groups. However, the study also found important variations in the susceptibility and relative significance of these risk factors by geographical location and race/ethnicity. This suggests that the relative significance of risk factors for stroke need to be studied at national levels, and by race and ethnicity where appropriate. Knowledge of geographic and race/ethnic specific significance of risk factors will inform more appropriate and effective primary prevention strategies in individual nations.

Stroke prevention needs to be a priority due to the enormity of its burden on individuals, families, and healthcare systems. Given that stroke is highly preventable, strategies for primary prevention must be a priority. There are two main currently used primary stroke prevention strategies: (1) high-risk, and (2) population-wide strategies.

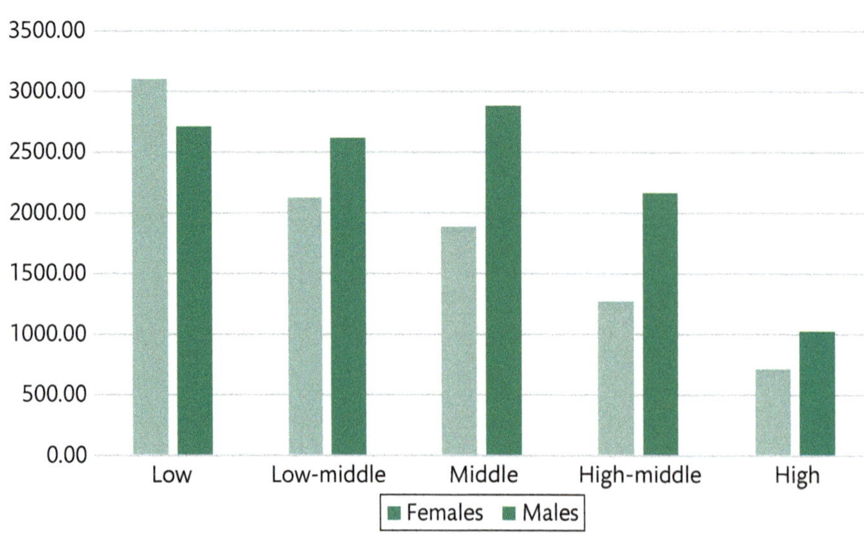

Fig. 19.9 Sex differences in DALY rates by SDI quintiles (per 100,000).

High-risk strategies

High-risk strategies are aimed at those individuals who are at a high risk of stroke and cardiovascular disease (usually defined as five-year risk ≥15%). This strategy may target multiple risk factors, and therefore is cost effective compared to strategies targeting single risk factors, especially if facilitated through primary healthcare services. The high-risk strategy for primary stroke prevention includes screening individuals to identify those with high absolute cardiovascular risk (including people with previous stroke/TIA or cardiovascular events), and prescription of medications for high blood pressure, diabetes, high cholesterol, and blood-thinning medications in the case of those with atrial fibrillation. Counselling for behaviour modification, such as stopping or reducing smoking and alcohol intake, increasing physical activity and eating a healthy, balanced diet are also recommended. However high-risk strategies need to be widely used, in order to have a significant impact.[14,20]

Population-wide strategies

Population-wide strategies aim to shift the overall risk in an entire population or community, through changes in health policy, legislation, economic measures, or education.[21] Common approaches for population-wide strategies are increased taxes on tobacco and sugary drinks, legislation to reduce sodium content in manufactured foods, and restricting sales of unhealthy foods in public canteens such as in schools and hospitals.[22] Several countries have successfully implemented these strategies by introducing taxes on tobacco, alcohol, and sugar.[23–26] Population-wide strategies have several advantages in that they are effective on whole populations at any level of risk, and focus determinants of risk factor distribution and not just the treatment of risk factors.[20]

Primary stroke prevention in low-middle SDI countries

As shown in Fig. 19.2 and 19.3, stroke incidence rates are highest in low and low-middle SDI countries, and these rates have not reduced significantly in the last three decades. Hence primary prevention of stroke is imperative in these regions. Significant disparities in stroke incidence rates and temporal trends have been previously shown, with incidence rates decreased in HICs by 42%, but increased by more than 100% in LMICs between 1970 and 2008.[27] These are likely to be a result of increases in prevalence of risk factors such as unhealthy diets and more sedentary lifestyles, leading to increased hypertension and diabetes, as shown in China,[28] and other regions.[29,30] Apart from the health-related burden of stroke, LICs and LMICs suffer a huge economic burden from stroke. For example, in China, the cost of hospital admissions for stroke is twice the yearly income of rural dwellers.[28]

There are several strategies that can be utilized to reduce the burden on stroke in low and low-middle SDI countries.[31] These include using STEPS Stroke, a surveillance approach recommended by the World Health Organization that has been shown to be feasible in LICs, where ideal population-based studies are difficult to conduct.[32] Screening, particularly at primary care level, is recommended as an effective means to identify individuals at increased risk of stroke, and for providing the opportunity to prescribe medications and offer lifestyle advice to reduce risk. Importantly, increasing the awareness of stroke, ways to control modifiable risk factors, including atrial fibrillation,[33] to reduce risk, are crucial in low SDI countries where awareness of, and therefore access to, preventative and post-stroke healthcare is particularly low.[34,35] The World Stroke Organization Global Stroke Services Guidelines and Action Plan is a clinical practice guideline that provides recommendations to augment stroke awareness, prevention, and treatment across the globe.[36] These guidelines also recommend action plans for those in low income regions with minimal resources to improve their outcomes.

Summary of Main Findings of GBD 2015

The GBD 2015 data provide the most recently updated estimates of stroke burden, and estimates of potentially modifiable risk factors attributable to stroke burden. These data show that in 2015 there remain disparities in stroke incidence rates by SDI. While incidence rates have shown a decline in other regions since 1990, this was not the case for low SDI countries. Females endure the greatest burden of stroke in low SDI countries. This disparity may be related to poorer access to preventative healthcare for females in poorer countries, combined with a greater exposure to household pollution, and increased psychosocial stress, and requires further investigation. Mortality rates have also remained high in low and low-middle SDI countries, and have surpassed rates in middle SDI countries, particularly since 2005. Low to middle SDI countries had the greatest burden of stroke in terms of DALY rates, with little change in these disparities seen since 1990.

The most significant modifiable risk factor contributing to stroke burden by far was high systolic blood pressure. The importance of a diet high in sodium and low in fruits unsurprisingly remained as the next most important contributors to stroke burden. A reduction in salt intake is associated with a reduction in blood pressure.[37,38] A recent meta-analysis found an association of high dietary fibre intake from fruits, vegetables, cereals, and water-soluble fibres with a reduced risk of ischaemic stroke.[39] The declining trend of the observed association of high systolic blood pressure with stroke-related DALYs is likely due to increased prescription and access to medication for hypertension control, particularly in high SDI countries.[40,41]

Conclusions and Future Implications

The GBD 2015 studies confirm previous findings that the global burden of stroke is high and increasing, particularly in countries with lowest income, and education levels but high fertility rates. However, the combined implementation of both ethnic specific population-wide and high-risk stroke prevention strategies has significant potential for reducing stroke incidence, disability, and mortality globally, including in low and low-middle SDI countries.

REFERENCES

1. DALYs GBD, Collaborators H. Global, regional, and national disability-adjusted life-years (DALYs) for 315 diseases and injuries and healthy life expectancy (HALE), 1990–2015: a systematic analysis for the Global Burden of Disease Study 2015. *Lancet.* 2016; 388: 1603–58.
2. Wang H, Naghavi M, Allen C, Barber RM, Bhutta ZA, Carter A, et al. Global, regional, and national life expectancy, all-cause

mortality, and cause-specific mortality for 249 causes of death, 1980–2015: a systematic analysis for the Global Burden of Disease Study 2015. *Lancet*. 2016; 388: 1459–1544.
3. Bamford J, Dennis M, Sandercock P, Burn J, Warlow C. The frequency, causes and timing of death within 30 days of a first stroke: the Oxfordshire Community Stroke Project. *Journal of Neurology, Neurosurgery & Psychiatry*. 1990; 53: 824–9.
4. Hankey GJ. Secondary stroke prevention. *Lancet Neurology*. 2014; 13: 178–94.
5. Ovbiagele B, Nguyen-Huynh MN. Stroke epidemiology: advancing our understanding of disease mechanism and therapy. *Neurotherapeutics*. 2011; 8: 319.
6. Paci M, Nannetti L, Dippolito P, Lombardi B. Outcomes from ischemic stroke subtypes classified by the Oxfordshire Community Stroke Project: a systematic review. *European Journal of Physical and Rehabilitation Medicine*. 2011; 47: 19–23.
7. Wardlaw JM. Differing risk factors and outcomes in ischemic stroke subtypes: Focus on lacunar stroke. *Future Neurology*. 2011; 6: 201–21.
8. Rathore SS, Hinn AR, Cooper LS, Tyroler HA, Rosamond WD. Characterization of incident stroke signs and symptoms. *Stroke*. 2002; 33: 2718–21.
9. Aho K, Harmsen P, Hatano S, Marquardsen J, Smirnov VE, Strasser T. Cerebrovascular disease in the community: results of a WHO collaborative study. *Bulletin of the World Health Organization*. 1980; 58: 113–30.
10. Roth GA, Johnson CO, Nguyen G, Naghavi M, Feigin VL, Murray CJL, et al. Methods for estimating the global burden of cerebrovascular diseases. *Neuroepidemiology*. 2015; 45: 146–51.
11. Lozano R, Naghavi M, Foreman K, Lim S, Shibuya K, Aboyans V, et al. Global and regional mortality from 235 causes of death for 20 age groups in 1990 and 2010: a systematic analysis for the Global Burden of Disease Study 2010. *Lancet*. 2013; 380: 2095–128.
12. Krishnamurthi RV, Moran AE, Forouzanfar MH, Bennett DA, Mensah GA, Lawes CMM, et al. The global burden of hemorrhagic stroke: a summary of findings from the GBD 2010 study. *Global Heart*. 2014; 9: 101–6.
13. Feigin VL, Roth GA, Naghavi M, Parmar P, Krishnamurthi R, Chugh S, et al. Global burden of stroke and risk factors in 188 countries, during 1990–2013: a systematic analysis for the Global Burden of Disease Study 2013. *Lancet Neurology*. 2016; 15: 913–24.
14. Feigin VL, Krishnamurthi R. Stroke is largely preventable across the globe: where to next? *Lancet*. 2016; 388(10046): 733–4.
15. Barker-Collo S, Bennett DA, Krishnamurthi RV, Parmar P, Feigin VL, Naghavi M, et al. Sex differences in stroke incidence, prevalence, mortality and disability-adjusted life years: Results from the global burden of disease study 2013. *Neuroepidemiology*. 2015; 45: 203–14.
16. Feigin VL, Forouzanfar MH, Krishnamurthi R, Mensah GA, Connor M, Bennett DA, et al. Global and regional burden of stroke during 1990–2010: Findings from the Global Burden of Disease Study 2010. *Lancet*. 2014; 383: 245–55.
17. Mozaffarian D, Benjamin EJ, Go AS, Arnett DK, Blaha MJ, Cushman M, et al. Executive summary: heart disease and stroke statistics—2016 update: a report from the American Heart Association. *Circulation*. 2016; 133: 447–54.
18. O'Donnell MJ, Xavier D, Liu L, Zhang H, Chin SL, Rao-Melacini P, et al. Risk factors for ischaemic and intracerebral haemorrhagic stroke in 22 countries (the INTERSTROKE study): a case-control study. *Lancet*. 2010; 376: 112–23.
19. O'Donnell MJ, Chin SL, Rangarajan S, Xavier D, Liu L, Zhang H, et al. Global and regional effects of potentially modifiable risk factors associated with acute stroke in 32 countries (INTERSTROKE): a case-control study. *Lancet*. 2016; 388: 761–75.
20. Emberson J, Whincup P, Morris R, Walker M, Ebrahim S. Evaluating the impact of population and high-risk strategies for the primary prevention of cardiovascular disease. *European Heart Journal*. 2004; 25: 484–91.
21. Gorelick PB, Farooq MU, Min J. Population-based approaches for reducing stroke risk. *Exp Rev Cardiovasc Ther*. 2015; 13: 49–56.
22. Appel LJ, Frohlich ED, Hall JE, Pearson TA, Sacco RL, Seals DR, et al. The importance of population-wide sodium reduction as a means to prevent cardiovascular disease and stroke. *Circulation*. 2011; 123: 1138–43.
23. Asma S, Warren W, Althomsons S, Wisotzky M, Woollery T, Henson R. Addressing the chronic disease burden with tobacco control programs. *Public Health Rep*. 2004; 119: 253–62.
24. Dilley JA, Harris JR, Boysun MJ, Reid TR. Program, policy, and price interventions for tobacco control: Quantifying the return on investment of a state tobacco control program. *American Journal of Public Health*. 2012; 102(2): e22–8.
25. Verguet S, Gauvreau CL, Mishra S, MacLennan M, Murphy SM, Brouwer ED, et al. The consequences of tobacco tax on household health and finances in rich and poor smokers in China: an extended cost-effectiveness analysis. *Lancet Global Health*. 2015; 3: 206–16.
26. Sánchez-Romero LM, Penko J, Coxson PG, Fernández A, Mason A, Moran AE, et al. Projected impact of Mexico's sugar-sweetened beverage tax policy on diabetes and cardiovascular disease: a modeling study. *PLOS Medicine*. 2016; 13.
27. Feigin VL, Lawes CM, Bennett DA, Barker-Collo SL, Parag V. Worldwide stroke incidence and early case fatality reported in 56 population-based studies: a systematic review. *Lancet Neurology*. 2009; 8: 355–69.
28. Liu L, Wang D, Lawrence Wong KS, Wang Y. Stroke and stroke care in China huge burden, significant workload, and a national priority. *Stroke*. 2011; 42: 3651–4.
29. Gupta R, Joshi P, Mohan V, Reddy KS, Yusuf S. Epidemiology and causation of coronary heart disease and stroke in India. *Heart*. 2008; 94: 16–26.
30. Kaul S, Bandaru VCSS, Suvarna A, Boddu DB. Stroke burden and risk factors in developing countries with special reference to India. *Journal of the Indian Medical Association*. 2009; 107: 358–70.
31. Yan LL, Li C, Chen J, Miranda JJ, Luo R, Bettger J, et al. Prevention, management, and rehabilitation of stroke in low- and middle-income countries. *eNeurological Sci*. 2016; 2: 21–30.
32. Truelsen T, Heuschmann P, Bonita R, Arjundas G, Dalal P, Damasceno A, et al. Standard method for developing stroke registers in low-income and middle-income countries: experiences from a feasibility study of a stepwise approach to stroke surveillance (STEPS Stroke). *Lancet Neurology*. 2007; 6: 134–9.
33. Murphy A, Banerjee A, Breithardt G, Camm AJ, Commerford P, Freedman B, et al. The Word Heart Federation roadmap for nonvalvular atrial fibrillation. *Global Heart*. 2017; 12(4): 273–84.
34. Mehndiratta P, Wasay M, Mehndiratta MM. Implications of female sex on stroke risk factors, care, outcome and rehabilitation: an Asian perspective. *Cerebrovascular Diseases*. 2015; 39: 302–8.

35. Modesti PA, Perruolo E, Parati G. Need for better blood pressure measurement in developing countries to improve prevention of cardiovascular disease. *Journal of Epidemiology*. 2015; 25: 91–8.
36. Lindsay P, Furie KL, Davis SM, Donnan GA, Norrving B. World stroke organization global stroke services guidelines and action plan. *International Journal of Stroke*. 2014; 9: 4–13.
37. Hankey GJ. Nutrition and the risk of stroke. *Lancet Neurology*. 2012; 11: 66–81.
38. He FJ, Pombo-Rodrigues S, MacGregor GA. Salt reduction in England from 2003 to 2011: its relationship to blood pressure, stroke and ischaemic heart disease mortality. *BMJ Open*. 2014; 4(4).
39. Li M, Cui F, Yang F, Huang X. Association between fiber intake and ischemic stroke risk: A meta-analysis of prospective studies. *International Journal of Clinical and Experimental Medicine*. 2017; 10: 4659–68.
40. Luepker RV, Steffen LM, Jacobs DR, Zhou X, Blackburn H. Trends in blood pressure and hypertension detection, treatment, and control 1980 to 2009: the Minnesota Heart Survey. *Circulation*. 2012; 126: 1852–7.
41. Koton S, Eizenberg Y, Tanne D, Grossman E. Trends in admission blood pressure and stroke outcome in patients with acute stroke and transient ischemic attack in a National Acute Stroke registry. *Journal of Hypertension*. 2016; 34: 316–22.

20

Stroke and TIA

Bo Norrving

Introduction

Tackling stroke requires availability of good epidemiological data (incidence, prevalence, case-fatality, and mortality), knowledge of risk factors, and understanding of the best means for prevention and treatment. In the most recent data on the global burden of stroke, it is the second commonest cause of death and the second largest cause of loss of DALYs,[1,2] indicating that stroke is a major global health concern. DALYs is the sum of YLLs) and YLDs.

Stroke is part of the cluster of non-communicable diseases (NCDs) that has increasingly come into focus not only in the medical system, but also among governmental and political bodies, as the world sees substantial changes in the pattern of diseases. In only a few decades, there has been a shift from infectious and nutritional disorders to NCDs such as stroke, heart disease, cancer, diabetes, and pulmonary disease.[1,2] All the core NCDs are highly prevalent, and they are highly preventable. The increase in stroke and other NCDs has been recognized as an important challenge for global economic development. In 2011, the United Nations (UN) adopted the resolution on prevention and control of NCDs,[3] a landmark event as it was the second time in history (preceded ten years earlier by the UN resolution on HIV/AIDS) that a medical topic was addressed at the UN General Assembly. More recently, health and NCDs were also included in the UN Sustainable Disease Goals 2015–2030, reinforcing the importance of stroke and NCDs for global health.[4] Stroke has been identified as one of the core NCDs for which actions are prioritized.[5]

The field of stroke has seen major progress in the possibilities in primary prevention and treatment, and secondary prevention, in only a few decades. Stroke is preventable, and treatable so that the disability and burden of stroke can be drastically reduced.[6] Prevention and treatment requires identification of risks in the individual and in the population, as well as recognition of stroke symptoms and rapid admission to hospital.

A further important warning sign for stroke is transient ischaemic attack (TIA). TIA carries a high imminent risk of stroke, that can be reduced by rapid therapy. Brief episodes of cerebral ischaemia (TIA) are important to recognize, and require urgent diagnosis and therapy to reduce the risk of stroke.[6]

The aim of this chapter is to provide information on the most current data on the epidemiology of stroke and TIA, as well as to summarize recent data on risk factors, and current actions in the medical sector and among governmental bodies to reduce the burden of stroke.

Definitions of Stroke and TIA

The classical WHO definition of stroke is: 'rapidly developing clinical signs of focal (or global) disturbance of cerebral function, with symptoms lasting 24 hours or longer or leading to death, with no apparent cause other than of vascular'.[7] Stroke is thus a *clinical* diagnosis. The diagnosis of stroke may be supported by neuroimaging findings, and neuroimaging is essential to determine if a stroke is caused by cerebral ischaemia, or by intracerebral haemorrhage or subarachnoid haemorrhage.

TIA was classically defined as a: 'brief episode of focal loss of brain function, thought to be due to ischaemia, that can usually be localized to that portion of the brain supplied by one vascular system (left or right carotid or vertebrobasilar system) and for which no other cause can be found'.[8] However, about 40% of patients with classically defined TIAs have signs of acute brain infarction on diffusion-weighted magnetic resonance imaging (dw-MRI).[9] A tissue-based definition of TIA: 'a transient episode of neurological dysfunction caused by focal brain or retinal ischaemia lasting up to 24 hours, without evidence of acute infarction' has therefore been introduced, and was adopted in the World Health Organization International Classification of Diseases (ICD) 11 revision, adopted by the World Health Assembly in 2018.[10] Stroke is defined: 'as an acute focal dysfunction of the brain of presumed vascular origin lasting longer than 24 hours, or of any duration if imaging or autopsy show focal infarction or haemorrhage relevant to the symptoms'. The identification of cerebral infarction in patients with brief episodes of neurological dysfunction requires imaging facilities, which will not be available in large parts of the world. To date, almost all research publications on epidemiology of stroke and TIA have used the classical time-based definition.

MRI examinations have revealed that silent cerebrovascular disease (silent cerebral infarcts and microbleeds) are common not only in patients with stroke and TIA, but also in the general population in proportions that increase with age.[11,12] Silent cerebral infarct is defined as a brain infarct that has not caused acute focal dysfunction of the brain, and silent microbleeds are defined analogously. It should be emphasized that silent cerebral infarcts and microbleeds are not included in the definition of stroke—the latter term is reserved for cerebrovascular disorders that cause acute neurological dysfunction. Today it is well recognized that silent cerebrovascular disease is not innocent, but an important determinant for cognitive impairment, dementia, micturition disorders, and gait disorders.

The Development of Stroke Epidemiology

The era of epidemiological stroke studies started in the mid-twentieth century with reports from small geographical areas and large variations in methodologies and reporting. Influential pioneers in the field were the Framingham study[13] and researchers at the Mayo Clinic in Rochester, Minnesota.[14] For a long period only reports from a very limited number of HICs were available. Studies from LMICs were almost non-existent.

An important large project was the WHO Multinational MONItoring of Determinants and Trends in CArdiovascular Disease (MONICA) Project which was the world's largest prospective study on cardiovascular disorders. In the stroke component, 34,715 individually validated stroke events were recorded in 14 populations in Europe, Siberia, and China.[15] The study demonstrated large variations in stroke incidence, mortality, and case-fatality. Differences could be linked to risk factors, socioeconomic factors, and quality of care. A limitation of the study is that for stroke only persons up to 70 years of age were included.

The MONICA project helped to establish more stringent criteria for stroke epidemiological studies, and identified elements that were critical for reliable and comparable results. These elements were further developed in defining criteria for 'the ideal stroke study', emphasizing the importance of complete, community-based case ascertainment, including strokes managed outside the hospital.[16,17] In a review of studies that fulfilled the proposed criteria, they found that comparable data did not exist for vast areas of the world, including Africa, Asia, and South America. This conclusion was also echoed in an important systematic review by Feigin et al. in 2003,[18] which found only modest geographical variation in incidence, prevalence, and case-fatality between populations, but again cautioned that data were very limited for many parts of the world.

In 2009, Feigin and co-workers[19] published a new systematic review of 56 population-based studies of the incidence and early case-fatality of stroke published from 1970 to 2008. This review demonstrated a divergent trend in stroke incidence rates over the past four decades, with a 42% decrease in stroke incidence in HICs and a greater than 100% increase in stroke incidence in LMICs. At the end of the study period, overall stroke incidence rates in LMICs for the first time exceeded the level of stroke incidence seen in HICs, by 20%. Another study from the same year demonstrated a ten-fold difference in rates of stroke mortality and DALY loss between the most-affected and the least-affected countries.[20] Rates of stroke mortality and DALY loss were highest in Eastern Europe, North Asia, Central Africa, and the South Pacific. National per capita income was the strongest predictor of mortality and DALY loss rates even after adjustment for cardiovascular risk factors. These two studies served as alarm bells on the seriousness of the development of stroke, in particular the very grave situation in LMICs which carried the highest burden of stroke.

The GBD project is an initiative that covers the burden for the world for all diseases, but which has had a profound influence in providing data on different epidemiological stroke metrics, and the comparison and ranking of stroke in comparison with other diseases. From its start in the early 1990s, the GBD had developed into a major international consortium of several thousand researchers in more than 50 countries. Updates are provided yearly. The GBD has developed a methodology to collect and model data, and provide estimates even for countries where data are limited. The GBD publications that refer to stroke are summarized in the present review.[21–26] Besides the GBD, risk factors for stroke have also been studied in the multicentre INTERSTROKE case-controlled study.[27,28]

Regular systematic analyses of all individual stroke epidemiological studies are featured in the Global Stroke Statistics series,[29,30] which uses a methodology different and complementary to that of the GBD.

Overview of the Current Overall Burden of Stroke, Including Trends

The burden of stroke has been delineated in several publications from the GBD project.[1,2,21–26] In 2015, stroke was the second most common cause of death worldwide, after ischaemic heart disease.[1] Stroke was also the second most common cause of disability (4.5% of DALYs from all cause after ischaemic heart disease (6.1%), having risen from fifth position in 1990 and third position in 2005).[2]

Detailed data on the burden of stroke were provided in the GBD 2010 and 2013 studies.[21–26] These reports confirmed a significant increase in the global stroke burden over the last two and a half decades. There were substantial geographical variations, with LMICs carrying the largest burden. The highest stroke DALYs and mortality rates in 2013 were observed in Russia and Eastern European countries, while stroke-related YLD rates were highest in North America and Western European countries and Japan.

Globally in 2013, there were almost 25.7 million stroke survivors (71% with IS), 6.5 million deaths from stroke (51% died from ischaemic stroke), 113 million DALYs due to stroke (58% due to ischaemic stroke), and 10.3 million new strokes (67% IS).[22] Most of the burden (69% incident strokes, 71% stroke deaths) affected LMICs. Whereas stroke mortality and DALYs rates have declined from 1990 to 2013, the absolute number of people who died from stroke, remained disabled from stroke (as measured by DALYs), affected by stroke (as measured by incidence of new strokes), or survived stroke have increased statistically significantly (1.4 to 1.8-fold for ischaemic stroke and 1.2 to 1.9-fold for haemorrhagic stroke). If these trends in stroke incidence, mortality, and DALYs continue, by 2030 there will be almost 12 million stroke deaths, 70 million stroke survivors, and more than 200 million DALYs lost globally.

The GBD 2013 Study also identified significant disparities in stroke burden between men and women, with men having consistently greater incidence of ischaemic stroke then women.[24] In both men and women, and for both ischaemic and haemorrhagic stroke, the number of incident and prevalent strokes was significantly greater in 2013 compared to 1990.

The GBD projects also identified important shifts in the age distributions of stroke. From 1990 to 2013 there were significant increases in prevalent cases, total deaths, and DALYs due to haemorrhagic and ischaemic stroke in younger adults aged 20–64.[23] The global prevalence of haemorrhagic stroke was 3.7 million cases and of ischaemic stroke 7.3 million cases. There were 1.5 million stroke deaths among younger adults, with 1.1 million from haemorrhagic stroke and 0.4 million from ischaemic stroke. Compared to 1990, there was a 20.1% decline in the number of total stroke deaths among younger adults in developed countries, but a 36.7% increase in developing countries. The total DALYs from all strokes in 20–64-year-olds were 51.0 million, almost half of the total DALYs from stroke over all. Globally there was a 24.4% increase in total DALYs for this age group, with a 20% increase in haemorrhagic stroke and a 37.3% increase in ischaemic stroke numbers. Trends of increasing incidence and mortality rates of stroke in young adults in HICs have also been reported from other studies.[31,32]

There is an increasing recognition that stroke in children, although much rarer than in adults, importantly contributes to the total burden of stroke, as children with stroke often survive with persistent disabilities. Data on stroke in children are sparse, but the GBD project estimated that in 2013, there were almost 100,000 prevalent cases of childhood ischaemic stroke and 68,000 prevalent cases of childhood haemorrhagic stroke.[25] There were about 33,000 deaths and 2.6 million DALYs due to childhood stroke in 2013 globally. The childhood stroke burden in terms of absolute numbers of prevalent strokes, deaths, and DALYs were much higher in developing countries.

The Global Stroke Statistics project collected and systematically reviewed specific single stroke studies on incidence, mortality, and case-fatality.[29,30] In the latest update, data on stroke incidence were available from 51 countries.[30] Some countries had data over many time periods. Since the previous review[29] there were new incidence studies from twelve countries, with four meeting pre-determined quality criteria. In these four studies, the incidence of stroke, adjusted to the WHO World standard population, ranged from 76 per 100,000 population per year in Australia (2009–10) up to 119 per 100,000 population per year in New Zealand (2011–12), with the latter being in those aged at least 15 years. The incidence of stroke, adjusted to World Health Organization World population, reported from the different studies is shown in Fig. 20.1.

The Global Stroke Statistics project used data on stroke mortality as reported in the most recent year to the WHO. Crude mortality was greatest in Kazakhstan, Bulgaria, and Greece. Countries with new mortality at the lower end of the spectrum included Qatar, Bahrain, and Kuwait. Age-adjusted mortality from stroke in the most recent year reported to the WHO is shown in Fig. 20.2. As can be seen, the data comes from different years, with some countries reporting data that is quite old. Data on both crude incidence and mortality were available from 29 countries. A strong positive association between incidence and mortality from stroke was observed,

Data on case-fatality were available in 42 studies in 22 countries, with large variations between countries. The greatest overall 28-day case-fatalities were observed in India at approximately 37–42% at 28 days, whereas the lowest case-fatality was observed in Dijon (2000–2004) at 10%. Overall 28-day and 30-day case-fatality of stroke in the different studies are shown in Fig. 20.3.

Risk Factors for Stroke

Data on incidence, prevalence, mortality, and DALYs are essential to have an understanding of the population impact of stroke and trends of development. However, for prevention efforts, it is essential to understand the risk factors that cause stroke, their relative importance, the possibility of modifying a risk factor, and the effects of intervention.

Whereas there have been a very large number of studies on risk factors for stroke, two recent studies stand out because of their importance for global health: the INTERSTROKE study,[27,28] and the GBD risk factor study.[26]

INTERSTROKE was a case-control study of cases with acute first stroke and controls with no history of stroke, matched for sex and age, and with the aim to calculate ORs and population-attributable risks (PARs) for the association of all stroke, ischaemic stroke, and intracerebral haemorrhagic stroke with selected risk factors. In the first publication from 2010,[27] data were available for 3000 cases and 3000 controls in 22 countries. The ten most important risk factors were: hypertension (PAR 34.6%); current smoking (18.9%); waist-to-hip ratio (26.5%); diet risk score (18.8%); regular physical activity (28.5%); diabetes mellitus (5.0%); alcohol intake (3.8%); psychosocial stress (4.6%) and depression (5.2%); cardiac causes (6.7%); and ratio of apolipoproteins B to A1 (24.9%). Collectively, these risk factors accounted for 88.1% of the PAR for all stroke, showing that there is a very large potential to prevent stroke as all the top risk factors are modifiable. Compared to a corresponding study for coronary heart disease (INTERHEART), the PAR for hypertension for stroke was almost twice that of coronary heart disease, demonstrating the singular importance of this risk factor for stroke.[33]

In a second publication,[28] the INTERSTROKE study had been much extended and included 26,919 patients (10,388 with ischaemic stroke and 3059 with intracerebral haemorrhage) and 13,472 controls, from 32 countries in Asia, America, Europe, Australia, the Middle East, and Africa. Compared to the first report, the findings of PAR for risk factors associated for all stroke were similar, with few differences in the ranking of the risk factors. Collectively, the top ten risk factors accounted for 90.7% of the PAR for all stroke worldwide. Importantly, this second extended study could demonstrate that the PAR was high not only for ischaemic stroke (91.5%) but also for intracerebral haemorrhage (87,1%). The findings were also consistent across regions (ranging from 82.7% in Africa to 97.4% in South-East Asia), sex (90.6% in men and in women), and age groups (92.2% in patients aged ≤55 years, 90.0% in patients aged >55 years). However, regional variations in the importance of individual risk factors were observed, related to variations in the magnitude of ORs and differences in prevalence of risk factors among regions. Hypertension was more associated with intracerebral haemorrhage than with ischaemic stroke, whereas current smoking, diabetes, apolipoproteins, and cardiac causes were more associated with ischaemic stroke.

The GBD study on the global burden of stroke and risk factors in 188 countries[26] used a different methodology to quantify stroke burden in terms of DALYs and report changes in burden attributable to 17 potentially modifiable behavioural, environmental and occupational, and metabolic risks or clusters of risks at the global, regional, and country levels from 1990 to 2013. The study showed that 90.5% of the global burden of stroke was attributable to the modifiable risk

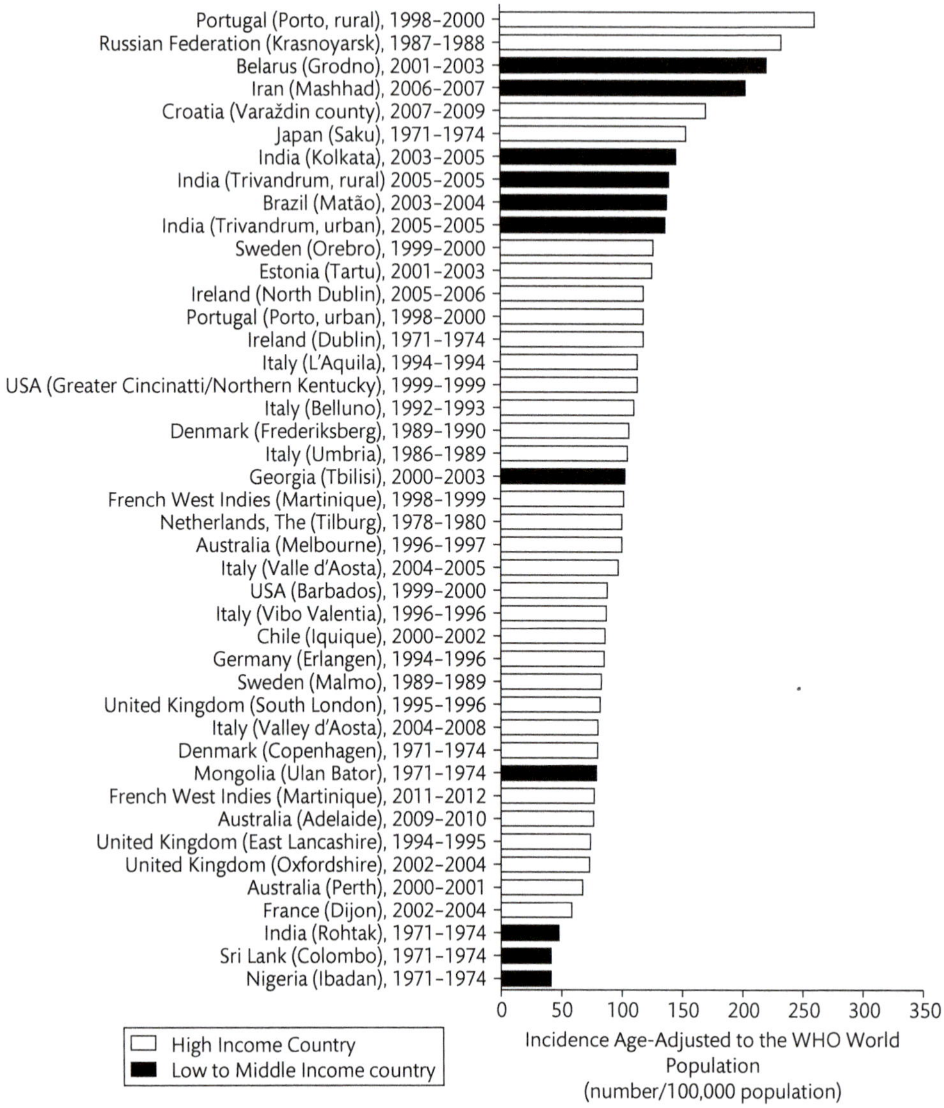

Fig. 20.1 Incidence of stroke, adjusted to World Health Organization World population.

Reproduced with permission from Thrift, A. G. et al. Global stroke statistics. *International Journal of Stroke*, 12(1): 13–32. Copyright © 2017, © SAGE Publications. DOI: 10.1177/1747493016676285.

factors analysed, including 74.2% to behavioural factors (smoking, poor diet, and low physical activity). Clusters of metabolic factors (high systolic blood pressure, high BMI, high fasting plasma glucose, high total cholesterol, and low glomerular filtration rate), and environmental factors (air pollution and lead exposure) were the second and third largest contributors to DALYs. This was the first time that air pollution emerged as one of the leading contributors to stroke burden worldwide, accounting for 29.2% of the stroke-related DALYs. The effect of air pollution was particularly high for LMICs (33.7%) compared to HICs (10.2%). Globally, the PAR of all risk factors to the burden of stroke increased with time (except for second-hand smoking and household air pollution from solid fuels) and varied significantly between countries and regions.

The GBD risk factor study was able to rank the importance of the different risk factors for individual countries and regions. A lower percentage of DALYs attributable to all risk factors combined was seen in African countries compared with other countries, which may be related to infectious and rheumatic heart diseases having a greater role as causes of stroke in Africa than in other countries.

Incidence of TIA

Compared to epidemiological studies on stroke, studies on incidence for TIA are much more sparse. The incidence of TIA is more difficult to study compared to stroke. Presumably, many people with transient neurological symptoms fail to seek medical care and are therefore not identified. This problem is present also in population-based studies that include patients referred to hospital, as well as those seen only in outpatient facilities. Furthermore, the diagnosis of TIA is often challenging, and there is substantial disagreement even between experts if a case meets TIA criteria or not. In clinical practice, the number of patients referred with suspected TIA outnumber those with a definitive TIA up to six-fold.[34]

The annual incidence of transient ischaemic attack per year in different populations ranges from 18 to 130 per 100,000 people (Fig. 20.4).[35] Part of this variation may be due to methodological issues on case ascertainment. Another cause may be differences related to background risk for cerebrovascular disease due to prevalence in risk factors in the population, and the use of primary and secondary

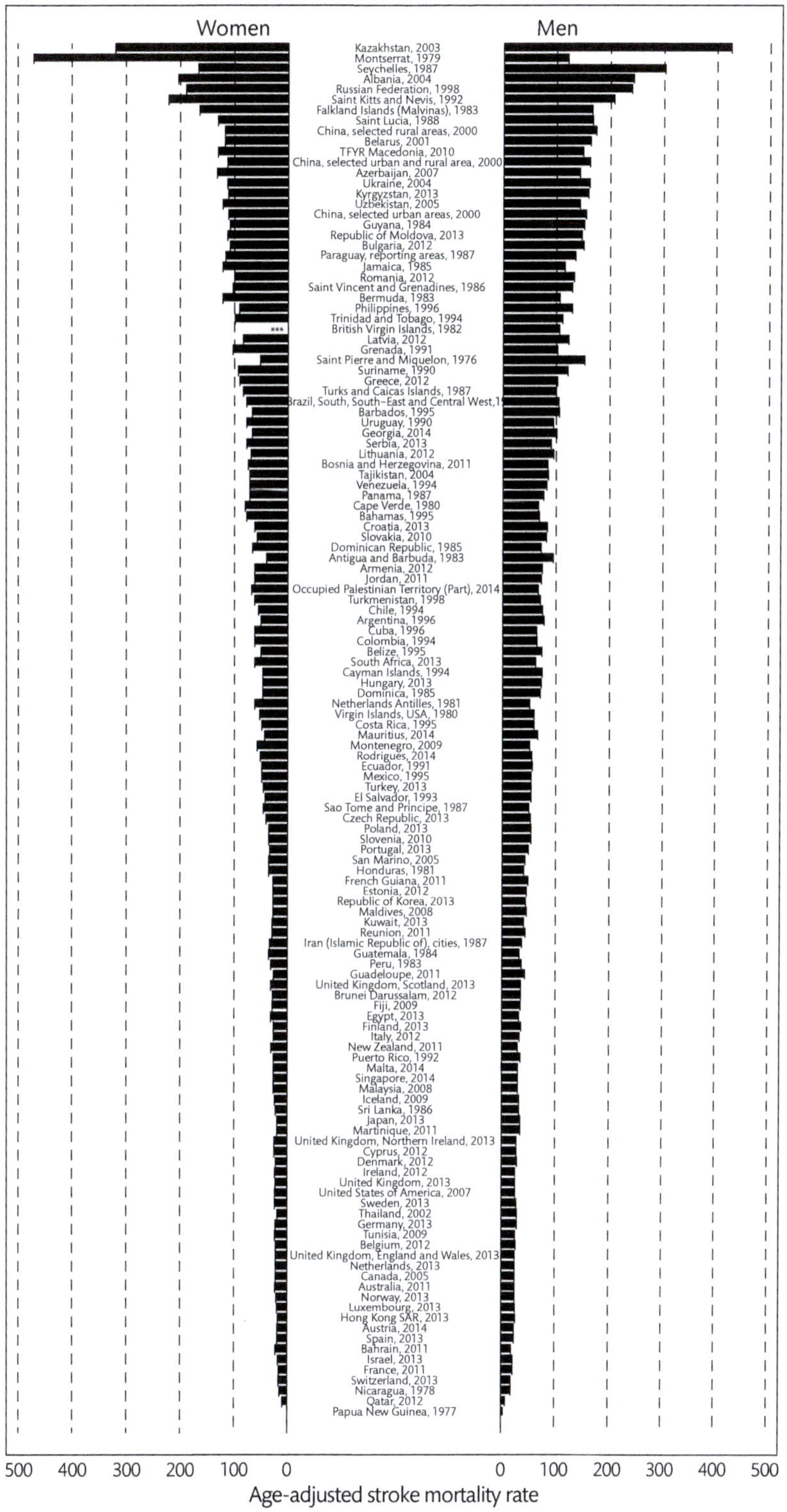

Fig. 20.2 Age-adjusted mortality from stroke in the most recent year reported to the WHO, ordered according to the average mortality for men and women. Note that mortality data for China are for selected regions only and represent <10% of all deaths in the country.

preventive treatments. Most studies report that patients with TIA are a few years younger than patients with ischaemic stroke. Furthermore, proportions of atrial fibrillation, previous stroke, and previous myocardial infarction are less common in TIA than in ischaemic stroke patients.

As described above, in almost all epidemiological TIA studies a time-based definition has been used, and the proportions investigated with MRI is very small. There is a gradual transition between TIA and mild ischaemic strokes, and the manifestations of cerebral ischaemia should be seen as a continuum rather than distinct

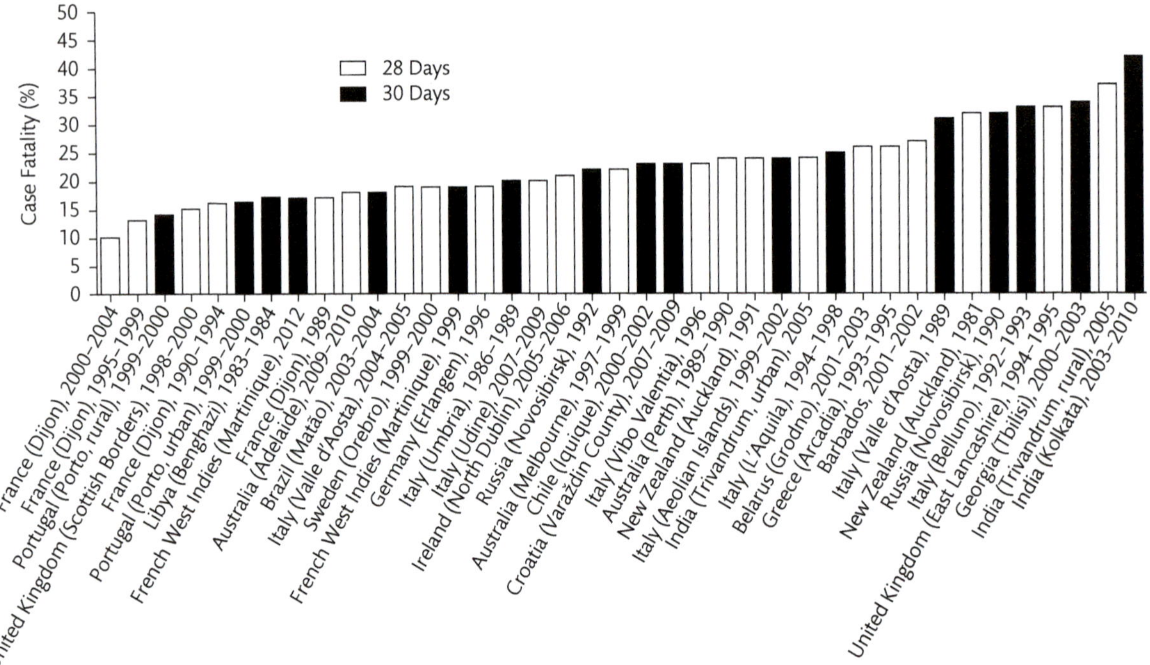

Fig. 20.3 Overall 28-day and 30-day case-fatality of stroke that are reported in countries.
Reproduced with permission from Thrift, A. G. et al. Global stroke statistics. *International Journal of Stroke*, 12(1): 13–32. Copyright © 2017, © SAGE Publications. DOI: 10.1177/1747493016676285.

separate entities. In a Danish study[36] of all patients admitted with TIA or acute ischaemic stroke in the Aarhus area, TIA accounted for 30%, and TIA and minor stroke combined accounted for 65% of all acute ischaemic cerebrovascular events.

Reducing the Burden of Stroke

The epidemiological data on stroke that have emerged during the last decade indicate the seriousness of the global burden of stroke at

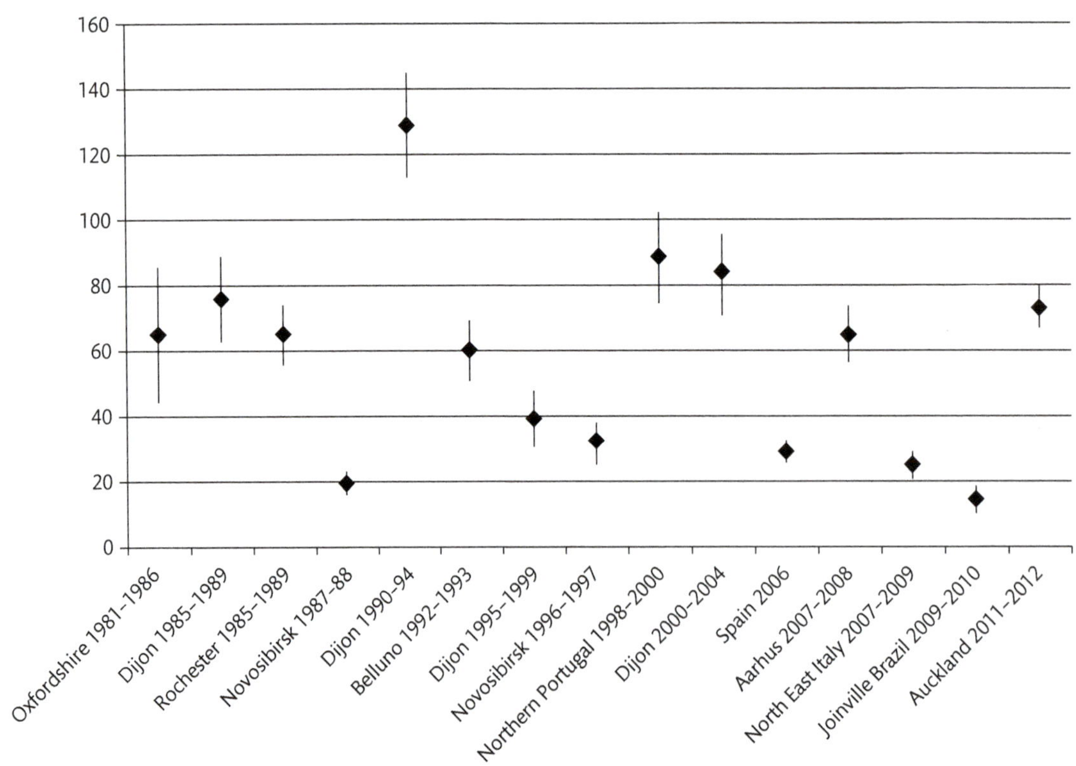

Fig. 20.4 Annual incidence of transient ischaemic attack per 100,000 people per year in different population, age standardized to the European population.
Reproduced with permission from Barber P.A., Krishnamurthi R., Parag V., et al; for the ARCOS IV Study Group. Incidence of Transient Ischemic Attack in Auckland, New Zealand, in 2011 to 2012. *Stroke*, 47:2183–2188. Copyright © 2016, Wolters Kluwer Health. DOI: https://doi.org/10.1161/STROKEAHA.116.014010.

present and as projected in the near future. An urgent need to change the course and reduce the burden of stroke has been recognized.[37] The actual burden of stroke is more severe than the data from the GBD indicate, as important long-term effects such as increasing risks of cognitive decline and dementia are not included in the estimates.

Foremost in reducing the burden of stroke is primary prevention. As described above, the main risk factors for stroke are well known and all are modifiable. Most of the risk factors coincide with the targets included in the WHO Global Action Plan on NCDs,[38] and apply also to prevention of all the major NCDs, not only to stroke. Primary stroke prevention should therefore not be a stand-alone silo, but part of the joint efforts of NCD prevention that are now ongoing. Stroke prevention has often been thought of as mainly a task by the health sector (primary care, hospitals), and the health system has the responsibility to identify risk factors that requires medical contacts for their detection and treatment (e.g. hypertension, atrial fibrillation), and to ensure proper treatment and secondary prevention for those affected by stroke or TIA. However, NCD prevention is a multisectorial task, with important responsibilities for governmental bodies and non-governmental organizations, besides the health sector. Governmental bodies have the power to influence lifestyle factors through legislation and taxation of tobacco, alcohol, and food content.[5,37] They are also able to influence physical activity, so that it becomes facilitated and is incorporated into the community structure through transportation and access to recreational areas. Ministries of health have the core responsibility for provision of adequate health services and installation of universal healthcare to cover primary and secondary prevention.

The INTERSTROKE and GBD studies showed that ten risk factors collectively explained (from their population-attributable risk) about 90% of all strokes.[26,28,29] It is uncertain what proportion of strokes is realistically preventable. It has been estimated that with effective actions on common lifestyle factors, about half of all strokes may be prevented.[39] This estimate does not include the effects of blood pressure control and stroke prevention in atrial fibrillation.

Implementation of primary prevention strategies based on the population-wide approach as well as the high-risk approach have been far from satisfactorily effective so far. There has been an inertia in governmental actions for population-wide health promotion, presumably from the barriers that these are political decisions that often meet resistance from the population/voters or from non-state actors (such as industry), and also often require substantial investments. There has been some progress in the high-risk approach, but screening for such high-risk individuals will only prevent a minority of cardiovascular events.[37,40] Recently, an additional strategy on prevention at any level of cardiovascular disease (CVD) risk, with the focus on behavioural risk factors, has been introduced.[40] Smartphone technologies, like the validated Stroke Riskometer app, may be applied for motivating and empowering people to reduce their risk of having a stroke/CVD, thus bridging the gap in the population-wide and high-risk prevention strategies.[40–42]

With the UN Sustainable Development Goals,[4] the interactions between stroke and poverty, climate, education, and other domains of the SDGs have been increasingly recognized. Reducing exposure to air pollution is not only an issue for the environment, but should also be one of the main priorities to reduce stroke burden in LMICs. Recent studies have also highlighted the close correlation between socioeconomical factors and NCDs, including stroke. The GBD project has reported a baseline analysis of the GBD 2015 dataset to measure the health-related sustainable development goals in 188 countries, and developed an index as a summary measure, the SDG index ranging from 0 (worst) to 100 (best).[43] In 2015, the median health-related SDG index was 59.3, and varied widely by country, ranging from 85.5 in Iceland to 20.4 in Central African Republic. An SDI, based on average income per person, educational attainment, and total fertility rate, was found to be a strong predictor of the health-related SDG index. Hence, there is a close correlation between overall health and NCDs and poverty, demonstrating the close links between the SDGs. Poverty contributes to stroke—and stroke can also contribute to poverty. This is particularly true in LMICs which do not have developed social security systems should a disabling disease occur. Stroke is a major cause of disability in the working age groups: according to the GBD project stroke ranks second in the overall disability burden in the 50–64 age group, third in the 45–49 age group, sixth in the 40–44 age group, and ninth in the 35–39 age group.[2]

It is uncertain whether the preventive effects demonstrated in HICs and MICs apply equally to countries with the lowest income. Risk factors for stroke and other cardiovascular diseases in the poorest billion of the world are different.[28,44] Infectious-related causes (e.g. rheumatic heart disease and HIV) and nutritional causes are important in these areas, along with a high proportion of hypertension being undetected and untreated. More research is needed on causes of stroke in the poorest areas.

Socioeconomical factors are also important with respect to stroke in deprived populations within HICs. These disparities are reflected not only in risk of stroke but also in short-term and long-term outcomes after stroke.[45] About half of these effects are estimated to be due to increased average levels of conventional risk factors (e.g. hypertension, hyperlipidaemia, excessive alcohol intake, smoking, obesity, and sedentary lifestyle) in populations with low socioeconomic status. There is emerging evidence that the effects of low income are not only related to the absolute level of income, but that large income differences within a country have damaging effects on health and social consequences.[46] In many HICs income inequality is increasing.

Primary prevention will avoid strokes, but the reduction in the burden of stroke treatments in the acute phase and later, as well as secondary prevention, are important to reduce the burden of stroke.[47] No less than one-third of all cerebrovascular events occur in persons who have had a previous stroke. Fortunately, effective therapies are available that can effectively reduce disability and death from stroke, and can prevent further strokes.[6] The World Stroke Organization has issued the world's first global stroke guidelines (The World Stroke Organization Global Stroke Services Guidelines and Action Plan) which lists essential components of care at different levels of services.[48] Whereas there are several quality of care registers in HICs,[49] data on the quality of services in LMICs are very limited. A new extension of the GBD Study showed heterogeneous patterns for the health services for individual diseases (including CVD and stroke) in given countries or territories, suggesting that few places have consistently achieved optimal healthcare access and quality across health-system functions and therapeutic areas.[50] A further issue is the recent demonstration that secondary preventive drugs were either not available or not affordable for a substantial proportion of patients in upper MICs, LMICs, and LICs.[51]

Conclusions and Further Directions

Epidemiological data on stroke show that the world is facing an epidemic of stroke of a magnitude that was not known only a decade ago. Despite stable incidence rates and declining mortality rates over the past two decades, the number of incident strokes, prevalent stroke survivors, DALYs lost due to stroke, and stroke-related deaths is increasing. Actions have been initiated both within the health system and from political and governmental bodies, since the stroke epidemic has important implications for public health and economies. In only a decade, stroke has moved from an anonymous position often invisible within the term 'cardiovascular disease' to the recognition that stroke is one of the core NCDs that require a stand-alone recognition and analysis. In the revision of the ICD 11 at WHO, all cerebrovascular diseases (stroke, TIA, silent cerebrovascular disease) were featured into a single block placed under Diseases of the Nervous System.[10] The second global cause of death and second global cause of lost DALYs should now receive the recognition that is warranted from the impact on global health.[1,2]

REFERENCES

1. GBD 2015 Mortality and Causes of Death Collaborators. Global, regional, and national life expectancy, all-cause mortality, and cause-specific mortality for 249 causes of death, 1980–2015: a systematic analysis for the Global Burden of Disease Study 2015. *Lancet*. 2016; 388: 1459–544.
2. GBD 2015 DALYs and HALE Collaborators. Global, regional, and national disability-adjusted life-years (DALYs) for 315 diseases and injuries and healthy life expectancy (HALE), 1990–2015: a systematic analysis for the Global Burden of Disease Study 2015. *Lancet*. 2016; 388: 1603–58.
3. United Nations General Assembly (2012). Resolution adopted by the General Assembly: 66/2: Political Declaration of the High-level Meeting of the General Assembly on the Prevention and Control of Non-communicable Diseases. Adopted September 19, 2011 (published 24 January 2012 edition). http://www.who.int/nmh/events/un_ncd_summit2011/political_declaration_en.pdf.
4. United Nations. Transforming our world: the 2030 Agenda for Sustainable Development. New York: United Nations, 2015. https://sustainabledevelopment.un.org/post2015/transformingourworld.
5. Beaglehole R, Bonita R, Horton R, et al. and Lancet NCD Action Group; NCD Alliance. Priority actions for the non-communicable disease crisis. *Lancet*. 2011; 377: 1438–47.
6. Hankey GJ. Stroke. *Lancet*. 2017; 389: 641–54.
7. WHO MONICA Project Investigators. The World Health Organization MONICA Project (Monitoring trends and determinants in cardiovascular disease). *J Clin Epidemiol*. 1988; 41: 105–114.
8. Special report from the National Institute of Neurological Disorders and Stroke. Classification of Cerebrovascular Disease. III. *Stroke*. 1990; 21: 637–76.
9. Redgrave JN, Coutts SB, Schultz UG, Briley D, Rothwell PM. Systematic review of associations between the presence of acute ischemic lesions on diffusion-weighted imaging and clinical predictors of early stroke risk after transient ischemic attack. *Stroke*. 2007; 38: 1482–8.
10. http://apps.who.int/classifications/icd11/browse/l-m/en#/http%3a%2f%2fid.who.int%2ficd%2fentity%2f1296093776.
11. Vermeer SE, Longstreth WT, Koudstaal PJ. Silent brain infarcts: a systematic review. *Lancet Neurology*. 2007; 6: 611–19.
12. Werring DJ (ed.). Cerebral Microbleeds. Pathophysiology to Clinical Practice. Cambridge: Cambridge University Press, 2011.
13. Wolf PA. Fifty years at Framingham: contributions to stroke epidemiology. *Adv Neurol*. 2003; 92: 165–72.
14. Whisnant JP, Fitzgibbons JP, Kurland LT, Sayre GP. Natural history of stroke in Rochester, Minnesota, 1945 through 1954. *Stroke*. 1971; 2: 11–22.
15. Asplund K. What MONICA told us about stroke. *Lancet Neurology*. 2005; 4: 64–8.
16. Sudlow CL, Warlow CP. Comparing stroke incidence worldwide: what makes studies comparable? *Stroke*. 1996; 27: 550–8.
17. Feigin V, Hoorn SV. How to study stroke incidence. *Lancet*. 2004; 363: 1920.
18. Feigin VL, Lawes CM, Bennett DA, Anderson CS. Stroke epidemiology: a review of population-based studies of incidence, prevalence, and case-fatality in the late 20th century. *Lancet Neurology*. 2003; 2: 43–53.
19. Feigin VL, Lawes CM, Bennett DA, Barker-Collo SL, Parag V. Worldwide stroke incidence and early case fatality reported in 56 population-based studies: a systematic review. *Lancet Neurology*. 2009; 8: 355–69.
20. Johnston SC, Mendis S, Mathers CD. Global variation in stroke burden and mortality: estimates from monitoring, surveillance, and modelling. *Lancet Neurology*. 2009; 8: 345–54.
21. Feigin VL, Forouzanfar MH, Krishnamurthi R, et al. and Global Burden of Diseases, Injuries, and Risk Factors Study 2010 (GBD 2010) and the GBD Stroke Experts Group. Global and regional burden of stroke during 1990–2010: findings from the Global Burden of Disease Study 2010. *Lancet*. 2014; 383: 245–54.
22. Feigin VL, Krishnamurthi RV, Parmar P, et al. and GBD 2013 Writing Group; GBD 2013 Stroke Panel Experts Group. Update on the Global Burden of Ischemic and Hemorrhagic Stroke in 1990–2013: The GBD 2013 Study. *Neuroepidemiology*. 2015; 45: 161–76.
23. Krishnamurthi RV, Moran AE, Feigin VL, et al. and GBD 2013 Stroke Panel Experts Group. Stroke prevalence, mortality and disability-adjusted life years in adults aged 20–64 years in 1990–2013: data from the Global Burden of Disease 2013 Study. *Neuroepidemiology*. 2015; 45: 190–202.
24. Barker-Collo S, Bennett DA, Krishnamurthi RV, et al. and GBD 2013 Writing Group; GBD 2013 Stroke Panel Experts Group. Sex differences in stroke incidence, prevalence, mortality and disability-adjusted life years: results from the Global Burden of Disease Study 2013. *Neuroepidemiology*. 2015; 45: 203–14.
25. Krishnamurthi RV, deVeber G, Feigin VL, et al. and GBD 2013 Stroke Panel Experts Group. Stroke prevalence, mortality and disability-adjusted life years in children and youth aged 0–19 years: data from the Global and Regional Burden of Stroke 2013. *Neuroepidemiology*. 2015; 45: 177–89.
26. Feigin VL, Roth GA, Naghavi M, et al. Global burden of stroke and risk factors in 188 countries, during 1990–2013: a systematic analysis for the Global Burden of Disease Study 2013. *Lancet Neurology*. 2016; 15: 913–24.
27. O'Donnell MJ, Xavier D, Liu L, et al. and INTERSTROKE Investigators. Risk factors for ischaemic and intracerebral haemorrhagic stroke in 22 countries (the INTERSTROKE Study): a case-control study. *Lancet*. 2010; 376: 112–23.
28. O'Donnell MJ, Chin SL, Rangarajan S, et al. INTERSTROKE investigators. Global and regional effects of potentially modifiable risk factors associated with acute stroke in 32

countries (INTERSTROKE): a case-control study. *Lancet*. 2016; 388(10046): 761–75.
29. Thrift AG, Cadilhac DA, Thayabaranathan T, et al. Global stroke statistics. *Int J Stroke* 2014; 9: 6–18.
30. Thrift AG, Thayabaranathan T, Howard G, Howard VJ, Rothwell PM, Feigin VL, et al. Global stroke statistics. *Int J Stroke*. 2017; 12: 13–32.
31. Giang KW, Björck L, Nielsen S, Novak M, Sandström TZ, Jern C, et al. Twenty-year trends in long-term mortality risk in 17,149 survivors of ischemic stroke less than 55 years of age. *Stroke*. 2013; 44: 3338–43.
32. Kissela BM, Khoury JC, Alwell K, Moomaw CJ, Woo D, Adeoye O, et al. Age at stroke: temporal trends in stroke incidence in a large, biracial population. *Neurology*. 2012; 79: 1781–7.
33. Yusuf S, Hawken S, Ounpuu S, Dans T, Avezum A, Lanas F, et al. and INTERHEART Study Investigators. Effect of potentially modifiable risk factors associated with myocardial infarction in 52 countries (the INTERHEART study): case-control study. *Lancet*. 2004; 364(9438): 937–52.
34. Giles MF, Rothwell PM. Substantial underestimation of the need for outpatient services for TIA and minor stroke. *Age Ageing*. 2007; 36: 676–80.
35. Barber PA, Krishnamurthi R, Parag V, et al. for the ARCOS IV Study Group. Incidence of transient ischemic attack in Auckland, New Zealand, in 2011 to 2012. *Stroke*. 2016; 47: 2183–8.
36. von Weitzel-Mudersbach P, Andersen G, Hundborg HH, Johnsen SP. Transient ischemic attack and minor stroke are the most common manifestations of acute cerebrovascular disease: a prospective, population-based study. The Aarhus TIA study. *Neuroepidemiology*. 2013; 40: 50–5.
37. Feigin VL, Norrving B, George MG, Foltz JL, Roth GA, Mensah GA. Prevention of stroke: a strategic global imperative. *Nat Rev Neurol*. 2016; 12 (9): 501–12.
38. WHO. World Health Organization Global Action Plan for the Prevention and Control of Noncommunicable Diseases 2013–2020. Available from: http://www.who.int/nmh/events/ncd_action_plan/en/.
39. Tikk K, Sookthai D, Monni S, Gross ML, Lichy C, Kloss M, et al. Primary preventive potential for stroke by avoidance of major lifestyle risk factors: the European Prospective Investigation into Cancer and Nutrition-Heidelberg cohort. *Stroke*. 2014; 45: 2041–6.
40. Feigin VL, Norrving B, Mensah GA. Primary prevention of cardiovascular disease through population-wide motivational strategies: insights from using smartphones in stroke prevention. *BMJ Global Health*. 2017; 2: e000306.
41. Feigin VL, Krishnamurthi R, Bhattacharjee R, et al. New strategy to reduce the global burden of stroke. *Stroke*. 2015; 46: 1740–7.
42. Parmar P, Krishnamurthi R, Ikram MA, et al. and Stroke Riskometer™ Collaboration Writing Group. The Stroke Riskometer™ App: validation of a data collection tool and stroke risk predictor. *Int J Stroke*. 2015; 10: 231–44.
43. GBD 2015 SDG Collaborators. Measuring the health-related Sustainable Development Goals in 188 countries: a baseline analysis from the Global Burden of Disease Study 2015. *Lancet*. 2016; 388: 1813–50.
44. Kwan GF, Bongani MM, Mocumbi AO, et al. Endemic cardiovascular diseases of the poorest billion. *Circulation*. 2016; 133: 2561–75.
45. Marshall IJ, Wang Y, Crichton S, McKevitt C, Rudd AG, Wolfe CD. The effects of socioeconomic status on stroke risk and outcomes. *Lancet Neurology*. 2015; 14: 1206–18.
46. Pickett KE, Wilkinson RG. Income inequality and health: a casual review. *Social Science & Medicine*. 2015; 128: 316–26.
47. Norrving B, Davis SM, Feigin VL, Mensah GA, Sacco RL, Varghese C. Stroke prevention worldwide—what could make it work? *Neuroepidemiology*. 2015; 45: 215–20.
48. Lindsay P, Furie KL, Davis SM, Donnan GA, Norrving B. World Stroke Organization global stroke services guidelines and action plan. *Int J Stroke*. 2014; 9(Suppl A100): 4–13.
49. Cadilhac DA, Kim J, Lannin NA, et al. National stroke registries for monitoring and improving the quality of hospital care: A systematic review. *Int J Stroke*. 2016; 11: 28–40.
50. GBD 2015 Health Care Access and Quality Collaborators. Healthcare Access and Quality Index based on mortality from causes amenable to personal health care in 195 countries and territories, 1990–2015: a novel analysis from the Global Burden of Disease Study 2015. *Lancet*. 2017; 390:231–266.
51. Khatib R, McKee M, Shannon H, et al. Availability and affordability of cardiovascular disease medicines and their effect on use in high-income, middle-income, and low-income countries: an analysis of the PURE study data. *Lancet*. 2015; 15: 61–9.

21

Small vessel disease

Fergus N Doubal, Anna Poggesi, Leonardo Pantoni, and Joanna M Wardlaw

Introduction

Cerebral small vessel disease (SVD) is the most prevalent neurological disorder,[1] significantly contributing to the worldwide burden of stroke and dementia. It is important to recognize that the term cerebral SVD encompasses a wide range of pathological, neuroradiological, and clinical features,[2,3] summarized in Fig. 21.1.

Fig. 21.1A depicts the two main types of small arteries and arterioles—superficial and deep perforators. Pathologically, cerebral SVD refers to a group of diseases that affect all vascular structures (ranging between 5 μm to 2 mm diameter) in the brain parenchyma or the subarachnoid space, thus including small arteries, arterioles, capillaries, venules, and small veins.[2,3] Many pathological conditions affect cerebral small vessels and one possible aetiopathogenic classification identifies arteriolosclerosis and cerebral amyloid angiopathy (either sporadic or hereditary) as the most prevalent subtypes, followed by inflammatory or immune-mediated and other forms (Fig. 21.1B). More recently, genetic forms of SVD have received attention, first because the number of recognized genetic conditions is increasing and second because diseases such as CADASIL may serve as models for sporadic SVD.[4]

Neuroimaging, particularly MRI, plays a critical role in defining cerebral SVD.[5] Small vessels cannot be easily visualized *in vivo*, so the parenchymal lesions that are thought to be caused by these vessel changes have been adopted as markers of SVD.[2] These lesions are heterogeneous and can include both ischaemic and haemorrhagic manifestations (Fig. 21.1C1 and C2). The mechanisms linking cerebral SVD with parenchymal damage, either ischaemic or haemorrhagic, are heterogeneous and hitherto incompletely understood. The vessel wall changes may lead to rupture of the vessel (and hence haemorrhagic SVD), structural restriction of the vessel lumen, or functional dysregulation of the blood vessel, which may lead to a state of chronic hypoperfusion and incomplete infarction or acute focal brain parenchymal necrosis.[2] However, while numerous cross-sectional studies demonstrate that cerebral blood flow (CBF) is reduced in patients with white matter hyperintensities (a common neuroimaging feature of SVD), there is little evidence from longitudinal studies that falling CBF leads to formation of WMH.[6] Thus, alternative explanations of the microvessel and brain tissue appearances have been proposed, which may act together with these mechanisms, amongst which blood brain barrier (BBB) dysfunction and endothelial dysfunction are nowadays considered pivotal mechanisms of the structural and functional brain-vessel alterations in SVD, with inflammatory and oxidative stress factors possibly playing an important role.[3,7] Lacunes (small 'holes' in the brain) and WMH are well-established imaging markers of cerebral SVD, but other radiological biomarkers such as perivascular spaces, cortical and white matter atrophy, cerebral microinfarcts, and microbleeds are also recognized as representing cerebral SVD. As many different names have been used for these SVD features over the years (the literature describes over 150 different terms for acute lacunar infarct), the nomenclature of SVD has been standardized by an international consensus statement.[5] In this chapter, we use this consensus terminology.

SVD has a huge impact on individual and social systems in the world's older populations, being highly prevalent, causing substantial cognitive and motor disabilities, representing one-fifth of all strokes, and contributing to up to 45% of dementias alone or mixed with AD. The clinical presentation of cerebral SVD can be acute, that is, stroke (ischaemic or haemorrhagic) or chronic, that is, cognitive decline, dementia, psychiatric, motor, or urinary disturbances (Fig. 21.1D).[8,9] SVD is a major determinant of disability, mortality, and poor prognosis.[8] This notwithstanding, data on prevention and treatment are still scarce. Among reasons for this lack of evidence is that most research conducted until now has focused on individual features of SVD rather than on the global SVD load, as well as under-recognition of SVD as a disease entity.

In the first section of this chapter, the imaging definition of SVD lesions and related epidemiological data, with particular focus on risk factors, are discussed. Subsequently we will highlight clinical presentations of cerebral SVD, before outlining future research directions.

Imaging Defined SVD Features and Their Risk Factors

After early 20th-century clinical-pathological studies and studies by Miller-Fisher, an explosion of interest in SVD took place in the 1980s with the introduction of neuroimaging, when it became

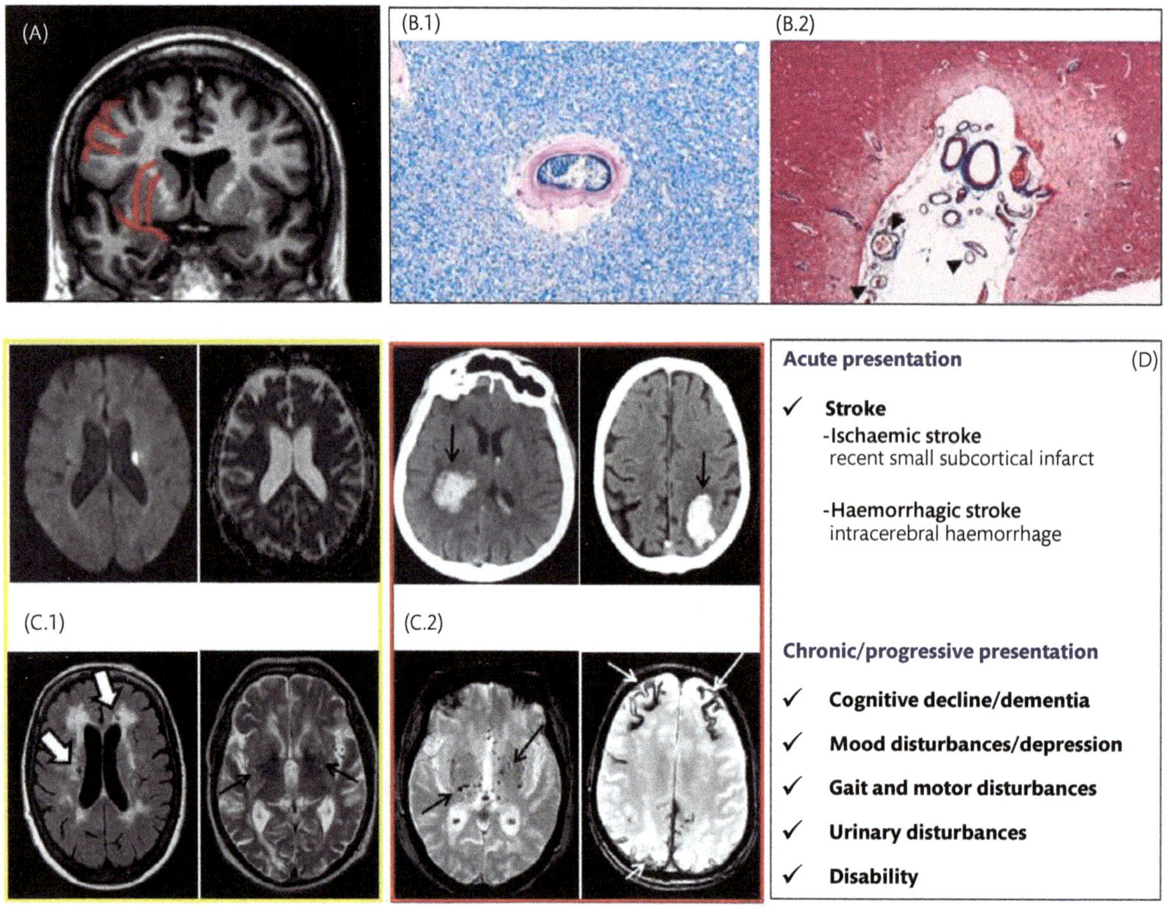

Fig. 21.1 Cerebral small vessel disease (SVD) definition.

Part A. Schematic representation of the two main types of small arteries and arterioles most commonly affected in SVD: superficial and deep perforating arterioles.

Part B. Pathological features of SVD. B.1 Lipoyalinosis (a diseased small vessel in the white matter; Luxol Fast Blue-PAS, 40X). B.2 Cerebral amyloid angiopathy (small vessels in the subarachnoid space: note the double barrel appearance of some; arrowheads: Masson's trichrome, 25X)

Part C. Neuroimaging features of SVD related brain parenchyma lesions.

C.1 Ischaemic lesions related to SVD. The upper figure shows diffusion weighted imaging sequences with related apparent diffusion coefficient images of a recent small subcortical infarct in the left centrum semiovale. The bottom of the figure shows FLAIR and T2-weighted sequences showing white matter hyperintensities (bilateral confluent lesions in the white matter of the centrum semiovale), lacunes (one in the right centrum semiovale and one in the left frontal lobe, open arrows), and dilated perivascular spaces (multiple small round or ovoid fluid-fulfilled spaces when in cross-section in the basal ganglia, thin arrows. Note that perivascular spaces appear linear when imaged in their long axis, e.g. in the centrum semiovale).

C.2 Haemorrhagic lesions related to SVD. The upper figure shows two examples of computed tomography of spontaneous intracerebral haemorrhage, one located in right deep brain structures (these are often attributed to hypertension, arrow), and the other in left fronto-parietal lobe reaching the cortex (these are often attributed to cerebral amyloid angiopathy, arrow). The bottom of the figure shows multiple small deeply located microbleeds (left, arrows) and disseminated superficial siderosis overlying the cortex (arrows) on T2*-weighted MRI sequences.

Part D. Clinical aspects related to SVD. The clinical course and presentation of SVD may be acute or chronic/progressive.

evident that changes located in the subcortical cerebral regions, particularly in the white matter, were frequent findings, especially in older subjects. White matter lesions, appearing as hypoattenuated areas, lacunes (small CSF-filled holes), a small proportion of acute small subcortical (or lacunar) infarcts, atrophy, and haemorrhages can all be detected by CT. Other features, such as perivascular spaces and microbleeds are not easily detected by CT. While the pathogenic interpretation of lacunes seen on CT was immediately ascribed to SVD, the initial link between white matter lesions and SVD was less clear.[10] With MRI, the spectrum of SVD parenchymal lesions has expanded, see Fig. 21.1B.

MRI appearances are described below.

WMH of presumed vascular origin Signal abnormality in the white matter appearing as hyperintensities on T2-weighted images such as fluid-attenuated inversion recovery, without cavitation (signal different from CSF). The size may be variable, from punctate to confluent hyperintensities.

Recent small subcortical infarct Neuroimaging evidence of recent infarction in the territory of one perforating arteriole, with imaging features or clinical symptoms consistent with a lesion occurring in the previous few weeks.

Lacune of presumed vascular origin A round or ovoid, subcortical, fluid-filled cavity (signal similar to CSF) of between 3 mm and about 15 mm in diameter, consistent with sequelae of a previous acute small subcortical infarct or haemorrhage (whether symptomatic or not) in the territory of one perforating arteriole.

Perivascular spaces Fluid-filled spaces that follow the typical course of a vessel as it goes through grey or white matter. The spaces have signal intensity similar to CSF on all sequences. Because they follow the course of penetrating vessels, they appear linear when imaged parallel to the course of the vessel, and round or ovoid, with a diameter generally smaller than 3 mm, when imaged perpendicular to the course of the vessel.

Brain atrophy Reduced brain volume that is not related to a specific macroscopic focal injury such as trauma or infarction.

Cerebral microbleed Small (generally 2–5 mm in diameter, but sometimes up to 10 mm) areas of signal void with associated blooming seen on T2*-weighted or SWI MRI which are sensitive to susceptibility effects.

Cerebral haemorrhage Occurring in the parenchyma, of any size, is increasingly attributed to underlying SVD.

Cortical superficial siderosis is now considered a subtype of SVD. This is described as well-defined, homogeneous hypointense curvilinear signal intensity (black) on T2*-GRE in the superficial layers of the cerebral cortex, within the subarachnoid space, or both. If there is corresponding signal hyperintensity in the subarachnoid space on proton density-weighted or FLAIR sequences (or hyperdense on CT) the term 'acute cortical subarachnoid haemorrhage' is recommended.[11]

For a full description and definition of the imaging findings of cerebral SVD see elsewhere.[5]

Large intracerebral haemorrhage can be easily detected by CT, and can be divided into those located in deep hemispheric areas (e.g. basal ganglia or thalami), cerebellum or pons, and those located in more superficial lobar areas. The former are typically associated with hypertension, while the latter are frequently associated with cerebral amyloid angiopathy.

The phenotypic expression of SVD is heterogenous and this variability is not fully explained by the severity of lesions depicted by conventional MRI. Accordingly, there is increasing focus on so-called *'invisible' SVD changes*, that is, those changes not, or only rarely, detected by conventional MRI, such as microinfarcts.[12] These microinfarcts, mainly located in the cortex, are very small (<1 mm) lesions, which may be detected at microscopic examination at autopsy or on high-field MRI.[12,13] Other advanced techniques such as magnetization transfer, diffusion tensor imaging, and spectroscopy can yield more in-depth information about the extent of tissue damage, its microstructural nature, and the underlying metabolic alterations. Therefore, attention has moved towards 'normal appearing white matter', which indeed may show altered white matter integrity and myelination. These invisible or 'pre-visible' changes show that altered interstitial fluid mobility and water content, which may be reversible, probably predate demyelination and axonal damage, which are less likely to be reversible and are probably a late-stage phenomenon.[14]

Available data focuses on individual neuroimaging features of cerebral SVD rather than on the global SVD burden. In general, prevalence data are available at a population level, in different patient groups, and in association with vascular risk factors. However, the amount of data available varies between different SVD lesion types. One common fact between all SVD lesion-types is the strong association with age, that is, their prevalence increases dramatically with age.[8]

WMH are the best recognized, commonest, and most studied feature of cerebral SVD and prevalent in the elderly,[15] although this prevalence of WMH varies and may reach 100%, depending on the study cohort under investigation, as well as technical factors.[2] Epidemiology has demonstrated important clues related to the pathogenesis and clinical significance of WMH, which are frequently associated with age and with other vascular risk factors, including hypertension, smoking, and diabetes.[2,16]

Lacunar strokes account for about one quarter of all ischaemic strokes, a proportion similar to that of cardioembolic and large vessel strokes. Furthermore, such small infarcts are not always associated with acute stroke symptoms, and these so-called silent infarcts are much more common than those associated with stroke.[17] In the general population, MRI studies have shown that silent infarcts, which are mainly subcortical infarcts, are present in more than a quarter of subjects aged 70 years or over, about five times more common than infarcts presenting with stroke.[18]

The prevalence of cerebral microbleeds increases if a higher field strength MRI scanner is used[19] and varies, depending on the cohort characteristics, from 5% in population-based studies to 34% in ischaemic stroke cohorts, and 61% in intracerebral haemorrhage stroke cohorts.[20] Given the strong association with intracerebral haemorrhage, microbleeds can be generally considered as the asymptomatic counterpart. Different aetiologic mechanisms may underlie different intracerebral haemorrhage, that is, cerebral amyloid angiopathy manifesting with lobar haemorrhages, versus age/hypertensive SVD manifesting with deep/infratentorial haemorrhage. In parallel with this distribution, microbleed location (lobar vs deep) is considered a major distinctive characteristic, indicating the different underlying type of SVD. In general, lobar ICH are more closely associated with predominantly lobar microbleeds than deep microbleeds (MB), and deep ICH are more closely associated with predominantly deep MB than lobar MB.[21] The risk factor profiles for microbleeds also differ according to location: deep/infratentorial microbleeds are more frequent in hypertensive subjects, and are associated with other markers of SVD, such as lacunar infarcts and WMH, while lobar microbleeds are more closely related to *APOE* allele genotype.[22] However these associations may not be as strong in routine practice as in focused research studies and more data using unconfounded diagnostic criteria are required to determine the strength of these associations.

For perivascular spaces, the same methodological considerations are applicable, for example the strength of the MRI scanner will influence the number of perivascular spaces seen. A recent study showed that perivascular spaces on 7T MRI are often found in a cohort of 50 community-dwelling individuals aged >40 years.[23] Others have reported frequent finding of PVS visible on T2 images even in much younger people at 1.5T if sensitive sequences are used. For example, we commonly see PVS in the basal ganglia or centrum semiovale in young healthy volunteers, although generally fewer than in older patients.[24] Interestingly, both at 7T and at 1.5T, the number of perivascular spaces were related to other imaging markers of SVD, but not to age or other vascular risk factors, suggesting that, due to the high sensitivity of the technique, 'non-pathological' spaces might be detected.[25] Perivascular spaces are indeed expressions of SVD,[26,27]and, similarly to microbleeds, their location, mainly in the white matter or in the basal ganglia, might indicate the presence of different types of SVD, cerebral amyloid angiopathy, or hypertensive-related SVD.[28] Little is known of the dynamics of 'normal' PVS and how they might change with time of day, hydration status, or episodes of systemic inflammation. Computational methods to assess PVS volume as well as count are now emerging, which will enhance studies of subtleties of disease processes leading to other SVD features and established brain damage.[29]

Very recently, we have learned that the presence of one or two microinfarcts in routinely sampled sections of a brain was speculated to indicate the presence of hundreds to thousands of these lesions in the entire brain.[30] From these estimates, microinfarcts become the most highly represented type of brain infarction, up to 15 times more frequent than clinically overt lacunar infarcts or lacunes.

Data are also very scanty on the possible ethnic differences in the prevalence of SVD neuroimaging features. Overall, the impression is that the high prevalence of these features in the general population and in the patient groups at higher risk is consistent across different world regions.[31] Specific data are, however, missing. One US study showed a higher prevalence of WMH in African-Americans and Hispanics as compared to white people.[32] Disease prevalence may also vary by geographical area but there is a lack of in-depth comparative studies investigating the prevalence in different world regions.

Considered globally, a substantial body of evidence suggests an association between cerebral SVD and traditional vascular risk factors, such as age, hypertension, diabetes, smoking, dyslipidaemia. Despite this evidence, the exact mechanisms linking traditional vascular risk factors and brain parenchyma lesions are complex and still not completely understood. A good example of such complexity is given by hypertension, considered a major risk factor for cerebral SVD. On one level, in small arteries, high blood pressure (BP) may be responsible for hypertrophic and/or eutrophic remodelling, reduced luminal diameter, increased resistance to flow, impaired autoregulation, and reduced tissue perfusion, but it is more difficult to reconcile interpretation of the available apparently inconsistent evidence relating elevated BP, systolic and/or diastolic, values with severity and progression of SVD.[3] Furthermore, in cross-sectional analyses of community dwelling individuals and patients with minor stroke, all common vascular risk factors combined (of which hypertension was the major one) only explained 2% of the variance in WMH in two samples[33] and objective evidence to support the proposed sequence of events described above is missing.[6,34] Also, accumulating data point to systemic and cranial vascular stiffening rather than absolute blood pressure levels as this is the feature most closely related to WMH severity.[35] One important consideration is that the effect of the exposure to the risk factor might change according to different age groups. Cross-sectional data from the Framingham Study showed that raised systolic BP has a negative effect on white-matter integrity and grey-matter volume in young adults, before the appearance of WMH,[36] while in elderly individuals, BP fluctuations might accentuate abnormalities of cerebral blood flow impairment and hypoperfusion.[37]

Another key element in the determination of the effect of hypertension is the effect that its treatment has on disease progression. Knowledge about longitudinal changes of SVD are now available for other SVD-related lesions beyond WMH.[38] Some of the evidence points to an association of hypertension and the quality of blood pressure control with WMH progression,[39,40] although in stroke cohorts, large randomized clinical trials failed to demonstrate a clear clinical benefit of hypertensive treatment, nor of optimal target BP value level, on both progression of WMH and stroke.[41,42] However, as the total risk resulting from the coexistence of high BP with other vascular risk factors is small,[33] the focus of future research should be on what else might account for the high unexplained variance in SVD.

Sporadic WMH has about 60–70% heritability, therefore genetic susceptibility is an obvious possibility, but other environmental (pollution), or dietary (salt), or lifestyle factors are relatively under-researched. It is beyond the scope of this chapter to cover the recent advances made in the field of genetics and SVD other than to emphasize this high heritability of WMH and other features suggests an important role for genetic studies of cerebral SVD. There are other recent publications and comprehensive reviews on this topic.[43,44]

Once again, it has to be noted that the level of evidence about the association between SVD and vascular risk factors is different for each of the single SVD-related brain lesions, and this issue might be overcome by the assessment of the total SVD load, instead of individual MRI SVD-related brain lesions. In this sense, the construct of a 'total SVD score' has recently been proposed and validated.[45] Together with traditional vascular risk factors, research is now focusing on other factors, such as salt intake, inflammation, and infective agents, that, as a common final pathway, may lead to endothelial and BBB dysfunction, thus contributing to SVD.[46]

While waiting for more data to disentangle the complex relationship between SVD and vascular risk factors, it will be important to treat modifiable vascular risk factors, according to guidelines, mainly by encouraging achievable lifestyle interventions, particularly smoking cessation, treatment of hypertension and diabetes, and lowering cholesterol. Future trials dedicated to prevent the development or progression of SVD are urgently needed, with some underway.[47]

Clinical Presentation of SVD

Introduction

Cerebral SVD is best defined radiologically and the heterogeneity of radiological abnormalities is reflected in the wide range of clinical manifestations of SVD.[2] Whilst there are numerous clinical associations with cerebral SVD, the increased use of clinical MRI (or even screening purposes) results in increased prevalence of patients presenting with asymptomatic cerebral SVD—that is to say, with no obvious overt clinical correlates to the SVD abnormalities apparent on brain scanning. One of the difficulties with describing clinical presentations of SVD is that although dementia results from SVD, SVD is not the only cause of dementia

(Alzheimer's disease [AD] and others also contribute) and this also applies to other clinical features of SVD. Because of this, the treating clinician needs to exercise caution in ascribing causation between brain scan appearances and symptoms when dealing with a patient with diffuse features of SVD. This section of the chapter will discuss the clinical presentations of SVD, the overlap with other neurological conditions, and also cover asymptomatic disease. As in the rest of the chapter the main focus of this section is on sporadic SVD rather than the important although less frequent SVD with known genetic causes.

Lacunar ischaemic stroke (recent small subcortical symptomatic infarct)

Cerebral SVD can result in a sudden focal neurological deficit, the clinical lacunar stroke syndrome which may result from an acute/recent small subcortical infarct or haemorrhage.[5] The clinical lacunar syndrome with underlying recent small subcortical infarct accounts for 25% of all ischaemic strokes.[48] Recent small subcortical infarcts occur subcortically in the basal ganglia, centrum semiovale, thalamus, internal capsule, or brainstem and their location can produce several classical lacunar syndromes, although as with many other diseases clinical-radiological correlation is imperfect,[49] and timely and detailed brain imaging is necessary to avoid misclassification of stroke.

Intracerebral haemorrhage

Worldwide, spontaneous intracerebral haemorrhage causes 9–27% of all stroke[50] with an increasing burden of disease between 1990 and 2010,[51] driven largely by an increasing burden in low and middle income countries (LMICs). The reported annual incidence of ICH is 24.6 per 100,000,[52] with a poor long-term prognosis (less than half survive one year and less than a third survive three years).[53]

Up to 85% of all ICH are caused by cerebral SVD. Traditionally, it was felt that deep ICH in the non-lobar regions (thalamus, brainstem, cerebellum, and basal ganglia) might be caused by a vasculopathy characterized by lipohyalinosis (historically considered to be associated with hypertension) and that lobar ICH are caused by cerebral amyloid angiopathy (abnormal deposition of beta amyloid in leptomeningeal and cortical blood vessels) whose hallmark is occipital lobar microbleeds seen on MRI brain imaging.[19] Certainly lobar ICH and non-lobar ICH may have differing risk factor profiles. In a large (n = 11,722) cohort of patients with vascular disease, age predicted lobar but not non-lobar haemorrhage and anticoagulant medication and male sex predicted non-lobar but not lobar haemorrhage.[54] There is emerging evidence to suggest that they have differing clinical outcomes—there is a lower one-year case-fatality after lobar than non-lobar haemorrhage after correcting for other known predictors of outcome (perhaps indicating that there are differing underlying SVD types causing each ICH subtype).[55] SVD not only causes ICH (and the significant associated comorbidity) but also predicts poorer outcome. In the INTERACT 2 trial, patients with concomitant brain imaging features of SVD have worse outcome following ICH than those without.[56] Similarly, in the large Third International Stroke Trial (IST-3) of rt-PA in acute ischaemic stroke, patients with more SVD features on CT at presentation had much worse outcomes than those without.[57]

Cognitive impairment and dementia

The estimated worldwide cost of dementia was US$818 billion in 2015.[58] Cerebral SVD causes vascular dementia, which is responsible for approximately 45% of all dementias. Furthermore there is increasing recognition of the vascular contribution to AD, suggesting that there may exist considerable overlap between these different disease states.[59] Patients with AD have evidence of cerebrovascular insults pathologically[60] and there is considerable overlap between shared (especially vascular) risk factors for both AD and vascular dementia.[61]

The link between cerebral SVD and cognition can be considered in two ways. The first relates to the patient who presents with dementia (progressive cognitive decline to the point that they are unable to manage their day-to-day activities). In this situation, the presence of cerebral SVD (or previous cerebral infarct or haemorrhage) is one of the key diagnostic markers of vascular dementia (or vascular cognitive impairment, a term used to emphasize that the deficit can be mild).[59] Despite the considerable overlap between pathological features and risk factors for AD and VCI[62] there are certain key differences in the cognitive profiles between the two. Cognition is a complex construct and can be subdivided into several key domains, including memory, language, attention, knowledge, judgement, planning, reasoning, and visuospatial awareness. Patients with AD typically present with memory problems as the predominant feature, whereas patients with VCI typically display deficits in a wider variety of domains but centred on executive functioning (the ability to plan and perform tasks using other cognitive domains).[63,64] It is important to use the correct test to find domain specific deficits—many tests of cognition (e.g. MMSE) are not good at detecting executive functioning deficits and it is possible that the vascular components of cognitive impairment have been under identified/represented generally.

The second method of considering the link between cSVD and cognition is to ask the question: 'Does this appearance of SVD on brain scanning have any cognitive implications for my patient either now or in the future?' Dealing with cross-sectional associations first, the presence of white matter lesions (or hyperintensities seen on MRI) versus similar patients without WMH is associated with decreased cognition in almost all patients groups.[65,66] Furthermore, illustrating the clinical importance to the patient, WMH predicted worse outcomes following stroke[57,67] and a systematic review and meta-analysis demonstrated that worse WMH predicted future stroke (HR 3.3, 95% CI 2.6–4.4, data from nine studies), dementia (HR 1.9, 1.3–2.8, 9 studies) and death (HR 2.0, 1.6–2.7, 8 studies).[8]

WMH are clearly important in clinical presentations with cognitive impairment, but their effect should not be considered in isolation as SVD causes a spectrum of changes that may act synergistically.[66] In non-cognitively impaired elderly individuals, lacunes, another common feature of SVD, are also associated with impaired executive functioning,[68] and speed and motor control.[69] Similarly, lacune number and volume predict poorer executive functioning in patients following lacunar stroke,[70] suggesting that their effect is not limited to healthy patients. In 1636 patients in the large SPS3 randomized trial, testing antiplatelet and blood pressure control regimes, 47% of all participants were classified as having mild cognitive impairment (MCI) at entry to the trial (in a study where having significant cognitive impairment was an exclusion to entry).[71] The importance of cognitive impairment in lacunar stroke is confirmed by a systematic review and meta-analysis that demonstrated 38% (95% CI 24–52%) of patients had MCI or dementia following lacunar stroke.[72] Therefore it is important to adopt a holistic approach when assessing the patient with cerebral SVD.

Of the remaining features of SVD, cerebral microbleeds predict worse performance on the MMSE and slower information processing.[73] Cognitive impairment in survivors of intracerebral haemorrhage is also common. A recent cohort study found that the incidence of dementia at six months after intracerebral haemorrhage was 14% (95% CI 10.0–19.3) and suggested that CAA may be a contributing factor as the rate was higher for patients with lobar ICH compared with those with non-lobar ICH (23.4%, 95% CI 14.6–33.3 vs 9.2%, 95% CI 5.1–14.7).[74] The burden of microbleeds was associated with cognitive impairment in a meta-analysis of 15 studies n = 3023.[75]

Gait instability/parkinsonism

Cerebral SVD can lead to gait instability and decreased mobility as well as what has been described as vascular parkinsonism. In the longitudinal Dutch Radboud University Nijmegen Diffusion tensor and Magnetic resonance imaging Cohort (RUN DMC) study of 431 patients, the presence of WMH and lacunar infarcts were both associated with decreased parameters of gait.[76] Gait abnormalities and unsteadiness or dizziness are common in the elderly. Cerebral SVD may play a role in non-specific presentations with dizziness. In a retrospective study of 122 patients, 22% of those with unexplained dizziness (where the cause could not be ascribed to other causes such as benign positional vertigo, postural hypotension, or other) had severe WMH (Fazekas 3) versus only 5% of an age-matched control group of patients with explained dizziness.[77]

The relationship between gait/mobility and cerebral SVD is complex, reflecting that several biological systems are required for successful walking. Moderate/severe WMH in the Leukoaraiosis and Disability in the Elderly study (LADIS) study predicted a decline in gait, but there was evidence of heterogeneity of responses between individuals, with a strong interaction between age and severity of WMH.[78] Gait impairment predicts mortality in SVD, again probably due to reflection of the decline in functioning of several different biological systems and not just the brain.[76] Patients with cerebral SVD may present with Parkinsonian symptoms and after brain scanning showing SVD be diagnosed with vascular parkinsonism.[79] The exact underlying pathophysiology of this condition is unclear, but it seems likely that it overlaps with cerebral SVD.[80]

Depression and mood disorders

Depression (and in particular DSM-IV-defined depressive symptoms) demonstrates a bidirectional association with vascular disease—depression is both a risk factor for and a sequelae of vascular disease. Depression related to vascular disease starts at older ages[81] and is important as it can be devastating to patients, families, and carers, and impede recovery from other illnesses, for example stroke. Depression has a post-stroke prevalence of approximately 30% and is predicted by cognitive impairment.[82,83] Cross-sectional analyses show that brain features of SVD are associated with prevalent depression and this is confirmed in some longitudinal studies,[84,85] but not all.[86] The LADIS study found that progression of WMH in outpatients predicted incidence of depression after multivariate analysis, including disability level.[87] Similarly, lacunar infarcts were associated with severity of depression in patients with symptomatic atherosclerosis.[88] The AGES-Reykjavik Trial of 1949 participants found that depression was common (10% of all participants) and that several features of SVD predicted a greater incidence of depression: WMH volume, subcortical infarcts (lacunes), enlarged perivascular spaces, and decreased brain volume.[84]

These findings represent static changes and possible mechanisms may underpin these associations. Two recent studies have used diffusion tensor imaging, an advanced technique which uses the diffusion of water molecules to determine white matter tract integrity to identify any changes associated with depression and SVD. The RUN DMC study showed decreased tract integrity in patients with SVD (correcting for factors including age) but this disappeared after WMH correction.[89] Path analysis in 101 lacunar stroke patients found an association between reduced fractional anisotropy and depression.[90] A meta-analysis of nine studies showed possible reduced neural network connectivity in patients with late-life depression.[91]

Disability and mortality

It is also important to consider the overall effect that SVD has on patients, including their level of functioning and independence. Having more WMH doubles the hazard ratio (HR 2.0, 95% CI 1.6–2.7) of death in a meta-analysis of eight studies.[8] The LADIS study further investigated brain features of SVD on MRI as predictors of decline in function (transition into institutionalized care) and death,[92] showing that in a large outpatient population aged 65–84 years old, having more severe WMH at inception predicted transition from no disability to disability or death over three years.[9]

Asymptomatic SVD

A proportion of patients will present with asymptomatic (or what is initially felt to be asymptomatic) SVD when they have brain scans for other reasons. Upon detailed cognitive or clinical assessment, deficits may be elicited. There is, however, minimal guidance on the best approach to take to the truly asymptomatic patient and most advocate a prudent primary prevention policy.

Summary

Cerebral SVD is common, causing a wide range of clinical manifestations that present with many different conditions to different healthcare services and healthcare professionals. This diversity makes recognizing and categorizing patients with cerebral SVD challenging, and both clinicians and researchers should be aware of this spectrum of presentation. Different subtypes of patients may need different investigation plans and treatments, but there is currently limited evidence to guide either of these.

Suggestions for Future Research

With the relatively recent advent of detailed brain imaging, we are only just beginning to recognize the full spectrum of radiological and clinical manifestations of cerebral SVD and the considerable impact of this disease on patients, carers, and society. The overarching aim of research should focus on identifying effective and appropriate prevention and treatment of SVD. The lack of effective treatments reflects an incomplete understanding of the underlying pathophysiology of cerebral SVD (including ignorance of the exact nature of the complex interactions between the individual components of SVD), incomplete knowledge about the range of impacts, clinical presentations, and longitudinal progression of the disease.

In order to address these issues, further studies should determine the pathology and sequence of events leading to overt SVD features on brain imaging, both those that lead to 'ischaemic' damage and to haemorrhage. This will help to determine the relative contributions of different types of small perforating arteriolar vasculopathy. A greater understanding of the complex relationships between known existing risk factors such as hypertension and the need to look for causes beyond traditional risk factors are both urgently required. There is limited understanding of the different prevalence and incidences between different world regions.

An increasing range of *in vivo* imaging techniques are being employed to study structure and function and, perhaps most excitingly, structure combined with function. High field 7T MRI is now demonstrating the presence of hitherto hard-to-detect-in-life lesions such as microinfarcts. Clearly, greater use of more detailed structural imaging in carefully characterized patients will reveal useful information. We would recommend adherence to published recommendations when reporting results of imaging research in SVD.[5] There is an argument for adopting the same standard terminology in routine clinical practice as well. Greater use of dynamic brain imaging to investigate cerebral blood flow, BBB permeability, vascular reactivity, and tissue structure (e.g. with diffusion tensor imaging) will provide information about underlying mechanisms. Exploiting the homology between retinal and brain microvasculatures, including with dynamic retinal vessel functional imaging, for example with scanning laser ophthalmoscopy, ocular computed tomography, and angiography will reveal information about microvessel structure and function to link with the brain changes. Additionally, many of these techniques may provide useful information as possible intermediary endpoints for use in clinical trials.

There is limited knowledge about rates of progression of this often insidious disease over longer time periods (above one year) pointing to a need for long-term serial clinical and neuroimaging assessments, which are also necessary to inform future trial design. Analysis of existing datasets to maximize use of available data is important,[93] but most previous studies simply did not collect sufficiently detailed data or characterize patients sufficiently to inform future practice. Improved patient characterization to stratify recurrent events and disease progression by age, presence, and type of symptoms, is critical. The clinical manifestations of cerebral SVD are varied, but hitherto the few studies in this area have generally used only fairly conventional outcome measures of recurrent stroke, other vascular endpoints, dependency, or death. It may be that these event rates are too low in SVD and that other measures such as depression, mobility, or cognition may be more patient centred and relevant to trials in this area. Further research is warranted to ascertain what matters to patients in terms of trial outcomes and which should be measured. There is an urgent need for randomized trials focusing on cerebral SVD. There are ongoing LACunar Intervention (LACI) trials, but more are required.

Patients with cerebral SVD present to different clinical specialties: psychiatry, gerontology, neurology, radiology, and general practice, and research up to now has reflected this heterogeneity of practice. There is increasing recognition of the vascular contribution to neurodegenerative disease such as AD and of the complex relationship between normal ageing, degeneration, and vascular disease. Elucidating these relationships will aid treatment discovery. In order to move away from concentrating on single aspects of a multifaceted disease, we recommend that researchers in these different fields work collaboratively in a multidisciplinary fashion to fully capture all aspects of this truly complex and serious disease.

REFERENCES

1. Thompson CS, Hakim AM. Living beyond our physiological means: small vessel disease of the brain is an expression of a systemic failure in arteriolar function: a unifying hypothesis. Stroke. 2009; 40: e322–e330.9.
2. Pantoni L, Fierini F, Poggesi A, et al. Impact of cerebral white matter changes on functionality in older adults: An overview of the LADIS Study results and future directions. Geriatr Gerontol Int. 2015; 15(Suppl1): 10–16.
3. Wardlaw JM, Smith C, Dichgans M. Mechanisms of sporadic cerebral small vessel disease: insights from neuroimaging. Lancet Neurology. 2013; 12: 483–97.
4. Chabriat H, Joutel, A, Dichgans M, Tournier-Lasserve, E, Bousser MG. CADASIL. Lancet Neurology. 2009; 8(7): 643–53.
5. Wardlaw JM, Smith EE, Biessels GJ, et al. STandards for ReportIng Vascular changes on nEuroimaging (STRIVE v1). Neuroimaging standards for research into small vessel disease and its contribution to ageing and neurodegeneration. Lancet Neurology. 2013; 12: 822–38.
6. Shi Y, Wardlaw J. Update on cerebral small vessel disease: a dynamic whole-brain disease. Stroke and Vascular Neurology. 2016;1(3):83–92.
7. Poggesi A, Pasi M, Pescini F, Pantoni L, Inzitari D. Circulating biologic markers of endothelial dysfunction in cerebral small vessel disease: A review. J Cereb Blood Flow Metab. 2016; 36: 72–94.
8. Debette S, Markus HS. The clinical importance of white matter hyperintensities on brain magnetic resonance imaging: systematic review and meta-analysis. BMJ. 2010; 341: c3666.
9. Inzitari D, Pracucci G, Poggesi A, et al. Changes in white matter as determinant of global functional decline in older independent outpatients: three year follow-up of LADIS study cohort. BMJ. 2009; 339: b2477.
10. Pantoni L, Garcia JH. Pathogenesis of leukoaraiosis: a review. Stroke. 1997; 28: 652–9.
11. Charidimou A, Pantoni L, Love S. The concept of sporadic cerebral small vessel disease: A road map on key definitions and current concepts. Int J Stroke. 2016; 11: 6–18.
12. Smith EE, Schneider JA, Wardlaw JM, Greenberg SM. Cerebral microinfarcts: the invisible lesions. Lancet Neurology. 2012; 11(3): 272–82.
13. vanVeluw SJ, Zwanenburg JJ, Engelen-Lee J, et al. In vivo detection of cerebral cortical microinfarcts with high-resolution 7T MRI. J Cereb Blood Flow Metab 2013; 33: 322–9.
14. Wardlaw JM, Valdés Hernández MC, Muñoz-Maniega S. What are white matter hyperintensities made of? Relevance to vascular cognitive impairment. J Am Heart Assoc. 2015; 4(6): 001140.

15. Ikram MA, van der Lugt A, Wiro J, et al. The Rotterdam Scan Study: design update 2016 and main findings. Eur J Epidemiol. 2015; 30: 1299–315.
16. Rincorn FR, Wright CB. Current pathophysiological concepts in cerebral small vessel disease. Front. Aging Neurosci. 2014; 6: 24.
17. Norrving B. Lacunar infarcts: no black holes in the brain are benign. Pract Neurol. 2008; 8(4): 222–8.
18. Vermeer S, Longstreth Jr WT, Koudstaal PJ. Silent brain infarcts: a systematic review. Lancet Neurology. 2007; 6: 611–19.
19. Greenberg SM, Vernooij MW, Cordonnier C, et al. Microbleed Study Group. Cerebral microbleeds: a guide to detection and interpretation. Lancet Neurology. 2009; 8: 165–74.
20. Cordonnier C, Al-Shahi Salman R, Wardlaw J. Spontaneous brain microbleeds: systematic review, subgroup analyses and standards for study design and reporting. Brain. 2007; 130: 1988–2003.
21. Lee SH, Bae HJ, Kwon SJ, et al. Cerebral microbleeds are regionally associated with intracerebral hemorrhage. Neurology. 2004; 62:72–6.
22. Vernooij MW, van der Lugt A, Ikram MA, et al. Prevalence and risk factors of cerebral microbleeds: the Rotterdam Scan Study. Neurology. 2008; 70: 1208–14.
23. Bouvy WH, Biessels GJ, Kuijf HJ, Kappelle LJ, Luijten PR, Zwanenburg JJ. Visualization of perivascular spaces and perforating arteries with 7 T magnetic resonance imaging. Invest Radiol. 2014; 49(5): 307–13.
24. Wiseman S, Bastin M, Jardine C, et al, Cerebral small vessel disease burden is increased in systemic lupus erythematosus. Stroke. 2016; 47(11): 2722–8.
25. Bouvy WH, Zwanenburg JJ, Reinink R, et al. Perivascular spaces on 7 Tesla brain MRI are related to markers of small vessel disease but not to age or cardiovascular risk factors. J Cereb Blood Flow Metab. 2016; 36: 1708–17.
26. Doubal FN, MacLullich AMJ, Ferguson KJ, Dennis MS, Wardlaw JM. Enlarged perivascular spaces on MRI are a feature of cerebral small vessel disease. Stroke. 2010; 41(3): 450–4.
27. Potter GM, Doubal FN, Jackson CA, et al. Enlarged perivascular spaces and cerebral small vessel disease. Int J Stroke. 2015; 10: 376–81.
28. Martinez-Ramirez S, Pontes-Neto OM, Dumas AP, et al. Topography of dilated perivascular spaces in subjects from a memory clinic cohort. Neurology. 2013; 80: 1551–6.
29. Aribisala BS, Wiseman S, Morris Z, et al. Circulating inflammatory markers are associated with MR visible perivascular spaces but not directly with white matter hyperintensities. Stroke. 2014; 45: 605–7.
30. Westover MB, Bianchi MT, Yang C, Schneider JA, Greenberg SM. Estimating cerebral microinfarct burden from autopsy samples. Neurology. 2013; 80: 1365–9.
31. Del Brutto OH, Mera RM, Del Brutto VJ, Zambrano M, Lama J. White matter hyperintensities of presumed vascular origin: a population-based study in rural Ecuador. Int J Stroke. 2015; 10: 372–5.
32. Brickman AM, Schupf N, Manly JJ, et al. Brain morphology in older African Americans, Caribbean Hispanics, and whites from northern Manhattan. Arch Neurol. 2008; 65: 1053–61.
33. Wardlaw JM, Allerhand M, Doubal FN, et al. Vascular risk factors, large-artery atheroma, and brain white matter hyperintensities. Neurology. 2014; 82: 1331–8.
34. Blair GW, Doubal FN, Thrippleton MJ, Marshall I, Wardlaw JM. Magnetic resonance imaging for assessment of cerebrovascular reactivity in cerebral small vessel disease: A systematic review. J Cereb Blood Flow Metab. 2016; 36(5): 833–41.
35. Aribisala BS, Morris Z, Eadie E, et al. Blood pressure, internal carotid artery flow parameters and age-related white matter hyperintensities. Hypertension. 2014; 63: 1011–18.
36. Maillard P, Seshadri S, Beiser A, et al. Effects of systolic blood pressure on white-matter integrity in young adults in the Framingham Heart Study: a cross-sectional study. Lancet Neurology. 2012; 11: 1039–47.
37. van Dijk EJ, Breteler MM, Schmidt R, et al. The association between blood pressure, hypertension, and cerebral white matter lesions: cardiovascular determinants of dementia study. Hypertension. 2004; 44(5): 625–30.
38. Schmidt R, Seiler S, Loitfelder M. Longitudinal change of small-vessel disease-related brain abnormalities. J Cereb Blood Flow Metab. 2016; 36: 26–39.
39. Dufouil C, deKersaint-Gilly A, Besançon V et al. Longitudinal study of blood pressure and white matter hyperintensities: the EVA MRI Cohort. Neurology. 2001; 56: 921–6.
40. Dufouil C, Chalmers J, Coskun O, et al. Effects of blood pressure lowering on cerebral white matter hyperintensities in patients with stroke. Circulation. 2005; 112: 1644–50.
41. Weber R, Weimar C, Blatchford J, et al. Telmisartan on top of antihypertensive treatment does not prevent progression of cerebral white matter lesions in the prevention regimen for effectively avoiding second strokes (PRoFESS) MRI substudy. Stroke. 2012; 43: 2336–42.
42. Benavente OR, Coffey CS, Conwit R, et al. Blood-pressure targets in patients with recent lacunar stroke: the SPS3 randomised trial. Lancet. 2013; 382: 507–15.
43. Traylor M, Rutten-Jacobs LC, Thijs V, et al. Genetic associations with white matter hyperintensities confer risk of lacunar stroke. Stroke. 2016; 47: 1174–9.
44. Martini SR, Williams SR, Moretti P, Woo D, Worrall B. A molecular/genetic approach to cerebral small-vessel disease: beyond aging and hypertension. Brain Circ. 2015: 1: 79–87.
45. Staals J, Makin S, Doubal F, Dennis M, Wardlaw J. Stroke subtype, vascular risk factors, and total MRI brain small-vessel disease burden. Neurology. 2014; 83: 1228–34.
46. Ihara M, Yamamoto Y. Emerging evidence for pathogenesis of sporadic cerebral small vessel disease. Stroke. 2016; 47: 554–60.
47. Scutt P, Blackburn D, Krishnan K, et al. Baseline characteristics, analysis plan and report on feasibility for the Prevention Of Decline in Cognition After Stroke Trial (PODCAST). Trials. 2015; 16: 509.
48. Adams HP, Bendixen BH, Kappelle LJ, et al. Classification of subtype of acute ischemic stroke. Definitions for use in a multicenter clinical trial. Stroke. 1993; 24(1): 35–41.
49. Mead GE, Lewis S, Wardlaw JM, Dennis MS, Warlow CP. Should computed tomography appearance of lacunar stroke influence patient management? J Neurol Neurosurg Psychiatry. 1999; 67: 682–4.
50. Feigin VL, Lawes CM, Bennett DA, Barker-Collo SL, Parag V. World- wide stroke incidence and early case fatality reported in 56 population-based studies: a systematic review. Lancet Neurology. 2009; 8: 355–69.
51. Feigin VL, Forouzanfar MH, Krishnamurthi R, et al. Global and regional burden of stroke during 1990–2010: findings from the Global Burden of Disease Study 2010. Lancet. 2014; 383: 245–54.
52. van Asch CJ, Luitse MJ, Rinkel GJ, et al. Incidence, case fatality, and functional outcome of intracerebral haemorrhage over time,

according to age, sex, and ethnic origin: a systematic review and meta-analysis. Lancet Neurology. 2010; 9: 167–76.
53. Poon M, Fonville AF, Salman RA. Long-term prognosis after intracerebral haemorrhage: systematic review and meta-analysis. J Neurol Neurosurg Psychiatry. 2014; 85: 660–7.
54. Kremer PHC, Jolink W, Kappelle LJ, et al. Risk factors for lobar and non-lobar intracerebral hemorrhage in patients with vascular disease. PLOS One. http://dx.doi.org/10.1371/journal.pone.0142338.
55. Samarasekera N, Fonville A, Lerpiniere C, et al. Influence of intracerebral hemorrhage location on incidence, characteristics, and outcome. Population-based study. Stroke. 2015; 46: 361–8.
56. Sato S, Delcourt C, Heeley E, et al. Significance of cerebral small-vessel disease in acute intracerebral hemorrhage. Stroke. 2016; 47: 701–7.
57. IST-3 collaborative group. Association between brain imaging signs, early and late outcomes, and response to intravenous alteplase after acute ischaemic stroke in the third International Stroke Trial (IST-3): Lancet Neurology. 2015; 14(5): 485–96.
58. World Alzheimer Report 2015: The global impact of dementia. https://www.alz.co.uk/research/world-report-2015.
59. Gorelick PB, Scuteri,A, Black SE, et al., Vascular contributions to cognitive impairment and dementia. Stroke. 2011; 42(9): 2672–713.
60. Snowdon DA, Nun Study. Healthy aging and dementia: findings from the Nun Study. Ann Intern Med. 2003; 139: 450–4.
61. Snyder H, Corriveau RA, Craft S, et al, Vascular contributions to cognitive impairment and dementia including Alzheimer's disease. Alzheimer's & Dementia. 2015; 11: 710–17.
62. Attems J, Jellinger KA. The overlap between vascular disease and Alzheimer's disease—lessons from pathology. BMC Medicine. 2014: 12: 206.
63. Yang FM, Grigorenko A, Tommet D, et al. AD pathology and cerebral infarctions are associated with memory and executive functioning one and five years before death. J Clin Exp Neuropsychol. 2013; 35(1): 24–34.
64. Wallin A, Nordlund A, Jonsson M, et al. Alzheimer's disease—subcortical vascular disease spectrum in a hospital-based setting: Overview of results from the Gothenburg MCI and dementia studies. J Cereb Blood Flow Metab. 2016; 36(1): 95–113.
65. Pantoni L, Poggesi A, Inzitari D. The relation between white-matter lesions and cognition. Curr Opin Neurol. 2007; 20(4): 390–7.
66. Prins ND, Scheltens P, White matter hyperintensities, cognitive impairment and dementia: an update. Nature Reviews Neurology. 2015; 11, 157–65.
67. Kang HJ, Stewart R, Park MS, et al. White matter hyperintensities and functional outcomes at 2 weeks and 1 year after stroke. Cerebrovasc Dis. 2013; 35(2): 138–45.
68. Carey CL, Kramer JH, Josephson SA, et al. Subcortical lacunes are associated with executive dysfunction in cognitively normal elderly. Stroke. 2008; 39(2): 397–402.
69. Benisty S, Gouw AA, Porcher R, et al. Location of lacunar infarcts correlates with cognition in a sample of non-disabled subjects with age-related white-matter changes. J Neurol Neurosurg Psychiatry. 2009; 80(5): 478–83.
70. Benjamin P, Lawrence AJ, Lambert C, et al. Strategic lacunes and their relationship to cognitive impairment in cerebral small vessel disease. Neuroimage Clin. 2014; 4: 828–37.
71. Jacova C, Pearce LA, Costello R, et al. Cognitive impairment in lacunar strokes: the SPS3 trial. Ann Neurol. 2012; 72(3): 351–62.
72. Makin SD, Turpin S, Dennis MS, Wardlaw JM. Cognitive impairment after lacunar stroke: systematic review and meta-analysis of incidence, prevalence and comparison with other stroke subtypes. J Neurol Neurosurg Psychiatry. 2013; 84(8): 893–900.
73. Poels MM, Ikram MA, van der Lugt A, et al. Cerebral microbleeds are associated with worse cognitive function: the Rotterdam Scan Study. Neurology. 2012; 78(5): 326–33.
74. Moulin S, Labreuche J,Bombois S, et al. Dementia risk after spontaneous intracerebral haemorrhage: a prospective cohort study. Lancet Neurology. 2016; 15: 820–9.
75. Wu RH, Feng C, Xu Y, Hua T, Liu XY, Fang M. Late-onset depression in the absence of stroke: associated with silent brain infarctions, microbleeds and lesion locations. Int J Med Sci. 2014; 11(6): 587–92.
76. van der Holst HM, van Uden IM, Tuladhar AM, et al. Factors associated with 8-year mortality in older patients with cerebral small vessel disease: RUN DMC Study. JAMA Neurol. 2016; 73: 402–9.
77. Ahmad H, Cerchiai N, Mancuso M, Casani AP, Bronstein AM. Are white matter abnormalities associated with 'unexplained dizziness'? J Neurol Sci. 2015: 4–7.
78. Kreisel SH, Blahak C, Bäzner H, et al. Deterioration of gait and balance over time: the effects of age-related white matter change. Cerebrovasc Dis. 2013; 35(6): 544–53.
79. Korczyn AD. Vascular parkinsonism—characteristics, pathogenesis and treatment. Nature Reviews Neurology. 2015; 11: 319–26.
80. Antonini A, Vitale C, Barone P, et al. The relationship between cerebral vascular disease and parkinsonism: The VADO study. Parkinsonism Relat Disord. 2012; 18(6): 775–80.
81. Herrmann LL, Le Masurier M, Ebmeier KP. White matter hyperintensities in late life depression: a systematic review. J Neurol Neurosurg Psychiatry. 2008; 79(6): 619–24.
82. Hackett ML, Köhler S, O'Brien J, Mead GE. Neuropsychiatric outcomes of stroke. Lancet Neurology. 2014; 13(5): 525–34.
83. Hackett ML, Anderson CS. Predictors of depression after stroke: a systematic review of observational studies. Stroke. 2005; 36: 2296–301.
84. van Sloten TT, Sigurdsson S, van Buchem MA, et al. Cerebral small vessel disease and association with higher incidence of depressive symptoms in a general elderly population: The AGES-Reykjavik Study. Am J Psychiatry. 2015; 172(6): 570–8.
85. Wu R, Feng C, Zhao Y, Jin AP, Fang M, Liu X. A meta-analysis of association between cerebral microbleeds and cognitive impairment. Med Sci Monit. 2014; 20: 2189–98.
86. Ikram MA, Luijendijk HJ, Vernooij MW, et al. Vascular brain disease and depression in the elderly. Epidemiology. 2010; 21(1): 78–81.
87. Firbank MJ, Teodorczuk A, van der Flier WM, et al. Relationship between progression of brain white matter changes and late-life depression: 3-year results from the LADIS Study. Br J Psychiatry. 2012; 201: 40–5.
88. Grool AM, Gerritsen L, Zuithoff NP, Mali WP, vanderGraaf Y, Geerlings MI. Lacunar infarcts in deep white matter are associated with higher and more fluctuating depressive symptoms during three years follow-up. Biol Psychiatry. 2013; 73(2): 169–76.
89. van Uden IW, Tuladhar AM, de Laat KF et al. White matter integrity and depressive symptoms in cerebral small vessel disease: The RUN DMC study. Am J Geriatr Psychiatry. 2014; 23(5): 525–35.

90. Brookes RL, Herbert V, Lawrence AJ, Morris RG, Markus HS. Depression in small-vessel disease relates to white matter ultrastructural damage, not disability. Neurology. 2014; 83(16): 1417–23.
91. Wen MC, Steffens DC, Chen MK, Zainal NH. Diffusion tensor imaging studies in late-life depression: systematic review and meta-analysis. Int J Geriatr Psychiatry. 2014; 29(12): 1173–84
92. Pantoni L, Fierini F, Poggesi A, et al. Impact of cerebral white matter changes on functionality in older adults: An overview of the LADIS Study results and future directions. Geriatr Gerontol Int. 2015; 15(Suppl1): 10–16.
93. METACOHORTS Consortium. METACOHORTS for the study of vascular disease and its contribution to cognitive decline and neurodegeneration. Alzheimer's Dement. 2016;12(12):1235–1249.

22

Migraine

Descriptive epidemiology and related neurobiology

Julio R Vieira and Richard B Lipton

Incidence

The incidence of migraine varies depending of multiple aspects, including age, sex, and the presence of aura[1]. At an earlier age (younger than age ten), migraine initially affects more boys than girls, with migraine with aura (MA) occurring at a younger age than migraine without aura (MO). The incidence of migraine with aura in boys is 14.1 compared to 3.5/1000 person-years at age 12–13 and the incidence of migraine without aura is 17.3 compared to 9.9/1000 person-years for migraine without aura[2]. Later in life, when puberty starts, this relationship changes and it becomes more common in women than men, with peak incidence for women ages 20–24 years at 18.2/1000 person-years and for men ages 15–19 at 6.2/1000 person-years.

The cumulative incidence in women is approximately 43% and for men 18%, with a variable annual incidence depending on the study selected, differing from 0.8% (women 1.5% and men 0.3%) to 2.38%/year (women 2.98% and men 1.93%).[3]

Prevalence

In 2015, there were approximately 958.8 million people in the world living with migraine.[4] There is a great variability in migraine prevalence depending on age, sex, and geographic location. The world's prevalence of migraine differs depending on geographic region, ranging from the lowest in Africa at 5%, to 15% in Europe,[5] with 12% overall prevalence in the USA. Worldwide migraine is more common in women, as seen in the USA, with 18% prevalence in US women compared to 6% in US men.[6,7] Prevalence also varies by age, with peak prevalence between ages 25–55 years, and sex prevalence ratio varying among female[8] and male from 1.5:1 at age 12–17 years old[7] to 3.25:1 at age 18–29[9] years old and peaking at 3.31:1 at ages 40–25 years old, then decreasing after menopause to 2.0:1. Migraine prevalence also varies depending on other aspects, including education, with prevalence amid university students varying from 11.3% in men and 21.7% in women, with overall prevalence of 16%. Moreover, prevalence also differs depending on sociodemographics, medical, neurological, and psychiatric comorbidities (See Table 22.1).

Prevalence of MA

Migraine aura are focal neurological symptoms that typically occur prior to the onset of a headache due to a phenomenon called cortical spreading depression. The prevalence of migraine with aura is approximately one-third of the migraineur population[10] and varies between visual, sensory, or motor symptoms, with predominantly 79% visual symptoms, 30% sensory, and up to 18% motor.[11] It can also present as diplopia, slurred speech, aphasia, dizziness, vertigo, and hemiparesis.

Prevalence of Chronic Migraine

The prevalence of migraine also varies according to headache frequency. Chronic migraine (CM) is typically defined as ≥15 headache days/month and has a global prevalence varying from 0% to 5.7%[12,13] depending on the study in question, which includes different definitions and different sample selections, contributing to the wide range in prevalence. The definition of chronic migraine differs throughout

Table 22.1 Migraine prevalence by sex and world region

	Overall	Men	Women
Global	11%	6%	14%
Africa	5%	3%	6%
Asia	9%	6%	11%
Europe	15%	7%	18%
Australia	N/A	N/A	22%
North America	13%	6%	18%
Central/South America	9%	4%	12%
US	12%	6%	18%

studies. One particular older criteria defines CM as chronic daily headache or near-daily headache with features of migraine with prevalence ranging from 0.86% to 2.4%; however, when utilizing the more modern and conservative definition of migraine occurring on ≥15 days/month, the prevalence estimates decreases from 0 to 0.7%. In the USA it varied from 0.91% to 4.1%.[13,14]

Paediatric Population

There are some differences in diagnostic criteria between adults and the paediatric population. It varies in duration, lasting from 2–72 hours, compared to at least 4 hours in adults. The location is more often bilateral than unilateral and switches sides. It is usually fronto-temporal, and possibly presents as abdominal pain with nausea and vomiting, instead of head pain. In younger children it can be manifested in a more subtle way due to limited communication, with features like photophobia and phonophobia manifesting as change in behaviour.[15] Beyond diagnostic criteria differences, there is also a difference in prevalence, varying between 3% and 10% in young children and increasing throughout adolescence when it can be as high as 20%.[16] Migraine prevalence in children varies quite a lot in relation to puberty, being initially more common in boys than girls prior to puberty and later on, after puberty there is a change and migraine becomes more common in girls than boys.[10]

Prevalence of Menstrual Migraine

Menstrual migraine is defined by the ICHD3 criteria as migraine attacks usually occurring on days -2 (2 days prior to menses) to +3 of menstruation in at least two out of three menstrual cycles. It is divided in pure menstrual migraine (PMM) and menstrually related migraine (MRM).[15] There is an enormous variability between the rates of MRM among studies depending on diagnostic criteria, research design, study sample population, and design of research methodology. It ranges from 3%[17] to 76%[18] of women with migraine. It is a very common occurrence, with diverse studies reporting that more than 50% of women with migraine had at least some association between menstrual cycle and migraine, with the peak incidence of migraine around menses and the lowest risk around the time of ovulation.[18] Peri-menstrual migraine attacks are reported by some studies, as well as suggested by clinical wisdom to have a longer duration, greater severity, have greater associated impairment, and are more difficult to treat than their counterpart migraine attacks occurring at other times of the month than around menses.[19] On the other hand peri-menopause also appears to be a source for increased attack frequency in women, with migraine during the peri-menopausal period, as shown by the American Migraine Prevalence and Prevention (AMPP) Study confirming a hormonal component in the variability of headache frequency.[20]

Burden of Migraine

Migraine is a debilitating disease with a potential colossal burden, which can affect not only the individual suffering from a migraine, but also family members, friends, employers, and society as a whole through direct and indirect costs.[21] The burden can occur both during attacks described as an ictal state, including the associated symptoms photophobia, phonophobia, nausea[22,23] and vomiting, as well as, between attacks called interically[24] with anxiety of a potential new attack and avoidance of many work-related and leisure-related activities due to fear of possibly causing or exacerbating an attack. This can lead to over treating the attacks, maybe even treating the pain before it starts, causing medication overuse and aggravating the cycle even more. Sometimes individuals can have an irrational fear and overreact when facing debilitating or potentially debilitating pain and assume the worse-case scenario called catastrophizing,[25] which by itself can be very debilitating. Migraine is onerous to individuals with the disorder, to their families, and to society.

Individual Burden

Globally, in 2015 there were almost 33 million DALYs lost due to migraine.[4,26] The burden of migraine at the individual level may be extremely severe.[27,28] It involves a potential personal disability, affecting multiple domains, including professional/education involving work and school, as well as personal, family, social, and leisure time. It can be associated with suboptimal performance at work, school, and at home, described as presenteeism,[13,14] which is when individuals are physically present; however, their performance and ability to relate to others is significantly affected due to a migraine preventing them from fully functioning. The impact of presenteeism can be even greater in people with chronic migraine and also among women who have migraine associated with menses.[29,30] Although presenteeism has been historically known, it is most likely under estimated.

Family Burden

The burden of migraine at the family level can also be enormous on family members, with migraineurs having difficulties in performing their routine responsibilities and chores, many times being unable to complete them. They can also miss multiple family gatherings and events, as well as miss or cancel vacations, which can have a financial impact beyond the social impact. Migraine can affect the mood and well-being of relationships between spouses, children, and other family members.[31]

Burden to Society

Headache is one of the most common reasons for seeking medical attention.[32] In the USA it is classified as being the fifth top reason to visit the emergency department overall and third among women ages 15–64 years old.[13] The highest prevalence of migraine occurs between the second and fifth decade of life, which is the period of time of the most productive years of an individual's life; therefore it can originate an excessive cost to society. These costs include a great reduction in productivity and lost working hours, accounting for 1.3% of years lost due to disability.[33] When accounting for just within the US alone, the expenditure employers have to absorb per

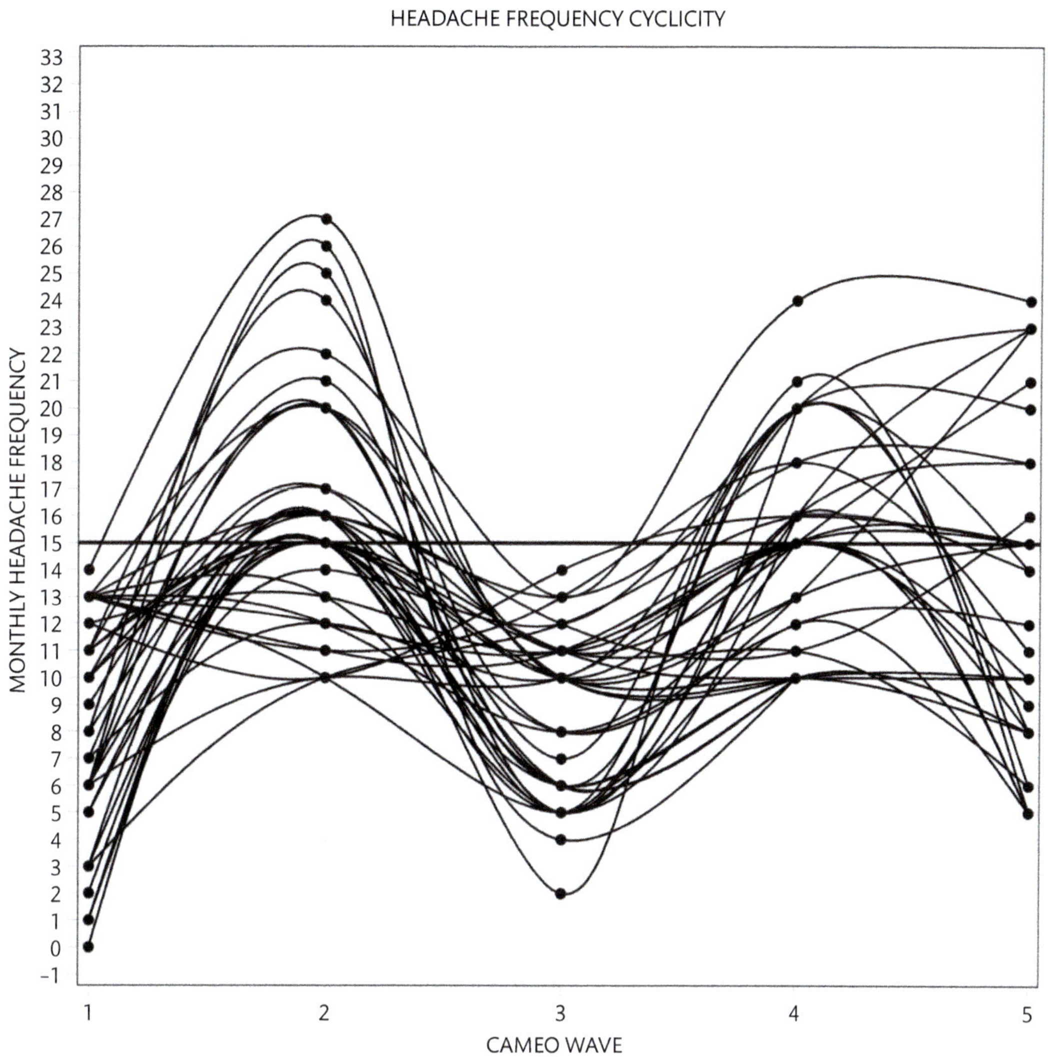

Fig. 22.1 Random sample from the CaMEO (Chronic Migraine Epidemiology and Outcomes) study showing the progression from a baseline EM to CM captured during follow up with subsequent remission back to EM. Cyclicity was common in the headache frequency trajectory both within persons (individual level) and between persons (population level).

year in indirect costs accounts for $13 billion dollars. When considering both direct and indirect costs, migraine is responsible for more global disability than any other single neurological condition.[34]

Natural History of Migraine

There is a natural cyclicity variability of the frequency of migraine attacks over time. These data were observed by both longitudinal population studies, as well as clinical experience. Among persons with baseline episodic migraine (EM) on year one, 2.5–3% of them will progress the next year and develop CM, 85% will continue to have EM the next year, and the remainder will no longer meet the criteria definition for migraine.[35] The two major studies to demonstrate this variability had some methodological differences with the Chronic Migraine Epidemiology and Outcomes (CaMEO) study measuring attacks at three-month intervals and the AMPP Study measuring it in annual intervals. Both studies demonstrated a high level of within person variability in headache days per month, which included fluid movement from HFEM (high frequency episodic migraine = 10–14 headache days per month) to CM (headache frequency ≥15 headache days per month) and vice versa (see Fig. 22.1). This variability can make diagnosis challenging.[36]

Migraine and Vascular Risk

There is a variable cardiovascular disease risk among persons with migraine and this risk depends on sex and migraine type (MA vs MO). According to the Women's Health Study (WHS), which is the largest population study of this relationship, women with MA have a two-fold increase in risk of ischaemic stroke, myocardial infarction, and all cause cardiovascular mortality when compared to those women without migraine.[37] However, the risk of cardiovascular events was not significantly increased among women with MO. One of the criticisms about the WHS is the way aura was defined, which was solely based on participant's answer of a single question about warnings, which precede a headache; therefore this definition may combine aura and prodrome. Subsequent studies when aura and prodrome were distinguished have reported an increase of cardiovascular events for both MA and MO.[38]

The Physician's Health Study reported that there was an increased risk of cardiovascular and cerebrovascular events in men with migraine; however, there was no distinction between MA and MO.[39]

Overall, migraine has not been shown to have an increased risk of myocardial infarction or cardiovascular death; however, MA has been associated with an increased risk of an ischaemic stroke by two-fold. In women who have MA, are younger than 45 years old, who also smoke and use oral contraceptives, there is an effect modification that can increase this risk exponentially by ten-fold. On the contrary, MO was not associated with increased risk of stroke. Despite the increased relative risk of stroke in women with MA, stroke remains a rare occurrence in young populations; therefore the absolute risk of stroke on the other hand is relatively low, with adjusted risk at 4.3/1,000 person-years for total stroke and 3.4/1,000 person-years for ischaemic stroke[40] (see Table 22.2).

Comorbidities

There are several comorbidities associated with migraine, including many neurologic, medical, and psychiatric conditions. Psychiatric comorbidities include depression and anxiety disorders between the most common conditions, despite others less common. Medical comorbidities include asthma, allergic rhinitis, cardiac diseases and events, and non-headache pain disorders, including temporomandibular joint disorder (TMD) and fibromyalgia among other conditions.[41] Neurologic comorbidities include epilepsy, stroke, restless legs syndrome (RLS), sleep disorders, ischaemic stroke, and multiple sclerosis (MS) most commonly, although there are other less common conditions as well.

The rates of comorbid conditions are higher in persons with CM, relative to EM and have been demonstrated in population-based studies as well as clinical studies. The AMPP Study and the International Burden of Illness Study reported that respondents with CM were more likely to have depression, anxiety, and chronic pain by approximately two-fold.

Table 22.2 Migraine with aura and risk of stroke

	Relative stroke risk RR (95% CI)	Absolute total stroke risk IR per 1000 person-year (95% CI)	Absolute ischaemic stroke risk IR per 1000 person-year (95% CI)
Migraine with Aura (MA)	RR = 2.16 (1.53-3.03)		
MA + women		IR = 4.3 (3.0-6.0)	IR = 3.4 (2.3-5.0)
MA + smoking	RR = 1.5 (1.1-2.3)		
MA + women + Smoking + OCP	RR = 10 (1.4-73.7)		

RR = relative risk, IR = incidence rate per 1000 women per year

Table 22.3 Risk factors for migraine progression to CM

Non-modifiable	Modifiable
Older age	Attack frequency at baseline
Female sex	Medication overuse
White race (US sample)	Cutaneous allodynia
Lower SES	Obesity
Low educational level	Depression
Genetic factors	Anxiety
Hx of head/neck injury	Chronic daily headache
Abuse/childhood maltreatment	Temporomandibular disorder
	Asthma

Persons with CM were also more likely to have vascular risk factors, including hypertension, diabetes, high cholesterol, and obesity, as well as respiratory disorders including asthma, bronchitis, and COPD.[42] Various theories have been suggested to interpret the underlying mechanisms that could possibly further develop comorbid conditions, including the idea that one disorder may cause the other, latent brain state models, shared environment, and shared genetic origins.[43–45]

Psychiatric Comorbidities

There are multiple psychiatric comorbidities associated with migraine, including depression, anxiety disorders, bipolar disorder, post-traumatic stress disorder, personality disorders, and suicide attempts.[46–48] The prevalence of major depression in participants with strict migraine on a large health-plan based study was 28.1%; in subjects with probable migraine[49] it was 19.5% compared with 10.3% of non-headache subjects. On a large population-based cohort study in Canada, there was a higher prevalence of major depression, bipolar disorder, panic disorder, and social phobia by at least two-fold in persons with migraine compared to those without migraine. This was also found on a large Norwegian study assessing persons with migraine, other non-migraine headache, and headache-free controls for depression and anxiety disorders.[50] When comparing persons with migraine to non-headache controls, the adjusted OR for depression was 1.9 (95% CI 1.6–2.3) and for anxiety it was 2.7 (95% CI 2.4–3.1). The adjusted ORs also increased as headache frequency increased, with participants having ≥15 migraine days/month having an adjusted OR of 6.4 (95% CI 4.4–9.3) for depression and 6.9 (95% CI 5.1–9.4) for anxiety. In the AMPP Study, respondents with CM were more likely to have depression, anxiety, and chronic pain than those with EM by approximately two-fold.[42] International studies also showed this similar pattern with increased rates of depression and anxiety among subjects with CM in Taiwan by almost four-fold higher.[51]

Neurologic Comorbidities

Migraine is linked to many neurological comorbidities including, epilepsy, MS, ischaemic stroke, cardiovascular diseases, and sleep disorders, among others.[52–55] The Epilepsy Comorbidities and Health Survey, including 172,959 adults, showed that the prevalence of migraine in persons with epilepsy was 27.9% (prevalence ratio, 1.36; 95% CI, 1.25–1.48).[56]

The Family Study of Columbia University reported an increased bi-directional risk between migraine and epilepsy by two-fold, which could potentially be due to shared genetic susceptibility and shared environment risk factors.[57] There is an increased risk of having an ischaemic stroke in persons with migraine,[58] particularly in women with MA. Increased pro-thrombotic states could also be a potential risk factor for the progression to CM among persons with EM.[61] Sleep disorders are comorbid with migraine, including breathing disorders (e.g. apnoea, snoring), insomnias, circadian rhythm disorders, and parasomnias. The National Comorbidity Survey-Replication study reported that migraineurs had greater difficulty initiating sleep by 2.2-fold, staying asleep by 2.8-fold, reported more early morning wakening by 2-fold and more daytime fatigue by 2.6-fold when compared to migraine-free controls.[62]

Like most comorbidities, sleep disorders are more frequent among persons with CM than in those with EM[63] and may be more severe in persons with higher migraine day frequency. Restless leg syndrome was also shown to be associated with migraine.[64–66] Subjects with migraine were shown to have an almost two-fold increased risk for RLS (adjusted OR 1.79; CI 1.00–3.19; P = 0.049) when compared to subjects without migraine in an Italian adult population study.[67] The Physicians' Health Study also reported an association between migraine and RLS in men with adjusted OR of 1.20 (95% CI 1.04–1.38).[68]

Multiple studies have shown an association between MS and migraine, with a two-fold increased rate of migraine in persons with MS. More often migraine develops in younger people with relapsing remitting type of MS.[69] On the other hand, a smaller percentage of tension-type headache more often affects persons of older age, more commonly males and individuals with secondary progressive MS.[70]

Medical Comorbidities

There are several medical comorbidities associated with migraine, including, but not limited to asthma, allergic rhinitis, cardiac diseases and events, and non-headache pain disorders, including TMD and fibromyalgia. In persons with EM, asthma confers a two-fold increased risk for the development of CM.[71] Among children, allergic rhinitis conferred a 3.2-fold higher risk of developing migraine compared to children without allergic rhinitis (11.4 vs 3.49 per 10,000 person years[72]). This risk was greater in boys than girls, and for younger children <6 years old. The pathophysiology of the association between asthma and migraine, as well as, allergic rhinitis and migraine are thought to be connected through the involvement of mast cells, histamine, and IgE.

Furthermore, other medical comorbidities include non-headache pain disorders like TMD with an increased odds of CM by an astounding 96-fold (OR = 95.9; 95% CI = 12.51–734.64) and seven-fold with EM (OR = 7.0; 3.45–14.22),[73] as well as sleep bruxism (only associated with CM (OR = 3.8; 1.83–7.84), but not EM), musculoskeletal pain, fibromyalgia, irritable bowel disease, Crohn's disease, and other conditions.[74–76]

Risk Factors for Progression to CM

In approximately 2.5–3% of patients with EM, there is an evolution with increased frequency and progression to CM over one year of follow-up. This progression is dependent of multiple risk factors described as modifiable and non-modifiable risk factors (See table 22.3).

Non-modifiable risk factors include: older age, female sex, white race (in a US sample),[77] lower socioeconomic status, low educational level, genetic factors, history of head and neck injury,[78] and abuse or childhood maltreatment.[6] Head trauma and traumatic brain injury are associated with 15% increased risk of chronic daily headache (CDH)[79] (which is an older definition based on headache frequency alone and includes chronic migraine among others).

Modifiable risk factors can be potentially minimized and grant a target for possible intervention. Potentially modifiable risk factors include:

(1) Attack frequency at baseline

This is one of the most critical risk factors for progression from EM to CM. The possibility of conversion from EM to CM is higher in people with HFEM than those with low frequency episodic migraine (LFEM (0–9 headache days/month)) even after adjusting for medication overuse. The increased hazard attributed to higher frequency could possibly be elucidated at least moderately by susceptibility to pain and central sensitization.[89]

(2) Medication overuse

In persons with EM, medication overuse is a powerful risk factor for the development of CM; however, its effects vary depending on the class of medication, days of use of the particular medication, and baseline headache frequency. In persons with EM, the use of either barbiturates or opioids confers a significant increased risk for progression to CM and the risk is dependent on the number of days of medication intake, increasing when medication is taken more frequently. Triptans have not shown to have an increased risk of CM onset; however, there was a trend towards increased risk of CM onset (OR 1.25; 95% CI 0.9–1.7). Similarly, NSAIDs were not a risk factor for overall development of CM (OR 0.85; 95% CI 0.63–1.17), although there was an interaction with headache days/month. In persons with less than ten headache days/month NSAIDs were protective. On the other hand, for persons with 10–14 headache days/month NSAIDs were a risk factor for the development of CM.[35]

(3) Cutaneous allodynia

CA affects 63–65% of persons with migraine[81] and it is a risk factor for the new development of CM.[61] It is associated with migraine frequency, duration, severity, disability, and migraine associated symptoms, and it has also been described as a possible symptom of psychiatric comorbidity.

(4) Obesity

Obesity is a very prevalent condition that is a risk factor for the exacerbation of migraine frequency and severity.[85] In the AMPP population-based study, morbid obese individuals more frequently had HFEM than their normal weight counterparts by 1.7-fold (10.4% vs 6.5% respectively; OR 1.74; 95% 1.41–1.93). Similarly, the prevalence of CM in a group of persons with severe obesity was more than two-fold higher than the comparison group with normal BMI.

(5) Depression
Persons with CM have a higher prevalence of depression than their EM counterparts by two-fold.[42] Depression also raises the risk for developing CM and this relationship magnitude is variable, depending on the severity of depression, with moderate depression increasing the risk by 2.5-fold and severe depression by 3.2-fold.

(6) Anxiety
Similarly, persons with CM also have a two-fold higher prevalence of anxiety than persons with EM. Persons with migraine and anxiety have an increased likelihood of developing CM by 53% when compared to persons with migraine and without anxiety.[46]

(7) Chronic daily headache (CDH)
Persons with CM are two times more likely to have chronic pain, including chronic daily headache among other types of pain. Persons with CDH are also more likely to snore when compared to controls.[86]

(8) Temporomandibular joint disorder
The prevalence of TMD in persons with CM is very prominent and can be as high as 80%. TMD has been shown to be associated with migraine chronification, allodynia, and CDH.[87]

(9) Asthma
Asthma is associated with increased risk of migraine chronification, conferring persons with EM a two-fold increased risk for the new development of CM.[71]

Factors Associated with CM Remission

Over two years of follow-up of participants with CM from the population based AMPP Study showed that there is a variability in frequency over time. Approximately one quarter (26%) of participants with CM returned to EM during that period of time. Roughly one-third (34%) of the group with CM at baseline had persistent CM over two years of follow-up, and 40% fluctuated from CM to EM and back to CM.

The associated disability was higher in those with persistent CM than when compared to those with remitted CM.[88] There were a couple of predictor factors associated with CM remission, including fewer headache days/month and the absence of CA. Surprisingly, there was a decrease in associated CM remission with the use of preventive medication; however, this relationship was likely confounded by high attack frequency and indication.

When modifying risk factors associated with CM, there was an improvement in headache frequency and severity shown by a few interventional studies including behavioural sleep modification in patients with poor sleep hygiene,[89] bariatric surgery in severely obese CM patients who achieved approximately 50% subsequent weight loss,[90] and onabotulinum toxin A in patients with CM and comorbid depression.[91]

Migraine Triggers

There are different exposure factors associated with an increased probability for the development of a migraine attack over a short period of time.[92] Those factors are described as triggers and can be either endogenous or exogenous. There is a gamut of frequently known triggers, which have a wide range of fluctuation both between and within person. Among 1750 patients with migraine from a clinic based study, 76% reported to have experienced triggered attacks of migraine. Those triggers were divided into different groups as very frequent 9%, frequent in 27%, and occasional in 40% of participants.[93] The most frequent triggers (from most common to least common) were stress (80%), hormones (65% women), missed meals (57%), weather (53%), sleep-related issues (50%), odours (44%), alcohol consumption (38%), heat (30%), and different foods (27%). The PAMINA study reported that menstruation was the strongest trigger, increasing likelihood of a migraine attack by up to 96%.[94] Additionally, tiredness, neck muscle tension,[95,96] psychic tension, noise, and odours were reported as triggers. On the other hand, days-off, consumption of beer, and relaxation after a period of stress appeared to be protective against a migraine attack. Another study at a tertiary headache centre in the USA found that 'let down', a phenomenon described as relaxation after stress was associated with a significant increase in migraine odds.[97]

This information might be advantageous in anticipating and possibly implementing an intervention to prevent potential attacks in those who have predictable and reliable triggers. Furthermore, protective factors such as healthy lifestyle habits may elevate the attack threshold and potentially help prevent future migraine attacks.[98]

Suboptimal Migraine Care and Consultation Patterns

Initial appropriate diagnosis of migraine is extremely important to achieving optimal migraine care for both EM and CM. The majority of US Headache Consortium therapies and migraine-specific pharmacologic therapies require a prescription; however, there is a disparity and suboptimal access to having previously consulted a healthcare professional (HCP). The American Migraine Study reported that 68% of female and 57% of male migraineurs expressed having consulted a HCP for headache.[99] In the AMPP Study, 45.5% of people with EM and headache-related disability had consulted a HCP for migraine in the previous year.[100] There are several predictors associated with potential migraine consultation including: (1) having health insurance; (2) higher levels of headache-related disability; and (3) greater reported headache pain intensity. In the CaMEO Study, among subjects with migraine, only 40.8% of participants with CM expressed to be consulting a HCP for migraine at the time of enrolment.[101] Participants with health insurance (OR 4.61; 95% CI 3.05–6.96), higher BMI (OR 1.01; 95% CI 1.00–1.03), increasing older age (OR 1.02; 95% CI 1.01–1.03), greater migraine-related disability (OR 1.02; 95% CI 1.00–1.04), and greater migraine symptom severity (OR 1.16; 95% CI 1.11–1.22) were more likely to have had consulted a HCP. However, only a mere 4.5% of participants had successfully achieved appropriate CM care, surpassing the three different obstacles to care defined as having consulted a HCP for migraine, received an accurate diagnosis, and been prescribed minimal acute and preventive pharmacologic treatments.

Barriers to Treatment

Acute migraine treatment

Despite approximately 90% of persons with migraine having access to acute therapies,[102] only the minority utilizes migraine-specific therapies including triptans[103,104] and/or dihydroergotamine.[105] An extensive amount of persons with migraine utilize opioids and other medications, which can lead to potential adverse outcomes, including dependence, overuse patterns,[106] and evolution from EM to CM.[35,107] In the AMPP Study, 92% of participants with EM used acute therapies for migraine;[108] nonetheless, only 36% used migraine-specific therapies: 18% used triptans, 12% used opioids, and 6% used barbiturates. Approximately 15.9% of participants with migraine were current opioid users and 13.8% were prior users.[107]

There were three required steps identified, which are associated with patients having access to migraine specific medications containing: (1) appropriate medical consultation; (2) an accurate diagnosis; and (3) an effective treatment regimen.[109] In the AMPP Study, among participants with migraine and moderate or greater headache-related disability, only 26% passed through the three steps to utilize the identified acute treatments.[100] Minimally appropriate care was more likely to be received by those with health insurance, higher household income, females, those with more severe migraine, and greater headache-related disability.

Compliance with consistently utilizing acute care for migraine appropriately is an extremely important issue. A US pharmacy claims database revealed that 53.8% of patients that were initially prescribed a particular triptan, did not persistently refill their prescription[110] for the medication in question. Out of those 40,982 patients, 7.4% switched to a different triptan, 25.5% discontinued prescription migraine therapy and two-thirds (67.1%) switched to a non-specific migraine medication including opioids and NSAIDs when the first medication refill was due.

Preventive migraine treatment

The purpose of utilizing preventive pharmacologic therapy for migraine is to attempt to decrease the frequency of migraine attacks or possibly eliminate them altogether, as well as to minimize the impact of migraine on headache-related disability or impact and health-related quality of life.

Despite the very common utilization of acute migraine therapy by most people when including both prescription based and over the counter medications, preventive medications are much less commonly used. In the AMPP Study, 43.3% of participants with migraine reported to have never used a migraine preventive medication. Interestingly enough, within that group, 32.4% met expert guideline criteria for considering preventive therapy (13.1%), or being offered (19.3%) preventive therapy.[102] In a study with adolescents, the issue was very similar, with roughly one-third of participants fitting criteria for the requirement of preventive therapy. However, just a mere 10–19% were presented with possible prevention therapy.[111] Certain barriers in the path to receiving suitable pharmacologic prescription preventive therapy were identified in the CaMEO Study following participants with CM. In this study, 40.8% of participants reported to have consulted with a HCP for headache evaluation. The likelihood of having consulted a HCP about migraine was higher for those who had health insurance, higher migraine symptom severity, greater migraine-related disability, and participants who were older.

Within that group, one quarter (24.6%) reported to have received a diagnosis of either CM or TM, and an absolute bare minimum of 4.4% reported to have been prescribed both acute and preventive prescription pharmacologic therapy for migraine, which is considered a minimally appropriate treatment. Those with higher migraine symptom severity, those who had consulted a specialist for migraine, and also females were more likely to receive an appropriate diagnosis of CM and TM. No compelling predictors associated with the appropriate use of prescription pharmacologic treatment were identified.

Migraine Neurobiology

Pathophysiology of migraine

Migraine is a chronic disorder with episodic attacks. The most prominent feature of migraine are the attacks of headache associated with various combinations of nausea, photophobia, phonophobia, osmophobia, and allodynia, among other features (ICHD).[15] Between attacks there is an enduring predisposition to attacks thought to take the form of brain hyper-excitability. Migraine aggregates within families and estimates from family studies and twin studies suggest that migraine is determined by genetic and environmental factors in approximately equal measure. Migraine, then, is a complex disorder, with multiple genetic and environmental determinants and a range of clinical phenotypes.[112]

Genetics

Despite its high heritability, most of the genetic variation in migraine remains to be explained. As with other complex disorders, there are a number of rare syndromes caused by well-characterized single gene mutations. Familial hemiplegic migraine has been linked to variants in a gene encoding for subunits of a neuronal calcium channel (*CACNA1A*), a glial sodium-potassium ATPase (*ATP1A2*), and a sodium channel (*SCN1A*). Variants in these genes have also been associated with sporadic hemiplegic migraine as well as more typical forms of migraine with aura and migraine without aura, reinforcing the hypothesis that familial hemiplegic migraine and more typical forms of migraine may share pathogenic underpinnings. Other mutations associated with rare forms of migraine include variants associated with vasculopathies and variants associated with familial advanced sleep phase syndrome.[114]

There are at least 38 genomic loci that have been associated with migraine[115,116] in population studies. These loci have tremendous functional diversity, highlighting the complexity and heterogeneity of migraine. There are several sets of genes associated with vascular biology and others associated with gastrointestinal function.

Pathophysiology

The life of a person with migraine is typically divided into five phases:[117] the premonitory phase,[92] the aura phase,[118] the headache phase,[119–122] the post-dromal phase, and the inter-ictal phase. The premonitory phase typically precedes headache onset by an hour to a day.[123] Typical features include changes in mood (depression, irritability, euphoria) and appetite, difficulty concentrating,[124,125] sensory sensitivity,[126,127] and yawning.[128,129] In both triggered and spontaneous migraine, PET[130,131] and MRI[132,133] revealed changes in function and connectivity of the hypothalamus,[134–140] well before head pain begins. The hypothalamus[141,142] is an appropriate localization for many premonitory features. Premonitory features occur in the majority of people with migraine.[128,129]

Auras are focal neurologic deficits that typically begin before headache but which may continue into the headache phase.[143] The classic aura of migraine is the scintillating scotoma comprised of positive features (zig-zag lines, flashing lights) and negative features (a greying out of vision or scotoma).[144,145] Aura features typically evolve slowly, over minutes or longer. Somatosensory[146] and motor auras are common. Somewhere between 15% and 30% of people with migraine meet criteria for migraine with aura.

The presumed substrate of migraine with aura is cortical spreading depression (CSD),[147] a wave of excitation, followed by a wave of inhibition that marches over the cortical mantle at the rate of 3 mm per second.[148] CSD is associated with an array of changes in experimental animals including ion shifts, activation of matrix metalloproteinases, and inflammatory changes,[149,150] as well as the closing of the perivascular spaces.[151] CSD may lead to depolarization of meningeal pain fibres and headache, though this remains controversial.

During the headache phase,[152] there is activation of the trigeminal pain pathway.[153–155] Emerging evidence suggests that calcitonin gene related peptide (CGRP), a peptide neurotransmitter, plays a primary role as a mediator of migraine pain. During migraine headaches, CGRP levels are elevated in blood[156,157] and they normalize after treatment with triptans. In persons with migraine, intravenous infusion of CGRP triggers migraine attacks. Treatments that target CGRP or its receptor have demonstrated effect as acute[158] or preventive treatments of migraine. Pituitary adenylate cyclase-activating polypeptide (PACAP)[159] is another peptide transmitter that may play a crucial role in migraine and may provide a target for future treatments.[160]

REFERENCES

1. Lipton RB, Sollars CM, Buse DC. Epidemiology, Progression, Prognosis, and Comorbidity of Migraine. In: Robbins MS, Grosberg BM, Lipton RB (eds). Headache. Oxford, UK: John Wiley & Sons, Ltd; 2013, pp64–87.
2. Linet MS, Stewart WF. Migraine headache: epidemiologic perspectives. Epidemiol Rev. 1984; 6: 107–39.
3. Lipton RB, Bigal ME, Hamelsky S, Scher AI. Headache: Epidemiology and Impact. In: Silberstein SD, Lipton RB, Dodick DW (eds). Wolff's Headache and Other Head Pain. New York: Oxford University Press, 2008. pp45–62.
4. Stewart WF, Wood C, Reed ML, et al. Cumulative lifetime migraine incidence in women and men. Cephalalgia. 2008; 28(11): 1170–8.
5. Stovner L, Hagen K, Jensen R, et al. The global burden of headache: a documentation of headache prevalence and disability worldwide. Cephalalgia. 2007; 27(3): 193–210.
6. Feigin VL, Vos T. Global, regional, and national burden of neurological disorders during 1990–2015: a systematic analysis for the Global Burden of Disease Study 2015. Lancet Neurology. 2017; 16(11): 877–97.
7. Buse DC, Loder EW, Gorman JA, et al. Sex differences in the prevalence, symptoms, and associated features of migraine, probable migraine and other severe headache: results of the American Migraine Prevalence and Prevention (AMPP) Study. Headache. 2013; 53(8): 1278–99.
8. Wang X, Zhou HB, Sun JM, et al. The prevalence of migraine in university students: a systematic review and meta-analysis. Eur J Neurol. 2016; 23(3): 464–75.
9. Robbins MS, Lipton RB. The epidemiology of primary headache disorders. Semin Neurol. 2010; 30(2): 107–19.
10. Stewart WF, Linet MS, Celentano DD, et al. Age- and sex-specific incidence rates of migraine with and without visual aura. Am J Epidemiol. 1991; 134(10): 1111–20.
11. Silberstein SD, Young WB. Migraine aura and prodrome. Semin Neurol. 1995; 15(2): 175–82.
12. Natoli JL, Manack A, Dean B, et al. Global prevalence of chronic migraine: a systematic review. Cephalalgia. 2010; 30(5): 599–609.
13. Smitherman TA, Burch R, Sheikh H, Loder E. The prevalence, impact, and treatment of migraine and severe headaches in the United States: a review of statistics from national surveillance studies. Headache. 2013; 53(3): 427–36.
14. Buse D, Manack A, Serrano D, et al. Headache impact of chronic and episodic migraine: results from the American Migraine Prevalence and Prevention study. Headache. 2012; 52(1): 3–17.
15. Headache Classification Committee of the International Headache Society (IHS). The International Classification of Headache Disorders (3rd edition) (beta version). Cephalalgia. 2013; 33(9): 629–808.
16. Barnes NP. Migraine headache in children. *BMJ Clin Evid.* 2011;2011:0318.
17. Stewart WF, Lipton RB, Liberman J. Variation in migraine prevalence by race. Neurology. 1996; 47(1): 52–9.
18. Lipton RB, Buse DC, Saiers J, et al. Frequency and burden of headache-related nausea: results from the American Migraine Prevalence and Prevention (AMPP) study. Headache. 2013; 53(1): 93–103.
19. Reed ML, Fanning KM, Serrano D, et al. Persistent frequent nausea is associated with progression to chronic migraine: AMPP study results. Headache. 2015; 55(1): 76–87.
20. Holroyd KA, Drew JB, Cottrell CK, et al. Impaired functioning and quality of life in severe migraine: the role of catastrophizing and associated symptoms. Cephalalgia. 2007; 27(10): 1156–65.
21. Lipton RB, Buse DC, Saiers J, et al. Healthcare resource utilization and direct costs associated with frequent nausea in episodic migraine: results from the American Migraine Prevalence and Prevention (AMPP) Study. J Med Econ. 2013; 16(4): 490–9.
22. Bigal ME, Ashina S, Burstein R, et al. Prevalence and characteristics of allodynia in headache sufferers: a population study. Neurology. 2008; 70(17): 1525–33.
23. Burstein R, Cutrer MF, Yarnitsky D. The development of cutaneous allodynia during a migraine attack clinical evidence for the sequential recruitment of spinal and supraspinal nociceptive neurons in migraine. Brain. 2000; 123(Pt 8): 1703–9.
24. Lipton RB, Bigal ME, Ashina S, et al. Cutaneous allodynia in the migraine population. Ann Neurol. 2008; 63(2): 148–58.
25. Bigal ME, Lipton RB. Modifiable risk factors for migraine progression. Headache: the journal of head and face pain. 2006; 46(9): 1334–43.
26. Burstein R, Collins B, Jakubowski M. Defeating migraine pain with triptans: a race against the development of cutaneous allodynia. Ann Neurol. 2004; 55(1): 19–26.

27. Buse DC, Rupnow MFT, Lipton RB. Assessing and managing all aspects of migraine: migraine attacks, migraine-related functional impairment, common comorbidities, and quality of life. Mayo Clinic Proceedings. 2009; 84(5): 422–35.
28. Pavlovic JM, Stewart WF, Bruce CA, et al. Burden of migraine related to menses: results from the AMPP study. J Headache Pain. 2015; 16(1): 24.
29. Buse DC, Manack AN, Fanning KM, et al. Chronic migraine prevalence, disability, and sociodemographic factors: results from the American Migraine Prevalence and Prevention Study. Headache. 2012; 52(10): 1456–70.
30. Buse DC, Scher AI, Dodick DW, et al. Impact of migraine on the family: perspectives of people with migraine and their spouse/domestic partner in the CaMEO Study. Mayo Clinic Proceedings. 2016; 91(5): 596–611.
31. Leonardi M, Steiner TJ, Scher AT, Lipton RB. The global burden of migraine: measuring disability in headache disorders with WHO's Classification of Functioning, Disability and Health (ICF). J Headache Pain. 2005; 6(6): 429–40.
32. World Health Organization. Headache disorders (Internet). WHO 2012; (Fact Sheet number 277) Available from: http://www.who.int/mediacentre/factsheets/fs277/en/
33. Murray CJL, Vos T, Lozano R, et al. Disability-adjusted life years (DALYs) for 291 diseases and injuries in 21 regions, 1990–2010: a systematic analysis for the Global Burden of Disease Study 2010. Lancet. 2012; 380(9859): 2197–223.
34. Scher AI, Bigal ME, Lipton RB. Comorbidity of migraine. Curr Opin Neurol. 2005; 18(3): 305–10.
35. Buse DC, Manack A, Serrano D, et al. Sociodemographic and comorbidity profiles of chronic migraine and episodic migraine sufferers. J Neurol Neurosurg Psychiatr. 2010; 81(4): 428–32.
36. Buse DC, Silberstein SD, Manack AN, et al. Psychiatric comorbidity of episodic and chronic migraine. J Neurol Neurosurg Psychiatry. 2012; 260(8): 1960–9.
37. Jette N, Patten S, Williams J, et al. Comorbidity of migraine and psychiatric disorders—a national population-based study. Headache: the journal of head and face pain. 2008; 48(4): 501–16.
38. Zwart JA, Dyb G, Hagen K, et al. Depression and anxiety disorders associated with headache frequency. The Nord-Trøndelag Health Study. European Journal of Neurology. 2003; 10(2): 147–52.
39. Chen Y-C, Tang C-H, Ng K, Wang S-J. Comorbidity profiles of chronic migraine sufferers in a national database in Taiwan. J Headache Pain. 2012; 13(4): 311–19.
40. Ottman R, Lipton RB, Ettinger AB, et al. Comorbidities of epilepsy: results from the Epilepsy Comorbidities and Health (EPIC) survey. Epilepsia. 2011; 52(2): 308–15.
41. Ottman R, Lipton RB. Comorbidity of migraine and epilepsy. Neurology. 1994; 44(11): 2105–10.
42. Katsarava Z, Weimar C. Migraine and stroke. Journal of the Neurological Sciences. 2010; 299(1): 42–4.
43. Donaghy M, Chang CL, Poulter N, European Collaborators of The World Health Organisation Collaborative Study of Cardiovascular Disease and Steroid Hormone Contraception. Duration, frequency, recency, and type of migraine and the risk of ischaemic stroke in women of childbearing age. J Neurol Neurosurg Psychiatr. 2002; 73(6): 747–50.
44. Schürks M, Rist PM, Bigal ME, et al. Migraine and cardiovascular disease: systematic review and meta-analysis. BMJ. 2009; 339: b3914.
45. Lateef T, Swanson S, Cui L, et al. Headaches and sleep problems among adults in the United States: findings from the National Comorbidity Survey-Replication study. Cephalalgia. 2011; 31(6): 648–53.
46. Kelman L, Rains JC. Headache and sleep: examination of sleep patterns and complaints in a large clinical sample of migraineurs. Headache: the journal of head and face pain. 2005; 45(7): 904–10.
47. Innes KE, Selfe TK, Agarwal P. Prevalence of restless legs syndrome in North American and Western European populations: a systematic review. Sleep Med. 2011; 12(7): 623–34.
48. Zanigni S, Giannini G, Melotti R, et al. Association between restless legs syndrome and migraine: a population-based study. Eur J Neurol. 2014; 21(9): 1205–10.
49. Winter AC, Schürks M, Berger K, et al. Migraine and restless legs syndrome in men. Cephalalgia. 2013; 33(2): 130–5.
50. Pakpoor J, Handel AE, Giovannoni G, et al. Meta-analysis of the relationship between multiple sclerosis and migraine. PLOS One. 2012; 7(9): e45295.
51. D'Amico D, La Mantia L, Rigamonti A, et al. Prevalence of primary headaches in people with multiple sclerosis. Cephalalgia. 2004; 24(11): 980–4.
52. Evans RW, de Tommaso M. Migraine and fibromyalgia. Headache. 2011; 51(2): 295–9.
53. Hagen K, Einarsen C, Zwart JA, et al. The co-occurrence of headache and musculoskeletal symptoms amongst 51,050 adults in Norway. European Journal of Neurology. 2002; 9(5): 527–33.
54. Fernandes G, Franco AL, Gonçalves DA, et al. Temporomandibular disorders, sleep bruxism, and primary headaches are mutually associated. J Orofac Pain. 2013; 27(1): 14–20.
55. Martin VT, Fanning KM, Serrano D, et al. Asthma is a risk factor for new onset chronic migraine: Results from the American migraine prevalence and prevention study. Headache. 2016; 56(1): 118–31.
56. Kurth T, Gaziano JM, Cook NR, et al. Migraine and risk of cardiovascular disease in women. JAMA. 2006; 296(3): 283–91.
57. Bigal ME, Kurth T, Santanello N, et al. Migraine and cardiovascular disease: a population-based study. Neurology. 2010; 74(8): 628–35.
58. Kurth T, Gaziano JM, Cook NR, et al. Migraine and risk of cardiovascular disease in men. Arch Intern Med. 2007; 167(8): 795–801.
59. Kurth T, Bubes V, Buring JE. Relative contribution of migraine with aura on stroke subtypes in women. Cephalalgia. 2013; 33(8 Suppl): 18–19.
60. Bigal ME, Serrano D, Buse D, et al. Acute migraine medications and evolution from episodic to chronic migraine: a longitudinal population-based study. Headache. 2008; 48(8): 1157–68.
61. Lipton RB. Seymour Solomon Lecture - Riding the Migraine Roller Coaster: Lessons for longitudinal Studies. 56th Annual Meeting of the American Headache Society (AHS), Los Angeles, CA 2014.
62. Couch JR, Lipton RB, Stewart WF, Scher AI. Head or neck injury increases the risk of chronic daily headache: a population-based study. Neurology. 2007; 69(11): 1169–77.
63. Buchgreitz L, Lyngberg AC, Bendtsen L, Jensen R. Frequency of headache is related to sensitization: a population study. Pain. 2006; 123(1–2): 19–27.
64. Bigal ME, Tsang A, Loder E, et al. Body mass index and episodic headaches: a population-based study. Arch Intern Med. 2007; 167(18):1 964–70.
65. Scher AI, Lipton RB, Stewart WF. Habitual snoring as a risk factor for chronic daily headache. Neurology. 2003; 60(8): 1366–8.

66. Gonçalves DAG, Bigal ME, Jales LCF, et al. Headache and symptoms of temporomandibular disorder: an epidemiological study. Headache. 2010; 50(2): 231–41.
67. Manack A, Buse DC, Serrano D, et al. Rates, predictors, and consequences of remission from chronic migraine to episodic migraine. Neurology. 2011; 76(8): 711–18.
68. Bond DS, Vithiananthan S, Nash JM, et al. Improvement of migraine headaches in severely obese patients after bariatric surgery. Neurology. 2011; 76(13): 1135–8.
69. Calhoun AH, Ford S. Behavioral sleep modification may revert transformed migraine to episodic migraine. Headache: the journal of head and face pain. 2007; 47(8): 1178–83.
70. Boudreau GP, Grosberg BM, McAllister PJ, et al. Prophylactic onabotulinumtoxinA in patients with chronic migraine and comorbid depression: An open-label, multicenter, pilot study of efficacy, safety and effect on headache-related disability, depression, and anxiety. Int J Gen Med. 2015; 9: 79–86.
71. Pavlovic JM, Buse DC, Sollars CM, et al. Trigger factors and premonitory features of migraine attacks: summary of studies. Headache. 2014; 54(10): 1670–9.
72. Kelman L. The triggers or precipitants of the acute migraine attack. Cephalalgia. 2007; 27(5): 394–402.
73. Wöber C, Brannath W, Schmidt K, et al. Prospective analysis of factors related to migraine attacks: the PAMINA study. Cephalalgia. 2007; 27(4): 304–14.
74. Lipton RB, Buse DC, Hall CB, et al. Reduction in perceived stress as a migraine trigger: testing the 'let-down headache' hypothesis. Neurology. 2014; 82(16): 1395–1401.
75. Lipton RB, Pavlovic JM, Haut SR, et al. Methodological issues in studying trigger factors and premonitory features of migraine. Headache. 2014; 54(10): 1661–9.
76. Couturier E, Bomhof M, Neven AK, van Duijn NP. Menstrual migraine in a representative Dutch population sample: prevalence, disability and treatment. Cephalalgia. 2003; 23(4): 302–8.
77. MacGregor EA, Hackshaw A. Prevalence of migraine on each day of the natural menstrual cycle. Neurology. 2004; 63(2): 351–3.
78. Pinkerman B, Holroyd K. Menstrual and nonmenstrual migraines differ in women with menstrually-related migraine. Cephalalgia. 2010; 30(10): 1187–94.
79. Martin VT, Pavlovic J, Fanning KM, et al. Perimenopause and menopause are associated with high frequency headache in women with migraine: Results of the American Migraine Prevalence and Prevention Study. Headache. 2016; 56(2): 292–305.
80. Lipton RB, Stewart WF, Simon D. Medical consultation for migraine: Results From the American Migraine Study. Headache. 1998; 38(2): 87–96.
81. Lipton RB, Serrano D, Holland S, et al. Barriers to the diagnosis and treatment of migraine: effects of sex, income, and headache features. Headache. 2013; 53(1): 81–92.
82. Dodick DW, Loder EW, Manack Adams A, et al. Assessing barriers to chronic migraine consultation, diagnosis, and treatment: Results From the Chronic Migraine Epidemiology and Outcomes (CaMEO) Study. Headache. 2016; 56(5): 821–34.
83. Lipton RB, Bigal ME, Diamond M, et al. Migraine prevalence, disease burden, and the need for preventive therapy. Neurology. 2007; 68(5): 343–9.
84. Bigal ME, Borucho S, Serrano D, Lipton RB. The acute treatment of episodic and chronic migraine in the USA. Cephalalgia. 2009; 29(8): 891–97.
85. Buse DC, Pearlman SH, Reed ML, et al. Opioid use and dependence among persons with migraine: Results of the AMPP Study. Headache. 2012; 52(1): 18–36.
86. Lipton RB, Buse DC, Serrano D, et al. Acute medication use patterns in episodic migraine: results of the American Migraine Prevalence and Prevention Study (AMPP). Cephalalgia. 2009; 29(suppl 1): 17.
87. Lipton RB, Amatniek JC, Ferrari MD, Gross M. Migraine. Identifying and removing barriers to care. Neurology. 1994; 44(6 Suppl 4): S63–8.
88. Katić BJ, Rajagopalan S, Ho TW, et al. Triptan persistency among newly initiated users in a pharmacy claims database. Cephalalgia. 2011; 31(4): 488–500.
89. Lipton RB, Bigal ME, Diamond M, et al. Migraine prevalence, disease burden, and the need for preventive therapy. Neurology. 2007; 68(5): 343–9.
90. Lewis DW, Diamond S, Scott D, Jones V. Prophylactic treatment of pediatric migraine. Headache: the journal of head and face pain. 2004; 44(3): 230–7.
91. Wang IC, Tsai JD, Lin CL, et al. Allergic rhinitis and associated risk of migraine among children: a nationwide population-based cohort study. Int Forum Allergy Rhinol. 2016 Mar; 6(3): 322–7.
92. Zhang N, Chen CF, Yu FY. Effects of pregabalin on central sensitization in patients with migraine. Int J Clin Pharmacol Ther. 2015; 53(4): 277–83.
93. GBD 2015 Disease and Injury Incidence and Prevalence Collaborators. Global, regional, and national incidence, prevalence, and years lived with disability for 310 diseases and injuries, 1990–2015: a systematic analysis for the Global Burden of Disease Study 2015. Lancet. 2016; 388: 1545–1602.
94. GBD 2016 Disease and Injury Incidence and Prevalence Collaborators. Global, regional, and national incidence, prevalence, and years lived with disability for 328 diseases and injuries for 195 countries, 1990–2016: a systematic analysis for the Global Burden of Disease Study 2016. Lancet. 2017; 390: 1211–59.
95. Steiner TJ, Stovner LJ, Vos T. GBD 2015: migraine is the third cause of disability in under 50s. J Headache Pain. 2016; 17: 104.
96. Headache Classification Committee of the International Headache Society (IHS). The International Classification of Headache Disorders (3rd edition) (beta version). Cephalalgia. 2013; 33: 629–808.
97. Hansen JM, Goadsby PJ, Charles AC. Variability of clinical features in attacks of migraine with aura. Cephalalgia. 2016; 36: 216–24.
98. Viana M, Sances G, Ghiotto N, et al. Variability of the characteristics of a migraine attack within patients. Cephalalgia. 2016; 36: 825–30.
99. Munksgaard SB, Bendtsen L, Jensen RH. Detoxification of medication-overuse headache by a multidisciplinary treatment programme is highly effective: a comparison of two consecutive treatment methods in an open-label design. Cephalalgia. 2012; 32: 834–44.
100. Hansen JM, Goadsby PJ, Charles A. Reduced efficacy of sumatriptan in migraine with aura vs without aura. Neurology. 2015; 84: 1880–5.
101. Amin FM, Asghar MS, Hougaard A, et al. Magnetic resonance angiography of intracranial and extracranial arteries in patients with spontaneous migraine without aura: a cross-sectional study. Lancet Neurology. 2013; 12: 454–61.

102. von Brevern M, Lempert T. Vestibular migraine. Handb Clin Neurol. 2016; 137: 301–16.
103. Nyholt DR, van den Maagdenberg AM. Genome-wide association studies in migraine: current state and route to follow. Curr Opin Neurol. 2016; 29: 302–8.
104. Sutherland HG, Griffiths LR. Genetics of migraine: insights into the molecular basis of migraine disorders. Headache. 2017; 57: 537–69.
105. Tan RY, Markus HS. CADASIL: migraine, encephalopathy, stroke and their inter-relationships. PLOS One. 2016; 11: e0157613.
106. Stam AH, Kothari PH, Shaikh A, et al. Retinal vasculopathy with cerebral leukoencephalopathy and systemic manifestations. Brain. 2016; 139: 2909–22.
107. Brennan KC, Bates EA, Shapiro RE, et al. Casein kinase Iδ mutations in familial migraine and advanced sleep phase. Sci Transl Med. 2013; 5: 183ra56,1–11.
108. Gormley P, Anttila V, Winsvold BS, et al. Meta-analysis of 375,000 individuals identifies 38 susceptibility loci for migraine. Nat Genet. 2016; 48: 856–66.
109. Yin P, Anttila V, Siewert KM, Palotie A, Davey Smith G, Voight BF. Serum calcium and risk of migraine: a Mendelian randomization study. Hum Mol Genet. 2017; 26: 820–8.
110. Charles A. The evolution of a migraine attack—a review of recent evidence. Headache. 2013; 53: 413–9.
111. Lampl C, Rudolph M, Deligianni CI, Mitsikostas DD. Neck pain in episodic migraine: premonitory symptom or part of the attack? J Headache Pain. 2015; 16: 566.
112. Schulte LH, Jürgens TP, May A. Photo-, osmo- and phonophobia in the premonitory phase of migraine: mistaking symptoms for triggers? J Headache Pain. 2015; 16: 14.
113. Karsan N, Prabhakar P, Goadsby PJ. Characterising the premonitory stage of migraine in children: a clinic-based study of 100 patients in a specialist headache service. J Headache Pain. 2016; 17: 94.
114. Laurell K, Artto V, Bendtsen L, et al. Premonitory symptoms in migraine: a cross-sectional study in 2714 persons. Cephalalgia. 2016; 36: 951–9.
115. Schwedt TJ, Zuniga L, Chong CD. Low heat pain thresholds in migraineurs between attacks. Cephalalgia. 2015; 35: 593–9.
116. Uglem M, Omland PM, Nilsen KB, et al. Does pain sensitivity change by migraine phase? A blinded longitudinal study. Cephalalgia. 2017(14): 1337–49.
117. Maniyar FH, Sprenger T, Monteith T, Schankin C, Goadsby PJ. Brain activations in the premonitory phase of nitroglycerin-triggered migraine attacks. Brain. 2014; 137: 232–41.
118. Schulte LH, May A. The migraine generator revisited: continuous scanning of the migraine cycle over 30 days and three spontaneous attacks. Brain. 2016; 139: 1987–93.
119. Maniyar FH, Sprenger T, Schankin C, Goadsby PJ. Photic hypersensitivity in the premonitory phase of migraine—a positron emission tomography study. Eur J Neurol. 2014; 21: 1178–83.
120. Maniyar FH, Sprenger T, Schankin C, Goadsby PJ. The origin of nausea in migraine—a PET study. J Headache Pain. 2014; 15: 84.
121. de Tommaso M, Ambrosini A, Brighina F, et al. Altered processing of sensory stimuli in patients with migraine. Nat Rev Neurol. 2014; 10: 144–55.
122. Hodkinson DJ, Wilcox SL, Veggeberg R, et al. Increased amplitude of thalamocortical low-frequency oscillations in patients with migraine. J Neurosci. 2016; 36: 8026–36.
123. Coppola G, Di Renzo A, Tinelli E, et al. Thalamo-cortical network activity between migraine attacks: insights from MRI-based microstructural and functional resting-state network correlation analysis. J Headache Pain. 2016; 17: 100.
124. Coppola G, Di Renzo A, Tinelli E, et al. Thalamo-cortical network activity during spontaneous migraine attacks. Neurology. 2016; 87: 2154–60.
125. Wang T, Chen N, Zhan W, et al. Altered effective connectivity of posterior thalamus in migraine with cutaneous allodynia: a resting-state fMRI study with Granger causality analysis. J Headache Pain. 2015; 17: 17.
126. Noseda R, Bernstein CA, Nir RR, et al. Migraine photophobia originating in cone-driven retinal pathways. Brain. 2016; 139: 1971–86.
127. Andreou AP, Holland PR, Akerman S, Summ O, Fredrick J, Goadsby PJ. Transcranial magnetic stimulation and potential cortical and trigeminothalamic mechanisms in migraine. Brain. 2016; 139: 2002–14.
128. Chong CD, Gaw N, Fu Y, Li J, Wu T, Schwedt TJ. Migraine classification using magnetic resonance imaging resting-state functional connectivity data. Cephalalgia. 2017; 37: 828–44.
129. Hougaard A, Amin FM, Larsson HB, Rostrup E, Ashina M. Increased intrinsic brain connectivity between pons and somatosensory cortex during attacks of migraine with aura. Hum Brain Mapp. 2017; 38: 2635–42.
130. Amin FM, Hougaard A, Magon S, et al. Change in brain network connectivity during PACAP38-induced migraine attacks: a resting-state functional MRI study. Neurology. 2016; 86: 180–7.
131. Tedeschi G, Russo A, Conte F, et al. Increased interictal visual network connectivity in patients with migraine with aura. Cephalalgia. 2016; 36: 139–47.
132. Niddam DM, Lai KL, Fuh JL, Chuang CY, Chen WT, Wang SJ. Reduced functional connectivity between salience and visual networks in migraine with aura. Cephalalgia. 2016; 36: 53–66.
133. Chen Z, Chen X, Liu M, Dong Z, Ma L, Yu S. Altered functional connectivity of amygdala underlying the neuromechanism of migraine pathogenesis. J Headache Pain. 2017; 18: 7.
134. Santangelo G, Russo A, Trojano L, et al. Cognitive dysfunctions and psychological symptoms in migraine without aura: a cross-sectional study. J Headache Pain. 2016; 17: 76.
135. Gil-Gouveia R, Oliveira AG, Martins IP. The impact of cognitive symptoms on migraine attack-related disability. Cephalalgia. 2016; 36: 422–30.
136. Ashina S, Bendtsen L, Lyngberg AC, Lipton RB, Hajiyeva N, Jensen R. Prevalence of neck pain in migraine and tension-type headache: a population study. Cephalalgia. 2015; 35: 211–19.
137. Florencio LL, Chaves TC, Carvalho GF, et al. Neck pain disability is related to the frequency of migraine attacks: a cross-sectional study. Headache. 2014; 54: 1203–10.
138. Viana M, Sances G, Terrazzino S, Sprenger T, Nappi G, Tassorelli C. When cervical pain is actually migraine: an observational study in 207 patients. Cephalalgia. 2018; 38(2): 383–8.
139. Goadsby PJ, Knight YE, Hoskin KL. Stimulation of the greater occipital nerve increases metabolic activity in the trigeminal nucleus caudalis and cervical dorsal horn of the cat. Pain. 1997; 73: 23–8.
140. Johnston MM, Jordan SE, Charles AC. Pain referral patterns of the C1 to C3 nerves: implications for headache disorders. Ann Neurol. 2013; 74: 145–8.

141. Kemp WJ 3rd, Tubbs RS, Cohen-Gadol AA. The innervation of the cranial dura mater: neurosurgical case correlates and a review of the literature. World Neurosurg. 2012; 78: 505–10.
142. Schueler M, Neuhuber WL, De Col R, Messlinger K. Innervation of rat and human dura mater and pericranial tissues in the parieto-temporal region by meningeal afferents. Headache. 2014; 54: 996–1009.
143. Takagi H, Umemoto T, for the ALICE (All-Literature Investigation of Cardiovascular Evidence) Group. A meta-analysis of case-control studies of the association of migraine and patent foramen ovale. J Cardiol. 2016; 67: 493–503.
144. Timm FP, Houle TT, Grabitz SD, et al. Migraine and risk of perioperative ischemic stroke and hospital readmission: hospital based registry study. BMJ. 2017; 356: i6635.
145. Li L, Schulz UG, Kuker W, Rothwell PM, for the Oxford Vascular Study. Age-specific association of migraine with cryptogenic TIA and stroke: population-based study. Neurology. 2015; 85: 1444–51.
146. Lin GY, Lin YK, Lee JT, et al. Prevalence of restless legs syndrome in migraine patients with and without aura: a cross-sectional, case-controlled study. J Headache Pain. 2016; 17: 97.
147. Schürks M, Winter A, Berger K, Kurth T. Migraine and restless legs syndrome: a systematic review. Cephalalgia. 2014; 34: 777–94.
148. Wang HI, Ho YC, Huang YP, Pan SL. Migraine is related to an increased risk of Parkinson's disease: a population-based, propensity score-matched, longitudinal follow-up study. Cephalalgia. 2016; 36: 1316–23.
149. Scher AI, Ross GW, Sigurdsson S, et al. Midlife migraine and late-life parkinsonism: AGES-Reykjavik study. Neurology. 2014; 83: 1246–52.
150. Saunders EF, Nazir R, Kamali M, et al. Gender differences, clinical correlates, and longitudinal outcome of bipolar disorder with comorbid migraine. J Clin Psychiatry. 2014; 75: 512–19.
151. Smitherman TA, Kolivas ED, Bailey JR. Panic disorder and migraine: comorbidity, mechanisms, and clinical implications. Headache. 2013; 53: 23–45.
152. Viana M, Sances G, Linde M, et al. Clinical features of migraine aura: results from a prospective diary-aided study. Cephalalgia. 2017; 37: 979–89.
153. Hansen JM, Baca SM, Vanvalkenburgh P, Charles A. Distinctive anatomical and physiological features of migraine aura revealed by 18 years of recording. Brain. 2013; 136: 3589–95.
154. Charles AC, Baca SM. Cortical spreading depression and migraine. Nat Rev Neurol. 2013; 9: 637–44.
155. Hartings JA, Shuttleworth CW, Kirov SA, et al. The continuum of spreading depolarizations in acute cortical lesion development: examining Leão's legacy. J Cereb Blood Flow Metab. 2017; 37: 1571–94.
156. Hansen JM, Lipton RB, Dodick DW, et al. Migraine headache is present in the aura phase: a prospective study. Neurology. 2012; 79: 2044–9.
157. Charles A. Migraine: a brain state. Curr Opin Neurol. 2013; 26: 235–9.
158. Schain AJ, Melo-Carrillo A, Strassman AM, Burstein R. Cortical spreading depression closes paravascular space and impairs glymphatic flow: implications for migraine headache. J Neurosci. 2017; 37: 2904–15.
159. Goadsby PJ, Edvinsson L, Ekman R. Vasoactive peptide release in the extracerebral circulation of humans during migraine headache. Ann Neurol. 1990; 28: 183–7.
160. Cernuda-Morollón E, Larrosa D, Ramón C, Vega J, Martínez-Camblor P, Pascual J. Interictal increase of CGRP levels in peripheral blood as a biomarker for chronic migraine. Neurology. 2013; 81: 1191–6.
161. Ashina M, Hansen JM, Olesen J. Pearls and pitfalls in human pharmacological models of migraine: 30 years' experience. Cephalalgia. 2013; 33: 540–53.
162. Marcus R, Goadsby PJ, Dodick D, Stock D, Manos G, Fischer TZ. BMS-927711 for the acute treatment of migraine: a double-blind, randomized, placebo controlled, dose-ranging trial. Cephalalgia. 2014; 34: 114–25.

SECTION 5
Neurology, neuropsychiatry, and phenomenology

23

The clinical spectrum of neurodegenerative disease

Moving beyond mild cognitive impairment

Stina Saunders, Graciela Muniz-Terrera, Tom C Russ, Craig W Ritchie, and Karen Ritchie

Introduction

There is a clinical tradition to try and apply a categorical *normal versus diseased* approach to describe the clinical outcomes to an insidious neurodegenerative disease process. This has led to the proposal of a three-stage decline: dementia (disease presence with cognitive and functional decline) is separated from an earlier prodromal phase (disease presence with only cognitive decline), and a preclinical phase (disease presence only). While a number of concepts have been proposed to describe this prodromal stage (e.g. historical overreviews), [1,2] MCI has been the most widely used in both research and clinical trials. In a clinical setting, however, there is a lack of consensus or confidence around the concept of MCI. MCI is generally defined as present when an individual manifests recent difficulties in at least one cognitive domain (memory, language or visuospatial functioning), but such that these difficulties do not significantly interfere with daily functioning. Such people commonly present to primary care with complaints of recall difficulties related to events, names and word-finding. MCI, however, does not satisfy standard requirements of a diagnosis, including an indication of shared aetiology, prognosis, or response to treatment and is therefore better thought of as a description rather than a diagnosis.

This chapter starts by examining how MCI has shifted historically from a classification originally intended for grouping high-risk residents in a care home to an individually-variable theoretical phase in a much longer-term disease process. The chapter then outlines what we currently know about the prevention of neurodegenerative disorders and how the accurate defining and identifying of the prodromal and preclinical phases of neurodegeneration might lead to strategies to prevent the decline of neurodegeneration and ultimately the development of dementia.

How symptoms lead to a diagnosis but do not necessarily inform the prognosis

An individual with minor cognitive impairment has been referred to by a variety of names over the last few decades. However, at the core of all these terms is the element of cognitive impairment, either reported by the individual themselves or the people close to them. The evidence that leads an individual to turn to his or her primary care doctor when they are worried about their cognition would indicate the need for further investigations by the GP or specialist memory assessment services. These are symptoms and signs relating to abnormalities in the individuals' cognitive performance. The issue with a categorical approach to MCI, however, comes from the vague understanding of how the symptoms and signs that would warrant a diagnosis might evolve over time. This chapter will illustrate how the current approaches in assessing MCI are inadequate and do not provide an evidence-based estimate of prognosis. Instead of being regarded as a diagnosis, MCI should be viewed as a stage on a continuum from intact cognitive function at one end to progressive neurodegeneration at the other.[3] Despite the prominence of cognitive test scores in the definition of the condition, it is insufficient to limit our consideration of MCI to a binary evaluation of cognitive dysfunction as *present* or *absent*. In fact, the fundamental difference between MCI and early dementia is not cognitive impairment *per se*, which is merely a question of degree, but rather the impact it has on the person's day-to-day functioning, this being largely preserved in MCI. The assessment of daily functioning, however, involves a more-or-less explicit value judgement, incorporating variability in expectation in what a person should be able to do as they get older. Within such a definition the difference between what a person can do, and what they have the opportunity to do, is often not clear. This has led to sociocultural bias in many functional assessment tests. The vigilance over what is expected of people over a certain age has also led to a heightened fear about risk, where people might seek help for any perceived deficits in cognition in mid to late life.[4] The value judgement and sociocultural context is at least partly responsible for the subjective aspects of assessing function in the current MCI criteria.

Historical Perspective on MCI

Reviewing the scientific literature around ageing reveals two distinct schools of thought that drive the underlying understanding and applicability of the concept of MCI. Broadly, the US based literature has conceptualized MCI as a pathological entity, whereas the European based-research has viewed MCI more as part of normal ageing. Today we define MCI as a state between a normal healthy state and dementia, indicated by relatively poor cognitive performance but functioning in daily life which is only mildly impaired (Winblad et al., 2004). This means that if an older person complains about his or her memory but has an otherwise normal general cognitive function, this person might be identified as having MCI after a series of assessments. This identification, though, is not accurate enough and sheds no light on the question of whether the problem will progress, remain the same, or improve. To begin, it is worth considering how the clinical spectrum of neurodegenerative disease has evolved historically.

A need to define MCI arising from a nursing home population

While MCI was first described in the 1990s (Flicker et al., 1991, Petersen et al., 1997), its historical origins go back to 1958 and the concept of benign senescent forgetfulness (BSF) (Kral, 1962). In the mid-1950s it was clear that older people in nursing homes have certain characteristics, which arise in the ageing process; this meant that nursing homes were looking for evidence-based recommendations to improve their resident's conditions.[1] The term MCI, therefore, originally arose from the need for a care home to classify some of their residents in a manner that would best benefit their individual differences and difficulties. The establishment that first paved the path for early neurodegenerative disease research was a specific care home in Canada; the residents were aged over 65 and were provided with food, shelter, and general medical care (Heinik, 2006). The care home's residents became the sample of VA Kral's ('Bertie') original works on BSF, the most widely cited predecessor of MCI. Kral, the Czech-Canadian psychiatrist and neurologist at the Montreal Hebrew Old People's Home, also concluded that the patients he studied were aware of their shortcomings and tried to compensate by circumvention, and might have been apologetic. They were also considered to have a relatively stable impairment. BSF referred to complaints of a persistent difficulty in recalling detail of relatively unimportant data and facts of an experience, commonly with accompanying depressive symptoms. BSF was differentiated from malignant senescent forgetfulness (MSF), a typical progressive amnestic syndrome, corresponding practically to today's AD, with or without a vascular component (Heinik, 2006). Interestingly, in the early days of defining what eventually would be known as MCI, BSF was not considered a pathology, or a risk factor for the development of dementia, but rather a continuum of memory changes as part of a normal ageing process.

Different positions on the ageing process

Over the following decades, the notion of BSF was replaced by more formal diagnostic criteria for non-dementia cognitive impairment by Crook et al. (1986) who referred to age-associated memory impairment (AAMI) in 1986 for the National Institute of Mental Health; they defined these changes as subjective complaints of memory loss in older people (aged over 50) verified by a decrement of at least one standard deviation on a formal memory test in comparison with means established for young adults (Ritchie, 2005). Around the same time, the Cambridge Mental Disorders of the Elderly Examination (CAMDEX) criteria was introduced, which referred to *minimal dementia* category in an attempt to characterize MCI as a high-risk group of progression to dementia (Roth et al., 1986). A few years after the suggestion of AAMI and CAMDEX, (Blackford RC., 1989) differentiated these classifications from the more severe state of late-life forgetfulness (LLF), defined as performance between one and two standard deviations below the mean on at least 50% of a battery of at least four tests. In collaboration with the International Psychogeriatric Association and the WHO Levy (Levy, 2005) subsequently proposed an alternative concept of ageing-associated cognitive decline (AACD) that considered the possibility of a wider range of cognitive functions as part of the pathology (attention, memory, learning, thinking, language, visuospatial function), and importantly also positioned that the deficit should be defined in reference to norms for older and not young adults. As the final step before the (Petersen et al., 1997) criteria of MCI, recognition by the major international classifications of disease of subclinical cognitive deterioration linked to the normal ageing process began with the appearance in (American Psychiatric Association (DSM-IV, 2000) of the concept of age-related cognitive decline (ARCD). The idea that mild memory issues are pathological introduced the possibility of developing pharmacological interventions for these complaints. So a move towards a separate clinical entity became more dominant that proposed a debatable set of symptoms and, despite a lack of understanding of how to measure these symptoms accurately, a prognosis of potential progression to AD. Following on, the ICD described MCD, and the DSM-IV proposed a similar entity, mild neurocognitive disorder (MNCD). In 1997, Graham et al. described cognitive impairment no dementia (CIND). Individuals with CIND, like MCD and MNCD, are considered to have cognitive impairment attributable to an underlying physical disorder, but may also have a 'circumscribed memory impairment', which is a modified form of AAMI (Ritchie, 2005).

Classifying types of MCI

Finally, Petersen et al. proposed diagnostic criteria for MCI for research purposes: complaints of defective memory, abnormal memory functioning for age on testing, with normal general cognitive functioning, and conserved ability to perform activities of daily living. It was concluded that individuals with MCI perform at least 1–1.5 standard deviations below the norm for age and education on standardized neuropsychiatric tests, but they carry out most daily activities satisfactorily (Sacuiu, 2016). However, it became evident that while some individuals who are identified as having MCI go on to develop dementia, some stay the same, and some improve, then all individuals who develop AD have passed through the MCI stage. Following on from that, MCI has since been the focus of extensive research as a proxy to AD. MCI syndromes are classified into amnestic and non-amnestic types—these terms refer to MCI where memory is affected or MCI where other cognitive domains rather than memory are affected (Winblad et al., 2004). However, largescale studies exploring the application of existing classifications of MCI and associated states have found that each MCI classification captures a unique group of individuals, with little concordance (Stephan et al., 2007). Over time, research focus has particularly moved to amnestic MCI, either as isolated memory impairment or with other cognitive domains only minimally affected (i.e. multiple domains amnestic MCI). It is becoming a common view that amnestic MCI is a stage on the neurodegenerative disease clinical spectrum, though non-amnestic MCI seems to have a heterogeneous underlying pathology that may not always be related to a specific neurodegenerative process (Sacuiu, 2016).

Current Understanding of MCI

Despite an incomplete understanding of the underlying pathology and prognosis of the condition, the term MCI has entered both research and clinical practice. MCI has even evolved to being referred to as Prodromal Alzheimer's Dementia (Dubois and Albert, 2004) or MCI due to AD (Jack et al., 2011). Considering MCI as a prodrome to AD has led to the investigation of risk factors to identify what predicts a progression to dementia.

Risks for MCI

There is growing acknowledgement that the whole life course is relevant to brain health (Kuh et al., 2013). An individual's experiences from all stages of life can increase or decrease their risk of cognitive decline, MCI, and dementia (Whalley et al., 2006). Indeed, even experiences before birth can have important and long-lasting effects. Muller et al. (2014) showed in the AGES-Reykjavik cohort that smaller size at birth (Ponderal index, which is considered an indicator of the intra-uterine environment) was associated with poorer cognitive function in individuals with no education. Further evidence for the importance of early life experience comes from the long-term follow up of the Lothian Birth Cohorts of 1921 and 1936 all of whom took part in national Scottish intelligence tests when they were 11 years old (Deary et al., 2011; Deary, Whalley & Starr, 2009). Childhood mental ability, which is itself influenced by previous experience, is associated with many subsequent developments, including cognitive ageing itself and even cross-sectional associations between intelligence and cortical thickness in later life (Karama et al., 2014).

Further, indirect evidence for the importance of early life factors for cognitive ageing comes from proxies for early life experience such as height (a marker for early-life illness, adversity, poorer nutrition, and psychosocial stress) or pulmonary function (which is affected by multiple insults, including smoking and illness), both of which are associated with greater cognitive decline and an increased risk of dementia (Russ et al., 2014; Russ et al., 2017). It has been found that for MCI, risk factors for conversion to dementia may be gender specific, with vascular risk factors being more predictive for men and neuropsychiatric symptoms for women (Modrego, 2006; Artero et al., 2008; Ritchie et al., 2010). Though population-based studies have concluded that the underlying mechanism by which vascular disease affects cognitive performance is poorly understood, Stephan et al. (2017) argue that the effects of each vascular condition on cognition might be related to their underlying pathogenesis as well as on the anatomical location of the vascular damage. Other risk factors reported to be associated with MCI are age, education, and carrying the e4 allele of the *APOE* gene (Tyas et al. in the Nun study, 2007).

Norton et al. (2014) conclude that around a third of AD cases worldwide might be attributable to potentially modifiable risk factors, the incidence might be reduced through improved access to education and use of effective methods targeted at reducing the prevalence of vascular risk factors (e.g. physical inactivity, smoking, midlife hypertension, midlife obesity, and diabetes) and depression. The modifiable risk factors proportion is corroborated in a recent review by Livingston et al. (2017) who recommend active treatment of hypertension in middle-aged (45–65 years) and older people (aged older than 65 years) without dementia and emphasize the protective factors against dementia risk, for example childhood education, exercise, maintaining social engagement, reducing smoking, and management of hearing loss, depression, and diabetes. However, much of the evidence for risk factors for developing MCI is extrapolated from either the *normal* cognitive ageing literature or the dementia literature. From the broader dementia literature, the 2014 World Alzheimer Report identified education, hypertension, and obesity as being robustly linked with dementia risk (Prince et al., 2014) (Fig. 23.1). Occupational status, late-life depression, smoking, diabetes, and hypercholesterolaemia were found to have

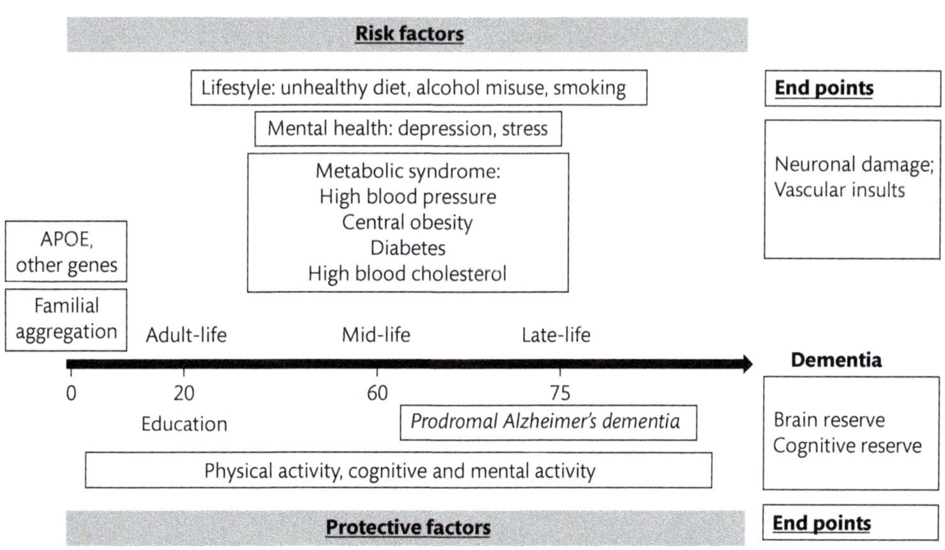

Fig. 23.1 Alzheimer's disease—a balance between life-long exposure to multiple risk and protective factors.

moderate levels of evidence. Of note, some of these risk and protective factors were more associated when they occurred at different stages in the life course. For example, smoking at any age is harmful, but depression seems to be particularly linked with dementia when it occurs in later life (for reasons which are not yet entirely clear). In order to clarify the fact that different exposures may have a different effect at different stages, Ben-Shlomo and Kuh (2002) specified different models of an exposure influencing risk: risk may be accumulated over time or a particular factor may influence risk only at a particular point in time (a critical period) or more at one point in time than at other times (a sensitive period).

In addition to these risk factors, some robustly linked, some less so, dementia risk is, of course, determined by genetic factors and gene-by-environment interactions. However, there is evidence that even in monozygotic twins discordant for dementia status (who are otherwise matched for age, sex, and genetic factors), dementia risk varies substantially by geographical location. The risk in the north of Sweden is two to three times higher than in the south, but patterns differ between men and women (Russ et al., 2015). The conclusion this leads to, since genetic variance has effectively been removed, is that environmental factors are likely to be important. Thus, geographical variation plays a key role in dementia risk. In the northern hemisphere, dementia mortality is higher in the north in a number of countries, but the pattern in the southern hemisphere is more complex (Russ et al., 2016). Following on from this research, there is at least moderate evidence implicating the following risk factors: air pollution; aluminium; silicon; selenium; pesticides; vitamin D deficiency; and electric and magnetic fields (Killin et al., 2016). Of these, factors of particular interest are air pollution and vitamin D deficiency (Underwood, 2017; Cacciottolo et al., 2017; Mokry et al., 2016).

Neuropsychological features and trajectories of MCI

As reviewed by Ritchie and Artero (2005), MCI affects principally episodic verbal memory and is distinguished from neurodegenerative disorders by a far slower progression, lesser impact on ability to perform activities of daily living, and the relative sparing of linguistic and visuospatial functions. It is, however, difficult to determine whether specific cognitive functions are differentially affected, or to characterize a *typical* neuropsychological profile. The principal problem in this context is that cognitive tests are not domain specific. Every test requires multiple cognitive processes and it is only through the application of multiple tests covering the same function administered over time that a discrete problem may be identified. For example, a person with an impairment in episodic memory will perform poorly on a recall task, but all persons performing poorly on such tasks may not all necessarily have a memory problem. This could occur for many other reasons: sensory impairment, attentional deficit, language impairment, misinterpretation of visual material. Moreover, cognitive dysfunction is not a stable and steadily progressing process. Cognitive performance fluctuates over time, particularly in relation to changes in health and fatigue. As a result, the profile of difficulties sampled may vary both across time and also according to which tests are chosen.

The prevalence over the age of 70 of MCI has been reported to be 14–18%, with a 6–10% yearly transition rate to dementia (as reviewed by Petersen et al., 2009) and a systematic review of longitudinal MCI studies has found the conversion rate to be 10% yearly (Bruscoli & Lovestone, 2004). The prevalence rates vary considerably depending on how MCI has been measured and whether comorbidities have been taken into account. In the COSMIC study, Sachdev et al. (2015) applied uniform criteria to a large international data set and found that this reduced the variation in MCI prevalence, resulting in 5.9% overall prevalence, though this increased with age but was unaffected by sex or the main races/ethnicities investigated (White and Chinese). There is evidence that in some cases, the cognitive impairment may either improve or remain stable over time (Roberts et al., 2014; Palmer et al., 2002; Ritchie et al., 2001). It has previously been found that ten years after being identified as having MCI, approximately 50% of individuals did not progress to dementia (Visser et al., 2006) having remained either stable or improving. Another longitudinal study looking at MCI conversion found that at 2.5-year follow up no MCI cases had converted to dementia and at 4.5 year follow up, most individuals had not converted to dementia (Marcos et al., 2016). The revised criteria for MCI (McKhann et al., 2011) allow for the inclusion of cognitive deficits other than memory functions and recognize that MCI may be associated with early and subtle changes in the ability to perform tasks of everyday living, providing an estimated prevalence of 16.6% and a yearly incidence of 0.06% in the general population (Artero et al., 2006). The conversion rates of MCI to AD has led to clinicians identifying MCI cases but providing ambiguous information as to what the condition means for the individual.

It is imperative to use multiple cognitive tests to capture deficits, and monitor any change of the disease course. As reviewed above, the revised criteria for MCI incorporates the possibility of changes in activities of daily living and alteration of non-amnesic cognitive functions. While modifications to the original algorithm have been found to better define subjects converting to dementia, results also point to the complexity of operationalizing this definition in terms of neuropsychological tests (Artero et al., 2006). Different cognitive tests are observed to give different results, with the common conclusion being that the measures are inadequate, rather than that the concept is too vague to operationalize (Ritchie and Ritchie, 2012b). A commonly used memory assessment method, the MMSE, is also used for differential diagnostics, although there is evidence that the MMSE cannot be used to screen for MCI as its sensitivity for MCI is only 18% (Nasreddine et al., 2005).

Ritchie et al. (2017a) examined associations between cognitive performance in a preclinical population of adults in midlife and various indicators of dementia risk. While these early findings cannot be used to explain the underlying causes between the associations, looking at a preclinical population, the authors found that a higher dementia risk score was associated with a small number of specific tests which have a strong spatial component, such as face name associations. Ritchie et al. (2018) examined allocentric (object to object) and egocentric (self to object) spatial processing in relation to future dementia risk in a middle-aged cohort and the authors concluded that allocentric rather than egocentric processing may be a potential indicator of risk for late-onset AD. Preliminary results from the baseline assessments of the PREVENT Dementia study (Ritchie and Ritchie 2012a; 2013) provide evidence for the cognitive changes in midlife for adults who are at high risk of late-onset AD. However, at a later stage, in a prodromal phase to dementia, it is common to see poor performance over a wider range of tests. It is essential that people with MCI are identified appropriately, as for a research criteria it would be vital that clinical trials include appropriately profiled participants to accurately determine whether a compound is effective and safe for the treatment of MCI (Ritchie and Ritchie, 2012b). Insensitive cognitive measures that are not able to detect slow disease progression to capture change using clinical markers may also lead to the negative results in neurodegenerative disease clinical trials to date.

Newer and more sensitive cognitive tests are administered using computers and often focus on a specific region of the brain. For example, the Four Mountains test is effective in identifying prodromal dementia which manifests as MCI (Chan et al., 2016). It focuses on allocentric spatial memory by altering the viewpoint, colours, and textures between the initially presented and target images. Allocentric spatial memory is a key function of the hippocampus, one of the earliest brain regions to be affected in Alzheimer's disease and impairment of hippocampal function predates the onset of dementia (Chan et al., 2016). Other newer developments in being able to detect neurodegenerative disorders early include the Capturing Changes in Cognition (Catch-Cog) study. Catch-Cog aims to develop and validate a composite measure combining cognition and function: the cognitive-functional composite (CFC), which is expected to be able to detect clinically relevant changes over time in early dementia stages of AD (Jutten et al., 2017).

MCI in memory clinics

Recent iterations of research criteria for the pre-dementia phases of AD have sought to incorporate both biomarkers and more specific cognitive tests to yield better prediction of conversion to dementia (Fig. 23.2). In essence, preclinical AD is thought of as having evidence of AD, but no overt symptoms, whereas Prodromal Alzheimer's Dementia (or MCI due to AD) is where there is both evidence of disease *and* cognitive symptoms though not sufficient to lead to functional impairment. Viewing MCI on the neurodegenerative disease spectrum as a proximal clinical prodrome to AD could lead to individuals who actually have a high risk of developing AD to be more accurately identified if additional specific tests were available and could be incorporated in a clinical assessment. The lack of success to modify the course of clinical symptoms through impacting on core AD pathologies (amyloid-β and tau) may be in part due to interventions being tested too late in the disease course. Improved identification of the prodrome to AD through better cognitive and biomarker evaluation would lead to high-risk strata of populations with both target disease and a high probability of clinical decline. Prevention research seeking to identify mechanisms for targeted risk reduction and accompanying pharmacological interventions is now attracting major funding and international collaborations (e.g. the European Prevention of Alzheimer's Dementia (EPAD) Programme that is described in more detail in the following sections) and will be key to finding a solution to the growing global dementia problem (Dementia Innovation Readiness Index, 2017).

In Prodromal Alzheimer's Dementia (Dubois, 2004) or MCI due to AD (Jack et al., 2011), the endorsement of the presence of the condition is made by inclusion of biomarker criteria, specific and sensitive to markers of underlying AD pathology. However, the validity of biomarkers may be far below clinical expectations and hopes (Ritchie et al., 2014; Ritchie et al., 2017b). Moreover, the quality of the diagnostic tests that are being used in clinical practice is poor, which leads to unreliable identification of MCI cases (Noel-Storr et al., 2012). There is a pervasive assumption that in dementia, early detection and diagnosis is beneficial by allowing planning, control, and access to interventions (Burns, 2012; Russ et al., 2012). But this argument makes an assumption that there is only a small false positive rate in identifying early dementia. Clearly, there are no benefits of predicting decline from the state of MCI to dementia if dementia does not manifest as this would lead to unnecessary anxiety for the individual.

Biomarkers (fluid and imaging): poor prognostic validity

Biomarkers are distinctive biological or biologically derived indicators of a process, event, or condition. Biomarkers in neurodegenerative disorders are principally either fluid markers, for example CSF, blood, urine, and saliva sampling, or observed through a range of structural and metabolic neuroimaging techniques. The pathology of AD includes neurofibrillary tangles and amyloid-β plaques, making these pathologies the underpinning entities of biomarkers which are at the centre for diagnostic test investigations. However, four recent Cochrane Diagnostic Test Accuracy reviews demonstrated that amyloid-β levels whether measured in CSF (Ritchie

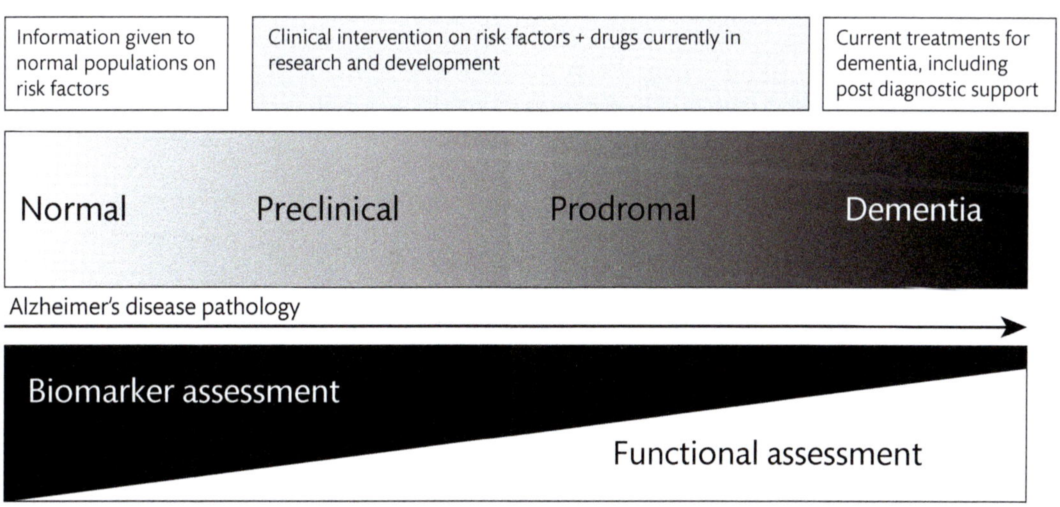

Fig. 23.2 Alzheimer's disease pathology and corresponding stages in assessments.

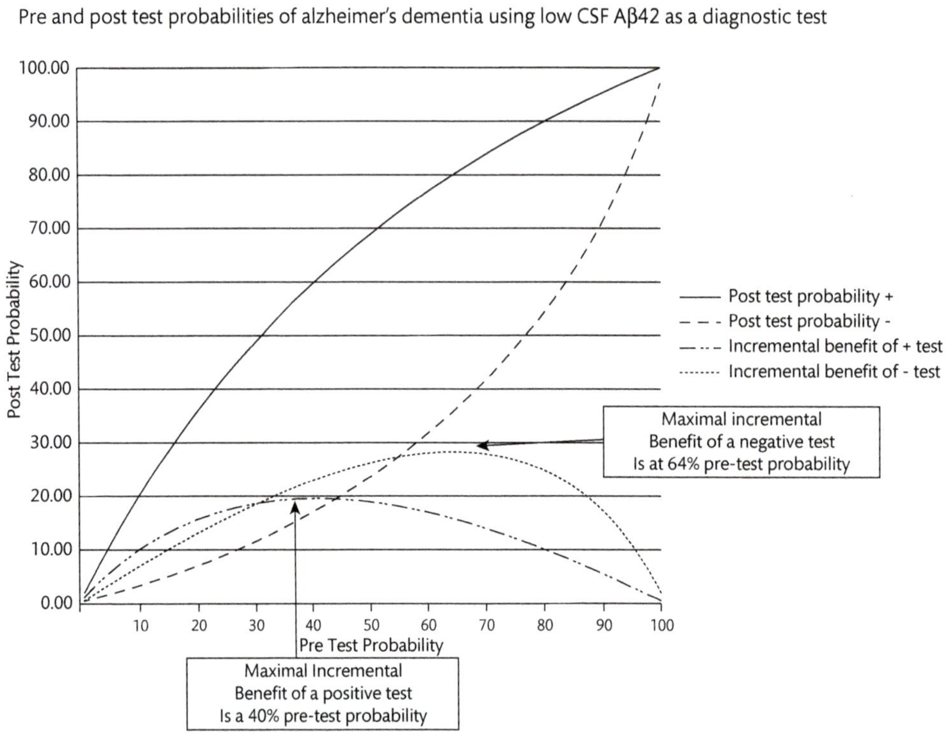

Fig. 23.3 Pre- and post- tests probabilities of Alzheimer's dementia using low CSF amyloid beta 42 as a diagnostic test (from Ritchie et al., 2014).

et al. 2014) or using PET imaging (Vacante et al. 2015; Zhang et al. 2014) had very low specificity, but better sensitivity for people with MCI subsequently developing AD. This suggests that while measuring amyloid-β levels is useful in accurately identifying individuals at risk, we are not currently able to use amyloid-β to delineate who, in the high-risk group, will progress on to dementia. From these reviews (Ritchie et al., 2014) it was possible to calculate the clinically meaningful Likelihood Ratios that allow the incremental benefit of the test to be determined. As single test and in combination (the amyloid-β/tau) ratio there was much greater benefit for a test being negative to rule out the possibility of decline to dementia compared to a positive test predicting decline (Fig. 23.3).

These data encourage the use of these tests in clinical trials to exclude people without AD pathology, but there remains a high probability that people who test positive do not decline to dementia. Clearly the next phase of diagnostic criteria will need to enhance further the use of multiple tests, incorporate risk factors in the models (e.g. age or *APOE* status), improve more sensitive measures of hippocampal function, and a sense or measure of intra-individual change between at least two but ideally three time points.

This research is ongoing (Ritchie et al., 2015), but is unlikely to yield clinically meaningful and applicable algorithms for at least another five years. Until then, clinical practice remains somewhat dependent on often quite subjective clinical judgements. The emerging reliance on biomarkers needs to be encouraged but clinicians must be cautious about over-valuing their utility in improving accuracy given quite small likelihood ratios. For now, the main reason for identifying MCI or any other prodromal phase of dementia could well be to help engage people in clinical research and offer pragmatic advice on lifestyle and health modifications which may have a beneficial effect on brain health.

In parallel to the development of fluid biomarkers, structural neuroimaging techniques with better resolution and the measurement of brain amyloid through PET imaging have made it possible to show in amnestic MCI both pathologic atrophy of the hippocampus regions and amyloid deposits in the cortex (Small et al., 2006; Schuff and Zhu, 2007; Mosconi et al., 2008). Consequently neuroimaging, which was previously used to exclude other causes of symptoms, has become an adjunct tool for AD diagnosis with PET scans and structural MRI scans being the most favoured either singly or in combination (Kogan et al., 2017). Stephan et al. (2012) studied brains from an unbiased population-based autopsy cohort (the Medical Research Council Cognitive Function and Ageing Study: MRC CFAS) and concluded that the neuropathology of MCI is complex, with 10% of MCI brains classified as normal, 10% as vascular disease, 10% as AD, and 40% as mixed AD/vascular disease (the remaining showing other pathologies). It is highly likely that the diagnosis of AD in the years before dementia occurs will very soon incorporate multi-modal testing of symptoms, risks, and biomarkers and this presumption needs to drive a shift in expertise, facilities, and expectation from healthcare providers (Ritchie et al., 2017a).

Future Directions of Neurodegenerative Diseases

The understanding that AD starts developing decades earlier when a person is outwardly healthy, corroborated by biomarker evidence and sensitive cognitive testing, forms the future approach to the neurodegenerative disease clinical spectrum. There needs to be a better specificity in the assessment of the condition to capture both the biological pathology as well as the early cognitive changes that act as a prodrome for dementia.

A need for modern statistical and analytical tools

In 2011 the NIA-AA workgroup updated the criteria for AD to reflect the period of 'preclinical' AD, when AD was present in the brain (and could theoretically be identified using biomarkers), but without clinical symptoms (Sperling et al. 2011). Individual, tailored, risk-factor modification is feasible if accurate probability models are developed which incorporate factors relevant to any given individual (Russ et al., 2016).

A move away from a single variable towards an integrative approach

The current medical model assesses MCI primarily on cognitive deficits. The future of MCI is to move away from a categorical approach and see MCI on the neurodegenerative disease spectrum. Prevention has been identified as a key approach to stopping MCI from progressing into dementia and a tailored model accounting for risk factors would enable determining of the earliest signs of neurodegenerative changes. In the current clinical practice, MCI is mainly considered based on memory deficits and possibly functional deficits if these are present; cognitive deficits would eventually manifest in functional deficits, though at a very early stage, the functional impairment would not yet be evident. As discussed above, the next step in better disease identification is adding the dimension of biomarkers in the assessment of neurodegenerative diseases; this would provide more accurate estimation of risk, factoring in biological changes. A significant move in neurodegenerative research has been focusing on the very early risk factors that contribute towards the development of AD and incorporating this knowledge into disease modelling. Understanding individual risk factors, such as genetic background, diet, and lifestyle factors would lead to an evidence-based approach to what contributes towards high risk. Finally, for early neurodegenerative disease identification, following individuals for a considerable period of time, rather than assessing them at one time point, would optimize risk prediction. The nuance is detecting these changes early, both in biomarkers and in cognitive functioning. In the PREVENT Dementia study, Ritchie et al. (2017a) looked at a population in their midlife and concluded that in a preclinical population, overall the traditional memory tests did not show an association between cognitive performance and later-life dementia risk. However, there was some evidence that the people at higher risk performed worse on tasks that measured specifically spatial awareness (Ritchie et al., 2017a). This raises the question of whether existing neuropsychological tests designed for detecting changes in older populations can be directly translated for use in younger individuals. The need for better testing in preclinical AD has also been identified by previous research (Ritchie et al., 2017c).

In a preclinical population, when incorporating biomarkers and neuroimaging in the detection of early pathology decades before the manifestation of any signs of dementia, it is evident that we need to look at an appropriate much more specific part of the brain. Many of the current studies use brain scanning methods that are not sensitive enough to the truly subtle brain changes that occur so long before dementia onset (Ritchie et al., 2017a).

These design considerations need to be accompanied by the use and development of adequate analytical tools that capture the multi-dimensional dynamics of the various operating processes, which are not accounted for in commonly used prediction models such as logistic regression or Cox models. Statistical models exist that improve these traditional analytical approaches, although these models are not commonly used in the medical literature. For instance, multivariate joint longitudinal survival models represent an exciting tool that acknowledges several of the desired features of these, needing new risk prediction models (Hickey et al., 2016). Furthermore, models need to capture and better explain the heterogeneity amongst individuals that we observe in clinical practice, acknowledging the existence of groups of individuals with diverse trajectories of change (Proust-Lima et al., 2007). Overlooking such heterogeneity may simply mask individuals at higher risk of disease, or fail to identify the group specific role of some risk factors.

Clinical trials to identify risk factors to prevent dementia

As reviewed above, targeting interventions at the stage where an individual already experiences memory problems is too late into the disease process and irreversible neurological damage has already occurred. As such, new AD studies focus on an earlier population including healthy volunteers from as early as midlife. If we are measuring change over time, potential decline, staying the same, or improvement, we need to be able to measure any such change accurately. The design of prevention trials poses an enormous challenge and risk for sponsors and while the majority of risk in any trial lies in whether the drug under study has the desired effect, failure to use appropriate tools for assessing cognitive and functional change adds the risk of missing interventions that work (Posner et al., 2017). It is important to use outcome measures that not only result in, for example, statistically significant change on a rating scale, but also translate into clinically meaningful improvement for the patient in current or future ability to perform cognitive tasks (Karlawish & Langa, 2016).

Ritchie and colleagues argue (Ritchie, 2017a) that cognitive changes may not only appear at the same time but also interact with the biological changes that occur decades before dementia manifests. This is vital as cognitive functioning is a central clinical concern and something that is monitored closely in dementia studies. Some of the newest dementia research, therefore, is targeted at a significantly younger, preclinical, age group. The world leading dementia prevention studies are currently EPAD (Ritchie et al., 2015) and the Global Alzheimer's Platform (GAP) (Cummings et al., 2016). These studies are based on the understanding that dementia is the last stage of an illness that starts developing far earlier in a life course when no symptoms of memory problems are expressed. Both EPAD and GAP recruit trial participants from existing parent cohorts, forming a new longitudinal cohort study.

The University of Edinburgh-led EPAD Longitudinal Cohort Study (LCS) (Fig. 23.4) is a public-private partnership funded by the Innovative Medicines Initiative. The EPAD LCS research participants are individuals over the age of 50 and the study is designed to build a cohort of 6000 healthy volunteers. Participants undergo phenotyping to collect a vast amount of baseline data including biological samples, neuroimaging, medical and family history, lifestyle

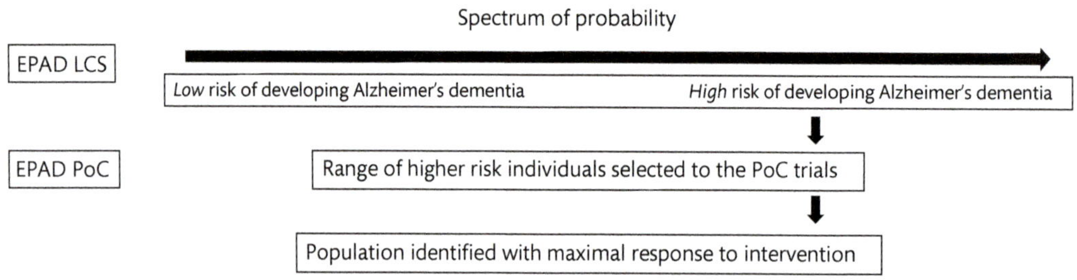

Fig. 23.4 Steps from disease modelling in EPAD LCS to PoC drug trials.
Source: data from Ritchie C.W., Molinuevo J.L., Truyen L., Satlin A., Van der Geyten S., Lovestone S. Development of interventions for the secondary prevention of Alzheimer's dementia: the European Prevention of Alzheimer's Dementia (EPAD) project. *The Lancet Psychiatry*. 2015;3, 179–186.

factors, and cognitive performance. This would allow stratifying individuals by their risk of decline and creating a spectrum of probability of individuals who, based on all the assessments carried out, would range from a low risk to a high risk of developing dementia. The LCS creates a *readiness cohort*, which feeds into the second pillar of the EPAD study, the Proof of Concept (PoC) trials. The PoC will enable adaptive drug trials to test novel interventions: targets for the drug can be modified and outcomes assessed accordingly. The adaptive trial design in the PoC would enable new drugs to be introduced into the EPAD trial machine regularly, stop drugs, which do not show an effect, or also combine the drugs tested. The process of recruiting participants into the LCS enables a much more specific eligibility for the PoC trials and reduces the high-screen failure rate we currently see in drug trials, and also allow for empirically derived disease models.

The PREVENT Dementia study (Ritchie & Ritchie 2012, 2013) is one of the cohorts that acts as a parent cohort for the EPAD study. PREVENT is a UK-based study of healthy volunteers in midlife looking to identify early risk factors of dementia that appear decades before any dementia symptoms occur. The study assessments focus on the biological and cognitive expression of AD and aims to inform the social, political, and ethical framework for applying risk screening and intervention programmes (Ritchie et al. 2013).

Conclusion

Arguably, memory and cognition are the key components in an individual's sense of self and the way they perceive themselves and the world around them. MCI can be a pre-dementia phase on the neurodegenerative disease clinical spectrum. If accurately identified, MCI is characterized by cognitive complaints (and possibly functional consequences) that might, or might not, progress on to dementia. However, its prognostic uncertainty leads us to question which methods should be employed to identify individuals at high risk of conversion to dementia which would allow us to ultimately intervene in the disease process.

Risk factors for MCI and for MCI conversion to dementia are reviewed in detail in the previous sections. We conclude that about a third of dementia risk remains unexplained—part of this may be due to environmental risk factors. Identifying the at-risk population by looking at a wide range of contributing factors, both lifestyle and biological, is vital to stop an individual from moving along the neurodegenerative disease spectrum into a symptomatic dementia phase. By the time a clear pattern of cognitive symptoms emerges and prodromal dementia can be clinically diagnosed according to current AD criteria, the AD pathology has already developed inside the brain, spreading neurofibrillary tangles and amyloid-β plaques.

The future for neurodegenerative disease is to incorporate accurate testing, disease modelling, and analytical tools to stratify at risk populations. This would allow us to developing interventions tailored to groups or even individuals: true precision medicine. The ultimate aim is, of course, preventing outwardly healthy or mildly impaired individuals from developing AD.

REFERENCES

Artero S, Petersen R, Touchon J, Ritchie K. Revised criteria for mild cognitive impairment: validation within a longitudinal population study. Dementia and Geriatric Cognitive Disorders. 2006; 22, 465–70.

American Psychiatric Association (DSM-IV 2000). *Diagnostic and Statistical Manual of Mental Disorders* (4th edition, text rev.). Washington, DC, American Psychiatric Association, 2000.

Ben-Shlomo Y, Kuh D. A life course approach to chronic disease epidemiology: conceptual models, empirical challenges and interdisciplinary perspectives. *International Journal of Epidemiology*. 2002; 31 (2): 285–93.

Bruscoli M, Lovestone S. Is MCI really just early dementia? A systematic review of conversion studies. Int Psychogeriatr. 2004; 16, 129–40.

Cacciottolo M, Wang X, Driscoll I, et al. Particulate air pollutants, APOE alleles and their contributions to cognitive impairment in older women and to amyloidogenesis in experimental models. *Translational Psychiatry*, 2017; 7(1): e1022.

Chan D, Gallaher LM, Moodley K, Minati L, Burgess N, Hartley T. The 4 Mountains Test: a short test of spatial memory with high sensitivity for the diagnosis of pre-dementia Alzheimer's disease. *Journal of Visualized Experiments: JoVE*. 2016; (116): 54454.

Cummings J, Aisen P, Barton R, et al. (2016). Re-engineering Alzheimer clinical trials: Global Alzheimer's Platform Network. Journal of Prevention of Alzheimer's Disease—JP Alzheimer's disease. 2016; 3: 114–20.

Deary IJ, Gow AJ, Pattie A, Starr JM. Cohort profile: the Lothian Birth Cohorts of 1921 and 1936. *International Journal of Epidemiology*. 2011; 41(6): 1576–84.

Deary IJ, Whalley LJ, Starr JM. *A Lifetime of Intelligence: Follow-Up Studies of the Scottish Mental Surveys of 1932 and 1947*. Washington DC: American Psychological Association, 2009.

Flicker C, Ferris FH, Reisberg B. Mild cognitive impairment in the elderly: predictors of dementia. Neurology. 1991; 41: 1006–9.

Graham JE, Rockwood K, Beattie EL, et al. Prevalence and severity of cognitive impairment with and without dementia in an elderly population. Lancet. 1997; 349: 1793–6.

Heinik J. VA Kral, the Montreal Hebrew Old People's Home, and benign senescent forgetfulness. History of Psychiatry, SAGE Publications. 2006; 17(3): 313–32.

Heinik J. VAKral and the origins of benign senescent forgetfulness and mild cognitive impairment. International Psychogeriatrics. 2010; 22(3): 395–402.

Henderson AS, Huppert FA. The problem of mild dementia. Psychol Med. 1984; 14: 5–11.

Hickey GL, Philipson P, Jorgensen A, Kolamunnage-Dona R. Joint modelling of time-to-event and multivariate longitudinal outcomes: recent developments and issues. *BMC Med Res Methodol.* 2016; 16: 117.

Jutten RJ, Harrison J, de Jong FJ, et al. A composite measure of cognitive and functional progression in Alzheimer's disease: design of the capturing changes in cognition study. *Alzheimer's & Dementia: Translational Research & Clinical Interventions.* 2017; 3(1): 130–8.

Karama S, Bastin ME, Murray C, et al. Childhood cognitive ability accounts for associations between cognitive ability and brain cortical thickness in old age. *Molecular Psychiatry.* 2014; 19(5): 555.

Karlawish J, Langa KM. Unfinished business in preventing Alzheimer disease. *JAMA Intern Med.* 2016; 176(12): 1739–40.

Killin LOJ, Starr JM, Shiue IJ, Russ TM. Environmental risk factors for dementia: a systematic review. BMC Geriatrics. 2016; 16: 175.

Kogan M, Jeong HS, Alzheimer's disease. In: Rakel D (ed.). Integrative Medicine (4th edition). Philadelphia, PA: Saunders Elsevier, 2017.

Kral VA. Senescent forgetfulness: benign and malignant. *Canadian Medical Association Journal.* 1962; 86: 257–60.

Kuh D, Cooper R, Hardy R, Richards M, Ben-Shlomo Y. (eds). *A Life Course Approach to Healthy Ageing.* Oxford: Oxford University Press, 2013.

Livingston et al. (2017). Dementia prevention, intervention, and care. The Lancet Commissions.

Marcos G, Santabárbara J, Lopez-Anton R, et al. and ZARADEMP Workgroup. Conversion to dementia in mild cognitive impairment diagnosed with DSM-5 criteria and with Petersen's criteria. Acta Psychiatr Scand. 2016; 133(5): 378–85.

McKhann GM, Knopman DS, Chertkow H, et al. The diagnosis of dementia due to Alzheimer's disease: recommendations from the National Institute on Aging-Alzheimer's Association workgroups on diagnostic guidelines for Alzheimer's disease. Alzheimer's Dement. 2011; 7: 263–9.

Mokry LE, Ross S, Morris JA, Manousaki D, Forgetta V, Richards JB. Genetically decreased vitamin D and risk of Alzheimer disease. *Neurology.* 2016; 87(24): 2567–74.

Muller M, Sigurdsson S, Kjartansson O, et al. Birth size and brain function 75 years later. *Pediatrics.* 2014; 134(4): 761–70.

Nasreddine ZS, Phillips NA, Bedirian V, et al. The Montreal Cognitive Assessment, MoCA: a brief screening tool for mild cognitive impairment. *J Am Geriatr Soc.* 2005; 53(4): 695–9.

National Institute for Health and Care Excellence NICE. Donepezil, Galantamine, Rivastigmine and Memantine for the Treatment of Alzheimer's Disease. London: NICE, 2011.

Norton S, Matthews FE, Barnes DE, Yafe K, Brayne C. Potential for primary prevention of Alzheimer's disease: an analysis of population-based data. Lancet Neurology. 2014; 13: 788–94.

Palmer K, Wang HX, Bäckman L, Winblad B, Fratiglioni L. Differential evolution of cognitive impairment in nondemented older persons: results from the Kungsholmen Project. Am J Psychiatry. 2002; 159(3): 436–42.

Petersen RC, Roberts RO, Knopman DS, et al. Mild cognitive impairment: ten years later. Arch Neurol. 2009; 66: 1447–55.

Prince M, Albanese E, Guerchet M, Prina M. *World Alzheimer Report 2014. Dementia and Risk Reduction: an Analysis of Protective and Modifiable Factors.* London: Alzheimer's Disease International, 2014.

Proust-Lima C, Letenneur L, Jacqmin-Gadda H. A nonlinear latent class model for joint analysis of multivariate longitudinal data and a binary outcome. *Stat Med.* 2007; 2229–45.

Richard E, Brayne C. Dementia: Mild cognitive impairment—not always what it seems.' Nat Rev Neurol. 2014; 10(3): 130–1.

Ritchie CW, Ritchie K. The PREVENT study: a prospective cohort study to identify mid-life biomarkers of late-onset Alzheimer's disease. BMJ Open 2. 2012.

Ritchie CW, Wells K, Ritchie K. The PREVENT research programme—a novel research programme to identify and manage midlife risk for dementia: the conceptual framework. Int Rev Psychiatry. 2013; 25: 748–54.

Ritchie CW, Smailagic N, Noel-Storr AH, et al. Plasma and cerebrospinal fluid amyloid beta for the diagnosis of Alzheimer's disease dementia and other dementias in people with mild cognitive impairment (MCI). *The Cochrane Library.* 2014.

Ritchie CW, Molinuevo JL, Truyen L, Satlin A, Van der Geyten S, Lovestone S. Development of interventions for the secondary prevention of Alzheimer's dementia: the European Prevention of Alzheimer's Dementia (EPAD) project. *Lancet Psychiatry.* 2015; 3: 179–86.

Ritchie CW, Smailagic N, Noel-Storr AH, Ukoumunne O, Ladds EC, Martin S. CSF tau and the CSF tau/ABeta ratio for the diagnosis of Alzheimer's disease dementia and other dementias in people with mild cognitive impairment (MCI). Cochrane Database of Systematic Reviews. 2017; (3): CD010803.

Ritchie K, Artero S, Touchon J. Classification Criteria for Mild Cognitive Impairment: a Population-Based Validation Study. MCI-AACD. 2001; 56(1): 37–42.

Ritchie K, Artero S. Mild cognitive impairment. A historical perspective. In: Burns A (ed.). Dementia. 2005.

Ritchie K, Ancelin ML, Beaino E, et al. Retrospective identification and characterization of mild cognitive impairment from a prospective population cohort. American Journal of Geriatric Psychiatry. 2010; 18(8): 692–700.

Ritchie K, Carriere I, Howett D, Su L, Hornberger M, O'Brien JT, et al. Allocentric and egocentric spatial processing in middle-aged adults at high risk of late-onset Alzheimer's disease: The PREVENT Dementia Study. Journal of Alzheimer's disease: JAD. 2018; 65(3): 885–96.

Ritchie K, Ritchie CW. Mild cognitive impairment (MCI) twenty years on. International Psychogeriatrics. 2012; 24(1): 1–5

Ritchie K, Carrière I, Su L, O'Brien JT, Lovestone S, Wells K, Ritchie CW. The mid-life cognitive profiles of adults at high risk of late-onset Alzheimer's disease: the PREVENT Study. Alzheimer's and Dementia. 2017; 13(10): 1089–97.

Ritchie K, Ropacki M, Albala B, Harrison J, Kaye J, Kramer J, et al. Recommended cognitive outcomes in preclinical Alzheimer's disease: Consensus statement from the European Prevention of Alzheimer's Dementia project. Alzheimer's & Dementia. 2017: 13(2): 186–95.

Roberts RO, Knopman DS, Mielke MM, et al. Higher risk of progression to dementia in mild cognitive impairment cases who revert to normal. *Neurology*. 2014; 82(4): 317–25. doi: 10.1212/WNL.0000000000000055. Epub 18 Dec 2013.

Roth M, Tym E, Mountjoy CQ, et al. CAMDEX: a standardised instrument for the diagnosis of mental disorder in the elderly, with special reference to the early detection of dementia. British Journal of Psychiatry. 1986; 149: 698–709.

Russ TC, Gatz M, Pedersen NL, et al. Geographical variation in dementia: examining the role of environmental factors in Sweden and Scotland. *Epidemiology*. 2015; 26(2): 263–70.

Russ TC, Ritchie WR, Ritchie K. Prevention of Alzheimer's disease and Alzheimer's dementia. In H. Chiu et al. (eds). Mental Health and Illness of the Elderly, Mental Health and Illness Worldwide. 2016.

Russ TC, Kivimäki M, Starr JM, Stamatakis E, Batty GD. Height in relation to dementia death: individual participant meta-analysis of 18 UK prospective cohort studies. *British Journal of Psychiatry*. 2014; 205(5): 348–54.

Russ, T. C., Kivimaki, M., & Batty, G. D. Respiratory Disease and Lower Pulmonary Function as Risk Factors for Dementia: A Systematic Review With Meta-analysis. *Chest*. (2020). doi:10.1016/j.chest.2019.12.012

Russ TC, Morling JR. Cholinesterase inhibitors for mild cognitive impairment. *Cochrane Database of Systematic Reviews*. 2012; 9.

Russ T, Murianni L, Icaza G, Slachevsky A, Starr J. Geographical Variation in dementia mortality in Italy, New Zealand, and Chile: the impact of latitude, vitamin D, and air pollution. Dementia and Geriatric Cognitive Disorders. 2016; 42(1–2): 31–41.

Sachdev PS, Lipnicki DM, Kochan NA, et al. The prevalence of mild cognitive impairment in diverse geographical and ethnocultural regions: the COSMIC Collaboration. PLOS One. 2015; 10(11).

Sacks C, Avorn J, Kesselheim A. The failure of solanezumab—how the FDA saved taxpayers billions. New England Journal of Medicine. 2017; 376 (18), 1706–8

Sacuiu, S. F. Chapter 8—Dementias. In M. J. Aminoff, F. Boller, & D. F. Swaab (Eds.), Handbook of Clinical Neurology (Vol. 138, pp. 123–151): Elsevier.

Saunders S, Ritchie K, Russ TC, Muniz-Terrera G, Ritchie CW. Evolution and future directions for the concept of mild cognitive impairment. International Psychogeriatrics. 2017: 1–4.

Schneider LSMF, Andreasen N, Feldman H, et al. Clinical trials and late-stage drug development for Alzheimer's disease: an appraisal from 1984 to 2014, J Intern Med. 2014; 275(3), 251–283

Sperling RA, Aisen PS, Beckett LA, et al. Toward defining the preclinical stages of Alzheimer's disease: recommendations from the National Institute on Aging-Alzheimer's Association workgroups on diagnostic guidelines for Alzheimer's disease. Alzheimer's Dement. 2011; 7: 280–292.

Stephan BC, Matthews FE, McKeith IG, Bond J, Brayne C. Medical Research Council Cognitive Function and Aging Study. 'Early cognitive change in the general population: how do different definitions work?' J Am Geriatr Soc. 2007; 55(10): 1534–40.

Stephan BC, Matthews FE, Hunter S, et al. Neuropathologicalprofile of mild cognitive impairment from a population perspec-tive. Alzheimer Dis Assoc Disord. 2012; 26: 205–12.

Stephan BCM, Minett T, Muniz-Terrera G, Harrison SL, Matthews FE, Brayne C. Neuropsychological profiles of vascular disease and risk of dementia: implications for defining vascular cognitive impairment no dementia (VCI-ND). Age and Ageing. 2017; 1–6.

Tyas SL, Salazar JC, Snowdon DA, Desrosiers MF, Riley KP, Mendiondo MS, et al. Transitions to mild cognitive impairments, dementia, and death: findings from the Nun Study. *American Journal of Epidemiology*. 2007; 165(11): 1231–8.

Underwood E. The polluted brain. *Science*. 2017; 355(6323): 342–5.

Visser PJ, Krester A, Jolles J, Verhey F. Ten-year risk of dementia in subjects with mild cognitive impairment. Neurology. 2006; 67: 1201–7.

Whalley LJ, Dick FD, McNeill G. A life-course approach to the aetiology of late-onset dementias. *Lancet Neurology*, 2006; 5(1): 87–96.

Winblad B, Palmer K, Kivipelto M, et al. Mild cognitive impairment-beyond controversies, towards a consensus: report of the International Working Group on Mild Cognitive Impairment. J Intern Med. 2004; 256: 240–6.

Zhang S, Smailagic N, Hyde C, et al. (11)CPIB-PET for the early diagnosis of Alzheimer's disease dementia and other dementias in people with mild cognitive impairment (MCI). Cochrane Database Syst Rev. 2014; 7: Cd010386.

Dementia Innovation Readiness Index by Global Coalition on Aging & Alzheimer 's disease International. (2017). http://www.globalcoalitiononaging.com/data/uploads/documents/gcoa-adi-dementia-index.pdf.

Blackford RC, riteria for diagnosing age-associated memory impairment: proposed improvement from the field. *Dev Neuropsychol.* 1989; 5: 295–306.

Crook T, Bartus RT, Ferris SH, Whitehouse P, Cohen GD, Gershon S. Age-associated memory impairment: Proposed diagnostic criteria and measures of clinical change—report of a national institute of mental health work group. *Developmental Neuropsychology.* 1986; 2: 261–76.

Dubois B, Albert ML. Amnestic MCI or prodromal Alzheimer's disease? *Lancet Neurology.* 2004; 3: 246–8.

Flicker C, Ferris SH, Reisberg B. Mild cognitive impairment in the elderly: predictors of dementia. *Neurology.* 1991; 41: 1006–9.

Graham JE, Rockwood K, Beattie BL, Eastwood R, Gauthier S, Tuokko H, et al. Prevalence and severity of cognitive impairment with and without dementia in an elderly population. *Lancet.* 1997; 349: 1793–6.

Heinik J. VA Kral and the Montreal Hebrew Old People's Home, and benign senescent forgetfulness. *History of Psychiatry.* 2006; 17: 313–32.

Heinik J. Kral VA, and the origins of benign senescent forgetfulness and mild cognitive impairment. *Int Psychogeriatr.* 2010; 22: 395–402.

Henderson AS, Huppert FA. The problem of mild dementia. *Psychol Med.* 1984; 14: 5–11.

Jack CR Jr, Vemuri P, Wiste HJ, Weigand SD, Aisen PS, Trojanowski J, et al. Evidence for ordering of Alzheimer disease biomarkers. *Arch Neurol.* 2011; 68, 1526–35.

Kral VA. Senescent forgetfulness: Benign and malignant. *Canadian Medical Association Journal.* 1962; 86: 257–60.

Levy R. Aging-Associated Cognitive Decline. *International Psychogeriatrics.* 2005; 6: 63–8.

Petersen RC, Smith GE, Waring SC, Ivnik RJ, Kokmen E, Tangelos EG. Aging, memory, and mild cognitive impairment. *Int Psychogeriatr.* 1997; 9(Suppl 1): 65–9.

Ritchie K, Artero S. *Mild cognitive impairment. A Historical Perspective.* 2005.

Roth M, Tym E, Mountjoy CQ, Huppert FA, Hendrie H, Verma S. et al. CAMDEX. A standardised instrument for the diagnosis of mental disorder in the elderly with special reference to the early detection of dementia. *Br J Psychiatry.* 1986; 49: 698–709.

Stephan BC, Matthews FE, Mckeith IG, Bond J, Brayne C. Early cognitive change in the general population: how do different definitions work? *J Am Geriatr Soc.* 2007; 55: 1534–40.

World Health Organization (ICD) *International Classification of Diseases and Related Health Problems* (10th revision). Geneva: World Health Organization, 1992.

Artero S, Ancelin M-L, Portet F, et al. Risk profiles for mild cognitive impairment and progression to dementia are gender specific. Journal of Neurology Neurosurgery and Psychiatry. 2008; 79; 979–84.

Ritchie K, Ancelin ML, Beaino E, et al. Retrospective identification and characterization of Mild Cognitive Impairment from a prospective population cohort. American Journal of Geriatric Psychiatry. 2010; 18: 692–700.

Ritchie K, Artero S. Mild Cognitive impairment: a historical perspective. In: Burns A, O'Brien J, Ames D (eds). Dementia. Oxford: Oxford University Press, 2005; reprinted 2010.

24

The epidemiology of apathy in neurological disorders

Sergio Starkstein, Bradleigh Hayhow, and Pierre Wibawa

Introduction

Apathy is defined as an independent psychiatric syndrome characterized by deficits in goal-directed behaviour, goal-directed cognitions, and the emotional concomitants of goal-directed behaviour.[1] Other definitions of apathy emphasize changes in emotional feeling and expression rather than in motivation.[2] In contemporary neuropsychiatry the motivation concept of apathy is the most commonly accepted for use in clinical settings and research studies.

The present chapter will discuss the epidemiology of apathy among the most common neurodegenerative disorders, such as AD, PD, and HD, as well as in acute neurological conditions such as stroke. We will examine the challenges in diagnosing apathy and review the different instruments currently in use. Finally, we will discuss specific phenomenological aspects of apathy in the above neurological disorders.

Diagnosis of Apathy in Neurological Disorders

The methodology for diagnosing psychiatric disorders in neurology includes three elements, namely structured psychiatric interviews, standardized diagnostic criteria, and severity rating scales. Thus, a diagnosis of apathy requires a formal neuropsychiatric assessment using an appropriate instrument, and the use of diagnostic criteria validated for each neurological condition. Rating scales should only be used to rate the severity of apathy and not to make a diagnosis. We shall now address what is available in neuropsychiatry in order to arrive at valid and reliable diagnoses.

Diagnostic criteria for apathy in neurological conditions

In the second half of the 20th century, Robert Marin was the first to conceptualize apathy as a syndrome consisting of loss of motivation as the main criterion, manifested by reductions in goal-directed behaviours (e.g. lack of effort, initiative, and productivity), reductions in goal-directed cognitions (e.g. decreased interests, lack of plans and goals, and lack of concern about one's own health and functional status), and reduced emotional concomitants of behaviours (e.g. flattened affect, emotional indifference, and restricted responses to important life events).[3] Other definitions of apathy have been proposed, stressing the emotional deficits, such as loss of feelings with blunting and flattening of affective response.[4] Levy and Dubois[5] defined apathy as a behavioural syndrome characterized by a quantitative reduction of self-generated voluntary and purposeful behaviours. They proposed 'emotional-affective', 'cognitive', and 'auto-activation' subtypes of apathy.

Apathy in Parkinson's Disease

Diagnosis of apathy in Parkinson's disease

One of the main diagnostic dilemmas in neuropsychiatry is how to distinguish apathy from anhedonia, depression, and cognitive deficits, in a reliable way. The Movement Disorders Society (MDS) organized a committee to identify instruments with the best psychometric attributes to diagnose and quantify the severity of apathy in PD.[6] A review of the clinimetric properties of apathy scales recommended the Apathy Scale (Box 24.1)[7] and the Lille Apathy Rating Scale[8] for use in PD. One of the main limitations when rating apathy in PD is the overlap with Parkinsonian symptoms, and the suggestion was made to use an 'inclusive' approach (i.e. all symptoms are scored, regardless of whether they overlap with motor symptoms) to increase diagnostic sensitivity. To standardize recollection bias the MDS committee also recommended apathy be assessed during the ON state (i.e. the state of maximal antiparkinsonian medication efficacy). Another diagnostic limitation is the assessment of apathy among patients with cognitive deficits. These patients may be assessed with the Dementia Apathy Interview and Rating Scale,[9] although this instrument has yet to be validated in PD. Another limitation to the assessment of apathy in PD is the lack of a clinical gold standard in terms of standardized diagnostic criteria or structured clinical interviews. Starkstein and Leentjens[10] proposed specific diagnostic criteria for apathy in PD (Box 24.2). These criteria were modified by a European group,[11] and validated for use in PD by Drijgers and co-workers.[12] A practical option is to use the UPDRS[13] item rating motivation to diagnose apathy. Starkstein and Merello[14] examined the psychometric attributes of the Motivation/Initiative item of the UPDRS to diagnose apathy, and found that a score of two or more had a sensitivity of 73% and a specificity

Box 24.1 Apathy Scale

1. Are you interested in learning new things?

   not at all   slightly   some   a lot

2. Does anything interest you?
3. Are you concerned about your condition?
4. Do you put much effort into things?
5. Are you always looking for something to do?
6. Do you have plans and goals for the future?
7. Do you have motivation?
8. Do you have the energy for daily activities?
9. Does someone have to tell you what to do each day?
10. Are you indifferent to things?
11. Are you unconcerned with many things?
12. Do you need a push to get started on things?
13. Are you neither happy nor sad, just in between?
14. Would you consider yourself apathetic?

Score key: For questions 1–8, *not at all* = 3 points *slightly* = 2; *some* = 1; a lot = 0. For questions 9–14, *not at all* = 0; *slightly* = 1; *some* = 2, *a lot* = 3

Scheme for converting ratings on the Apathy Scale to specific criteria for apathy

Item A of the Starkstein-Leentjens[13] diagnostic criteria (i.e. lack of motivation) was scored positive whenever there was a score of 2 (i.e. slightly) or 3 (i.e. not at all) on item 7 of the Apathy Scale (Does he/she have motivation?).

Diminished goal-directed behaviour was scored positive whenever there was a score of 2 or 3 on items 4 (Does the patient put much effort into things? slightly or not at all) or 9 of the Apathy Scale (Does someone have to tell the patient what to do each day? most of the time or always).

Diminished goal-directed cognition was scored positive whenever there was a score of 2 or 3 on items 1 (Is the patient interested in learning new things? slightly or not at all) or 2 of the Apathy Scale (Does anything interest the patient? slightly or not at all).

Diminished concomitants of goal-directed behaviour was scored positive whenever there was a score of 2 or 3 on item 10 (Is the patient indifferent to things? most of the time or always) or 13 of the Apathy Scale (Is the patient neither happy nor sad, just in-between, no matter what happens? most of the time or always).

Box 24.2 Diagnostic criteria for apathy

A. Lack of motivation relative to the patient's previous level of functioning or the standards of his or her age and culture as indicated either by subjective account or observation by others.

B. Presence **for at least four weeks during most of the day**, of at least one symptom belonging to each of the following three domains:

Diminished goal-directed behaviour

1. Lack of effort or energy to perform everyday activities.
2. Dependency on prompts from others to structure everyday activities.

Diminished goal-directed cognition

3. Lack of interest in learning new things, or in new experiences.
4. Lack of concern about one's personal problems.

Diminished concomitants of goal-directed behaviour

5. Unchanging or flat affect
6. Lack of emotional responsivity to positive or negative events.

C. The symptoms cause clinically significant distress or impairment in social, occupational, or other important areas of functioning.

D. The symptoms are not due to diminished level of consciousness or the direct physiological effects of a substance.

of 65%. For patients with moderate-severe PD the specificity was higher when using a cut-off score of three points. Thus, this UPDRS item may be used as a screen for apathy in PD, but should be followed by more comprehensive diagnostic assessments.

Frequency of apathy in Parkinson's disease

Apathy has been reported to range from 7% to 70% in PD.[15] This wide discrepancy is related to methodological factors. The highest frequencies of apathy have been reported from studies including patients from movement disorders clinics,[16] whilst studies that included patients recruited from the community reported lower frequencies.[17] Using the Apathy Scale, Starkstein and co-workers reported apathy in 32% of a consecutive series of 50 patients with PD attending a movement disorders clinic. Similar frequencies were reported from a study assessing PD patients from another movement disorder clinic.[7] Aarsland and co-workers[18] carried out an incidence study of apathy in PD and diagnosed apathy in 27% of 175 patients and in 23% of drug-naive patients. When patients with dementia or depression were excluded, the incidence of apathy decreased to 5%.[7] In a more recent longitudinal study, Pedersen and co-workers reported that 49% of 75 patients with no apathy at baseline developed apathy during a four-year follow-up period.[15] This finding strongly suggests that most patients with PD will develop apathy at some stage during the progression of the illness.

Correlates of apathy in Parkinson's disease

One of the most vexing questions is how to separate apathy from depression on clinical grounds. A task force organized by the National Institute of Neurological Disorders and Stroke and National Institute of Mental Health (NINDS/NIMH) suggested that loss of interest should not be used to diagnose depression in PD.[19] On the other hand, recent studies suggest that loss of interest is an intrinsic component of depression in PD and should not be excluded from the diagnostic criteria.[20] Kirsch-Darrow and co-workers[21] reported apathy in the absence of depression in 28% of a large series of PD patients. Contrasting evidence was provided by Starkstein and co-workers in a study that included a consecutive series of 166 patients with PD.[20] Using the Apathy Scale and standardized diagnostic criteria, they diagnosed apathy in 32% of the patients, but about two-thirds of patients with apathy were also depressed.

Dementia is another frequent correlate of apathy in PD. Dujardin and co-workers[22] reported apathy in 56% of PD patients with dementia as compared to 9% of patients without dementia. Similar results were reported by Starkstein and co-workers,[23] who found apathy in 47% with dementia. Moreover, only 3% of patients had apathy in the absence of depression or dementia. In an 18-month follow-up study Dujardin and co-workers[24] found that eight of twenty patients with apathy at baseline developed dementia at follow-up compared to only one patient without apathy at baseline, demonstrating that apathy is a significant predictor of dementia in PD. Drijgers and co-workers[12] reported a frequency of apathy of 11% among PD patients with neither dementia nor depression.

In conclusion, about 3–15% of PD patients may show apathy in the absence of depression or dementia, suggesting that neither of them is necessary to produce apathy in PD. The fact that many PD patients with depression or dementia have no apathy further suggests that depression and dementia are not sufficient to produce apathy in PD.

Mechanism of apathy in Parkinson's disease

The mechanism of apathy in PD seems to be multifactorial. Whilst most patients have comorbid depression and/or dementia, 5–10% of patients in cross-sectional studies have apathy only. Dujardin et al. suggested that apathy in PD may be a predictor or even an incipient symptom of dementia.[25] Ready and co-workers[26] found a significant association between apathy and testosterone levels, but this association was not replicated in a more recent study.[27]

Levy and Czernecki[28] suggested that the mechanism of apathy in PD may be related to deficits in basal ganglia-prefrontal cortical interaction in the context of reduced dopamine (DA) levels. Among PD patients undergoing deep brain stimulation in the subthalamic nucleus (DBS-STN) Le Jeune and co-workers[29] reported significant correlations between higher apathy scores and low metabolic activity in the cingulate and left fronto-medial cortex. Thobois and co-workers[30] found greater DA denervation in the orbitofrontal, dorsolateral prefrontal and anterior cingulate cortices, left thalamus, globus pallidus, and right temporal lobe among PD patients with apathy when compared to PD patients without apathy.

Apathy and deep brain stimulation

Apathy has been recognized as a frequent sequel of DBS-STN.[31] Two types of apathy after DBS have been described: the first is a transient state of loss of motivation that occurs in the early stages after DBS, which may result from reducing the dose of levodopa;[32] whereas a second type runs a more protracted course and is independent of levodopa dose.[33]

There are conflicting results on the frequency and mechanism of post-DBS apathy. Czernecki and co-workers[34] reported a significant improvement in apathy for patients on STN stimulation and concomitant levodopa therapy. In a small open label study, these investigators used the dopaminergic agonist ropinirole in eight patients who developed apathy and the withdrawal of levodopa after successful DBS-STN[35] and found significant improvements in seven of the eight patients. Different outcomes were reported by Drapier and co-workers[33] who found that 30% of PD patients developed apathy after DBS-STN. They were unable to replicate a significant association between the severity of apathy and levodopa dose, and suggested that post-DBS apathy may result from a more central stimulation in patients with apathy with diffusion of the stimulus to the medial limbic sections of the STN. Further studies are needed to clarify the frequency and mechanism of apathy after DBS-STN, and to examine whether new targets have a different relationship with this behavioural condition.

Treatment of apathy in Parkinson's disease

The efficacy of psychotropic medication or psychotherapy to reduce apathy in PD has rarely been examined. Several small case series provided early evidence for the efficacy of DA to treat apathy in PD.[36,37] A recent open-label study using ropinirole[35] showed a significant decrease in apathy scores after six months of treatment, without relevant side effects or changes on motor scores. This effect was not specific to apathy, as patients also showed mood improvement. A recent randomized controlled trial examined the efficacy of the selective noradrenaline reuptake inhibitor atomoxetine for depression and apathy in PD, but results were negative.[38] Finally, a recent study demonstrated the efficacy of the D2/D3 agonist piribedil for treating post-DBS apathy.[39]

Apathy in Alzheimer's Disease

Phenomenology and assessment of depression in Alzheimer's disease

Several instruments have been validated to measure the severity of apathy in AD. Marin and co-workers[1] developed the Apathy Evaluation Scale (AES), which consists of a self-rated, clinician-rated, and informant-rated version. Starkstein and co-workers[7] adapted the AES into a 14-item scale which was validated for use in AD. The Neuropsychiatric Inventory (NPI)[40] is a multidimensional instrument assessed with caregivers, which examines the presence of apathy together with nine other behavioural and emotional domains. The Dementia Apathy Review and Rating[9] has been specifically designed to assess apathy in dementia, and examines changes in motivation, emotional responsiveness, and engagement. More recently, Starkstein and co-workers[41] validated the Structured Clinical Interview for Apathy (SCIA) to assess apathy in AD in a standardized way. The SCIA includes specific questions assessing the domains of lack of motivation, lack of effort to perform daily activities, dependency on others to structure activities, lack of interest in learning new activities, lack of concern, blunted affect, and poor emotional response.

Frequency of apathy in Alzheimer's disease

Few studies have examined the frequency of apathy in AD using adequate psychiatric instruments. Starkstein and co-workers[42] diagnosed apathy in 37% of a series of 319 patients using the Apathy Scale. Apathy was also present in 32% of patients with major depression but no dementia, and in none of an age-comparable group of healthy controls. About two-thirds of AD patients with apathy had comorbid (major or minor) depression. The progression of apathy in AD has been rarely examined. Starkstein and co-workers[42] reported the frequency of apathy to increase from 14% at the stage of very mild dementia to 61% in the stage of severe dementia, which suggests that most patients with AD will suffer from apathy during the course of their illness.

Clinical correlates of apathy in Alzheimer's disease

Cross-sectional studies have demonstrated that apathy is significantly associated with more severe impairments in activities of daily living (ADLs) and cognitive function, older age, and poorer insight.[42] Whilst apathy in AD is significantly associated with major depression, the association with minor depression is four times lower.[42] Starkstein and co-workers[42] reported that non-depressed patients with apathy had similar depression scores to AD patients with neither apathy nor depression, suggesting that apathy may not inflate depression scores in AD in the absence of syndromal depression.

In a 1–4-year follow-up study, Starkstein and co-workers[43] found apathy to be a significant predictor of depression. Moreover, those patients who developed apathy during the follow-up period had a significantly greater cognitive and functional decline than AD patients without apathy. Boyle and co-workers[44] replicated the finding of a significant association between apathy and more severe functional deficits. Recent studies suggest that apathy may be a significant predictor of conversion from mild cognitive impairment (MCI) to AD. Robert and co-workers[45,46] reported that after a one-year follow-up, 15% of individuals with MCI and apathy converted to AD compared to just 7% of MCI individuals without apathy. This finding can also be construed as suggesting that apathy is an early manifestation of AD, even before functional deficits become evident.

Treatment of apathy in Alzheimer's disease

There is little evidence that pharmacological or psychotherapeutic treatment improves apathy in AD. Several studies using acetylcholinesterase inhibitors have reported improvements on NPI apathy scores,[47–49] but the findings are limited by the fact that some of the studies were retrospective or open-label, and none investigated apathy as the main outcome measure. Whilst small case open-label studies suggested the efficacy of methylphenidate to treat apathy in AD,[50] appropriate RCTs have yet to be carried out. Similar findings and limitations apply to treatment with dopaminergic agonists.[51] A recent RCT in a small sample of AD patients demonstrated that listening to live interactive music may be an effective treatment for apathy.[52] There is also preliminary evidence that multisensory stimulation, and controlled time and attention techniques may reduce apathy in late stages of dementia.[53,54]

Apathy in Huntington's Disease

Phenomenology and assessment of apathy in Huntington's disease

Several apathy scales have been used in the HD population,[55] including the Apathy Scale, the AES, NPI, the Frontal System Behavioural Scale, and the Lille Apathy Rating Scale. A recent revision of the Unified Huntington Disease Rating Scale has included a section rating apathy in the Problem Behaviours Assessment (PBA) section.[56] Apathy assessment in PBA is limited to the severity and frequency of the syndrome. Consequently, various dimensions of apathy are not evaluated and can impact on the correlations with other apathy instruments. In a study of 34 HD patients, Naarding and colleagues reported moderate correlation between the PBA the behavioural domain of the AES ($r = 0.50$, $p<0.001$) but a weak relationship with the cognitive and emotional domains.[57] The authors concluded that the cognitive component of the AES may be more representative for studying apathy in the HD population.

Frequency of apathy in Huntington's disease

The prevalence of apathy in HD varies, and depends on the assessment methods and cut-off scores. One study reported a prevalence as high as 76%[58] but a more recent and larger study reported a much lower cumulative prevalence of 11% in the early stages, increasing to 55% in the final stages of HD.[59] Apathy seems to peak around the phenoconversion period with prevalence up to 64%.[60] This peak may be attributed to mood changes, as manifested by a positive correlation between apathy and likelihood of proceeding with a genetic testing.[61] In a two-year follow-up of 34 HD subjects, 41% of apathy remitted and there was a 14% incidence of new onset apathy.[62] Persistent apathy is associated with older age and longer disease duration. The natural remission of apathy remains debatable as it may be related to fluctuations in depression.

Clinical correlates of apathy in Huntington's disease

Similar to other neurodegenerative disease, apathy is associated with older age, more severe cognitive and motor impairment, use of psychotrophic medications, more severe functional impairment, and reduced cerebral reserve, as demonstrated by structural imaging in HD.[59,63–65] There are also independent correlations with male gender, obsessive-compulsive behaviour, and previous history of depression and suicide attempt. For cognition, apathy is associated with worse performance on MMSE and symbol digit modalities.[62]

Recent longitudinal studies in HD have yielded structural imaging and various clinical measures as reliable markers of phenoconversion and disease progression. In TRACK-HD, a 36-month cohort study of 366 individuals, apathy was the only significant neuropsychiatric predictor across the prodromal and early stages of HD.[64] Compared to the control group, more severe brain atrophy in those at a higher risk of phenoconversion correlates with a modest increase of apathy (0.34 points; 95% CI 0.02–0.66, $p = 0.038$. Effect size = 0.424), as well as a greater motor and cognitive impairment. A recent study of over a thousand premanifest HD patients identified apathy as a robust marker of disease onset (likelihood ratio test 80.71, $p<0.001$).[65] Atrophy of the putamen, caudate, and accumbens were the most reliable markers of phenoconversion. Impaired recognition of negative emotions and other facets of unawareness have also been associated with apathy in HD.[64,66–68] The former has been associated with limbic atrophy and compensatory hyperactivity.[69]

Mechanism of apathy in Huntington's disease

Although several studies showed significant correlations between apathy and atrophy in various brain structures, there is limited evidence for a neural correlate of apathy in HD. In a group comparison, apathy was associated with reduced structural connectivity in the orbitofrontal cortex,[70] a region implicated with the affective-emotional component of apathy.[71–74] As with PD, the association between apathy and striatal hypodopaminergic state has been replicated in HD with DOPA-PET and 11C-raclopride PET imaging.[75,76]

Treatment of apathy in Huntington's disease

There are current guidelines for the treatment of apathy in HD.[77] Pagonabarraga and colleagues have conceptualized the treatment of apathy into four domains: emotional-affective, reward deficiency, executive function, and auto-activation, which they have proposed correspond to pathogenic dysfunction in the orbitomedial prefrontal cortex, accumbens, dorsolateral-caudate, and basal ganglia, respectively.[71] Despite these potential targets, there are no RCTs to support the benefits of psychotropic agents for the treatment of apathy in HD. Potential useful agents include cholinesterase inhibitors, stimulants, dopaminergic agonists, and antidepressants. Rasagiline has been reported to improve apathy in two HD cases with parkinsonism.[78] The beneficial effects of bupropion have been reported in other neurological conditions.

Apathy after Stroke

Phenomenology and assessment of apathy after stroke

While there is no diagnosis-specific assessment tool for post-stroke apathy, the majority of published studies utilized either the Apathy Scale,[7] the AES,[1] or the NPI.[40] Because of its timeframe, the NPI is only suitable for use in the post-acute stage (>15 days), whereas the Apathy Scale and AES can be applied at any stage. All three scales have been used in hospital, rehabilitation, and community settings.

Frequency of apathy after stroke

Apathy after stroke is common and can occur in the acute, subacute, and chronic stages of recovery. In a meta-analysis of 19 studies including 2221 patients, Caeiro and colleagues[79] calculated a pooled-post stroke apathy rate of 36.3% (95% CI 30.3–42.8), indicating that post-stroke apathy may be even more common than post-stroke depression, the frequency of which was recently estimated by Hackett and colleagues[80] to be around 31% (95% CI 28–35).

Clinical correlates of apathy after stroke

Post-stroke apathy is more common in older patients[79] and more likely to be associated with poor rehabilitation outcomes,[81] decreased patient quality of life, and increased caregiver burden and distress.[82] There is an overall association with both depression (OR 2.29; 95% CI 1.41–4.23) and cognitive impairment (OR 2.90; 95% CI 1.09–7.72),[79] but the strength of the relationship with depression depends upon the time frame in which they are assessed. In a case-control study of 94 consecutive acute stroke patients compared to 50 acute coronary syndrome patients, Caeiro and colleagues[83] demonstrated that post-stroke apathy and depression could be disassociated, and only co-occurred in a minority of acute stroke patients. Brodaty and colleagues[84] arrived at a similar conclusion in their clinical assessment of 135 ischaemic stroke patients at 3–6 months, but in a subsequent study of 106 stroke patients they found that apathy and depression were significantly correlated at 12 months (OR 7.75; 95% CI 2.6–23.13) and that dementia at index assessment was a common risk factor for both (OR 12.45; 95% CI 2.98–23.13 and OR 10.35; 95% CI 2.84–27.32).[85] In addition to being more common, cognitive impairment is also more severe in apathetic patients.[86]

Mechanism of apathy after stroke

A number of studies have investigated the role of stroke location and aetiology in relation to apathy, but no robust findings have been generated by systematic reviews.[79,87]

The strongest evidence for a specific neuroanatomical contribution to post-stroke apathy comes from a neuroimaging study conducted by Kang and Kim[88] in which 43 apathetic patients in a consecutive series of 100 patients with anterior cerebral artery infarcts had significantly more frequent damage to the superior frontal gyrus ($p < 0.001$), frontal pole ($p = 0.002$), or cingulate gyrus ($p = 0.003$) than stroke patients without apathy. Brodaty and colleagues associated post-stroke apathy with right frontal lesions,[84] but Hama and colleagues found that the severity of apathy symptoms could be related to damage to the bilateral basal ganglia, but not the frontal lobes.[89] Bhatia and Marsden reported an association between apathy with unilateral lesions of the caudate,[90] while Tang and colleagues described an association between apathy and pontine infarcts.[91]

White matter lesions may also play a role in the mediation of post-stroke apathy. Starkstein and Manes reported a significant association between apathy and lesions in the internal capsule and the pallidal and nigral output to the thalamus.[92] Yao and colleagues reported a higher frequency of hypertension and deep white matter lesions with apathetic behaviour in clinically healthy older subjects.[93]

The heterogeneity of these findings have led several research groups to explore anatomically diverse disruptions to functional brain networks as the underlying mechanism for the development of post-stroke apathy,[94–96] linking them to neuropsychological models such as pathogenic reward insensitivity.[97]

Treatment of apathy after stroke

While there have been no randomized controlled trials of treatments in which apathy has been the primary outcome, several studies have reported improvements in apathy in the course of related investigations. For instance, Robinson and colleagues[98] conducted a 12-week randomized double-blind placebo-controlled trial of nefiracetam for post-stroke depression in which no significant treatment effect was found for the primary outcome after 12 weeks, but in which a secondary analysis[99] revealed a significant improvement in apathy associated with post-stroke depression at 900 mg/day compared to nefiracetam 600 mg/day or placebo. These findings were not replicated in a recent small RCT.[100] In another small open-label pilot study exploring the effect of acetylcholinesterase inhibitors on functional stroke recovery, Whyte and colleagues[101] demonstrated a significant improvement in FIM motor score and an associated improvement in apathy in patients receiving donepezil (maximum dose 10 mg/day) compared to patients receiving galantamine (maximum dose 24 mg/day) or historical controls.

A secondary analysis of a RCT using escitalopram or problem-solving therapy to prevent post-stroke depression demonstrated that escitalopram was significantly more effective than placebo to prevent post-stroke apathy.[102]

In conclusion, the management and prevention of post-stroke apathy has only been examined in small, preliminary studies, and larger RCTs with a longer follow-up are indicated.

Conclusions

Apathy is a common finding in both neurodegenerative conditions and stroke. Apathy is present in about one-third of patients with PD. Whereas the frequency of apathy is higher among patients with more severe parkinsonism; about 20% of drug-naive individuals were reported to have apathy. Most PD patients with apathy had comorbid depression or incipient dementia. Apathy has been described in patients undergoing DBS-STN, but both the frequency and mechanism are yet to be clarified. Apathy is also frequent in AD, with a strong association between frequency and severity of dementia. Whereas some AD patients with apathy have concomitant depression, others have poor awareness of their behavioural problems. The treatment of apathy in PD and AD is still unclear, and results from randomized controlled trials are still awaited. Apathy is also frequent in HD, but the mechanism and management of this comorbid condition requires further study. Finally, apathy is a frequent finding after stroke, and has a negative impact upon recovery. A recent study suggests that the antidepressant escitalopram may be effective in preventing post-stroke apathy, and this interesting finding is in need of replication.

REFERENCES

1. Marin RS. Apathy: a neuropsychiatric syndrome. Journal of Neuropsychiatry & Clinical Neurosciences. 1991; 3: 243–54.
2. van Reekum R, Stuss DT, Ostrander L. Apathy: why care? Journal of Neuropsychiatry & Clinical Neurosciences. 2005; 17: 7–19.
3. Marin RS. Differential diagnosis and classification of apathy. American Journal of Psychiatry. 1990; 147: 22–30.
4. Sims A. Symptoms in the Mind. China: Saunders, 2003.
5. Levy R, Dubois B. Apathy and the functional anatomy of the prefrontal cortex-basal ganglia circuits. Cerebral Cortex. 2006; 16: 916–28.
6. Leentjens AF, Dujardin K, Marsh L, et al. Apathy and anhedonia rating scales in Parkinson's disease: critique and recommendations. Movement Disorders. 2008; 23: 2004–14.
7. Starkstein SE, Mayberg HS, Preziosi TJ, Andrezejewski P, Leiguarda R, Robinson RG. Reliability, validity, and clinical correlates of apathy in Parkinson's disease. Journal of Neuropsychiatry & Clinical Neurosciences. 1992; 4: 134–9.
8. Dujardin K, Sockeel P, Delliaux M, Destee A, Defebvre L. The Lille Apathy Rating Scale: validation of a caregiver-based version. Movement Disorders. 2008; 23: 845–9.
9. Strauss ME, Sperry SD. An informant-based assessment of apathy in Alzheimer disease. Neuropsychiatry, Neuropsychology, & Behavioral Neurology. 2002; 15: 176–83.
10. Starkstein S, Leentjens AF. The nosological position of apathy in clinical practice. Journal of Neurology, Neurosurgery & Psychiatry. 2008; 79: 1088–92.
11. Benoit M, Berrut G, Doussaint J, et al. Apathy and depression in mild Alzheimer's disease: a cross-sectional study using diagnostic criteria. Journal of Alzheimer's Disease. 2012; 31: 325–34.
12. Drijgers RL, Dujardin K, Reijnders JS, Defebvre L, Leentjens AF. Validation of diagnostic criteria for apathy in Parkinson's disease. Parkinsonism Relat Disord. 2010; 16: 656–60.
13. Fahn S, Elton E. Unified Parkinson's disease rating scale. In: Fahn S, Marsden CD, Goldstein M, Calne CD (eds). Recent Developments in Parkinson's Disease. Florham Park, NJ: Macmillan, 1987. pp153–63.
14. Starkstein SE, Merello M. The unified Parkinson's disease rating scale: Validation study of the mentation, behavior, and mood section. Movement Disorders. 2007; 22: 2156–61.
15. Pedersen KF, Alves G, Aarsland D, Larsen JP. Occurrence and risk factors for apathy in Parkinson disease: a 4-year prospective longitudinal study. Journal of Neurology Neurosurgery and Psychiatry. 2009; 80: 1279–82.
16. Starkstein SE, Leentjens AF. The nosological position of apathy in clinical practice. Journal of Neurology, Neurosurgery & Psychiatry. 2008; 79: 1088–92.
17. Pedersen KF, Larsen JP, Alves G, Aarsland D. Prevalence and clinical correlates of apathy in Parkinson's disease: a community-based study. Parkinsonism & Related Disorders. 2009; 15: 295–99.
18. Aarsland D, Bronnick K, Alves G, et al. The spectrum of neuropsychiatric symptoms in patients with early untreated Parkinson's disease. Journal of Neurology Neurosurgery and Psychiatry. 2009; 80: 928–30.
19. Marsh L, McDonald WM, Cummings J, Ravina B. Provisional diagnostic criteria for depression in Parkinson's disease: report of an NINDS/NIMH Work Group. Mov Disord. 2006; 21: 148–58.
20. Starkstein S, Dragovic M, Jorge R, et al. Diagnostic criteria for depression in Parkinson's disease: a study of symptom patterns using latent class analysis. Mov Disord. 2011; 26: 2239–45.
21. Kirsch-Darrow L, Fernandez HF, Marsiske M, Okun MS, Bowers D. Dissociating apathy and depression in Parkinson disease. Neurology. 2006; 67: 33–8.
22. Dujardin K, Sockeel P, Devos D, Defebvre L, Destee A. Apathy: Its characteristics in Parkinson's disease. Neurology. 2006; 66: A210.
23. Starkstein SE, Merello M, Jorge R, Brockman S, Bruce D, Power B. The Syndromal Validity and Nosological Position of Apathy in Parkinson's Disease. Movement Disorders. 2009; 24: 1211–16.
24. Dujardin K, Sockeel P, Delliaux M, Destee A, Defebvre L. Apathy May Herald Cognitive Decline and Dementia in Parkinson's Disease. Movement Disorders. 2009; 24: 2391–7.
25. Dujardin K, Delliaux M, Dernoncourt C, Sockeel P, Defebvre L. Apathy: A predictive factor of dementia in Parkinson's disease. Movement Disorders. 2009; 24: S296.
26. Ready RE, Friedman J, Grace J, Fernandez H. Testosterone deficiency and apathy in Parkinson's disease: a pilot study.[see comment]. Journal of Neurology, Neurosurgery & Psychiatry. 2004; 75: 1323–6.
27. Kenangil G, Orken DN, Ur E, Forta H, Celik M. The relation of testosterone levels with fatigue and apathy in Parkinson's disease. Clin Neurol Neurosur. 2009; 111: 412–14.
28. Levy R, Czernecki V. Apathy and the basal ganglia. Journal of Neurology. 2006; 253: 54–61.
29. Le Jeune F, Drapier D, Bourguignon A, et al. Subthalamic nucleus stimulation in Parkinson disease induces apathy A PET study. Neurology. 2009; 73: 1746–51.
30. Thobois S, Ardouin C, Lhommee E, et al. Non-motor dopamine withdrawal syndrome after surgery for Parkinson's disease: predictors and underlying mesolimbic denervation. Brain. 2010; 133: 1111–27.
31. Bronstein JM, Tagliati M, Alterman RL, et al. Deep brain stimulation for Parkinson disease: an expert consensus and review of key issues. Arch Neurol. 2011; 68: 165.
32. Voon V, Kubu C, Krack P, Houeto JL, Troster AI. Deep brain stimulation: Neuropsychological and neuropsychiatric issues. Movement Disorders. 2006; 21: S305–27.
33. Drapier D, Drapier S, Sauleau P, et al. Does subthalamic nucleus stimulation induce apathy in Parkinson's disease? Journal of Neurology. 2006; 253: 1083–91.
34. Czernecki V, Pillon B, Houeto JL, et al. Does bilateral stimulation of the subthalamic nucleus aggravate apathy in Parkinson's disease? Journal of Neurology Neurosurgery and Psychiatry. 2005; 76: 775–9.
35. Czernecki V, Schupbach M, Yaici S, et al. Apathy following subthalamic stimulation in Parkinson disease: A dopamine responsive symptom. Movement Disorders. 2008; 23: 964–9.
36. Chatterjee A, Fahn S. Methylphenidate treats apathy in Parkinson's disease. Journal of Neuropsychiatry & Clinical Neurosciences. 2002; 14: 461–2.
37. Czernecki V, Pillon B, Houeto JL, Pochon JB, Levy R, Dubois B. Motivation, reward, and Parkinson's disease: influence of dopatherapy. Neuropsychologia. 2002; 40: 2257–67.

38. Weintraub D, Mavandadi S, Mamikonyan E, et al. Atomoxetine for depression and other neuropsychiatric symptoms in Parkinson disease. Neurology. 2010; 75: 448–55.
39. Thobois S, Lhommee E, Klinger H, et al. Parkinsonian apathy responds to dopaminergic stimulation of D2/D3 receptors with piribedil. Brain. 2013; 136: 1568–77.
40. Cummings JL. The Neuropsychiatric Inventory: assessing psychopathology in dementia patients. Neurology. 1997; 48(suppl 6): S10–16.
41. Starkstein SE, Ingram L, Garau ML, Mizrahi R. On the overlap between apathy and depression in dementia. Journal of Neurology, Neurosurgery & Psychiatry. 2005; 76: 1070–74.
42. Starkstein SE, Petracca G, Chemerinski E, Kremer J. Syndromic validity of apathy in Alzheimer's disease. American Journal of Psychiatry. 2001; 158: 872–7.
43. Starkstein SE, Jorge R, Mizrahi R, Robinson RG. A prospective longitudinal study of apathy in Alzheimer's disease. Journal of Neurology, Neurosurgery, and Psychiatry. 2006; 77: 8–11.
44. Boyle PA, Malloy PF, Salloway S, Cahn-Weiner DA, Cohen R, Cummings JL. Executive dysfunction and apathy predict functional impairment in Alzheimer disease. American Journal of Geriatric Psychiatry. 2003; 11: 214–21.
45. Robert PH, Berr C, Volteau M, et al. Apathy in patients with mild cognitive impairment and the risk of developing dementia of Alzheimer's disease: a one-year follow-up study. Clin Neurol Neurosurg. 2006; 108: 733–6.
46. Robert PH, Darcourt G, Koulibaly MP, et al. Lack of initiative and interest in Alzheimer's disease: a single photon emission computed tomography study. European Journal of Neurology. 2006; 13: 729–35.
47. Cummings JL, Koumaras B, Chen M, Mirski D. Effects of rivastigmine treatment on the neuropsychiatric and behavioral disturbances of nursing home residents with moderate to severe probable Alzheimer's disease: A 26-week, multicenter, open-label study. American Journal of Geriatric Pharmacotherapy. 2005; 3: 137–48.
48. Cummings JL, Nadel A, Masterman D, Cyrus PA. Efficacy of metrifonate in improving the psychiatric and behavioral disturbances of patients with Alzheimer's disease. Journal of Geriatric Psychiatry & Neurology. 2001; 14: 101–8.
49. Herrmann N, Rabheru K, Wang J, Binder C. Galantamine treatment of problematic behavior in Alzheimer disease: post-hoc analysis of pooled data from three large trials. American Journal of Geriatric Psychiatry. 2005; 13: 527–34.
50. Galynker I, Prikhojan A, Phillips E, Focseneanu M, Ieronimo C, Rosenthal R. Negative symptoms in stroke patients and length of hospital stay. Journal of Nervous & Mental Disease. 1997; 185: 616–21.
51. Erkulwater S, Pillai R. Amantadine and the end-stage dementia of Alzheimer's type. Southern Medical Journal. 1989; 82: 550–4.
52. Holmes C, Knights A, Dean C, Hodkinson S, Hopkins V. Keep music live: music and the alleviation of apathy in dementia subjects. International Psychogeriatrics. 2006; 18: 623–30.
53. Politis AM, Vozzella S, Mayer LS, Onyike CU, Baker AS, Lyketsos CG. A randomized, controlled, clinical trial of activity therapy for apathy in patients with dementia residing in long-term care. International Journal of Geriatric Psychiatry. 2004; 19: 1087–94.
54. Verkaik R, Nuyen J, Schellevis F, Francke A. The relationship between severity of Alzheimer's disease and prevalence of comorbid depressive symptoms and depression: a systematic review. International Journal of Geriatric Psychiatry. 2007; 22: 1063–86.
55. Mestre TA, van Duijn E, Davis AM, et al. Rating scales for behavioral symptoms in Huntington's disease: Critique and recommendations. Mov Disord. 2016; 31: 1466–78.
56. Kingma EM, van Duijn E, Timman R, van der Mast RC, Roos RA. Behavioural problems in Huntington's disease using the Problem Behaviours Assessment. Gen Hosp Psychiatry. 2008; 30: 155–61.
57. Naarding P, Janzing JG, Eling P, van der Werf S, Kremer B. Apathy is not depression in Huntington's disease. J Neuropsychiatry and Clin Neurosci. 2009; 21: 266–70.
58. van Duijn E, Kingma EM, van der Mast RC. Psychopathology in verified Huntington's disease gene carriers. J Neuropsychiatry Clin Neurosci. 2007; 19: 441–48.
59. van Duijn E, Craufurd D, Hubers AA, et al. Neuropsychiatric symptoms in a European Huntington's disease cohort (REGISTRY). J Neurol Neurosurg Psychiatry. 2014; 85: 1411–8.
60. Martinez-Horta S, Perez-Perez J, van Duijn E, et al. Neuropsychiatric symptoms are very common in premanifest and early stage Huntington's Disease. Parkinsonism & Related Disorders. 2016; 25: 58–64.
61. Quaid KA, Eberly SW, Kayson-Rubin E, Oakes D, Shoulson I. Factors related to genetic testing in adults at risk for Huntington disease: the prospective Huntington at-risk observational study (PHAROS). Clinical Genetics. 2016; 91(6): 824–31.
62. Reedeker N, Bouwens JA, van Duijn E, Giltay EJ, Roos RA, van der Mast RC. Incidence, course, and predictors of apathy in Huntington's disease: a two-year prospective study. J Neuropsychiatry Clin Neurosci. 2011; 23: 434–41.
63. Thompson JC, Snowden JS, Craufurd D, Neary D. Behavior in Huntington's disease: dissociating cognition-based and mood-based changes. J Neuropsychiatry Clin Neurosci. 2002; 14: 37–43.
64. Tabrizi SJ, Scahill RI, Owen G, et al. Predictors of phenotypic progression and disease onset in premanifest and early-stage Huntington's disease in the TRACK-HD study: analysis of 36-month observational data. Lancet Neurology. 2013; 12: 637–49.
65. Paulsen JS, Long JD, Johnson HJ, et al. Clinical and biomarker changes in premanifest Huntington disease show trial feasibility: a decade of the PREDICT-HD Study. Frontiers in Aging Neuroscience. 2014; 6: 78.
66. Duff K, Paulsen JS, Beglinger LJ, et al. 'Frontal' behaviors before the diagnosis of Huntington's disease and their relationship to markers of disease progression: evidence of early lack of awareness. J Neuropsychiatry Clin Neurosci. 2010; 22: 196–207.
67. McCusker E, Loy CT. The many facets of unawareness in Huntington disease. Tremor and other Hyperkinetic Movements (New York, NY). 2014; 4: 257.
68. Johnson SA, Stout JC, Solomon AC, et al. Beyond disgust: impaired recognition of negative emotions prior to diagnosis in Huntington's disease. Brain. 2007; 130: 1732–44.
69. Dogan I, Sass C, Mirzazade S, et al. Neural correlates of impaired emotion processing in manifest Huntington's disease. Social Cognitive and Affective Neuroscience. 2014; 9: 671–80.
70. Delmaire C, Dumas EM, Sharman MA, et al. The structural correlates of functional deficits in early Huntington's disease. Hum Brain Mapp. 2013; 34: 2141–53.
71. Pagonabarraga J, Kulisevsky J, Strafella AP, Krack P. Apathy in Parkinson's disease: clinical features, neural substrates, diagnosis, and treatment. Lancet Neurology. 2015; 14: 518–31.

72. Levy R, Dubois B. Apathy and the functional anatomy of the prefrontal cortex-basal ganglia circuits. Cerebral Cortex. 2006; 16(7): 916–28.
73. Elliott R. Executive functions and their disorders. British Medical Bulletin. 2003; 65: 49–59.
74. Tremblay L, Schultz W. Relative reward preference in primate orbitofrontal cortex. Nature. 1999; 398: 704–8.
75. van Oostrom JC, Dekker M, Willemsen AT, de Jong BM, Roos RA, Leenders KL. Changes in striatal dopamine D2 receptor binding in pre-clinical Huntington's disease. Eur J Neurol. 2009; 16: 226–31.
76. Ginovart N, Lundin A, Farde L, et al. PET study of the pre- and post-synaptic dopaminergic markers for the neurodegenerative process in Huntington's disease. Brain. 1997; 120 (Pt 3): 503–14.
77. Krishnamoorthy A, Craufurd D. Treatment of apathy in Huntington's disease and other movement disorders. Current Treatment Options in Neurology. 2011; 13: 508–19.
78. Perez-Perez J, Martinez-Horta S, Pagonabarraga J, Carceller M, Kulisevsky J. Rasagiline for the treatment of parkinsonism in Huntington's disease. Parkinsonism & Related Disorders. 2015; 21: 340–2.
79. Caeiro L, Ferro JM, Costa J. Apathy secondary to stroke: a systematic review and meta-analysis. Cerebrovasc Dis. 2013; 35: 23–39.
80. Hackett ML, Pickles K. Part I: frequency of depression after stroke: an updated systematic review and meta-analysis of observational studies. International Journal of Stroke: official journal of the International Stroke Society. 2014; 9: 1017–25.
81. Hama S, Yamashita H, Shigenobu M, et al. Depression or apathy and functional recovery after stroke. International Journal of Geriatric Psychiatry. 2007; 22: 1046–51.
82. Tang WK, Lau CG, Mok V, Ungvari GS, Wong KS. Apathy and health-related quality of life in stroke. Arch Phys Med Rehabil. 2014; 95: 857–61.
83. Caeiro L, Ferro JM, Figueira ML. Apathy in acute stroke patients. Eur J Neurol. 2012; 19: 291–7.
84. Brodaty H, Sachdev PS, Withall A, Altendorf A, Valenzuela MJ, Lorentz L. Frequency and clinical, neuropsychological and neuroimaging correlates of apathy following stroke—the Sydney Stroke Study. Psychological Medicine. 2005; 35: 1707–16.
85. Withall A, Brodaty H, Altendorf A, Sachdev PS. A longitudinal study examining the independence of apathy and depression after stroke: the Sydney Stroke Study. Int Psychogeriatr. 2011; 23: 264–73.
86. van Almenkerk S, Smalbrugge M, Depla MF, Eefsting JA, Hertogh CM. Apathy among institutionalized stroke patients: prevalence and clinical correlates. American Journal of Geriatric Psychiatry: official journal of the American Association for Geriatric Psychiatry. 2015; 23: 180–8.
87. van Dalen JW, Moll van Charante EP, Nederkoorn PJ, van Gool WA, Richard E. Poststroke apathy. Stroke. 2013; 44: 851–60.
88. Kang SY, Kim JS. Anterior cerebral artery infarction: stroke mechanism and clinical-imaging study in 100 patients. Neurology. 2008; 70: 2386–93.
89. Hama S, Yamashita H, Shigenobu M, et al. Post-stroke affective or apathetic depression and lesion location: left frontal lobe and bilateral basal ganglia. Eur Arch Psychiatry Clin Neurosci. 2007; 257: 149–52.
90. Bhatia KP, Marsden CD. The behavioural and motor consequences of focal lesions of the basal ganglia in man. Brain. 1994; 117: 859–76.
91. Tang WK, Chen YK, Liang HJ, et al. Location of infarcts and apathy in ischemic stroke. Cerebrovasc Dis. 2013; 35: 566–71.
92. Starkstein SE, Manes F. Apathy and depression following stroke. CNS Spectr. 2000; 5: 43–50.
93. Yao H, Takashima Y, Mori T, et al. Hypertension and white matter lesions are independently associated with apathetic behavior in healthy elderly subjects: the Sefuri brain MRI study. Hypertens Res. 2009; 32: 586–90.
94. Yang S, Hua P, Shang X, et al. Deficiency of brain structural sub-network underlying post-ischaemic stroke apathy. Eur J Neurol. 2015; 22: 341–7.
95. Murakami T, Hama S, Yamashita H, et al. Neuroanatomic pathways associated with poststroke affective and apathetic depression. American Journal of Geriatric Psychiatry: official journal of the American Association for Geriatric Psychiatry. 2013; 21: 840–47.
96. Siegel JS, Snyder AZ, Metcalf NV, et al. The circuitry of abulia: insights from functional connectivity MRI. Neuroimage Clin. 2014; 6: 320–26.
97. Rochat L, Van der Linden M, Renaud O, et al. Poor reward sensitivity and apathy after stroke: implication of basal ganglia. Neurology. 2013; 81: 1674–80.
98. Robinson RG, Jorge RE, Clarence-Smith K. Double-blind randomized treatment of poststroke depression using nefiracetam. Journal of Neuropsychiatry & Clinical Neurosciences. 2008; 20: 178–84.
99. Robinson RG, Jorge R, Clarence-Smith K, Starkstein SE. Double-bind treatment of apathy in patients with poststroke depression using nefiracetam. Journal of Neurology, Neurosurgery & Psychiatry. 2009; 21(2): 144–51.
100. Starkstein SE, Brockman S, Hatch KK, et al. A randomized, placebo-controlled, double-blind efficacy study of nefiracetam to treat poststroke apathy. Journal of Stroke and Cerebrovascular Diseases: the official journal of National Stroke Association. 2016; 25: 1119–27.
101. Whyte EM, Lenze EJ, Butters M, et al. An open-label pilot study of acetylcholinesterase inhibitors to promote functional recovery in elderly cognitively impaired stroke patients. Cerebrovascular Diseases. 2008; 26: 317–21.
102. Mikami K, Jorge RE, Moser DJ, et al. Prevention of poststroke apathy using escitalopram or problem-solving therapy. Am J Geriatr Psychiatry. 2013; 21: 855–62.

25

Behavioural and psychological symptoms of dementia

Rianne van der Linde and Tom Dening

Introduction

BPSD are present in 80% of people with dementia,[1,2,3,4] and are also seen in the older population without dementia.[5] They include apathy, depressive symptoms, anxiety, irritability, agitation, psychotic symptoms, sleep problems, wandering, and elation. BPSD impact upon quality of life of older people and their carers, and influence prescribing and use of services.[6,7] BPSD are sometimes also referred to as neuropsychiatric symptoms of dementia.[8] This seems to be interchangeable so this chapter will refer mainly to BPSD. This chapter discusses the history and conceptual basis of BPSD; their clinical features and associated factors; and their course and outcome.

History

Non-cognitive symptoms were an important feature of the first description of AD,[9,10] including unpredictable behaviour, paranoia, and auditory hallucinations. The patient described, Mrs Deter, became jealous towards her husband, sometimes felt that someone wanted to kill her, and sometimes shouted wildly.

However, until the 1970s, AD was seen as extremely rare and confined to young patients. The term 'senile dementia' was used to describe cognitive decline in older people, and was thought to be caused by atherosclerosis. During this period there was little focus on non-cognitive features as they did not fit the theory that dementia is exaggerated ageing.

After it was concluded that the clinical and pathological manifestations of presenile and senile dementia are almost identical,[11] new definitions of dementia in the DSMMD and new criteria for diagnosis were followed by an interest in non-cognitive manifestations.[12,13] Comprehensive dementia rating scales, for example the Blessed Dementia Scale and the Sandoz Clinical Assessment Geriatric Scale[14,15] include BPSD items. Instruments specifically to measure behavioural problems were developed in the 1980s, most notably the BEHAVE-AD by Reisberg et al. in 1987.[16] In 1994, the Neuropsychiatric Inventory (NPI) was published by Cummings et al.[17] Using these new instruments, BPSD were measured in large epidemiological studies such as the Cache County Study.[18]

The term 'Behavioural and Psychological Symptoms of Dementia' was introduced by the International Psychogeriatric Association (IPA) in 1996 at the Consensus Conference of the IPA Task Force on Behavioral Disturbances of Dementia.[19] BPSD were defined as: 'Symptoms of disturbed perception, thought content, mood or behaviour that frequently occur in patients with dementia'. This includes a range of symptoms: apathy, depression, anxiety, irritability, aggression, non-aggressive agitation, hallucination, persecution, misidentification, sleep problems, wandering, elation, disinhibition, and appetite and eating disorders, as shown in Table 25.1.

International diagnostic criteria such as ICD10, DSMIV, and DSM5 recognize the occurrence of symptoms like delusions or depression. BPSD occur across the various subtypes of dementia. For example, they are important in the diagnosis of dementia with Lewy bodies, with visual hallucinations being a core feature and REM sleep behaviour disorder being a suggestive feature.[20] By definition, BPSD are to the forefront in the behavioural variant of FTD.[21]

In recent years, there has been increasing interest in how such factors as the environment and pain, for example, can trigger the expression of BPSD.[22] There has been a move away from a primarily pharmacological approach to management because of concerns about the safety of antipsychotic drugs, which were often used for the treatment of BPSD.[23] Non-pharmacological treatments are regarded as the usual first-line approach, with evidence of efficacy for at least some techniques.[24]

Clinical Features of BPSD

BPSD are a very mixed group of phenomena, with some (e.g. depression and anxiety) largely defined by subjective mental state, and others (e.g. irritability, disinhibition, aggression) being defined by third party observations. Sleep and appetite disorders relate to physiological functioning. The criteria that are applied in clinical practice are quite variable and some terms, for example agitation, are notoriously unreliable as different observers may mean very different things.

Table 25.1 Definitions of BPS

Symptom	Definition
Apathy	Loss of interest, lack of motivation, little energy
Depressive symptoms	Feeling sad or depressed, can include tearfulness, being in low spirits, negative view of future, death wish
Anxiety	Very nervous, worried or frightened, bodily features of anxiety
Irritability	Gets irritated or easily disturbed, can include sudden flashes of anger, changeable mood or being impatient
Aggression	Uncooperative or hard to handle, can include shouting, kicking, hitting, throwing, or other aggressive behaviours
Non-aggressive agitation	Being restless, for example fidgeting, pacing, difficulty sitting still, doing things over and over again, picking at things or other repetitive activities
Hallucinations	Seeing, hearing, smelling, feeling, or tasting things that others do not
Persecution/delusions	Beliefs that are not true, can include the belief that family members are not who they say they are, that their house is not their home, that people are laughing at them, or that others are planning to harm them
Misidentification	Imagination plays tricks, can include the belief that special messages are being sent, that their mind or body is being controlled or difficulty telling difference between people
Sleep problems	Difficulty sleeping, being up at night, can include difficulty falling asleep or staying asleep, problems with falling asleep during the day, wandering at night or waking too early
Wandering	Getting lost or wandering
Elation	Too cheerful or too happy, abnormally good mood, can include bouts of laughter, infectious gaiety, laughing at things others do not find funny
Disinhibition	Acting impulsively, doing embarrassing things, can include talking to strangers as if they know them, saying insensitive things, making sexual remarks, talking openly about very private matters, touching or hugging
Appetite and eating disorders	Change in appetite, weight or eating habits or change in the type of food that is preferred

Source: data from Savva G.M. et al. Prevalence, correlates and course of behavioural and psychological symptoms of dementia in the population. *Br J Psychiatry.* 2009;194(3):212–9; data from Cummings J.L. The Neuropsychiatric Inventory: comprehensive assessment of psychopathology in dementia. *Neurology.* 1994;44(12):2308–14.

Apathy

Apathy has various definitions, varying as to their emphasis on (lack of) feelings, thoughts, or behaviours. It is clearly not a unitary phenomenon. Levy and Dubois suggested three components of apathy: 'emotional-affective', 'cognitive', and 'auto-activation', each with a distinct underlying neural substrate.[25] These correspond to lack of feeling, lack of interest, and lack of (initiating) behaviour. An apathy measurement scale, the Dimensional Apathy Scale, is available although it does not seem to have been applied to dementia yet.[26]

Apathy may be present to some degree early in the course of dementia, when it can be difficult to detect, for example if it is regarded as merely the effects of getting older and losing previous interests. It can be mistaken for other things, for example in the case of social withdrawal, because hearing loss or aphasia makes social conversation difficult. As dementia progresses, apathy often becomes more prominent. It is the source of much frustration to carers since, on the face of it, the person with dementia may appear perfectly capable of undertaking a task like making a cup of tea yet they seem to choose not to do it unless encouraged. This may be interpreted as wilfulness or stubbornness, whereas in fact the person is genuinely unable to initiate the task.

Apathy is frequently confused with depression, though it is not really a mood disorder. This is because of some overlap in the clinical picture, for example slowness or self-neglect, and also because the two problems may co-occur.

Depression and anxiety

Depression is a common feature of dementia, which may reflect the individual's assessment of their own situation and/or the direct effects of the pathological process on brain circuits. In early dementia, the approach to diagnosis and treatment is much the same as in people who do not have dementia. People with mild dementia will be able to report on their mood or to complete rating scales. In severe dementia, the capacity of the person to describe and report on their mood may be lost, and the probability of depression depends on observation and behaviour change, for example being tearful or having the characteristic facial expression of depression with furrowed brow and downcast gaze. Negative thoughts about the future are common and, especially among very old people with dementia, there are often limited expectations of the future. People in their tenth decade often have an ambiguous attitude towards continuing to live ('I have lived long enough'); however, overt suicidal intent and acts of self-harm are not more likely to occur in people with dementia.

There may also be a labile affect with the person being readily moved to sudden crying (or, less often, laughing), but, in the absence of prolonged low mood, this is distinct from depression. Emotionalism of this kind, sometimes referred to as pseudobulbar affect, is common across a range of neurodegenerative conditions.[27]

Depression has a complex relationship with dementia as it may be the first manifestation of it, especially if it occurs for the first time in late life.[28] Whether depression in earlier life is a true independent risk factor for dementia seems less likely.[29] It has been found that midlife stress is associated with higher rates of dementia later on, which may be mediated through social and lifestyle factors.[30]

Anxiety has also been associated with an increased incidence of dementia[31] and this is likely to be a prodromal symptom. Anxiety is commonly observed but not much studied, probably as it is often comorbid with other disorders, especially depression. In moderate to severe dementia, it may be difficult to distinguish clinically between anxiety and agitation. However, evidence suggests that they are distinct constructs. For example, a factor analysis study[32] found that anxiety loaded with depression, and agitation with other psychomotor features.

Irritability, aggression, agitation, and wandering

These form a miscellaneous group of altered behaviours. Irritability can be a prominent feature of depression, so it is worth considering the latter if someone seems especially irritable. Aggression is generally subdivided into verbal and physical manifestations but what constitutes aggressive behaviour is open to differing interpretations.

Hence, estimated prevalence figures vary markedly. Verbal aggression includes shouting or swearing; physical aggression includes punching, kicking, biting, throwing things, or hitting with objects such as walking sticks. Whether the aggression has to be sustained or repeated and to what extent is highly variable. Apparently aggressive behaviour is often observed in the context of intimate personal care, where the person with dementia misinterprets the intentions of the caregiver as being threatening and thus lashes out in self-defence.

Agitation, like apathy, is a complicated phenomenon with both motor and emotional aspects. A useful definition is: excessive physical activity with the feeling of inner tension.[33] Examples of motor disturbance include hand movements (fidgeting, wringing, rubbing, picking), vocalization (e.g. calling out), and evidence of restlessness such as pacing up and down. Emotional features include overwhelming subjective feelings of anxiety and distress. It is important to consider that there may be a specific and remediable problem causing the agitation, such as pain, hunger, or side effects of medication. The International Psychogeriatric Association has proposed some consensus criteria,[34] though these seem to conflate agitation and aggression to some extent, which may not be very helpful.

Wandering is a frankly unsatisfactory term that covers various types of behaviour. Alternative terms like purposeful walking are sometimes used, as it often argued that 'wandering' implies aimlessness. Some people with dementia are very restless and unable to sit down, in which case this is a form of agitation. Sometimes a person with dementia is simply trying to get outside, for example they may be disorientated and think they need to be going home even if, in some instances, they are there already. Other people labelled as 'wanderers' turn out to be people who habitually took a lot of exercise and are frustrated by their lack of liberty to access fresh air.[35]

Hallucinations, delusions, and misidentification

Psychotic symptoms are not uncommon in dementia and seem to increase in frequency with the severity of the dementia. Hallucinations may occur in any sensory modality though visual hallucinations are most commonly reported. However, it is difficult to be precise as to the true frequency of hallucinations for two reasons. One is that it is sometimes difficult to separate what is a true hallucination from what is a misperceived sensory input, for example someone with visual loss and dementia may easily misperceive an object, such as a piece of furniture, for a person in the room. The other reason is that, in severe dementia, the occurrence of a hallucination can only be inferred from observation, for example the person talking to hallucinatory figures.

Some people with visual or hearing sensory impairment but minimal, if any cognitive impairment, present with vivid hallucinations in the affected modality. When associated with visual hallucinations, this condition is referred to as the Charles Bonnet syndrome[36] and is relevant mainly as it does not indicate that the person has dementia or other serious mental pathology.

The delusions seen in dementia tend to originate from gaps in the person's memory. For example, it is common to make accusations that an item has been stolen when it is not in its usual place. Following from this, the person with dementia may then secrete the item somewhere else, which compounds the problem, as they may forget where the hiding place is. In other situations, there may be delusional beliefs about intruders even in the absence of any signs of forced entry. Sometimes people with dementia may come to believe that people are conspiring against them. Of course, by this stage there may well be a co-ordinated care plan or even safeguarding measures if they are deemed to be vulnerable, so in one sense they may not be wrong in this belief.

Misidentification of other people is also quite common. This is variable, from simply forgetting someone's name or getting it wrong, to situations where the person with dementia is convinced that (say) their spouse is an imposter. In this latter case, the situation may become dangerous, since to have a delusion of this kind is obviously very frightening. Another common misidentification is getting the generations of the family muddled up, for example mistaking your daughter for your wife as your daughter is now at the age that you best remember your wife, or she looks rather like your wife does in the wedding photograph on the mantelpiece. People with dementia may also misidentify their own reflection (in a mirror, window, or TV screen) or they may confuse people on television with reality, and start trying to interact with them. It is also possible to misidentify a place, which may take the form of insisting that your house is not, in fact, your home.

Sleep problems

The commonest sleep-related problems seen in the context of dementia are insomnia, altered circadian rhythm, excessive daytime sleepiness, and REM sleep behaviour disorder (RBD). Also common in older people generally, are obstructive sleep apnoea and sleep-related movement disorders (restless legs). Insomnia, altered circadian rhythm, and daytime sleepiness may co-exist since, if a person with dementia has an inactive and understimulating day, they may readily doze off during the day, with consequent adverse effects on night-time sleeping. Alternatively, if they develop insomnia related to depression or pain, for example, they may be trying to catch up during the day. This may eventually result in them being more awake at night than during the day, a stressful situation for anyone living with them.

RBD is dramatic, although the diagnosis is quite often overlooked. Usually REM sleep is associated with muscle atonia but if this does not happen, a person's dreams are associated with physical enactments such as shouting, kicking, and lashing out. Both the person and anyone sleeping with them may be at risk of injury. RBD is much commoner in men and is associated with Parkinson's disease, multisystem atrophy, and DLB. RBD may precede the diagnosis of DLB by several years[37] so its occurrence should alert clinicians to this possibility.

Elation and disinhibition

Elation is relatively uncommon and so, too, is mania. People with severe agitation may have a degree of hyperactivity resembling mania, and also the distinction between mania and delirium can be hard to make. Among the various changes in personality that may be seen in dementia, a person may become less inhibited, for example becoming blunt and tactless in their social manner. There may also be profound changes in eating behaviour:[38] eating excessive amounts; cramming food into the mouth; eating non-food items such as plants; or eating only sweet foods. Sexual disinhibition may also occur, including flirtatiousness, preoccupations with pornography, and attempting sexual acts. Simply undressing in the middle of a room is not necessarily sexual in nature and may merely reflect disorientation.

BPSD in different types of dementia

As mentioned above, certain BPSD are suggestive of certain types of dementia, for example visual hallucinations and RBD suggest the diagnosis of DLB, but they are not specific to the condition. Behavioural variant FTD is characterized mainly by changes in behaviour and personality. Various combinations of disinhibition and apathy may be seen, along with diminished social skills, especially sympathy and/or empathy. Any of the features described above may be seen in AD. There is little to differentiate BPSD in AD versus vascular dementia, except the latter may produce more instability of mood and sometimes marked apathy if there is extensive subcortical vascular damage. However, it is also the case, especially in older people with dementia, that mixed forms of pathology are common,[39] and this also reduces the specificity of any BPSD profile.

BPS without dementia, and mild behavioural impairment

It is also important to consider that BPS are not restricted to people with dementia but may occur in significant numbers of the non-demented population. Numerous studies have reported prevalence figures for BPS in people with MCI: see Apostolova and Cummings, and Monastero et al. for reviews.[5,40] Prevalence rates varied between 35% to 85%, depending on factors such as the site of sampling (hospital vs community), criteria for MCI, and the behavioural measures used. A more recent review of community-based studies[41] found a lower range of prevalences (13–66%). Van der Linde et al. studied a community-based sample of 1781 people aged 65 and over.[42] MCI was subdivided according to whether there was memory impairment alone (amnestic; A-MCI), non-memory impairment (N-MCI), or a mixed picture of both forms of impairment (M-MCI). Most types of BPS were more common in those with more severe cognitive impairment and subjective memory complaints were an independent predictor of reported symptoms.

The important question is whether BPS in people with either MCI or no cognitive impairment are useful predictors of progressing to an eventual diagnosis of dementia. This has been most often investigated in relation to depression, presumably as depression is the commonest BPS. Most, but not all, studies have found that the presence of depression carries a higher risk of progressing from MCI to dementia,[5] especially if agitation is also a feature.[43] Rosenberg et al. reported a hazard ratio of 1.37 (95% CI = 1.17–1.84) with an annual conversion rate of 25% for MCI with BPS into dementia.[44]

The past few years has seen the introduction of the term mild behavioural impairment (MBI) to describe the appearance of psychiatric symptoms and behavioural changes in later life that may be predictive of subsequent dementia. The original use of MBI was by analogy with MCI; that is, to describe those individuals with BPS but no cognitive changes.[45] In the hospital setting described by Taragano et al., MBI was more predictive of subsequent FTD, whereas MCI tended to lead to AD.[45] However, more recently, MBI has been proposed as an umbrella term that subsumes MCI[46] and research diagnostic criteria have been proposed for further evaluation. The value of this concept therefore remains to be seen.

Two areas that do not seem to be much considered in the literature are, first, the relationship with general psychological morbidity in the population, and, second, the description of neuropsychiatric symptoms related to other neurological conditions. First, psychological symptoms, such as depression and anxiety, are common in the population at all ages. The notion of BPS or MBI rests on the idea that the symptoms are related to the underlying brain pathology and, indeed, the proposed MBI criteria,[46] state that 'the behavioural or personality changes are not attributable to another current psychiatric disorder, traumatic, or general medical causes, or the physiological effects of a substance or medication'. It is not, however, clear how this judgement is to be made. Second, numerous other disorders affecting the brain have neuropsychiatric symptoms but the term BPS seems to be limited to dementia. This must be a matter of convention rather than science, since there is no logical reason why we should not speak (for example) of BPSHD or BPSMS, in relation to HD or MS, respectively.

Prevalence

BPSD are common, with around 80% of people with dementia reported to show at least one symptom.[1,2,3,4] However, any prevalence figure is an approximation as it depends both on the measures used and the population studied: this may vary in terms of the proportion of people with severe dementia, who are likely to have higher rates of certain BPSD. Fig. 25.1 shows the prevalence of BPSD in studies in various settings: the general population, memory clinic, and care homes. Apathy, depression, and irritability were most prevalent, whereas elation and hallucinations were reported less often. As might be expected, population-based studies had lower prevalences of most symptoms. The memory clinic study[1] reported the highest prevalence of apathy, depression, and anxiety; and the care home study[4] reported the highest prevalence of agitation. BPS are also seen in people without dementia and in those with MCI.[5,42,47]

Instruments to Measure Symptoms

Over 80 different instruments have been used to measure BPS in people with dementia or in older people.[48] Table 25.2 summarizes the characteristics and quality of the ten most commonly used instruments.

The NPI[17] has become the most widely used instrument[49] (see Fig. 25.2) and now dominates the market, for example being used in over 90% of European countries.[50] Use of other instruments has relatively declined in this time. The NPI is informant-based and studies investigating its reliability have shown good results. Compared to other instruments, it is broader and shorter, measuring ten or twelve symptoms using one question for each, with seven or eight additional subsidiary questions if the behaviour is present. This makes it easy to use when requiring a broad overview of the presence of BPSD, but it provides less detail, with only one question to assess if the symptom is present or not.

When requiring detailed information on a single symptom, symptom-specific scales such as the Cornell Scale for Depression in Dementia[51] may be more appropriate. Other observational instruments, including the non-cognitive subscale of the Alzheimer Disease Assessment Scale (ADAS),[57] Ryden Aggression Scale (RAS),[60] or Agitated Behaviour Mapping Instrument (ABMI),[61]

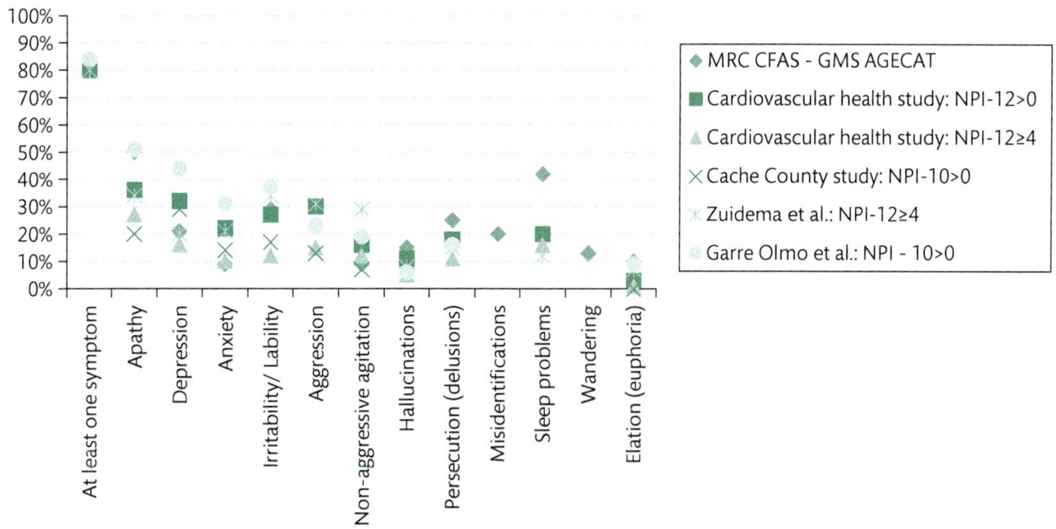

	MRC CFAS[1]	Cardiovascular health study[2]		Cache County study[3]	Zuidema et al.[4]	Garre Olmo et al.[5]
Population	Population-based	Population-based		Population-based (religious population)	Care homes	Memory clinic
Country	UK	USA		USA	Netherlands	Spain
n	587	362		408	1322	491
Age (mean)	82	77		83	83	75
% female	70	63		62	80	70.9
BPS measurement	GMS AGECAT	NPI-12 >0	NPI-12 ≥4	NPI-10>0	NPI-12≥4	NPI-10>0

1. (Savva et al. 2009)[47] 2. (Lyketsos et al. 2002)[2] 3. (Steinberg et al. 2008)[3] 4. (Zuidema et al. 2007)[4] 5. (Garre-Olmo et al. 2010)[1]

GMS AGECAT, Geriatric Mental State Examination Automated Geriatric Examination for Computer Assisted Taxonomy; MRC CFAS, Medical Research Council Cognitive Function and Ageing Study; NPI, Neuropsychiatric Inventory.

Fig. 25.1 Prevalence of BPS in dementia.

may add valuable information. The wide use of NPI increases comparability between studies, which is desirable to combine evidence on potential risk factors and the effect of treatments. Comparing prevalence rates across populations can only be achieved if similar instruments are employed.[5]

Thus, in practice, the NPI should form the core of any battery, but the specific research question should be carefully scrutinized to ensure that the question is adequately addressed. The choice of instrument will be influenced by the symptoms of interest, the population, the quality of the instrument, the amount of detail required, the time frame, other relevant components of the instrument, and practical issues such as time constraints.

In publications, researchers should report characteristics of the instrument as these can influence results. There are several difficulties in measuring BPSD that may influence findings, for example:

- Differences in visibility of symptoms:

  For example, irritability can be challenging for caregivers and is likely to be noticed, while caregivers may overlook depressive or anxiety symptoms.
- No clear definitions of symptoms and how they may overlap:

  Distinguishing between BPSD and cognitive symptoms and between individual BPSD is not always clear, for example is a misidentification a cognitive or non-cognitive problem?
- Little information is available on cut-off points to decide if a symptom is present or absent.
- BPSD are often unstable over time and may occur on some days but not on others.
- Under reporting by the person with dementia:

  For example, the obvious problems with spoken language, but also their willingness to report something may be influenced by such factors as the living situation and the relationship between the person with dementia and an informant.[62]

Grouping of Symptoms

Traditionally, authors have focused on single symptoms, such as depression. However, since the introduction of BPSD and the availability of instruments such as the NPI it has become more common to study a wider range of symptoms.

Certain symptoms, such as depression and anxiety, are frequently seen together and may have similar aetiology. Therefore, it is suggested that groups of correlated symptoms should be studied together. The US FDA considered that BPSD is too broad a target for treatment and proposed instead to 'identify and define unique psychiatric/behavioural syndromes'.[63] A consensus of the European Alzheimer's Disease Consortium concluded that there is clinical

Table 25.2 Summary of the characteristics and quality of the instruments

Name	BPSD	Detail	Length	Quality investigated*	Setting	Interview	Severity/ frequency
Dementia							
NPI (Cummings et al. 1994)[17]	Broad	Low	Short	Low	3	Informant	Both, distress
BEHAVE-AD (Reisberg et al. 1987)[16]	Medium	Medium	Medium	High	3	Informant	Severity
CERAD-BRSD (Tariot et al. 1995)[52]	Broad	High	Long	Low	2, 3	Informant	Severity
BMDS (Greene et al. 1982)[53]	Medium	Medium	Medium	Low	2	Informant	Frequency
CUSPAD (Devanand et al. 1992)[54]	Medium	Medium	Medium	Medium	1	Informant	Severity
DBDS (Baumgarten et al. 1990)[55]	Medium	Medium	Medium	Low	2	Informant	Frequency
Including cognition							
Dementia							
RMBPC (Teri et al. 1992)[56]	Narrow	Medium	Medium	–	–	Informant	Frequency
ADAS-noncog (Mohs et al. 1983)[57]	Medium	Medium	Short	–	–	Observation	Severity
Older adults							
CAMDEX (Roth et al. 1986)[58]	Medium	Low	Long	–	–	Informant	Dichotomous
GMS/AGECAT (Copeland et al. 1976)[58]	Broad	Low	Long	–	–	Participant or informant	Dichotomous

BPSD, Behavioural and psychological symptoms of dementia

BPSD: narrow: 1-3 symptoms, medium 4-8 symptoms, broad 9-10 symptoms; **Detail**: Low: dichotomous or only one question per symptom Medium: more than one response option and more than one question per symptoms High: more than one response option and consistently more than two/three questions per symptom; **Length**: of total instrument, short: ≤20, medium 21-35, >35 long; **Quality**: Low: Reliability and/or validity not investigated by independent researchers, Medium: One independent study investigated reliability and/or validity, High: >1 independent study investigated reliability and/or validity; **Setting:** Reliability and/or validity studied in 1: primary care, 2: secondary care, 3: tertiary care

ADAS, Alzheimer's Disease Assessment Scale; BEHAVE-AD, Behavioural Pathology in Alzheimer's Disease scale; BMDS, Behaviour and Mood Disturbance Scale; CAMDEX, Cambridge Mental Disorders of the Elderly Examination; CERAD-BRSD, Behaviour Rating Scale for Dementia of the Consortium to Establish a Registry for Alzheimer's Disease; CUSPAD, Columbia University Scale for Psychopathology in Alzheimer's disease; DBDS, Dementia Behaviour Disturbance Scale; GMS AGECAT, Geriatric Mental State Examination (GMS) Automated Geriatric Examination for Computer Assisted Taxonomy (AGECAT); NPI, Neuropsychiatric Inventory; RMBPC, Revised Memory and problems checklist behaviour.

Adapted from van der Linde R.M., Dening T., Matthews F.E., and Brayne C. Grouping of behavioural and psychological symptoms of dementia. *International Journal of Geriatric Psychiatry* 29(6): 562–568.

evidence for groups within BPSD and therefore it is more appropriate to examine interventions for groups of symptoms rather than individual symptoms.[64] It is argued that these grouped symptoms may share common biological mechanisms, so that therefore similar treatments will be effective within a symptom group. Grouping of symptoms is important not only for taxonomy and research but also for everyday clinical practice, in terms of communication between clinicians, patients, and families, and to set clear goals for therapeutic efforts.

Symptom clusters may be identified using clinical experience and judgement, with careful observation of which symptoms seem to hang together in the patients seen in a clinic. Statistical approaches include measuring correlations between individual symptoms in groups of patients or more complex multivariate approaches that explore the patterns of correlated variables (e.g. symptoms) and group them into 'factors' or 'clusters'. Cluster analysis and latent class analysis group patients based on their symptom profile, leading to non-overlapping clusters of patients. In contrast, factor analysis and principal component analysis group symptoms rather than patients, and an individual patient may have more than one factor of symptoms, while an individual symptom may appear in more than one factor.

Published studies have usually identified the following symptom groups: affective symptoms (including depressive symptoms and anxiety), psychosis (including delusions and hallucinations), hyperactivity (sometimes named agitation or psychomotor symptoms, including irritability, agitation or aggression, and aberrant motor behaviour), and euphoria.[65] Similar findings emerged from studies using the NPI and those using other instruments. Apathy did not consistently load into any one group, sometimes grouping with affective symptoms or otherwise independently.

Grouping methods allow similar symptoms to be studied together, which might strengthen results and may point to common factors in their aetiology and treatment. However, much of the individual variability of the symptoms cannot be explained by the symptom groups. Taking into account the advantages and disadvantages of each of these methods, authors should carefully address their research question and hypotheses to decide if symptoms should be studied in groups or individually. In similar fashion, clinicians assessing patients and developing strategies for treatment need to consider each symptom in its own right but also be aware of their interrelations. The symptom groups seem robust enough to be used in future research in BPSD and it will be important to explore if they do share a common aetiology, course, and response to treatment.

Causes

The causes of BPSD are multifactorial, with a combination of neurobiological, genetic, social, psychological, and environmental factors.

Biological

Biological factors associated with BPSD include neurotransmitter changes, genetic factors, loss of structure and function in the brain,

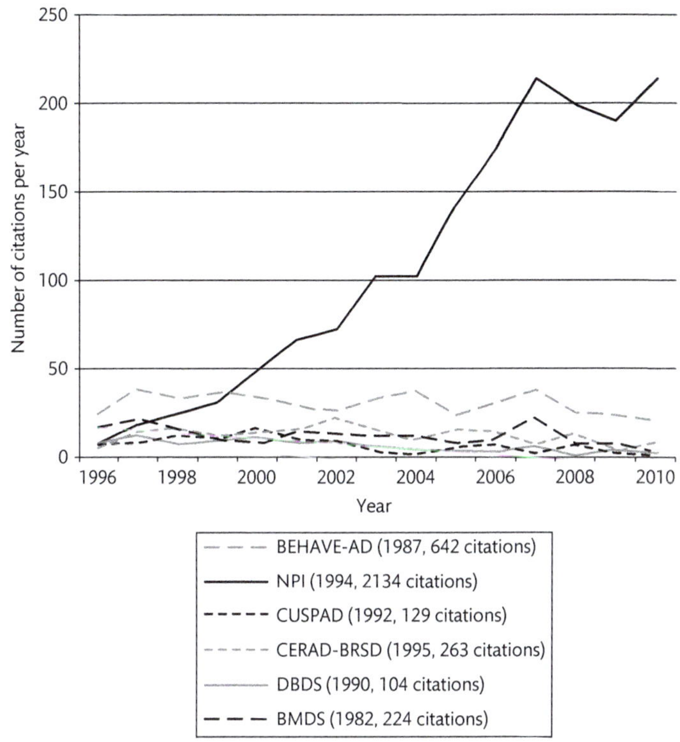

Fig. 25.2 Number of citations per year over time of the most commonly used instruments to measure BPSD in dementia.

Reproduced with permission from Van der Linde R.M. Instruments to measure behavioural and psychological symptoms of dementia. *Int J Methods Psychiatr Res*, 23(1):69–98. Copyright © 2014 John Wiley & Sons, Ltd. DOI: https://doi.org/10.1002/mpr.1414

and hormonal changes. Different neurotransmitter systems are likely to be implicated in different groups of BPSD.[66] For example, reduced activity of serotonin (5-hydroxytryptamine, 5HT) is suggested to underlie impulsive aggression, though the evidence comes mainly from forensic rather than dementia studies. However, there is also evidence of a correlation between noradrenergic cell loss and aggression in dementia,[67] suggesting possible involvement of noradrenergic dysfunction too. Depression is likely to involve monoamine neurotransmitter pathways, though evidence to support this is less strong than in depression occurring in the absence of dementia. Depression in DLB may be associated with greater serotonin depletion than in AD.[68] Anatomically, both AD and depression are associated with hippocampal atrophy.[69] The subtypes of apathy (lack of feeling, interest, and behaviour)[25] are each likely to result from the distribution of pathology in the basal ganglia, prefrontal cortex, and related neuronal circuits. Psychotic symptoms such as delusions and hallucinations appear to result from cholinergic deficits in AD and DLB, along with dysfunction in dopamine systems.

Numerous genetic studies have investigated links with BPSD. These have mainly looked at genes coding for APOE and genes related to monoamine function, such as serotonin receptors, serotonin transport, catechol-O-methyltransferase, and dopamine transmission. Findings have been generally inconsistent,[70] which reflects in part the difficulty of seeking genetic roots for complex behaviours, but also methodological issues such as variations in diagnostic criteria and criteria for BPSD, what population and which symptoms are studied, and the size and power of the study.

Hormones may be involved in various manifestations of BPSD. For example, cortisol is associated with hippocampal atrophy and dementia progression,[71] and also depression. Increased cortisol is also related to stress and insomnia, but the direction of causation may be unclear. Hormones involved in appetite regulation, such as agouti-related peptide, contribute to hyperphagia seen in behavioural variant FTD.[72]

Finally, physical health issues are frequently associated with BPSD, notably pain.[73] Pain is common in older people with dementia and may be due to various comorbid conditions, but it is difficult to assess and may remain undetected.[74] Irritability has especially been associated with pain, but pain may also trigger the expression of other BPSD, for example apathy and depression. Other health-related triggers of BPSD include dehydration, hunger, vision, or hearing problems, cardiovascular disease, infections, or adverse effects from medication.[75,76,77]

Psychological, social, and environmental

It is important not to assume that BPSD are simply a consequence of the dementia. Psychosocial factors, including some present since early life, are strongly associated with BPSD. These include female sex, low social interaction, low social class, previous and family history of psychiatric disorder, and poor physical health.[77,78,79]

Personality before the onset of dementia has been associated with the presence of BPSD.[80,81,82] For example, neuroticism has been associated with anxiety, and agreeableness has been negatively associated with agitation and irritability.[80] Dementia has been associated with changes in personality that may occur alongside, or may precede, development of BPSD. Dementia is associated with an increase in neuroticism, and a decrease in extraversion, openness, agreeableness, and conscientiousness.[83] Thus, BPSD may be affected by pre-existing personality traits,[84] but also the dementia process may itself cause certain personality changes, for example blunting of interpersonal skills in FTD.

BPSD may occur in reaction to the cognitive decline associated with dementia. Awareness of cognitive decline could trigger various emotional responses, including depression and anxiety. Indeed, sometimes symptoms may arise prior to the diagnosis of dementia being made as a person struggles to make sense of their experiences or due to a sense of rising fear that something is seriously wrong.

Other psychosocial factors that have been associated with BPSD include confusion, boredom (lack of entertainment or too little social contact), lack of self-esteem, stressful life events and bereavement, lack of dignity, and the relation with the caregiver (including caregiver distress, poor interpersonal interactions, and caregiver intrusion in personal space).[77,79,85] As well as understimulation, overstimulation may also be a problem, especially in care homes or hospitals, where the environment can be noisy and chaotic. For example, turning off televisions and lowering voices can help reduce agitation and the use of restraints, and changing the visual environment to obscure exits can reduce residents' attempts to leave the building.[86]

Protective factors and interventions

More attention should be paid to what factors protect people with dementia from developing BPSD, such as their own personal resilience. Most research on resilience has either focused on cognitive resilience or the resilience of informal carers. However, there are exceptions. Harris et al. used a longitudinal cohort followed since childhood to demonstrate how, perhaps surprisingly, early life stresses predicted higher resilience in later life.[86] Studies drawing directly on the experiences of people with dementia have indicated the importance of the person remaining at the centre of their own personal stage ('narrative citizenship') and involved with social networks.[88,89] Thus, irrespective of potential causal factors, the behaviours within BPSD may be modified by a person's relationships and attitudes, by his/her environment or by behavioural, social, or cognitive interventions.[90]

Impact and burden

BPSD are associated with caregiver burden,[91] cognitive decline,[5] and mortality,[92] and they contribute to considerable financial costs.[93] BPSD are also associated with disability; people with BPSD function at a lower level than those without.[94] If symptoms can be ameliorated or removed, the person's functional level is likely to improve.

Most care received by older people is provided by informal carers, including spouse, family members, or friends,[95] who often find BPSD more demanding to cope with than cognitive decline or physical disability. BPSD have been significantly associated with burden, distress, and depression amongst caregivers.[91] Factors that lead caregivers to regard behaviour as 'challenging', and therefore stressful, include declining communication and a sense of losing the relationship with the person who has dementia; misperceptions of the behaviour and how it may transgress social norms; and an underlying assumption that the person with dementia is losing their identity and personhood.[96]

Longitudinal Course

Describing the course of BPSD helps patients and care providers to understand what may happen and to plan for the future. The pattern of BPSD throughout the course of dementia needs to be well understood in order to identify when and how possible interventions should optimally be delivered.

Cross-sectional studies have shown that BPSD can occur at any time during the development of dementia. BPSD prevalence may increase from mild to severe dementia, while others suggest a non-linear course, with the highest prevalence seen in the intermediate stages of disease.[97,98] BPSD may persist or may be episodic over time, and this may differ between symptoms.

As an example, a large population-based study of people aged over 65, with interviews every 2–4 years over a follow-up period of over 16 years (MRC CFAS) showed that most BPSD were persistent (wandering, apathy, misidentification, depression, and anxiety showing the highest persistence). Some symptoms were more likely to develop than others (apathy, sleep problems, depression, irritability, and wandering were most likely), and BPSD were associated with mortality.[99] Low cognitive function and dementia were associated with development of symptoms.

Our systematic review of longitudinal studies of BPSD confirmed that many BPSD are common and relatively persistent in individuals with dementia.[100] There were differences between the course of different symptoms: hyperactivity and apathy showed high persistence and incidence; depression and anxiety showed low or moderate persistence and moderate incidence; and psychotic symptoms showed low persistence and a moderate or low incidence. Studies of the association between BPSD and cognitive function suggest that in those without dementia, the presence of depression is associated with subsequent cognitive decline. In people with dementia, psychosis, hyperactivity, agitation, and physical aggression are all associated with more rapid cognitive decline.

However, the prevalence of symptoms varied widely across the studies and these differences may be associated with study design, for example setting, dementia severity, mean age, and BPSD measurement. Large differences were also seen in the reported persistence and incidence of symptoms.

Principles of Treatment and Management

Details of treatment and management of BPSD are beyond the scope of this chapter. The main principle is that non-pharmacological approaches should be considered ahead of prescribing medication. Contemporary person-centred care is, however, more likely to consider BPSD within the context of good care as a whole, aiming to prevent the development of distressed behaviour.[101] Numerous interventions have been proposed, including reality orientation, cognitive stimulation, arts therapies, aromatherapy, environmental changes, and behavioural management techniques. The evidence base on these is variable, although there are several relevant Cochrane reviews;[102] however, many of these find that the quality of trials reviewed is relatively low. Most interventions that are effective appear to be related to improving the communication skills and person-centred focus of informal carers and/or care staff.[24]

As regards medication, the main issue has been concern over excessive prescribing of antipsychotic drugs to control symptoms such as agitation, for which they are not licensed. This is because of adverse effects, such as increased mortality[103] and cognitive decline.[104] Discontinuing antipsychotics is useful, but apparently only alongside other measures, such as increased social interaction or exercise.[105] Antidepressants are frequently prescribed, either for mood changes or for other BPSD, such as agitation. Evidence that antidepressants are effective in depression related to dementia is limited[106] and perhaps limited to short periods only.[107] Cholinesterase inhibitors seem to help with improving attention, but are not effective in treating agitation.[108] Any prescribing for BPSD needs to consider whether such treatment is actually necessary and also consider other factors such as comorbid medical conditions and other drugs being taken by the patient.

Discussion: the Concept of BPSD

BPSD has been with us as a concept for over 20 years. Its biggest strength has been to introduce an internationally defined term that has concentrated the minds of researchers and clinicians. The limitations of BPSD are two-fold: (1) the adequacy of the term to cover the non-cognitive aspects of dementia, and (2) criticism that the whole concept is too medical and deterministic in nature and that alternative ways of looking at behaviour are more helpful.

In relation to the first issue, the elements of BPSD are clearly very mixed phenomena that lie in all domains of mental life and life in the real world too. A unifying term like BPSD seems to imply that they can be reduced into a single quality, or even that BPSD is a 'thing', which of course it is not. As well as this, BPSD has come to be regarded almost as a checklist, governed by the symptoms that have been set out in Table 25.1 and discussed in that section of the chapter. This is reinforced by the use of standard instruments such as the NPI.[17] The disadvantage of the current position is that it represents a closed glossary, that is, that certain terms are officially sanctioned but other ways of looking at the person's experience or behaviour are not. A good example is 'emotionalism' which doesn't fit readily into our list of BPSD or into the NPI, even though the phenomenon of being easily moved to tears is not uncommon. Alternatively, a term like 'aggression' includes a range of different behaviours, which may include hitting out, biting, scratching, throwing objects, or sexual assaults. These may have different causes and different meanings, which in turn require different remedies. Labelling them together with a single term implies a degree of homogeneity that may be unwarranted.

The major criticism of BPSD is, however, that the concept takes too narrow a focus of the observed phenomena and the personal experience of the individual, emphasizing the neurological basis of the changes in emotion, thinking, and behaviour. This can imply that BPSD are biologically determined and perhaps, therefore, that interventions should be pharmacological. However, the field of dementia care has been transformed by the influence of person-centred approaches, originating from social psychology.[109] From this perspective, behaviours are seen primarily as attempts to communicate, so interventions are focused on understanding the needs of the person and what they are trying to say. Therefore, there is much more emphasis on understanding behaviour and meeting the underlying need(s) that may be driving it. There is a rejection of some of the terms used in the BPSD paradigm, for example 'wandering' becomes 'walking with purpose'. Thus, any account of how to manage 'behaviours that challenge' always begins by stressing the importance of non-pharmacological approaches.

The question therefore arises as to whether BPSD will survive as a term that is used in the future. Despite its limitations, it remains a convenient means of symptom grouping so long as we remain conscious of its heterogeneity and we acknowledge alternative frames of reference.

Conclusion

BPSD are common. Many occur as dementia progresses. Several are persistent. Apathy is recognized as particularly challenging as it is highly prevalent and persistent, limits the quality of people's lives, and is stressful for carers. It is therefore seen as a priority area for future research and interventions.[110]

REFERENCES

1. Garre-Olmo J, Lopez-Pousa S, Vilalta-Franch J, de Gracia BM, Vilarrasa AB. Grouping and trajectories of the neuropsychiatric symptoms in patients with Alzheimer's disease, part I: symptom clusters. *Journal of Alzheimer's Disease*. 2010; 22(4): 1157–67.
2. Lyketsos CG, Lopez O, Jones B, Fitzpatrick AL, Breitner J, DeKosky S. Prevalence of neuropsychiatric symptoms in dementia and mild cognitive impairment: results from the cardiovascular health study. *Journal of the American Medical Association*. 2002; 288(12): 1475–83.
3. Steinberg M, Shao H, Zandi P, Lyketsos CG, Welsh-Bohmer KA, Norton MC, et al. Point and 5-year period prevalence of neuropsychiatric symptoms in dementia: the Cache County Study. *International Journal of Geriatric Psychiatry*. 2008; 23(2): 170–7.
4. Zuidema SU, Derksen E, Verhey FR, Koopmans RT. Prevalence of neuropsychiatric symptoms in a large sample of Dutch nursing home patients with dementia. *International Journal of Geriatric Psychiatry*. 2007; 22(7): 632–8.
5. Monastero R, Mangialasche F, Camarda C, Ercolani S, Camarda R. A systematic review of neuropsychiatric symptoms in mild cognitive impairment. *Journal of Alzheimer's Disease*. 2009; 18(1): 11–30.
6. Department of Health. 2009. Living well with dementia: a National Dementia Strategy. https://assets.publishing.service.gov.uk/government/uploads/system/uploads/attachment_data/file/168220/dh_094051.pdf.
7. National Institute for Health and Clinical Excellence. *Dementia—Supporting people with dementia and their carers in health and social care*. National Institute for Health and Clinical Excellence: Clinical Guideline 42, 2006.
8. Lyketsos CG, Carrillo MC, Ryan JM, Khachaturian AS, Trzepacz P, Amatniek J, et al. Neuropsychiatric symptoms in Alzheimer's disease. *Alzheimer's Dement*. 20011; 7(5): 532–9.
9. Alzheimer A. Über einen eigenartigen schweren Er Krankungsprozeb der Himrinde. *Neurologisches Centralblatt*. 1906; 23: 1129–36.
10. Maurer K, Volk S, Gerbaldo H. Auguste D and Alzheimer's disease. *Lancet*. 1997; 349(9064): 1546–9.
11. Katzman R, Terry RD, Bick KL. *Alzheimer's Disease: Senile Dementia and Related Disorders*. New York: Raven Press, 1978.
12. Burns A, Jacoby R, Levy R. Psychiatric phenomena in Alzheimer's disease. III: Disorders of mood. *Br J Psychiatry*. 1990; 157: 81–4.
13. Burns A, Jacoby R, Levy R. Psychiatric phenomena in Alzheimer's disease. IV: Disorders of behaviour. *Br J Psychiatry*. 1990; 157: 86–94.
14. Blessed G, Tomlinson BE, Roth M. The association between quantitative measures of dementia and of senile change in the cerebral grey matter of elderly subjects. *Br J Psychiatry*. 1968; 114(512): 797–811.
15. Venn RD. The Sandoz Clinical Assessment-Geriatric (SCAG) scale. A general-purpose psychogeriatric rating scale. *Gerontology*. 1983; 29(3): 185–98.
16. Reisberg B, Borenstein J, Salob SP, Ferris SH, Franssen E, Georgotas A. Behavioral symptoms in Alzheimer's disease: phenomenology and treatment. *Journal of Clinical Psychiatry*. 1987; 48(Suppl): 9–15.
17. Cummings JL, Mega M, Gray K, Rosenberg-Thompson S, Carusi DA, Gornbein J. The Neuropsychiatric Inventory: comprehensive assessment of psychopathology in dementia. *Neurology*. 1994; 44(12): 2308–14.
18. Lyketsos CG, Steinberg M, Tschanz JT, Norton MC, Steffens DC, Breitner JC. Mental and behavioral disturbances in dementia: findings from the Cache County Study on Memory in Aging. *American Journal of Psychiatry*. 2000; 157(5): 708–14.
19. Finkel SI, Costa e Silva, Cohen G, Miller S, Sartorius N. Behavioral and psychological signs and symptoms of dementia: a consensus statement on current knowledge and implications for research and treatment. *International Psychogeriatrics*. 1996; 8(Suppl 3): 497–500.

20. McKeith IG, Dickson DW, Lowe J, Emre M, O'Brien JT, Feldman H, et al. Diagnosis and management of dementia with Lewy bodies: third report of the DLB Consortium. *Neurology*. 2005; 65(12): 1863–72.
21. Rascovsky K, Hodges JR, Knopman D, Mendez MF, Kramer JH, Neuhaus J, et al. Sensitivity of revised diagnostic criteria for the behavioural variant of frontotemporal dementia. *Brain*. 2001; 134(Pt 9): 2456–77.
22. Corbett A, Husebo B, Malcangio M, Staniland A, Cohen-Mansfield J, Aarsland D, et al. Assessment and treatment of pain in people with dementia. *Nat Rev Neurol*. 2011; 8(5): 264–74.
23. Banerjee S. *The Use of Antipsychotic Medication for People with Dementia: Time for Action*. London: Department of Health, 2009.
24. Livingston G, Kelly L, Lewis-Holmes E, Baio G, Morris S, Patel N, et al. Non-pharmacological interventions for agitation in dementia: systematic review of randomised controlled trials. *Br J Psychiatry*. 2014; 205(6): 436–42.
25. Levy R, Dubois B. Apathy and the functional anatomy of the prefrontal cortex-basal ganglia circuits. *Cereb Cortex*. 2006; 16(7): 916–928.
26. Radakovic R, Abrahams S. Developing a new apathy measurement scale: Dimensional Apathy Scale. *Psychiatry Res*. 2014; 219(3): 658–63.
27. Work SS, Colamonico JA, Bradley WG, Kaye RE. Pseudobulbar affect: an under-recognized and under-treated neurological disorder. *Adv Ther*. 2011; 28(7): 586–601.
28. Diniz BS, Butters MA, Albert SM, Dew MA, Reynolds CF, III. Late-life depression and risk of vascular dementia and Alzheimer's disease: systematic review and meta-analysis of community-based cohort studies. *Br J Psychiatry*. 2013; 202(5): 329–35.
29. Heser K, Bleckwenn M, Wiese B, Mamone S, Riedel-Heller SG, Stein J, et al. Late-Life depressive symptoms and lifetime history of major depression: cognitive deficits are largely due to incipient dementia rather than depression. *J Alzheimer's Dis*. 2016; 54(1): 185–99.
30. Johansson L, Guo X, Waern M, Ostling S, Gustafson D, Bengtsson C, et al. Midlife psychological stress and risk of dementia: a 35-year longitudinal population study. *Brain*. 2010; 133(Pt 8): 2217–24.
31. Gulpers B, Ramakers I, Hamel R, Kohler S, Oude VR, Verhey F. Anxiety as a predictor for cognitive decline and dementia: a systematic review and meta-analysis. *Am J Geriatr Psychiatry*. 2016; 24(10): 823–42.
32. Spalletta G, Musicco M, Padovani A, Rozzini L, Perri R, Fadda L, et al. Neuropsychiatric symptoms and syndromes in a large cohort of newly diagnosed, untreated patients with Alzheimer disease. *Am J Geriatr Psychiatry*. 2010; 18(11): 1026–35.
33. Sandilyan MB, Dening T. Signs and symptoms of dementia. *Nurs Stand*. 2015; 29(41): 42–51.
34. Cummings J, Mintzer J, Brodaty H, Sano M, Banerjee S, Devanand DP, et al. Agitation in cognitive disorders: International Psychogeriatric Association provisional consensus clinical and research definition. *Int Psychogeriatr*. 2015; 27(1): 7–17.
35. Argyle E, Dening T, Bartlett P. Space, the final frontier: outdoor access for people living with dementia. *Aging Ment Health*. 2017; 21(10): 1005–6.
36. Nair AG, Nair AG, Shah BR, Gandhi RA. Seeing the unseen: Charles Bonnet syndrome revisited. *Psychogeriatrics*. 2015; 15(3): 204–8.
37. Marchand DG, Montplaisir J, Postuma RB, Rahayel S, Gagnon JF. Detecting the cognitive prodrome of dementia with Lewy bodies: A prospective study of REM sleep behavior disorder. *Sleep*. 2017; 40(1): zsw014.
38. Cipriani G, Carlesi C, Lucetti C, Danti S, Nuti A. Eating behaviors and dietary changes in patients with dementia. *Am J Alzheimer's Dis Other Demen*. 2016; 31(8): 706–16.
39. Brayne C, Richardson K, Matthews FE, Fleming J, Hunter S, Xuereb JH, et al. Neuropathological correlates of dementia in over-80-year-old brain donors from the population-based Cambridge city over-75s cohort (CC75C) study. *J Alzheimer's Dis*. 2009; 18(3): 645–58.
40. Apostolova LG, Cummings JL. Neuropsychiatric manifestations in mild cognitive impairment: A systematic review of the literature. *Dementia and Geriatric Cognitive Disorders*. 2008; 25(2): 115–26.
41. Kohler CA, Magalhaes TF, Oliveira JM, Alves GS, Knochel C, Oertel-Knochel V, et al. Neuropsychiatric Disturbances in Mild Cognitive Impairment (MCI): A Systematic Review of Population-Based Studies. *Curr Alzheimer Res*. 2016; 13(10): 1066–82.
42. van der Linde R, Stephan BC, Matthews FE, Brayne C, Savva GM. Behavioural and psychological symptoms in the older population without dementia—relationship with socio-demographics, health and cognition. *BMC Geriatrics*. 2010; 10(1): 87.
43. Van der Mussele S, Fransen E, Struyfs H, Luyckx J, Marien P, Saerens J, et al. Depression in mild cognitive impairment is associated with progression to Alzheimer's disease: a longitudinal study. *J Alzheimer's Dis*. 2014; 42(4): 1239–50.
44. Rosenberg PB, Mielke MM, Appleby BS, Oh ES, Geda YE, Lyketsos CG. The association of neuropsychiatric symptoms in MCI with incident dementia and Alzheimer disease. *Am J Geriatr Psychiatry*. 2013; 21(7): 685–95.
45. Taragano FE, Allegri RF, Krupitzki H, Sarasola DR, Serrano CM, Lon L, et al. Mild behavioral impairment and risk of dementia: a prospective cohort study of 358 patients. *J Clin Psychiatry*. 2009; 70(4): 584–92.
46. Ismail Z, Smith EE, Geda Y, Sultzer D, Brodaty H, Smith G, et al. Neuropsychiatric symptoms as early manifestations of emergent dementia: Provisional diagnostic criteria for mild behavioral impairment. *Alzheimer's Dement*. 2016; 12(2): 195–202.
47. Savva GM, Zaccai J, Matthews FE, Davidson JE, McKeith I, Brayne C. Prevalence, correlates and course of behavioural and psychological symptoms of dementia in the population. *British Journal of Psychiatry*. 2009; 194(3): 212–19.
48. Van der Linde R.M. Instruments to measure behavioural and psychological symptoms of dementia. *Int J Methods Psychiatr Res*, 23(1):69–98. Copyright © 2014 John Wiley & Sons, Ltd. DOI: https://doi. org/10.1002/mpr.1414
49. van der Linde R, Stephan B, Dening T, Brayne C. Instruments to measure behavioural and psychological symptoms of dementia: changing use over time. *International Journal of Geriatric Psychiatry*. 2013; 28(4): 433–435.
50. Maruta C, Guerreiro M, de MA, Hort J, Scheltens P. The use of neuropsychological tests across Europe: the need for a consensus in the use of assessment tools for dementia. *European Journal of Neurology*. 2011; 18(2): 279–85.
51. Alexopoulos GS, Abrams RC, Young RC, Shamoian CA. Cornell Scale for Depression in Dementia. *Biological Psychiatry*. 1998; 23(3): 271–84.
52. Tariot PN, Mack JL, Patterson MB, Edland SD, Weiner MF, Fillenbaum G, et al. The Behavior Rating Scale for Dementia of

the Consortium to Establish a Registry for Alzheimer's Disease. The Behavioral Pathology Committee of the Consortium to Establish a Registry for Alzheimer's Disease. *American Journal of Psychiatry*. 1995; 152(9): 1349–57.

53. Greene JG, Smith R, Gardiner M, Timbury GC. Measuring behavioural disturbance of elderly demented patients in the community and its effects on relatives: a factor analytic study. *Age and Ageing*. 1982; 11(2): 121–6.
54. Devanand DP, Miller L, Richards M, Marder K, Bell K, Mayeux R, et al. The Columbia University Scale for Psychopathology in Alzheimer's disease. *Archives of Neurology*. 1992; 49(4): 371–6.
55. Baumgarten M, Becker R, Gauthier S. Validity and reliability of the dementia behavior disturbance scale. *Journal of the American Geriatrics Society*. 1990; 38(3): 221–6.
56. Teri L, Truax P, Logsdon R, Uomoto J, Zarit S, Vitaliano PP. Assessment of behavioral problems in dementia: the revised memory and behavior problems checklist. *Psychology and Aging*.1992; 7(4): 622–31.
57. Mohs RC, Rosen WG, Davis KL. The Alzheimer's disease assessment scale: an instrument for assessing treatment efficacy. *Psychopharmacology Bulletin*. 1983; 19(3): 448–450.
58. Roth M, Tym E, Mountjoy CQ, Huppert FA, Hendrie H, Verma S, CAMDEX. A standardised instrument for the diagnosis of mental disorder in the elderly with special reference to the early detection of dementia. *Br J Psychiatry* 1986; 149: 698–709.
59. Copeland JR, Kelleher MJ, Kellett JM, Gourlay AJ, Gurland BJ, Fleiss JL, et al. A semi-structured clinical interview for the assessment of diagnosis and mental state in the elderly: the Geriatric Mental State Schedule. I. Development and reliability. *Psychological Medicine*. 1976; 6(3): 439–49.
60. Ryden MB. Aggressive behavior in persons with dementia who live in the community. *Alzheimer Disease and Associated Disorders*. 1988; 2(4): 342–55.
61. Cohen-Mansfield J, Marx MS, Rosenthal AS. 1989. A description of agitation in a nursing home. *Journals of Gerontology* 44(3): M77–M84.
62. Ready RE, Ott BR, Grace J. Validity of informant reports about AD and MCI patients' memory. *Alzheimer Disease and Associated Disorders*. 2004; 18(1): 11–16.
63. FDA. *Division of Neuropharmacological Drug Products (DNDP) Issues Paper for March 9, 2000 Meeting of the Psychopharmacological Drugs Advisory Committee Meeting on the Various Psychiatric and Behavioral Disturbances Associated with Dementia*. US Food and Drug Administration, 2000.
64. Robert PH, Verhey FRJ, Byrne EJ, Hurt C, De Deyn PP, Nobili F, et al. Grouping for behavioral and psychological symptoms in dementia: Clinical and biological aspects. Consensus paper of the European Alzheimer disease consortium. *European Psychiatry*. 2005; 20(7): 490–6.
65. van der Linde RM, Dening T, Matthews FE, Brayne C. Grouping of behavioural and psychological symptoms of dementia. *International Journal of Geriatric Psychiatry*. 2014; 29(6): 562–8.
66. Wint D, Cummings J. Neuropsychiatric Aspects of Cognitive Impairment. Oxford: Oxford University Press, 2016. pp197–208.
67. Matthews KL, Chen CP, Esiri MM, Keene J, Minger SL, Francis PT. Noradrenergic changes, aggressive behavior, and cognition in patients with dementia. *Biol Psychiatry*. 2002; 51(5): 407–16.
68. Vermeiren Y, Van DD, Aerts T, Engelborghs S, Martin JJ, De Deyn PP. The monoaminergic footprint of depression and psychosis in dementia with Lewy bodies compared to Alzheimer's disease. *Alzheimer's Res Ther*. 2015; 7(1): 7.
69. Sawyer K, Corsentino E, Sachs-Ericsson N, Steffens DC. Depression, hippocampal volume changes, and cognitive decline in a clinical sample of older depressed outpatients and non-depressed controls. *Aging Ment Health*. 2012; 16(6): 753–62.
70. Flirski M, Sobow T, Kloszewska I. Behavioural genetics of Alzheimer's disease: a comprehensive review. *Arch Med Sci*. 2011; 7(2): 195–210.
71. Csernansky JG, Dong H, Fagan AM, Wang L, Xiong C, Holtzman DM, et al. Plasma cortisol and progression of dementia in subjects with Alzheimer-type dementia. *Am J Psychiatry*. 2006; 163(12): 2164–9.
72. Ahmed RM, Latheef S, Bartley L, Irish M, Halliday GM, Kiernan MC, et al. Eating behavior in frontotemporal dementia: Peripheral hormones vs hypothalamic pathology. *Neurology*. 2015; 85(15): 1310–17.
73. Husebo BS, Ballard C, Aarsland D. Pain treatment of agitation in patients with dementia: a systematic review. *International Journal of Geriatric Psychiatry*. 2011; 26(10): 1012–1018.
74. Corbett A, Husebo B, Malcangio M, Staniland A, Cohen-Mansfield J, Aarsland D, et al. Assessment and treatment of pain in people with dementia. *Nature Reviews Neurology*. 2012; 8(5): 264–74.
75. Ballard C, Corbett A, Chitramohan R, Aarsland D. Management of agitation and aggression associated with Alzheimer's disease: controversies and possible solutions. *Current Opinion in Psychiatry*. 2009; 22(6): 532–40.
76. Ballard CG, Gauthier S, Cummings JL, Brodaty H, Grossberg GT, Robert P, et al. Management of agitation and aggression associated with Alzheimer disease. *Nature Reviews Neurology*. 2009; 5(5): 245–55.
77. Vink D, Aartsen MJ, Schoevers RA. Risk factors for anxiety and depression in the elderly: A review. *Journal of Affective Disorders*. 2008; 106(1-2): 29–44.
78. Ropacki SA, Jeste DV. Epidemiology of and risk factors for psychosis of Alzheimer's disease: a review of 55 studies published from 1990 to 2003. *American Journal of Psychiatry*. 2005; 162(11): 2022–30.
79. Zuidema S, Koopmans R, Verhey F. Prevalence and predictors of neuropsychiatric symptoms in cognitively impaired nursing home patients. *Journal of Geriatric Psychiatry and Neurology*. 2007; 20(1): 41–9.
80. Archer N, Brown RG, Reeves SJ, Boothby H, Nicholas H, Foy C, et al. Premorbid personality and behavioral and psychological symptoms in probable Alzheimer disease. *American Journal of Geriatric Psychiatry* 2007; 15(3): 202–13.
81. Low LF, Brodaty H, Draper B. A study of premorbid personality and behavioural and psychological symptoms of dementia in nursing home residents. *International Journal of Geriatric Psychiatry*. 2002; 17(8): 779–83.
82. Meins W. Impact of personality on behavioral and psychological symptoms of dementia. *International Psychogeriatrics*. 2000; 12(Suppl 1): 107–9.
83. Robins Wahlin TB, Byrne GJ. Personality changes in Alzheimer's disease: a systematic review. *International Journal of Geriatric Psychiatry*. 2011; 26(10): 1019–29.
84. Prior J, Abraham R, Nicholas H, Chan T, Vanvlymen J, Lovestone S, et al. Are premorbid abnormal personality traits associated with behavioural and psychological symptoms in dementia? *Int J Geriatr Psychiatry*. 2016; 31(9): 1050–55.
85. Orrell M, Bebbington P. Life events and senile dementia. Affective symptoms. *Br J Psychiatry*. 1995; 166(5): 613–20.

86. Livingston G, Johnston K, Katona C, Paton J, Lyketsos CG. Systematic review of psychological approaches to the management of neuropsychiatric symptoms of dementia. *American Journal of Psychiatry*. 2005; 162(11): 1996–2021.
87. Harris MA, Brett CE, Starr JM, Deary IJ, McIntosh AM. Early-life predictors of resilience and related outcomes up to 66 years later in the 6-day sample of the 1947 Scottish mental survey. *Soc Psychiatry Psychiatr Epidemiol*. 2016; 51(5): 659–68.
88. Angus J, Bowen-Osborne S. A self-narrative of life-long disability: a reflection on resilience and living with dementia. *Dementia (London)*. 2014; 13(2): 147–59.
89. Clarke CL, Bailey C. Narrative citizenship, resilience and inclusion with dementia: On the inside or on the outside of physical and social places. *Dementia (London)*. 2016; 15(3): 434–52.
90. Spector A, Orrell MW. Using a biopsychosocial model of dementia as a tool to guide clinical practice. *International Psychogeriatrics*. 2010; 22(6): 957–65.
91. Black W, Almeida OP. A systematic review of the association between the Behavioral and Psychological Symptoms of Dementia and burden of care. *International Psychogeriatrics*. 2004; 16(3): 295–315.
92. Todd S, Barr S, Roberts M, Passmore AP. Survival in dementia and predictors of mortality: a review. *International Journal of Geriatric Psychiatry*. 2013; 28(11): 1109–24.
93. Beeri MS, Werner P, Davidson M, Noy S. The cost of behavioral and psychological symptoms of dementia (BPSD) in community dwelling Alzheimer's disease patients. *International Journal of Geriatric Psychiatry*. 2002; 17(5): 403–8.
94. Brody JA. An epidemiologist views senile dementia—facts and fragments. *Am J Epidemiol*. 1982; 115(2): 155–62.
95. Bond J, Farrow G, Gregson BA, Bamford C, Buck D, McNamee P, et al. Informal caregiving for frail older people at home and in long-term care institutions: who are the key supporters? *Health & Social Care in the Community*. 1999; 7(6): 434–444.
96. Feast A, Orrell M, Charlesworth G, Melunsky N, Poland F, Moniz-Cook E. Behavioural and psychological symptoms in dementia and the challenges for family carers: systematic review. *Br J Psychiatry*. 2016; 208(5): 429–34.
97. Lovheim H, Sandman PO, Karlsson S, Gustafson Y. Behavioral and psychological symptoms of dementia in relation to level of cognitive impairment. *International Psychogeriatrics*. 2008; 20(4): 777–89.
98. Purandare N, Allen NHP, Burns A. Behavioural and psychological symptoms of dementia. *Reviews in Clinical Gerontology*. 2000; 10(3): 245–60.
99. van der Linde RM, Matthews FE, Dening T, Brayne C. Patterns and persistence of behavioural and psychological symptoms in those with cognitive impairment: the importance of apathy. *Int J Geriatr Psychiatry*. 2017; 32(3): 306–15.
100. van der Linde RM, Dening T, Stephan BC, Prina AM, Evans E, Brayne C. Longitudinal course of behavioural and psychological symptoms of dementia: systematic review. *Br J Psychiatry*. 2016; 209(5): 366–77.
101. Brooker D, Latham I. *Person-Centred Dementia Care* (2nd edition). London: Jessica Kingsley, 2015.
102. James I, Fossey J. Nonpharmacological Interventions in Care Homes. Oxford: Oxford University Press, 2013. pp269–81.
103. Ballard C, Hanney ML, Theodoulou M, Douglas S, McShane R, Kossakowski K, et al. The dementia antipsychotic withdrawal trial (DART-AD): long-term follow-up of a randomised placebo-controlled trial. *Lancet Neurology*. 2009; 8(2): 151–7.
104. Vigen CL, Mack WJ, Keefe RS, Sano M, Sultzer DL, Stroup TS, et al. Cognitive effects of atypical antipsychotic medications in patients with Alzheimer's disease: outcomes from CATIE-AD. *Am J Psychiatry*. 2011; 168(8): 831–9.
105. Ballard C, Orrell M, YongZhong S, Moniz-Cook E, Stafford J, Whittaker R, et al. Impact of antipsychotic review and nonpharmacological intervention on antipsychotic use, neuropsychiatric symptoms, and mortality in people with dementia living in nursing homes: a factorial cluster-randomized controlled trial by the Well-Being and Health for People With Dementia (WHELD) Program. *Am J Psychiatry*. 2016; 173(3): 252–62.
106. Bains J, Birks J, Dening T. Antidepressants for treating depression in dementia. *Cochrane Database Syst Rev*. 2002; 4: CD003944.
107. Banerjee S, Hellier J, Dewey M, Romeo R, Ballard C, Baldwin R, et al. Sertraline or mirtazapine for depression in dementia (HTA-SADD): a randomised, multicentre, double-blind, placebo-controlled trial. *Lancet*. 2011; 378(9789): 403–11.
108. Howard RJ, Juszczak E, Ballard CG, Bentham P, Brown RG, Bullock R, et al. Donepezil for the treatment of agitation in Alzheimer's disease. *N Engl J Med*. 2007; 357(14): 1382–92.
109. Kitwood T. *Dementia Reconsidered: The Person Comes First*. Open University Press: Buckingham, 1997.
110. Lanctot KL, Aguera-Ortiz L, Brodaty H, Francis PT, Geda YE, Ismail Z, et al. Apathy associated with neurocognitive disorders: recent progress and future directions. *Alzheimer's Dement*. 2017; 13(1): 84–100.

26 Delirium

Daniel Davis, Sarah Richardson, and Esteban Sepulveda

Introduction

Delirium is an acute neuropsychiatric syndrome characterized by fluctuating inattention, changes in level of arousal, and other cognitive and perceptual deficits in the context of acute illness. Delirium is common in hospital, affecting more than one in five older inpatients.[1] As well as causing distress among patients, carers, and healthcare staff,[2] delirium results in excess treatment costs of an additional £13,000 per hospitalization.[3] Critically, delirium is independently associated with poor outcomes, including increased risk of mortality[4] and dementia.[5]

Despite the considerable patient impact, delirium is generally under-researched, well out of proportion to its prevalence. This chapter discusses the descriptive epidemiology of delirium, including methodological issues around case ascertainment in different population and clinical settings. There remains a lack of epidemiological research in the field, but there is potential for observational longitudinal studies to address key questions on the population impact of delirium and its role in punctuating trajectories of cognitive decline.

Case Ascertainment

Defining delirium

The word delirium itself is derived from the Latin 'de-lira', meaning to go out of the furrow, first used by Celsus in the 1st century AD.[6] Earlier descriptions of the syndrome were recorded by Hippocrates, who used multiple terms to describe the mental abnormalities caused by fever, poisoning, or head trauma including *phrenitis* (a state of frenzy) and *lethargus* (inertia and dulling of senses).[6]

The first formal classification only emerged with the third edition of the American Psychiatric Association's DSM (DSM-III) in 1980. This definition has subsequently evolved (DSM-5 shown in Box 26.1). The alternative nosology from the ICD definition (World Health Organization) differs from the various iterations of DSM, and several studies show how use of a given reference standard affects prevalence estimates.[7–9] However, it is probably the case that there has been insufficient field work to empirically quantify these problems with the stability of classifications over time and secular trends in how criteria are operationalized.

Validity studies on the diagnostic criteria in delirium

Valid diagnostic criteria are vital for delirium classification, determining both management and prognosis.[10] However, when reference standards drift over time, further iterations result in different proportions of a given population being diagnosed with delirium. An early study exploring the validity of DSM-III-R criteria found it to be more restrictive than DSM-III, but less so than ICD-10.[11] Later studies showed the simpler criteria in DSM-IV enhanced its inclusiveness over ICD-10.[12] In comparing DSM-III, DSM-III-R, DSM-IV, and ICD-10 in a sample of older patients from acute wards and nursing homes, 31% met any criteria, but only 6% met all four.[13] Reference standards with more detailed specifications identified lower proportions with delirium (DSM-IV 25%; DSM-III-R 20%; DSM-III 19%; ICD-10 10%), also seen in more recent comparative studies using DSM-5 criteria (Fig. 26.1).[9] When stratifying between general hospital patients and nursing home residents, DSM-III-R was more inclusive in the latter than DSM-IV. These observations have been generally replicated in a range of settings.[14–16] The performance of a given reference standard itself is a function of the underlying population tested. For delirium, this issue is greatly compounded by its frequent co-existence with other neurocognitive disorders.

With respect to delirium superimposed on dementia (DSD), there is no specific guidance for the application of delirium criteria in the context of pre-existing dementia. DSD is therefore generally evaluated with instruments used for diagnosing delirium alone.[17] This is problematic given that many of these tools rely on cognitive tests, which may be abnormal in both dementia and delirium.[18,19] Moreover, the extent to which these tools were validated in populations with comorbid dementia is often not reported. DSM–IV first tried to differentiate delirium and dementia by adding an item describing 'change in cognition or alteration of perception that cannot be accounted for by a previous dementia'. Therefore, there is a reliance on the demonstration of acute change from the patient's baseline, itself dependent on the reliability of an informant to provide an accurate collateral history. If this is not available in acute or research settings, there is a risk of delaying diagnosis or missing delirium altogether under the assumption that cognitive abnormalities are due to underlying dementia rather than delirium. This emphasizes the need for studies prospectively characterizing baseline cognitive status in delirium research, along with the need

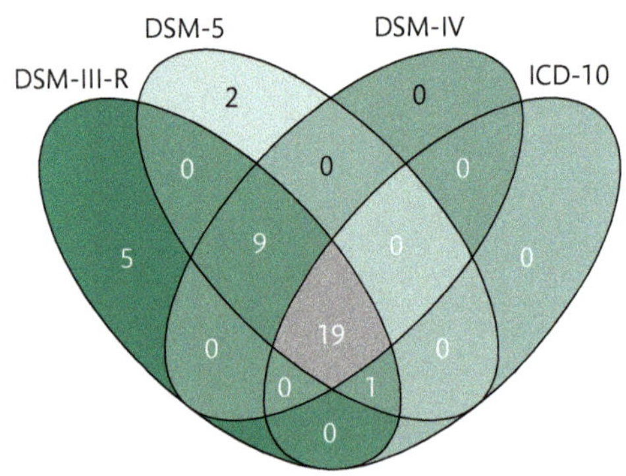

Fig. 26.1 Different diagnostic overlaps for four classifications in 36 patients with delirium in a cohort of 125 patients, 85 of whom had dementia.

Reproduced with permission from Sepulveda E, Franco JG, Trzepacz PT, Gaviria AM, Vinuelas E, Palma J, Ferre G, Grau I, Vilella E. Performance of the Delirium Rating Scale-Revised-98 Against Different Delirium Diagnostic Criteria in a Population With a High Prevalence of Dementia. *Psychosomatics*, 56(5): 530–41. Copyright © 2015 The Academy of Psychosomatic Medicine. Published by Elsevier Inc. All rights reserved. DOI: https://doi.org/10.1016/j.psym.2015.03.005.

for further research regarding the detection of delirium in people with dementia. It is not known whether it is possible to distinguish the two in a cross-sectional assessment, but some studies, focusing largely on testing attention and measuring level of arousal, suggest that this might be possible.[20–22]

If there is a fundamental difficulty with multiple reference standards identifying different sets of individuals with delirium, then there is a need for an agnostic approach to field test a range of delirium symptoms and relate these to prognostic outcomes. From the outset, nosology studies would need to be performed in populations with a wide range of diagnostic severity and complexity, and in the context of other neuropsychiatric disorders, especially dementia.[18,23] Categorizing features could be facilitated by cluster analysis without the constraint of an a priori diagnostic system.[24] As such, an empirically-based reference standard could claim primacy as well as offer better clinical utility.

Operationalizing the definition

It is clear that operationalization of delirium criteria present challenges. Inter-rater reliability studies measuring agreement have themselves been shown to be dependent on the reference criteria used. In general, when comparing kappa values for DSM-IIIR, DSM-IV, DSM-5, and ICD-10 criteria, DSM-5 performed the best (0.73) and ICD-10 the worst (0.57).[25] Performance of all criteria, but especially DSM-IIIR, has been shown to be poorer in the subset of those with dementia.[9,26]

As with any set of clinical criteria, definitions require operationalization through a history from the individual and collateral sources, physical examination, laboratory and other investigations, and assessor judgement. The DSM guidance notes notwithstanding, there are few examples of how to apply an individual diagnostic item for specific circumstances and in general, publications from the literature rarely specify the procedures used for case ascertainment.[27] In a survey of validation studies for new delirium instruments, most did not report how the delirium reference standards were actually applied, and 27% apparently did so without formal cognitive testing (i.e. using global clinical impression).[27] Of note, 15% of studies excluded patients who were too drowsy or declined to participate in delirium evaluation. This is problematic because altered arousal and drowsiness may itself be part of the impairment (clouding) of consciousness integral to the delirium presentation.

Here we use DSM-5 to demonstrate some of the issues around operationalization for delirium. The idea of impaired consciousness is a consistent feature of most delirium classifications, even if DSM-5 describes this as: 'disturbance in ... alertness (reduced orientation to the environment)'. *Impairment of consciousness* might be conceptually (even philosophically) complex, but with respect to delirium there is the specific implication that these are deficits arising through acute illness. Consciousness can be regarded as having two components, namely *level* and *content*. These are hierarchically related such that *content* of consciousness can only be tested if *level* of consciousness is sufficient. Overall, these can be considered as being on an arousal-attention axis (where arousal broadly relates to *level* and attention deficits relate to *content*).

What are the implications for delirium ascertainment if a patient's mental state cannot be assessed with formal cognitive tests? DSM-5 only offers brief guidance on diagnosing delirium when a patient's level of arousal is so impaired that they are deemed 'untestable' (Fig. 26.2). Not accounting for these patients would introduce substantial bias.[28] As above, considering arousal and attention to be on a spectrum leads to an inclusive approach whereby the inability to engage in cognitive testing or interview is considered severe inattention for the purposes of delirium diagnosis (insofar as this is precipitated by an acute illness).[29] Nonetheless, little research specifically evaluates the diagnostic accuracy of tests for inattention in delirium, thresholds for how they should be scored, and whether they vary in the context of underlying dementia or depression (see Fig. 26.3).[19]

DSM-5 presented a new issue with respect to variation in delirium ascertainment. The first empirical data found DSM-5 to be less inclusive than DSM-IV, explained mainly by the interpretation of the term 'attention and awareness'.[7] A *strict* interpretation involved both attention and awareness alteration having to be present for the first criterion and both acute onset and fluctuation having to be present for the second criterion.[30] For the *relaxed* interpretation, only inattention was required for the first criterion and either acute onset or fluctuation for the second criterion. They found the *strict*

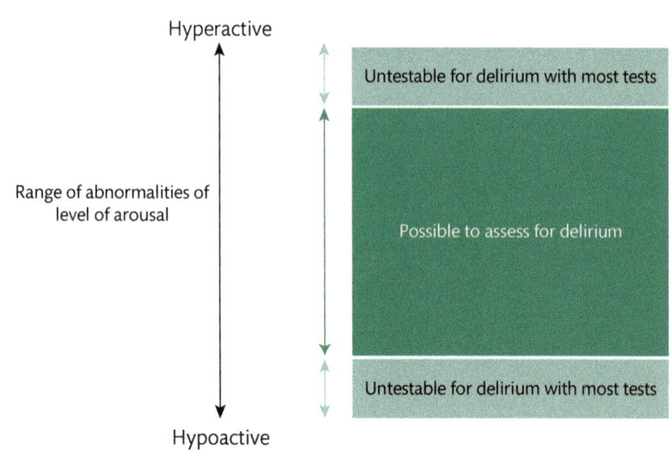

Fig. 26.2 Patients with very deranged level of arousal are unable to complete most of the tests used to assess for delirium.

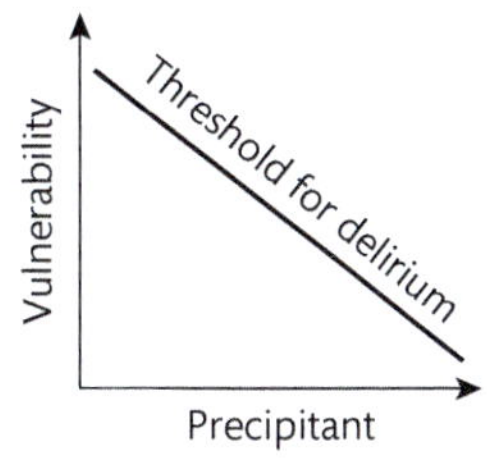

Fig. 26.3 The threshold for delirium depends on both vulnerability and the precipitant.

DSM-5 to coincide with the DSM-IV in only 53% of cases, with sensitivity of 30% and specificity of 99%, but the *relaxed* interpretation obtained a concordance of 91% (improving sensitivity to 89% and with specificity of 96%).[30]

Fluctuations are highly specific to delirium and required to fulfil Criterion B of DSM-5. However, this feature makes ascertainment more challenging, with scores from delirium instruments varying in severity during the course of the day. Due to the practical difficulties and burden of multiple assessments, both clinical and research ascertainment relies on obtaining information about the preceding few hours from an informant. The best method of capturing such information has not been evaluated. Fluctuations also make the assessment of inter-rater reliability by multiple assessors an additional concern.

Uncertainty also exists regarding Criterion E, which states that there must be evidence of an underlying medical disorder without specifying the level of evidence required. Delirium occurs as a result of a wide range of aetiological precipitants, including infections, medications, surgery, trauma, dehydration, constipation, pain, and a change of environment. There are often multiple causes and in 10% of cases, the aetiology is not apparent even after detailed evaluation.[31] It is not known whether the precipitant affects the phenomenological presentation or longer term outcomes.

Subtyping delirium on motor or arousal presentations

The original terms described by Hippocrates, *phrenitis* and *lethargicus*, now respectively correspond to *hyperactive delirium*, where patients are often more agitated and constantly moving, and *hypoactive delirium*, characterized by a reduced number and frequency of movements.[32] With the fluctuating nature of delirium, many patients present with a mixed picture when examined longitudinally. The pathophysiological basis of these contrasting clinical phenotypes remains elusive and it is possible that the treatment and outcomes of each may differ, emphasizing the need to reliably differentiate these subtypes in research studies.[33] These contrasting clinical phenotypes also mean that finding one particular test that can be used to detect all delirium in all settings is probably not appropriate or practical.[34] Additionally, many of the scores used to measure delirium severity tend to be biased towards hyperactive delirium due to the challenges of demonstrating features such as perceptual disturbances, delusions, and disorganized thinking in patients with hypoactive delirium due to their reduced level of arousal.

Summary: case ascertainment

Standardizing a definition of delirium is essential to ensure consistent case ascertainment in future research and comparability of studies. The optimal operationalization of DSM-5 for delirium is currently unclear but will require reliable and valid tests of inattention, cognition and neuropsychiatric symptoms with guidance regarding delirium status when individuals are unable to complete the tests due to advanced dementia or substantially abnormal levels of arousal. Validated methods of recording level of arousal and capturing the temporal nature of acute change are required. Until these are available, one method of improving case ascertainment of delirium in research studies is to record the components of DSM-5 and submit these descriptions to a consensus panel to determine whether delirium is present or absent. The literature also needs more detailed reporting of procedures for arriving at case ascertainment, their inter-rater reliability, and the processes they used to capture information from patients unable to participate in formal testing.

Epidemiology

Epidemiological studies in whole populations are lacking, despite the potential to answer questions of clinical significance. As discussed above, without a clear, operationalizable reference standard, the descriptive epidemiology of delirium is difficult to estimate reliably.

Community

Estimates of delirium point prevalence are lowest in community-based samples: under 0.5–1.3% for older people, with the highest rates in the oldest old (90 years and over) and those with concomitant dementia.[35–37] In a population sample of those aged 85 years and older, delirium was reported in 100 per 1000 persons surviving at three-year follow-up.[38,39]

Prevalence estimates in nursing homes and post-acute care range from 6.5% to 16%,[40–42] with higher rates identified (27–70% depending on the diagnostic system) in those with dementia[16] and physical comorbidity.[43] In a study of 261 consecutive outpatients with dementia in a memory clinic, 19% had evidence of delirium (average DRS-R98 scores 18.5; SD 5.0), with the highest proportion seen in those with vascular dementia (34%) and DLB (32%).[44]

Hospital

In an acute general hospital setting, one of the most comprehensive studies estimated a point prevalence of 19.3% among adult inpatients.[45] However, there is an important difference between wards, with the highest proportions seen on geriatric medical wards (prevalence range from 10% to 68% and incidence rates from 3% to 29%)[46–48] and intensive care units (45–87%).[49] The prevalence in orthopaedic wards ranged from 29% to 41%,[45,50] while the prevalence in general surgical wards was 7.2%,[45] with an incidence of 15–34% for older surgical patients.[51] In the emergency department, delirium prevails in older patients in a range of 7–10%.[52] A systematic review of prospective studies of delirium in adult palliative care inpatients found an incidence ranging from 3% to 45%, increasing to 59–88% in the weeks or hours preceding death.[53]

Misidentification and under-diagnosis

Despite delirium being common in a variety of settings and having important consequences for patients, their family, and health systems, it is frequently under-diagnosed. In a study of an acute general hospital in Ireland, only 44% of patients with delirium had 'delirium' or one of its synonyms documented in the case notes.[54] These figures were similar in geriatric medicine wards,[8] but even higher in the emergency department, where nearly three-quarters of cases remained undiagnosed.[55,56] This under-recognition of delirium has been associated with higher mortality and poorer functional recovery at hospital discharge and after six months,[35,57] underlining the importance of improving diagnostic methods for delirium and their implementation by healthcare professionals into routine clinical practice.

Outcomes

Mortality

Most studies consistently indicate an association with higher mortality in a variety of clinical settings. A meta-analysis of seven studies, including a total of 2957 participants in hospital or post-acute care facilities with a mean follow-up of 22.7 months (range 3–48 months) found that participants with delirium had an increased risk of death compared with controls (HR, 1.95, 95% CI, 1.51–2.52).[4] This association has also been demonstrated in critical care[58] and palliative care settings.[59]

The extent to which these associations are explained by underlying acute illness or chronic comorbidity has not been fully quantified. Generally, observational studies adjust for chronic comorbidity or acute illness, though none have accounted for both. Therefore, an important unanswered question is whether the association remains independent of acute *and* chronic health factors that might otherwise drive mortality.[60] Indeed, a more nuanced understanding of delirium and mortality is relevant given the proposal that the relationship may be bimodal.[61] That is, while delirium may have catastrophic outcomes in some patients, for others it may be an early indicator of acute illness leading to earlier recognition and treatment, perhaps even being protective.

General health/institutionalization

There are wider effects on general health as a consequence of delirium. Delirium increases rehabilitation needs,[62] and may be complicated by pressure sores and aspiration pneumonia.[5] In a study of 278 men and women aged 75 years and over, admitted acutely to a general medical service in a hospital in south Wales, delirium was associated with significantly increased lengths of stay (mean 13.1 days without delirium and 26.1 days with delirium) and significantly higher rates of residential or nursing home placement in the two years following admission.[63] Other studies have shown that functional decline is more common following delirium,[38,46,64] along with higher rates of readmission.[65] Overall, these associations are more pronounced in patients with underlying dementia.[66]

Cognitive impairment

Delirium is a strong predictor of new-onset dementia as well as acceleration of existing cognitive decline. In a population-based study of 553 participants aged 85 years and over, delirium increased the risk of incident dementia (OR 8.7, 95% CI 2.1–35).[38] Delirium was also associated with worsening dementia severity (OR 3.1, 95% CI 1.5–6.3) as well as deterioration in global function score (OR 2.8, 95% CI 1.4–5.5). On brain autopsy, it was found that the relationship did not appear to be mediated by classical neuropathologies associated with dementia. Similar findings have been demonstrated in other cohorts.[67]

Acute hospitalization itself has been shown to adversely affect trajectories of cognitive decline, even when delirium has not been specifically ascertained.[68–70] Multiple animal models of neurodegeneration have also shown that systemic inflammation exacerbates pathology[71,72] and accelerates functional decline over longer time periods.[73,74] This implies that delirium and/or its causes contribute to the overall burden of dementia. Nonetheless, the attributable fraction of delirium on future cognitive impairment is itself likely to be a function of the underlying pre-morbid cognitive impairment. In this way, delirium may have least impact when there is little or no prior cognitive impairment (no long-term decline) or when dementia is advanced (little further decline possible) compared with intermediate states of prior chronic cognitive impairment when catastrophic further decline is possible.

Conclusion

Despite being first described more than 2000 years ago, delirium remains poorly characterized as a clinical and epidemiological entity. Measuring the neuropsychiatric features is still problematic and the mechanisms are largely unknown. Much of the existing research is limited by a lack of standardization, which is underlined by the challenge of agreeing the boundaries for psychiatric symptoms. This is particularly the case where delirium presents in the context of other neurocognitive disorders. However, approaching delirium as a marker of acute brain injury—presenting as changes in level and content of consciousness—has been an important recent change in perspective. While there are estimates of delirium prevalence in several clinical and population settings, little work has described the cumulative incidence of delirium in cohort studies. Prospectively ascertaining delirium in longitudinal samples as it punctuates trajectories of cognitive decline would start addressing questions of major significance to patients, their families and the population as a whole.

REFERENCES

1. Bellelli G, Morandi A, Di Santo SG, Mazzone A, Cherubini A, Mossello E, et al. 'Delirium Day': a nationwide point prevalence study of delirium in older hospitalized patients using an easy standardized diagnostic tool. *BMC Medicine*. 2016; 14(1): 1–12.
2. Partridge JS, Martin FC, Harari D, Dhesi JK. The delirium experience: what is the effect on patients, relatives and staff and what can be done to modify this? *International Journal of Geriatric Psychiatry*. 2013; 28: 804–12.
3. Akunne A, Murthy L, Young J. Cost-effectiveness of multi-component interventions to prevent delirium in older people admitted to medical wards. *Age and Ageing*. 2012: 41(3): 285–91.
4. Witlox J, Eurelings LS, de Jonghe JF, Kalisvaart KJ, Eikelenboom P, van Gool WA. Delirium in elderly patients and the risk of postdischarge mortality, institutionalization, and dementia: a meta-analysis. *JAMA*. 2010; 304(4): 443–51.

5. Fong TG, Davis D, Growdon ME, Albuquerque A, Inouye SK. The interface between delirium and dementia in elderly adults. *Lancet Neurology.* 2015; 14(8): 823–32.
6. Adamis D, Treloar A, Martin FC, Macdonald AJ. A brief review of the history of delirium as a mental disorder. *History of Psychiatry.* 2007; 18(72 Pt 4): 459–69.
7. Adamis D, Rooney S, Meagher D, Mulligan O, McCarthy G. A comparison of delirium diagnosis in elderly medical inpatients using the CAM, DRS-R98, DSM-IV and DSM-5 criteria. *International Psychogeriatrics.* 2015; 27(6): 883–9.
8. Laurila JV, Pitkala KH, Strandberg TE, Tilvis RS. Impact of different diagnostic criteria on prognosis of delirium: a prospective study. *Dementia and Geriatric Cognitive Disorders.* 2004; 18(3–4): 240–4.
9. Sepulveda E, Franco JG, Trzepacz PT, Gaviria AM, Vinuelas E, Palma J, et al. Performance of the delirium rating scale-revised-98 against different delirium diagnostic criteria in a population with a high prevalence of dementia. *Psychosomatics.* 2015; 56(5): 530–41.
10. Regier DA, Kuhl EA, Kupfer DJ. The DSM-5: classification and criteria changes. *World Psychiatry.* 2013; 12(2): 92–8.
11. Liptzin B, Levkoff SE, Cleary PD, Pilgrim DM, Reilly CH, Albert M, et al. An empirical study of diagnostic criteria for delirium. *Am J Psychiatry.* 1991; 148(4): 454–7.
12. Laurila JV, Pitkala KH, Strandberg TE, Tilvis RS. Delirium among patients with and without dementia: does the diagnosis according to the DSM-IV differ from the previous classifications? *International Journal of Geriatric Psychiatry.* 2004; 19(3): 271–7.
13. Laurila JV, Pitkala KH, Strandberg TE, Tilvis RS. The impact of different diagnostic criteria on prevalence rates for delirium. *Dementia and Geriatric Cognitive Disorders.* 2003; 16(3): 156–62.
14. Cole MG, Dendukuri N, McCusker J, Han L. An empirical study of different diagnostic criteria for delirium among elderly medical inpatients. *Journal of Neuropsychiatry and Clinical Neurosciences.* 2003; 15(2): 200–7.
15. Kazmierski J, Kowman M, Banach M, Fendler W, Okonski P, Banys A, et al. Incidence and predictors of delirium after cardiac surgery: results from the IPDACS Study. *Journal of Psychosomatic Research.* 2010; 69(2): 179–85.
16. Voyer P, Richard S, Doucet L, Carmichael P-H. Detecting delirium and subsyndromal delirium using different diagnostic criteria among demented long-term care residents. *Journal of the American Medical Directors Association.* 2009; 10(3): 181–8.
17. Morandi A, McCurley J, Vasilevskis EE, Fick DM, Bellelli G, Lee P, et al. Tools to detect delirium superimposed on dementia: a systematic review. *J Am Geriatr Soc.* 2012; 60: 2005–13.
18. Meagher DJ, Leonard M, Donnelly S, Conroy M, Saunders J, Trzepacz PT. A comparison of neuropsychiatric and cognitive profiles in delirium, dementia, comorbid delirium-dementia and cognitively intact controls. *Journal of Neurology, Neurosurgery and Psychiatry.* 2010; 81(8): 876–81.
19. Tieges Z, Brown LJE, MacLullich AMJ. Objective assessment of attention in delirium: a narrative review. *International Journal of Geriatric Psychiatry.* 2014; 29(12): 1185–97.
20. Brown LJE, Ferner HS, Robertson J, Mills NL, Pessotto R, Deary IJ, et al. Differential effects of delirium on fluid and crystallized cognitive abilities. *Archives of Gerontology and Geriatrics.* 2011; 52(2): 153–8.
21. Chester JG, Harrington MB, Rudolph JL. Serial administration of a modified richmond agitation and sedation scale for delirium screening. *J Hosp Med.* 2012; 7: 450–3.
22. Tieges Z, McGrath A, Hall RJ, Maclullich AM. Abnormal level of arousal as a predictor of delirium and inattention: an exploratory study. *American Journal of Geriatric Psychiatry: official journal of the American Association for Geriatric Psychiatry.* 2013; 21(12): 1244–53.
23. Davis DHJ, Kreisel SH, Muniz Terrera G, Hall AJ, Morandi A, Boustani M, et al. The epidemiology of delirium: challenges and opportunities for population studies. *American Journal of Geriatric Psychiatry: official journal of the American Association for Geriatric Psychiatry.* 2013; 21(12): 1173–89.
24. Franco JG, Trzepacz PT, Meagher DJ, Kean J, Lee Y, Kim JL, et al. Three core domains of delirium validated using exploratory and confirmatory factor analyses. *Psychosomatics.* 2013; 54(3): 227–38.
25. Sepulveda E, Franco JG, Trzepacz PT, Gaviria AM, Meagher DJ, Palma J, et al. Delirium diagnosis defined by cluster analysis of symptoms versus diagnosis by DSM and ICD criteria: diagnostic accuracy study. *BMC Psychiatry.* 2016; 16: 167.
26. Malt UF, Huyse FJ, Herzog T, Lobo A, Rijssenbeek AJ. The ECLW Collaborative Study: III. Training and reliability of ICD-10 psychiatric diagnoses in the general hospital setting—an investigation of 220 consultants from 14 European countries. European Consultation Liaison Workgroup. *Journal of Psychosomatic Research.* 1996; 41(5): 451–63.
27. Neufeld KJ. Delirium classification by the Diagnostic and Statistical Manual—a moving target. *International Psychogeriatrics.* 2015; 27(6): 881–2.
28. Jackson TA, MacLullich AMJ, Gladman JRF, Lord JM, Sheehan B. Undiagnosed long-term cognitive impairment in acutely hospitalised older medical patients with delirium: a prospective cohort study. *Age and Ageing.* 2016; 45(4): 493–9.
29. European Delirium Association, American Delirium Society: The DSM-5 criteria, level of arousal and delirium diagnosis: inclusiveness is safer. *BMC Medicine.* 2014; 12: 141.
30. Davis D, Barnes L, Stephan B, MacLullich A, Meagher D, Copeland J, et al. The descriptive epidemiology of delirium symptoms in a large population-based cohort study: results from the Medical Research Council Cognitive Function and Ageing Study (MRC CFAS). *BMC Geriatrics.* 2014; 14(1): 87.
31. Meagher DJ, Maclullich AM, Laurila JV. Defining delirium for the International Classification of Diseases, 11th Revision. *Journal of Psychosomatic Research* 2008; 65(3): 207–14.
32. Lipowski ZJ. Transient cognitive disorders (delirium, acute confusional states) in the elderly. *Am J Psychiatry.* 1983; 140(11): 1426–36.
33. Meagher D. Motor subtypes of delirium: Past, present and future. *International Review of Psychiatry.* 2009; 21(1): 59–73.
34. Voyer P, Champoux N, Desrosiers J, Landreville P, Monette J, Savoie M, et al. Assessment of inattention in the context of delirium screening: one size does not fit all! *International Psychogeriatrics.* 2016; 28(8): 1293–301.
35. Andrew MK, Freter SH, Rockwood K. Prevalence and outcomes of delirium in community and non-acute care settings in people without dementia: A report from the Canadian study of health and aging. *BMC Medicine.* 2006; 4: 15.
36. Vilalta-Franch J, Llinas-Regla J, Lopez-Pousa S, Garre-Olmo J. Prevalence and evolution of delirium in a community population of 70 years and older. *Actas Esp Psiquiatr.* 2009; 37(1): 27–33.
37. Folstein MF, Bassett SS, Romanoski AJ, Nestadt G. The epidemiology of delirium in the community: the Eastern Baltimore Mental Health Survey. *Int Psychogeriatr.* 1991; 3(2): 169–76.

38. Davis DH, Muniz Terrera G, Keage H, Rahkonen T, Oinas M, Matthews FE, et al. Delirium is a strong risk factor for dementia in the oldest-old: a population-based cohort study. *Brain: a Journal of Neurology*. 2012; 135(Pt 9): 2809–16.
39. Rahkonen T, Eloniemi-Sulkava U, Halonen P, Verkkoniemi A, Niinisto L, Notkola IL, et al. Delirium in the non-demented oldest old in the general population: risk factors and prognosis. *International Journal of Geriatric Psychiatry*. 2001; 16(4): 415–21.
40. Boorsma M, Joling KJ, Frijters DH, Ribbe ME, Nijpels G, van Hout HP. The prevalence, incidence and risk factors for delirium in Dutch nursing homes and residential care homes. *Int J Geriatr Psychiatry*. 2012; 27(7): 709–15.
41. Kiely DK, Bergmann MA, Jones RN, Murphy KM, Orav EJ, Marcanotnio ER. Characteristics associated with delirium persistence among newly admitted post-acute facility patients. *J Gerontol A Biol Sci Med Sci*. 2004; 59(4): 344–9.
42. von Gunten A, Mosimann UP. Delirium upon admission to Swiss nursing homes: a cross-sectional study. *Swiss Med Wkly*. 2010; 140(25–26): 376–81.
43. McCusker J, Cole MG, Voyer P, Monette J, Champoux N, Ciampi A, et al. Prevalence and incidence of delirium in long-term care. *Int J Geriatr Psychiatry*. 2011; 26(11): 1152–61.
44. Hasegawa N, Hashimoto M, Yuuki S, Honda K, Yatabe Y, Araki K, et al. Prevalence of delirium among outpatients with dementia. *International Psychogeriatrics*. 2013; 25(11): 1877–83.
45. Ryan DJ, O'Regan NA, Caoimh RO, Clare J, O'Connor M, Leonard M, et al. Delirium in an adult acute hospital population: predictors, prevalence and detection. *BMJ Open*. 2013; 3(1): e001772.
46. Buurman BM, Hoogerduijn JG, de Haan R, Abu-Hanna A, Lagaay AM, Verhaar HJ, et al. Geriatric conditions in acutely hospitalized older patients: prevalence and one-year survival and functional decline. *PLOS One*. 2011; 6(11): e26951.
47. Eeles EMP, Hubbard RE, White SV, O'Mahoney S, Savva GM, Bayer AJ. Hospital use, institutionalisation and mortality associated with delirium. *Age and Ageing*. 2010; 39: 470–5.
48. Siddiqi N, House AO, Holmes JD. Occurrence and outcome of delirium in medical in-patients: a systematic literature review. *Age and Ageing*. 2006; 35: 350–64.
49. Jackson P, Khan A. Delirium in critically ill patients. *Crit Care Clin*. 2015; 31(3): 589–603.
50. Albrecht JS, Marcantonio ER, Roffey DM, Orwig D, Magaziner J, Terrin M, et al. Stability of postoperative delirium psychomotor subtypes in individuals with hip fracture. *J Am Geriatr Soc*. 2015; 63(5): 970–6.
51. de Castro SM, Unlu C, Tuynman JB, Honig A, van Wagensveld BA, Steller EP, et al. Incidence and risk factors of delirium in the elderly general surgical patient. *Am J Surg*. 2014; 208(1): 26–32.
52. Han JH, Zimmerman EE, Cutler N, Schnelle J, Morandi A, Dittus RS, et al. Delirium in older emergency department patients: recognition, risk factors, and psychomotor subtypes. *Academic Emergency Medicine*. 2009; 16(3): 193–200.
53. Hosie A, Davidson PM, Agar M, Sanderson CR, Phillips J. Delirium prevalence, incidence, and implications for screening in specialist palliative care inpatient settings: a systematic review. *Palliative Medicine*. 2013; 27: 486–98.
54. Kuhn E, Du X, McGrath K, Coveney S, O'Regan N, Richardson S, et al. Validation of a consensus method for identifying delirium from hospital records. *PLOS One*. 2014; 9(11): e111823.
55. Collins N, Blanchard MR, Tookman A, Sampson EL. Detection of delirium in the acute hospital. *Age Ageing*. 2010; 39(1): 131–5.
56. Han JH, Shintani A, Eden S, Morandi A, Solberg LM, Schnelle J, et al. Delirium in the emergency department: an independent predictor of death within six months. *Annals of Emergency Medicine*. 2010; 56(3): 244–52.
57. Kakuma R, du Fort GG, Arsenault L, Perrault A, Platt RW, Monette J, et al. Delirium in older emergency department patients discharged home: effect on survival. *J Am Geriatr Soc*. 2003; 51(4): 443–50.
58. Salluh JI, Wang H, Schneider EB, Nagaraja N, Yenokyan G, Damluji A, et al. Outcome of delirium in critically ill patients: systematic review and meta-analysis. *BMJ*. 2015; 350: h2538.
59. Lawlor PG, Gagnon B, Mancini IL, Pereira JL, Hanson J, Suarez-Almazor ME, et al. Occurrence, causes, and outcome of delirium in patients with advanced cancer: a prospective study. *Archives of Internal Medicine*. 2000; 160(6): 786–94.
60. Bellelli G, Frisoni GB, Turco R, Lucchi E, Magnifico F, Trabucchi M. Delirium superimposed on dementia predicts 12-month survival in elderly patients discharged from a postacute rehabilitation facility. *J Gerontol A Biol Sci Med Sci*. 2007; 62(11): 1306–9.
61. Jackson TA, Wilson D, Richardson S, Lord JM. Predicting outcome in older hospital patients with delirium: a systematic literature review. *Int J Geriatr Psychiatry*. 2016; 31(4): 392–9.
62. Morandi A, Davis D, Fick DM, Turco R, Boustani M, Lucchi E, et al. Delirium superimposed on dementia strongly predicts worse outcomes in older rehabilitation inpatients. *Journal of the American Medical Directors Association*. 2014; 15(5): 349–54.
63. Eeles EM, Hubbard RE, White SV, O'Mahony MS, Savva GM, Bayer AJ. Hospital use, institutionalisation and mortality associated with delirium. *Age Ageing*. 2010; 39(4): 470–5.
64. Marcantonio ER, Simon SE, Bergmann MA, Jones RN, Murphy KM, Morris JN. Delirium symptoms in post-acute care: prevalent, persistent, and associated with poor functional recovery. *J Am Geriatr Soc*. 2003; 51(1): 4–9.
65. Marcantonio ER, Kiely DK, Simon SE, John Orav E, Jones RN, Murphy KM, et al. Outcomes of older people admitted to postacute facilities with delirium. *J Am Geriatr Soc*. 2005; 53(6): 963–9.
66. Fong TG, Jones RN, Marcantonio ER, Tommet D, Gross AL, Habtemariam D, et al. Adverse outcomes after hospitalization and delirium in persons with Alzheimer disease. *Ann Intern Med*. 2012; 156(12): 848–56, W296.
67. Davis DH, Muniz-Terrera G, Keage HA, Stephan BC, Fleming J, Ince PG, et al. Association of delirium with cognitive decline in late life: a neuropathologic study of 3 population-based cohort studies. *JAMA Psychiatry*. 2017; 74(3): 244–51.
68. Ehlenbach WJ, Hough CL, Crane PK, Haneuse SJ, Carson SS, Curtis JR, et al. Association between acute care and critical illness hospitalization and cognitive function in older adults. *JAMA*. 2010; 303(8): 763–70.
69. Wilson RS, Hebert LE, Scherr PA, Dong X, Leurgens SE, Evans DA. Cognitive decline after hospitalization in a community population of older persons. *Neurology*. 2012; 78(13): 950–6.
70. Mathews SB, Arnold SE, Epperson CN. Hospitalization and cognitive decline: Can the nature of the relationship be deciphered? *American Journal of Geriatric Psychiatry: Official Journal of the American Association for Geriatric Psychiatry*. 2014; 22(5): 465–80.

71. Cunningham C, Wilcockson DC, Campion S, Lunnon K, Perry VH. Central and systemic endotoxin challenges exacerbate the local inflammatory response and increase neuronal death during chronic neurodegeneration. *J Neurosci.* 2005; 25(40): 9275–84.
72. Kitazawa M, Oddo S, Yamasaki TR, Green KN, LaFerla FM. Lipopolysaccharide-induced inflammation exacerbates tau pathology by a cyclin-dependent kinase 5-mediated pathway in a transgenic model of Alzheimer's disease. *Journal of Neuroscience: the official journal of the Society for Neuroscience.* 2005; 25(39): 8843–53.
73. Cunningham C, Campion S, Lunnon K, Murray CL, Woods JF, Deacon RM, et al. Systemic inflammation induces acute behavioral and cognitive changes and accelerates neurodegenerative disease. *Biol Psychiatry.* 2009; 65(4): 304–12.
74. Cerejeira J, Firmino H, Vaz-Serra A, Mukaetova-Ladinska EB. The neuroinflammatory hypothesis of delirium. *Acta Neuropathol (Berl).* 2010; 119(6): 737–54.

27

Methods and approaches to examining the interface of late-life depression and dementia

Mirjam I Geerlings

Introduction: Dementia

As a result of increased life expectancy, the size of the older population will double from 10% currently to 20% in 2050. This implies fundamental changes to the population structure. For the first time in history, the number of people aged 60 years or older will outnumber those of children (www.un.org). These changes are likely to have a profound influence on individuals' lives. The shift in population characteristics will also have tremendous impact on healthcare and society because age-related diseases will increase with it, of which dementia will be the most important.[1,2]

Dementia is a clinical syndrome characterized by progressive memory impairment and "decline" may be better here in other cognitive domains, such as orientation in time and place, planning, judgement, language, and performing routine tasks.[3,4] When dementia progresses, it leads to loss of autonomy and independence,[5] with an increased risk of death.[6,7]

The most common causes of dementia are AD, accounting for about 70% of all dementia cases,[8,9] and cerebrovascular disease[10] or the co-existence of these two.[11] Pathologically, dementia is characterized by accumulation of neurofibrillary tangles, amyloid plaques, and cerebral infarctions.[10,12] Because dementia is a clinical syndrome, definite diagnosis of the disease can only be confirmed post-mortem.[4]

With increasing age, prevalence and incidence of dementia increase exponentially.[8,13–17] At age 85 years and older, >30% of the population may have AD.[17] It has been estimated that >35 million persons had dementia worldwide in 2010, a number that increased to >45 million in 2015,[18] and this number will increase to 115–140 million persons in 2050.[18,19] Dementia may become the third leading cause of death after heart disease and cancer.[6,7] In Europe, dementia ranks second for all brain disorders with respect to total economic costs, with mood disorders ranking first. Costs for dementia were estimated to be >800 billion US dollars worldwide in 2015 and are expected to increase.[18] The greatest majority of these costs result from direct non-medical costs, such as nursing homes.[2] Although recent reports suggest that the prevalence and incidence of dementia may be declining,[20] the increase in the older population will still confront us with great challenges in the next decades, one of which will be to maintain cognitive functioning in later life.

Co-occurrence of Depression and Dementia

Non-cognitive symptoms, such as changes in mood and personality, are also frequently seen in patients with dementia[21–23] and are the most important contributor to the burden of disease; quality of life is reduced, not only of patients but also of caregivers, leading to increased healthcare and societal costs.[24] Non-cognitive symptoms are also associated with poorer outcome, including misuse of medication, earlier hospitalization, and increased risk of death.[24]

One of the most common non-cognitive symptoms in dementia, particularly in AD, is depression. It has been estimated that 30–50% of patients with AD have clinically relevant depressive symptoms or clinical depression.[25,26] To compare, clinically relevant depressive symptoms are present in 10–15% of older persons without dementia, and a diagnosis of major depressive disorder (MDD) in older persons without dementia is estimated to occur in 2–3%.[27,28]

Depression and dementia not only frequently co-occur, they also show a temporal relationship. Many prospective studies have shown that depression occurring later in life, that is, late-life depression, increases the risk of future dementia, including AD and vascular dementia.[29–34] Overall, this risk has consistently been estimated to be two times higher for persons with late-life depression compared to those without depression for all-cause dementia, while it is less consistent for AD and vascular dementia. One meta-analysis showed somewhat higher estimates for vascular dementia than for AD,[32] and another meta-analysis found no difference between AD and vascular dementia.[33] It has been estimated that 10–15% of dementia cases may be attributable to depression, which is more than estimated for cardiovascular risk factors.[35] If depression

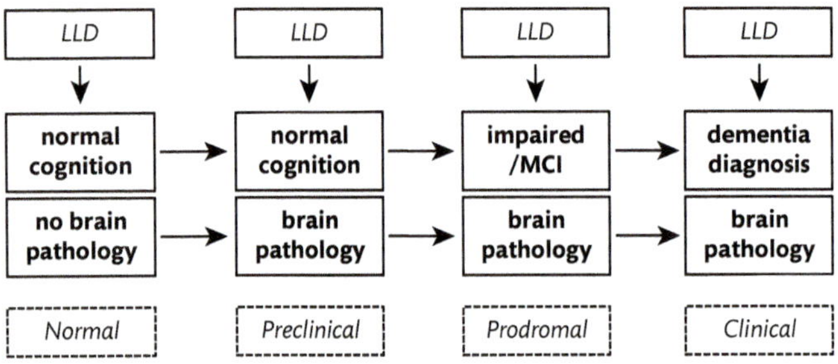

Fig. 27.1 Different stages at which late-life depression (LLD) may influence risk of dementia.

is a causal contributor to dementia, it would make depression a timely and important candidate for preventive or therapeutic intervention, particularly given the disappointing results of clinical trials targeting amyloid beta that have raised renewed interest in environmental risk factors for dementia.[36] However, the relationship is not straightforward, partly because the neurobiological mechanisms underlying the relation between late-life depression and dementia are not fully understood, partly because late-life depression can exert its influence at different stages of the dementia disease process (Fig. 27.1).

Neurotoxicity Hypothesis

The observation that depression increases the risk of future dementia has led to the hypothesis that depression is causally related to development of dementia in some persons. The prevailing causal hypothesis to explain the relation between late-life depression and risk of dementia is the *neurotoxicity hypothesis*,[37] which has also been referred to as the 'glucocorticoid-cascade hypothesis',[38] originating mainly from animal studies but also, at least indirectly, supported by studies in humans. Animal studies have shown that severe stress has neurotoxic effects on the hippocampus,[39–41] and observational studies have shown that late-life depression is associated with hyperactivity of the hypothalamic-pituitary-adrenal (HPA) axis[42,43] and with hippocampal volume reduction.[44] Also, in humans higher levels of cortisol have been found to be related to neurodegeneration[44–46] and poorer cognitive functioning over time,[47] particularly in participants carrying the APOE-4 allele,[48] which is the main genetic risk factor for AD. Because hippocampal volume atrophy is associated with increased risk of dementia and AD, even in older persons with normal cognition,[49] and the HPA axis is inhibited by the hippocampus,[50] a cascade is hypothesized to occur in which age-associated hippocampal atrophy would lead to diminished ability of the hippocampus to inhibit cortisol and, in turn, further atrophy of the hippocampus as a result of neurotoxic effects of glucocorticoids,[51] eventually leading to development of clinical dementia (Fig. 27.2).[31,46] Importantly, while this hypothesis has dominated the field of epidemiology studying the interface of depression and dementia, there are no studies that have examined the relationship between late-life depression, HPA axis functioning, hippocampal atrophy, and risk of dementia within one study and using a prospective design.[44] Convincing support for this hypothesis is thus not available and needs further investigation.

Vascular Hypothesis

Another frequently proposed explanation for the relationship between late-life depression and dementia is the *vascular hypothesis*,[52,53] stating that depression precedes dementia through small vessel ischaemic changes in mood-regulating brain areas,[54–57] originating from clinical and epidemiological studies that depression may increase the risk of cardiovascular disease,[58–60] and that cardiovascular risk factors and vascular brain pathology may play an important role in the aetiology of dementia.[34,61–64] Consistent with the 'vascular depression' hypothesis,[65,66] late-life depression is associated with vascular lesions as seen on brain MRI, including white matter hyperintensities and lacunar infarcts,[55] and with specific cognitive deficits, including problems with attention and executive functioning.[67] The direction of causation is more ambiguous in this hypothesis.[67] Depression may lead to dementia through its risk on vascular disease and vascular brain pathology, but depression and dementia may also be co-occurring as a result of vascular disease and vascular brain pathology. To what extent late-life depression is a cause or a consequence of vascular risk has not been fully elucidated, but studies suggest a bi-directional relationship.[68–71] While it may seem that the neurotoxicity hypothesis and the vascular hypothesis explain separate underlying processes, they likely influence each other or interact (Fig. 27.3). For instance, it is known that in AD small vessel lesions are frequent findings in the brain[72] and HPA axis hyperactivity may lead to increased risk of vascular disease through, for instance, inflammatory processes.[73]

Cause or Consequence?

The observation that late-life depression increases dementia risk does not necessarily mean that it is a causal factor for the onset of dementia. Because of the long preclinical phase of dementia development, late-life depression may represent a preclinical or prodromal phase of dementia development, and not be a true risk factor of the disease, even if it occurs many years before the

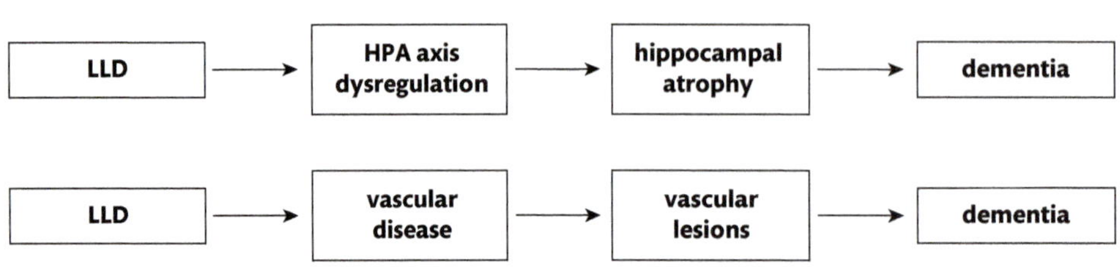

Fig. 27.2 Two main hypothesized pathways (neurotoxicity and vascular) through which late-life depression (LLD) contributes to risk of dementia.

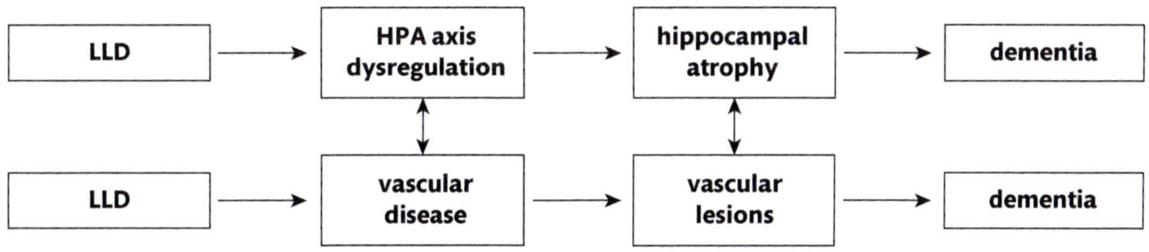

Fig. 27.3 Two main hypothesized pathways (neurotoxicity and vascular) through which late-life depression (LLD) contributes to risk of dementia. This figure shows that the hypothesized underlying mechanisms may interact.

clinical diagnosis of AD (Fig. 27.4). In general, a prodromal stage of dementia is more likely if late-life depression occurs with onset close to dementia diagnosis, while depression more than 15 years prior to dementia diagnosis may be a risk factor. Findings from longitudinal studies are that the risk of dementia became stronger with longer time interval between depression and clinical onset of AD,[30,74] that a dose-response relationship existed between number of previous depressive episodes and AD risk,[75] and that the risk for dementia was stronger for early-onset depression compared with late-onset depression.[76] Other studies, however, have found that the association became stronger with a shorter interval between the diagnoses of depression and dementia[77–79] and these findings have been interpreted as being supportive of the hypothesis that depression is a prodromal factor of dementia. It should be noted that an alternative explanation for these latter findings is that late-life depression and dementia share common causes and therefore occur close in time.

Trajectories of Depressive Symptoms

Another approach to increase our understanding of the relationship between late-life depression and dementia is to study trajectories of depressive symptoms or episodes over time before the development of dementia—as opposed to one measurement further or closer in time before dementia diagnosis. In a large population-based study of older persons without dementia, at the start of the study, ten-year trajectories of depressive symptoms before dementia diagnosis were examined. It was observed that older persons with an increase in depressive symptoms over time had an increased risk of developing dementia, including AD, compared to those with a trajectory of low levels of depressive symptoms.[80] Another large population-based study with 28 years of follow-up observed that there was no increased risk for dementia between 28 years and ten years before dementia diagnosis, while depressive symptoms up to ten years before diagnosis increased the risk of dementia, with a stronger association with shorter interval between measurement of depressive symptoms and dementia diagnosis.[81] These studies suggest that depressive symptoms are more likely a prodromal factor, or that they share common causes, than a causal factor in the development of dementia. They also elegantly show that the interpretation of cause or consequence depends on the timing of measurement of depressive symptoms.

Neurobiological Substrates

Many studies investigated the relationship between late-life depression and neurobiological substrates in older populations without dementia or cognitive impairment. Studies have shown that late-life depression is associated with smaller hippocampal volume[44,82] and with white matter hyperintensities[55] in persons without dementia. Further, there is some evidence that HPA axis dysregulation is associated with reduced hippocampal volume[44] in older persons without dementia, and HPA axis dysregulation has been observed in late-life depression.[43] Advantages of this approach are that the relationship between late-life depression and underlying neurobiological substrates is studied before dementia onset, and that these studies shed light on potential underlying mechanisms. A limitation is that dementia outcomes are not included in this approach. Another issue that limits the interpretation of these findings is that the greatest majority of existing studies are cross-sectional, and it is therefore not clear to what extent late-life depression is a cause

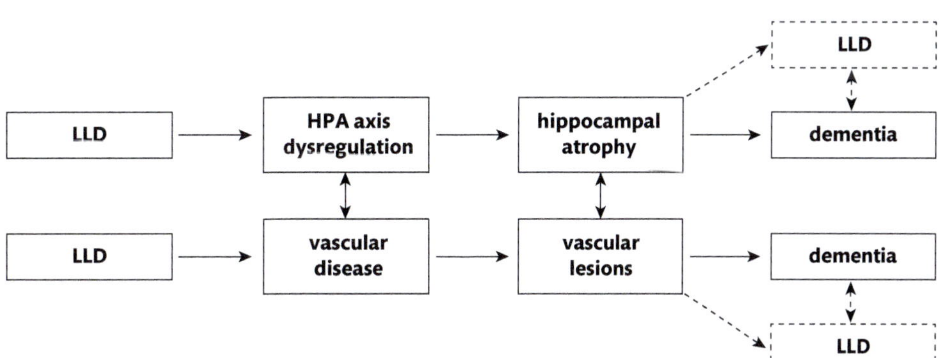

Fig. 27.4 Two main hypothesized pathways (neurotoxicity and vascular) through which late-life depression (LLD) contributes to risk of dementia. The dotted lines indicate that LLD may also be a consequence of (underlying mechanisms of) dementia.

of HPA axis dysfunctioning, hippocampal volume reduction, and increase in white matter hyperintensities. Indeed, more recent evidence suggests that pre-existing smaller hippocampal volume may be a susceptibility factor for depression.[83–85]

Prospective studies that investigated hippocampal volume decline over time associated with depression and, vice versa, the onset of depression associated with hippocampal volume, are relatively scarce and reported ambiguous results. In one prospective population-based study, depressive symptoms were associated with greater decline in hippocampal volume,[86] but not in another,[87] and only in women in another study.[88] In the first study, hippocampal volume was not associated with incident depression,[86] while in two other studies smaller hippocampal volume was associated with an increase in depressive symptoms over time.[89,90] With respect to the temporal relationship between white matter hyperintensities and late-life depression, results of a meta-analysis showed a small but statistically significantly increased risk for incidence of depression in persons with more white matter hyperintensities.[91]

Design, Sample Size, Confounding

Apart from the fact that most studies examining neurobiological correlates of late-life depression are cross-sectional, other methodological issues also need to be considered when interpreting existing evidence. One is the study design. In general, case-control studies found stronger relationships between late-life depression and hippocampal volume reduction than cohort studies, as was found in a meta-analysis.[44] One explanation for this difference is that a greater contrast between cases and controls exists with respect to hippocampal volume, because the effect estimate was also stronger when a clinical diagnosis was used to identify persons with late-life depression as opposed to a symptom questionnaire. Case-control studies almost invariably select patients based on clinical diagnoses. Compared to cohort studies, case-control studies are thus more likely to include true cases or more severe cases of depression. However, another explanation is that the effect size in case-control studies is overestimated. Case-control studies are prone to selection bias and the effect size is overestimated, for instance if very healthy controls, with healthy brains, are selectively over-represented, or if more severely depressed cases are selectively over-represented.

Confounding is another issue, particularly in existing case-control studies. Most case-control studies match cases and controls on age and sex, and do not further adjust for potential confounders such as cardiovascular risk factors.[44] Perhaps more important, in case-control studies the majority of patients with MDD included are on antidepressant medication, while the controls are not,[44] and observed differences in hippocampal volume between cases and controls may be explained, not by the depression itself but by the effects of medication. While it may be problematic to properly control for antidepressants or to include representative cases without antidepressants use,[92] studies should at least report the medication history of patients included.

Another issue is sample size. The meta-analysis also showed that the effect estimates were stronger for studies with sample size of fewer than 100 participants, while no relationship between late-life depression and hippocampal volume was observed in studies that had a total sample size of >=100.[44] Other factors that showed stronger effect estimates were: the setting, with studies using inpatients and/or outpatients showing stronger associations than community-based studies; the quality of studies, with studies of lower quality showing stronger associations; and segmentation method, with studies using manual segmentation of the hippocampus showing stronger associations than studies using automated segmentation.[44] Whereas sample size appeared to be the factor that explained most of the heterogeneity, it should be noted that most other factors that moderated the effect size tend to cluster together, that is, case-control design, inpatients and outpatients, clinical diagnosis, smaller sample size, and studies with lower quality, which makes them difficult to disentangle. It is thus important that studies take these factors into consideration and preferably combine the strengths of both designs by using a community-dwelling cohort design, a clinical diagnosis, including lifetime history, of late-life depression, and a large sample size such that a sufficiently large number of depression cases are obtained.

Definition and Measurement of Late-life Depression

Another methodological issue when studying the relationship between depression and dementia is the measurement and definition of late-life depression. Late-life depression is used for a clinical diagnosis of MDD but also for scores above a cut-off on a certain depressive symptom questionnaire.[27,93] Also, some studies define late-life depression based on one or two questions[94] or a depressive symptom questionnaire in combination with the use of antidepressant medication.[95,96] These different assessments of late-life depression can result in different relationships with dementia and underlying brain abnormalities. A meta-analysis showed that a clinical diagnosis of MDD was more strongly associated with hippocampal volume reduction in older persons without dementia than late-life depression based on a symptom questionnaire.[44] Similarly, another meta-analysis showed that a clinical diagnosis showed a stronger association with dementia incidence.[33] Interestingly, this latter study also showed that the association was stronger when a more stringent cut-off score on depressive symptom questionnaires was used.[33]

Early Onset vs Late Onset Depression

The definition of late-life depression includes depression occurring later in life, including first episodes as well as recurring episodes. To investigate the history of depressive episodes, a distinction is often made between late-onset depression (LOD) and early-onset depression (EOD). EOD is defined as a first onset of depression earlier in life, and LOD as a first onset later in life. This differentiation can give important insights into the role of late-life depression in the aetiology of dementia and neurobiological correlates. For instance, based on the neurotoxicity hypothesis it would be predicted that particularly early-onset depression is associated with more severe hippocampal atrophy and risk of AD[76] because of longer exposure to neurotoxic high levels of glucocorticoids.[97] However, a meta-analysis showed that particularly late-onset depression was related to smaller hippocampal volumes.[44] Consistent with this, a study in community-dwelling older persons without dementia found that current depression, but not past depression, was associated with volume reduction in brain tissue regions, including the hippocampus.[98] Also, late-onset depression has been associated with more white matter hyperintensities compared to early-onset depression,[55] but late-onset depression has also been found to increase risk of AD, while recurrent early-onset depression has been found to increase vascular dementia.[54] This may seem contradictory but may partly be explained by the age cut-off used in studies to define late-onset and early onset depression. This cut-off varies between 45 and 60 years, which may be a critical period in life when the first brain changes occur that may lead to dementia 20 years later.[44] The early-onset vs late-onset distinction thus does not capture the heterogeneity in history of depressive episodes. Relatively few older persons have a first onset of depression[98] and the majority of older persons with a history of depressive episodes may have a wide variety of histories, that potentially have different aetiologies and risk factor profiles. Some may have had a first depressive episode at 20 years of age that did not recur until age 60, while others may have had a course of multiple chronic or intermittent episodes. Adding to this, at older age the risk factor profile of early-onset depression may have changed due to selective survival and may have become more different or similar in aetiology than late-onset depression. This may lead to biased associations with dementia risk or underlying brain changes.[44] While the latter issue is difficult to prevent, it is important that studies obtain a detailed history of depressive episodes, including the age of onset but also whether DSM criteria are fulfilled, and duration and number of episodes. Still, most observational studies that have dementia as the outcome of interest do not have a detailed clinical interview on history of depressive episodes and base the history on one or two questions.[76] This may result in misclassification of depression in the past, not only because recollection from the past in general is prone to misclassification and persons who are depressed at time of interview may differentially—better or worse—remember previous depressive episodes relative to those not depressed at time of interview, but also because one or two depressive symptoms do not define a depression.

Subtypes and Symptom Profiles of Depression

The heterogeneity of depression has become a research focus of interest in recent years,[52,69,99] and has given new insights into the aetiology of depression that can be relevant to increasing our understanding of the relationship between depression and dementia. For instance, the subtypes of melancholic and atypical depression have differential relationships with metabolic, inflammatory, and neuroendocrine systems.[100] Further, evidence exists that specific symptom profiles of late-life depression have differential relationships with underlying brain changes, also in the absence of a diagnosis of MDD. For instance, motivational symptoms, including anhedonia, energy loss, psychomotor retardation, and executive dysfunction, have been associated with vascular brain lesions in fronto-subcortical brain regions, consistent with the vascular depression hypothesis[101–104] and showing that location of vascular lesions is important.[56,102,105] To what extent mood symptoms are associated with specific vascular or neurodegenerative brain changes is less clear.[103] Interestingly, apathy-related symptoms are also associated with neurodegenerative brain changes, including brain volume reductions in grey matter and normal white matter.[104] These studies indicate that there are subtypes of depression or clusters of depressive symptoms that are associated with specific biological and neuroimaging factors. However, very few studies have examined this in combination with dementia outcomes.[54,76] Also, the identification of subtypes of late-life depression is heavily focused on diagnostic subclassification,[106–108] and the possibility that symptoms of late-life depression do not fulfil clinical criteria[104] or other dimensional depression profiles related to dementia risk needs further investigation.

Microstructural Brain Abnormalities

Conventional imaging techniques usually visualize the hippocampus as a unitary structure. However, the hippocampus consists of several anatomically different subfields with distinct cellular and molecular characteristics: the subiculum, the four Cornu Ammonis sections (CA 1-4), and the dentate gyrus, that may differentially be affected by ageing and disease.[109] Furthermore, conventional imaging techniques capture later stages of pathology because they are limited to visualizing very small brain lesions and volume loss in very small brain (sub)structures that may represent the earliest stages of disease development. Advances in high field MRI techniques such as 7 tesla MRI, have made it possible to visualize microstructural and microvascular brain changes in great detail,[110–117] and these techniques can be used to identify novel neuroimaging markers of late-life depression and dementia. This gives the opportunity to investigate to what extent differential relationships exist between late-life depression, cognitive functioning, and *in vivo* markers of Alzheimer and vascular pathology at the earliest stages of the disease. The increasing availability of high field MRI and automated segmentation programmes for hippocampal subfields[111,118] and vascular lesions[116,119] make it feasible to incorporate these techniques in larger studies. While this is an exciting and promising development, there are many challenges to overcome. For instance, with respect to hippocampal subfields, many different MRI protocols and segmentation programmes are used, and the anatomical landmarks and definition of hippocampal subfields need to be harmonized.[113,120] Also, much of the existing evidence for differential effects of hippocampal subfields on aging and disease originate from animal and *ex vivo* studies[109] and there is a lack of *in vivo* studies in human populations.

Conclusion

While a firm relationship between late-life depression and dementia has been established, the exact nature of this relationship is still not well understood. This chapter discussed some methodological issues that can give guidance to advance studies of the interface between depression and dementia. Most likely, multiple pathways exist through which depression and dementia are related.[108] Depression may be a risk factor, a preclinical or a prodromal symptom, or shared risk factors may explain the co-occurrence, depending on the depression subtype or symptom profile with its associated neurobiological substrate. To identify these pathways, detailed measurements of depression history, underlying neurobiological mechanisms, and trajectories to dementia development are needed. Only then subgroups of persons, that have different relationships with dementia development, can be identified. Identifying these subgroups may help in finding new strategies to adequately treat the depression, to prevent or delay the clinical expression of dementia, or to learn to cope with the disease. Given the enormous burden that depression and dementia have on individuals' life and society, this may have profound impact on well-being of individuals and the ageing population.

REFERENCES

1. Thies W, Bleiler L. Alzheimer's disease facts and figures. Alzheimer's Dement. 2013; 9(2): 208–45.
2. Olesen J, Gustavsson A, Svensson M, Wittchen HU, Jonsson B. The economic cost of brain disorders in Europe. Eur J Neurol. 2012; 19(1): 155–62.
3. Cummings JL, Cole G. Alzheimer disease. JAMA. 2002; 287(18): 2335–8.
4. Ballard C, Gauthier S, Corbett A, Brayne C, Aarsland D, Jones E. Alzheimer's disease. Lancet. 2011; 377(9770): 1019–31.
5. McLaughlin T, Feldman H, Fillit H, et al. Dependence as a unifying construct in defining Alzheimer's disease severity. Alzheimer's Dement. 2010; 6(6): 482–93.
6. Weuve J, Hebert LE, Scherr PA, Evans DA. Deaths in the United States among persons with Alzheimer's disease (2010–2050). Alzheimer's Dement. 2014; 10(2): e40–6.
7. James BD, Leurgans SE, Hebert LE, Scherr PA, Yaffe K, Bennett DA. Contribution of Alzheimer disease to mortality in the United States. Neurology. 2014; 82(12): 1045–50.
8. Ott A, Breteler MMB, van Harskamp F, et al. Prevalence of Alzheimer's disease and vascular dementia: association with education. The Rotterdam Study. BMJ. 1995; 310(6985): 970–3.
9. Ruitenberg A, Ott A, van Swieten JC, Hofman A, Breteler MMB. Incidence of dementia: does gender make a difference? Neurobiol Aging. 2001; 22(4): 575–80.
10. White L, Petrovitch H, Hardman J, et al. Cerebrovascular pathology and dementia in autopsied Honolulu-Asia Aging Study participants. Ann NY Acad Sci. 2002; 977: 9–23.
11. Langa KM, Foster NL, Larson EB. Mixed dementia: emerging concepts and therapeutic implications. JAMA. 2004; 292(23): 2901–8.
12. Braak H, Braak E. Neuropathological staging of Alzheimer-related changes. Acta Neuropathol. 1991; 82(4): 239–59.
13. Ott A, Breteler MMB, van Harskamp F, Stijnen T, Hofman A. Incidence and risk of dementia. The Rotterdam Study. Am J Epidemiol. 1998; 147(6): 574–80.
14. Launer LJ, Andersen K, Dewey ME, et al. Rates and risk factors for dementia and Alzheimer's disease: results from EURODEM pooled analyses. EURODEM Incidence Research Group and Work Groups. European Studies of Dementia. Neurology. 1999; 52(1): 78–84.
15. Ganguli M, Dodge HH, Chen P, Belle S, DeKosky ST. Ten-year incidence of dementia in a rural elderly US community population: the MoVIES Project. Neurology. 2000; 54(5): 1109–16.
16. Hebert LE, Scherr PA, Bienias JL, Bennett DA, Evans DA. Alzheimer disease in the US population: prevalence estimates using the 2000 census. Arch Neurol. 2003; 60(8): 1119–22.
17. Hebert LE, Weuve J, Scherr PA, Evans DA. Alzheimer disease in the United States (2010–2050) estimated using the 2010 census. Neurology. 2013; 80(19): 1778–83.
18. Livingston G, Sommerlad A, Orgeta V, et al. Dementia prevention, intervention, and care. Lancet. 2017; 13(10): 579–80.
19. Prince M, Bryce R, Albanese E, Wimo A, Ribeiro W, Ferri CP. The global prevalence of dementia: a systematic review and metaanalysis. Alzheimer's Dement. 2013; 9(1): 63–75 e2.
20. Larson EB, Yaffe K, Langa KM. New insights into the dementia epidemic. N Engl J Med. 2013; 369(24): 2275–7.
21. Lyketsos CG, Lopez O, Jones B, Fitzpatrick AL, Breitner J, DeKosky S. Prevalence of neuropsychiatric symptoms in dementia and mild cognitive impairment: results from the cardiovascular health study. JAMA. 2002; 288(12): 1475–83.
22. Aalten P, Verhey FR, Boziki M, et al. Neuropsychiatric syndromes in dementia. Results from the European Alzheimer Disease Consortium: part I. Dement Geriatr Cogn Disord. 2007; 24(6): 457–63.
23. Aalten P, Verhey FR, Boziki M, et al. Consistency of neuropsychiatric syndromes across dementias: results from the European Alzheimer Disease Consortium. Part II. Dement Geriatr Cogn Disord. 2008; 25(1): 1–8.
24. van der Linde RM, Stephan BC, Savva GM, Dening T, Brayne C. Systematic reviews on behavioural and psychological symptoms in the older or demented population. Alz Res Ther. 2012; 4(4):28.
25. Lee HB, Lyketsos CG. Depression in Alzheimer's disease: heterogeneity and related issues. Biol Psychiatry. 2003; 54(3): 353–62.
26. Lyketsos CG, Lee HB. Diagnosis and treatment of depression in Alzheimer's disease. A practical update for the clinician. Dement Geriatr Cogn Disord. 2004; 17(1–2): 55–64.
27. Beekman AT, Copeland JR, Prince MJ. Review of community prevalence of depression in later life. Br J Psychiatry. 1999; 174: 307–11.
28. Kessler RC, Birnbaum H, Bromet E, Hwang I, Sampson N, Shahly V. Age differences in major depression: results from the National Comorbidity Survey Replication (NCS-R). Psychol Med. 2010; 40(2): 225–37.
29. Jorm AF. History of depression as a risk factor for dementia: an updated review. Aust N Z J Psychiatry. 2001; 35(6): 776–81.
30. Ownby RL, Crocco E, Acevedo A, John V, Loewenstein D. Depression and risk for Alzheimer disease: systematic review, meta-analysis, and metaregression analysis. Arch Gen Psychiatry. 2006; 63(5): 530–38.
31. Byers AL, Yaffe K. Depression and risk of developing dementia. Nat Rev Neurol. 2011; 7(6): 323–31.
32. Diniz BS, Butters MA, Albert SM, Dew MA, Reynolds CF, 3rd. Late-life depression and risk of vascular dementia and Alzheimer's disease: systematic review and meta-analysis of community-based cohort studies. Br J Psychiatry. 2013; 202(5): 329–35.
33. Cherbuin N, Kim S, Anstey KJ. Dementia risk estimates associated with measures of depression: a systematic review and meta-analysis. BMJ Open. 2015; 5(12): e008853.
34. Bellou V, Belbasis L, Tzoulaki I, Middleton LT, Ioannidis JP, Evangelou E. Systematic evaluation of the associations between environmental risk factors and dementia: An umbrella review of systematic reviews and meta-analyses. Alzheimer's Dement. 2017; 13(4): 406–18.
35. Barnes DE, Yaffe K. The projected effect of risk factor reduction on Alzheimer's disease prevalence. Lancet Neurology. 2011; 10(9): 819–28.
36. Salloway S, Sperling R, Fox NC, *et al.* Two phase 3 trials of bapineuzumab in mild-to-moderate Alzheimer's disease. New Eng J Med. 2014; 370(4): 322–33.

37. Lupien SJ, McEwen BS, Gunnar MR, Heim C. Effects of stress throughout the lifespan on the brain, behaviour and cognition. Nat Rev Neurosci. 2009; 10(6): 434–45.
38. Sapolsky RM, Krey LC, McEwen BS. The neuroendocrinology of stress and aging: the glucocorticoid cascade hypothesis. Endocr Rev. 1986; 7(3): 284–301.
39. Park CR, Zoladz PR, Conrad CD, Fleshner M, Diamond DM. Acute predator stress impairs the consolidation and retrieval of hippocampus-dependent memory in male and female rats. Learn Mem. 2008; 15(4): 271–80.
40. Kim JJ, Song EY, Kosten TA. Stress effects in the hippocampus: synaptic plasticity and memory. Stress. 2006; 9(1): 1–11.
41. McEwen BS. Plasticity of the hippocampus: adaptation to chronic stress and allostatic load. Ann N Y Acad Sci. 2001; 933: 265–77.
42. Stetler C, Miller GE. Depression and hypothalamic-pituitary-adrenal activation: a quantitative summary of four decades of research. Psychosom Med. 2011; 73(2): 114–26.
43. Belvederi Murri M, Pariante C, Mondelli V, et al. HPA axis and aging in depression: systematic review and meta-analysis. Psychoneuroendocrinology. 2014; 41: 46–62.
44. Geerlings MI, Gerritsen L. Late-life depression, hippocampal volumes, and hypothalamic-pituitary-adrenal axis regulation: a systematic review and meta-analysis. Biol Psychiatry. 2017; 82(5): 339–50.
45. Ennis GE, An Y, Resnick SM, Ferrucci L, O'Brien RJ, Moffat SD. Long-term cortisol measures predict Alzheimer disease risk. Neurology. 2017; 88(4): 371–8.
46. Geerlings MI, Sigurdsson S, Eiriksdottir G, et al. Salivary cortisol, brain volumes, and cognition in community-dwelling elderly without dementia. Neurology. 2015; 85: 976–83.
47. Comijs HC, Gerritsen L, Penninx BW, Bremmer MA, Deeg DJ, Geerlings MI. The association between serum cortisol and cognitive decline in older persons. Am J Geriatr Psychiatry. 2010; 18(1): 42–50.
48. Gerritsen L, Comijs HC, Deeg DJ, Penninx BW, Geerlings MI. Salivary cortisol, APOE-epsilon4 allele and cognitive decline in a prospective study of older persons. Neurobiol Aging. 2011; 32(9): 1615–25.
49. den Heijer T, Geerlings MI, Hoebeek FE, Hofman A, Koudstaal PJ, Breteler MM. Use of hippocampal and amygdalar volumes on magnetic resonance imaging to predict dementia in cognitively intact elderly people. Arch Gen Psychiatry. 2006; 63(1): 57–62.
50. Jacobson L, Sapolsky R. The role of the hippocampus in feedback regulation of the hypothalamic- pituitary-adrenocortical axis. Endocr Rev. 1991; 12(2): 118–34.
51. Sapolsky RM. Glucocorticoids and hippocampal atrophy in neuropsychiatric disorders. Arch Gen Psychiatry. 2000; 57(10): 925–35.
52. Disabato BM, Sheline YI. Biological basis of late life depression. Curr Psychiatry Rep. 2012; 14(4): 273–9.
53. Krishnan KR, Hays JC, Blazer DG. MRI-defined vascular depression. Am J Psychiatry. 1997; 154(4): 497–501.
54. Barnes DE, Yaffe K, Byers AL, McCormick M, Schaefer C, Whitmer RA. Midlife vs late-life depressive symptoms and risk of dementia: differential effects for Alzheimer disease and vascular dementia. Arch Gen Psychiatry. 2012; 69(5): 493–8.
55. Herrmann LL, Le Masurier M, Ebmeier KP. White matter hyperintensities in late life depression: a systematic review. J Neurol Neurosurg Psychiatry. 2008; 79(6): 619–24.
56. Taylor WD, Aizenstein HJ, Alexopoulos GS. The vascular depression hypothesis: mechanisms linking vascular disease with depression. Mol Psychiatry. 2013; 18(9): 963–74.
57. Vu NQ, Aizenstein HJ. Depression in the elderly: brain correlates, neuropsychological findings, and role of vascular lesion load. Curr Opin Neurol. 2013; 26(6): 656–61.
58. Hemingway H, Marmot M. Evidence based cardiology: psychosocial factors in the aetiology and prognosis of coronary heart disease. Systematic review of prospective cohort studies. BMJ. 1999; 318(7196): 1460–7.
59. Lett HS, Blumenthal JA, Babyak MA, et al. Depression as a risk factor for coronary artery disease: evidence, mechanisms, and treatment. Psychosom Med. 2004; 66(3): 305–15.
60. Wulsin LR, Singal BM. Do depressive symptoms increase the risk for the onset of coronary disease? A systematic quantitative review. Psychosom Med. 2003; 65(2): 201–10.
61. Breteler MMB. Vascular risk factors for Alzheimer's disease: an epidemiologic perspective. Neurobiol Aging. 2000; 21(2): 153–60.
62. Vermeer SE, Prins ND, den Heijer T, Hofman A, Koudstaal PJ, Breteler MM. Silent brain infarcts and the risk of dementia and cognitive decline. N Engl J Med. 2003; 348(13): 1215–22.
63. Luchsinger JA, Mayeux R. Cardiovascular risk factors and Alzheimer's disease. Curr Atheroscler Rep. 2004; 6(4): 261–6.
64. Power MC, Weuve J, Gagne JJ, McQueen MB, Viswanathan A, Blacker D. The association between blood pressure and incident Alzheimer disease: a systematic review and meta-analysis. Epidemiology. 2011; 22(5): 646–59.
65. Alexopoulos GS, Meyers BS, Young RC, Campbell S, Silbersweig D, Charlson M. 'Vascular depression' hypothesis. Arch Gen Psychiatry. 1997; 54(10): 915–22.
66. Alexopoulos GS. The vascular depression hypothesis: 10 years later. Biol Psychiatry. 2006; 60(12): 1304–5.
67. Aizenstein HJ, Baskys A, Boldrini M, *et al.* Vascular depression consensus report—a critical update. BMC Med. 2016; 14(1): 161.
68. Alexopoulos GS. Vascular disease, depression, and dementia. J Am Geriatr Soc. 2003; 51(8):1178–1180.
69. Penninx BW, Milaneschi Y, Lamers F, Vogelzangs N. Understanding the somatic consequences of depression: biological mechanisms and the role of depression symptom profile. BMC Med. 2013; 11: 129.
70. Frasure-Smith N, Lesperance F, Talajic M. Depression and 18-month prognosis after myocardial infarction. Circulation. 1995; 91(4): 999–1005.
71. Lichtman JH, Bigger JT, Jr., Blumenthal JA, et al. Depression and coronary heart disease: recommendations for screening, referral, and treatment: a science advisory from the American Heart Association Prevention Committee of the Council on Cardiovascular Nursing, Council on Clinical Cardiology, Council on Epidemiology and Prevention, and Interdisciplinary Council on Quality of Care and Outcomes Research: endorsed by the American Psychiatric Association. Circulation. 2008; 118(17): 1768–75.
72. Prins ND, Scheltens P. White matter hyperintensities, cognitive impairment and dementia: an update. Nat Rev Neurol. 2015; 11(3): 157–65.
73. Smekal A, Vaclavik J. Adipokines and cardiovascular disease: A comprehensive review. Biomed Pap Med Fac Univ Palacky Olomouc Czech Repub. 2017; 161(1): 31–40.
74. Saczynski JS, Beiser A, Seshadri S, Auerbach S, Wolf PA, Au R. Depressive symptoms and risk of dementia: the Framingham Heart Study. Neurology. 2010; 75(1): 35–41.

75. Dotson VM, Beydoun MA, Zonderman AB. Recurrent depressive symptoms and the incidence of dementia and mild cognitive impairment. Neurology. 2010; 75(1): 27–34.
76. Geerlings MI, den Heijer T, Koudstaal PJ, Hofman A, Breteler MM. History of depression, depressive symptoms, and medial temporal lobe atrophy and the risk of Alzheimer disease. Neurology. 2008; 70(15): 1258–64.
77. Karlsson IK, Bennet AM, Ploner A, et al. Apolipoprotein E epsilon4 genotype and the temporal relationship between depression and dementia. Neurobiol Aging. 2015; 36(4): 1751–6.
78. Brommelhoff JA, Gatz M, Johansson B, McArdle JJ, Fratiglioni L, Pedersen NL. Depression as a risk factor or prodromal feature for dementia? Findings in a population-based sample of Swedish twins. Psychol Aging. 2009; 24(2):373–84.
79. Mirza SS, de Bruijn RF, Direk N, et al. Depressive symptoms predict incident dementia during short- but not long-term follow-up period. Alzheimer's Dement. 2014; 10(5 Suppl): S323–S9 e1.
80. Mirza SS, Wolters FJ, Swanson SA, et al. 10-year trajectories of depressive symptoms and risk of dementia: a population-based study. Lancet Psychiatry. 2016; 3(7): 628–35.
81. Singh-Manoux A, Dugravot A, Fournier A, et al. Trajectories of depressive symptoms before diagnosis of dementia: a 28-year follow-up study. JAMA Psychiatry. 2017; 74(7): 712–18.
82. Sexton CE, Mackay CE, Ebmeier KP. A systematic review and meta-analysis of magnetic resonance imaging studies in late-life depression. Am J Geriatr Psychiatry. 2013; 21(2): 184–95.
83. Rao U, Chen LA, Bidesi AS, Shad MU, Thomas MA, Hammen CL. Hippocampal changes associated with early-life adversity and vulnerability to depression. Biol Psychiatry. 2010; 67(4): 357–64.
84. Taylor WD, McQuoid DR, Payne ME, Zannas AS, MacFall JR, Steffens DC. Hippocampus atrophy and the longitudinal course of late-life depression. Am J Geriatr Psychiatry. 2014; 22(12): 1504–12.
85. Chen MC, Hamilton JP, Gotlib IH. Decreased hippocampal volume in healthy girls at risk of depression. Arch Gen Psychiatry. 2010; 67(3): 270–6.
86. den Heijer T, Tiemeier H, Luijendijk HJ, et al. A study of the bidirectional association between hippocampal volume on magnetic resonance imaging and depression in the elderly. Biol Psychiatry. 2011; 70(2): 191–7.
87. Dotson VM, Davatzikos C, Kraut MA, Resnick SM. Depressive symptoms and brain volumes in older adults: a longitudinal magnetic resonance imaging study. J Psychiatr Neurosci. 2009; 34(5): 367–75.
88. Elbejjani M, Fuhrer R, Abrahamowicz M, et al. Depression, depressive symptoms, and rate of hippocampal atrophy in a longitudinal cohort of older men and women. Psychol Med. 2015; 45(9): 1931–44.
89. Buddeke J, Kooistra M, Zuithoff NP, et al. Hippocampal volume and the course of depressive symptoms over eight years of follow-up. Acta Psychiatr Scand. 2017; 135(1): 78–86.
90. Elbejjani M, Fuhrer R, Abrahamowicz M, et al. Hippocampal atrophy and subsequent depressive symptoms in older men and women: results from a 10-year prospective cohort. Am J Epidemiol. 2014; 180(4): 385–93.
91. van Agtmaal MJM, Houben A, Pouwer F, Stehouwer CDA, Schram MT. Association of microvascular dysfunction with late-life depression: a systematic review and meta-analysis. JAMA Psychiatry. 2017; 74(7): 729–39.
92. Bianchi R, Laurent E. Late-Life depression, cortisol, and the hippocampus: on the need to consider depressive, hippocampal, and pharmacological complexities. Biol Psychiatry. 2018; 83(1): e23–24.
93. Beekman AT, Deeg DJ, van Tilburg T, Smit JH, Hooijer C, Van Tilburg W. Major and minor depression in later life: a study of prevalence and risk factors. J Affect Disord. 1995; 36(1–2): 65–75.
94. Gerritsen L, Comijs HC, van der Graaf Y, Knoops AJ, Penninx BW, Geerlings MI. Depression, hypothalamic pituitary adrenal axis, and hippocampal and entorhinal cortex volumes-the SMART Medea study. Biol Psychiatry. 2011; 70(4): 373–80.
95. Geerlings MI, Brickman AM, Schupf N, et al. Depressive symptoms, antidepressant use, and brain volumes on mri in a population-based cohort of old persons without dementia. J Alzheimer's Dis. 2012; 30(1): 75–82.
96. van Uden IW, van Norden AG, de Laat KF, et al. Depressive symptoms and amygdala volume in elderly with cerebral small vessel disease: The RUN DMC Study. J Aging Res. 2011; 647869.
97. Lupien SJ, Maheu F, Tu M, Fiocco A, Schramek TE. The effects of stress and stress hormones on human cognition: Implications for the field of brain and cognition. Brain Cogn. 2007; 65(3): 209–37.
98. Geerlings MI, Sigurdsson S, Eiriksdottir G, et al. Associations of current and remitted major depressive disorder with brain atrophy: the AGES-Reykjavik Study. Psychol Med. 2013; 43(2): 317–28.
99. Baune BT, Stuart M, Gilmour A, et al. The relationship between subtypes of depression and cardiovascular disease: a systematic review of biological models. Transl Psychiatry. 2012; 2: e92.
100. Lamers F, Vogelzangs N, Merikangas KR, de Jonge P, Beekman AT, Penninx BW. Evidence for a differential role of HPA-axis function, inflammation and metabolic syndrome in melancholic versus atypical depression. Mol Psychiatry. 2013; 18(6): 692–9.
101. Krishnan KR, Taylor WD, McQuoid DR, et al. Clinical characteristics of magnetic resonance imaging-defined subcortical ischemic depression. Biol Psychiatry. 2004; 55(4): 390–7.
102. Grool AM, Gerritsen L, Zuithoff NP, Mali WP, van der Graaf Y, Geerlings MI. Lacunar infarcts in deep white matter are associated with higher and more fluctuating depressive symptoms during three years follow-up. Biol Psychiatry. 2013; 73(2): 169–76.
103. Grool AM, van der Graaf Y, Mali WP, Witkamp TD, Vincken KL, Geerlings MI. Location and progression of cerebral small-vessel disease and atrophy, and depressive symptom profiles: the Second Manifestations of ARTerial disease (SMART)-Medea study. Psychol Med. 2012; 42(2): 359–70.
104. Grool AM, Geerlings MI, Sigurdsson S, et al. Structural MRI correlates of apathy symptoms in older persons without dementia: AGES-Reykjavik Study. Neurology. 2014; 82(18): 1628–35.
105. Grool AM, van der Graaf Y, Mali WP, Geerlings MI. Location of cerebrovascular and degenerative changes, depressive symptoms and cognitive functioning in later life: the SMART-Medea study. J Neurol Neurosurg Psychiatry. 2011; 82(10): 1093–1100.
106. Xekardaki A, Santos M, Hof P, Kovari E, Bouras C, Giannakopoulos P. Neuropathological substrates and structural changes in late-life depression: the impact of vascular burden. Acta Neuropathol. 2012; 124(4): 453–64.
107. Santos M, Xekardaki A, Kovari E, Gold G, Bouras C, Giannakopoulos P. Microvascular pathology in late-life depression. J Neurol Sci. 2012; 322(1–2): 46–9.
108. Butters MA, Young JB, Lopez O, et al. Pathways linking late-life depression to persistent cognitive impairment and dementia. Dialogues Clin Neurosci. 2008; 10(3): 345–57.

109. Small SA, Schobel SA, Buxton RB, Witter MP, Barnes CA. A pathophysiological framework of hippocampal dysfunction in ageing and disease. Nat Rev Neurosci. 2011; 12(10): 585–601.
110. Ghaznawi R, de Bresser J, van der Graaf Y, et al. Detection and characterization of small infarcts in the caudate nucleus on 7 Tesla MRI: The SMART-MR study. J Cereb Blood Flow Metab. 2018; 38(9): 1609–17.
111. Wisse LE, Kuijf HJ, Honingh AM, et al. Automated hippocampal subfield segmentation at 7T MRI. AJNR Am J Neuroradiol. 2016; 37(6):1050–7.
112. Bouvy WH, Zwanenburg JJ, Reinink R, et al. Perivascular spaces on 7 Tesla brain MRI are related to markers of small vessel disease but not to age or cardiovascular risk factors. J Cereb Blood Flow Metab. 2016; 36(10): 1708–17.
113. Yushkevich PA, Amaral RS, Augustinack JC, et al. Quantitative comparison of 21 protocols for labeling hippocampal subfields and parahippocampal subregions in in vivo MRI: towards a harmonized segmentation protocol. Neuroimage. 2015; 111: 526–41.
114. van Veluw SJ, Jolink WM, Hendrikse J, et al. Cortical microinfarcts on 7T MRI in patients with spontaneous intracerebral hemorrhage. J Cereb Blood Flow Metab. 2014; 34(7): 1104–6.
115. Wisse LE, Gerritsen L, Zwanenburg JJ, et al. Subfields of the hippocampal formation at 7 T MRI: in vivo volumetric assessment. Neuroimage. 2012; 61(4): 1043–9.
116. Kuijf HJ, de Bresser J, Geerlings MI, et al. Efficient detection of cerebral microbleeds on 7.0 T MR images using the radial symmetry transform. Neuroimage. 2012; 59(3): 2266– 73.
117. Conijn MM, Hoogduin JM, van der Graaf Y, Hendrikse J, Luijten PR, Geerlings MI. Microbleeds, lacunar infarcts, white matter lesions and cerebrovascular reactivity—a 7 T study. Neuroimage. 2012; 59(2): 950–6.
118. Giuliano A, Donatelli G, Cosottini M, Tosetti M, Retico A, Fantacci ME. Hippocampal subfields at ultra high field MRI: An overview of segmentation and measurement methods. Hippocampus. 2017; 27(5): 481–94.
119. Kuijf HJ, Bouvy WH, Zwanenburg JJ, et al. Quantification of deep medullary veins at 7 T brain MRI. Eur Radiol. 2016: 26(10): 3412–8.
120. Wisse LEM, Daugherty AM, Olsen RK, et al. A harmonized segmentation protocol for hippocampal and parahippocampal subregions: Why do we need one and what are the key goals? Hippocampus. 2017; 27(1):3–11.

28

Epidemiology of schizophrenia and related disorders

Assen Jablensky, Hannah E Jongsma, James B Kirkbride, and Peter B Jones

Introduction

Epidemiological research into schizophrenia has had a long and productive history over many decades, since Kraepelin's formulation of the disease concept of *dementia praecox* in 1896 and the renaming of the disorder as *schizophrenia* by Bleuler in 1911.[1] Being a counterpart to clinical and biological research, the focus of epidemiology is on the population frequency of the disorder and the distribution of its incidence, prevalence, course, outcome, and associated risk factors. The hallmark of the 'classical' epidemiological method is the referral of a counting measure (numerator) of the occurrence of a disorder and any associated characteristics to a population base (denominator), yielding its epidemiological 'signature' which enables the testing of hypotheses about risk factors and causes. The epidemiology of schizophrenia and other psychotic disorders aims to address three essential questions: (1) does the incidence, manifestations, and course of these disorders vary in relation to factors of the physical and social environment? (2) who is at risk and what forces determine or influence the risk of developing schizophrenia or other psychotic disorders? (3) can epidemiological research contribute to the understanding of the aetiology of psychotic disorders and their prevention?

While epidemiological investigations to address these questions have been conducted for over a century, they are still encountering difficulties related to the nature of the disease concept of schizophrenia. Recurring problems include the dependence of the diagnosis on self-reported subjective experience; the clinical and genetic heterogeneity of the disorder; the absence of validated biological markers; and its tenuous delineation from other psychotic disorders and bipolar affective disorder. Although the ICD-10 and DSM-V criteria have clinical utility, a resolution of these difficulties is currently provided by the schizophrenia spectrum concept that embraces schizophrenia, schizoaffective disorder, schizotypal disorder, and acute transient psychotic disorders. One further challenge is creating valid and reliable nosological entities of disorder, warranting clinical intervention, which differentiate 'healthy' from 'disordered' populations.

Psychotic phenomena in the general population are relatively common,[2] may be very brief, and usually do not persist or warrant clinical intervention. As such, it has been proposed that psychotic phenomena exist more as dimensional constructs, as reflected in the recently revised DSM-V, rather than as binary (present/absent) diagnoses. Nonetheless, it remains both clinically and aetiologically important to be able to target appropriate treatment and prevention to groups whose symptomatology presents sufficient distress, disability, or disruption to impact their lives. Classification systems, such as ICD-10 and DSM-V, although not perfect, present evidence-based attempts to draw these nosological lines according to a set of agreed, standardized criteria. Notwithstanding the outstanding classificatory issues, there is at present a broad consensus that schizophrenia is a genetically complex disease, with variants and mutations in multiple genes and gene networks, as well as with a significant neurodevelopmental and environmental contribution to its phenotypic expression. The findings of epidemiological research provide a useful background for the interpretation of genetic, neurobiological, and social research, as well as aiding clinicians in making evidence-based diagnostic and treatment decisions.

In this chapter we survey a broad range of findings that jointly outline the composite epidemiological profile of schizophrenia and its spectrum. In the second section we outline the major historical milestones in the epidemiology of psychotic disorders. Next, in the third section, we review the main findings with respect to the incidence (new) and prevalence (total) burden of such disorders worldwide. In the fourth section we review the major risk factors which have been identified for psychotic disorders, and the strength of evidence to support these. We also discuss major public health issues surrounding, course, outcome, and mortality in people who develop a psychotic disorder, before presenting our concluding remarks on the direction of psychiatric epidemiology in this field in the section entitled Future Prospects.

Historical 'Milestones' of Epidemiological Research into Psychotic Disorders

Measuring the burden—or disease frequency—of psychotic disorders in the population is a challenging issue in psychiatric epidemiology. Studies of incidence—the rate of new cases in a defined population over a defined period—require large samples, or relatively long time periods of observation, given the absolutely rarity of psychotic disorders (in England for example, the pooled incidence of all adult-onset (16–64 years) psychotic disorders has been placed at 31.7 new cases per 100,000 people per year).[3]

The most accurate method of estimating the true incidence of psychotic disorder in the population would be to identify all new cases wherever they may occur in the community. However, since it is impractical to contact and screen every person in a population, the gold standard for estimating true incidence rates typically involves establishing a case ascertainment procedure which monitors several informal or formal potential points of contact for psychosis. This may include primary and secondary healthcare providers, religious organizations, charitable and government welfare providers, and the police and judicial system. Because it is often argued that the severity of a first episode of psychosis (FEP) is sufficiently severe to warrant mental healthcare at some point—even when an untreated disorder may be longstanding—many incidence studies may restrict case ascertainment to those coming into contact with secondary mental healthcare services, which may lead to the estimation of 'treated' incidence rates which are assumed to sufficiently approximate the true underlying incidence of disorder in the population. The validity of this methodology is open to debate, and may lead to issues when inferring differences in treated incidence rates between groups of aetiological importance, if this methodology has introduced differential case ascertainment between the groups under study.

Prevalence studies—which estimate the total burden of psychotic disorder in a population at a given point, or over a given period, are typically ascertained via household surveys.[4,5,6] While such studies use sampling strategies which lead to the identification of representative samples for many psychiatric conditions, this methodology may lead to an underestimation of the prevalence of psychotic disorders,[7] since people with such conditions may be less likely to respond to household surveys as a function of paranoia or other related symptoms often inherent to the disorder.

The various case finding strategies employed in the early epidemiological studies of psychoses fall into three categories: (1) birth cohort studies; (2) surveys of whole communities; and (3) population sample surveys. *Birth cohort studies* were first introduced by Klemperer,[8] who selected a random sample of 1000 individuals from the birth register of Munich but succeeded in tracing and examining only about 30% of them. This approach was used with greater success by Fremming,[9] who collected life history data on 92% of the 5500 persons born on the island of Bornholm during 1883–7. In Iceland, Helgason[10] compiled a cohort of all 5395 individuals born 1895–97 who had survived into adulthood and traced their life history and psychiatric data until 1957 from admission records and interviews. A further step was taken during the 1990s when this approach encompassed national, general population birth cohorts established for reasons other than psychiatric research, including the study of many physical and mental health outcomes over the life course.[11] Linked to means of identifying psychiatric outcomes, nested case control studies within these cohorts have illuminated questions of aetiology and mechanism, particularly in a developmental context.[12] *Surveys of whole communities* involving a census and personal interviewing of every adult person were pioneered by Brugger[13,14] in small rural towns in Thuringia and Bavaria. However, the major share of such studies took place in the Scandinavian countries, owing to their excellent population statistics.[15,16] A special variety of the comprehensive survey was the *prospective repeat survey*, of which the Lundby study in Sweden[17,18] and Böök's re-examinations of the entire population of a North Swedish genetic isolate[20,21] remain as the best examples. *Population sample surveys* involved the selection of random samples of individuals without regard to their health, and the collection of data on the mental morbidity of all of their first-degree relatives.[16,21,22] The most striking finding of all of these study designs was the relatively good agreement across studies between prevalence estimates, incidence rates, and morbid risk of schizophrenia—regardless of the ongoing arguments about its definition and diagnostic boundaries. Thus, in most population studies the point prevalence of schizophrenia was estimated within the range of 1.4–4.6 per 1000.[23] Incidence rates were reported within the range of 17–57 per 100,000 per year, and morbid risk for the general population between 0.36% and 1.87%. In addition, repeat surveys of the same population using very similar designs suggested the possibility of a real decrease of the morbid risk for schizophrenia during the 30 or more years separating the individual studies,[24] although other studies have found the rate of all non-affective psychoses may be relatively stable over time.[25]

The data on the frequency of schizophrenia in different communities are probably among the best documented evidence of early psychiatric epidemiology. However, their interpretation at the time was contentious. On one hand, the similarity of prevalence, incidence, and expectancy rates of schizophrenia in different populations was seen as evidence favouring a predominantly genetic (Mendelian) causation of the disorder. On the other hand, a hypothesis proposed by Böök,[20] but never properly tested, proposed that the operation of an environmental aetiological factor would be manifested in disproportionately elevated morbid risks for the siblings, parents, and children of schizophrenia patients, particularly in settings characterized by higher than average incidence of schizophrenia and some sort of social upheaval.

Generally, past epidemiological research has demonstrated that psychotic disorders, including schizophrenia, are ubiquitous (no human group, society, or culture has been convincingly shown to be free of such disorders), although more recent literature has identified pronounced—and replicable—heterogeneity in risk,[26] between and within populations (see the next two sections). Furthermore, it has shown that the phenomenology and natural history of these disorders appear to be less uniform than current classifications and diagnostic concepts tend to assume. This provides evidence that many aspects of the enduring burden of psychotic disorders are the result of adverse social reactions to the phenomena of illness, rather than intrinsic characteristics of the disease process. This suggests that much of the disability associated with schizophrenia and related disorders can be contained, reduced, or even prevented.

The Current State of Neuropsychiatric Epidemiology of Psychotic Disorders

Incidence

The ubiquity of schizophrenia and other psychotic disorders worldwide should not be confused with uniformity in their distribution. In the early epidemiological evidence presented in the previous section, variation in the *incidence rate* of schizophrenia across studies was more than three-fold, implying that social or biological factors might lead to the exact rate at which psychotic disorders manifest in different populations. The identification of these features—whether genetic, social, or environmental—would also be important for understanding the aetiology of these disorders. Early epidemiological studies which focused on the micro-level geographical distribution of psychotic disorders across neighbourhoods within cities, observed strong social and spatial gradients in incidence, with cases over-represented from more socially deprived and socially fragmented or isolated areas.[27–30] During the latter half of the 20th century interest grew in comparing the global distribution, incidence, course, and outcome of schizophrenia and other psychotic disorders using a standardized methodology. Such advances were a critical exercise in benchmarking the occurrence and manifestation of psychotic disorders globally,[31–33] and in conducting multisite studies in different countries using a singular methodology, in an attempt to minimize biases which may have been introduced in comparing incidence rates from different studies, which used different case finding approaches, inclusion criteria, estimation of the population at-risk, and diagnostic instruments.

Following a successful pilot study in the 1960s, the WHO set out to conduct an even more ambitious international comparison of cross-cultural variation in incidence rates and course in the late 1970s, the WHO "10-country" study.[33] This study encompassed twelve centres in ten countries, including both urban and rural settings, and developed and developing nations, under an umbrella methodology. Case finding was based on the gold standard for epidemiological research, and included:

(1) Defined geographical catchment areas from which cases and the population at-risk were estimated.
(2) Standardized inclusion criteria, including restrictions on age (15–54), minimum residency in the catchment (six months) and first contact with a 'helping agency' for suspected psychosis of recent onset (12 months).
(3) Defined case ascertainment period (two years).
(4) Exclusion of people presenting with psychotic disorders of organic origin.
(5) Standardized diagnostic assessment, assessed for reliability, using clinical information (obtained from the Present State Examination[34]) to produce comparable, that is, standardized diagnoses across settings via a computerized diagnostic algorithm known as CATEGO.
(6) Use of a 'leakage' protocol, to return to all participating agencies and any others to identify potentially missed cases during the initial screen.
(7) Training and inter-centre reliability estimates across all instruments used in the study.

Such was the rigour of the WHO ten-country study, that data quality assurance meant that only seven of the original twelve sites were deemed appropriate to provide incidence rate comparisons. The WHO ten-country study[33] found that incidence rates of narrowly-defined schizophrenia varied across these centres from 7 (Aarhus, Denmark) to 14 (Nottingham, UK) per 100,000 population at-risk, while a broader definition was associated with more variation, ranging from 16 (Honolulu, Hawaii, USA) to 35 (rural Chandigarh, India) per 100,000 population at-risk, respectively. Although these studies suggested a two-fold variation in rates globally, consistent with earlier studies,[23] findings of the WHO ten-country study were popularly misinterpreted as evidence of a uniform distribution of psychosis incidence worldwide. Inspection of incidence rates from the study, based on four diagnostic categories from the broadest to narrowest definitions of schizophrenia, actually revealed statistically significant ($p<0.001$) variation in incidence across all but the narrowest definition of schizophrenia (CATEGO: 'S+') for men, and similarly strong evidence for women in the two broadest CATEGO classes of psychotic disorder. Subsequently the earlier, erroneous interpretation of these findings have been challenged by carefully conducted systematic reviews which reveal substantial variation in the incidence of non-affective psychotic disorders between populations.[3,26,35]

The decade following the publication of the WHO findings almost completely eschewed further investigation into global variation in the incidence of psychotic disorders, and ushered in technological breakthroughs in the hunt for what some presumed would be a singular genetic cause, which penetrated populations with such uniform regularity that it led some influential thinkers[36] to state that: 'The evidence points to the singular conclusion that, contrary to almost any other common condition, the incidence of schizophrenia is independent of the environment and a characteristic of human populations. Perhaps it is the human condition.'

This view was not, of course, held by all. Many suggested that the genetic architecture leading to psychosis would be as exquisitely complicated and heterogeneous,[37–39] as it has thus far proved to be.[40] Indeed, one common feature of the genetic and epidemiological landscape of psychotic disorders is the marked heterogeneity in risk at multiple levels of causation.

During the late 1990s and first decade of the 21st century important epidemiological findings built an evidence base which strongly suggested that the incidence of psychotic disorders was not equally distributed in the population (see section entitle Future Prospects for an overview). Of particular note, the Aetiology and Ethnicity in Schizophrenia and Other Psychoses (AESOP) study[41–43] sought to estimate first contact incidence rates of psychotic disorder, in an ambitious study to provide definitive estimates of epidemiological risk, and investigate the neural, biological, and social correlates of excess risks experienced in some population groups, most notably amongst people of black Caribbean and black African ethnicity living in England.[44] The study used a similar case finding design to the WHO 10-country study to investigate variation in incidence in three settings in England over a two-year case ascertainment period: south-east London, Nottinghamshire, and Bristol (over the first nine months of this period). The authors found variation between[43] and within settings,[45] such that rates tended to be higher in more urban, socially fragmented, and densely populated regions of the catchment areas;[46] findings which could not be explained by differences in the age, sex, or ethnic composition of the population in those areas.

Other seminal epidemiological studies of schizophrenia have used longitudinal or cohort designs—the gold standard for observational epidemiology—to investigate the association between urban living and risk of disorder.[47,48] Unlike previous studies, which estimated psychosis incidence close to the time of presentation to healthcare services, these longitudinal studies—often utilizing routinely collected register-based data on the entire population of a nation—were able to investigate the association between schizophrenia risk in adulthood and urban birth[48] and upbringing.[47] These designs overcame some weaknesses of the more conventional 'first contact' designs above.[33,43] Notably, the longitudinal nature of these studies ensured that the exposure under investigation (urban living) occurred temporally before the outcome (schizophrenia) in these studies, all but excluding the possibility that any association between the two factors could be attributed to people with schizophrenia moving into more urban settings as a result (i.e. consequence) of their disorder, known in epidemiology as reverse causation.

This process, also termed *social drift*, has long been thought to play a role in the unequal distribution of psychotic disorders in the population, since people who begin to develop psychotic symptoms eventually leading to disorder may also be more likely to become unemployed, drop out of school, or struggle to afford access to better quality housing. While there is some evidence that this process exists as an unwanted and even preventable consequence of psychosis onset,[49,50] the pioneering work by Lewis et al.[47] in Sweden and Mortensen et al.[48] in Denmark suggested that this type of social drift could not explain the longitudinal association between urban birth or upbringing and later risk of schizophrenia. Moreover, these study designs were also able to adjust for several potential confounders—alternative explanations—of the relationship between urban birth and upbringing and later psychosis risk, including family history of psychiatric disorder, family income, parental divorce, paternal age and even, in one study,[47] cannabis use; the relationship between urban living and future schizophrenia risk persisted.

More recently, in the first major international comparison of the incidence of psychotic disorders in the 40 years since the WHO ten-country study, the European Network of National Schizophrenia Networks Studying Gene-Environment Interactions (EU-GEI) study has reported over an eight-fold variation in the incidence of psychotic disorders across 17 centres in 6 countries, including the UK, France, Netherlands, Spain, Italy, and Brazil.[51] As in earlier first contact designs, the study employed a comprehensive approach to identifying all new cases of potential psychotic disorder presenting to mental health services in defined catchment areas. Although, unlike earlier first contact designs,[33,43] the study did not systematically include a leakage methodology, it extended previous knowledge by showing substantial international variation in incidence which could not be explained by age, sex, or ethnic differences between settings. Here, rates were substantially higher in three major northern European cities (London, Amsterdam, and Paris) than in southern European cities (Madrid, Barcelona, and Palermo) or rural catchment areas. Furthermore, the study investigated whether a range of putative risk factors measured at the ecological (i.e. setting) level were correlated with variation in incidence.

In univariable analyses, greater incidence across settings was predicted by higher levels of social isolation (percentage of people living alone), lower unemployment, and lower levels of home ownership, for which only the latter persisted in fully adjusted analyses (see Fig. 28.1). These results raise the possibility that the level of socio-economic instability or disadvantage, or other closely-correlated factors* in a population may predict the incidence of psychotic disorders, though further research is required to understand the causal implications of such associations (see the next section).

Several well-conducted systematic reviews have synthesized all the available evidence on variation in incidence rates of psychotic disorders between people and places published over the last 70 years.[3,26,35] All these reviews have concluded that the incidence of non-affective psychotic disorders vary along both these dimensions. In general, the affective psychoses (including bipolar disorder and severe depression with psychotic features) seem to show less variation with regard to place,[35] and have a somewhat different age-sex distribution to non-affective psychoses (see the next section),

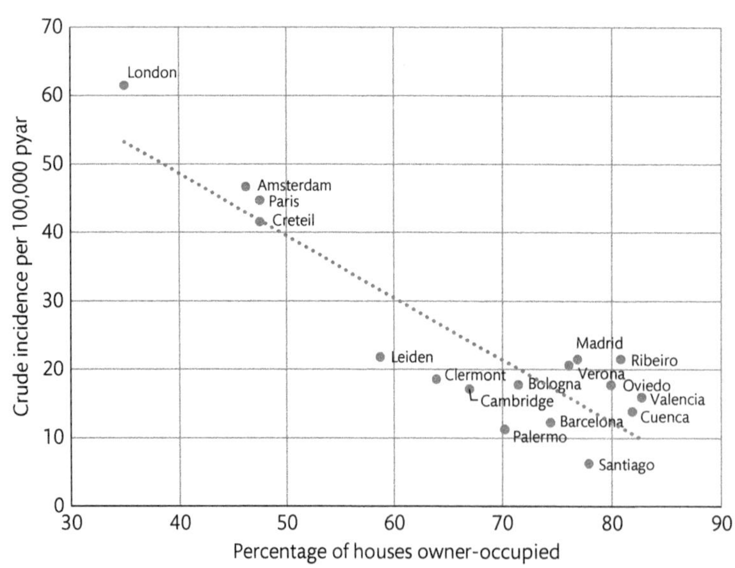

Fig. 28.1 Correlation between crude incidence of psychotic disorders and proportion of owner-occupied homes across 17 settings in the EU-GEI study.[51]

Legend: crude incidence rates are plotted per 100,000 person-years at risk. Percentage of home ownership is plotted along the x-axis. Correlation between crude incidence rates and % owner-occupied homes was -0.79.

Adapted from Jongsma H.E., Gayer-Anderson, C., Lasalvia, A. et al. Treated Incidence of Psychotic Disorders in the Multinational EU-GEI Study. *JAMA Psychiatry*, 75(1): 36–46.

suggesting that while these disorders share some genetic[52] and environmental origins,[42] they may also differ in their exact aetiology.[53,54]

Prevalence

While epidemiological studies of incidence can provide rich information about variation of psychotic disorders, and even clues as to their aetiology, they typically rely on first-contact or register-based designs to ascertain caseloads. Thus, most such studies, even those that work closely with a range of help-seeking agencies to identify cases missed by initial screening procedures, formally provide estimates of the *treated* incidence of psychotic disorder. Whether this rate is close to the true rate of disorder in the underlying population will depend both on the severity of the illness (with more severe illnesses more likely to come into contact with care services) and the design of the case ascertainment phase of the study. Because the absolute incidence of psychotic disorders is typically low (placed at around 31.7 new case per 100,000 in a review of English rates published between 1950–2009[3]) it is prohibitively expensive to design truly population-based surveys (e.g. via household surveys and screening) to establish the true, population-based incidence of psychotic disorders. Here, however, surveys to establish the prevalence of psychotic disorders in the population are more feasible, though not without challenges. Prevalence—the proportion of people in a given population over a given time period with a new or existing occurrence of disorder—is an essential measure of establishing overall psychiatric morbidity between and within populations. Prevalence is typically estimated at a given point in time (*point prevalence*), over a given period (i.e. *period prevalence;* when over a year typically denoted as *annual prevalence*) or over the entire life course (*lifetime prevalence*).

Several major studies of the prevalence of psychotic and other psychiatric disorders have been made. Amongst these, two in the USA, the Epidemiological Catchment Area (ECA) study and the National Comorbidity Surveys (NCS) have provided estimates of the lifetime and period prevalence of broadly defined schizophrenia. The ECA study, based on a representative sample of over 18,000 adults living in private households or institutionalized settings in five US cities (New Haven, Baltimore, St Louis, Durham, and Los Angeles), used the Diagnostic Interview Schedule (DIS) to estimate the prevalence of major psychiatric disorders according to DSM-III criteria at the beginning of the 1980s.[55] Lifetime prevalence estimates of schizophrenia spectrum disorders were published for three of these sites (New Haven, Baltimore, and St Louis),[56] which were found to vary from 1.1% in St Louis (Missouri) to 2.0% in New Haven (Connecticut).

The lifetime prevalence of non-affective psychosis in the first NCS study, based on a representative sample of over 8000 Americans aged 15–54 living in non-institutionalized settings in the 48 contiguous states of the USA, was placed at 2.2%, with lifetime prevalence of schizophrenia estimated to be 1.3%.[5] These prevalence estimates, which used a similar diagnostic algorithm to the ECA study, were somewhat higher than estimates based on clinical diagnoses alone (0.7% and 0.2%, respectively, for non-affective psychoses and schizophrenia), and highlight the important issue surrounding methods of assessment used in epidemiological studies. Kendler and colleagues[5] went on to show that clinician-rated diagnoses tended to agree poorly with computerized diagnoses based on the DIS in the NCS studies.

Concerned by the high sensitivity and low specificity of the DIS instrument used in the earlier ECA and NCS studies,[55,57] the NCS-R replication study used tighter screening criteria in the WHO's Composite International Diagnostic Interview (CIDI 3.0) in an attempt to minimize the introduction of false positive cases to estimate prevalence.[7] In a representative sample of 9000 respondents aged 18 and older, the lifetime prevalence of non-affective disorders using the CIDI was much smaller, estimated as 0.5%.[7] This variation highlights the importance of using carefully designed epidemiological studies which use well-validated screening and follow-up assessments to make psychiatric (particularly, here, psychotic) diagnoses.

In a systematic review of the available literature, Saha et al.[58] observed that the median lifetime prevalence of schizophrenia, identified from 29 unique estimates, was placed at 0.4% (10–90th percentile: 0.2–1.2%), but they reported that better quality studies tended to find higher estimates. Moreover, until recently, the scientific community has tended to prioritize understanding of the lifetime prevalence of schizophrenia, or other related non-affective psychotic disorders, over the affective psychosis. In both the ECA and NCS (and NCS-R) studies the lifetime prevalence of manic episodes, for example, has been placed at between 0.6% (Baltimore, ECA,[56]) and 1.6%.[57]

In addition to the aforementioned design issues which may have a bearing on prevalence estimates, other issues may also affect variation in lifetime prevalence, as observed, including the age, sex, and ethnic composition of the underlying population at risk, level of urbanization or other factors such as deprivation, which may affect the burden of disorder in different populations. One further substantive problem inherent in many household survey designs is response or ascertainment bias. This problem is particularly pertinent in the estimation of the prevalence of psychotic disorders, whereby people with paranoid beliefs or suspicious thoughts may be less likely to respond to survey invitations. This could lead to the substantial underestimation of the prevalence of psychotic disorders.

While analytical methods to weight estimates by survey non-response exist, these are chiefly to recover representative prevalence estimates and confidence intervals by adjusting the distribution of parameters of interest (say, age or sex) in the sample, based on known values of these distributions in the target population (i.e. *post-stratification*). Such methods do not necessarily resolve the issue of whether non-responders to a survey were more likely to have the outcome of interest, precisely because the value of this estimate in the target population is unknown, and the object of interest to be estimated.

One novel methodology to partially overcome these issues utilized a hybrid household survey design with linkage to national population registers in Finland.[59] Thus, in this study of over 8000 participants, of whom 93% took part, people who screened positive for potential psychosis were invited for re-interview to confirm the presence of diagnosis via the CIDI. For those who refused or could not be contacted, the study had permission to examine evidence of a history of a diagnosis for psychotic disorder in the Finnish hospital registers. Using this method, the lifetime prevalence of any psychotic disorder, including bipolar disorders, rose from 3.06% to 3.48%, with total figures for all non-affective psychoses and schizophrenia only, placed at 1.44% and 0.87%, respectively. This design is likely to provide closer insights into the true prevalence of psychotic disorders, albeit in a particular context (i.e. Finland).

Alternatively, we may look to other epidemiological designs, such as cohort studies, to estimate the lifetime (and other) morbid risk of psychotic disorders. *Lifetime prevalence* estimates the proportion of all people with the disorder of interest at a given point in time. Necessarily, its estimate depends on survival, since people who have died prior to this point will not contribute to lifetime prevalence.

In contrast, *morbid risk* (sometimes referred to as *disease expectancy*) estimates the proportion of the population who will experience the disorder of interest at some point in their lifetime. In this respect, morbid risk is similar to *lifetime risk*, a measure of *cumulative incidence*, which estimates the proportion of people alive and disease free at a certain point in time (typically, birth) who will subsequently experience the disorder over their lifetime. Morbid risks of broadly-defined schizophrenia in the WHO ten-country study[33] for the population aged 15–54 years ranged from 0.5% in Honolulu (Hawaii, USA) to 1.72% in rural Chandigarh (India). Saha and colleagues[58] observed similar variation in their review of the international literature. They reported a median morbid risk of 0.72% for schizophrenia (10–90th percentile: 0.31–2.71%), based on 27 estimates.

The Impact of Epidemiological Research

Aetiology

Age and sex

While schizophrenia onset can start at almost any age,[72] over 70% of cases will occur between early adolescence and before 35 years old.[43,60] This finding has had a substantial impact on the provision of EIP services in several countries.[61] Although childhood-onset schizophrenia (onset before age 12) and late-onset schizophrenia (onset after age 50) have lower incidences, they appear to present with similar clinical features and risk factors that characterize schizophrenia arising in young adults;[62,63] nonetheless, psychotic disorganization symptoms may be more common in early onset cases while systematized paranoid delusions predominate in late onset cases.[64]

It remains unclear whether this robust age-at-onset distribution comprises variation determined by random genetic, developmental, or environmental effects unique to the individual,[5] or whether the apparent continuum masks underlying discontinuities. At younger ages, typically before 35 years old, rates of schizophrenia and other non-affective psychoses are twice as common in men than women, although the peak in risk for both sexes probably occurs before 20 years old.[60] Nonetheless, attenuated or even inverted sex effects, that is, a female preponderance of cases in younger age groups, has been consistently reported from India[65,66] and China,[67] and these findings have received little recent attention.

Generally, in the mid-forties incidence rates for men and women become more similar, or even higher amongst women. This later peak for women, robustly demonstrated in a meta-analytic approach[68] coincides with the menopausal epoch, which may be associated with biopsychosocial changes, including a possible cessation of a neuroprotective role of oestrogen around this time.[69,70] In very late onset psychosis (after age 60 years old) cohort studies suggest a higher cumulated lifetime risk in women, compared to men.[71,72]

Genetic factors

The genetic risk for psychotic disorders is complex and, with the exception of rare syndromes such as 22q11 deletion syndrome,[73–75] involves a large number of genes each carrying a small effect size.[76–78] Schizophrenia, for instance, is highly heritable, with 50% monozygotic twin concordance.[79] Recent advances in genetic research, particularly the increased availability and decreased cost of carrying out GWASs, mean that understanding of genetics of psychotic disorders has improved substantially.[80] Yet, heritability is considered complex and non-Mendelian.[81] There is also considerable overlap in genetic risk between schizophrenia and bipolar I[76,82] and other psychiatric disorders.[83]

The landmark meta-analysis of GWASs in schizophrenia identified 108 independently associated loci,[40] which each explained a very small part of the genetic variance. With larger samples becoming available for GWAS the number of loci identified will increase.[84] The largest meta-analysis of bipolar-I GWASs has established 56 independently associated loci across five regions,[85] and further study estimates there might be as many as 105 loci,[86] but these have not yet been discovered (largely, due to the large sample sizes needed for such discoveries).

A common way of combining these genetic loci with small effect sizes and improving predictive ability is via so-called polygenic risk scores (PRSs; a weighted sum of genetic variance of disease risk). The PRS for schizophrenia is derived from the aforementioned meta-analysis of GWASs[40] and contains genes for known neurobiological mechanisms involved in psychosis, such as dopamine-2 receptors,[87] genes involved in glutamatergic neurotransmission and synaptic plasticity,[88] and genes involved in immune function—also implicated in psychosis.[89]

Nonetheless, PRS is no panacea: current PRS for schizophrenia is thought to explain only about 8% of the total variance in genetic predisposition to schizophrenia, with the remainder most likely explained by, as of yet, undiscovered genetic loci, rare variants, and gene-gene and gene-environment interactions.[77] It is also susceptible to population stratification effects whereby allele frequency differences between cases and controls are due to systematic genetic ancestry differences and spurious disease correlations,[90] although it is possible to control for such effects to an extent. PRS for schizophrenia scores are beginning to be used in population-based epidemiological studies, in at least three ways. First, and most classically, it has been possible to examine whether greater PRS for schizophrenia was associated with psychotic experiences and disorders in population-based samples. For example, Vassos and colleagues[80] suggested that PRS for schizophrenia had good discriminant validity to distinguish between first episode psychosis cases and controls of European ancestry, and to predict diagnoses of schizophrenia amongst the control group. PRS scores currently lack validity in people of non-European ancestry. Curiously, data from a longitudinal, population-based birth cohort (the Avon Longitudinal Study of Parents and Children (ALSPAC) study) found that PRS scores were not predictive of psychotic experiences in adolescence, although they did predict negative symptoms associated with schizophrenia, as well as anxiety.[91]

This leads to the second potential use of PRS scores. In the same study, PRS for schizophrenia significantly predicted depressive symptoms, thus providing confirmation of the likely polygenic basis of generalized psychiatric morbidity. Genetic and family risk of a range of neurodevelopmental and psychiatric disorders are known to predict the full spectrum of mental health outcomes,[52,92,93] and PRS for schizophrenia are highly predictive of, and share overlap with, genes for bipolar disorder.[94] Schizophrenia PRS has also been associated with lower cognitive ability, though it appears to explain less of the genetic variance here than for schizophrenia.[95]

Finally, and perhaps most interestingly, PRS may allow us to test causal inference about putative relationships between environmental risk factors and psychiatric outcomes, including schizophrenia. For example, evidence that PRS for schizophrenia are associated with known risk factors for schizophrenia such as cannabis use, or urban living, may suggest that genetic factors are implicated in both the development of psychosis, and independently, the choice to smoke cannabis or live in a more urban environment. Such gene-environment correlation could imply that unmeasured genetic confounders are the causal drivers of the association between factors previously presumed to be solely environmental and subsequent schizophrenia risk. While this is still an emerging literature, some, though not all, early examples support the possibility that higher PRS for schizophrenia predicts exposure to both cannabis use and urban living.[95,96] Larger studies, free of selection biases, with even better characterized genetic and environmental measures are still required to elucidate the main, interactive, and potentially mediating effects of these variables on schizophrenia risk. This includes the PRS for any disorder, which is also liable to change as studies become larger and technologically improved.[84] Recent evidence suggests that even when controlling for PRS for schizophrenia, associations between urban birth and adolescent psychotic experiences in the general population remain evident.*

Substance use

Concern about the harmful effects of un-prescribed drugs on the mental state has a long history. Some substances, such as amphetamine, can lead to a psychotic state in virtually all users in a dose-dependent manner as part of intoxication. Others, such as alcohol, have aspects of the schizophrenia syndrome as part of relatively rare states associated with chronic, heavy use. Much focus has been placed on the role of cannabis (marijuana, hashish, etc.) that has, for at least a century, attracted particular attention.

It is clear that use of alcohol and cannabis alongside other drugs is common in people with schizophrenia. For instance, the Australian Survey of High Impact Psychosis[97] collected nationally representative data on 1825 people with psychotic illness, mainly schizophrenia. Alcohol and substance abuse or dependence were common, with lifetime prevalence of 51% and 55%, respectively.[97] It is accepted that drug use, particularly cannabis, can complicate the management of schizophrenia, but whether or not it can cause the disorder in those otherwise at the same risk as the healthy population has been contentious for at least a century, with the Indian Hemp Drugs Commission Report, completed in 1894, concluding that the evidence was nuanced.[98]

As in many investigations of personal risk factors and schizophrenia, the question of cause and effect is hard to answer with surveys and case control designs, some of which indicate that people with schizophrenia may stop using the drug around onset of psychosis.[99,100] Furthermore, the question as to whether cannabis can lead to schizophrenia remotely, after the acute effects of intoxication have settled, is complicated by the recognition of a dependence syndrome, particularly for preparations of cannabis containing higher levels of pro- versus anti-psychotic components that are increasingly available.[101]

Recent epidemiological data, again relying on birth cohort designs, indicates that there is an elevated risk associated with cannabis consumption, particularly in the early teenage years. Andreasson et al.[102] contributed a seminal study of military conscripts in Sweden and demonstrated an increased risk of schizophrenia in those who reported cannabis use by age 18 years of age; a systematic review including further cohort studies confirmed a modestly increased increase in risk.[103] Nevertheless, the public health implications remain unclear.[104] The prevalence of use and potency of cannabis is increasing in many countries, while it remains a moot point as to whether incidence of schizophrenia is increasing, the *sine qua non* of a causal association between the two. While an increasing number of US states, Canada, and Uruguay are legalizing cannabis use, with a variety of preparations and potencies available, the debate on causality[105,106] will continue. It remains crucial that relevant epidemiological data continue to be scrupulously collected while natural experiments are underway.

Neurodevelopmental issues and milestones

Psychotic disorders are thought to have important neurodevelopmental factors in their origin,[107] and risk factors for development of psychosis can be identified *in utero*. Severe maternal malnutrition[108] and prenatal exposure to infection increase risk of later disorder.[109] Obstetric complications and other perinatal hazards such as complications in pregnancy, abnormal foetal growth and complications during labour,[119,111] markers of disordered motor development and neurodevelopment in childhood,[112–114] and cognitive problems predating the onset of disorder[115] have also been associated with increased risk of disorder. High educational attainment in childhood is considered protective against the development of psychosis,[116,117] and study authors have suggested this might link to neurodevelopmental origins of disorder and the existence of a 'cognitive reserve' which increases available coping strategies.[116] These developmental risk factors for schizophrenia appear to act in a dose-response manner, arguing against a specific developmental subtype of schizophrenia.

Childhood trauma

Childhood adversities are also strongly associated with later psychosis risk,[118–120] including emotional, psychological abuse, physical and sexual abuse, neglect, peer victimization, and bullying.[120] A longitudinal study (n<1,000 adolescents) suggested a bidirectional relation between childhood trauma and psychotic experiences in adolescence: trauma both predicted these experiences and later trauma was a consequence of them. After accounting for this bidirectionality, trauma was still strongly predictive of psychotic experiences in a dose-response relationship, suggesting a causal role.[121] Trauma characterized by intention to harm (maltreatment, bullying) was particularly associated with increased psychotic symptoms in a longitudinal twin study,[121] and people experiencing more than one type of trauma (poly-victimization) are particularly at risk of adverse outcomes.[121,122] This poly-victimization is common, as is re-victimization of maltreated children in adulthood.[123]

Research into childhood maltreatment is often done by either prospective informant-reports or retrospective self-reports, and neither of these are perfect. Informant reports may lead to underestimation of the prevalence of childhood maltreatment, and self-report might be subject to memory or recall bias (cases might be more likely to remember maltreatment than controls). Recent research from the E-Risk study (the longitudinal twin study mentioned above) suggests that these measure largely non-overlapping populations (people who say they experienced childhood maltreatment are not considered to be maltreated by key informants) and those who self-report maltreatment appear most at risk of adverse mental health outcomes.[124]

Inflammation

An emerging body of evidence is accumulating regarding the association between inflammation and psychiatric illness including schizophrenia. Early pointers to this association, that may have considerable therapeutic impact, included the increased risk of schizophrenia following pandemic infections such as the global 1918 influenza outbreak.[125] While there is now clear evidence that a pro-inflammatory state exists during acute episodes of depression and psychosis, and that conventional psychiatric treatments normalize cytokine levels, circulating protein markers of infection,[126] the direction of causality in this association was not, until recently, clear.

Khandaker and colleagues[89] demonstrated that higher childhood inflammatory markers (interleukin 6 and C-reactive protein) were associated with depression, psychotic experiences, and psychotic disorder in young adulthood,[89,127] indicating a potential causal or pathogenic role for inflammation; this was later supported through a Mendelian randomization approach.[128] In addition to illuminating the mechanism through which causal factors may operate, this may illuminate the sometimes lethal comorbidity between schizophrenia cardiovascular disease and metabolic disorders.[89] There is also interest in the adaptive immune response and schizophrenia,[129] with auto-antibodies to neuronal surface antigens (largely neurotransmitter receptors) being demonstrated in 5–10% of people with first episode psychosis.[130] Randomized controlled trials of immune therapy for this group will establish whether or not this represents stratification of schizophrenia based on a cause, and echoes robust and long-standing epidemiological evidence of associations between the disorder and a variety of auto-immune disorders.[131]

Urban living

Neighbourhood-level risk factors have long been associated with the incidence of psychotic disorders, and appear to hold some specificity to non-affective psychotic disorders.[35] Limited evidence of a role in the affective psychosis[132] points towards possible mechanisms which are specific to non-affective psychotic disorders, such as the possibility that cognitive impairments or early developmental delays (see above) interact with exposure to neighbourhood social adversities. This research tenet started in the early 20th century, with Faris and Dunham's seminal work in Chicago.[133] They established that neighbourhoods with increased residential mobility and percentage of African-Americans and those of no fixed abode faced an increased incidence of psychosis.[133]

This work was later replicated in Bristol,[27] Nottingham,[30] and Mannheim in Germany,[134] amongst others. More recent studies have used advances in multilevel modelling[135] and spatial epidemiology[45,136] to show that environmental-level variance in non-affective psychosis risk remains even after accounting for compositional characteristics of the people within those areas, such as lower socioeconomic status, minority position (see below), or younger age. While neighbourhoods typically explain less than 10% of the variance in schizophrenia and other psychoses,[135] this effect seems to be relatively robust.

Most such multilevel studies have focused on the role of socio-environmental factors, finding support for exposures such as population density,[47,48,137] deprivation,[136,138] inequality,[136,139] low social cohesion,[140] crime rates,[140] social fragmentation,[142,143] and ethnic density: the size of a particular ethnic group in proportion to the total population in a specified area.[144] A low ethnic density is hypothesized to be associated with increased incidence of psychotic disorders in ethnic minorities.[145,146] It is thought that a high ethnic density is associated with strong support networks, alleviating the effects of discrimination.[146] Results of recent epidemiological investigations are mixed: some studies established a relationship,[145,147,148] but others showed a more nuanced picture of differential effects of ethnic density by ethnic group.[136] Non-social environmental risk factors for psychosis have received less attention to date, but factors such as air pollution, noise, and vitamin D deficiencies, to which urban populations may be more likely to be exposed ,have also been proposed as potential risk factors for psychosis; little evidence currently supports these findings,[149] but this may be due to difficulties in reliably and validly measuring such exposures.

Interestingly, these patterns of association are beginning to be replicated in both non-clinical samples of adolescent psychotic symptoms,[150–152] and in social neuroscience,[153–155] suggesting that exposure to adverse environmental factors over the early life course may lead to tangible changes in key brain regions known to be associated with the continuum of risk of psychotic experiences. Nonetheless, many, though not all,[47,48,132] of epidemiological studies investigating neighbourhood risk factors have been cross-sectional, meaning any observed association could at least partially be due to downward social drift whereby individuals in the prodromal stages of disorder move to neighbourhoods with higher levels of the exposure of interest. Prospectively collected longitudinal studies have shown that urban birth and upbringing [47,48] are associated with future risk of schizophrenia, meaning that the association cannot be fully attributable to social drift of individuals in the early stages of psychosis. Nonetheless, recent advances in the availability of genetic data (see above) and causal inference techniques in epidemiology[156] have suggested that some risk factors, including urban upbringing, might be subject to a degree of gene-environment selection. Here, individuals with a higher genetic risk of schizophrenia might be more likely to move to more densely populated areas,[156,157] or alternatively might be more likely to develop a substance use issues[158] which precipitate a downward social cascade.

Moreover, recent research has shone further light onto the role of urban factors in the onset of psychotic disorders across the world. In the 17-centre EU-GEI incidence study,[51] an eight-fold variation in rates across Europe and Brazil was not simply explained by population density; instead urban-rural differences were found in northern European countries (the UK, Netherlands) but not their southern counterparts (Spain, Italy). Instead, the strongest predictor of inter-centre variation in rates was owner-occupancy, a strong marker of social stability, not urbanicity per se. This finding accords with recent research in East Anglia[137] which shows that higher rates of psychosis exist in more deprived and fragmented rural populations, suggesting urbanicity alone may be one of a set of socio-environmental markers which alter incidence.

The importance of local context in driving environmental associations with psychosis risk may also be borne out in emerging evidence from LMICs. For example, in a recent large meta-analysis of World Health Survey data from 42 LMIC settings,[159] no overall effect of urban-rural living was found on the prevalence of psychotic experiences or disorder, though high between-country heterogeneity highlights the importance of measuring specific contextual factors which may drive rates in some, but not all urban environments. In a population survey of Chinese men, urban birth was a stronger predictor of psychotic symptoms in adulthood than current urban residency.[160]

Migration and ethnicity

One of the most consistent epidemiological findings in the epidemiology of psychotic disorders is the excess risk experienced by migrants and their descendants. This finding is long-established,[161] and well replicated.[162,163] Excess rates in some migrant and minority group (such as those of black Caribbean and African origin in the UK[3,164] and elsewhere[165–167]) may be up to five times greater than in the majority white population, making this one of the greatest structural and cultural injustices in public mental health. There are no reasons to assume this increased incidence is an artefact of demographics, as incidence is still higher after adjusting for age and sex[42] and socio-economic status.[46,168] Moreover, rates do not appear to be elevated in the countries of origin from which migrant groups originated,[161,169–171] though further research in more diverse settings is needed on this topic, or due to selective emigration of people predisposed to psychosis.[172,173]

These findings argue strongly against a genetic explanation for excess rates in many black and ethnic minority (BME) groups. Furthermore, whilst it appears to be true that there are, for instance, ethnic differences in pathways to care[174,175] and worse treatment when accessing mental health services,[175–180] there is little evidence that there are systemic racist diagnostic biases (at least, not concerning black Caribbeans in the UK).[181,182]

Timing of exposure to such effects may be important, although it is not currently clear at which age migration conveys the greatest risk, but childhood appears to be a key time. A Dutch study showed that an earlier age of migration (0–4 years) is associated with the highest risk,[183] whereas a Danish study demonstrated that in immigrants from the developed world, those who migrated aged 10–14 appeared to be at a similarly high risk,[184] and findings from East Anglia indicated that those who migrated during childhood (5–12 years) carried the highest risk.[168] Interestingly, internal migration—measured via greater residential instability in childhood and adolescence also has independent effects on later psychosis risk,[185,186] though this may also extend to other psychiatric disorders.[189]

Observations that the relative increase in psychosis risk is highly correlated with visible minority status[163] and perceived levels of discrimination[188] have led authors to investigate whether exposure to a range of pre-migratory and post-migratory social adversities increases psychosis risk amongst migrants and their descendants. Refugees are likely to be at increased risk of psychosis compared with the general migrant population,[189,190] and this is thought to be due to a combination of increased exposure to pre-migratory stressors and a more traumatic migration experience (although post-migratory factors may also play a role).[191] Post-migratory stressors may also play a role.

Several studies have found support for an ethnic density effect in psychosis,[192,193] whereby BME risk is conditional upon the proportion of people from one's ethnic group living in the neighbourhood. Although this finding could be explained by differential help-seeking and case ascertainment, one possibility is that greater social support from people with more similar social, economic and cultural backgrounds, or immigrant experiences, buffers against psychosis risk. Interestingly, in healthy volunteers, recent social neuroscience has shown that ethnic density results in lower activation of amygdala activity during stress responses.[155] Migrant and minority groups may face exposure to a range of increased social stressors relevant to psychosis risk,[194] and more longitudinal research is required to understand the pathways through which exposure to social adversities over the life course may disproportionately increase psychosis risk for these groups.

Course and outcome

While schizophrenia is largely defined on the basis of abnormal mental phenomena, disability in terms of restricted everyday activities and social functioning may be driven as much by cognitive dysfunction and so-called negative features as it is by the key diagnostic components of the syndrome. Studies investigating the long-term course and outcome of psychotic disorders for many years focused on prevalent cases with a diagnosis of schizophrenia or non-affective psychosis[195] where the degree of chronicity required to merit an operational diagnosis of schizophrenia heavily conditioned the outcomes achieved. This approach systematically excludes those developing a psychotic syndrome but who recover promptly and may bias our view towards a poorer outcome, skewing our understanding of the true long-term prognosis of these.[196,197] We may have been too pessimistic about outcome and so give an overly gloomy answer to questions family members ask about outcome when their relative first seeks help.[198]

The WHO ten-country study follow-up in people 12–26 years after diagnosis[197] demonstrated good symptomatic outcomes in over half of those with schizophrenia and other psychotic disorders. Indeed, the report was titled 'Recovery From Schizophrenia: An International Perspective'. Kraepelin's assertion of the deteriorating course of schizophrenia as its hallmark appears inconsistent with such data, and a likely consequence of the individuals with chronic conditions on which his descriptions relied;[199] modern models of course and outcome need to incorporate notions of remission and recovery.[200]

As the results of the WHO study show, the answer to the question as to what might happen after onset of schizophrenia or a first episode of any psychosis is anything, from complete recovery to a relapsing and remitting or even chronic course of psychosis over many years. Unfortunately, while *symptomatic* recovery is possible for some, the outcomes of schizophrenia in terms of the *social* and *functional* spheres are discrepant and often poor. For instance, Morgan et al.[201] followed up over ten years the AESOP study described above in terms of incidence. Symptomatic outcome was generally good. Three-quarters of participants experienced at least one period of sustained remission a decade after onset; at follow-up 141 (46%) had been symptom free for at least two years. In contrast, most (72%) had been unemployed for more than 75% of the follow-up period. This emphasizes the importance of considering a broad range of outcomes, and the factors that may determine the facets of outcome that are of importance in everyday life that may not see symptoms of psychosis as core.

Mortality

Although the effects of schizophrenia and other psychotic disorders on premature mortality have been known for over 175 years,[202] it is only relatively recently that this issue has returned to public prominence. Farr[202] demonstrated a six-fold excess of deaths among asylum inmates, compared with the general population of England and Wales. He concluded—obliquely—that a lack of medical supervision and treatment was to blame. Nearly two centuries later, studies still provide compelling evidence for excess mortality associated with psychosis, culminating in reduced life expectancy estimates for people with serious mental illness of between 10–25 years.[203–205] In a systematic review of 37 studies emanating from 25 different countries, Saha et al.[58] calculated a median standardized mortality ratio (SMR) of 2.58 for all-cause mortality in schizophrenia patients. Using the UK's General Practice Research Database, Osborn et al.[206] estimated a hazard ratio (HR) of 3.22 for increased risk of death from coronary heart disease and stroke in people with severe mental illness that could not be wholly explained by antipsychotic medication, smoking, or social deprivation. Unnatural causes apart, there is a nearly five-fold increase (SMR 4.68) of 'avoidable' natural deaths, due to hypertension, cerebrovascular disease, and smoking-related disease.[207] The phenomenon of 'sudden unexplained death' among schizophrenic patients[208] may also be related to cardiotoxic effects of antipsychotic drugs, especially in patients receiving more than one antipsychotic concurrently.[203,209,210]

Unnatural causes, including suicide (particularly in the early phase of illness),[211] accidents, and homicide (particularly high risk in men with schizophrenia), accounted for 25% of all deaths of people with psychoses over a 20-year period, according to a study based on the Danish Psychiatric Case Register.[212] In recent decades, the suicide rate in schizophrenia patients has become at least equal to, or possibly higher, than the suicide rate in major depression (SMR 9.60 in males, 6.80 in females).[213] Data from Scotland[214] and Australia[215] point to an increasing suicide rate in schizophrenia patients, mostly within the first year after discharge from hospital. Several risk factors have been suggested as relatively specific to suicide in schizophrenia suicide: being young and male, the experience of a disabling mental illness with multiple relapses and remissions, awareness of the deteriorating course of the condition, comorbid substance use, and loss of faith in treatment.[211,216,217] These recent findings have led to the notion of a persistent 'mortality gap' between people with schizophrenia and the general population,[218] leading to calls for parity of esteem in the treatment for (and research into) mental as compared with physical illness.[219]

Future Prospects

The epidemiology of schizophrenia and other psychotic disorders has a set of distinct features which provided important clues for aetiology and information for the provision, care, treatment, and intervention for people at risk of, or who experience first episode psychosis. As we have highlighted in this chapter, the causes of psychosis are likely to be multifaceted and complex, probably invoking multiple genetic, biological, and environmental risk factors and pathways which may lead to the onset of alterations in perception, beliefs, and cognitive schema which give rise to psychotic symptoms and in some cases, the persistence of disorder.

The most recent epidemiological data reveals a particularly challenging landscape, whereby established environmental risk factors for psychosis, including urban living and cannabis use, may be under a degree of genetic control.[156,220] This has not been universally replicated,[221] and such environmental factors appear to have independent effects on psychosis risk.[96,222] Many of these risk factors for schizophrenia and other psychotic disorders appear to begin early in life, consistent with current socio-neurodevelopmental theories of disorder.[107,223,224] Life course epidemiological approaches have been critical in elucidating some of these factors.[48,112,225] However, psychiatric epidemiology needs to adapt to both the realistic complexity of neuropsychiatric disorders and the availability of modern causal inference methods in epidemiology[226,227] if progress in the identification of the risk factors and pathways which lead to psychosis are to be fully understood and ameliorated at a population level.

Part of the solution to these problems will be the development of sufficiently powered, modern birth cohorts with well-characterized, reliable, and validated psychiatric outcomes over the life course. Such cohorts would need to collect information on a range of genetic, biological, and environmental measures over early childhood and adolescence—the period at which most mental health disorders, including psychosis, emerge—and acknowledge the multitude of individual, familial, school-based, and societal and cultural layers through which risk and protective factors may influence mental health.[228–230] Such samples may need to be huge in order to have sufficient statistical power to investigate interactive effects and, to constrain this, they will need to draw on as well as contribute to basic science investigations of causal heterogeneity. These goals are ambitious, but no more so than the large investments made in psychiatric genetics and neuroscience over the past three decades that must now incorporate environmental measures. Integrating a population-based understanding of psychotic disorders with these two domains will yield fruitful insights into their aetiology.

REFERENCES

1. Bleuler E. *Dementia Praecox Oder Gruppe Der Schizophrenien.* Tubingen: Diskord, 1911.
2. Van Os J, Reininghaus U. Psychosis as a transdiagnostic and extended phenotype in the general population. *World Psychiatry.* 2016; 15: 118–24.
3. Kirkbride JB, Errazuriz A, Croudace TJ, et al. Incidence of schizophrenia and other psychoses in England, 1950–2009: A systematic review and meta-analyses. *PLOS One.* 2012; 7: e31660.
4. Regier DA, Boyd JH, Burke Jr JD, et al. One-month prevalence of mental disorders in the United States. Based on five Epidemiologic Catchment Area sites. *Arch Gen Psychiatry.* 1988; 45: 977–86.
5. Kendler KS, Gallagher TJ, Abelson JM, et al. Lifetime prevalence, demographic risk factors, and diagnostic validity of nonaffective

psychosis as assessed in a US community sample. The National Comorbidity Survey. *Arch Gen Psychiatry.* 1996; 53: 1022–31.
6. McManus S, Bebbington PE, Jenkins R, et al. *Mental Health and Wellbeing in England: Adult Psychiatric Morbidity Survey 2014 Executive Summary*. Leeds: NHS Digital, 2016.
7. Kessler RC, Birnbaum H, Demler O, et al. The prevalence and correlates of nonaffective psychosis in the national comorbidity survey replication (NCS-R). *Biol Psychiatry.* 2005; 58: 668–76.
8. Klemperer J. Zur Belastungsstatistik der Durchschnittsbevölk erung: Psychosenhäufigkeit unter 1000 stichprobenmäßig aus den Geburtsregistern der Stadt München (Jahrgang 1881–1890) ausgelesenen Probanden. *Zeitschrift für die gesamte Neurol und Psychiatr.* 1933; 146: 277–316.
9. Fremming K. *Sygdomsrisikoen for Sindslidelser Og Andre Sjaelelige Abnormtilstande in Den Danske Gennemsnitsbefolkning.* London: Munksgaard, 1947.
10. Helgason T. Epidemiology of mental disorders in Iceland. A psychiatric and demographic investigation of 5395 Icelanders. *Acta Psychiatr Scand.* 1964; 40: (Suppl 173): 1+.
11. Mann A. The evolving face of psychiatric epidemiology. *Br J Psychiatry.* 1997; 171: 314–18.
12. Colman I, Jones PB. Birth cohort studies in psychiatry: beginning at the beginning. *Psychol Med.* 2004; 34: 1375–83.
13. Brugger C. Versuch einer Geisteskrankenzahlung in Turingen. *J Neurol Psychiatry.* 1931; 133: 252–390.
14. Brugger C. Psychiatrische Ergebnisse einer medizinischen, anthropologischen und soziologischen Bevolkerungsuntersuchung. *Zschr Ges Neurol Psychiatr.* 1933; 146.
15. Strömgren E. Beiträge zur psychiatrischen Erblehre, auf Grund von Untersuchungen an einer Inselbevölkerung. *Acta Psychiatr Neurol Scand.* 1938; Suppl. 19.
16. Sjögren T. Genetic-statistical and psychiatric investigations of a West Swedish population. *Acta Psychiatr Neurol Scand.* 1948; Suppl. 52.
17. Esson-Moller E, Larsson H, Uddenberg CE, et al. Individual traits and morbidity in a Swedish rural population. *Acta Psychiatr Neurol Scand Suppl.* 1956; 100: 1–160.
18. Hagnell O. *A Prospective Study of the Incidence of Mental Disorder*. Stockholm: Scand Univ Books, Svenska Bokförlaget/Norstedts-Bonniers, 1966.
19. Hagnell O. The incidence and duration of episodes of mental illness in a total population. In: Hare EH, Wing JK (eds). *Psychiatric Epidemiology*. Lund: Oxford University Press, 1970. pp213–24.
20. Böök JA. A genetic and neuropsychiatric investigation of a North-Swedish population. with special regard to schizophrenia and mental deficiency. *Acta Genet Stat Med.* 1953; 4: 1–100.
21. Böök JA, Wettererg L, Modrzewska K. Schizophrenia in a North Swedish geographical isolate, 1900–77: epidemiology, genetics and biochemistry. *Clin Genet.* 1978; 14: 373–94.
22. Rüdin E. *Studien Über Vererbung Und Entstehung Geistiger Störungen*. London: Springer, 1916.
23. Jablensky A. Epidemiology of schizophrenia: the global burden of disease and disability. *Eur Arch Psychiatry Clin Neurosci.* 2000; 250: 274–85.
24. Eagles JM. Is schizophrenia disappearing? *Br J Psychiatry.* 1991; 158: 834–5.
25. Kirkbride JB, Croudace T, Brewin J, et al. Is the incidence of psychotic disorder in decline? Epidemiological evidence from two decades of research. *Int J Epidemiol.* 2009; 38: 1255–64.
26. McGrath J, Saha S, Welham J. et al. A systematic review of the incidence of schizophrenia: the distribution of rates and the influence of sex, urbanicity, migrant status and methodology. *BMC Med.* 2004; 2: 1–22.
27. Hare EH. Mental illness and social conditions in Bristol. *J Ment Sci.* 1956; 102: 349–57.
28. Faris R, Dunham H. Ecology of Mental Disorders in Urban Areas. Chicago: Chicago University Press, 1969.
29. Häfner H, Reimann H, Immich H, et al. Inzidenz seelischer Erkrankungen in Mannheim 1965. *Soc Psychiatr.* 1969; 4: 127–35.
30. Giggs JA, Cooper JE. Ecological structure and the distribution of schizophrenia and affective psychoses in Nottingham. *Br J Psychiatry.* 1987; 151: 627–33.
31. Baudiš P, Matesová A, Škoda C, et al. A comparison of first admissions of Mania in Prague, Aarhus and London—A transcultural study linked up with the International Pilot Study of Schizophrenia of WHO. *Soc Psychiatry.* 1977; 12: 185–93.
32. Sartorius N, Jablensky A, Korten A, et al. Early manifestations and first-contact incidence of schizophrenia in different cultures. A preliminary report on the initial evaluation phase of the WHO Collaborative Study on determinants of outcome of severe mental disorders. *Psychol Med.* 1986; 16: 909–28.
33. Jablensky A, Sartorius N, Ernberg G, et al. *Schizophrenia: Manifestations, Incidence and Course in Different Cultures A World Health Organization Ten-Country Study*. Psychological Medicine. Monograph Supplement.1992; 20: 1–97. http://www.journals.cambridge.org/abstract_S0264180100000904
34. Wing JK, Cooper JE, Sartorius N. *The Measurement and Classification of Psychiatric Symptoms*. Cambridge & London: Cambridge University Press, 1974.
35. March D, Hatch SL, Morgan C, et al. Psychosis and Place. *Epidemiol Rev.* 2008; 30: 84–100.
36. Crow TJ. Schizophrenia as the price that homo sapiens pays for language: a resolution of the central paradox in the origin of the species. *Brain Res Rev.* 2000; 31: 118–29.
37. Gottesman II, Shields J. A polygenic theory of schizophrenia. *Proc Natl Acad Sci U S A.* 1967; 58: 199–205.
38. Risch N, Rao DC. Genetic linkage and complex diseases, with special reference to psychiatric disorders. *Genet Epidemiol.* 1990; 7: 3–16.
39. McGuffin P, Owen M, Farmer A. Genetic basis of schizophrenia. *Lancet.* 1995; 346: 678–82.
40. Ripke S, Neale BM, Corvin A, et al. Biological insights from 108 schizophrenia-associated genetic loci. *Nature.* 2014; 511: 421–7.
41. Lloyd T, Kennedy N, Fearon P, et al. Incidence of bipolar affective disorder in three UK cities: Results from the ÆSOP study. *Br J Psychiatry.* 2005; 186: 126–131.
42. Fearon P, Kirkbride JB, Morgan C, et al. Incidence of schizophrenia and other psychoses in ethnic minority groups: results from the MRC AESOP Study. *Psychol Med.* 2006; 36: 1541–50.
43. Kirkbride JB, Fearon P, Morgan C, et al. Heterogeneity in incidence rates of schizophrenia and other psychotic syndromes: findings from the 3-center AeSOP study. *Arch Gen Psychiatry.* 2006; 63: 250–8.
44. Harrison G, Owens D, Holton A, et al. A prospective study of severe mental disorder in Afro-Caribbean patients. *Psychol Med.* 1988; 18: 643–57.
45. Kirkbride JB, Fearon P, Morgan C, et al. Neighbourhood variation in the incidence of psychotic disorders in Southeast London. *Soc Psychiatry Psychiatr Epidemiol.* 2007; 42: 438–45.

46. Kirkbride JB, Barker D, Cowden F, et al. Psychoses, ethnicity and socio-economic status. *Br J Psychiatry.* 2008; 193: 18–24.
47. Lewis G, David A, Andreasson S, et al. Schizophrenia and city life. *Lancet.* 1992; 340: 137–40.
48. Mortensen PB, Pedersen CB, Westergaard T, et al. Effects of family history and place and season of birth on the risk of schizophrenia. *N Engl J Med.* 1999; 340: 603–8.
49. Goldberg EM, Morrison SL. Schizophrenia and Social Class. *Br J Psychiatry.* 1963; 109.
50. Ngamini Ngui A, Cohen AA, Courteau J, et al. Does elapsed time between first diagnosis of schizophrenia and migration between health territories vary by place of residence? A survival analysis approach. *Heal Place.* 2013; 20: 66–74.
51. Jongsma HE, Gayer-Anderson C, Lasalvia A, et al. Treated incidence of psychotic disorders in the multinational EU-GEI Study. *JAMA Psychiatry.* 2018; 75: 36–46.
52. Lee SH, Ripke S, Neale BM, et al. Genetic relationship between five psychiatric disorders estimated from genome-wide SNPs. *Nat Genet.* 2013; 45: 984–94.
53. Murray RM, Sham P, Van Os J, et al. A developmental model for similarities and dissimilarities between schizophrenia and bipolar disorder. *Schizophr Res.* 2004; 71: 405–16.
54. Kaymaz N, Krabbendam L, de Graaf R, et al. Evidence that the urban environment specifically impacts on the psychotic but not the affective dimension of bipolar disorder. *Soc Psychiatry Psychiatr Epidemiol.* 2006; 41: 679–85.
55. Regier DA, Myers JK, Kramer M, et al. The NIMH Epidemiologic Catchment Area program. Historical context, major objectives, and study population characteristics. *Arch Gen Psychiatry.* 1984; 41: 934–41.
56. Robins LN, Helzer JE, Weissman MM, et al. Lifetime prevalence of specific psychiatric disorders in three sites. *Arch Gen Psychiatry.* 1984; 41: 949.
57. Kessler RC, McGonagle KA, Zhao S, et al. Lifetime and 12-month prevalence of DSM-III-R psychiatric disorders in the United States. Results from the National Comorbidity Survey. *Arch Gen Psychiatry.* 1994; 51: 8–19.
58. Saha S, Chant D, Welham J, et al. A systematic review of the prevalence of schizophrenia. *PLOS Med.* 2005; 2: e141.
59. Perälä J, Suvisaari J, Saarni SI, et al. Lifetime prevalence of psychotic and bipolar I disorders in a general population. *Arch Gen Psychiatry.* 2007; 64: 19–28.
60. Kirkbride JB, Hameed Y, Ankireddypalli G, et al. The epidemiology of first-episode psychosis in early intervention in psychosis services: findings from the Social Epidemiology of Psychoses in East Anglia [SEPEA] Study. *Am J Psychiatry.* 2017; 174: 143–53.
61. Csillag C, Nordentoft M, Mizuno M, et al. Early intervention services in psychosis: from evidence to wide implementation. *Early Interv Psychiatry.* 2016; 10: 540–546.
62. Brodaty H, Sachdev P, Rose N, et al. Schizophrenia with onset after age 50 years. I: Phenomenology and risk factors. *Br J Psychiatry.* 1999; 175: 410–15.
63. Nicolson R, Rapoport JL. Childhood-onset schizophrenia: rare but worth studying. *Biol Psychiatry.* 1999; 46: 1418–28.
64. Häfner H, Löffler W, Riecher-Rössler A, et al. Schizophrenia and delusions in middle aged and elderly patients. Epidemiology and etiological hypothesis. *Nervenarzt* 2001; 72: 347–57.
65. Murthy G V, Janakiramaiah N, Gangadhar BN, et al. Sex difference in age at onset of schizophrenia: discrepant findings from India. *Acta Psychiatr Scand.* 1998; 97: 321–5.
66. Gangadhar BN, Panner Selvan C, Subbakrishna DK, et al. Age-at-onset and schizophrenia: reversed gender effect. *Acta Psychiatr Scand.* 2002; 105: 317–19.
67. Phillips MR, Yang G, Li S, et al. Suicide and the unique prevalence pattern of schizophrenia in mainland China: a retrospective observational study. *Lancet.* 2004; 364: 1062–8.
68. Jackson D, Kirkbride J, Croudace T, et al. Meta-analytic approaches to determine gender differences in the age-incidence characteristics of schizophrenia and related psychoses. *Int J Methods Psychiatr Res.* 2013; 22(1): 36–45.
69. Häfner H, Riecher-Rossler A, An Der Heiden W, et al. Generating and testing a causal explanation of the gender difference in age at first onset of schizophrenia. *Psychol Med.* 1993; 23: 925–40.
70. Chua WLLC, Izquierdo de Santiago A, Kulkarni J, et al. Estrogen for schizophrenia. *Cochrane Database Syst Rev.* 2005; DOI: 10.1002/14651858.CD004719.pub2.
71. Helgason T, Magnússon H. The first 80 years of life. A psychiatric epidemiological study. *Acta Psychiatr Scand Suppl.* 1989; 348: 85–94; discussion 167–78.
72. Stafford J, Howard R, Kirkbride JB. The incidence of very late-onset psychotic disorders: a systematic review and meta-analysis, 1960–2016. *Psychol Med.* 2018; 48: 1775–86.
73. Bassett AS, Chow EWC, AbdelMalik P, et al. The schizophrenia phenotype in 22q11 deletion syndrome. *Am J Psychiatry.* 2003; 160: 1580–6.
74. Bassett AS, Chow EWC, Husted J, et al. Clinical features of 78 adults with 22q11 deletion syndrome. *Am J Med Genet Part A.* 2005; 138A: 307–13.
75. Baker KD, Skuse DH. Adolescents and young adults with 22q11 deletion syndrome: psychopathology in an at-risk group. *Br J Psychiatry.* 2005; 186.
76. Craddock N, Sklar P. Bipolar disorder 1: Genetics of bipolar disorder. *Lancet.* 2013; 381: 1654–62.
77. Harrison PJ. Recent genetic findings in schizophrenia and their therapeutic relevance. *J Psychopharmacol.* 2015; 29: 85–96.
78. Schizophrenia Working Group of the Psychiatric Genomic Consortium, 2015. https://pubmed.ncbi.nlm.nih.gov/25056061-biological-insights-from-108-schizophrenia-associated-genetic-loci/.
79. Dean L, Pratt V Mcleod H, et al. *Schizophrenia.* National Center for Biotechnology Information (US), 2012. https://pubmed.ncbi.nlm.nih.gov/28520342-schizophrenia/.
80. Vassos E, Di Forti M, Coleman J, et al. An examination of polygenic score risk prediction in individuals with first-episode psychosis. *Biol Psychiatry.* 2017; 81: 470–7.
81. Giegling I, Hosak L, Mössner R, et al. Genetics of schizophrenia: A consensus paper of the WFSBP Task Force on Genetics. *World J Biol Psychiatry.* 2017: 1–14.
82. International Schizophrenia Consortium. Common polygenic variation contributes to risk of schizophrenia and bipolar disorder. *Nature.* 2009; 460: 748–52.
83. Cross-Disorder Group of the Psychiatric Genetics Consortium. Identification of risk loci with shared effects on five major psychiatric disorders: a genome-wide analysis. *Lancet.* 2013; 381: 1371–9.
84. Pardiñas AF, Holmans P, Pocklington AJ, et al. Common schizophrenia alleles are enriched in mutation-intolerant genes and in regions under strong background selection. *Nat Genet.* 2018; 50: 381–9.
85. Mühleisen TW, Leber M, Schulze TG, et al. Genome-wide association study reveals two new risk loci for bipolar disorder. *Nat Commun.* 2014; 5: DOI: 10.1038/ncomms4339.

86. Chen DT, Jiang X, Akula N. et al. Genome-wide association study meta-analysis of European and Asian-ancestry samples identifies three novel loci associated with bipolar disorder. *Mol Psychiatry.* 2013; 18: 195–205.
87. Howes OD, McCutcheon R, Owen MJ, et al. the role of genes, stress, and dopamine in the development of schizophrenia. *Biol Psychiatry.* 2017; 81: 9–20.
88. Howes OD, Kapur S. A neurobiological hypothesis for the classification of schizophrenia: type A (hyperdopaminergic) and type B (normodopaminergic). *Br J Psychiatry.* 2014; 205: 1–3.
89. Khandaker GM, Pearson RM, Zammit S, et al. Association of serum interleukin 6 and C-reactive protein in childhood with depression and psychosis in young adult life. *JAMA Psychiatry.* 2014; 71: 1121–8.
90. Price AL, Patterson NJ, Plenge RM, et al. Principal components analysis corrects for stratification in genome-wide association studies. *Nat Genet.* 2006; 38: 904–9.
91. Jones HJ, Stergiakouli E, Tansey KE, et al. Phenotypic Manifestation of Genetic Risk for Schizophrenia During Adolescence in the General Population. *JAMA Psychiatry.* 2016; 73: 221.
92. Dean K, Stevens H, Mortensen PB, et al. Full spectrum of psychiatric outcomes among offspring with parental history of mental disorder. *Arch Gen Psychiatry.* 2010; 67: 822.
93. Mistry S, Harrison JR, Smith DJ, et al. The use of polygenic risk scores to identify phenotypes associated with genetic risk of schizophrenia: Systematic review. *Schizophr Res.* 2018; 197: 2–8.
94. Neale BM, Sklar P. Genetic analysis of schizophrenia and bipolar disorder reveals polygenicity but also suggests new directions for molecular interrogation. *Curr Opin Neurobiol.* 2015; 30: 131–8.
95. Sariaslan A, Fazel S, D'Onofrio BM, et al. Schizophrenia and subsequent neighborhood deprivation: revisiting the social drift hypothesis using population, twin and molecular genetic data. *Transl Psychiatry.* 2016; 6: e796.
96. Paksarian D, Trabjerg BB, Merikangas KR, et al. The role of genetic liability in the association of urbanicity at birth and during upbringing with schizophrenia in Denmark. *Psychol Med.* 2018; 48: 305–14.
97. Morgan VA, Waterreus A, Carr V, et al. Responding to challenges for people with psychotic illness: Updated evidence from the Survey of High Impact Psychosis. *Aust N Z J Psychiatry.* 2017; 51: 124–40.
98. Indian Hemp Drugs Commission Report of the Indian Hemp Drugs Commission 1893–1894. Simla: Government Central Printing Office; 1894.
99. McGuire PK, Jones P, Harvey I, et al. Cannabis and acute psychosis. *Schizophr Res.* 1994; 13: 161–7.
100. Dekker N, de Haan L, van den Berg S, et al. Cessation of cannabis use by patients with recent-onset schizophrenia and related disorders. *Psychopharmacol Bull.* 2008; 41: 142–53.
101. ElSohly MA, Mehmedic Z, Foster S, et al. Changes in cannabis potency over the last 2 decades (1995–2014): analysis of current data in the United States. *Biol Psychiatry.* 2016; 79: 613–19.
102. Andreasson S, Allebeck P, Engstrom A, et al. Cannabis and schizophrenia. A longitudinal study of Swedish conscripts. *Lancet.* 1987; 2: 1483–6.
103. Moore THM, Zammit S, Lingford-Hughes A, et al. Cannabis use and risk of psychotic or affective mental health outcomes: a systematic review. *Lancet.* 2007; 370: 319–28.
104. Hickman M, Vickerman P, MacLeod J, et al. If cannabis caused schizophrenia—How many cannabis users may need to be prevented in order to prevent one case of schizophrenia? England and Wales calculations. *Addiction.* 2009; 104: 1856–61.
105. Hill M. Perspective: Be clear about the real risks. *Nature.* 2015; 525: S14.
106. Murray RM, Quigley H, Quattrone D, et al. Traditional marijuana, high-potency cannabis and synthetic cannabinoids: increasing risk for psychosis. *World Psychiatry.* 2016; 15: 195–204.
107. Howes OD, Murray RM. Schizophrenia: an integrated sociodevelopmental-cognitive model. *Lancet.* 2014; 383:1677–87.
108. Susser ES, Lin SP. Schizophrenia after prenatal exposure to the Dutch Hunger Winter of 1944–1945. *Arch Gen Psychiatry.* 1992; 49: 983–8.
109. Khandaker GM, Zimbron J, Lewis G, et al. Prenatal maternal infection, neurodevelopment and adult schizophrenia: A systematic review of population-based studies. *Psychol Med.* 2013; 43: 239–57.
110. Brown AS, Derkits EJ. Prenatal infection and schizophrenia: a review of epidemiologic and translational studies. *Am J Psychiatry.* 2010; 167: 261–80.
111. Cannon M, Jones PB, Murray RM. Obstetric complications and schizophrenia: historical and meta-analytic review. *Am J Psychiatry.* 2002; 159: 1080–92.
112. Jones P, Rodgers B, Murray R, et al. Child development risk factors for adult schizophrenia in the British 1946 birth cohort. *Lancet.* 1994; 344: 1398–402.
113. Bramon E, Walshe M, Mcdonald C, et al. Dermatoglyphics and schizophrenia: A meta-analysis and investigation of the impact of obstetric complications upon a–b ridge count. *Schizophr Res.* 2005; 75: 399–404.
114. Filatova S, Koivumaa-Honkanen H, Hirvonen N, et al. Early motor developmental milestones and schizophrenia: A systematic review and meta-analysis. *Schizophr Res.* 2017; 188: 13–20.
115. Reichenberg A, Caspi A, Harrington H, et al. Static and Dynamic Cognitive Deficits in Childhood Preceding Adult Schizophrenia: A 30-year Study. *Am J Psychiatry.* 2010; 167: 160–9.
116. Khandaker GM, Stochl J, Zammit S, et al. A population-based longitudinal study of childhood neurodevelopmental disorders, IQ and subsequent risk of psychotic experiences in adolescence. *Psychol Med.* 2014; 44: 3229–38.
117. Khandaker GM, Barnett JH, White IR, et al. A quantitative meta-analysis of population-based studies of premorbid intelligence and schizophrenia. *Schizophr Res.* 2011; 132: 220–7.
118. Bendall S, Jackson HJ, Hulbert CA, et al. Childhood trauma and psychotic disorders: a systematic, critical review of the evidence. *Schizophr Bull.* 2008; 34: 568–79.
119. Matheson SL, Shepherd AM, Pinchbeck RM, et al. Childhood adversity in schizophrenia: a systematic meta-analysis. *Psychol Med.* 2013; 43: 225–238.
120. Varese F, Smeets F, Drukker M, et al. Childhood adversities increase the risk of psychosis: a meta-analysis of patient-control, prospective- and cross-sectional cohort studies. *Schizophr Bull.* 2012; 38: 661–71.
121. Kelleher I, Keeley H, Corcoran P, et al. Childhood trauma and psychosis in a prospective cohort study: cause, effect, and directionality. *Am J Psychiatry.* 2013; 170: 734–41.
122. Arseneault L, Cannon M, Fisher HL, et al. Childhood trauma and children's emerging psychotic symptoms: a genetically sensitive longitudinal cohort study. *Am J Psychiatry.* 2011; 168: 65–72.

123. Fisher HL, Caspi A, Moffitt TE, et al. Measuring adolescents' exposure to victimization: The Environmental Risk (E-Risk) Longitudinal Twin Study. *Dev Psychopathol.* 2015; 27: 1399–416.
124. Newbury JB, Arseneault L, Moffitt TE, et al. Measuring childhood maltreatment to predict early-adult psychopathology: Comparison of prospective informant-reports and retrospective self-reports. *J Psychiatr Res.* 2018; 96: 57–64.
125. Menninger KA. Influenza and schizophrenia. An analysis of post-influenzal "dementia precox," as of 1918, and five years later further studies of the psychiatric aspects of influenza. 1926. *Am J Psychiatry.* 1994; 151: 182–7.
126. Köhler CA, Freitas TH, Stubbs B, et al. Peripheral alterations in cytokine and chemokine levels after antidepressant drug treatment for major depressive disorder: systematic review and meta-analysis. *Mol Neurobiol.* 2017; 55: 4195–206.
127. Khandaker GM, Zammit S, Lewis G, et al. A population-based study of atopic disorders and inflammatory markers in childhood before psychotic experiences in adolescence. *Schizophr Res.* 2014; 152: 139–45.
128. Khandaker GM, Zammit S, Burgess S, et al. Association between a functional interleukin 6 receptor genetic variant and risk of depression and psychosis in a population-based birth cohort. *Brain Behav Immun.* 2018; 69: 264–72.
129. Khandaker GM, Cousins L, Deakin J, et al. Inflammation and immunity in schizophrenia: implications for pathophysiology and treatment. *Lancet Psychiatry.* 2015; 2: 258–70.
130. Lennox BR, Palmer-Cooper EC, Pollak T, et al. Prevalence and clinical characteristics of serum neuronal cell surface antibodies in first-episode psychosis: a case-control study. *Lancet Psychiatry.* 2017; 4: 42–8.
131. Benros ME, Eaton WW, Mortensen PB. The Epidemiologic Evidence Linking Autoimmune Diseases and Psychosis. *Biol Psychiatry.* 2014; 75: 300–6.
132. Pedersen CB, Mortensen PB. Urbanicity during upbringing and bipolar affective disorders in Denmark. *Bipolar Disord.* 2006; 8: 242–7.
133. Faris R, Dunham H. *Mental Disorders in Urban Areas: An Ecological Study of Schizophrenia and Other Psychoses.* Chicago: University of Chicago Press, 1939.
134. Weyerer S, Häfner H. The stability of the ecological distribution of the incidence of treated mental disorders in the city of Mannheim. *Soc Psychiatry Psychiatr Epidemiol.* 1989; 24: 57–62.
135. Zammit S, Lewis G, Rasbash J, et al. Individuals, schools, and neighborhood: a multilevel longitudinal study of variation in incidence of psychotic disorders. *Arch Gen Psychiatry.* 2010; 67: 914–22.
136. Kirkbride JB, Jones PB, Ullrich S, et al. Social deprivation, inequality, and the neighborhood-level incidence of psychotic syndromes in East London. *Schizophr Bull.* 2014; 40: 169–80.
137. Richardson L, Hameed Y, Perez J, et al. Association of environment with the risk of developing psychotic disorders in rural populations: Findings from the social epidemiology of psychoses in east anglia study. *JAMA Psychiatry* 2018; 75: 75–83.
138. Lasalvia A, Bonetto C, Tosato S, et al. First-contact incidence of psychosis in north-eastern Italy: influence of age, gender, immigration and socioeconomic deprivation. *Br J Psychiatry.* 2014; 205: 127–34.
139. Burns JK, Esterhuizen T. Poverty, inequality and the treated incidence of first-episode psychosis: an ecological study from South Africa. *Soc Psychiatry Psychiatr Epidemiol.* 2008; 43: 331–5.
140. Kirkbride JB, Morgan C, Fearon P, et al. Neighbourhood-level effects on psychoses: re-examining the role of context. *Psychol Med.* 2007; 37: 1413–25.
141. Bhavsar V, Boydell J, Murray R, et al. Identifying aspects of neighbourhood deprivation associated with increased incidence of schizophrenia. *Schizophr Res.* 2014; 156: 115–21.
142. Allardyce J, Gilmour H, Atkinson J, et al. Social fragmentation, deprivation and urbanicity: Relation to first-admission rates for psychoses. *Br J Psychiatry.* 2005; 187: 401–6.
143. Veling W, Susser E, Selten J-P, et al. Social disorganization of neighborhoods and incidence of psychotic disorders: a 7-year first-contact incidence study. *Psychol Med.* 2015; 45: 1789–98.
144. Bhugra D, Gupta S, Bhui K, et al. WPA guidance on mental health and mental health care in migrants. *World Psychiatry.* 2011; 10: 2–10.
145. Boydell J, Van Os J, Lambri M, et al. Incidence of schizophrenia in south-east London between 1965 and 1997. *Br J Psychiatry.* 2003; 182: 45–9.
146. Bécares L, Nazroo J, Stafford M. The buffering effects of ethnic density on experienced racism and health. *Heal Place.* 2009; 15: 670–8.
147. Schofield P, Ashworth M, Jones R. Ethnic isolation and psychosis: re-examining the ethnic density effect. *Psychol Med.* 2011; 41: 1263–9.
148. Veling W, Susser E, van Os J, et al. Ethnic density of neighborhoods and incidence of psychotic disorders among immigrants. *Am J Psychiatry.* 2008; 165: 66–73.
149. Pedersen C, Mortensen P. Urbanization and traffic related exposures as risk factors for schizophrenia. *BMC Psychiatry.* 2006; 6: 2.
150. Newbury J, Arseneault L, Caspi A, et al. Why Are children in urban neighborhoods at increased risk for psychotic symptoms? Findings from a UK Longitudinal Cohort Study. *Schizophr Bull.* 2016; 42: 1372–83.
151. Newbury J, Arseneault L, Caspi A *et al.* Cumulative Effects of Neighborhood social adversity and personal crime victimization on adolescent psychotic experiences. *Schizophr Bull.* 2018; 44: 348–358.
152. Solmi F, Colman I, Weeks M, et al. Trajectories of neighborhood cohesion in childhood, and psychotic and depressive symptoms at age 13 and 18 years. *J Am Acad Child Adolesc Psychiatry.* 2017; 56: 570–7.
153. Lederbogen F, Kirsch P, Haddad L, et al. City living and urban upbringing affect neural social stress processing in humans. *Nature.* 2011; 474: 498–501.
154. Haddad L, Schafer A, Streit F, et al. Brain structure correlates of urban upbringing, an environmental risk factor for schizophrenia. *Schizophr Bull.* 2014; 41: 115–122.
155. McCutcheon R, Bloomfield MAP, Dahoun T, et al. Amygdala reactivity in ethnic minorities and its relationship to the social environment: an fMRI study. *Psychol Med.* 2018: 1–8.
156. Sariaslan A, Larsson H, D'Onofrio B, et al. Does population density and neighborhood deprivation predict schizophrenia? A nationwide Swedish family-based study of 2.4 million individuals. *Schizophr Bull.* 2015; 41: 494–502.
157. Colodro-Conde L, Couvy-Duchesne B, Whitfield JB, et al. Association Between Population Density and Genetic Risk for Schizophrenia. *JAMA Psychiatry.* 2018; 75: 901–910.
158. Hartz SM, Horton AC, Oehlert M, et al. Association between substance use disorder and polygenic liability to schizophrenia. *Biol Psychiatry.* 2017; 82: 709–15.

159. DeVylder JE, Kelleher I, Lalane M, et al. Association of urbanicity with psychosis in low- and middle-income countries. *JAMA Psychiatry.* 2018; 75: 678–686.
160. Coid JW, Hu J, Kallis C, et al. Urban birth, urban living, and work migrancy: differential effects on psychotic experiences among young Chinese men. *Schizophr Bull.* 2018; 44: 1123–1132.
161. Ødegaard Ø. Emigration and insanity. *Acta Psychiatr Neurol.* 1932; Supp: 1–206.
162. Cantor-Graae E, Selten J-PP. Schizophrenia and migration: A meta-analysis and review. *Am J Psychiatry.* 2005; 162: 12–24.
163. Bourque F, Van Der Ven E, Malla A. A meta-analysis of the risk for psychotic disorders among first- and second-generation immigrants. *Psychol Med.* 2011; 41: 897–910.
164. Tortelli A, Errazuriz A, Croudace T, et al. Schizophrenia and other psychotic disorders in Caribbean-born migrants and their descendants in England: systematic review and meta-analysis of incidence rates, 1950–2013. *Soc Psychiatry Psychiatr Epidemiol.* 2015; 50: 1039–55.
165. Tortelli A, Morgan C, Szoke A, et al. Different rates of first admissions for psychosis in migrant groups in Paris. *Soc Psychiatry Psychiatr Epidemiol.* 2014; 49: 1103–9.
166. Zolkowska K, Cantor-Graae E, McNeil TF. Increased rates of psychosis among immigrants to Sweden: is migration a risk factor for psychosis? *Psychol Med.* 2001; 31: 669–78.
167. Dykxhoorn J, Hollander A-C, Lewis G, et al. Does risk of schizophrenia, schizoaffective, and bipolar disorders vary by migrant status, age-at-migration, and region of origin? A national cohort study of 1.8 million people. *Psychol Med.* 2019; 49(14): 2354–63.
168. Kirkbride JB, Hameed Y, Ioannidis K, et al. Ethnic minority status, age-at-immigration and psychosis risk in rural environments: evidence from the SEPEA study. *Schizophr Bull.* 2017; 43: 1251–61.
169. Hickling FW, Rodgers-Johnson P. The incidence of first contact schizophrenia in Jamaica. *Br J Psychiatry.* 1995; 167: 193–196.
170. Bhugra D, Hilwig M, Hossein B, et al. First-contact incidence rates of schizophrenia in Trinidad and one-year follow-up. *Br J Psychiatry.* 1996; 169: 587–92.
171. Mahy GE, Mallett R, Leff J, et al. First-contact incidence rate of schizophrenia on Barbados. *Br J Psychiatry.* 1999; 175: 28–33.
172. Selten J-P, Cantor-Graae E, Slaets J, et al. Odegaard's selection hypothesis revisited: schizophrenia in Surinamese immigrants to the Netherlands. *Am J Psychiatry.* 2002; 159: 669–71.
173. van der Ven E, Dalman C, Wicks S, et al. Testing Ødegaard's selective migration hypothesis: a longitudinal cohort study of risk factors for non-affective psychotic disorders among prospective emigrants. *Psychol Med.* 2015; 45: 727–34.
174. Morgan C, Mallett R, Hutchinson G, et al. Negative pathways to psychiatric care and ethnicity: the bridge between social science and psychiatry. *Soc Sci Med.* 2004; 58: 739–52.
175. Morgan C, Mallett MR, Hutchinson G, et al. Pathways to care and ethnicity II. Source of referral and help-seeking: Report from the ÆSOP study. *Br J Psychiatry.* 2005; 186: 290–6.
176. Morgan C, Mallett MR, Hutchinson G, et al. Pathways to care and ethnicity I. Sample characteristics and compulsory admission: Report from the AESOP study. *Br J Psychiatry.* 2005; 186: 281–9.
177. Koffman J, Fulop NJ, Pashley D, et al. Ethnicity and use of acute psychiatric beds: one-day survey in north and south Thames regions. *Br J Psychiatry.* 1997; 171: 238–41.
178. Takei N, Persaud R, Woodruff P, et al. First episodes of psychosis in Afro-Caribbean and White people. An 18-year follow-up population-based study. *Br J Psychiatry.* 1998; 172: 147–53.
179. Kuno E, Rothbard AB. Racial disparities in antipsychotic prescription patterns for patients with schizophrenia. *Am J Psychiatry.* 2002; 159: 567–72.
180. Mallinger JB, Fisher SG, Brown T, et al. Racial disparities in the use of second-generation antipsychotics for the treatment of schizophrenia. *Psychiatr Serv.* 2006; 57: 133–6.
181. Lewis G, Croft-Jeffreys C, David A. Are British psychiatrists racist?. *Br J Psychiatry.* 1990; 157: 410–15.
182. Hickling FW, McKenzie K, Mullen R, et al. A Jamaican psychiatrist evaluates diagnoses at a London psychiatric hospital. *Br J Psychiatry.* 1999; 175: 283–5.
183. Veling W, Hoek HW, Selten JP, et al. Age at migration and future risk of psychotic disorders among immigrants in the Netherlands: A 7-year incidence study. *Am J Psychiatry.* 2011; 168: 1278–85.
184. Pedersen CB, Cantor-Graae E. Age at migration and risk of schizophrenia among immigrants in Denmark: A 25-year incidence study. *Am J Psychiatry.* 2012; 169: 1117–18.
185. Price C, Dalman C, Zammit S, et al. Residential mobility and non-affective psychosis over the life course in 1.4 m young people in Sweden. *JAMA Psychiatry.* 2018; 75(11): 1128–36.
186. Paksarian D, Eaton WW, Mortensen PB, et al. Childhood residential mobility, schizophrenia, and bipolar disorder: a population-based study in Denmark. *Schizophr Bull.* 2015; 41: 346–54.
187. Mok PLH, Webb RT, Appleby L, et al. Full spectrum of mental disorders linked with childhood residential mobility. *J Psychiatr Res.* 2016; 78: 57–64.
188. Veling W, Selten J-P, Susser E, et al. Discrimination and the incidence of psychotic disorders among ethnic minorities in the Netherlands. *Int J Epidemiol.* 2007; 36: 761–8.
189. Anderson KK, Cheng J, Susser E, et al. Incidence of psychotic disorders among first-generation immigrants and refugees in Ontario. *CMAJ.* 2015; 187: E279–E286.
190. Hollander A-C, Dal H, Lewis G, et al. Refugee migration and risk of schizophrenia and other non-affective psychoses: cohort study of 1.3 million people in Sweden. *BMJ.* 2016; 352: i1030.
191. Rechel B, Mladovsky P, Ingleby D, et al. Migration and health in an increasingly diverse Europe. *Lancet.* 2013; 381: 1235–45.
192. Boydell J, van Os J, McKenzie K, et al. Incidence of schizophrenia in ethnic minorities in London: ecological study into interactions with environment. *Br Med J.* 2001; 323: 1336–8.
193. Kirkbride JB, Boydell J, Ploubidis GB, et al. Testing the association between the incidence of schizophrenia and social capital in an urban area. *Psychol Med.* 2008; 38: 1083–94.
194. Hjern A, Wicks S, Dalman C. Social adversity contributes to high morbidity in psychoses in immigrants -a national cohort study of two generations of Swedish residents. *Psychol Med.* 2004; 34: 1025–33.
195. Hegarty JD, Baldessarini RJ, Tohen M, et al. One hundred years of schizophrenia: a meta-analysis of the outcome literature. *Am J Psychiatry.* 1994; 151: 1409–16.
196. Cohen P, Cohen J. The clinician's illusion. *Arch Gen Psychiatry.* 1984; 41: 1178–82.
197. Hopper K, Harrison G, Janca A, et al. *Recovery from Schizophrenia: an International Perspective: a Report from the WHO Collaborative Project, the International Study of Schizophrenia.* New York: Oxford University Press, 2007.

198. Revier CJ, Reininghaus U, Dutta R, et al. Ten-Year outcomes of first-episode psychoses in the MRC AESOP-10 study. *J Nerv Ment Dis.* 2015; 203: 379–86.
199. Jablensky A. The diagnostic concept of schizophrenia: its history, evolution, and future prospects. *Dialogues Clin Neurosci.* 2010; 12: 271–87.
200. Barber ME. Recovery as the new medical model for psychiatry. *Psychiatr Serv.* 2012; 63: 277–9.
201. Morgan C, Lappin J, Heslin M, et al. Reappraising the long-term course and outcome of psychotic disorders: the AESOP-10 study. *Psychol Med.* 2014; 44: 2713–26.
202. Farr W. Report on the mortality of lunatics. *Lancet.* 1841; 36: 332–5.
203. Tiihonen J, Lönnqvist J, Wahlbeck K, et al. 11-year follow-up of mortality in patients with schizophrenia: a population-based cohort study (FIN11 study). *Lancet.* 2009; 374: 620–7.
204. Laursen TM, Munk-Olsen T, Vestergaard M. Life expectancy and cardiovascular mortality in persons with schizophrenia. *Curr Opin Psychiatry.* 2012; 25: 83–8. 10.1097/YCO.0b013e32835035ca.
205. Laursen TM, Wahlbeck K, Hällgren J, et al. Life expectancy and death by diseases of the circulatory system in patients with bipolar disorder or schizophrenia in the Nordic countries. *PLOS One.* 2013; 8: e67133.
206. Osborn DPJ, Levy G, Nazareth I, et al. Relative risk of cardiovascular and cancer mortality in people with severe mental illness from the United Kingdom's General Practice Research Database. *Arch Gen Psychiatry.* 2007; 64: 242.
207. Brown S, Inskip H, Barraclough B. Causes of the excess mortality of schizophrenia. *Br J Psychiatry.* 2000; 177: 212–17.
208. Appleby L, Thomas S, Ferrier N, et al. Sudden unexplained death in psychiatric in-patients. *Br J Psychiatry.* 2000; 176: 405–6.
209. Waddington JL, Youssef HA, Kinsella A. Mortality in schizophrenia. Antipsychotic polypharmacy and absence of adjunctive anticholinergics over the course of a 10-year prospective study. *Br J Psychiatry.* 1998; 173: 325–9.
210. Joukamaa M, Heliövaara M, Knekt P, et al. Schizophrenia, neuroleptic medication and mortality. *Br J Psychiatry.* 2006; 188: 122–7.
211. Simon GE, Stewart C, Yarborough BJ. et al. Mortality rates after the first diagnosis of psychotic disorder in adolescents and young adults. *JAMA Psychiatry.* 2018; 75: 254.
212. Hiroeh U, Appleby L, Mortensen PB, et al. Death by homicide, suicide, and other unnatural causes in people with mental illness: a population-based study. *Lancet.* 2001; 358: 2110–12.
213. Mortensen PB, Juel K. Mortality and causes of death in first admitted schizophrenic patients. *Br J Psychiatry.* 1993; 163: 183–9.
214. Geddes JR, Juszczak ED. Period trends in rate of suicide in first 28 days after discharge from psychiatric hospital in Scotland, 1968–92. *BMJ.* 1995; 311: 357.
215. Lawrence D, Holman CD, Jablensky AV, et al. Increasing rates of suicide in Western Australian psychiatric patients: a record linkage study. *Acta Psychiatr Scand.* 2001; 104: 443–51.
216. Caldwell CB, Gottesman II. Schizophrenics kill themselves too: a review of risk factors for suicide. *Schizophr Bull.* 1990; 16: 571–89.
217. Hawton K, Sutton L, Haw C, et al. Schizophrenia and suicide: Systematic review of risk factors. *Br J Psychiatry.* 2005; 187: 9–20.
218. Chwastiak LA, Tek C. The unchanging mortality gap for people with schizophrenia. *Lancet.* 2009; 374: 590–2.
219. Royal College of Psychiatrists. Whole person care: from rhetoric to reality, 2013. https://www.basw.co.uk/system/files/resources/basw_103627-6_0.pdf.
220. Power RA, Verweij KJH, Zuhair M, et al. Genetic predisposition to schizophrenia associated with increased use of cannabis. *Mol Psychiatry.* 2014; 19: 1201–4.
221. French L, Gray C, Leonard G, et al. Early Cannabis Use, Polygenic Risk Score for Schizophrenia and Brain Maturation in Adolescence. *JAMA Psychiatry.* 2015; 72: 1002.
222. Solmi F, Lewis G, Kirkbride JB. Neighbourhood characteristics at birth and positive and negative psychotic symptoms in adolescence: findings from the ALSPAC birth cohort. 2018: DOI: 10.17605/OSF.IO/NMH9Y.
223. Howes OD, Kapur S. The dopamine hypothesis of schizophrenia: Version III—the final common pathway. *Schizophr Bull.* 2009; 35: 549–62.
224. Morgan C, Charalambides M, Hutchinson G, et al. Migration, ethnicity, and psychosis: toward a sociodevelopmental model. *Schizophr Bull.* 2010; 36: 655–664.
225. Susser E, Hoek HW, Brown A. Neurodevelopmental disorders after prenatal famine: The story of the Dutch Famine Study. *Am J Epidemiol.* 1998; 147: 213–16.
226. Kendler KS. The structure of psychiatric science. *Am J Psychiatry.* 2014; 171: 931–8.
227. Petersen ML, van der Laan MJ. Causal models and learning from data. *Epidemiology.* 2014; 25: 418–26.
228. Susser E, Schwartz S, Morabia A. Eco-epidemiology. In: Susser E, Schwartz S, Morabia A, et al. (eds). *Psychiatric Epidemiology.* Oxford: Oxford University Press, 2006.
229. Susser M, Susser E. Choosing a future for epidemiology: I. Eras and paradigms. *Am J Public Health.* 1996; 86: 668–73.
230. Susser M, Susser E. Choosing a future for epidemiology: II. From black box to Chinese boxes and eco-epidemiology. *Am J Public Health.* 1996; 86: 674–7.

SECTION 6

Other key neurological conditions

29

Multiple sclerosis

Descriptive epidemiology and related neurobiology

Elisabeth Gulowsen Celius

Descriptive Epidemiology

Multiple sclerosis (MS) is a progressive disease affecting the central nervous system. The onset is usually in young adulthood and it is the most common cause of non-traumatic disability in young adults. The aetiology is unknown, but a genetic predisposition causing autoimmunity and demyelination is confirmed.[1] Most probably an unknown, possibly environmental factor, leads to the triggering of the immune system in predisposed individuals.

Prevalence

The prevalence of a disease is defined as the number of cases with a defined disease in a defined cohort at a given time point. The methods used for case ascertainment varies considerably from door-to-door-surveys to population registries. Thus, the quality of the studies is highly variable with especially smaller studies characterized by wide confidence intervals.[2] Differences in ethnicity, age and gender distribution, access to healthcare and availability of diagnostic tools, migration, socioeconomic status, and environmental factors may all influence the prevalence of the disease.

Studies of the prevalence of MS may also be hampered by the use of different criteria for the diagnosis of the disease over time.[3–10] Inclusion of only definite or also possible cases according to the different criteria, as well as differences in access to healthcare, including MRI and analysis of the cerebrospinal fluid, will influence the number of patients diagnosed. The diagnosis of MS relies on diagnostic criteria, making MS the most probable diagnosis in absence of other more likely causes and there are a number of misdiagnoses.[11,12] Also, the access to analysis of antibodies like aquaporin-4 (AQP-4) and anti-myelin oligodendrocyte (anti-MOG) antibodies constituting variants of MS varies.[13–15] Whether neuromyelitis optica spectrum disorder (NMOSD) defined by the AQP-4 antibodies is a variant or subgroup of MS is still to be determined.[16,17]

It has been recognized for decades that MS is unevenly distributed around the world. The prevalence is increasing with increasing latitude in both hemispheres,[18] but it has also been questioned if confounding factors may explain this latitude gradient.[19,20] The highest prevalence is found in Northern Europe, North America, Australia, and New Zealand.[2] The 'Viking theory' has been proposed, suggesting that genetic mutations caused the disease in Scandinavia around year AD 1000, and then the disease was spread by the Vikings, explaining the higher incidence in populations of European ancestry around the world.[21]

Europe

The prevalence of MS in the Nordic countries, Scotland, the Orkneys, and Northern Ireland is about 200/100,000 and among the highest in the world.[22–24] Within Norway there is no latitude gradient,[22] but in neighbouring Sweden an increase in prevalence with increasing latitude has been shown.[25] The prevalence in central Europe is 61–148/100,000, and in southern Europe 15–151/100,000.[2] In Sardinia, clusters with a prevalence resembling northern Europe and significantly higher than mainland Italy has been described.[26] From eastern Europe studies are emerging, and the figures do so far resemble those of central and southern Europe.[2]

North America

In the USA only a few studies have been conducted. In the Olmsted County in Minnesota a prevalence of 191/100,000 has been reported and in Lubbock, Texas 39.9/100,000, thus in line with a north-south gradient. The high prevalence in the mid-west may be caused by the high prevalence of people of Scandinavian descent.[27] Canada has been more extensively investigated, with the highest reported prevalence from Saskatoon of 298/100,000 and the lowest from Newfoundland of 56/100,000.[27] A population-based study of the province of British Columbia in Canada showed an increase in the prevalence over time up to 179/100,000.[28]

Latin and South America

In the Caribbean, only Martinique and Guadeloupe has been investigated, with a prevalence of 19/100,000 and 9/100,000.[27] The prevalence in Ecuador, Panama, and Columbia ranges from 0.7–6.5/100,000 and is not different from the Caribbean.[27,29] In South America, studies in the southern Argentinian Patagonia yielded a prevalence of 172/100,000.[27] In Brazil the few studies showed a gradient from 1.3/100,000 in the north to 18/100,000 in the south, and it has been suggested that this latitude gradient could be explained by the European and especially North-Italian immigration to the southern and south-eastern part of Brazil.[30]

Africa

Prevalence studies in Africa are scarce, one study of a region in South Africa showed a much higher prevalence among white (25/100,000) compared to blacks (0.2/100,000) and Indians (7/100,000).[31] The white population is of European descent and this may explain the higher disease susceptibility. Older and small studies have shown a low prevalence of 6–15/100,000 in northern Africa.[32]

Asia

In Asia most studies have been performed in the Middle East and the Far East, showing a prevalence of 20–60/100,000 in the Middle East and between 0.8/100,000 in China and 10.8/100,000 in Japan.[33] The prevalence of MS in Arabs varies between 3.4 and 42/100,000 and between 7.8 and 42/100,000 in Palestinians.[34] The prevalence is higher among Palestinians living in Kuwait and Jordan compared to the Arab population in these countries.[35] Jews and Arabs born and living in an Arab country prior to migration to Israel have half the prevalence of MS compared to Israeli and American-European born Arabs and Jews.[36]

India is a country of numerous different races and a huge diversity in religion, culture, and language. Also, migration from both the Middle East and across the Himalaya adds to the diversity. The prevalence ranges from 1.33 to 58/100,000 depending on region and ethnicity, with the highest prevalence of 58/100,000 in the Parsi from Pune and 21–26/100,000 in Parsi from Mumbai.[37] The Parsi are believed to have migrated from Iran and this may explain the higher prevalence in this group compared to other ethnic groups in the same regions.

New Zealand and Australia

The prevalence in Australia and New Zealand varies, but recent studies have shown an increase in prevalence and figures of 73–124/100,000.[38,39]

Racial differences in prevalence

In Europe the prevalence among ethnic minorities differs from the majority, with a markedly lower prevalence among Gypsies in Bulgaria[40] and the Sami in Norway.[41] In Malta the prevalence among Maltese-born inhabitants is significantly lower compared to mainly European non-Maltese born inhabitants.[42] Hispanics in Texas, USA showed a lower prevalence of than non-Hispanics in the same region.[43] Israeli-born and American European-born Jews in Israel have twice the prevalence of Arabs and Jews born in Israel or living in an Arab country prior to migration to Israel.[36] Palestinians in Jordan and Kuwait have a higher prevalence than the general population in these countries.[35] In Canada, the aboriginal population shows a significantly lower prevalence compared to the non-aboriginal population living in the same area,[44–46] but the higher than expected prevalence in a native population has been suggested as the result of European ancestors in the native population.[47] The prevalence in migrants from the Middle East living in Norway, Sweden, and British Columbia, Canada, is higher than expected from their home countries, but lower than the population in their new countries.[48–50]

Increasing prevalence

The increasing prevalence may be the result of better case ascertainment with repeated surveys,[23] changes in diagnostic criteria, earlier diagnosis, better access to healthcare, and new disease-modifying treatments prompting earlier diagnosis.[51] The main reason is probably the general increase in life expectancy that has occurred over the last decades.[52] In addition, migration may influence the prevalence rates in many regions.[28,53] Thus, the increased prevalence may not only be the result of increased risk of disease, but is often partly explained by this.

The age of onset, onset symptoms, and relative distribution of relapsing and progressive disease course seems to be relatively uniform across the world. A study of non-western immigrants to a high-risk Nordic environment showed a lower age at onset among first-generation and an even lower age among the second-generation immigrants, indicating that environmental factors may modify disease onset in susceptible individuals;[53] this is also observed in immigrants from North Africa to France.[54] MS in Japan was previously dominated by the optico-spinal form (neuromyelitis optica, NMO), but in recent years incident cases in Japan are changing towards the relapsing remitting disease observed in the European/American population.[55]

The female to male ratio is changing, with an increasing number of female cases and a ratio of 2.5–3:1, but this may at least partly be explained by increased life expectancy in the population and predominantly among females.[2]

Incidence

The incidence of a disease is defined as the number of newly diagnosed cases in a defined population and time span, usually a geographically defined area and over a time span of one year.

The highest incidences of 7–12/100,000/year are found in the regions with the highest prevalence such as the Nordic countries and in Canada.[28,56] The increased incidence observed in many regions may, in addition to a possible true increase in the disease, be explained by repeated surveys, advances in diagnostics, and recognition of the disease.[23,56–58]

Disease course

Several studies have shown increasing incidence of relapsing-remitting disease, whereas the incidence of patients with primary progressive disease seems to be stable.[59] This may in part be due to changes in definitions over time drifting away from the traditional subdivision in relapsing remitting and primary progressive disease and towards dividing patients according to disease activity.[60] Increasing availability of MRI scanners has also increased the number of active lesions detected even in patients with clinically stable disease, and may be one reason why the proportion of patients with primary progressive disease has been reduced in some areas.[61] The lack of treatment options in progressive MS may also contribute to the lower rate of newly diagnosed progressive patients in order to have the option to consider treatment.

Time Trends

There has been a change in diagnostic criteria from the early Schumacher criteria intended for research in 1965,[8] to the most recent McDonald criteria with emphasis on MRI, published in 2011 and intended for use both in research and in clinical practice and revised in 2017.[3,6] The changing definitions of disease with earlier diagnosis will inevitably lead to changes in incidence, as will also the change in accessibility to healthcare and inclusion of MRI in the diagnostic work up throughout the world over the last decades. The term 'radiologically isolated syndrome' has been introduced to describe asymptomatic patients with MRI findings suggestive of demyelinating disease, but further studies are needed to understand these findings.[62]

Repeated surveys have been performed in some areas, showing in the majority of studies an increase over the years, but some studies have also shown a fluctuating pattern.[63,64] The female to male ratio in MS has increased over the years;[23,56,59,65,66] this seems attributable to a higher increase in risk in females compared to males. Several factors have been discussed as possible exogenous factors affecting the susceptibility, such as increased use of hormonal contraceptives, reduced number of childbirths, and the increase in smoking habits among females. The incidence of progressive disease in males and females are similar and have been stable over time.[59] From Canada the incidence figures were stable and the increase in the female ratio could be explained by the longer survival of females in the population compared to males;[28] similar corrections have not been performed in the majority of the other studies. In Denmark, inclusion in the MS registry has been mandatory since 1948; the incidence in women has almost doubled over 60 years whereas the increase is only moderate in men.[56] The increase is for both men and women most pronounced in the older age groups, indicating, at least partly, better case ascertainment.

Environmental Risk Factors

Repeated surveys of MS prevalence and incidence in the Faroe Islands suggested an 'epidemic' after the placement of British troops during the Second World War and this was interpreted as MS being a related to an infection introduced by the British troops.[67] Most probably the increased incidence was caused by the thorough investigation performed at intervals, but the possibility of an infection causing MS has so far not been completely abandoned.

Infectious diseases have decreased in the western world since the beginning of the 19th century, and in the same time we have observed an increase in autoimmune diseases.[68] The reduction in infections have prompted the question of whether increasing hygienic standards is responsible for the increase in autoimmune diseases (among them MS): the hygiene hypothesis.[69] In line with the hygiene hypothesis a decreased risk of MS is observed in patients having had a dog or cat in the household during childhood.[70,71] Some studies have shown no effect of having older siblings or attending daycare in childhood,[72] but others have shown an increased risk with increasing number of older siblings.[73–77] Childhood infections seem not to influence the late risk of developing MS.[78]

Clustering of residence has been associated with lower age at onset and thus seen as a sign of an environmental agent in the disease aetiology,[79,80] but this has not been confirmed in further studies.

Studies have shown an increased risk of MS among patients born in the month of May compared with November in the northern hemisphere and the reverse pattern in the southern part of Australia and New Zealand,[81] but others have not confirmed this association.[82] The possible month of birth association has been attributed to the decreased levels of vitamin D during the winter season, and recent studies of vitamin D levels in newborn babies later aquiring MS shows an increased risk with low concentrations of vitamin D.[83] Studies of nurses at school later acquiring MS have shown lower levels of vitamin D compared to those who do not,[84] but this may well be a consequence of the disease as the onset of the disease may be years before the clinical symptoms become evident. In line with this theory, the observation of lower bone mineral density in patients with a clinically isolated syndrome and in newly diagnosed patients may point to factors influencing for many years before MS is diagnosed.[85] Similarly, the increased body weight observed in patients at younger age later diagnosed with MS may be a consequence of clinically silent disease for many years[86] and is in accordance with the recently shown increase in use of healthcare prior to diagnosis.[87] Smoking seems consistently to increase the risk of MS,[88,89] and especially in patients carrying certain genetic risk alleles.[90] In addition, some studies also showed increased disease severity in smokers.[91]

Presence of the HLA-DRB1*15 is associated with female gender and younger age at onset.[92–94] The role of HLA-genes in increasing MS risk also applies for smoking and/or obesity, with significantly increased risk.[90,95] Also, for the infection with Epstein-Barr virus the risk is increased if you carry the HLA risk alleles.[96] So far these studies have been carried out in mainly Caucasian populations, and it remains to be seen if similar associations can be replicated in other ethnic groups. The association between genes and disease severity and disease course has shown diverging results and no firm conclusions can be made.

Genetic Risk Factors in Population-based Studies

Based on prevalence figures the individual risk of MS in northern Europe and North America is around 0.1%. The familial recurrence risk has been estimated to approximately 20%, with an increase by 2–4% in first-degree relatives.[97–99] Twin studies show a five-fold increased risk in monozygotic twins compared to dizygotic (25% vs 5% concordance rate), implying the role of a genetic susceptibility factor.[100,101] The prevalence of MS among adoptees is similar to the general population and this is a strong argument for genetics being more important than environment for the familial aggregation of MS.[99] A study based on the Swedish national registry estimated the impact of heritability on MS risk to 0.64 and shared environment to 0.01.[102] Similar studies have not been performed in other parts of the world with lower prevalence figures and in other ethnic populations.

Migration studies

Based on earlier studies it was suggested that migration before puberty led to acquiring the risk of the new homeland, whereas migrating after puberty meant keeping the risk of the childhood country.[103] Recent migration studies indicate that the risk may differ depending on both country of origin and destination. Immigrants from eastern Asia seem to keep their risk of MS from their home country at least for the first generation, whereas first-generation immigrants from Africa and the Middle East seem to acquire an intermediate risk.[49,104,105] Thus, the risk may be modulated by ethnic differences, that is, the genetics may in addition to environmental factors modulate the susceptibility. There are few studies of acceptable size on population genetics, but the international MS genetics collaboration showed differences in the genetic composition according to country of origin even across the relatively homogenous Western Europe, USA and Australia.[1]

Studies of genetic risk variants have not confirmed any association between different gene variants and disease severity.[1,106] On the other hand several studies have shown that ethnicity affects the disease severity, implying that genetic factors may modulate severity. African-Americans compared to non-African Americans, Brazilians of African ancestry compared to Brazilians of non-African ancestry, native North Americans compared to Caucasians and non-western immigrants compared to the western/Caucasian population in Norway shows a more severe disease course.[53,107–109]

Studies of MS risk in migrants are complicated as only a few are population based, and the migrating population may differ from the population in the country of origin regarding ethnicity, health, and socioeconomic factors. Even with these objections, migrant studies may add valuable information in differentiating between genetics and environment.

Prognosis, Including Mortality

A reduction in life expectancy of about six years has been reported, but recent studies show a significant improvement in survival,[23,28] although this difference disappears in a Canadian, Norwegian, and Danish study when the general increase in life expectancy in the total population is taken into consideration.[52,110,111] The proposed increase in survival in many regions has been interpreted as a result of better symptomatic treatment options, but a similar increase is also seen in the general population. Whether the life expectancy will increase due to new and more potent disease-modifying drugs remains to be seen in the years to come. The recent study based on the Danish MS registry from 1950 onwards shows that the decline in excess mortality started decades before MRI and new diagnostic criteria came in use, and also decades before the use of disease-modifying drugs.[52] Thus, there seems to be a change in the disease prognosis independent of diagnostics and treatment.

Younger age at onset, female sex, relapsing-remitting disease course, and initial symptoms like paraesthesia and optic neuritis have been associated with longer survival,[112–114] but younger age at onset has also been associated with younger age at attainment of disability milestones in some studies.[115] A shorter time between onset and diagnosis predicts a more aggressive disease[116] and complete recovery from relapses is more common in younger patients and associated with a better prognosis.[117] Several studies have shown a more rapid progression of disability in patients with a primary progressive disease course compared to patients with a relapsing remitting disease course, but when addressing mortality there is no difference in age at death.[110,111]

A recent systematic review of modifiable risk factors could not identify any factor with significant impact on the risk of progression, but pointed to the need for more powered studies to explore vitamin D supplementations, physical exercise, and smoking cessation.[118,119]

Future Directions

Studies of prevalence and incidence are an important tool in dissecting the aetiology and distribution of MS. Differences between different geographical areas and changes over time, as well as studies of ethnic differences may point to environmental factors of importance for both disease susceptibility and disease progression. Furthermore, studies of ethnic differences may help in studying the relative contribution of genetic and environmental factors. Future studies should apply age and sex standardization to make comparisons possible both across regions and also over time. The studies should be large, use multiple sources of notification, validated diagnostic criteria, and strict definitions of disease characteristics.[120] There is a high need for studies of the natural course of the disease, as existing studies are from pre-treatment times and probably not applicable to today's patient population. The cost associated with MS is high,[121] and also in the context of future planning of healthcare to patients with MS, epidemiological studies are important.

REFERENCES

1. Sawcer S, Hellenthal G, Pirinen M, Spencer CC, Patsopoulos NA, Moutsianas L, et al. Genetic risk and a primary role for cell-mediated immune mechanisms in multiple sclerosis. Nature. 2011; 476(7359): 214–19.
2. Kingwell E, Marriott JJ, Jette N, Pringsheim T, Makhani N, Morrow SA, et al. Incidence and prevalence of multiple sclerosis in Europe: a systematic review. BMC Neurol. 2013; 13: 128.
3. Polman CH, Reingold SC, Banwell B, Clanet M, Cohen JA, Filippi M, et al. Diagnostic criteria for multiple sclerosis: 2010 revisions to the McDonald criteria. Ann Neurol. 2011; 69(2): 292–302.
4. Polman CH, Reingold SC, Edan G, Filippi M, Hartung HP, Kappos L, et al. Diagnostic criteria for multiple sclerosis: 2005 revisions to the 'McDonald Criteria'. Ann Neurol. 2005; 58(6): 840–6.
5. Poser CM, Paty DW, Scheinberg L, McDonald WI, Davis FA, Ebers GC, et al. New diagnostic criteria for multiple sclerosis: guidelines for research protocols. Ann Neurol. 1983; 13(3): 227–31.
6. Thompson AJ, Banwell BL, Barkhof F, Carroll WM, Coetzee T, Comi G, et al. Diagnosis of multiple sclerosis: 2017 revisions of the McDonald criteria. Lancet Neurology. 2018; 17(2): 162–73.
7. Rose AS, Ellison GW, Myers LW, Tourtellotte WW. Criteria for the clinical diagnosis of multiple sclerosis. Neurology. 1976; 26(6 pt 2): 20–22.

8. Schumacher GA, Beebe G, Kibler RF, Kurland LT, Kurtzke JF, McDowell F, et al. Problems of experimental trials of therapy in multiple sclerosis: report by the panel on the evaluation of experimental trials of therapy in multiple sclerosis. Ann NY Acad Sci. 1965; 122: 552–68.
9. McAlpine D. The benign form of multiple sclerosis. A study based on 241 cases seen within three years of onset and followed up until the tenth year or more of the disease. Brain. 1961; 84: 186–203.
10. Allison RS, Millar JH. Prevalence of disseminated sclerosis in Northern Ireland. Ulster Med J. 1954; 23(Suppl. 2): 1–27.
11. Howard J, Trevick S, Younger DS. Epidemiology of multiple sclerosis. Neurol Clin. 2016; 34(4): 919–39.
12. Solomon AJ, Bourdette DN, Cross AH, Applebee A, Skidd PM, Howard DB, et al. The contemporary spectrum of multiple sclerosis misdiagnosis: A multicenter study. Neurology. 2016; 87(13):1393–9.
13. Bukhari W, Prain KM, Waters P, Woodhall M, O'Gorman CM, Clarke L, et al. Incidence and prevalence of NMOSD in Australia and New Zealand. J Neurol Neurosurg Psychiatry. 2017; 88(8): 632–8.
14. Flanagan EP, Cabre P, Weinshenker BG, St Sauver J, Jacobson DJ, Majed M, et al. Epidemiology of aquaporin-4 autoimmunity and neuromyelitis optica spectrum. Ann Neurol. 2016; 79(5): 775–83.
15. Poser CM, Brinar VV. The accuracy of prevalence rates of multiple sclerosis: a critical review. Neuroepidemiology. 2007; 29(3–4): 150–5.
16. Lennon VA, Wingerchuk DM, Kryzer TJ, Pittock SJ, Lucchinetti CF, Fujihara K, et al. A serum autoantibody marker of neuromyelitis optica: distinction from multiple sclerosis. Lancet. 2004; 364(9451): 2106–12.
17. Weinshenker BG, Wingerchuk DM. Neuromyelitis spectrum disorders. Mayo Clin Proc. 2017; 92(4): 663–79.
18. Simpson S, Jr, Blizzard L, Otahal P, Van der Mei I, Taylor B. Latitude is significantly associated with the prevalence of multiple sclerosis: a meta-analysis. J Neurol Neurosurg Psychiatry. 2011; 82(10):1132–41.
19. Zivadinov R, Iona L, Monti-Bragadin L, Bosco A, Jurjevic A, Taus C, et al. The use of standardized incidence and prevalence rates in epidemiological studies on multiple sclerosis. A meta-analysis study. Neuroepidemiology. 2003; 22(1): 65–74.
20. Alonso A, Hernan MA. Temporal trends in the incidence of multiple sclerosis: a systematic review. Neurology. 2008; 71(2): 129–35.
21. Poser CM. The epidemiology of multiple sclerosis: a general overview. Ann Neurol. 1994; 36(Suppl 2): S180–93.
22. Berg-Hansen P, Moen SM, Harbo HF, Celius EG. High prevalence and no latitude gradient of multiple sclerosis in Norway. Mult Scler. 2014; 20(13): 1780–2.
23. Koch-Henriksen N, Sorensen PS. The changing demographic pattern of multiple sclerosis epidemiology. Lancet Neurology. 2010; 9(5): 520–32.
24. Svenningsson A, Salzer J, Vagberg M, Sundstrom P, Svenningsson A. Increasing prevalence of multiple sclerosis in Vasterbotten County of Sweden. Acta Neurol Scand. 2015; 132(6): 389–94.
25. Ahlgren C, Oden A, Lycke J. High nationwide prevalence of multiple sclerosis in Sweden. Mult Scler. 2011; 17(8): 901–8.
26. Nicoletti A, Patti F, Lo Fermo S, Sorbello V, Reggio E, Maimone D, et al. Possible increasing risk of multiple sclerosis in Catania, Sicily. Neurology. 2005; 65(8): 1259–63.
27. Evans C, Beland SG, Kulaga S, Wolfson C, Kingwell E, Marriott J, et al. Incidence and prevalence of multiple sclerosis in the Americas: a systematic review. Neuroepidemiology. 2013; 40(3): 195–210.
28. Kingwell E, Zhu F, Marrie RA, Fisk JD, Wolfson C, Warren S, et al. High incidence and increasing prevalence of multiple sclerosis in British Columbia, Canada: findings from over two decades (1991–2010). J Neurol. 2015; 262(10): 2352–63.
29. Cristiano E, Rojas J, Romano M, Frider N, Machnicki G, Giunta D, et al. The epidemiology of multiple sclerosis in Latin America and the Caribbean: a systematic review. Mult Scler. 2013; 19(7): 844–54.
30. Comini-Frota ER, Brum DG, Kaimen-Maciel DR, Fragoso YD, Barreira AA, Donadi EA. Frequency of reported European ancestry among multiple sclerosis patients from four cities in the southern and southeastern regions of Brazil. Clin Neurol Neurosurg. 2013; 115(9): 1642–6.
31. Bhigjee AI, Moodley K, Ramkissoon K. Multiple sclerosis in KwaZulu Natal, South Africa: an epidemiological and clinical study. Mult Scler. 2007; 13(9): 1095–9.
32. Rosati G. The prevalence of multiple sclerosis in the world: an update. Neurol Sci. 2001; 22(2): 117–39.
33. Makhani N, Morrow SA, Fisk J, Evans C, Beland SG, Kulaga S, et al. MS incidence and prevalence in Africa, Asia, Australia and New Zealand: A systematic review. Multiple Sclerosis and Related Disorders. 2014; 3(1): 48–60.
34. Benamer HT, Ahmed ES, Al-Din AS, Grosset DG. Frequency and clinical patterns of multiple sclerosis in Arab countries: a systematic review. J Neurol Sci. 2009; 278(1–2): 1–4.
35. al-Din AS, Khogali M, Poser CM, al-Nassar KE, Shakir R, Hussain J, et al. Epidemiology of multiple sclerosis in Arabs in Kuwait: a comparative study between Kuwaitis and Palestinians. J Neurol Sci. 1990; 100(1–2): 137–41.
36. Alter M, Kahana E, Zilber N, Miller A. Multiple sclerosis frequency in Israel's diverse populations. Neurology. 2006; 66(7): 1061–6.
37. Zahoor I, Haq E. Multiple sclerosis in India: Iceberg or volcano. J Neuroimmunol. 2017; 307: 27–30.
38. Ribbons K, Lea R, Tiedeman C, Mackenzie L, Lechner-Scott J. Ongoing increase in incidence and prevalence of multiple sclerosis in Newcastle, Australia: A 50-year study. Mult Scler. 2017; 23(8): 1063–71.
39. Taylor BV, Pearson JF, Clarke G, Mason DF, Abernethy DA, Willoughby E, et al. MS prevalence in New Zealand, an ethnically and latitudinally diverse country. Mult Scler. 2010; 16(12): 1422–31.
40. Milanov I, Topalov N, Kmetski T. Prevalence of multiple sclerosis in Gypsies and Bulgarians. Neuroepidemiology. 1999; 18(4): 218–22.
41. Harbo HF, Utsi E, Lorentzen AR, Kampman MT, Celius EG, Myhr KM, et al. Low frequency of the disease-associated DRB1*15-DQB1*06 haplotype may contribute to the low prevalence of multiple sclerosis in Sami. Tissue Antigens. 2007; 69(4): 299–304.
42. Dean G, Elian M, de Bono AG, Asciak RP, Vella N, Mifsud V, et al. Multiple sclerosis in Malta in 1999: an update. J Neurol Neurosurg Psychiatry. 2002; 73(3): 256–260.
43. Williamson DM, Henry JP, Schiffer R, Wagner L. Prevalence of multiple sclerosis in 19 Texas counties, 1998-2000. J Environ Health. 2007; 69(10): 41–5.
44. Svenson LW, Warren S, Warren KG, Metz LM, Patten SB, Schopflocher DP. Prevalence of multiple sclerosis in

First Nations people of Alberta. Can J Neurol Sci. 2007; 34(2): 175–80.
45. Warren S, Svenson LW, Warren KG, Metz LM, Patten SB, Schopflocher DP. Incidence of multiple sclerosis among First Nations people in Alberta, Canada. Neuroepidemiology. 2007; 28(1): 21–7.
46. Mirsattari SM, Johnston JB, McKenna R, Del Bigio MR, Orr P, Ross RT, et al. Aboriginals with multiple sclerosis: HLA types and predominance of neuromyelitis optica. Neurology. 2001; 56(3): 317–23.
47. Correa E, Paredes V, Martinez B. Prevalence of multiple sclerosis in Latin America and its relationship with European migration. Multiple Sclerosis Journal—Experimental, Translational and Clinical. 2016; 2: 2055217316666407.
48. Berg-Hansen P, Moen SM, Sandvik L, Harbo HF, Bakken IJ, Stoltenberg C, et al. Prevalence of multiple sclerosis among immigrants in Norway. Mult Scler. 2015; 21(6): 695–702.
49. Ahlgren C, Lycke J, Oden A, Andersen O. High risk of MS in Iranian immigrants in Gothenburg, Sweden. Mult Scler. 2010; 16(9): 1079–82.
50. Guimond C, Lee JD, Ramagopalan SV, Dyment DA, Hanwell H, Giovannoni G, et al. Multiple sclerosis in the Iranian immigrant population of BC, Canada: prevalence and risk factors. Mult Scler. 2014; 20(9): 1182–8.
51. Comi G, Radaelli M, Soelberg Sorensen P. Evolving concepts in the treatment of relapsing multiple sclerosis. Lancet. 2017; 389(10076): 1347–56.
52. Koch-Henriksen N, Laursen B, Stenager E, Magyari M. Excess mortality among patients with multiple sclerosis in Denmark has dropped significantly over the past six decades: a population-based study. J Neurol Neurosurg Psychiatry. 2017; 88(8): 626–31.
53. Berg-Hansen P, Smestad C, Sandvik L, Harbo HF, Celius EG. Increased disease severity in non-Western immigrants with multiple sclerosis in Oslo, Norway. Eur J Neurol. 2013; 20(12): 1546–52.
54. Kurtzke JF, Delasnerie-Laupretre N, Wallin MT. Multiple sclerosis in North African migrants to France. Acta Neurol Scand. 1998; 98(5): 302–9.
55. Houzen H, Kondo K, Horiuchi K, Niino M. Consistent increase in the prevalence and female ratio of multiple sclerosis over 15 years in northern Japan. Eur J Neurol. 2018; 25(2): 334–9.
56. Koch-Henriksen N, Thygesen LC, Stenager E, Laursen B, Magyari M. Incidence of MS has increased markedly over six decades in Denmark particularly with late onset and in women. Neurology. 2018; 90(22): e1954–e63.
57. Marrie RA, Cutter G, Tyry T, Hadjimichael O, Campagnolo D, Vollmer T. Changes in the ascertainment of multiple sclerosis. Neurology. 2005; 65(7): 1066–70.
58. Inglese M. Multiple sclerosis: new insights and trends. AJNR Am J Neuroradiol. 2006; 27(5): 954–7.
59. Celius EG, Smestad C. Change in sex ratio, disease course and age at diagnosis in Oslo MS patients through seven decades. Acta Neurol Scand Suppl. 2009(189): 27–9.
60. Lublin FD, Reingold SC, Cohen JA, Cutter GR, Sorensen PS, Thompson AJ, et al. Defining the clinical course of multiple sclerosis: the 2013 revisions. Neurology. 2014; 83(3): 278–86.
61. Westerlind H, Stawiarz L, Fink K, Hillert J, Manouchehrinia A. A significant decrease in diagnosis of primary progressive multiple sclerosis: a cohort study. Mult Scler. 2016; 22(8): 1071–9.
62. Lebrun C. The radiologically isolated syndrome. Rev Neurol (Paris). 2015; 171(10): 698–706.
63. Lund C, Nakken KO, Edland A, Celius EG. Multiple sclerosis and seizures: incidence and prevalence over 40 years. Acta Neurol Scand. 2014; 130(6): 368–73.
64. Edland A, Nyland H, Riise T, Larsen JP. Epidemiology of multiple sclerosis in the county of Vestfold, eastern Norway: incidence and prevalence calculations. Acta Neurol Scand. 1996; 93(2–3): 104–9.
65. Orton SM, Ramagopalan SV, Brocklebank D, Herrera BM, Dyment DA, Yee IM, et al. Effect of immigration on multiple sclerosis sex ratio in Canada: the Canadian Collaborative Study. J Neurol Neurosurg Psychiatry. 2010; 81(1): 31–6.
66. Westerlind H, Bostrom I, Stawiarz L, Landtblom AM, Almqvist C, Hillert J. New data identify an increasing sex ratio of multiple sclerosis in Sweden. Mult Scler. 2014; 20(12): 1578–83.
67. Kurtzke JF, Hyllested K. MS epidemiology in Faroe Islands. Riv Neurol. 1987; 57(2): 77–87.
68. Bach JF. The effect of infections on susceptibility to autoimmune and allergic diseases. N Engl J Med. 2002; 347(12): 911–20.
69. Wendel-Haga M, Celius EG. Is the hygiene hypothesis relevant for the risk of multiple sclerosis? Acta Neurol Scand. 2017; 136(Suppl 201): 26–30.
70. Gustavsen MW, Page CM, Moen SM, Bjolgerud A, Berg-Hansen P, Nygaard GO, et al. Environmental exposures and the risk of multiple sclerosis investigated in a Norwegian case-control study. BMC Neurol. 2014; 14: 196.
71. Ghadirian P, Dadgostar B, Azani R, Maisonneuve P. A case-control study of the association between socio-demographic, lifestyle and medical history factors and multiple sclerosis. Can J Public Health. 2001; 92(4): 281–5.
72. Sadovnick AD, Yee IM, Ebers GC. Multiple sclerosis and birth order: a longitudinal cohort study. Lancet Neurology. 2005; 4(10): 611–17.
73. Ponsonby AL, van der Mei I, Dwyer T, Blizzard L, Taylor B, Kemp A. Birth order, infection in early life, and multiple sclerosis. Lancet Neurology. 2005; 4(12): 793– 4; author reply 5.
74. Montgomery SM, Lambe M, Olsson T, Ekbom A. Parental age, family size, and risk of multiple sclerosis. Epidemiology. 2004; 15(6): 717–23.
75. Ahlgren C, Andersen O. No major birth order effect on the risk of multiple sclerosis. Neuroepidemiology. 2005; 24(1–2): 38–41.
76. Conradi S, Malzahn U, Schroter F, Paul F, Quill S, Spruth E, et al. Environmental factors in early childhood are associated with multiple sclerosis: a case-control study. BMC Neurol. 2011; 11: 123.
77. Bager P, Nielsen NM, Bihrmann K, Frisch M, Wohlfart J, Koch-Henriksen N, et al. Sibship characteristics and risk of multiple sclerosis: a nationwide cohort study in Denmark. Am J Epidemiol. 2006; 163(12): 1112–17.
78. Ascherio A, Munger KL. Environmental risk factors for multiple sclerosis. Part I: the role of infection. Ann Neurol. 2007; 61(4): 288–99.
79. Riise T, Gronning M, Klauber MR, Barrett-Connor E, Nyland H, Albrektsen G. Clustering of residence of multiple sclerosis patients at age 13 to 20 years in Hordaland, Norway. Am J Epidemiol. 1991; 133(9): 932–9.
80. Riise T, Klauber MR. Relationship between the degree of individual space-time clustering and age at onset of disease among multiple sclerosis patients. Int J Epidemiol. 1992; 21(3): 528–32.
81. Willer CJ, Dyment DA, Sadovnick AD, Rothwell PM, Murray TJ, Ebers GC. Timing of birth and risk of multiple sclerosis: population based study. BMJ. 2005; 330(7483): 120.

82. Eliasdottir O, Hildeman A, Longfils M, Nerman O, Lycke J. A nationwide survey of the influence of month of birth on the risk of developing multiple sclerosis in Sweden and Iceland. J Neurol. 2018; 265(1): 108–14.
83. Nielsen NM, Munger KL, Koch-Henriksen N, Hougaard DM, Magyari M, Jorgensen KT, et al. Neonatal vitamin D status and risk of multiple sclerosis: a population-based case-control study. Neurology. 2017; 88(1): 44–51.
84. Mirzaei F, Michels KB, Munger K, O'Reilly E, Chitnis T, Forman MR, et al. Gestational vitamin D and the risk of multiple sclerosis in offspring. Ann Neurol. 2011; 70(1): 30–40.
85. Moen SM, Celius EG, Sandvik L, Nordsletten L, Eriksen EF, Holmoy T. Low bone mass in newly diagnosed multiple sclerosis and clinically isolated syndrome. Neurology. 2011; 77(2): 151–7.
86. Hedstrom AK, Olsson T, Alfredsson L. High body mass index before age 20 is associated with increased risk for multiple sclerosis in both men and women. Mult Scler. 2012; 18(9): 1334–6.
87. Wijnands JMA, Kingwell E, Zhu F, Zhao Y, Hogg T, Stadnyk K, et al. Health-care use before a first demyelinating event suggestive of a multiple sclerosis prodrome: a matched cohort study. Lancet Neurology. 2017; 16(6): 445–51.
88. Hedstrom AK, Baarnhielm M, Olsson T, Alfredsson L. Exposure to environmental tobacco smoke is associated with increased risk for multiple sclerosis. Mult Scler. 2011; 17(7): 788–93.
89. Hedstrom AK, Baarnhielm M, Olsson T, Alfredsson L. Tobacco smoking, but not Swedish snuff use, increases the risk of multiple sclerosis. Neurology. 2009; 73(9): 696–701.
90. Hedstrom AK, Sundqvist E, Baarnhielm M, Nordin N, Hillert J, Kockum I, et al. Smoking and two human leukocyte antigen genes interact to increase the risk for multiple sclerosis. Brain. 2011; 134(Pt 3): 653–64.
91. Healy BC, Ali EN, Guttmann CR, Chitnis T, Glanz BI, Buckle G, et al. Smoking and disease progression in multiple sclerosis. Arch Neurol. 2009; 66(7): 858–64.
92. Celius EG, Harbo HF, Egeland T, Vartdal F, Vandvik B, Spurkiand A. Sex and age at diagnosis are correlated with the HLA-DR2, DQ6 haplotype in multiple sclerosis. J Neurol Sci. 2000; 178(2): 132–5.
93. Masterman T, Ligers A, Olsson T, Andersson M, Olerup O, Hillert J. HLA-DR15 is associated with lower age at onset in multiple sclerosis. Ann Neurol. 2000; 48(2): 211–19.
94. Hensiek AE, Sawcer SJ, Feakes R, Deans J, Mander A, Akesson E, et al. HLA-DR 15 is associated with female sex and younger age at diagnosis in multiple sclerosis. J Neurol Neurosurg Psychiatry. 2002; 72(2): 184–7.
95. Hedstrom AK, Lima Bomfim I, Barcellos L, Gianfrancesco M, Schaefer C, Kockum I, et al. Interaction between adolescent obesity and HLA risk genes in the etiology of multiple sclerosis. Neurology. 2014; 82(10): 865–72.
96. Sundqvist E, Sundstrom P, Linden M, Hedstrom AK, Aloisi F, Hillert J, et al. Epstein-Barr virus and multiple sclerosis: interaction with HLA. Genes Immun. 2012; 13(1): 14–20.
97. Westerlind H, Imrell K, Ramanujam R, Myhr KM, Celius EG, Harbo HF, et al. Identity-by-descent mapping in a Scandinavian multiple sclerosis cohort. Eur J Hum Genet. 2015; 23(5): 688–92.
98. Compston A, Coles A. Multiple sclerosis. Lancet. 2008; 372(9648): 1502–17.
99. Dyment DA, Ebers GC, Sadovnick AD. Genetics of multiple sclerosis. Lancet Neurology. 2004; 3(2): 104–10.
100. Willer CJ, Dyment DA, Risch NJ, Sadovnick AD, Ebers GC. Twin concordance and sibling recurrence rates in multiple sclerosis. Proc Natl Acad Sci USA. 2003; 100(22): 12877–82.
101. Mumford CJ, Wood NW, Kellar-Wood H, Thorpe JW, Miller DH, Compston DA. The British Isles survey of multiple sclerosis in twins. Neurology. 1994; 44(1): 11–15.
102. Westerlind H, Ramanujam R, Uvehag D, Kuja-Halkola R, Boman M, Bottai M, et al. Modest familial risks for multiple sclerosis: a registry-based study of the population of Sweden. Brain. 2014; 137(Pt 3): 770–8.
103. Gale CR, Martyn CN. Migrant studies in multiple sclerosis. Prog Neurobiol. 1995; 47(4–5): 425–48.
104. Smestad C, Sandvik L, Holmoy T, Harbo HF, Celius EG. Marked differences in prevalence of multiple sclerosis between ethnic groups in Oslo, Norway. J Neurol. 2008; 255(1): 49–55.
105. Guimond C, Dyment DA, Ramagopalan SV, Giovannoni G, Criscuoli M, Yee IM, et al. Prevalence of MS in Iranian immigrants to British Columbia, Canada. J Neurol. 2010; 257(4): 667–8.
106. George MF, Briggs FB, Shao X, Gianfrancesco MA, Kockum I, Harbo HF, et al. Multiple sclerosis risk loci and disease severity in 7125 individuals from 10 studies. Neurology Genetics. 2016; 2(4): e87.
107. Cree BA, Khan O, Bourdette D, Goodin DS, Cohen JA, Marrie RA, et al. Clinical characteristics of African Americans vs Caucasian Americans with multiple sclerosis. Neurology. 2004; 63(11): 2039–45.
108. Saeedi J, Rieckmann P, Yee I, Tremlett H. Characteristics of multiple sclerosis in aboriginals living in British Columbia, Canada. Mult Scler. 2012; 18(9): 1239–43.
109. Weinstock-Guttman B, Jacobs LD, Brownscheidle CM, Baier M, Rea DF, Apatoff BR, et al. Multiple sclerosis characteristics in African American patients in the New York State Multiple Sclerosis Consortium. Mult Scler. 2003; 9(3): 293–8.
110. Smestad C, Sandvik L, Celius EG. Excess mortality and cause of death in a cohort of Norwegian multiple sclerosis patients. Mult Scler. 2009; 15(11): 1263–70.
111. Kingwell E, van der Kop M, Zhao Y, Shirani A, Zhu F, Oger J, et al. Relative mortality and survival in multiple sclerosis: findings from British Columbia, Canada. J Neurol Neurosurg Psychiatry. 2012; 83(1): 61–6.
112. Phadke JG. Survival pattern and cause of death in patients with multiple sclerosis: results from an epidemiological survey in north east Scotland. J Neurol Neurosurg Psychiatry. 1987; 50(5): 523–31.
113. Sumelahti ML, Tienari PJ, Wikstrom J, Salminen TM, Hakama M. Survival of multiple sclerosis in Finland between 1964 and 1993. Mult Scler. 2002; 8(4): 350–5.
114. Bronnum-Hansen H, Koch-Henriksen N, Stenager E. Trends in survival and cause of death in Danish patients with multiple sclerosis. Brain. 2004; 127(Pt 4): 844–50.
115. Confavreux C, Vukusic S. Age at disability milestones in multiple sclerosis. Brain. 2006; 129(Pt 3): 595–605.
116. Signori A, Izquierdo G, Lugaresi A, Hupperts R, Grand'Maison F, Sola P, et al. Long-term disability trajectories in primary progressive MS patients: A latent class growth analysis. Mult Scler. 2018; 24(5): 642–52.
117. Cossburn M, Ingram G, Hirst C, Ben-Shlomo Y, Pickersgill TP, Robertson NP. Age at onset as a determinant of presenting phenotype and initial relapse recovery in multiple sclerosis. Mult Scler. 2012; 18(1): 45–54.

118. Hempel S, Graham GD, Fu N, Estrada E, Chen AY, Miake-Lye I, et al. A systematic review of modifiable risk factors in the progression of multiple sclerosis. Mult Scler. 2017; 23(4): 525–33.
119. Hempel S, Graham GD, Fu N, Estrada E, Chen AY, Miake-Lye I, et al. A systematic review of the effects of modifiable risk factor interventions on the progression of multiple sclerosis. Mult Scler. 2017; 23(4): 513–24.
120. Simpson S, Jr, Taylor BV. The Scandinavian paradox revisited: Editorial comment on Berg-Hansen et al. 'High prevalence and no latitude gradient of multiple sclerosis in Norway'. Mult Scler. 2014; 20(13): 1675–7.
121. Kobelt G, Thompson A, Berg J, Gannedahl M, Eriksson J. New insights into the burden and costs of multiple sclerosis in Europe. Mult Scler. 2017: 1352458517694432.

30 Myasthenia gravis

Anne Taraldsen Heldal and Nils Erik Gilhus

Introduction

Myasthenia gravis (MG) is a rare neuromuscular autoimmune disease, the cause of which remains unknown.[1] However, what is well established is the role of pathogenic circulating antibodies targeting the nicotinic acetylcholine receptor and other functionally linked molecules in the post-synaptic cell membrane. Occurring in all races, in both genders, of all ages, MG has evolved from being a severe disease with a mortality of 70%,[2] to in most cases being a disease that can be effectively treated. As a result of optimal treatment, the disease can be managed satisfactorily in most instances with a relatively good long-term prognosis, although slightly shorter survival compared to the general population.[3] While the pathology of this disease is well known, the aetiology of MG is still poorly understood. Epidemiologic research is one of the main methods to gain understanding and provide clues to the aetiology of this disease.

In this chapter we will outline the main aspects of MG epidemiology and the cutting edge of the field. Finally, we will discuss challenging future aspects of MG research.

Epidemiological research seeks to: '(1) describe health status by measuring disease frequency, distribution and trends; (2) know who becomes ill, what are the specific characteristics of cases, where and when these cases occur; (3) explain disease aetiology; (4) control the spread of specific diseases and their effects, by setting up preventive measures, improving prognosis and/or quality of life, and reducing mortality and other devastating complications.'[4] In MG research for the last decades, all these points have been applied. Disease frequency has been measured by calculating prevalence and incidence of MG, the distribution of the disease, and trends of incidence over decades have been studied, thereby trying to explain aetiological factors. Prognosis and mortality have been markedly changed so that MG patients today can expect overall a good long-term prognosis.

Prevalence and Incidence

As mentioned above, two concepts are essential in epidemiological research: prevalence and incidence.

Prevalence can be defined as 'the probability that an individual in a population will be a case at time t'.[5] A more practical definition of prevalence is to define it as the proportion of the population that has a disease at a set time point, point prevalence. Prevalence is a crucial estimator to gain an understanding of how many patients live with MG at a given time and enables comparing frequency of a disease among regions or countries. To know the prevalence of a certain disease is also useful for long-range healthcare planning, organizing health services for the disease, and for distribution of research and clinical competence of the disease.

Incidence can be expressed as a rate providing a measure of the occurrence of new disease cases per person-time unit.[5] Another incidence measure is the incidence proportion, which gives the proportion of the population that develops the disease during a specific period of time. Incidence per year is the most common way to refer to time when studying MG either as a rate or as a proportion. A reason for this is that life-expectancy in MG is now approximately the same as in the general population in most western countries.[6] Thus the denominator, which for the incidence rate is the number of persons under surveillance multiplied by one (one year), equals the general population, resulting in the incidence rate and incidence proportion being two concepts measuring the same number of new incident cases.

Prevalence-incidence ratio is interesting to study over time because it can reveal a change in the disease dynamics: if incidence is high relative to prevalence of a disease, it shows that this disease has a low survival rate or alternatively that the patients are cured. If incidence is low compared to the prevalence, it shows that the survival rate is high, or it can be a result of improved detection of the disease. MG has a high prevalence and a low incidence. The prevalence-incidence ratio has increased over the last decades,[7] suggesting an improving MG treatment and survival with subsequently increasing life-expectancy. The other explanation is the improved detection; it is, for example, most likely that case-ascertainment has improved during the time periods covered by the epidemiologic studies conducted in Norway. Moreover, there have been demographic changes in most western countries with an ageing population and lower birth rates.

MG prevalence and incidence can be calculated from different sources, most often either hospital-based or population-based studies. Calculations from hospitals or specialist centres usually suffer from selection and information bias. In such studies more patients tend to be severely affected and to be young, whereas there is a risk of missing milder and older patients with MG. Children in some hospital studies are not included because they are treated in a separate unit. Some MG patients go undiagnosed, especially if there are no detected muscle antibodies or only ocular symptoms. In population-based studies calculations are provided on the complete disease spectrum in unselected and defined denominator populations. Reviewing MG epidemiology from studies worldwide often reveals methodological differences, making a unified and internationally relevant description of the disease difficult. When evaluating MG epidemiological literature, it is important to be aware of what populations the calculations are drawn from and any subsequent biases.

In the last 60 years a large number of MG epidemiological studies have been performed in more than 40 different countries worldwide (Table 30.1). Reported MG prevalence has increased over time from 15 per million in 1951[8] to 260 per million in 2016.[9] Despite variations, there is a significant trend towards an increase in MG prevalence over time. This increase can in part be explained by increased survival for MG patients, and in part by population cohorts with more elderly people and less children. In Norway, three recently published studies reported prevalence of 131, 138, and 145 per million respectively,[10–12] and with a good concordance for two of the databases used.[13] From publications during the last five years, the MG prevalence has ranged between 112 and 260 per million.[9,14–18]

Reported annual MG incidence has also increased from 4.0 in the period 1951–1981,[19] to a report of 24.9 per million in 2012.[16] Published MG incidence during the last five years has ranged between 6.3 and 24.9 per million.[9,14–16,18] The increasing incidence can be explained by several factors. First, case-finding has improved due to the advent and increasing use of the acetylcholine receptor (AChR) antibody assay. Worldwide, the MG incidence doubled after 1976, when the first version of the modern AChR-antibody assay was described and introduced.[7] Furthermore, the healthcare system and neurological services have improved greatly during the last decades. This has probably led to a lower threshold for neurological examinations and a subsequent increased case ascertainment. Both in rich and poor countries the number of AChR antibody tests undertaken is steadily increasing.

There is evidence for MG previously having been underdiagnosed, in the elderly in particular. The clinical signs in MG are harder to assess correctly in this age group. Symptoms such as slurred speech,

Table 30.1 Overview over some incidence and prevalence studies published during the last 13 years

Country	Region/ nationwide	Year of publication	Study period	MG antibody subgroup	Case-finding method	Incidence (per million)	Prevalence (per million)
Portugal[14]	North Portugal	2016	2013	Total	Hospital databases and pyridostigmine registries	6.3	112
Korea[15]	Nationwide	2016	2010-2014	Total	Health insurance review and assessment data	6.9	104-130
Canada[9]	Ontario	2016	1996-2013	Total	Administrative health data sources	28	166-320
South Africa[31]	Nationwide	2015	2011-2012	AChR-antibody positive	Positive AChR-antibody laboratory data	8.3	
Sweden[32]	Nationwide	2015	2005-2010	Total	Swedish health and population registers		248
Norway[12]	Nationwide	2015	1994-2014	Total	Hospital databases		138
Denmark[27]	Nationwide	2013	1996-2009	Total	National registry of MG and pyridostigmine database	9.2	
Serbia[33]	Belgrade	2013	1979-2008	Total	Hospital records and the Belgrade MG registry	13.3	188.3
Australia[16]	Nationwide	2012	2009	Total	National prescribing database	25	117
Italy[17]	Pavia	2012	1995-2008	Total	Hospital registries		240
Italy[18]	Trento	2011	2005-2009	Total	Hospital and GP registries, AChR serology registries and pyridostigmine database		
Taiwan[34]	Nationwide	2010	2000-2007	Total	National health insurance research database	21	84-140
Norway[10]	Nationwide	2010	2004-2007	Total	Norwegian prescription database	16	131
Norway[11]	Nationwide	2009	1995-2008	AChR-antibody positive	AChR-antibody database	7.2	115.5
USA[35]	Nationwide	2009	2000-2005	Total	Nationwide inpatient sample database	10	
South Africa[36]	Capetown	2007	2003-2005	AChR-antibody positive	AChR-antibody database	11.2	
Denmark[37]	Eastern Denmark	2005	1970-1999	Total	Regional hospital registries	8.3	
Estonia[38]	Nationwide	2003	1997-1999	Total	Hospital databases and AChR-antibody laboratory data		78

difficulty in swallowing, and dysphagia, have many potential explanations in elderly people.[20–23] In addition, elderly patients have more comorbidity than younger patients, which can complicate the correct identification of the symptoms. Moreover, ocular symptoms such as ptosis and diplopia are common clinical signs at MG onset and are easier to detect in a more youthful appearance. Ptosis can be difficult to spot in the elderly because of a decrease in the total eyelid area with sagging of the lower eyelids, as a result of ageing. Macular degeneration or cataract formation can impede the detection of diplopia.[24] More patients are diagnosed with MG today than previously because of enhanced awareness of MG in the elderly.[23,24]

With an ageing population, an increase in new MG cases is expected as this group are at higher risk of acquiring MG. When comparing two studies from Norway from 1984 and 2008, respectively, twice as many patients had their first-time positive AChR-antibody test (anti-AChR MG) after 50 years of age in the latter study.[11] In the study from 1984, the calculated incidence rate was in contrast found to be higher for those with onset before 50 years versus those with onset after 50 years of age (2.9 per million versus 1.1 per million).[19] The higher incidence among the elderly in recent years is also clearly shown in two epidemiological studies from Italy conducted within the same geographical region, with a similar study design and with a 20-year interval between the studies. The increase in incidence was mainly due to an increase of male patients, with MG onset after age 50 years.[18] Enhanced awareness about late-onset MG and increased longevity in the general population with more MG patients diagnosed among the elderly are the main causes of the increased MG incidence.[11,18,23,25–27]

It is a striking observation that in several studies the MG incidence peaks in the group aged 70–80 years old, and then falls off markedly.[10,11,23,28] This could in theory be explained by missing the diagnosis in some of the very elderly. In addition, Vincent et al.[23] discussed two other explanations. The peak can be a cohort effect, where people represented in the peak have been exposed to a particular environmental exposure, increasing their risk for developing MG. However, this explanation requires a very short time of duration of susceptibility of the exposure and a very long fixed duration from exposure to MG development. This explanation fits poorly, as the short time of rise and fall for the incidence peak happens in several populations. It could alternatively be that the steep fall in the incidence represents a competing risk for those patients at risk for developing MG. It could be that these patients are at higher risk than the general population for developing some other fatal disease. This is unlikely as it has to be very strongly associated with the risk of developing MG, and a risk strictly limited to the very elderly.[23]

As discussed above, the increase in MG incidence demonstrated in many studies is mainly caused by an increase in the proportion of patients with onset after 50 years of age.[7] The immunological differences between early and late-onset MG, suggest that these subgroups are different disease entities. The majority of early-onset anti-AChR MG patients have hyperplastic thymus with lymphocytic infiltrates and germinal centres similar to those found in lymph nodes. The thymus contains all components necessary for a development of an immune response, supporting an intrathymic pathogenesis involved in the immune response in early-onset MG.[29] Late-onset MG usually lacks the thymic abnormalities, and the mechanisms of autosensitization to AChRs in this subgroup are unclear. Their HLA-profile differs, and titres of circulating AChR-antibodies are lower in late-onset MG than in early-onset MG. Antibodies to striated muscle antigens outside the neuromuscular junction are more often found in late-onset MG, while autoimmune comorbidity is more uncommon in this subgroup.[30] These aspects can explain why a genuine increase in late-onset MG may occur even if this is not true for early-onset MG and other MG subgroups.

Gender Characteristics

The MG incidence was for many years described with a peak in the 2nd and 3rd decade for women, and peaking in the 6th and 7th decade for men.[28,39] In recent years, studies have demonstrated a two-peaked MG incidence for women, and with a ratio close to 1:1 in the 6th and 7th decade (Fig. 30.1).[10,11,14,18] Other studies have not identified any early peak for women,[16,34] but a steady increase in MG incidence and a peak for both genders in the 6th and 7th decade (Fig. 30.2). In a systematic review of epidemiological

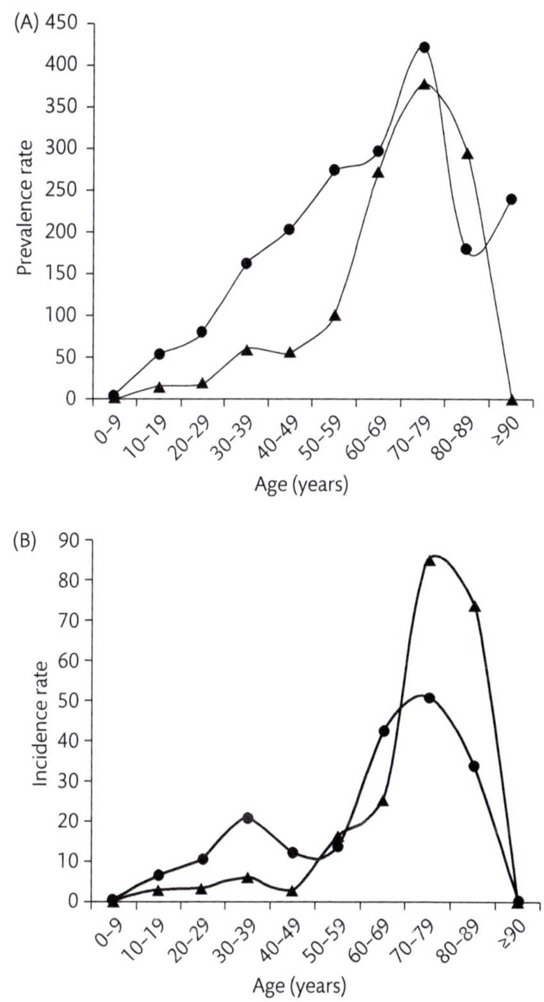

Fig. 30.1 Age and sex specific distribution of myasthenia gravis in Norway demonstrating a bimodal pattern. (A) prevalence, (B) incidence. Circles = women; triangles = men. Rates are per million inhabitants.

Reproduced with permission from Andersen JB, et al. Myasthenia gravis requiring pyridostigmine treatment in a national population cohort. *EurJN*. 17(12): 1445–50. Copyright © 2010 The Author(s). European Journal of Neurology © 2010 EFNS. DOI: https://doi.org/10.1111/j.1468-1331.2010.03089.x.

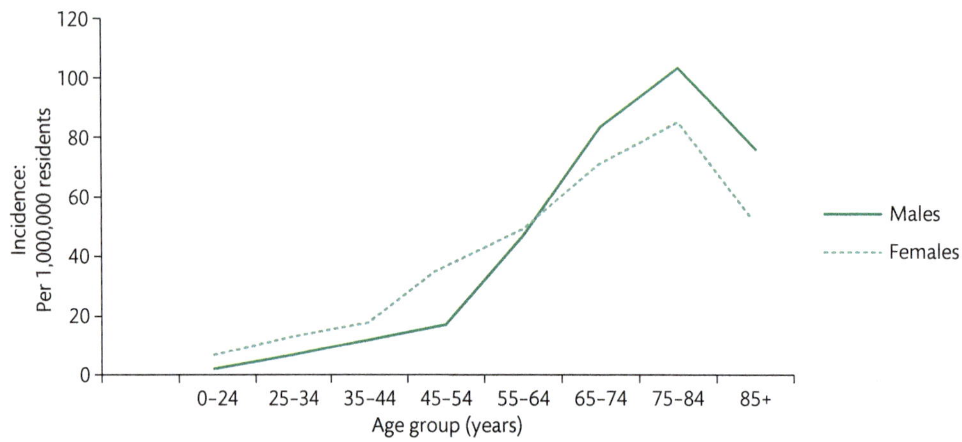

INCIDENCE	Number of cases	Population at risk	Crude rate (95% CI)	Standardized rate (95% CI)*
Female	306	10,986,535	27.9 (24.8–31.2)	21.6 (19.2–24.2)
Male	239	10,888,385	21.9 (19.3–24.9)	16.7 (14.6–18.9)
Total	545	21,874,920	24.9 (22.9–27.1)	19.1 (17.5–20.8)

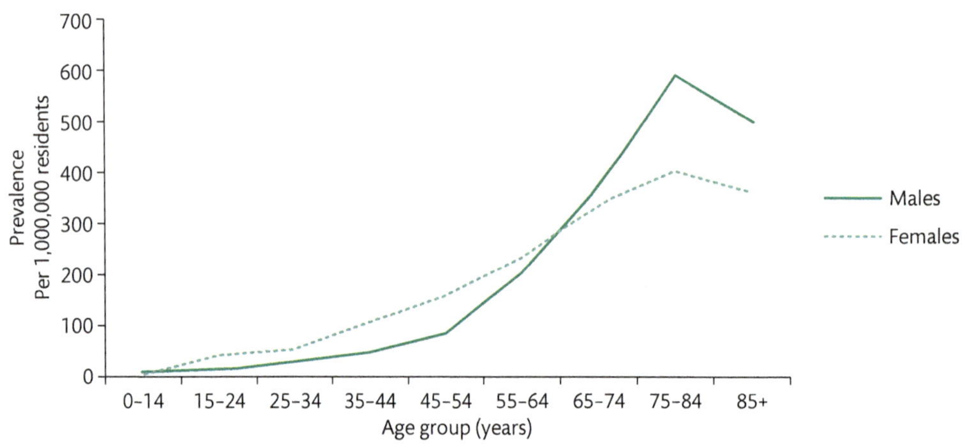

PREVALENCE	Number of cases	Population at risk	Crude rate (95% CI)	Standardized rate (95% CI)*
Female	1433	10,986,535	130.4 (123.8–137.7)	98.2 (93.0–103.6)
Male	1141	10,888,385	104.8 (98.8–111.1)	78.1 (73.6–82.8)
Total	2574	21,874,920	117.7 (113.2–122.3)	87.8 (84.3–91.3)

*Directly age-standardized to WHO world population

Fig. 30.2 Age and sex specific distribution of myasthenia gravis in Australia with an age-dependent increase in both sexes, and with a peak in the 7th decade.

Reproduced with permission from Gattellari M, et al. A national epidemiological study of Myasthenia Gravis in Australia. *EurJN*. 19(11): 1413–20. © 2012 The Author(s) European Journal of Neurology © 2012 EFNS. DOI: https://doi.org/10.1111/j.1468-1331.2012.03698.x.

studies of MG, the bimodal pattern for women was observed in 5 of 14 studies.[7] This pattern was in particular found in studies from Scandinavia, the UK, and Italy. The frequency of older individuals with MG and with MG debut in old age is probably greater than previously thought for both genders.[23,40,41]

Mortality

The mortality rate is a measurement in epidemiology for characterizing the number of deaths within a given population scaled to the size of that population, per unit of time.[42] Most epidemiological studies on MG have evaluated incidence and prevalence. Only a few studies have tried to calculate mortality.[2,3,28,40,43] Studies from the 1990s and earlier showed an increased mortality in MG. With improved diagnostics combined with effective treatment with immunosuppressive drugs, one should expect a decrease in mortality. However, a nationwide Danish study from 2016 containing anti-AChR MG patients, still found an excess mortality of 1.41 compared to the general population covering the period 1985–2005.[3] This is particularly the case during the first few years after diagnosis, and more so in women than in men. It is still important to bear in mind the markedly reduced mortality compared to before corticosteroids and other immunosuppressive drugs were introduced decades ago. It has been suggested that the still increased mortality rate in the first years after diagnosis could in part be due to severe respiratory problems and delayed diagnostics. A Norwegian study from 2006 looking at causes of death in MG patients 1951–2001, found a higher risk of respiratory tract disease in MG patients compared with a matched control group.[44] Deaths among men were in the Norwegian study more commonly related to respiratory tract disease before 1996 than after 1996, reflecting the improved MG therapy. They did not find any differences in the risk of respiratory tract disease at the age of over 70 years. However, in the Danish study, age remained an independent risk factor for mortality in MG, especially among patients older than 50 years.[35,43]

The mortality rate of MG has improved greatly from above 40% in the 1960s to less than 5% today,[45,46] presumably because of improvements in respiratory care and availability of treatment options, including plasma exchange and intravenous immunoglobulin. In addition, myasthenic crisis occurs much more rarely today than some years ago, due to more effective treatment and earlier diagnosis.

Ten to fifteen per cent of MG patients have a thymoma. Patients with MG and thymoma tend to have a more complicated clinical course and often a less favourable prognosis.[47] There are few studies on mortality rate in this subgroup, but a study from 1989 with 5–10 years follow-up, showed that 20% died within the study period.[48]

There is an increased risk of comorbidity for MG patients, especially for other autoimmune diseases, and varying between the MG subgroups.[49–51] A systematic review from 2011 found a pooled estimate of 13% for a coexisting autoimmune disease for MG.[52] For the early onset MG subgroup, there is a higher frequency of a second autoimmune disorder compared to patients with late onset MG.[32] However, the latter subgroup also has an increased risk for an autoimmune disease compared with control populations.[51]

Various Auto-antibodies Causing MG

MG patients should today always be defined into subgroups, as MG is regarded as a heterogeneous autoimmune disease with a post-synaptic defect of neuromuscular transmission as the common feature. Several auto-antibodies that can cause MG have been discovered during the last decades. The major pathologic antibodies in MG target AChR and MuSK (muscle-specific tyrosine kinase). Antibodies can also target other end-plate proteins (LRP4, rapsyn) and proteins outside the neuromuscular junction and involved in muscle contraction and excitation-contraction coupling (titin, myofibrillar proteins, ryanodine receptor) (Table 30.2).

In approximately 85% of cases, MG is caused by AChR-antibodies with affinity for the nicotinic AChRs in skeletal muscle.[53,54] AChR positive MG is the most studied subgroup of MG, this also being true for epidemiology, as a method for detection of AChR-antibodies assays was developed in 1976.[55] When AChR-antibody assays were introduced, it would have been expected that the variation in MG incidence would be reduced. However, there is no evidence for this, although the MG incidence rates increased significantly, with approximately a doubling after the introduction of this assay.[7] MuSK antibodies are detected in up to 5% of the MG patients.[56] This percentage varies among populations. MuSK is a neuromuscular junction protein co-localized with AChR at the post-synaptic membrane. The protein is important in the maintenance of the normal functionality of the neuromuscular junction by mediating clustering of AChRs.[30] MuSK-antibodies are not detected in AChR-antibody positive patients.[57] In Europe, anti-MuSK MG patients are most frequently found between the latitudes 30° and 50°N.[58] Up to 60% of non-AChR MG patients in Italy have a detectable concentration of MuSK-antibodies.[59] In contrast, there have been only very few reports of anti-MuSK MG patients in northern countries such as Norway.[60] An association between MuSK-antibody concentration and disease severity has been seen,[61] in contrast to the findings for AChR-antibodies.

Table 30.2 Myasthenia gravis antibody and subgroup characteristics. MG should be separated into several subgroups, reflecting pathogenesis and different considerations prior to therapeutic choices. Agrin-associated myasthenia gravis might emerge as a new entity. MG epidemiology should be subgroup specific [63,64]

Subgroup	Immune respons	Thymus pathological changes
Early onset (<50 yrs)	AChR-antibodies	Hyperplasia
Late onset (>50 yrs)	AChR-antibodies	Normal or hyperplasia
Thymoma	AChR-antibodies	Lymphoepithelioma
Ocular	Variable	Normal
Anti-MuSK MG	MuSK-antibodies	Normal
Anti-LRP4 MG	LRP4-antibodies	Normal
Antibody-negative MG	Unknown	Normal or hyperplasia

AChR = acetylcholine receptor. MuSK = muscle specific kinase. LRP4 = lipoprotein-related protein 4.

Source: data from Meriggioli M.N. and Sanders D.B. Muscle autoantibodies in myasthenia gravis: beyond diagnosis? *Expert Rev Clin Immunol*, 2012; 8(5): 427–438; data from Behin A. and Le Panse R. New Pathways and Therapeutic Targets in Autoimmune Myasthenia Gravis. *J Neuromuscul Dis*. 2018; 5(3): 265–277.

In approximately 60% of patients negative for both AChR- and MuSK-antibodies, low affinity AChR-antibodies have been identified. These antibodies can be detected using cell-based assays and direct immunofluorescence.[62] Unfortunately, these methods have not yet been commercially introduced. The antibodies are still likely to be pathogenic because of the high density of AChRs at the neuromuscular junction, and because the antibodies are of the IgG1 class and activate complement.[58]

There is a lack of formal reporting of the epidemiology of MG with no known antibodies and MG with antibodies other than those against AChR or MuSK. These MG subgroups might be more challenging to identify either because there is no antibody to use as a diagnostic marker, or no commercialized technique being available for antibody analysis. In addition, these subgroups have usually milder symptoms that do not always lead to specialist consultation or a correct diagnosis of MG. More detailed knowledge of the distinct disease subgroups within the MG phenotypic spectrum and examination of their individual frequencies and demographics are important aspects of MG epidemiology and research because it should bring important clues to aetiology of MG and contribute to optimize the treatment for each MG subgroup.

Genetic Epidemiology

The use of the term 'genetic epidemiology' emerged in the mid-1980s as a new scientific field and can be defined as: 'the study of the aetiology, distribution, and control of disease in groups of relatives and of inherited causes of disease in populations'.[65] The aetiology of acquired MG is complex and obviously includes a combination of both genetic and environmental risk factors (Fig. 30.3). In congenital myasthenia, a non-immune condition, mutations in different genes encoding molecules functionally important in the neuromuscular junction cause changes in muscle strength. Unlike congenital myasthenia, genetic factors alone are not sufficient for the development of disease in autoimmune MG. The underlying predisposing role of genes is still not well understood. In the 1970s, genes within the human leukocyte antigen locus (HLA) were discovered as the most important genetic risk factor for MG.[66–68] Since then, several studies have aimed to identify candidate genes in MG subgroups. The HLA locus remains to be the most strongly associated with the disease.[69] The main risk allele for early-onset MG is HLA-*B*08,[69] but also HLA class II region DRB1*16 is positively associated with early-onset MG.[70] HLA class II DRB1*0701 is negatively associated with early-onset MG. Late-onset MG is associated with HLA DRB1*15:0. Regarding non-HLA genes, early onset MG has been associated with the PTPN22*R620W risk allele, which is common in humoral autoimmune disorders.[71] Polymorphisms at *CHRNA1*, encoding for the α-subunit of the AChR, are strongly associated with early onset MG patients.[70,72] One of these *CHRNA1* SNPs interacts with the autoimmune regulator, AIRE, and so may affect thymic tolerance induction. Anti-MuSK MG has been associated with HLA class II DRB1*14, DRB1*16 and DQB1*05.[73–75]

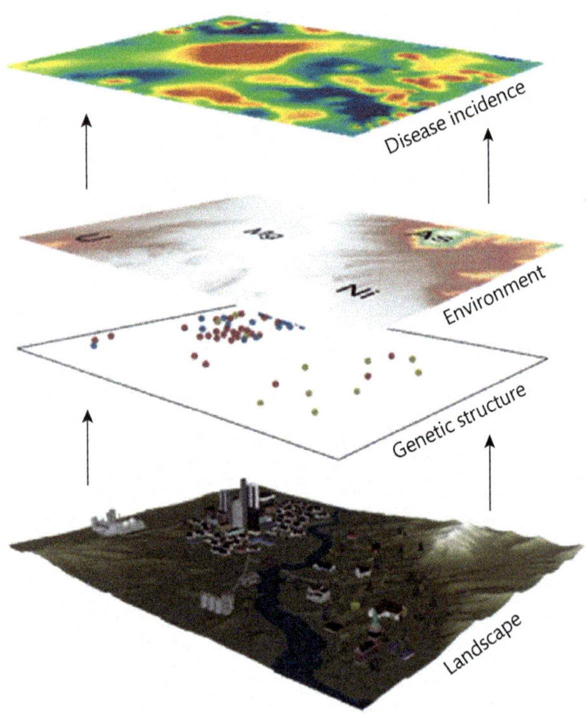

Fig. 30.3 The complex aetiology of autoimmune diseases illustrating the interaction between the landscape, the genetic susceptibility of a disease, local environmental exposures, and the spatial pattern of disease rates (colour plate).

Reproduced with permission from Sloan CD, et al. Ecogeographic genetic epidemiology. *Genet Epidemiol.* 33(4): 281–9. © 2008 Wiley-Liss, Inc. DOI: https://doi.org/10.1002/gepi.20386.

In MG the predisposing genetic factors are probably acting through minor changes in multiple genes, called SNPs. Minor changes in the products of those genes seem to be involved in the pathogenesis of the disease.[76]

GWASs have become an important approach in genetic epidemiology for identifying susceptibility genes for complex traits. A sample of DNA from each participant in such a study is examined using SNPs arrays. High-power computing capacity allows analysis of a large number of genes in a very large number of patients with a particular disease and control individuals without having to preselect candidate genes of interest. As a result, the genetic risk factors in the development of autoimmune diseases have been increasingly identified.[77]

The GWAS approach is called 'phenotype-first' since the study group is identified through clinical symptoms, as opposed to 'genotype-first'. The first successful study for genetic disease risk using GWAS was published in 2005.[78] The first GWAS study on MG was published in 2012.[70] A GWAS study was recently performed on anti- AChR MG, revealing new insights on genetic risk factors on this disease.[79] The study confirmed evidence that early and late-onset anti-AChR MG represent two distinct conditions, but with overlapping genetic risk factors. Susceptibility loci for AChR antibody-positive myasthenia gravis were identified at CTLA4, HLA-DRB1/HLA-DQA1, and TNFRSF11A. Several new loci that drive susceptibility to develop MG were identified.

The GWAS approach is well known in MS. In MS, more than 110 candidate variants have been identified, the vast majority of genes being involved in the immune system, in particular T cells.[80] MS is now firmly established as an autoimmune disease.

Migration and Epidemiology

Human migration can be defined as: 'Movement of people to a new area or country in order to find work or better living conditions'.[81] The purpose of migration may be permanent or semi-permanent residence and can be voluntary and non-voluntary. An example of semi-permanent residence is seasonal movements of labourers. Migration occurs in a large variety of scales: between continents, between countries within a continent, and between regions within countries. In national MG research, it is most relevant to study permanent migration from other countries and continents. However, one of the most significant patterns of migration has been rural to urban migration. In countries where the gap between the rural and urban way of living is large, this kind of migration will be interesting to study. Migration can change the epidemiology of MG and provide new insights into the genetic and environmental risk factors of MG. Assuming that the main migrational flows are from countries and areas with insufficient diagnostics of MG, this will influence the incidence of MG. It will be important to study changes in MG susceptibility within migrating social or ethnic groups over time. To compare incidence and prevalence of MG from the same ethnic or social group according to age at migration, length of time since migration, and first or second generation will provide information regarding the relative influence of genes and environment. Infections, smoking, D-vitamins, and pollutants are examples of environmental factors that may influence MG probability. Exposure to these factors will usually change over time and particularly with migration.

Epidemiological studies which consider migration will face several major methodological and analytical challenges. Such challenges will constitute a considerable amount of noise in the analysis of the impact of migration. One main problem is to define ethnicity since this is a complex anthropological concept and can be based on linguistic, national, racial, regional, or religious group identity.[82] Furthermore, using ethnicity risks underplaying variables like socioeconomic status, urban versus rural background, and social organization, for instance related to marriage traditions. Immigrants may be a selected group compared to non-immigrants. Those that emigrate may be in better general health, have higher education, have more financial support, be younger, and often include a preponderance of males.

There are variations both between different migrating groups, and within the same migration group located in different geographical areas, for example regarding how they interact with their new society. A further challenge when considering migration is that it raises issues that lie outside the field of knowledge of most medical scholars. An obvious remedy for this would be to include co-authors with a background in relevant social sciences, such as sociology, anthropology, and political sciences. Findings and methodology of epidemiological studies of migration may be used for political aims in debates concerning the general impact of migration on society. A poor understanding of the complexities of defining and using terms like ethnicity causes a risk of misuse. Well-performed studies and a well-balanced and sound evaluation of the results should for the same reasons be highly important for society. Most countries that people migrate from have poor or non-existent health registries; hence there is no reliable data on MG epidemiology from these countries. It may also be difficult to collect medical data, socioeconomic status, and ethnicity because of juridical barriers and ethical concerns. For example, it is illegal to register ethnicity in all databases in Norway. Often, the only alternative for data collection is by self-reporting. This may be challenging because of language, low participation rates, and complicated follow-up.

In 2011, a Norwegian study that aimed to investigate geographical distribution of anti-AChR MG in Norway was published.[26] The study used an AChR-antibody positive test as a proxy for MG. One laboratory in Norway performed all AChR antibody assays and had been doing so since 1983. Every suspected MG case was tested. This provided an opportunity to study a large nationwide population using one database and with a very specific test for anti-AChR MG. One main hypothesis was that the MG prevalence in the Sami population would be lower than in the main population. Since ethnicity is illegal to register, there is no official Sami registry in Norway. Because of this, the precise population size is impossible to estimate. Another complicating factor is how a Sami is defined. According to the Sami Act, the definition of being a Sami depends on a combination of subjective and language criteria. It is not dependent on geographical area or lifestyle. The subjective criteria mean, at least theoretically, that it is possible to switch between being a Sami or not during a lifetime. Perhaps because of this it was not possible to disclose any epidemiological differences between the Norwegian and the Sami population. The epidemiological study of MG in Norway provides an example of how complicated it is to study variations between and within social and ethnic groups.

Conclusions and Future Directions

Robust methods and high-quality data are necessary to make accurate epidemiological estimates of MG-populations. Correct figures for incidence, prevalence, and mortality in well-defined MG populations over time, should give clues to the aetiology. MG is a heterogeneous disease with variation in pathogenesis and aetiology between well-defined subgroups.

An important way of creating robust methods and good-quality data is to develop large population-based patient registries. In Norway, several national health registries have been established. National health registries provide an opportunity to conduct epidemiological research on a complete, nationwide population. These registries represent an opportunity for studying health problems in complete populations, with enhanced power and less bias. The studies are also less time and cost consuming for the individual researcher. Linkage of different health registries is important to reveal new insights by combining information. The Norwegian Prescription Database is one example of a national health registry from which data on MG incidence and prevalence has been obtained.[10]

Nationwide registries covering whole populations are emerging in many countries, providing a sound basis for epidemiological studies. The validity of the databases used in epidemiological studies is crucial. It is important to clarify whether the wide variations in reported MG prevalence and incidence are due to methodological issues or actual differences in unselected populations. The trend has been towards a decreasing heterogeneity with enhanced study quality.[7] National registries should allow investigating MG epidemiology over time, to examine trends in the same population with unchanged methodology, thus giving important clues to aetiologic factors.

In well-developed health systems, AChR- and MuSK-antibodies are routinely tested for in suspected MG cases. Antibody and biomarker studies will be expanded in the future. Diagnosing precisely the different MG subgroups will improve MG epidemiology and give better clues to genetic and environmental causative factors. Some MG subgroups are probably more influenced by genetic factors, while others are more susceptible to environmental factors. Mapping different MG subgroups will also support the personalized treatment for individual MG patients.

Migration should be a major issue in future epidemiological studies of MG, as it can provide new insights into genetic and environmental causative factors. Migration studies need highly specialized and multidisciplinary expertise.

REFERENCES

1. Jayam Trouth A, Dabi A, Solieman N, Kurukumbi M, Kalyanam J. Myasthenia gravis: a review. Autoimmune Diseases. 2012; 2012: 874680.
2. Grob D, Brunner N, Namba T, Pagala M. Lifetime course of myasthenia gravis. Muscle & Nerve. 2008; 37(2): 141–9.
3. Hansen JS, Danielsen DH, Somnier FE, Froslev T, Jakobsen J, Johnsen SP, et al. Mortality in myasthenia gravis: A nationwide population-based follow-up study in Denmark. Muscle & Nerve. 2016; 53(1): 73–7.
4. de la Paz MP, Villaverde-Hueso A, Alonso V, Janos S, Zurriaga O, Pollan M, et al. Rare diseases epidemiology research.

Advances in Experimental Medicine and Biology. 2010; 686: 17–39.
5. Hennekens CH, Buring JE, Mayrent SL. Epidemiology in Medicine (1st edition). Boston: Little, Brown, 1987. ppxv, 383.
6. Posada de la Paz M, Groft SC. Rare Diseases Epidemiology. Dordrecht; New York: Springer, 2010. pp. xxii, 542.
7. Carr AS, Cardwell CR, McCarron PO, McConville J. A systematic review of population based epidemiological studies in Myasthenia Gravis. BMC Neurology. 2010; 10: 46.
8. Storm-Mathisen A. Epidemiological and prognostical aspects of myasthenia gravis in Norway. Annals of the New York Academy of Sciences. 1966; 135(1): 431–5.
9. Breiner A, Widdifield J, Katzberg HD, Barnett C, Bril V, Tu K. Epidemiology of myasthenia gravis in Ontario, Canada. Neuromuscular Disorders: NMD. 2016; 26(1): 41–6.
10. Andersen JB, Engeland A, Owe JF, Gilhus NE. Myasthenia gravis requiring pyridostigmine treatment in a national population cohort. European Journal of Neurology: the official journal of the European Federation of Neurological Societies. 2010; 17(12): 1445–50.
11. Heldal AT, Owe JF, Gilhus NE, Romi F. Seropositive myasthenia gravis: a nationwide epidemiologic study. Neurology. 2009; 73(2): 150–1.
12. Boldingh MI, Maniaol AH, Brunborg C, Dekker L, Heldal AT, Lipka AF, et al. Geographical distribution of myasthenia gravis in Northern Europe—results from a population-based study from two countries. Neuroepidemiology. 2015; 44(4): 221–31.
13. Andersen JB, Heldal AT, Engeland A, Gilhus NE. Myasthenia gravis epidemiology in a national cohort; combining multiple disease registries. Acta Neurologica Scandinavica Supplementum. 2014(198): 26–31.
14. Santos E, Coutinho E, Moreira I, Silva AM, Lopes D, Costa H, et al. Epidemiology of myasthenia gravis in northern Portugal: Frequency estimates and clinical epidemiological distribution of cases. Muscle & Nerve. 2016; 54(3): 413–21.
15. Lee HS, Lee HS, Shin HY, Choi YC, Kim SM. The epidemiology of myasthenia gravis in Korea. Yonsei Med J. 2016; 57(2): 419–25.
16. Gattellari M, Goumas C, Worthington JM. A national epidemiological study of Myasthenia Gravis in Australia. European Journal of Neurology: the official journal of the European Federation of Neurological Societies. 2012; 19(11): 1413–20.
17. Montomoli C, Citterio A, Piccolo G, Cioccale R, Ferretti VV, Fratti C, et al. Epidemiology and geographical variation of myasthenia gravis in the province of Pavia, Italy. Neuroepidemiology. 2012; 38(2): 100–5.
18. Pallaver F, Riviera AP, Piffer S, Ricciardi R, Roni R, Orrico D, et al. Change in myasthenia gravis epidemiology in Trento, Italy, after twenty years. Neuroepidemiology. 2011; 36(4): 282–7.
19. Storm-Mathisen A. Epidemiology of myasthenia gravis in Norway. Acta Neurologica Scandinavica. 1984; 70(4): 274–84.
20. Ejma M, Koszewicz M, Podemski R, Marianska K, Budrewicz S, Turek T. Anatomical variation of the vertebral artery clinically mimicking myasthenia gravis. Neurological Sciences: official journal of the Italian Neurological Society and of the Italian Society of Clinical Neurophysiology. 2011; 32(4): 715–17.
21. Libman R, Benson R, Einberg K. Myasthenia mimicking vertebrobasilar stroke. Journal of Neurology. 2002; 249(11): 1512–14.
22. Montero-Odasso M. Dysphonia as first symptom of late-onset myasthenia gravis. Journal of General Internal Medicine. 2006; 21(6): C4–6.
23. Vincent A, Clover L, Buckley C, Grimley Evans J, Rothwell PM, Survey UKMG. Evidence of underdiagnosis of myasthenia gravis in older people. Journal of Neurology, Neurosurgery, and Psychiatry. 2003; 74(8): 1105–8.
24. Aarli JA. Myasthenia gravis in the elderly: Is it different? *Annals of the New York Academy of Sciences*. 2008; 1132: 238–43.
25. Phillips LH, 2nd, Torner JC. Epidemiologic evidence for a changing natural history of myasthenia gravis. Neurology. 1996; 47(5): 1233–8.
26. Heldal AT, Eide GE, Gilhus NE, Romi F. Geographical distribution of a seropositive myasthenia gravis population. Muscle & Nerve. 2012; 45(6): 815–19.
27. Pedersen EG, Hallas J, Hansen K, Jensen PE, Gaist D. Late-onset myasthenia not on the increase: a nationwide register study in Denmark, 1996-2009. European Journal of Neurology: the official journal of the European Federation of Neurological Societies. 2013; 20(2): 309–14.
28. Poulas K, Tsibri E, Kokla A, Papanastasiou D, Tsouloufis T, Marinou M, et al. Epidemiology of seropositive myasthenia gravis in Greece. Journal of Neurology, Neurosurgery, and Psychiatry. 2001; 71(3): 352–6.
29. Klein R, Marx A, Strobel P, Schalke B, Nix W, Willcox N. Autoimmune associations and auto-antibody screening show focused recognition in patient subgroups with generalized myasthenia gravis. Human Immunology. 2013; 74(9): 1184–93.
30. Meriggioli MN, Sanders DB. Autoimmune myasthenia gravis: emerging clinical and biological heterogeneity. Lancet Neurology. 2009; 8(5): 475–90.
31. Mombaur B, Lesosky MR, Liebenberg L, Vreede H, Heckmann JM. Incidence of acetylcholine receptor-antibody-positive myasthenia gravis in South Africa. Muscle & Nerve. 2015; 51(4): 533–7.
32. Fang F, Sveinsson O, Thormar G, Granqvist M, Askling J, Lundberg IE, et al. The autoimmune spectrum of myasthenia gravis: a Swedish population-based study. J Intern Med. 2015; 277(5): 594–604.
33. Lavrnic D, Basta I, Rakocevic-Stojanovic V, Stevic Z, Peric S, Nikolic A, et al. Epidemiological study of adult-onset myasthenia gravis in the area of Belgrade (Serbia) in the period 1979–2008. Neuroepidemiology. 2013; 40(3): 190–4.
34. Lai CH, Tseng HF. Nationwide population-based epidemiological study of myasthenia gravis in taiwan. Neuroepidemiology. 2010; 35(1): 66–71.
35. Alshekhlee A, Miles JD, Katirji B, Preston DC, Kaminski HJ. Incidence and mortality rates of myasthenia gravis and myasthenic crisis in US hospitals. Neurology. 2009; 72(18): 1548–54.
36. Bateman KJ, Schinkel M, Little F, Liebenberg L, Vincent A, Heckmann JM. Incidence of seropositive myasthenia gravis in Cape Town and South Africa. S Afr Med J. 2007; 97(10): 959–62.
37. Somnier FE. Increasing incidence of late-onset anti-AChR antibody-seropositive myasthenia gravis. Neurology. 2005; 65(6): 928–30.
38. Oopik M, Kaasik AE, Jakobsen J. A population based epidemiological study on myasthenia gravis in Estonia. Journal of Neurology, Neurosurgery, and Psychiatry. 2003; 74(12): 1638–43.
39. Drachman DB. Myasthenia gravis. New England Journal of Medicine. 1994; 330(25): 1797–1810.
40. Somnier FE, Keiding N, Paulson OB. Epidemiology of myasthenia gravis in Denmark. A longitudinal and comprehensive population survey. *Archives of Neurology*. 1991; 48(7): 733–9.

41. Guidetti D, Sabadini R, Bondavalli M, Cavalletti S, Lodesani M, Mantegazza R, et al. Epidemiological study of myasthenia gravis in the province of Reggio Emilia, Italy. European Journal of Epidemiology. 1998; 14(4): 381–7.
42. A Dictionary of Epidemiology, Porta, Miquel (ed.), Oxford University Press, 2008: 61.
43. Christensen PB, Jensen TS, Tsiropoulos I, Sorensen T, Kjaer M, Hojer-Pedersen E, et al. Mortality and survival in myasthenia gravis: a Danish population-based study. Journal of Neurology, Neurosurgery, and Psychiatry. 1998; 64(1): 78–83.
44. Owe JF, Daltveit AK, Gilhus NE. Causes of death among patients with myasthenia gravis in Norway between 1951 and 2001. Journal of Neurology, Neurosurgery, and Psychiatry. 2006; 77(2): 203–7.
45. Wendell LC, Levine JM. Myasthenic crisis. Neurohospitalist. 2011; 1(1): 16–22.
46. Cohen MS, Younger D. Aspects of the natural history of myasthenia gravis: crisis and death. Annals of the New York Academy of Sciences. 1981; 377: 670–7.
47. Beydoun SR, Gong H, Ashikian N, Rison RA. Myasthenia gravis associated with invasive malignant thymoma: two case reports and a review of the literature. J Med Case Rep. 2014; 8: 340.
48. Maggi G, Casadio C, Cavallo A, Cianci R, Molinatti M, Ruffini E. Thymectomy in myasthenia gravis. Results of 662 cases operated upon in 15 years. Eur J Cardiothorac Surg. 1989; 3(6): 504–9; discussion 10–1.
49. Andersen JB, Owe JF, Engeland A, Gilhus NE. Total drug treatment and comorbidity in myasthenia gravis: a population-based cohort study. European Journal of Neurology: the official journal of the European Federation of Neurological Societies. 2014; 21(7): 948–55.
50. Gilhus NE, Nacu A, Andersen JB, Owe JF. Myasthenia gravis and risks for comorbidity. European Journal of Neurology: the official journal of the European Federation of Neurological Societies. 2015; 22(1): 17–23.
51. Nacu A, Andersen JB, Lisnic V, Owe JF, Gilhus NE. Complicating autoimmune diseases in myasthenia gravis: a review. Autoimmunity. 2015; 48(6): 362–8.
52. Mao ZF, Yang LX, Mo XA, Qin C, Lai YR, He NY, et al. Frequency of autoimmune diseases in myasthenia gravis: a systematic review. Int J Neurosci. 2011; 121(3): 121–9.
53. Vincent A, Newsom-Davis J. Acetylcholine receptor antibody as a diagnostic test for myasthenia gravis: results in 153 validated cases and 2967 diagnostic assays. Journal of Neurology, Neurosurgery, and Psychiatry. 1985; 48(12): 1246–52.
54. Lindstrom JM, Seybold ME, Lennon VA, Whittingham S, Duane DD. Antibody to acetylcholine receptor in myasthenia gravis. Prevalence, clinical correlates, and diagnostic value. Neurology. 1976; 26(11): 1054–9.
55. Lindstrom JM, Einarson BL, Lennon VA, Seybold ME. Pathological mechanisms in experimental autoimmune myasthenia gravis. I. Immunogenicity of syngeneic muscle acetylcholine receptor and quantitative extraction of receptor and antibody-receptor complexes from muscles of rats with experimental automimmune myasthenia gravis. Journal of Experimental Medicine. 1976; 144(3): 726–38.
56. Reddel SW, Morsch M, Phillips WD. Clinical and scientific aspects of muscle-specific tyrosine kinase-related myasthenia gravis. Current Opinion in Neurology. 2014; 27(5): 558–65.
57. Guptill JT, Sanders DB, Evoli A. Anti-MuSK antibody myasthenia gravis: clinical findings and response to treatment in two large cohorts. Muscle & Nerve. 2011; 44(1): 36–40.
58. Leite MI, Jacob S, Viegas S, Cossins J, Clover L, Morgan BP, et al. IgG1 antibodies to acetylcholine receptors in 'seronegative' myasthenia gravis. Brain: a Journal of Neurology. 2008; 131(Pt 7): 1940–52.
59. Scuderi F, Marino M, Colonna L, Mannella F, Evoli A, Provenzano C, et al. Anti-p110 auto-antibodies identify a subtype of 'seronegative' myasthenia gravis with prominent oculobulbar involvement. Laboratory Investigation; a journal of technical methods and pathology. 2002; 82(9): 1139–46.
60. Tsonis AI, Zisimopoulou P, Lazaridis K, Tzartos J, Matsigkou E, Zouvelou V, et al. MuSK auto-antibodies in myasthenia gravis detected by cell based assay--A multinational study. Journal of Neuroimmunology. 2015; 284: 10–17.
61. Bartoccioni E, Scuderi F, Minicuci GM, Marino M, Ciaraffa F, Evoli A. Anti-MuSK antibodies: correlation with myasthenia gravis severity. Neurology. 2006; 67(3): 505–7.
62. Vincent A, Waters P, Leite MI, Jacobson L, Koneczny I, Cossins J, et al. Antibodies identified by cell-based assays in myasthenia gravis and associated diseases. Annals of the New York Academy of Sciences. 2012; 1274: 92–8.
63. Gilhus NE, Verschuuren JJ. Myasthenia gravis: subgroup classifications—Authors' reply. Lancet Neurology. 2016; 15(4): 357–8.
64. Gilhus NE, Skeie GO, Romi F, Lazaridis K, Zisimopoulou P, Tzartos S. Myasthenia gravis—auto-antibody characteristics and their implications for therapy. Nature Reviews Neurology. 2016; 12(5): 259–68.
65. Kaprio J. Science, medicine, and the future. Genetic epidemiology. BMJ. 2000; 320(7244): 1257–9.
66. Compston DA, Vincent A, Newsom-Davis J, Batchelor JR. Clinical, pathological, HLA antigen and immunological evidence for disease heterogeneity in myasthenia gravis. Brain: a Journal of Neurology. 1980; 103(3): 579–601.
67. Pirskanen R. Genetic associations between myasthenia gravis and the HL-A system. Journal of Neurology, Neurosurgery, and Psychiatry. 1976; 39(1): 23–33.
68. Feltkamp TE, van den Berg-Loonen PM, Nijenhuis LE, Engelfriet CP, van Rossum AL, van Loghem JJ, et al. Myasthenia gravis, auto-antibodies, and HL-A antigens. Br Med J. 1974; 1(5899): 131–3.
69. Maniaol AH, Elsais A, Lorentzen AR, Owe JF, Viken MK, Saether H, et al. Late onset myasthenia gravis is associated with HLA DRB1*15:01 in the Norwegian population. PLOS One. 2012; 7(5): e36603.
70. Gregersen PK, Kosoy R, Lee AT, Lamb J, Sussman J, McKee D, et al. Risk for myasthenia gravis maps to a (151) Pro→Ala change in TNIP1 and to human leukocyte antigen-B*08. Annals of Neurology. 2012; 72(6): 927–35.
71. Vandiedonck C, Capdevielle C, Giraud M, Krumeich S, Jais JP, Eymard B, et al. Association of the PTPN22*R620W polymorphism with autoimmune myasthenia gravis. Annals of Neurology. 2006; 59(2): 404–7.
72. Giraud M, Taubert R, Vandiedonck C, Ke X, Levi-Strauss M, Pagani F, et al. An IRF8-binding promoter variant and AIRE control CHRNA1 promiscuous expression in thymus. Nature. 2007; 448(7156): 934–7.
73. Saruhan-Direskeneli G, Hughes T, Yilmaz V, Durmus H, Adler A, Alahgholi-Hajibehzad M, et al. Genetic heterogeneity within the HLA region in MG. Clin Immunol. 2016: 166–7.
74. Alahgholi-Hajibehzad M, Yilmaz V, Gulsen-Parman Y, Aysal F, Oflazer P, Deymeer F, et al. Association of HLA-DRB1 *14, -DRB1 *16 and -DQB1 *05 with MuSK-myasthenia

gravis in patients from Turkey. Human Immunology. 2013; 74(12): 1633–5.
75. Nikolic AV, Andric ZP, Simonovic RB, Rakocevic Stojanovic VM, Basta IZ, Bojic SD, et al. High frequency of DQB1*05 and absolute absence of DRB1*13 in muscle-specific tyrosine kinase positive myasthenia gravis. European Journal of Neurology: the official journal of the European Federation of Neurological Societies. 2015; 22(1): 59–63.
76. Lisak RP, Barcellos L. New insights into the genetics of autoimmune myasthenia gravis: an evolving story. JAMA Neurology. 2015; 72(4): 386–7.
77. Kochi Y. Genetics of autoimmune diseases: perspectives from genome-wide association studies. Int Immunol. 2016; 28(4): 155–61.
78. Klein RJ, Zeiss C, Chew EY, Tsai JY, Sackler RS, Haynes C, et al. Complement factor H polymorphism in age-related macular degeneration. Science. 2005; 308(5720): 385–9.
79. Renton AE, Pliner HA, Provenzano C, Evoli A, Ricciardi R, Nalls MA, et al. A genome-wide association study of myasthenia gravis. JAMA Neurology. 2015; 72(4): 396–404.
80. Lin X, Deng FY, Lu X, Lei SF. Susceptibility genes for multiple sclerosis identified in a gene-based genome-wide association study. J Clin Neurol. 2015; 11(4): 311–18.
81. Stevenson A. *Oxford Dictionary of English* (3rd edition). New York: Oxford University Press, 2010. pp. xxii, 2069.
82. Ashmore RD, Jussim LJ, Wilder D. *Social Identity, Intergroup Conflict, And Conflict Reduction*. Oxford; New York: Oxford University Press, 2001. pp. xii, 270.

31

Epilepsy

Ettore Beghi, Giorgia Giussani, and Torbjorn Tomson

Introduction

Epilepsy is a chronic disease affecting both sexes and all ages, with worldwide distribution. The 2010 GBD study ranked epilepsy as the second most burdensome neurological disorder in terms of DALYs.[1] Epilepsy is a symptom complex arising from altered brain function, which may be secondary to a variety of structural or functional injuries to the CNS. The cardinal manifestations of epilepsy are the *epileptic seizures*, which are recurrent paroxysmal events characterized by stereotyped behavioural alterations reflecting the neural mechanisms involved by the epileptic process. In most cases, the disease can be diagnosed through a careful history or by the observation of a seizure. The interictal electroencephalogram (EEG) is of limited value in making the diagnosis, as its sensitivity is only 44% and the specificity is 80%.[2] Although an aetiologic agent can be identified in several instances, in about half of cases the cause is unknown.

The differential diagnosis of epilepsy encompasses a number of clinical conditions characterized by transient alteration of consciousness and/or behaviour, which may explain the possibility of false-positive and false-negative diagnoses. These limitations, along with the differing distribution of some environmental risk factors, are possible explanations of the heterogeneous frequency, course, and consequences of the disease in the world. To overcome at least in part these limitations, several data for this chapter have been obtained from the Rochester Epidemiology Project, a comprehensive medical records linkage system established in 1966 and covering the entire population residing in Olmsted County, Minnesota, USA.[3]

Definitions of Seizures and Epilepsy

While all people with epilepsy experience seizures, not all individuals with seizures have epilepsy. Epileptic seizures may occur in the context of an acute CNS insult (structural, systemic, toxic, or metabolic). These events (*provoked* or *acute symptomatic seizures*) are intended as an acute manifestation of the insult and may not recur when the underlying cause has been removed or the acute phase has elapsed.[4] According to the International League Against Epilepsy (ILAE), epilepsy is a disease of the brain defined by any of the following conditions: (1) at least two unprovoked (or reflex) seizures occurring >24 hours apart; (2) one unprovoked (or reflex) seizure and a probability of further seizures similar to the general recurrence risk (at least 60%) after two unprovoked seizures, occurring over the next ten years; (3) diagnosis of an epilepsy syndrome.[5] An *unprovoked seizure* is a seizure occurring within 24 hours in a person aged one month or older, in the absence of precipitating factors. Unprovoked seizures include events occurring in the absence of a recognized aetiological or risk factor (*idiopathic and cryptogenic seizures*), in patients with antecedent stable (non-progressing) CNS insults (*remote symptomatic seizures*), or in those with progressive CNS abnormalities such as brain tumours, genetic, metabolic, or degenerative conditions (*progressive symptomatic seizures*). Unprovoked seizures may be single or recurrent. *Status epilepticus* (SE) is an epileptic seizure that is sufficiently prolonged or repeated at sufficiently brief intervals so as to produce an unvarying and enduring epileptic condition. SE can have long-term consequences, including neuronal injury or death and alteration of neuronal networks, depending on the type and duration of seizures. A new diagnostic classification of SE has been recently proposed.[6]

Sudden unexpected death in epilepsy (SUDEP) is the sudden, unexpected, witnessed or unwitnessed, non-traumatic, and non-drowning death in patients with epilepsy, with or without evidence for a seizure and excluding documented SE, in which post-mortem examination does not reveal a toxicologic or anatomic cause of death.[7] In most cases, SUDEP is triggered by a seizure, and seizure-induced cardio-respiratory alterations are a plausible hypothesis.

The ILAE classification of the epileptic seizures and the epilepsies have been updated recently, following the major scientific advances on the underlying mechanisms that have taken place in the last decades.[8,9]

These definitions are relevant to the interpretation of the main epidemiological indexes when comparing past, present, and future studies. As the information available for epidemiologic studies of epilepsy depends on which definitions were used, the ILAE Epidemiology Commission[10] proposed the use of various degrees of diagnostic certainty for case definition: (1) *Definite*, with clear evidence of recurrent unprovoked seizures (a) and primary documentation by someone trained in the recognition of epilepsy (b);

(2) *Probable*, with other sources of information meeting criterion (a) or (b); *Suspect*, when information provided is inadequate to confirm or refute the diagnosis of epilepsy.

Although epilepsy is, by definition, a chronic clinical condition, patients may achieve seizure remission at variable intervals after the onset of seizures. *Epilepsy in remission with treatment* is defined by the absence of seizures for at least five years in patients still receiving anti-epileptic drugs (AEDs). *Epilepsy in remission without treatment (terminal remission)* is seizure remission for at least five years in patients off medications at time of ascertainment.[11] These cases are included in the so-called *inactive epilepsy*. By contrast, *active epilepsy* is defined as being treated with AEDs or having at least one seizure in the preceding 2–5 years regardless of treatment.[10] *Drug resistant epilepsy* is defined as failure to obtain seizure control after adequate trials of two tolerated, appropriately chosen, and used antiepileptic drug schedules (whether as monotherapies or in combination) to achieve sustained seizure freedom.[12]

Sources of Cases and Study Designs

As with other clinical conditions, the results of the epidemiological studies in epilepsy must be interpreted in the light of methodological differences and the quality of published reports. Checklists and accompanying guidelines have been developed to assess the methodological quality of incidence and prevalence studies.[13,14] These checklists should facilitate international comparisons. Details on the healthcare systems must be provided to identify the most reliable sources of cases. The investigation of multiple sources is required to optimize case ascertainment. Definition of cases is required, referring to widely accepted diagnostic criteria and standardized severity scales. Administrative health data are a valuable source of epidemiological findings because they are obtained from large representative population samples, are routinely collected, and can be obtained at almost no cost. However, before they can be used as disease tracers, administrative data need to be validated to test the accuracy of the information.

Incidence of Epilepsy and Unprovoked Seizures

The worldwide annual incidence of unprovoked seizures ranges from 33 to 198 per 100,000[15] and the annual incidence of epilepsy from 24 to 190 per 100,000. The overall incidence of epilepsy in HICs ranges from 24 and 71.0 per 100,000 per year (Table 31.1).[16–46] In LMICs the incidence of the disease is higher (Table 31.2)[47–63] and is up to 190 per 100,000. In a systematic review and meta-analysis of 48 incidence studies, the pooled incidence rate of epilepsy was 61.4 per 100,000 person-years (95% CI 50.7–74.4).[64] The corresponding figures for HICs and LMICs were 48.9 (95% CI 39.0–61.1) and 139.0 (95% CI 69.4–278.2). This higher incidence in LMICs can be explained by a greater exposure to perinatal risk factors, infections, and traumatic brain injury and the different structure of the populations at risk which, in these countries, is characterized by the predominance of young individuals and by premature mortality.

In HICs epilepsy tends to affect mostly individuals at the two extremes of the age spectrum. In the residents of Rochester, Minnesota, USA, from 1935 through to 1984, the incidence of the disease was 86 per 100,000 per year in the first year of age. It tended to decrease to about 23–31 per 100,000 in individuals aged 30–59 years, and increased thereafter, up to 180 per 100,000 in the 85+ year age class.[65] The peak in the elderly was not detected in several LICs, where the disease peaked in children. This may depend on the age structure of the population and a possible under-ascertainment of the disease in older individuals.

Table 31.1 Incidence (per 100,000 per year) of epilepsy in high-income countries

Country	Age	Incidence range	Notes
Canada[1]	Children	46.0	
Denmark[2]	All ages	68.8	
Estonia[3,4]	All ages	35.4–45.0	
Finland[5–9]	All ages	24.0–124.0	Higher rates in infants
France[10]	All ages	44.0	
Germany[11]	Children	60.3	
Iceland[12,13]	All ages	33.3–46.5	
Italy[14–17]	All ages	32.5–57.0	Higher rates in children
Japan[18]	All ages	24–53	Higher rates in older ages
Norway[19,20]	All ages	32.8–42.0	Higher rates in children
Serbia[21]	Children	650.0	Cumulative incidence
Sweden[22,23]	All ages	50.0–56.0	
Switzerland[24]	All ages	71.0	
United Kingdom[25,26]	All ages	46.0–70.1	Higher rates in infants
United States[27–30]	All ages	35.0–71.0	Higher rates in administrative data
Faroe Islands[31]	All ages	42.0	
The Netherlands[32]	>13 years old	29.5	

The incidence of epilepsy has been reported to be slightly higher in men than in women both in HICs and in LMICs,[64] although this finding does not attain statistical significance. The different distribution of epilepsy in men and women can be explained by the genetic background, the prevalence of the commonest risk factors in the two sexes, and the concealment of the disease in women for sociocultural reasons.

Age-specific incidence rates of epilepsy tend to decrease with time in the youngest age groups and to increase in the elderly. The decreased incidence in the youngest individuals can be explained by the improvement of perinatal care and the control of infectious diseases, while the increased incidence in the elderly can be attributed to the increased life expectancy (followed by the increase of age-related epileptogenic conditions, like stroke and degenerative CNS disorders) and to an increased ascertainment of the disease in this age group.

In population-based studies focal seizures are the predominant pattern both in children and in adults. In a systematic review of incidence studies, the median seizure-specific incidence rate was 30.4

Table 31.2 Incidence (per 100,000 per year) of epilepsy in low/middle income countries

Country	Age	Incidence range	Notes
Burkina-Faso[32]	All ages	83.0	
Chile[33]	All ages	113.0	
Ecuador[34]	All ages	122.0–190.0	Urban and rural area, reasons for this difference not identified
Ethiopia[35]	All ages	64.0	
India[36]	All ages	49.3	
Tanzania[37]	All ages	81.1	
Uganda[38]	All ages	215.0	
China[39]	All ages	35.0	
Kenya[40,41]	All ages	39.16–187.0	Lower rates in women and higher rates in children
Egypt[42]	All ages	43.14	
Benin[43]	All ages	10.5	
Martinique[44]	All ages	64.1	
Sub-Saharan Africa[45]	All ages	81.7	
Latin America[46]	All ages	77.7–190	
Honduras[47]	All ages	92.7	
Togo[48]	Children	102.1	

per 100,000 per year (range 10.6–60.8) for focal seizures and 19.6 per 100,000 per year for generalized seizures (range 5.6–72.1).[15] In the Rochester, Minnesota population, complex partial seizures were the predominating pattern (36%), followed by generalized tonic-clonic (23%), simple partial (14%), other generalized (8%), partial unknown (7%), absence (6%), myoclonic (3%), and unclassified (3%).[65] In the same population, the predominant mode of onset in children and adolescents was focal (68%), followed by generalized/bilateral onset (23%), and spasms (3%).[66] In contrast to industrialized countries, in most LICs the predominant seizure pattern is represented by tonic-clonic seizures. This tends to reflect a relative under-ascertainment of the other seizure types because of lack of recognition and their minor impact on quality of life. Incidence of SE has been found to vary from 6.8 to 41 per 100,000 per year with a bimodal distribution (peaks in children less than one year and the elderly).[67]

Few studies provide information on the variability of the incidence of epilepsy when comparing different races and ethnic groups. In one such study done in a multi-ethnic population enrolled in an urban Health Maintenance Organization, the ethnicity-specific OR for the first unprovoked seizure, by using non-Hispanic whites as referent, was 1.04 (95% CI 0.73–1.49) for African Americans, 0.97 (95% CI 0.64–1.48) for Hispanics, and 0.25 (95% CI 0.08–0.84) for Asian Americans.[68]

In the Rochester, Minnesota population, cryptogenic focal epilepsies were the commonest epilepsy syndrome in newly diagnosed patients (17.5 cases per 100,000 per year), followed by symptomatic focal epilepsies (17.2), undetermined epilepsies (9.7), symptomatic/cryptogenic epilepsies (4.0), idiopathic generalized epilepsies (3.7), and idiopathic focal epilepsies (0.2).[69] Different figures were reported in a prospective population-based study in Iceland,[70] where higher percentages were found for idiopathic focal epilepsies (5.4% vs 1.3% in Rochester) and idiopathic generalized epilepsies (10.2% vs 5.7%) and lower percentages were found for symptomatic focal epilepsies (25.2% vs 33.8%), cryptogenic focal epilepsies (26.5% vs 34.4% and generalized symptomatic epilepsies (0.3% vs 3.8%). The differences can be explained by difficulties with use of the syndrome classification in population-based studies. In a population-based study in children in the Rochester population, age at onset was significantly correlated with aetiology. A structural/metabolic aetiology was significantly more likely in children with seizure onset before 12 months of age. Conversely, a genetic aetiology was much more likely with older age at onset.[66] A specific epilepsy syndrome could be detected in 28% of cases at first diagnosis and in 29% at last follow-up. In Bordeaux, France, the incidence was 15.3 per 100,000 for focal epilepsies (idiopathic 1.7; symptomatic 13.6), 6.7 per 100,000 for generalized epilepsies (idiopathic 5.6; symptomatic 1.1), and 1.9 per 100,000 for undetermined epilepsies.[71] Some of the differences between the US and the French study can be explained by accuracy in case ascertainment, selection bias, and inclusion (in the French study) of patients with a single seizure. The most remarkable difference was found for undetermined epilepsies, which reflects a more or less stringent application of the ILAE syndromic classification and the limitations of this classification for epidemiological purposes. There are numerous reports of the incidence of specific syndromes, with differing rates depending on the target population, the diagnostic criteria, and sample size.

The incidence of epilepsy is higher in the lower socio-economic classes, shown by comparing HICs and LMICs and, within the same population, in people of differing ethnic origin.[72]

The incidence of acute symptomatic seizures is 29–39 per 100,000 per year.[73] Men seem at higher risk than women, depending on the differing distribution of the underlying epileptogenic conditions in the two sexes. Acute symptomatic seizures predominate in the youngest age class (less than one year of age) and, to a lesser extent, in the elderly. Traumatic brain injury, cerebrovascular disease, drug withdrawal, infection, and metabolic insults are the commonest causes.

In a study exploring a 50-year period, the age-adjusted incidence of a first unprovoked seizure was 61 per 100,000 person-years, which was approximately 33% higher than the incidence of epilepsy in the same community.[65] In the Rochester, Minnesota population, the cumulative incidence of epilepsy through age 74 years was 3.0%, of all unprovoked seizures was 4.1%, and of any convulsive disorder approached 10%.[74] The incidence was close to 10% when acute symptomatic seizures were also included.

Prevalence of Epilepsy

The overall prevalence of epilepsy ranges from 2.7 to 104.97 per 1000 population, although in the majority of the published reports the rate of active epilepsy varied from 4 to 8 per 1000. The prevalence of active epilepsy is generally lower in HICs (Table 31.3)[17–19,22,32,33,36–38,43,45,75–111] than in LMICs

Table 31.3 Prevalence (per 1000) of active epilepsy in high-income countries

Country	Age	Prevalence range	Notes
Australia[49]	All ages	4.4	
Denmark[2]	All ages	6.0	
Estonia[3,4]	All ages	3.6-5.3	Lower ratios in children and higher in adults
France[50]	Adults	5.4	
Finland[7,51,52]	All ages	3.2-6.3	Lower ratios in children
Iceland[53]	All ages	4.8	
Italy[17,54-57]	All ages	3.0*-7.9	*Aeolian Islands
Japan[18]	All ages	2.7-40.0	Lower ratios in children and higher in older ages
Norway[59-60]	All ages	5.1-6.5	Lower ratios in children
Poland[61]	>16 years	3.7	
Spain[62-64]	All ages	4.1-6.3	Higher ratios in adolescents
Sweden[22,23,65,66]	All ages	4.2-8.8	Lower ratios in children
The Netherlands[67]	Adults and elderly	9.0	
United Kingdom[26,68-72]	All ages	4.0-8.0	
USA[28,73-77]	All ages	7.2*-21.0	*Only adults in Georgia and in Tennessee
Taiwan[78,79]	All ages	2.7*-4.2	Lower ratios in adults
Canada[80-82]	All ages	4.03-5.5	
Saudi Arabia[83]	All ages	6.5	
Croatia[84]	All ages	10.9	
Faroe Islands[30]	All ages	7.6	
Lithuania[85]	Children	4.2	
Albania[86]	All ages	14.2	
Serbia[21]	Children	6.5	

(Table 31.4),[48,49,52,57,60-62,112-169] which may reflect a lower prevalence of selected risk factors (mostly infection and trauma), a more stringent case verification, and the exclusion of isolated provoked and unprovoked seizures. In a systematic review and meta-analysis of 197 prevalence studies, the point prevalence of active epilepsy was 6.4 per 1000 (95% CI 5.6–7.3) and the lifetime prevalence was 7.6 per 1000 (95% CI 6.2–9.4).[8] The prevalence was lowest in infancy and tended to increase with age, with a peak at 20–29 years and a subsequent decrease. Both lifetime and active period prevalence were higher in LMICs than in HICs, but the difference for active epilepsy was not significant. These differences can be mostly explained by the differing distribution of the risk factors and the shorter life expectancy in the latter.

As with incidence, the prevalence of epilepsy tends to prevail in men.[8] However, this finding is not consistent across studies and, with few exceptions, is not statistically significant. In multi-racial populations, the lifetime prevalence of epilepsy prevailed in blacks compared to whites (7.5 vs 5.9 per 1000), but among whites the prevalence was higher in Hispanics than in non-Hispanics (7.5 vs 4.7 per 1000).[170] Ethnic and racial differences and different sociocultural environments may explain the heterogeneity of the figures.

Focal seizures are commoner than generalized seizures both in children and adults. In prevalence studies in adults from HICs, focal seizures were reported in 55–60% of cases, generalized seizures in 26–32%, and unclassifiable seizures in 8–17%. Different figures are present for children (36–66%, 30–62%, and 2–4%), mostly depending on a different distribution of epilepsy syndromes, and for LMICs (11–55%, 26–86%, and 0–19% respectively), as a consequence of a less accurate diagnostic ascertainment of minor seizures (other than generalized tonic-clonic).[171]

The prevalence of epilepsy syndromes has been mostly studied in children and adolescents from Baltic and Scandinavian countries.[171] In Estonia, the prevalence of idiopathic epilepsies in children was 1.2 per 1000, and that of cryptogenic epilepsies was 1.0 per 1000. In Lithuania, focal epilepsies in children were the commonest syndromic category (2.3 per 1000), followed by generalized epilepsies (1.3 per 1000), and undetermined epilepsies (0.6 per 1000). Focal epilepsies were the predominant syndromic category in 41–54% of cases from Sweden, Finland, and Norway, followed by generalized (37–48%) and unclassified (5–10%). In these countries, idiopathic focal epilepsy with centro-temporal spikes was 5–17%, absence epilepsy 6–8%, juvenile myoclonic epilepsy 1–5%, West syndrome 0.5–8%, and Lennox-Gastaut syndrome 2–6%.

Socioeconomic background affects the frequency of epilepsy both in HICs and in LMICs.[72] A strong correlation was detected between the prevalence of epilepsy and social deprivation, defined by unemployment, no car in the household, overcrowded households, and households not occupied by the owner.

Trends in Unprovoked Seizures and Epilepsy

Secular trends in unprovoked seizures were investigated in the Rochester, Minnesota population during the period 1935–84.[65,172] There was no significant difference in the age-adjusted annual incidence over time. However, significant trends were found in age-specific incidence. The most pronounced was a decrease in the incidence of unprovoked seizures in children aged less than ten years in the period 1935–74 (from 79.4 to 41.6 per 100,000) and an increase in the period 1975–84 (to 55.4 per 100,000). In contrast, the incidence increased with time in the elderly, mostly in the last decade (up to 253.2 per 100,000). A similar decrease in the incidence of childhood epilepsy was found in a Swedish population-based study.[173] The increased incidence in the elderly is consistent with a study in Finland.[174] In a UK population of 6000 persons followed for ten years,[175] the lifetime prevalence of one or more afebrile seizures was 20.3 per 1000 in 1983 and 21.0 per 1000 in 1993, but the prevalence of active epilepsy was highest in the elderly (6.0 per 1000 in patients 60 years or older) and decreased from 5.3 to 4.3 per 1000. In the same population, the annual incidence, measured by first hospital attendance, declined from 152.4 to 60.9 per 100,000 in children (less than 20 years). The corresponding decline in the entire sample was from 75.0 to 48.3 per 100,000. The decreased incidence in children has been confirmed by others[29] and can be interpreted as a result of better prenatal care and immunization programmes, while the increased incidence in the Rochester, Minnesota study was explained by improved survivorship of children with neurological complications, including seizures. An increased case ascertainment cannot be likewise excluded, as indicated by a Finnish study that found an

Table 31.4 Prevalence (per 1000) of active epilepsy in low-middle income countries

Country	Age	Prevalence range	Notes
Bolivia[86]	All ages	11.1	
Chile[33]	All ages	17.7	
Ecuador[34,87–88]	All ages	6.7–22.6	Higher ratios in migrant populations
Ethiopia[89]	All ages	5.2–29.46	Higher ratios in the Zay Society after a door-to-door survey
India[90–92]	All ages	4.9–7.0	Higher ratios in children
Pakistan[93,94]	All ages	7.0–9.98	
Panama[95]	All ages	22.0–57.0	Lower ratios in Panama City populations than in the Caribbean Coast
Tanzania[37,96,97]	All ages	2.9–8.7	Lower ratios in adults and higher in a door-to-door survey
Tunisia[98]	All ages	4.0	
Brazil[99–101]	All ages	5.1–8.2 active 13.0 lifetime	
Colombia[102–104]	All ages	10.3 active 19.5 lifetime	
China[105–111]	All ages	1.5–4.4 active 23.5 lifetime	Lower ratios in adults with active convulsive epilepsy
Guatemala[112–113]	All ages	5.8–18.0*	Higher ratios in two rural Guatemalan communities
Libya[114]	All ages	2.3	
Korea[115]	All ages	2.4	
Turkey[116–123]	All ages	2.5–8.6	Lower ratios in adolescents and higher rates in children
Egypt[42,124]	All ages	2.1–6.9	Lower ratios in adults
Iran[125]	All ages	7.9	
Georgia[126]	All ages	8.8	
Peru[127]	Adults	15.3–35.6	Lower ratios in the urban group, middle ratios in the rural group, higher ratios in migrant group.
Kenya[128–139]	All ages	2.6–11.0	Lower ratios in active convulsive epilepsy, higher ratios in children
South Africa[130]	All ages	7.0	
Nigeria[131]	All ages	4.7–20.8	Lower ratios in the rural community and higher ratios in the semi-rural community
Sub-Saharan Africa[45,132]	All ages	7.0–14.8	
Senagal[133]	All ages	14.2	
Cambodia[134]	All ages	5.8	
Benin[135,136]	All ages	8.2–12.7*	*Capture-recapture method in rural community Lower ratios in ≥15 years
Burkina Faso[137]	All ages	45.0	Lifetime
Azebaijan[138]	All ages	9.0	
Gambia[139]	All ages	4.9	Lifetime
Latin America[46]	All ages	6.0–43.2	Lifetime
Zambia[140]	All ages	12.5	
Togo[141]	All ages	15.7	
Nepal[142]	All ages	7.3	
Honduras[47]	All ages	15.4	
Cameroon[143]	All ages	104.97	

increased incidence of the disease from the 1960s to the 1990s.[21] The increasing incidence of unprovoked seizures and epilepsy in the elderly was confirmed by others[17] and can be explained by increased life expectancy and better case ascertainment in this age group. A similar explanation can be given for the increasing incidence of SE in the USA.[176]

There is no evidence that SMRs and mortality rates have changed significantly over time in Europe and North America.[177] In contrast, in the UK all epilepsy deaths significantly decreased from 2001 to 2013, predominantly due to a decrease in SE mortality,[178] which suggests that early and aggressive treatment of SE may be a positive prognostic indicator. An increase in mortality rates was also documented in Taiwan during the period 1971–2005, attributed by the authors to poor quality of treatment.[179]

Aetiology of Epilepsy

The burden of comorbidity in epilepsy is high.[180] Several somatic and psychiatric comorbidities tend to prevail significantly in people with epilepsy when compared to the general population.[181,182] Several mechanisms can explain the association between epilepsy and a number of comorbidities, including causal relation, shared risk factors, and bidirectional effects. Factors clearly associated with the development of epilepsy must be identified before accepting the concept of a causal association between a brain insult and the occurrence of epileptic seizures. First, the timing of the seizure(s) must be identified, to separate acute symptomatic from unprovoked seizures. Second, the frequency and spectrum of epilepsy and putative aetiological factors in the general population must be assessed to define the fraction of epilepsies associated with a given risk factor and the risk of epilepsy attributable to that factor. Third, the accuracy and validity of the diagnostic work-up must be considered. Fourth, evidence of a causal relationship should be produced to exclude the possibility of a chance association even in the presence of a well-established aetiological factor. This requires the satisfaction of specific criteria, including temporal sequence, strength and consistency of association, biological gradient, and plausibility.

The ILAE proposes classification into six different categories: structural, genetic, infectious, metabolic, immune, as well as an unknown aetiological group.[9]

In incidence studies, the proportion of cases with documented aetiology has been reported to vary from 13.7% in Ethiopia to 51.6% in Poland.[183] The differences are mostly explained by the structure of the population at risk, the prevalence of the aetiological factors in the local environment, the study design, and the extent of the diagnostic ascertainment. In the Rochester, Minnesota population, epilepsy was idiopathic/cryptogenic in about two-thirds of patients. The commonest aetiological factors included cerebrovascular disease (10.9%), congenital neurological disorders (8.0%), trauma (5.5%), neoplasm (4.1%), degenerative disorders (3.5%), and infection (2.5%).[65] Aetiological factors varied significantly with age, congenital disorders being most common in children aged less than 14 years and cerebrovascular disorders in the elderly.

At least in part, the risk of epilepsy is accounted for by genetic factors. Despite the increasing pace of gene discovery in the epilepsies, the contribution of specific genes still needs to be elucidated. In epidemiology, the role of the genetic components has been mostly explored by studies of familial aggregation of epilepsy, studies on paternal and maternal transmission, and twin studies. However, these studies suffer from methodological limitations, including referral and reporting biases, small sample size, ambiguous disease definition, and lack of controls.[184] Siblings and offspring of patients with epilepsy have a two to three-fold increased risk in developing epilepsy. In offspring of patients with epilepsy, the cumulative incidence of unprovoked seizures to age 25 is about 6%, as opposed to 1–2% of the general population. The risk of seizures among offspring of mothers with epilepsy exceeds that of offspring of fathers with epilepsy. If a proband has an early age at onset of seizures, there is an increased risk of seizures among siblings and offspring. The risk of unprovoked seizures is highest among siblings of probands with generalized epilepsy and is related to seizure type (mostly tonic-clonic or absence) and EEG abnormalities (mostly generalized spike and slow wave patterns). Twin studies show a higher concordance for epilepsy in monozygotic compared to dizygotic twin pairs.

In the only comprehensive study in first-degree relatives of probands with epilepsy,[185] the cumulative incidence of the disease to age 40 years was 4.7%, accounting for a three-fold increased risk (measured by the standardized incidence ratio, SIR) compared to the general population. A significantly increased risk was found for idiopathic generalized epilepsy (SIR 5.0; 95% CI 3.2–7.4), generalized epilepsy due to structural-metabolic causes (SIR 3.9; 95% CI 1.0–8.2), and focal epilepsy (SIR 4.8; 95% CI 1.6–9.9). A five-fold increased incidence of epilepsy was found in the offspring of female probands, restricted to focal epilepsy. The results of this and other epidemiological studies providing heritability estimates support the concept that epilepsy has a robust genetic component.

Although the role of pre- and perinatal risk factors in the aetiology of epilepsy seems established, most of the studies provide inconsistent findings and indicate, at best, a moderate association. These results may be explained by the use of differing definitions of pre- and perinatal factors, the study populations, the methods of ascertainment of the cause-effect relationship, and the sample size.

Learning disability and cerebral palsy are markers of brain dysfunction, which explains the significant association with epilepsy. In a systematic review of 38 studies, the pooled prevalence among people with intellectual disabilities was 22.2% (95% CI 19.6–25.1) with increase with the disability level.[186] In the US National Collaborative Perinatal Project, a study following newborns prospectively up to age seven, epilepsy occurred in 34% of children with cerebral palsy and cerebral palsy was present in 19% of children developing epilepsy.[187] In this cohort, the risk of learning disability was 5.5 times higher among children developing epilepsy following a febrile seizure than in children with a febrile seizure alone. Epilepsy was more common in individuals with severe or profound learning disability compared to mild to moderate learning disability.[184]

CNS infections are a worldwide risk factor for epilepsy involving all ages. In the Rochester, Minnesota population, survivors of a CNS infection had a three-fold increased risk of epilepsy.[188] The risk was highest during the first five years after infection and tended to decrease thereafter, but it remained elevated up to 15 years. The risk was highest with encephalitis (16.2), followed by bacterial meningitis (4.2), and aseptic meningitis (2.3, non-significant). Acute symptomatic seizures greatly affected the risk of subsequent unprovoked seizures and epilepsy. As encephalitis and bacterial meningitis are more prevalent in infants, children, and young adults, most post-infectious epilepsies tend to occur in these individuals. There is no clear epidemiological evidence for immunizations to be considered risk factors for epilepsy.

In LMICs, where infectious diseases are commoner than in HICs, cysticercosis, malaria, and HIV/AIDS were reported among the commonest infectious agents,[189] with higher prevalence in rural compared to urban areas. In these countries, mostly in South America, neurocysticercosis is a major cause of epilepsy.[190]

Dementia is a significant and increasing economic burden across the world. The disease is the leading cause of dependence in older adults worldwide. According to the 2010 GBD report, the DALYs attributable to AD and other dementias doubled in the past 20 years, and dementia is estimated as the major driver in late life.[1] Although there are indications that the incidence of dementia is declining in HICs,[191] the dementia-attributable DALYs are going to increase for the longer survival with dementia and the increasing incidence of the disease in LMICs, where life expectancy is increasing, and resources for the provision of healthcare for older adults are limited or unavailable.

Patients with AD are at increased risk of seizures and epilepsy.[192] There is, however, considerable variability in the reported prevalence and incidence of seizures in patients with AD, with lifetime prevalence rates ranging from 1.5% to 64%.[192] Compared to non-demented individuals matched for age and sex, patients with AD have a six-fold risk of unprovoked seizures and people with other types of dementia have an eight-fold risk.[193] Generalized tonic-clonic (including myoclonus) seizures are the most commonly reported type. In the UK, the prevalence ratio of AD in people with and without epilepsy was 8.0.[194] The cumulative incidence of unprovoked seizures was 7.7% in a cohort of patients with mild AD by seven years of follow-up.[195] In this group, independent predictors of unprovoked seizures were younger age, African-American ethnicity, more severe dementia, and focal epileptiform EEG activity.

Stroke is a major cause of worldwide disability. The burden of ischaemic and haemorrhagic stroke has increased significantly in the last decades, in terms of incidence, mortality, and DALYs.[196] In patients with ischaemic stroke, the cumulative incidence is 2–33% for acute symptomatic seizures, 3–67% for unprovoked seizures, and 2–4% for recurrent unprovoked seizures.[197] Cortical site, severity, and size of the lesion are independent predictors of acute symptomatic seizures in ischaemic stroke. In a US population-based study, acute symptomatic seizures occurred in 6% of patients with ischaemic stroke.[198] In patients with acute symptomatic seizures, cerebral infarcts were more likely located in the anterior hemisphere (OR 4.0; 95% CI 1.2–13.7). There was an inverse correlation between age and risk of seizures with a peak in patients aged less than 55 years. The risks were higher after recurrent stroke.

Compared to ischaemic stroke, haemorrhagic stroke (subarachnoid haemorrhage and, to a lesser extent, primary intracerebral haemorrhage) are followed by a higher risk of seizures. In the Oxfordshire Community Stroke Project, the cumulative probability of seizures after a first stroke was about 6% at one year and rose to 11% at 5 years, with significant differences across stroke subtypes (cerebral infarction 4 and 10%; primary cerebral haemorrhage 20 and 26%; subarachnoid haemorrhage 22 and 34%).[199] Acute symptomatic seizures (onset seizures) occurred in 2.1% of cases during the first 24 hours.

In the civilian population, traumatic brain injury (TBI) is one of the most common types of injury. The annual incidence of TBI in HICs is about 200 per 100,000.[200] Even higher incidence rates are expected in LMICs. TBI can be followed by acute and chronic complications, including seizures and epilepsy. In a large US population-based study, five years after concussion, the cumulative probability of post-traumatic epilepsy was 0.7% after mild injuries, 1.2% after moderate injuries, and 10% after severe injuries.[201] The risk was highest during the first year and diminished during the ensuing years. After ten years, only severe injuries still exhibited an increased risk of seizures. The 30-year cumulative incidence of seizures was 2.1% for mild injuries, 4.2% for moderate injuries, and 16.7% for severe injuries. In military series, the highest risk of post-traumatic epilepsy occurred following missile wounds with brain volume loss. Unprovoked seizures were reported in up to 41% of the veterans involved in the Vietnam Head Injury Study.[202] Additional risk factors include focal neurological signs, haematoma, the presence of metal fragments, and the location of the lesion. Risk factors for acute symptomatic seizures include acute intracerebral haematoma (especially subdural haematoma), younger age, increased severity of brain injury, and chronic alcoholism.[203] Risk factors for unprovoked seizures include acute symptomatic seizures, brain contusion, intracerebral haematoma (especially subdural haematoma), increased severity of brain injury, and age 65 years or older.

There are virtually no data on epilepsy in patients with tumours from population-based studies. The incidence of tumours in people with epilepsy is about 4%.[204] The epileptogenicity of tumours is related to their grade and location. Seizures are more often the presenting symptoms in low-grade tumours than in rapidly invasive tumours. Individuals with tumours in the centro-temporo-parietal region have the highest incidence of epilepsy. Epilepsy is more frequent in patients with superficial and cortical tumours than those with deep and non-cortical tumours. Although most seizures caused by brain tumours are focal and associated with abnormal clinical and electrophysiological changes, sensitivity and specificity of seizure type, neurological examination, and EEG are no higher in brain tumours than in other causes of epilepsy.

Prognosis of Epilepsy

The design of an ideal study on the prognosis of epilepsy should have the following pre-requisites: (1) a well-defined inception cohort; (2) a prospective follow-up; (3) standard definitions of prognostic predictors and outcome measures; (4) adequate duration of follow-up and minimization of drop-outs. Most of the differences among studies on the prognosis of epilepsy can be explained by the different design (retrospective or prospective; community-based or clinic-based), the target population (children and/or adults), the timing of enrolment (interval between onset seizure and admission), the type of seizure, the length of follow-up, and the use of antiepileptic drugs.

The overall prognosis of epilepsy is favourable in most patients. Reports from several LMICs (where patients with epilepsy are largely untreated) give prevalence and remission rates overlapping with those of HICs.[205] As in most LMICs the incidence of epilepsy is higher than in HICs and increased mortality can explain only in part the difference between incidence and prevalence, spontaneous remission of seizures is a meaningful explanation. In addition, contrary to the old reports, studies done in the last 30 years in newly diagnosed patients have consistently shown that 55–68% of cases tend to achieve prolonged seizure remission (Table 31.5).[41,49,162,206–218] However, in a long-term, population-based study done in patients with childhood-onset epilepsy, different remission patterns were seen. Half of the patients entered terminal remission, without relapse and one-fifth after relapse. One-third had a bad outcome in terms of persistent seizures after

Table 31.5 Population-based studies on the prognosis of epilepsy

Country	Age	%(duration) remission
Finland[144]	Children	48% (5 yr) at 37 years 61% (5 yr) at 45 years
United Kingdom[26,145-147]	All ages	47% (5 yr) at 11.8 years 71% (5 yr) and 54% (tr) at 7.1 years 86% (3 yr), 68%/5 yr), 68% (3 yr), 54% (5 yr) at 9 years 95% (1 yr), 47% (5 yr) at 6 years
United States[148,149]	All ages	76% (5 yr) at 20 years In children 95% (1 yr), 92% (2 yr), 89% (3 yr), and 81% (5 yr) at 10 years
Japan[150]	Children	62.8% (5 yr) at 18.9 years
Sweden[151]	All ages	In children 75.6% at 10 years In adults 68,64, and 58% (1, 3, and 5 yr) from 1985-87 to 1996
Holland[152]	Children	71% terminal remission at 14.8 years
Italy[153]	All ages	92% (2 yr) and 78% (3 yr) at 5 years 59.7% (2 yr sustained-r) at 20 years 42.6% (5 yr sustained-r) at 20 years
Canada[154]	Children	71% (1–4yr) at 8.1 years
Japan[155]	All ages	56, 59 and 62% (terminal remission) at 10, 5, and 3 years
Bolivia[156]	All ages	43.7% (5 yr) at 10 years
Benin[136]	All ages	45% (total seizure remission) at 18 months
Ecuador[34]	All ages	21% (complete) at 4 years

remission or without any remission.[219] These patterns have been confirmed in part by others.[211,215,220,221]

The risk of relapse of a first unprovoked seizure has been reported to range from 23 to 71%.[222] Population-based studies provided more homogeneous relapse rates at one year (36–37%) and two years (43–45%). In a systematic review of 16 reports, the average recurrence risk was 51% (95% CI 49–53%).[223] After a first unprovoked seizure, the probability of a relapse decreases with time. About 50% of recurrences occur within six months of the initial seizure and 76–96% within two years. A documented aetiology of the seizure and an abnormal (epileptiform and/or slow) EEG pattern are the two most consistent predictors of recurrence. The pooled two-year recurrence risk is lowest for an idiopathic or cryptogenic first seizure with a normal EEG (24%; 95% CI 19–29%), intermediate for a remote symptomatic seizure (48%; 95% CI 34–62%) with normal EEG *or* an idiopathic/cryptogenic seizure with an abnormal EEG (48%; 95% CI 40–55%), and highest with a remote symptomatic seizure with an abnormal EEG (65%; 95% CI 55–76%). Interictal EEG epileptiform abnormalities tend to be associated with a higher risk of seizure recurrence than non-epileptiform abnormalities. Seizures occurring during sleep are associated with a higher risk of recurrence both in children and in adults. Focal seizures are also correlated with a higher risk of recurrent seizures, even after controlling for aetiology and EEG abnormalities. A positive correlation between seizure relapse and family history of seizures has been confirmed in patients with idiopathic or cryptogenic first seizures. History of prior acute symptomatic seizures has been occasionally found to increase the risk of relapse, while evidence is inconclusive or lacking for sex, age, and status epilepticus.

The prognosis of untreated epilepsy can be assessed only in LICs where epilepsy is largely untreated (treatment gap ranging from 70 to 94%).[224] In a population-based study done in Ecuador the cumulative annual incidence rate was 190 per 100,000 and the prevalence rate of active epilepsy was 7 per 1000, which implies a remission rate of at least 50%.[49] Similar prevalence rates of active epilepsy were found in other countries.[225,226] These findings lend support to the hypothesis that spontaneous remission of epilepsy is a common event.

Treatment of epilepsy is generally started at the time of diagnosis, which is most frequently made when at least two unprovoked seizures have occurred. In fact, after a second unprovoked seizure, the risk of a third seizure has been estimated as 73% and the risk of a fourth seizure as 76%.[227] Population-based studies on the long-term prognosis of treated epilepsy report a 58–65% cumulative five-year remission rate at ten years.[205] This number rises to about 70% by 20 years following seizure onset.

Aetiology of epilepsy is by far the strongest prognostic predictor for seizure recurrence in patients with epilepsy. Idiopathic epilepsy has a better chance of seizure remission than symptomatic or cryptogenic epilepsy. In the Rochester, Minnesota population, symptomatic epilepsies had a significantly lower chance of five-year remission compared to idiopathic epilepsies (30 vs 42% at 15 years) and patients with neurological dysfunction present at birth had the lowest chance of remission.[228] Lower remission rates in patients with symptomatic epilepsies were found in several European countries.[205] Other indicators of five-year remission in the Rochester, Minnesota study included absence of EEG epileptiform abnormalities (OR 1.6) and absence of generalized tonic-clonic seizures. In the National General Practice Study of Epilepsy (NGPSE), the only independent predictor of one-year and two-year remission was the number of seizures experienced by the patient after the first seizure.[228]

As proposed by Sander,[229] epilepsy syndromes can be classified into four different prognostic groups: (1) excellent prognosis (about 20–30% of the total) with high probability of spontaneous remission; these include neonatal seizures, benign focal epilepsies, benign myoclonic epilepsy in infancy, and epilepsies provoked by specific modes of activation; (2) good prognosis (about 30–40%) with easy pharmacological control and possibility of spontaneous remission; these include infantile absence epilepsy, epilepsies with GTC seizures secondary to specific conditions, and some focal epilepsies; (3) uncertain prognosis (about 10–20%), which may respond to drugs, but tend to relapse after treatment withdrawal; these include juvenile myoclonic epilepsy, and most focal epilepsies (symptomatic or cryptogenic); (4) bad prognosis (about 20%) in which seizures tend to recur despite intensive treatment; these include epilepsies associated with congenital neurological defects, progressive neurological disorders, and some symptomatic or cryptogenic focal epilepsies.

Mortality of Epilepsy

The epidemiological approach to epilepsy mortality depends on the accuracy of the information on the causes of death and the survey methods.[230] For a more precise calculation of the mortality attributable to epilepsy, studies should be population-based, large, and

Table 31.6 Community-based studies of mortality in epilepsy in high-income countries

Country	Age	Mortality measures	Notes
Canada[157]	Children	SMR 7.5	
Finland[158,159]	All ages	SMR 6.4* HR 3.21	*Children
Estonia[160]	Adults	SMR 2.6	
Denmark[161]	<35 years old	HR 11.9	
Iceland[162,163]	All ages	SMR 1.6 W 0.79 M 2.25	
Poland[164]	All ages	SMR 1.8	
Sweden[165,166]	All ages	SMR 2.5–3.6*	*≥15 years old
United Kingdom[145,147,167,168]	All ages	SMR 2.1–3.0	
USA[169–172]	All ages	SMR 1.7–7.54*	Children

SMR = Standardized Mortality Ratio.

involve incident patients. Significant differences in mortality rates are expected when comparing incidence-based and prevalence-based studies. Patients with epilepsy should be assessed separately from patients with a first unprovoked seizure. Also, children, adults, and persons with acute symptomatic seizures and with unprovoked seizures should be examined separately.

The mortality rate of epilepsy ranges from 1 to 8 per 100,000 population per year, but international vital statistics give annual mortality rates of 1–2 per 100,000.[181]

Based on population-based studies investigating mortality in HICs, the SMR for incident unprovoked seizures or epilepsy was found to range from 1.6 to 3.0.[231] In prospective and retrospective incidence cohorts, the SMR for epilepsy ranges from 1.6 to 5.3 in children and adults (Table 31.6).[207,209,232–247]

Mortality of Epilepsy in Selected Clinical Conditions

In Gironde, France, the SMR was 9.3 (95% CI 7.9–10.9).[248] The SMR was 4.1 (95% CI 2.5–6.2) for unprovoked seizures, 6.5 (95% CI 3.8–10.5) for remote symptomatic seizures, 10.1 (95% CI 8.1–12.4) for acute symptomatic seizures, and 19.8 (95% CI 14.0–27.3) for seizures secondary to progressive neurological conditions. There were no deaths in patients with idiopathic seizures and mortality was not increased in patients with cryptogenic seizures (SMR 1.6; 95% CI 0.4–4.1). These figures were comparable to those from other population-based studies. Mortality risk was higher with remote symptomatic aetiology and age younger than 60.

In a retrospective US population-based cohort study, the 30-day mortality of a first episode of status epilepticus was 19%, 89% of deaths occurring with non-febrile acute symptomatic seizures. In the same population, 40% of patients surviving the first 30 days after the seizure died within the ensuing ten years.[249] The SMR was 2.8 (95% CI 2.1–3.5) and was significantly elevated in symptomatic SE. While patients with idiopathic/cryptogenic status epilepticus had no increased risk of death than the general population. Age, duration of SE, seizure type, and aetiology were independent predictors of mortality.

In HICs, patients with symptomatic epilepsy have an SMR ranging from 2.2 to 4.3.[231] Patients with a CNS lesion presumed to be present at birth present the highest mortality, with an SMR up to 50. Mortality is greater both in men and in women. There is an inverse correlation between SMR and age. The highest mortality in children may be explained by the rate expected in the general population, which is lowest in children, and by the higher proportion of neuro-deficits in this age group. There is also an inverse correlation between SMR and duration of epilepsy during the first years of disease, perhaps due to the mortality of the underlying cause. Generalized tonic-clonic and myoclonic seizures, but not absence seizures, have been associated with the highest mortality. The SMR in patients with focal seizures is still elevated, but at a lower extent. Status epilepticus is associated with a significant short-term mortality. In prospective population-based studies, the case-fatality ratio ranged from 21 to 33%.[250]

Accident-related deaths (drowning, falls) are common in patients with epilepsy and range between 1 and 6% of all deaths, with SMR ranging between 2.0 and 5.6.[231] Patients with epilepsy are reported to be at higher risk of suicide than the general population (SMR 2.6–5.0).

While seizure-related mortality is rare in new onset epilepsy, the pattern of mortality in patients with chronic epilepsy is high. SUDEP is the commonest cause of spontaneous mortality in people with epilepsy. While the incidence of SUDEP is about 0.35 cases/1000

Table 31.7 Community-based studies of mortality in epilepsy in low-middle income countries

Country	Population	Mortality measures	Notes
Bolivia[156]	All ages	SMR 1.34	
China[173,174]	All ages	SMR 2.9–4.9	Lower rates in a follow-up survey and higher rates in a prospective study
Kenya[175]	All ages	SMR 6.5	
Benin[43]	All ages	Mortality rate 22.2 per 1000	
Argentina[176]	All ages	SMR 2.45	
Uganda[177]	All ages	SMR 7.2	
India[178, 179]	All ages	SMR 0.76–2.58*	Lower ratio in a postal and telephone survey among the Parsi community and higher ratio in a two-stage door-to-door survey of a stratified random sample in Kolkata
Cameroon[180]	All ages	Mortality rate 28.9 per 1000	
Mali[178]	All ages	Mortality rate 34.9 per 1000	
Taiwan[181]	All ages	Mortality ratio 0.8 per 100,000	
Ecuador[178]	All ages	SMR 6.3	
Martinica[178]	All ages	SMR 4.25	

SMR = Standardized Mortality Ratio.

person-years in population-based incidence cohort of epilepsy,[251] in these populations, the incidence is 1–2/1000 person-years and is highest with severe, refractory seizures (3–9/1000).[252] The risk factors for SUDEP include young age at onset, gender, increased frequency of generalized tonic-clonic seizures, use of polytherapy, duration of epilepsy, and symptomatic aetiology.[253]

In patients undergoing epilepsy surgery, the SMR was found to range from 4.5 to 32. However, most studies have found no association between AEDs and SUDEP.[254]

In LMICs, the annual mortality rate in people with epilepsy is higher than in HICs and ranges from 9.7 to 45.1 deaths per 1000, with a median SMR of 2.6 (range 1.3–7.2) (Table 31.7).[58,218,255–264] Median SMRs are slightly higher in men than in women (SMR 5.0 vs 4.5) and relatively higher in children and adolescents, patients with symptomatic epilepsies, and those reporting less adherence to treatment. The main causes of death in people with epilepsy living in LMICs include those directly attributable to epilepsy, which yield a mean proportional mortality ratio (PMR) of 27.3% (range 5–75.5%) derived from population-based studies. These direct causes comprise SE, with reported PMRs ranging from 5 to 56.6%, and SUDEP, with reported PMRs ranging from 1 to 18.9%. Other causes of death include drowning, head injury, and burns. Epilepsy in LMICs carries a significantly greater premature mortality, as in HICs, but in these countries the excess mortality is more likely associated with lack of access to medical facilities and preventable causes.

Conclusions and Future Directions

The world population is growing, primarily in resource-poor countries, and life expectancy is increasing worldwide. These findings, along with an improvement of the prevention of risk factors for several acute and chronic diseases and the amelioration of sanitary measures, will have profound effects on the epidemiology of epilepsy. The growth of the population and the ageing process will result in the increase of the incidence, prevalence, and mortality of epilepsy and, consequently, in an increased burden of the disease worldwide. This increase may be, however, counterbalanced by a decrease in the number of cases due to infectious or metabolic diseases associated with poor education and sanitation, both reflections of a low socioeconomic status.

In 2016, a report from the GBD collaborators was published on the burden of neurological disorders[265] showing a significant decrease in epilepsy deaths and DALY rates between 1990 and 2016, while the age-standardized prevalence rate remained stable. In that period there was an increasing incidence of epilepsy in the elderly. A total of 45.9 million cases of all-active epilepsy was estimated in 2016. Of these, 24.0 million had active idiopathic epilepsy. A high prevalence of epilepsy was still found in LMICs, partly accounted for by the greater number of cases with communicable causes.

The results of future epidemiological studies will be significantly affected by the use of the new ILAE classification of seizures and epilepsy.[8,9] The inclusion of patients with only one seizure will result in a significant increase in the incidence of the disease even though the diagnosis should be made only in patients with a first seizure thought to be at high risk of relapse. The inclusion of these cases will have effects on the gap between the lifetime prevalence of epilepsy (that will probably increase) and the prevalence of active epilepsy (that will remain unchanged) because of the increasing number of cases unlikely to relapse.

The use of more and more sophisticated diagnostic tests will probably determine a decrease in the proportion of cases with epilepsy due to unknown causes. This includes the growing impact of genetic tests and their interactions with old and new environmental factors.[266] The effects of treatments on the prognosis of the disease must also be considered. Although the present drugs are unlikely to modify the outcome of epilepsy,[267] future compounds with different mechanisms of action might be successful.

This complex and evolving scenario indicates the need of future epidemiological investigations of epilepsy to assess the real burden of the disease and the effects of the changing structure of world population, along with the efficacy of preventive and therapeutic measures.

REFERENCES

1. Murray CJ, Vos T, Lozano R, et al. Disability-adjusted life years (DALYs) for 291 diseases and injuries in 21 regions, 1990–2010: A systematic analysis of the Global Burden of Disease study 2010. Lancet. 2012; 380(9859): 2197–223.
2. Bouma HK, Labos C, Gore GC, Wolfson C, Keezer MR. The diagnostic accuracy of routine electroencephalography after a first unprovoked seizure. Eur J Neurol. 2016; 23(3): 455–63.
3. Rocca WA, Yawn BP, St Sauver JL, et al. History of the Rochester Epidemiology Project: Half a century of medical records linkage in a US population. Mayo Clin Proc. 2012; 87(12): 1202–13.
4. Beghi E, Carpio A, Forsgren L, et al. Recommendation for a definition of acute symptomatic seizure. Epilepsia. 2010; 51(4): 671–5.
5. Fisher RS, Acevedo C, Arzimanoglou A, et al. ILAE official report: a practical clinical definition of epilepsy. Epilepsia. 2014; 55(4): 475–82.
6. Trinka E, Cock H, Hesdorffer D, et al. A definition and classification of status epilepticus—Report of the ILAE Task Force on Classification of Status Epilepticus. Epilepsia. 2015; 56(10): 1515–23.
7. Nashef L, So EL, Ryvlin P, Tomson T. Unifying the definitions of sudden unexpected death in epilepsy. Epilepsia. 2012; 53(2): 227–33.
8. Fisher RS, Cross JH, French JA, et al. Operational classification of seizure types by the International League Against Epilepsy: Position Paper of the ILAE Commission for Classification and Terminology. Epilepsia. 2017; 58(4): 522–30.
9. Scheffer IE, Berkovic S, Capovilla G, et al. ILAE classification of the epilepsies: Position paper of the ILAE Commission for Classification and Terminology. Epilepsia. 2017; 58(4): 512–21.
10. Thurman DJ, Beghi E, Begley CE, et al. Standards for epidemiologic studies and surveillance of epilepsy. Epilepsia. 2011; 52 (Suppl 7): 2–26.
11. Commission on Epidemiology and Prognosis, International League Against Epilepsy. Guidelines for epidemiologic studies on epilepsy. Epilepsia. 1993; 34(4): 592–6.
12. Kwan P, Arzimanoglou A, Berg AT, et al. Definition of drug resistant epilepsy: consensus proposal by the ad hoc Task Force of the ILAE Commission on Therapeutic Strategies. Epilepsia. 2010; 51(6): 1069–77.
13. Bennett DA, Brayne C, Feigin VL, et al. Development of the standards of reporting of neurological disorders (STROND)

checklist: a guideline for the reporting of incidence and prevalence studies in neuroepidemiology. Eur J Epidemiol. 2015; 30(7): 569–76.
14. Bennett DA, Brayne C, Feigin VL, et al. Explanation and elaboration of the standards of reporting of neurological disorders checklist: a guideline for the reporting of incidence and prevalence studies in neuroepidemiology. Neuroepidemiology. 2015; 45(2): 113–37.
15. Kotsopoulos IAW, van Mrode T, Kessels FGH, de Krom MCTFM, Knottnerus JA. Systematic review and meta-analysis of incidence studies of epilepsy and unprovoked seizures. Epilepsia. 2002; 42(11): 1402–9.
16. Camfield CS, Camfield PR, Gordon K, Wirrell E, Dooley JM. Incidence of epilepsy in childhood and adolescence: a population-based study in Nova Scotia from 1977 to 1985. Epilepsia. 1996; 37(1): 19–23.
17. Christensen J, Vestergaard M, Pedersen MG, Pedersen CB, Olsen J, Sidenius P. Incidence and prevalence of epilepsy in Denmark. Epilepsy Res. 2007; 76(1): 60–65.
18. Beilmann A, Napa A, Hämarik M, Sööt A, Talvik I, Talvik T. Incidence of childhood epilepsy in Estonia. Brain Dev. 1999; 21(3): 166–74.
19. Oun A, Haldre S, Mägi M. Incidence of adult epilepsy in Estonia. Acta Neurol Scand. 2003; 108(4): 245–51.
20. Gaily E, Lommi M, Lapatto R, Lehesjoki AE. Incidence and outcome of epilepsy syndromes with onset in the first year of life: A retrospective population-based study. Epilepsia. 2016; 57(10): 1594–1601.
21. Saarinen MM, Sillanpää M, Schmidt D, Virta LJ. Long-term changes in the incidence of childhood epilepsy. A population study from Finland. Epilepsy Behav. 2016; 58: 81–5.
22. Keränen T, Riekkinen PJ, Sillanpää M. Incidence and prevalence of epilepsy in adults in eastern Finland. Epilepsia. 1989; 30(4): 413–21.
23. Sillanpää M, Jalava M, Kaleva O, Shinnar S. Long-term prognosis of seizures with onset in childhood. N Engl J Med. 1998; 338(24): 1715–22.
24. Sillanpää M, Schmidt D. Natural history of treated childhood-onset epilepsy: prospective, long-term population-based study. Brain. 2006; 129: 617–24.
25. Loiseau J, Loiseau P, Guyot M, Duche B, Dartigues J-F, Aublet B. Survey of seizure disorders in French southwest. I. Incidence of epileptic syndromes. Epilepsia. 1990; 31: 391–6.
26. Freitag CM, May TW, Pfäfflin M, König S, Rating D. Incidence of epilepsies and epileptic syndromes in children and adolescents: a population-based prospective study in Germany. Epilepsia. 2001; 42(8): 979–85.
27. Olafsson E, Hauser WA, Ludvigsson P, Gudmundsson G. Incidence of epilepsy in rural Iceland: a population-based study. Epilepsia. 1996; 37(10): 951–5.
28. Olafsson E, Ludvigsson P, Gudmundsson G, Hesdorffer D, Kjartansson O, Hauser WA. Incidence of unprovoked seizures and epilepsy in Iceland and assessment of the epilepsy syndrome classification: a prospective study. Lancet Neurology. 2005; 4(10): 627–34.
29. Casetta I, Pugliatti M, Faggioli R, Cesnik E, Simioni V, Bencivelli D, et al. Incidence of childhood and adolescence epilepsy: a community-based prospective study in the province of Ferrara and in Copparo, Italy, 1996–2005. Eur J Neurol. 2012; 19(2): 312–16.
30. Cesnik E, Pedelini F, Faggioli R, Monetti VC, Granieri E, Casetta I. Incidence of epilepsy in Ferrara, Italy. Neurol Sci. 2013; 34(12): 2167–72.
31. Giussani G, Franchi C, Messina P, et al. Prevalence and incidence of epilepsy in a well-defined population of Northern Italy. Epilepsia. 2014; 55(10): 1526–33.
32. Granieri E, Rosati G, Tola R, et al. A descriptive study of epilepsy in the district of Copparo, Italy, 1964-1978. Epilepsia. 1983; 24(4): 502–14.
33. Nakano H, Inoue Y. Epidemiology and cause of epilepsy. Nihon Rinsho. 2014; 72(5): 785–9.
34. de Graaf AS. Epidemiological aspects of epilepsy in northern Norway. Epilepsia. 1974; 15(3): 291–9.
35. Breivik N, Reiher T. Epilepsy in children in the Sunnmøre District. Tidsskr Nor Laegeforen. 2008; 128(18): 2049–51.
36. Pavlovic M, Jarebinski M, Pekmezovic T, Levic Z. Seizure disorders in preschool children in a Serbian district. Neuroepidemiology. 1998; 17(2): 105–10.
37. Forsgren L. Prevalence of epilepsy in adults in northern Sweden. Epilepsia. 1992; 33(3): 450–8.
38. Brorson LO, Wranne L. Long-term prognosis in childhood epilepsy: survival and seizure prognosis. Epilepsia. 1987; 28(4): 324–30.
39. Jallon P, Goumaz M, Haenggeli C, Morabia A. Incidence of first epileptic seizures in the canton of Geneva, Switzerland. Epilepsia. 1997; 38(5): 547–52.
40. Eltze CM, Chong WK, Cox T, et al. A population-based study of newly diagnosed epilepsy in infants. Epilepsia. 2013; 54(3): 437–45.
41. MacDonald BK, Cockerell OC, Sander JW, Shorvon SD. The incidence and lifetime prevalence of neurological disorders in a prospective community-based study in the UK. Brain. 2000; 123 (Pt 4): 665–76.
42. Hauser WA, Annegers JF, Kurland LT. Incidence of epilepsy and unprovoked seizures in Rochester, Minnesota: 1935–1984. Epilepsia. 1993; 34(3): 453–68.
43. Holden EW, Thanh Nguyen H, Grossman E, et al. Estimating prevalence, incidence, and disease-related mortality for patients with epilepsy in managed care organizations. Epilepsia. 2005; 46(2): 311–19.
44. Zarrelli MM, Beghi E, Rocca WA, Hauser WA. Incidence of epileptic syndromes in Rochester, Minnesota: 1980–1984. Epilepsia. 1999; 40(12): 1708–14.
45. Joensen P. Prevalence, incidence, and classification of epilepsy in the Faroes. Acta Neurol Scand. 1986; 74(2): 150–5.
46. Kotsopoulos I, de Krom M, Kessels F, et al. Incidence of epilepsy and predictive factors of epileptic and non-epileptic seizures. Seizure. 2005; 14(3): 175–82.
47. Debouverie M, Kabore J. Epidémiologie de l'épilepsie au Burkina Faso. In: Dumas M, Giordano C, Gentillini F (eds). Neurologie Tropicale. Paris: John Libbey Eurotex, 1993. pp57–61.
48. Lavados J, Germain L, Morales A, Campero M, Lavados P. A descriptive study of epilepsy in the district of El Salvador, Chile, 1984–1988. Acta Neurol Scand. 1992; 85(4): 249–56.
49. Placencia M, Shorvon SD, Paredes V, et al. Epileptic seizures in an Andean region of Ecuador. Incidence and prevalence and regional variation. Brain. 1992; 115(Pt 3): 771–82.
50. Tekle-Haimanot R, Forsgren L, Ekstedt J. Incidence of epilepsy in rural central Ethiopia. Epilepsia. 1997; 38(5): 541–6.
51. Mani KS, Rangan G, Srinivas HV, Kalyanasundaram S, Narendran S, Reddy AK. The Yelandur study: a community-based approach to epilepsy in rural South India—epidemiological aspects. Seizure. 1998; 7(4): 281–8.
52. Winkler AS, Kerschbaumsteiner K, Stelzhammer B, Meindl M, Kaaya J, Schmutzhard E. Prevalence, incidence, and clinical

characteristics of epilepsy--a community-based door-to-door study in northern Tanzania. Epilepsia. 2009; 50(10): 2310–13.
53. Kaiser C, Asaba G, Leichsenring M, Kabagambe G. High incidence of epilepsy related to onchocerciasis in West Uganda. Epilepsy Res. 1998; 30(3): 247–51.
54. Li SC, Schoenberg BS, Wang CC, Cheng XM, Zhou SS, Bolis CL. Epidemiology of epilepsy in urban areas of the People's Republic of China. Epilepsia. 198; 26(5): 391–4.
55. Ibinda F, Wagner RG, Bertram MY, et al. Burden of epilepsy in rural Kenya measured in disability-adjusted life years. Epilepsia. 2014; 55(10): 1626–33.
56. Mung'ala-Odera V, White S, Meehan R, et al. Prevalence, incidence and risk factors of epilepsy in older children in rural Kenya. Seizure. 2008; 17(5): 396–404.
57. El Tallawy HN, Farghaly WM, Rageh TA, et al. Epidemiology of major neurological disorders project in Al Kharga district, New Valley, Egypt. Neuroepidemiology. 2010; 35(4): 291–7.
58. Houinato D, Yemadje LP, Glitho G, et al. Epidemiology of epilepsy in rural Benin: prevalence, incidence, mortality, and follow-up. Epilepsia. 2013; 54(4): 757–63.
59. Jallon P, Smadja D, Cabre P, Le Mab G, Bazin M. EPIMART: prospective incidence study of epileptic seizures in newly referred patients in a French Carribean island (Martinique). Epilepsia. 1999; 40(8): 1103–9.
60. Ba-Diop A, Marin B, Druet-Cabanac M, Ngoungou EB, Newton CR, Preux PM. Epidemiology, causes, and treatment of epilepsy in sub-Saharan Africa. Lancet Neurology. 2014; 13(10): 1029–44.
61. Burneo JG, Tellez-Zenteno J, Wiebe S. Understanding the burden of epilepsy in Latin America: a systematic review of its prevalence and incidence. Epilepsy Res. 2005; 66(1–3): 63–74.
62. Medina MT, Durón RM, Martínez L, et al. Prevalence, incidence, and etiology of epilepsies in rural Honduras: the Salamá Study. Epilepsia. 2005; 46(1): 124–31.
63. Dogui M, Jallon P, Tamallah JB, et al. Episousse: incidence of newly presenting seizures in children in the Region of Sousse, Tunisia. Epilepsia. 2003; 44(11): 1441–4.
64. Fiest KM, Sauro KM, Wiebe S, et al. Prevalence and incidence of epilepsy. A systematic review and meta-analysis of international studies. Neurology. 2017; 88: 1–8.
65. Hauser WA, Annegers JF, Kurland LT. Incidence of epilepsy and unprovoked seizures in Rochester, Minnesota: 1935–1984. Epilepsia. 1993; 34(3): 453–68.
66. Wirrell EC, Grossardt BR, Wong-Kisiel LC, Nickels KC. Incidence and classification of new-onset epilepsy and epilepsy syndromes in children in Olmsted County, Minnesota from 1980 to 2004: a population-based study. Epilepsy Res. 2011; 95(1–2): 110–18.
67. Chin RFM, Neville BGR, Scott RC. A systematic review of the epidemiology of status epilepticus. Eur J Neurol. 2004; 11(12): 800–10.
68. Annegers JF, Dubinsky S, Pasternak Coan S, Newmark ME, Roht L. The incidence of epilepsy and unprovoked seizures in multi-ethnic, urban Health Maintenance Organizations. Epilepsia. 1999; 40(4): 502–6.
69. Zarrelli MM, Beghi E, Rocca WA, Hauser WA. Incidence of epileptic syndromes in Rochester, Minnesota: 1980–1984. Epilepsia. 1999; 40(12): 1708–14.
70. Olafsson E, Ludvigsson P, Gudmundsson G, et al. Incidence of unprovoked seizures and epilepsy in Iceland and assessment of the epilepsy syndrome classification: a prospective study. Lancet Neurology. 2005; 1(10): 627–34.
71. Loiseau J, Loiseau P, Guyot M, Duche B, Dartigues J-F, Aublet B. Survey of seizure disorders in the French southwest. I. Incidence of epileptic syndromes. Epilepsia. 1990; 31(4): 391–6.
72. Beghi E, Hesdorffer D. Prevalence of epilepsy—an unknown quantity. Epilepsia. 2014; 55(7): 963–7.
73. Hauser WA, Beghi E. First seizure definitions and worldwide incidence and mortality. Epilepsia. 2008; 49(Suppl 1): 8–12.
74. Hauser WA, Annegers JF, Rocca WA. Descriptive epidemiology of epilepsy: contributions of population-based studies from Rochester, Minnesota. Mayo Clin Proc. 1996; 71(6): 576–86.
75. D'Souza WJ, Quinn SJ, Fryer JL, et al. The prevalence and demographic distribution of treated epilepsy: a community-based study in Tasmania, Australia. Acta Neurol Scand. 2012; 125(2): 96–104.
76. Picot MC, Baldy-Moulinier M, Daurès JP, et al. The prevalence of epilepsy and pharmacoresistant epilepsy in adults: a population-based study in a Western European country. Epilepsia. 2008; 49(7): 1230–8.
77. Sillanpää M. Medico-social prognosis of children with epilepsy. Epidemiological study and analysis of 245 patients. Acta Paediatr Scand Suppl. 1973; 237: 3–104.
78. Eriksson KJ, Koivikko MJ. Prevalence, classification, and severity of epilepsy and epileptic syndromes in children. Epilepsia. 1997; 38(12): 1275–82.
79. Olafsson E, Hauser WA. Prevalence of epilepsy in rural Iceland: a population-based study. Epilepsia. 1999; 40(11): 1529–34.
80. Gallitto G, Serra S, La Spina P, et al. Prevalence and characteristics of epilepsy in the Aeolian islands. Epilepsia. 2005; 46(11): 1828–35.
81. Cossu P, Deriu MG, Casetta I, et al. Epilepsy in Sardinia, insular Italy: a population-based prevalence study. Neuroepidemiology. 2012; 39(1): 19–26.
82. Giussani G, Canelli V, Bianchi E, et al. A population-based study of active and drug-resistant epilepsies in Northern Italy. Epilepsy Behav. 2016; 55: 30–7.
83. Giussani G, Cricelli C, Mazzoleni F, et al. Prevalence and incidence of epilepsy in Italy based on a nationwide database. Neuroepidemiology. 2014; 43(3–4): 228–32.
84. Oka E, Ohtsuka Y, Yoshinaga H, Murakami N, Kobayashi K, Ogino T. Prevalence of childhood epilepsy and distribution of epileptic syndromes: a population-based survey in Okayama, Japan. Epilepsia. 2006; 47(3): 626–30.
85. Waaler PE, Blom BH, Skeidsvoll H, Mykletun A. Prevalence, classification, and severity of epilepsy in children in western Norway. Epilepsia. 2000; 41(7): 802–10.
86. Syvertsen M, Nakken KO, Edland A, Hansen G, Hellum MK, Koht J. Prevalence and etiology of epilepsy in a Norwegian county: a population based study. Epilepsia. 2015; 56(5): 699–706.
87. Bilikiewicz A, Matkowski K, Przybysz K, et al. Epidemiology and psychopathology of epileptics in Bydgoszca Province registered between 1976 and 1980. Psychiatr Neurol Med Psychol (Leipz). 1988; 40(1): 9–15.
88. Luengo A, Parra J, Colás J, et al. Prevalence of epilepsy in north-east Madrid. J Neurol. 2001; 248(9): 762–7.
89. Benavente I, Rubio E, Morales C, Tajada N, Tamargo P. Prevalence of epilepsy amongst adolescents in Huesca, Spain: a community-based study. Eur J Neurol. 2009; 16(10): 1138–43.
90. Garcia-Martin G, Perez-Errazquin F, Chamorro-Muñoz MI, Romero-Acebal M, Martin-Reyes G, Dawid-Milner MS. Prevalence and clinical characteristics of epilepsy in the South of Spain. Epilepsy Res. 2012; 102(1–2): 100–8.
91. Sidenvall R, Forsgren L, Heijbel J. Prevalence and characteristics of epilepsy in children in northern Sweden. Seizure. 1996; 5(2): 139–46.

92. Bolin K, Berggren F, Landtblom AM. Prevalence and cost of epilepsy in Sweden—a register-based approach. Acta Neurol Scand. 2015; 131(1): 37–44.
93. de la Court A, Breteler MM, Meinardi H, Hauser WA, Hofman A. Prevalence of epilepsy in the elderly: the Rotterdam Study. Epilepsia. 1996; 37(2): 141–7.
94. Goodridge DM, Shorvon SD. Epileptic seizures in a population of 6000. II: Treatment and prognosis. Br Med J (Clin Res Ed). 1983; 287(6393): 645–7.
95. Wallace H, Shorvon S, Tallis R. Age-specific incidence and prevalence rates of treated epilepsy in an unselected population of 2,052,922 and age-specific fertility rates of women with epilepsy. Lancet. 1998; 352(9145): 1970–3.
96. Wright J, Pickard N, Whitfield A, Hakin N. A population-based study of the prevalence, clinical characteristics and effect of ethnicity in epilepsy. Seizure. 2000; 9(5): 309–13.
97. Gaitatzis A, Sander JW. The mortality of epilepsy revisited. Epileptic Disord. 2004; 6: 3–13.
98. Steer S, Pickrell WO, Kerr MP, Thomas RH. Epilepsy prevalence and socioeconomic deprivation in England. Epilepsia. 2014; 55(10): 1634–41.
99. Hauser WA, Annegers JF, Kurland LT. Prevalence of epilepsy in Rochester, Minnesota: 1940–1980. Epilepsia. 1991; 32(4): 429–45.
100. Kobau R, DiIorio CA, Price PH, et al. Prevalence of epilepsy and health status of adults with epilepsy in Georgia and Tennessee: Behavioral Risk Factor Surveillance System, 2002. Epilepsy Behav. 2004; 5(3): 358–66.
101. Chong J, Hesdorffer DC, Thurman DJ, et al The prevalence of epilepsy along the Arizona-Mexico border. Epilepsy Res. 2013; 105(1–2): 206–15.
102. Ablah E, Hesdorffer DC, Liu Y, et al. Prevalence of epilepsy in rural Kansas. Epilepsy Res. 2014; 108(4): 792–801.
103. Chen CC, Chen TF, Hwang YC, et al. Population-based survey on prevalence of adult patients with epilepsy in Taiwan (Keelung community-based integrated screening no. 12). Epilepsy Res. 2006; 72(1): 67–74.
104. Hsieh LP, Huang CY. Prevalence of treated epilepsy in western medicine among the adult population in Taiwan: a study conducted using antiepileptic drug prescription data. Epilepsy Res. 2008; 80(2–3): 114–18.
105. Tellez-Zenteno JF, Pondal-Sordo M, Matijevic S, Wiebe S. National and regional prevalence of self-reported epilepsy in Canada. Epilepsia. 2004; 45(12): 1623–9.
106. Prasad AN, Sang X, Corbett BA, Burneo JG. Prevalence of childhood epilepsy in Canada. Can J Neurol Sci. 2011; 38(5): 719–22.
107. Schiariti V, Farrell K, Houbé JS, Lisonkova S. Period prevalence of epilepsy in children in BC: a population-based study. Can J Neurol Sci. 2009; 36(1): 36–41.
108. Al Rajeh S, Awada A, Bademosi O, Ogunniyi A. The prevalence of epilepsy and other seizure disorders in an Arab population: a community-based study. Seizure. 2001; 10(6): 410–14.
109. Josipovic-Jelic Z, Sonicki Z, Soljan I, Demarin V, and Collaborative Group for Study of Epilepsy Epidemiology in Sibenik-Knin County, Croatia. Prevalence and socioeconomic aspects of epilepsy in the Croatian county of Sibenik-Knin: community-based survey. Epilepsy Behav. 2011; 20(4): 686–90.
110. Endziniene M, Pauza V, Miseviciene I. Prevalence of childhood epilepsy in Kaunas, Lithuania. Brain Dev. 1997; 19(6): 379–87.
111. Kruja J, Beghi E, Zerbi D, et al. High prevalence of major neurological disorders in two Albanian communities: results of a door-to-door survey. Neuroepidemiology. 2012; 38(3): 138–47.
112. Nicoletti A, Reggio A, Bartoloni A, et al. Prevalence of epilepsy in rural Bolivia: a door-to-door survey. Neurology. 1999; 53(9): 2064–9.
113. Cruz ME, Schantz PM, Cruz I, et al. Epilepsy and neurocysticercosis in an Andean community. Int J Epidemiol. 1999; 28(4): 799–803.
114. Del Brutto OH, Santibáñez R, Idrovo L, et al. Epilepsy and neurocysticercosis in Atahualpa: a door-to-door survey in rural coastal Ecuador. Epilepsia. 2005; 46(4): 583–7.
115. Tekle-Haimanot R, Forsgren L, Abebe M, et al. Clinical and electroencephalographic characteristics of epilepsy in rural Ethiopia: a community-based study. Epilepsy Res. 1990; 7(3): 230–9.
116. Radhakrishnan K, Pandian JD, Santhoshkumar T, et al. Prevalence, knowledge, attitude, and practice of epilepsy in Kerala, South India. Epilepsia. 2000; 41(8): 1027–35.
117. Banerjee TK, Hazra A, Biswas A, et al. Neurological disorders in children and adolescents. Indian J Pediatr. 2009; 76(2): 139–46.
118. Pandey S, Singhi P, Bharti B. Prevalence and treatment gap in childhood epilepsy in a north Indian city: a community-based study. J Trop Pediatr. 2014; 60(2): 118–23.
119. Aziz H, Güvener A, Akhtar SW, Hasan KZ. Comparative epidemiology of epilepsy in Pakistan and Turkey: population-based studies using identical protocols. Epilepsia. 1997; 38(6): 716–22.
120. Malik MA, Akram RM, Tarar MA, Sultan A. Childhood epilepsy. J Coll Physicians Surg Pak. 2011; 21(2): 74–8.
121. Gracia F, de Lao SL, Castillo L, et al. Epidemiology of epilepsy in Guaymi Indians from Bocas del Toro Province, Republic of Panama. Epilepsia. 1990; 31(6): 718–23.
122. Dent W, Helbok R, Matuja WB, Scheunemann S, Schmutzhard E. Prevalence of active epilepsy in a rural area in South Tanzania: a door-to-door survey. Epilepsia. 2005; 46(12): 1963–9.
123. Hunter E, Rogathi J, Chigudu S, et al. Prevalence of active epilepsy in rural Tanzania: a large community-based survey in an adult population. Seizure. 2012; 21(9): 691–8.
124. Attia-Romdhane N, Mrabet A, Ben Hamida M. Prevalence of epilepsy in Kelibia, Tunisia. Epilepsia. 1993; 34(6): 1028–32.
125. Marino Jr R, Cukiert A, Pinho E. Epidemiological aspects of epilepsy in S. Paulo, Brazil. In: Wolf P, ed. Advances in Epileptology—XVIth Epilepsy International Symposium. New York: Raven Press, 1987.
126. Gomes Md Mda M, Zeitoune RG, Kropf LA, Beeck Ed Eda S. A house-to-house survey of epileptic seizures in an urban community of Rio de Janeiro, Brazil. Arq Neuropsiquiatr. 2002; 60(3-B): 708–11.
127. Borges MA, Min LL, Guerreiro CA, et al. Urban prevalence of epilepsy: populational study in São José do Rio Preto, a medium-sized city in Brazil. Arq Neuropsiquiatr. 2004; 62(2A): 199–204.
128. Gomez JG, Arciniegas E, Torres J. Prevalence of epilepsy in Bogota, Colombia. Neurology. 1978; 28(1): 90–94.
129. Pradilla G, Vesga BE, Leon-Sarmiento FE, et al. Neuroepidemiology in the eastern region of Colombia. Rev Neurol. 2002; 34(11): 1035–43.

130. Velez A, Eslava-Cobos J. Epilepsy in Colombia: epidemiologic profile and classification of epileptic seizures and syndromes. Epilepsia. 2006; 47(1): 193–201.
131. Li SC, Schoenberg BS, Wang CC, Cheng XM, Zhou SS, Bolis CL. Epidemiology of epilepsy in urban areas of the People's Republic of China. Epilepsia. 1985; 26(5): 391–4.
132. Kwong KL, Chak WK, Wong SN, So KT. Epidemiology of childhood epilepsy in a cohort of 309 Chinese children. Pediatr Neurol. 2001; 24(4): 276–82.
133. Wang WZ, Wu JZ, Wang DS, et al. The prevalence and treatment gap in epilepsy in China: an ILAE/IBE/WHO study. Neurology. 2003; 60(9): 1544–5.
134. Fong GC, Kwan P, Hui AC, Lui CH, Fong JK, Wong V. An epidemiological study of epilepsy in Hong Kong SAR, China. Seizure. 2008; 17(5): 457–64.
135. Zhao YH, Zhang Q, Long N, et al. Prevalence of epilepsy and alcohol-related risk in Zayul County, Tibet Autonomous Region in China: an initial survey. Epilepsy Behav. 2010; 19(4): 635–8.
136. Hu J, Si Y, Zhou D, et al. Prevalence and treatment gap of active convulsive epilepsy: a large community-based survey in rural West China. Seizure. 2014; 23(5): 333–7.
137. Pi X, Zhou L, Cui L, et al. Prevalence and clinical characteristics of active epilepsy in southern Han Chinese. Seizure. 2014; 23(8): 636–40.
138. Mendizabal JE, Salguero LF. Prevalence of epilepsy in a rural community of Guatemala. Epilepsia. 1996; 37(4): 373–6.
139. Garcia-Noval J, Moreno E, de Mata F, et al. An epidemiological study of epilepsy and epileptic seizures in two rural Guatemalan communities. Ann Trop Med Parasitol. 2001; 95(2): 167–75.
140. Sridharan R, Radhakrishnan K, Ashok PP, Mousa ME. Epidemiological and clinical study of epilepsy in Benghazi, Libya. Epilepsia. 1986; 27(1): 60–65.
141. Lee SY, Jung KY, Lee IK, et al. Prevalence of treated epilepsy in Korea based on national health insurance data. J Korean Med Sci. 2012; 27(3): 285–90.
142. Aziz H, Güvener A, Akhtar SW, Hasan KZ. Comparative epidemiology of epilepsy in Pakistan and Turkey: population-based studies using identical protocols. Epilepsia. 1997; 38(6): 716–22.
143. Karaagaç N, Yeni SN, Senocak M, et al. Prevalence of epilepsy in Silivri, a rural area of Turkey. Epilepsia. 1999; 40(5): 637–42.
144. Onal AE, Tumerdem Y, Ozturk MK, et al. Epilepsy prevalence in a rural area in Istanbul. Seizure. 2002; 11(6): 397–401.
145. Aydin A, Ergor A, Ergor G, Dirik E. The prevalence of epilepsy amongst school children in Izmir, Turkey. Seizure. 2002; 11(6): 392–6.
146. Huseyinoglu N, Ozben S, Arhan E, Palanci Y, Gunes N. Prevalence and risk factors of epilepsy among school children in eastern Turkey. Pediatr Neurol. 2012; 47(1): 13–18.
147. Velioglu SK, Bakirdemir M, Can G, Topbas M. Prevalence of epilepsy in northeast Turkey. Epileptic Disord. 2010; 12(1): 22–37.
148. Canpolat M, Kumandas S, Poyrazoglu HG, Gumus H, Elmali F, Per H. Prevalence and risk factors of epilepsy among school children in Kayseri City Center, an urban area in Central Anatolia, Turkey. Seizure. 2014; 23(9): 708–16.
149. Ozkan A, Degirmenci Y, Bakar C, Karaman HI. The prevalance of epilepsy among college students in Canakkale, Turkey. Acta Clin Croat. 2015; 54(1): 14–18.
150. Farghaly WM, El-Tallawy HN, Rageh TA et al. Epidemiology of uncontrolled epilepsy in the Al-Kharga District, New Valley, Egypt. Seizure. 2013; 22: 611–16.
151. Ebrahimi H, Shafa M, Hakimzadeh Asl S. Prevalence of active epilepsy in Kerman, Iran: a house-based survey. Acta Neurol Taiwan. 2012; 21(3): 115–24.
152. Lomidze G, Kasradze S, Kvernadze D, et al. The prevalence and treatment gap of epilepsy in Tbilisi, Georgia. Epilepsy Res. 2012; 98(2–3): 123–9.
153. Gonzales I, Miranda JJ, Rodriguez S, et al. Seizures, cysticercosis and rural-to-urban migration: the PERU MIGRANT study. Trop Med Int Health. 2015; 20(4): 546–52.
154. Mung'ala-Odera V, White S, Meehan R, et al. Prevalence, incidence and risk factors of epilepsy in older children in rural Kenya. Seizure. 2008; 17(5): 396–404.
155. Ibinda F, Wagner RG, Bertram MY, et al. Burden of epilepsy in rural Kenya measured in disability-adjusted life years. Epilepsia. 2014; 55(10): 1626–33.
156. Wagner RG, Ngugi AK, Twine R, et al. Prevalence and risk factors for active convulsive epilepsy in rural northeast South Africa. Epilepsy Res. 2014; 108(4): 782–91.
157. Osakwe C, Otte WM, Alo C. Epilepsy prevalence, potential causes and social beliefs in Ebonyi State and Benue State, Nigeria. Epilepsy Res. 2014; 108(2): 316–26.
158. Ngugi AK, Bottomley C, Kleinschmidt I, et al. Prevalence of active convulsive epilepsy in sub-Saharan Africa and associated risk factors: cross-sectional and case-control studies. Lancet Neurology. 2013; 12(3): 253–63.
159. Ndoye NF, Sow AD, Diop AG, et al. Prevalence of epilepsy its treatment gap and knowledge, attitude and practice of its population in sub-urban Senegal an ILAE/IBE/WHO study. Seizure. 2005; 14(2): 106–11.
160. Preux PM, Chea K, Chamroeun H, et al. First-ever, door-to-door cross-sectional representative study in Prey Veng province (Cambodia). Epilepsia. 2011; 52(8): 1382–7.
161. Yemadje LP, Houinato D, Boumédiène F, Ngoungou EB, Preux PM, Druet-Cabanac M. Prevalence of epilepsy in the 15 years and older in Benin: a door-to-door nationwide survey. Epilepsy Res. 2012; 99(3): 318–26.
162. Houinato D, Yemadje LP, Glitho G, et al. Epidemiology of epilepsy in rural Benin: prevalence, incidence, mortality, and follow-up. Epilepsia. 2013; 54(4): 757–63.
163. Nitiéma P, Carabin H, Hounton S, et al. Prevalence case-control study of epilepsy in three Burkina Faso villages. Acta Neurol Scand. 2012; 126(4): 270–8.
164. Magalov SI, Hasanov NF, Azizova NX, et al. The prevalence of epilepsy in the Nakhichevan Autonomous Republic of Azerbaijan. CNS Neurol Disord Drug Targets. 2012; 11(2): 102–9.
165. Coleman R, Loppy L, Walraven G. The treatment gap and primary health care for people with epilepsy in rural Gambia. Bull World Health Organ. 2002; 80(5): 378–83.
166. Birbeck GL, Kalichi EM. Epilepsy prevalence in rural Zambia: a door-to-door survey. Trop Med Int Health. 2004; 9(1): 92–5.
167. Balogou AA, Grunitzky EK, Belo M, et al. Management of epilepsy patients in Batamariba district, Togo. Acta Neurol Scand. 2007; 116(4): 211–16.
168. Rajbhandari KC. Epilepsy in Nepal. Can J Neurol Sci. 2004; 31(2): 257–60.
169. Prischich F, De Rinaldis M, Bruno F, et al. High prevalence of epilepsy in a village in the Littoral Province of Cameroon. Epilepsy Res. 2008; 82(2–3): 200–10.

170. Kelvin EA, Hesdorffer DC, Bagiella E, et al. Prevalence of self-reported epilepsy in a multiracial and multiethnic community in New York City. Epilepsy Res. 2007; 77(2–3): 141–50.
171. Forsgren L. Epidemiology and prognosis of epilepsy and ita treatment. In: Shorvon S, Perucca E, Fish D, Dodson E (eds). The Treatment of Epilepsy (2nd edition). Malden, MA: Blackwell Publishing, 2004. pp21–42.
172. Annegers JF, Hauser WA, Lee JR, Rocca WA. Secular trends and birth cohort effects in unprovoked seizures: Rochester, Minnesota 1935–1984. Epilepsia. 1995; 36(6): 575–9.
173. Sidenvall R, Forsgren L, Blomquist HK, Heijbel J. A community-based prospective incidence study of epileptic seizures in children. Acta Paediatr. 1993; 82(1): 60–65.
174. Sillanpää M, Lastunen S, Helenius H, Schmidt D. Regional differences and secular trends in the incidence of epilepsy in Finland: a nationwide 23-year registry study. Epilepsia. 2011; 52(10): 1857–67.
175. Cockerell OC, Eckle I, Goodridge DM, Sander JW, Shorvon SD. Epilepsy in a population of 6000 re-examined: secular trends in first attendance rates, prevalence, and prognosis. J Neurol Neurosurg Psychiatry. 1995; 58(5): 570–6.
176. Dham BS, Hunter K, Rincon F. The epidemiology of status epilepticus in the United States. Neurocrit Care. 2014; 20(3): 476–83.
177. Neligan A, Bell GS, Shorvon SD, Sander JW. Temporal trends in the mortality of people with epilepsy: a review. Epilepsia. 2010; 51(11): 2241–6.
178. Neligan A, Walker MC. Falling status epilepticus mortality rates in England and Wales: 2001–2013? Epilepsia. 2016; 57(7): e121–e124.
179. Chang YH, Li CY, Tung TH, Tsai JJ, Lu TH. Age-period-cohort analysis of mortality from epilepsy in Taiwan, 1971–2005. Seizure. 2011; 20(3): 240–3.
180. Keezer MR, Sisodiya SM, Sander JW. Comorbidities of epilepsy: Current concepts and future perspectives. Lancet Neurology. 2016; 15(1): 106–15.
181. Gaitatzis A, Sander JW. The mortality of epilepsy revisited. Epileptic Disord. 2004; 6: 3–13.
182. LaFrance WC Jr, Kanner AM, Hermann B. Psychiatric comorbidities in epilepsy. Int Rev Neurobiol. 2008; 83: 347–83.
183. Beghi E. Aetiology of epilepsy. In: Shorvon S, Perucca E, Fish D, Dodson E (eds). The Treatment of Epilepsy (2nd edition). Malden, MA: Blackwell Publishing, 2004. pp50–63.
184. Hauser WA, Hesdorffer DC. Genetics. In: Epilepsy: Frequency, Causes and Consequences. New York: Demos Publications, 1990. pp93–118.
185. Peljto AL, Barker-Cummings C, Vasoli VM, et al. Familial risk of epilepsy: a population-based study. Brain. 2014; 137(Pt 3): 795–805.
186. Robertson J, Hatton C, Emerson E, Baines S. Prevalence of epilepsy among people with intellectual disabilities: A systematic review. Seizure. 2015; 29(1): 46–62.
187. Nelson KB, Ellenberg JH. Predisposing and causative factors in childhood epilepsy. Epilepsia. 1987; 28(Suppl 1): S16–24.
188. Annegers JF, Hauser WA, Beghi E, Nicolosi A, Kurland LT. The risk of unprovoked seizures after encephalitis and meningitis. Neurology. 1988; 38(9): 1407–10.
189. Walsh S, Donnan J, Fortin Y, et al. A systematic review of the risks factors associated with the onset and natural progression of epilepsy. Neurotoxicology. 2017; 61: 64–77.
190. Ndimubanzi PC, Carabin H, Budke CM, et al. A systematic review of the frequency of neurocysticercosis with a focus on people with epilepsy. PLOS Negl Trop Dis. 2010; 4: e870.
191. Prince M, G-C Ali, Guerchet M, et al. Recent global trends in the prevalence and incidence of dementia, and survival with dementia. Alzheimer's Res Ther. 2016; 8: 23.
192. Friedman D, Honig LS, Scarmeas N Seizures and epilepsy in Alzheimer's disease. CNS Neurosci Ther. 2012; 18(4): 285–94.
193. Hesdorffer DC, Hauser WA, Annegers JF, Kokmen E, Rocca WA. Dementia and adult-onset unprovoked seizures. Neurology. 1996; 46(3): 727–30.
194. Gaitatzis A, Sisodiya SM, Sander JW. The somatic comorbidity of epilepsy: A weighty but often unrecognized burden. Epilepsia. 2012; 53(8): 1282–93.
195. Amatniek JC, Hauser WA, DelCastillo-Castaneda C, et al. Incidence and predictors of seizures in patients with Alzheimer's disease. Epilepsia. 2006; 47(5): 867–72.
196. Krishnamurti RV, Feigin VL, Forouzanfar MH, et al. Global and regional burden of first-ever ischaemic and haemorrhagic stroke during 1990–2010: Findings from the Global Burden of Disease Study 2010. Lancet Glob Health. 2013; 1: e259–81.
197. Camilo O, Goldstein LB. Seizures and epilepsy after ischemic stroke. Stroke. 2004; 35(5): 1769–75.
198. So EL, Annegers JF, Hause WA, O'Bien PC, Whisnant JP. Population-based study of seizure disorders after cerebral infarction. Neurology. 1995; 46: 350–355.
199. Burn J, Dennis M, Bamford J, Sandercock P, Wade D, Warlow C. Epileptic seizures after a first stroke: the Oxfordshire Community Stroke Project. BMJ. 1997; 13; 315(7122): 1582–7.
200. Bruns J Jr, Hauser WA. The epidemiology of traumatic brain injury: a review. Epilepsia. 2003; 44(Suppl 10): 2–10.
201. Annegers JF, Hauser WA, Coan SP, Rocca WA. A population-based study of seizures after traumatic brain injuries. N Engl J Med. 1998; 338(1): 20–24.
202. Caveness WF, Meirowsky AM, Rish BL, et al. The nature of post-traumatic epilepsy. J Neurosurg. 1979; 50: 545–53.
203. Frey LC. Epidemiology of post-traumatic epilepsy. Epilepsia. 2003; 44(Suppl 10): 11–17.
204. van Breemen MSM, Wilms EB, Vecht CJ. Epilepsy in patients with brain tumours: Epidemiology, mechanisms, and management. Lancet Neurology. 2007; 6(5): 421–30.
205. Beghi E, Giussani G, Sander JW. The natural history and prognosis of epilepsy. Epileptic Disord. 2015; 17(3): 243–53.
206. Sillanpää M, Saarinen M, Schmidt D. Clinical conditions of long-term cure in childhood-onset epilepsy: a 45-year follow-up study. Epilepsy Behav. 2014; 37: 49–53.
207. Lhatoo SD, Sander JW, Shorvon SD. The dynamics of drug treatment in epilepsy: an observational study in an unselected population-based cohort with newly diagnosed epilepsy followed up prospectively over 11–14 years. J Neurol Neurosurg Psychiatry. 2001; 71: 632–7.
208. Cockerell OC, Eckle I, Goodridge DM, Sander JW, Shorvon SD. Epilepsy in a population of 6000 re-examined: secular trends in first attendance rates, prevalence, and prognosis. J Neurol Neurosurg Psychiatry. 1995; 58(5): 570–6.
209. Cockerell OC, Johnson AL, Sander JW, Shorvon SD. Prognosis of epilepsy: a review and further analysis of the first nine years of the British National General Practice Study of Epilepsy, a prospective population-based study. Epilepsia. 1997; 38(1): 31–46.

210. Annegers JF, Hauser WA, Elveback LR. Remission of seizures and relapse in patients with epilepsy. Epilepsia. 1979; 20(6): 729–37.
211. Berg AT, Rychlik K. The course of childhood-onset epilepsy over the first two decades; A prospective, longitudinal study. Epilepsia. 2015; 56(1): 40–48.
212. Wakamoto H, Nagao H, Hayashi M, Morimoto T. Long-term medical, educational, and social prognoses of childhood-onset epilepsy: a population-based study in a rural district of Japan. Brain Dev. 2000; 22(4): 246–55.
213. Jonsson P, Eeg-Olofsson O. 10-year outcome of childhood epilepsy in well-functioning children and adolescents. Eur J Paediatr Neurol. 2011; 15(4): 331–7.
214. Geerts A, Arts WF, Stroink H, et al. Course and outcome of childhood epilepsy: a 15-year follow-up of the Dutch Study of Epilepsy in Childhood. Epilepsia. 2010; 51(7): 1189–97.
215. Giussani G, Canelli V, Bianchi E, et al. Long-term prognosis of epilepsy, prognostic patterns and drug resistance: a population-based study. Eur J Neurol. 2016; 23(7): 1218–27.
216. Camfield P, Camfield C. The frequency of intractable seizures after stopping AEDs in seizure-free children with epilepsy. Neurology. 2005; 64(6): 973–5.
217. Okuma T, Kumashiro H. Natural history and prognosis of epilepsy: report of a multi-institutional study in Japan. The group for the study of prognosis of epilepsy in Japan. Epilepsia. 1981; 22(1): 35–53.
218. Nicoletti A, Sofia V, Vitale G, et al. Natural history and mortality of chronic epilepsy in an untreated population of rural Bolivia: a follow-up after 10 years. Epilepsia. 2009; 50(10): 2199–206.
219. Sillanpää M, Schmidt D. Natural history of treated childhood-onset epilepsy: prospective, long-term population-based study. Brain. 2006; 129(Pt 3): 617–24.
220. Brodie MJ, Barry SJ, Bamagous GA, Norrie JD, Kwan P. Patterns of treatment response in newly diagnosed epilepsy. Neurology. 2012; 78(20): 1548–54.
221. Shorvon SD, Goodridge DM. Longitudinal cohort studies of the prognosis of epilepsy: contribution of the National General Practice Study of Epilepsy and other studies. Brain. 2013; 136(Pt 11): 3497–510.
222. Beghi E. Prognosis of first seizure. In: Jallon P (ed.) Prognosis of Epilepsies. Montrouge: John Libbey Eurotext, 2003. pp21–28.
223. Berg AT, Shinnar S. The risk of seizure recurrence following a first unprovoked seizure: a quantitative review. Neurology. 1991; 41(7): 965–72.
224. Mbuba CK, Ngugi AK, Newton CR, Carter JA. The epilepsy treatment gap in developing countries: a systematic review of the magnitude, causes, and intervention strategies. Epilepsia. 2008; 49(9): 1491–503.
225. Watts AE. The natural history of untreated epilepsy in a rural community in Africa. Epilepsia. 1992; 33(3): 464–8.
226. Nicoletti A, Sofia V, Vitale G, et al. Natural history and mortality of chronic epilepsy in an untreated population of rural Bolivia: a follow-up after 10 years. Epilepsia. 2009; 50(10): 2199–206.
227. Hauser WA, Rich SS, Lee JR, Annegers JF, Anderson VE. Risk of recurrent seizures after two unprovoked seizures. N Engl J Med. 1998; 338(7): 429–34.
228. MacDonald BK, Johnson AL, Goodridge DM, Cockerell OC, Sander JW, Shorvon SD. Factors predicting prognosis of epilepsy after presentation with seizures. Ann Neurol. 2000; 48(6): 833–41.
229. Sander JW. Some aspects of prognosis in the epilepsies: a review. Epilepsia. 1993; 34(6): 1007–16.
230. Tomson T, Forsgren L. Mortality studies in epilepsy. In: Jallon P (ed.), Prognosis of Epilepsies. Montrouge: John Libbey Eurotext, 2003. pp12–20.
231. Thurman DJ, Logroscino G, Beghi E, et al. The burden of premature mortality of epilepsy in high-income countries: a systematic review from the Mortality Task Force of the International League Against Epilepsy. Epilepsia. 2017; 58(1): 17–26.
232. Camfield CS, Camfield PR, Veugelers PJ. Death in children with epilepsy: a population-based study. Lancet. 2002; 359(9321): 1891–5.
233. Sillanpää M, Shinnar S. SUDEP and other causes of mortality in childhood-onset epilepsy. Epilepsy Behav. 2013; 28(2): 24–55.
234. Nevalainen O, Raitanen J, Ansakorpi H, Artama M, Isojärvi J, Auvinen A. Long-term mortality risk by cause of death in newly diagnosed patients with epilepsy in Finland: a nationwide register-based study. Eur J Epidemiol. 2013; 28(12): 981–90.
235. Rakitin A, Liik M, Oun A, Haldre S. Mortality risk in adults with newly diagnosed and chronic epilepsy: a population-based study. Eur J Neurol. 2011; 18(3): 465–70.
236. Holst AG, Winkel BG, Risgaard B, et al. Epilepsy and risk of death and sudden unexpected death in the young: a nationwide study. Epilepsia. 2013; 54(9): 1613–20.
237. Olafsson E, Hallgrimsson JT, Hauser WA, Ludvigsson P, Gudmundsson G. Pregnancies of women with epilepsy: a population-based study in Iceland. Epilepsia. 1998; 39(8): 887–92.
238. Rafnsson V, Ólafsson E, Hauser WA, Gudmundsson G. Cause-specific mortality in adults with unprovoked seizures. Neuroepidemiology. 2001; 20: 232–6.
239. Zieliński JJ. Epilepsy and mortality rate and cause of death. Epilepsia.1974; 15(2): 191–201.
240. Nilsson L, Tomson T, Farahmand BY, Diwan V, Persson PG. Cause-specific mortality in epilepsy: a cohort study of more than 9000 patients once hospitalized for epilepsy. Epilepsia. 1997; 38(10): 1062–8.
241. Lindsten H, Nyström L, Forsgren L. Mortality risk in an adult cohort with a newly diagnosed unprovoked epileptic seizure: a population-based study. Epilepsia. 2000; 41(11): 1469–73.
242. Morgan CL, Kerr MP. Epilepsy and mortality: a record linkage study in a U.K. population. Epilepsia. 2002; 43(10): 1251–5.
243. Neligan A, Bell GS, Sander JW, Shorvon SD. How refractory is refractory epilepsy? Patterns of relapse and remission in people with refractory epilepsy. Epilepsy Res. 2011; 96(3): 225–30.
244. Hauser WA, Annegers JF, Elveback LR. Mortality in patients with epilepsy. Epilepsia. 1980; 21(4): 399–412.
245. Berg AT, Shinnar S, Testa FM, Levy SR, Smith SN, Beckerman B. Mortality in childhood-onset epilepsy. Arch Pediatr Adolesc Med. 2004; 158(12): 1147–52.
246. Benn EK, Hauser WA, Shih T, et al. Estimating the incidence of first unprovoked seizure and newly diagnosed epilepsy in the low-income urban community of Northern Manhattan, New York City. Epilepsia. 2008; 49(8): 1431–9.
247. Nickels KC, Grossardt BR, Wirrell EC. Epilepsy-related mortality is low in children: a 30-year population-based study in Olmsted County, MN. Epilepsia. 2012; 53(12): 2164–71.

248. Loiseau J, Picot MC, Loiseau P. Short-term mortality after a first epileptic seizure: a population-based study. Epilepsia. 1999; 40(10): 1388–92.
249. Logroscino G, Hesdorffer DC, Cascino G, Annegers JF, Hauser WA. Time trends in incidence, mortality, and case-fatality after first episode of status epilepticus. Epilepsia. 2001; 42(8): 1031–5.
250. Logroscino G, Hesdorffer DC, Cascino G, et al. Mortality after a first episode of status epilepticus in the United States and Europe. Epilepsia. 2005; 46(Suppl 11): 46–8.
251. Ficker DM, So EL, Shen WK, et al. Population-based study of the incidence of sudden unexplained death in epilepsy. Neurology. 1998; 51(5): 1270–4.
252. Tomson T, Walczak T, Sillanpaa M, Sander JW. Sudden unexpected death in epilepsy: a review of incidence and risk factors. Epilepsia. 2005; 46(Suppl 11): 54–61.
253. Hesdorffer DC, Tomson T, Benn E, et al. Combined analysis of risk factors for SUDEP. Epilepsia. 2011; 52(6): 1150–9.
254. Hesdorffer DC, Tomson T, Benn E, et al. Do antiepileptic drugs or generalized tonic-clonic seizure frequency increase SUDEP risk? A combined analysis. Epilepsia. 2012; 53(2): 249–52.
255. Levira F, Thurman DJ, Sander JW, et al. Premature mortality of epilepsy in low- and middle-income countries: a systematic review from the Mortality Task Force of the International League Against Epilepsy. Epilepsia. 2017; 58(1): 6–16.
256. Mu J, Liu L, Zhang Q, et al. Causes of death among people with convulsive epilepsy in rural West China: a prospective study. Neurology. 2011; 77(2): 132–7.
257. Ding D, Wang W, Wu J, et al. Premature mortality risk in people with convulsive epilepsy: long follow-up of a cohort in rural China. Epilepsia. 2013; 54(3): 512–17.
258. Ngugi AK, Bottomley C, Fegan G, et al. Premature mortality in active convulsive epilepsy in rural Kenya: causes and associated factors. Neurology. 2014; 82(7): 582–9.
259. Kochen S, Melcon MO. Prognosis of epilepsy in a community-based study: 8 years of follow-up in an Argentine community. Acta Neurol Scand. 2005; 112(6): 370–4.
260. Kaiser C, Asaba G, Kasoro S, Rubaale T, Kabagambe G, Mbabazi M. Mortality from epilepsy in an onchocerciasis-endemic area in West Uganda. Trans R Soc Trop Med Hyg. 2007; 101(1): 48–55.
261. Carpio A, Bharucha NE, Jallon P, et al. Mortality of epilepsy in developing countries. Epilepsia. 2005; 46(Suppl 11): 28–32.
262. Banerjee TK, Ray BK, Das SK, et al. A longitudinal study of epilepsy in Kolkata, India. Epilepsia. 2010; 51(12): 2384–91.
263. Kamgno J, Pion SD, Boussinesq M. Demographic impact of epilepsy in Africa: results of a 10-year cohort study in a rural area of Cameroon. Epilepsia. 2003; 44(7): 956–63.
264. Tsai JJ. Mortality of epilepsy from national vital statistics and University epilepsy clinic in Taiwan. Epilepsia. 2005; 46(Suppl 11): 8–10.
265. GBD 2016 Epilepsy Collaborators. Global, regional, and national burden of epilepsy, 1990–2016: a systematic analysis for the Global Burden of Disease Study 2016. Lancet Neurology. 2019; 18(4): 357–75.
266. Thomas RH, Berkovic SF The hidden genetics of epilepsy-a clinically important new paradigm. Nat Rev Neurol. 2014; 10(5): 283–92.
267. Schmidt D, Sillanpää M. Prevention of epilepsy: issues and innovations. Curr Neurol Neurosci Rep. 2016; 16(11): 95.

32

Neuropathies

Descriptive epidemiology and related neurobiology

Ettore Beghi, Giorgia Giussani, and Marco Poloni

Introduction

Peripheral neuropathies are most frequently a component of a variety of acute and chronic diseases and injuries, with a wide spectrum of manifestations that range from subclinical entities to severe, disabling conditions. Peripheral neuropathies include diseases of the roots, plexuses, and nerves in various combinations that, by definition, are categorized as symmetric polyneuropathies, mononeuropathies, multifocal neuropathies, and radiculopathies. Sensory symptoms (numbness, paresthesia, pain), muscle weakness and/or autonomic signs in the distribution of the affected nerve(s) are the main complaints. Pain or pain sensitivity can be also present as a result of maladaptive changes occurring in injured sensory nerves.[1] The underlying pathogenic mechanisms of these conditions are diverse, and include an array of molecular and cellular contributions involving cytokines and other inflammatory mediators, changes in ion channels and neurotransmitters, and changes in intracellular signalling and structures.[2] Molecular motor proteins, that play a significant role in intracellular transport in neurons and control neuronal function, morphogenesis, and survival, are also involved.[3] Mechanical injuries (entrapment neuropathies) are additional factors, sometimes superimposed on other biological mechanisms. Genetic predisposition cannot be excluded to explain the response of the peripheral nerves to the structural and/or metabolic effects of the underlying diseases or environmental injuries.

Peripheral neuropathies represent a challenge for descriptive epidemiology for several reasons. First of all, the incidence and prevalence are preferably calculated in patients with the underlying cause (e.g. diabetes, environmental toxins). The diagnosis rests on differing criteria, ranging from simple detection of symptoms of peripheral nerve impairment to accurate electrophysiological investigation of the somatic and autonomic functions. Then, given the wide spectrum of severity, incidence and prevalence may vary according to the sensitivity and specificity of the diagnostic criteria. Last, the accuracy of the diagnosis may depend on the background of the investigator and, for multicentre studies, may depend on the extent of the inter-rater agreement. For these reasons, there are only a limited number of prevalence studies and even fewer incidence studies. A further complication is the low frequency of several peripheral neuropathies, which makes epidemiological investigation difficult unless large populations at risk are made available. For these reasons, descriptive epidemiology of peripheral neuropathies in the general population is based on very few reports (see below) and on a limited number of reviews[4,5] and book chapters.[6,7] This chapter provides an overview of studies investigating the prevalence and incidence of polyneuropathy in the general population and of the commonest peripheral neuropathies of various origins.

Peripheral Neuropathies in the General Population

The detection of peripheral neuropathies in the general population is generally based on a two-step screening procedure. A screening questionnaire is used to identify individuals with symptoms and/or signs suggesting peripheral nerve involvement. Individuals screening positive are then assessed by a specialist with or without electrophysiological testing. Community studies on the prevalence and incidence of polyneuropathy were performed in several resource-rich and resource-poor countries (Table 32.1).[8–21] The latter were door-to-door surveys using the WHO protocol, specifically designed for countries with limited resources.[8–13] In these studies, the prevalence of polyneuropathy ranged from 0.84 to 9 per 1000.

The prevalence and general characteristics of chronic symmetric symptomatic polyneuropathy were assessed in two elderly populations in Varese, Northern Italy, and San Giovanni Rotondo, Southern Italy.[15] Individuals aged 55 years or older, seen in office consultations by local general practitioners (GPs) were screened for neuropathic symptoms. Persons screening positive were assessed by a neurologist who confirmed the diagnosis of probable polyneuropathy in the presence of at least one among bilateral impairment

Table 32.1 Prevalence/incidence of polyneuropathy in population-based samples

Author, year	Study area	Source of cases (population)	Diagnostic criteria	N. of patients	Incidence/Prevalence (per 1000)	Risk factors
Cruz, 1985[8]	Quitonga, Ecuador	Door-to-door survey (1113, all ages)	WHO protocol	399	P, 9	NA
Osuntokun, 1987[9]	Igbo-Ora, Nigeria	Door-to-door survey (18,954, all ages)	WHO protocol	48	P, 2.5 Tropical 1.9 Diabetic 0.1 Nutritional 0.1 Hereditary 0.1 Idiopathic 1.9	NA
Cruz Gutierrez-del-Olmo, 1989[10]	Madrid, Spain	Door-to-door survey (961, all ages)	WHO protocol	7	P, 7.3 Diabetic 2.1 Alcoholic 2.1 Idiopathic 3.1	NA
Longe, 1989[11]	Udo, Nigeria	Door-to-door survey (2925, all ages)	WHO protocol	5	P, 1.4	NA
Bharucha, 1991[12]	Parsi community, Mumbai, India	Door-to-door survey (14,010)	Modified WHO protocol	334	P 2.4 per 1000 Diabetic 3.7 Toxic 0.4 Inflammatory 0.3 Hereditary 0.1 Idiopathic 2.1	Diabetes
Al Rajeh, 1993[13]	Thugbah, Saudi Arabia	Door-to-door survey (22,630, all ages)	Modified WHO protocol	19	P, 0.84	NA
IGPSG, 1995 Beghi, 1998[14,15]	Varese & San Giovanni Rotondo, Italy	General practitioners' lists (31,685, age 55+)	Screening symptoms & neurological examination	307	P, 36 (Varese) P, 33 (San Giovanni Rotondo)	Older age, diabetes, alcoholism, liver disease, tumor
Mygland & Monstad, 2001[16]	Vest-Agder, Norway	Population register (155,464, all ages)	Clinical and electrophysiological Immunofixation electrophoresis	192	P, 1.23 (total) CIDP 7.7 Paraproteinemia 0.05 RA 0.01 Sjogren 0.04 Sarcoidosis 0.02 Lyme 0.006 Paraneoplastic 0.02 Diabetic 0.23 Vitamin deficiency 0.05 Alcohol & toxic 0.20 Hereditary 0.15 Cryptogenic 0.26	NA
Baldereschi, 2007[17]	Eight municipalities, Italy	Stratified random samples (1784, age 65–84)	Self-reported symptoms & neurological examination		P, 70 I, 7.9	Older age, diabetes
Kruja, 2012[18]	Tirana (urban) & Saranda (rural), Albania	Door-to-door survey (9869)	Same as IGPSG	321	P, 39.8 (Tirana) P, 25.2 (Saranda)	NA
Kandil, 2012[19]	Assiut, Egypt	Door-to-door survey (42,234, all ages)	Modified WHO protocol	1343	P, 31.8 (total) Urban 18.4 Rural 37.9 Diabetic 5.71 Uremic 0.21 Hepatic 0.14 Hypothyroidism 0.12 Idiopathic 0.92	NA
Hoffman, 2015[20]	Olmsted County, US	Rochester Epidemiology Project (148,201, all ages)	ICD-9 CM administrative codes	2,892	P, 16.6	Diabetes
Hanewinckel, 2016b[21]	Rotterdam district, the Netherlands	Screening (1310, age 45+)	Interviews & medical records	72	P, 55	Diabetes

IGPSG = Italian General Practitioner Study Group; P = Prevalence; I = Incidence; NA = Not available.

of strength, sensation, or deep tendon reflexes. The age and sex-adjusted prevalence of probable polyneuropathy was 36 per 1000 in Varese and 33 per 1000 in San Giovanni Rotondo and increased with age. Diabetes was the commonest risk factor. The prevalence and incidence of distal symmetric neuropathy was investigated in individuals aged 65–84 years from seven Italian municipalities in population-based samples seen at study entry and after three years.[17] The diagnosis was made on clinical grounds. The study provided an adjusted prevalence of 70 per 1000 and an adjusted annual incidence of 7.9 per 1000 person-years. In a US study on the burden and mortality of patients with polyneuropathy using a records-linkage system and ICD-9CM diagnostic codes, the overall prevalence of polyneuropathy was 1.66% and rose to 6.6% in individuals older than 60 years.[20] Diabetic polyneuropathy was the most common specific subtype (38.2%). Multiple comorbidities were found associated with polyneuropathy after adjusting for diabetes co-occurrence. These included, among others, peripheral vascular, pulmonary, and renal diseases. The participants in the population-based Rotterdam Study were screened to investigate the prevalence and risk factors of polyneuropathy in individuals aged 55 years or older.[21] Polyneuropathy was diagnosed by a consensus panel based on symptoms, neurological examination, and nerve conduction studies. Age-adjusted prevalence was 5.5%. The disease prevailed in men and increased with age. Diabetes was the commonest risk factor. In a door-to-door survey screening a variety of neurological disorders in an urban and a rural Albanian community (Tirana and Saranda), polyneuropathy was found in 32 per 1000 population, with differences between the two study areas (Tirana, 40; Saranda, 25).[18] The differing prevalence across countries can be largely explained by differences in the size and age of the study population, in the screening methods, and in the diagnostic criteria (with special reference to the use of nerve conduction tests). Diabetes was consistently found as the predominating risk factor. The differences in resource-poor countries can also be explained by the differing life expectancy.

Diabetic Neuropathy

Diabetes mellitus is a fairly common disease worldwide. The GBD collaborators found a 0.9% age-adjusted prevalence and an increasing number of DALYs in the period 2005–2015.[22] Diabetic neuropathy is the most common type of polyneuropathy and the prevailing neuropathic syndrome in persons with diabetes.[23] Demyelination and axonal degeneration are established hallmarks of the pathology of diabetic neuropathy. Neurovascular dysfunction is a key finding caused by metabolic and molecular mechanisms, including glucose and lipid imbalances and insulin resistance, interconnected via oxidative stress, inflammation, and altered gene expression.[24] Additional abnormalities include alterations in the expression of neurotrophins and limited changes in muscle fibre size and capillary density.[25] Diabetic polyneuropathy is defined as a 'symmetrical, length-dependent sensorimotor polyneuropathy attributable to metabolic and microvessel alterations as a result of chronic hyperglycaemia exposure and cardiovascular risk covariates'.[26] Less common neuropathic syndromes include cranial mononeuropathies and focal neuropathies. In a cross-sectional and longitudinal study of diabetic neuropathies among the Rochester, Minnesota residents,[27] 66% of insulin-dependent diabetic patients had a peripheral neuropathy (polyneuropathy, 54%; carpal tunnel syndrome, asymptomatic, 22%, and symptomatic, 11%; autonomic neuropathy, 7%, and other varieties, 3%). Fifty-nine per cent of non-insulin-dependent diabetic patients had a peripheral neuropathy and the corresponding percentages were 45%, 29%, 6%, 5%, and 3%. Several studies investigated the prevalence of polyneuropathy in individuals with diabetes, reporting differing ratios (2–47.3%). The differences can be largely explained by the diversity of sources, screening methods, populations at risk, disease duration, and diagnostic criteria (Table 32.2).[27–33]

The incidence of diabetic neuropathy has been less frequently investigated. In a community-based retrospective study of people with maturity-onset diabetes, 4% of cases developed peripheral neuropathy within 5 years of diagnosis and 15% within 20 years.[28] Symmetric polyneuropathy was the predominating phenotype. Poor glycaemic control, disease duration, and age are the most consistent risk factors. In a more recent study done in 13 general practices in the UK,[33] incident cases of neurological disorders were ascertained prospectively using multiple screening sources. The age and sex-adjusted annual incidence of diabetic polyneuropathy was 54 per 100,000 and the lifetime prevalence was 2 per 1000.

Pain is a common symptom. In a population-based sample of patients with type 2 diabetes, the prevalence of painful neuropathy was 26.4%.[34] A study in the UK using the General Practice Research Database reported an annual incidence of painful diabetic neuropathy of 15.3 per 100,000, with an increasing trend during the study period (11 years).[35] The prevalence of painful diabetic neuropathy has been found to range from 10.9% to 26.4% in different studies,[34,36,37] In a Finnish study in newly diagnosed patients with non-insulin-dependent diabetes followed for ten years, the prevalence of painful neuropathy (assessed with clinical criteria and electrodiagnostic studies) was 7% at baseline and increased to 20% at the end of follow-up.[32] Age, diabetes type, disease duration, and glycaemic control can explain in part the differences in reported rates and ratios. However, sources, screening measures, diagnostic criteria, and attrition can have a major role.

Inflammatory Neuropathies

Inflammatory neuropathies represent 2–16% of all polyneuropathies in hospital-based studies.[23] These neuropathies can present as subacute motor polyneuropathies, with frequent sensory and cranial nerve involvement, or as chronic polyneuropathies, with a relapsing-remitting or a progressive course. While the epidemiology of the subacute form (acute inflammatory polyradiculoneuropathy or Guillain-Barre syndrome) has been extensively investigated, data on the chronic form (chronic inflammatory demyelinating polyradiculoneuropathy) are sparse.

Acute inflammatory polyradiculoneuropathy

The Guillain-Barre syndrome (GBS) is an acute or subacute condition characterized by a rapidly increasing weakness in the limbs and/or the cranial nerves, associated with reduction or loss of deep tendon reflexes and, in most cases, typical CSF and electrodiagnostic

Table 32.2 Prevalence/incidence of diabetic neuropathy in different populations

Author, year	Study area	Source of cases (population)	Diagnostic criteria	N. of patients	Prevalence/Incidence per year	Risk factors
Palumbo, 1978[28]	Rochester, MN, USA	Medical records (approx 55,000)	Sensory symptoms and/or signs	1028 patients with NIDDM, age >30	P 3% at time of diabetes diagnosis P 20% after 20 years	NA
Franklin, 1990[29]	San Luis Valley, CO, USA	Screening Neurological examination	2/3 among sensory symptoms, sensory or motor signs, reduced/absent DTR	279 patients with NIDDM	P 27.8%	Older age, male sex, poor glucose tolerance, duration of diabetes
Dyck, 1993[27]	Rochester, MN, USA	Medical records (approx 65,000)	National Diabetes Data Group criteria	870 patients with IDDM/NIDDM	P 60.4% (all neuropathy); P 47.3% (distal polyneuropathy)	NA
Harris, 1993[30]	USA	Structured interview (84,572)	Sensory symptoms, altered touch/temperature perception in hands/feet	2405 patients with diabetes	P 30% (IDDM) 37% (NIDDM)	Mexican-American, duration of diabetes, poor glycaemic control, hypertension
Savettieri, 1993[31]	Two Sicilian municipalities, Italy	Door-to-door survey (14,540)	Neuropathic symptoms, clinical findings	27	P 2.7 per 1000	NA
Partanen, 1995[32]	Kuopio county, Finland	NA	Clinical criteria & electrodiagnostic studies	133 patients, age 45–64 with NIDDM	P 8.3% at diagnosis P 41.9% after 10 years	Poor glycaemic control
MacDonald, 2000[33]	London, UK	General practice records (100,230)	Assessment by neurologist	NA	Lifetime P 2 per 1,000 I 54 per 100,000	NA

IDDM = Insulin-dependent diabetes mellitus; NIDDM = Non insulin-dependent diabetes mellitus; NA = Not available.

abnormalities. The disease is the result of an immune-mediated process due to the generation of autoantibodies and inflammatory cells cross-reacting with epitopes on roots and peripheral nerves, resulting in myelin and axonal damage (molecular mimicry). The immune response is triggered by various antigenic stimuli represented by viral or bacterial infections. Exposure to *Campylobacter jejuni* and several vaccines have been implicated. The progression of the clinical deficit peaks in 2–4 weeks. Signs and symptoms tend to subside in the following weeks to months, depending on the severity of the clinical and electrophysiological findings. The outcome of the disease is favourable, but up to 20% of cases have persisting deficits at six months and 3–7% die during the acute phase. Although GBS has a typical clinical picture in the majority of cases, two major forms (demyelinating and axonal) and a variety of variants have been identified. The epidemiology, pathophysiology, clinical picture of the typical form and its variants, course, and treatments of the disease have been recently reviewed.[38]

The incidence of GBS has been assessed in several resource-rich and resource-poor countries but most studies were performed in Europe and North America (Fig. 32.1). These studies have been the object of a systematic review and meta-analysis that, based on the critical appraisal of 13 published reports and 1643 cases, provided a crude incidence ranging from 0.81 to 1.89 cases per 100,000 person-years.[39] The incidence of the disease was higher in males than in females (relative risk 1.78; 95% CI 1.36–2.33) and increased with age, from 0.62 per 100,000 among 0–9-year-olds to 2.66 per 100,000 among 80–89-year-olds. There is no consistent seasonal pattern, but only a modest increase of the disease in winter than in summer (relative risk, 1.14, 96% CI 1.02–1.27), not evident in all geographic areas, as shown in a systematic review with a cohort study done in the UK.[40] In China the disease has been found to peak in the summer months, present as an axonal neuropathy, and affect predominantly children and young adults.[41] However, the authors concluded that this was a distinctive syndrome, distinguishable from poliomyelitis and GBS. While the incidence of GBS is consistently low, with fairly modest variations in resource-rich countries, where the demyelinating type is predominant, data from resource-poor countries are variable, reflecting differences in diagnostic criteria, ascertainment methods, and, not least, population structure.[42]

Since the GBS outbreak at the time of the 1976 swine flu vaccination programme,[43] vaccination campaigns have been extensively monitored in the USA and in other countries. Most studies did not show an association between vaccine administration and GBS.[44] However, some studies found small but significantly increased risks of GBS in the six weeks following the administration of the influenza vaccine. Risks were 1.45 (95% CI 1.05–1.99) in Canada;[45] 1.7 (95% CI 1.0–2.8) in the USA;[46] and 3.8 (95% CI 1.3–10.5) in Italy.[47] The Italian study was performed at the time of the H1N1 (a virus of swine origin) influenza pandemic. In that study, a self-controlled case series analysis found a relative risk of 2.1 (95% CI 1.1, 3.9). A small but still significantly increased risk (2.35; 95% CI 1.42–4.01) was confirmed in the USA by a meta-analysis of six adverse event monitoring systems during the H1N1 vaccination campaign.[48] However, studies using a case-centred or a self-controlled design showed that the risk of GBS following infections, including influenza, exceeds the risk following influenza vaccination.[44] According to these results the attributable risk of GBS in adults ranges from 1 to 5 GBS cases per 1,000,000 vaccinations.

GBS has also been associated with other viral infections. The most recent refers to the Zika virus infection. This topic has been recently reviewed.[49] In summary, the first GBS cases have been reported in 2014 in French Polynesia, A case-control study describing clinical

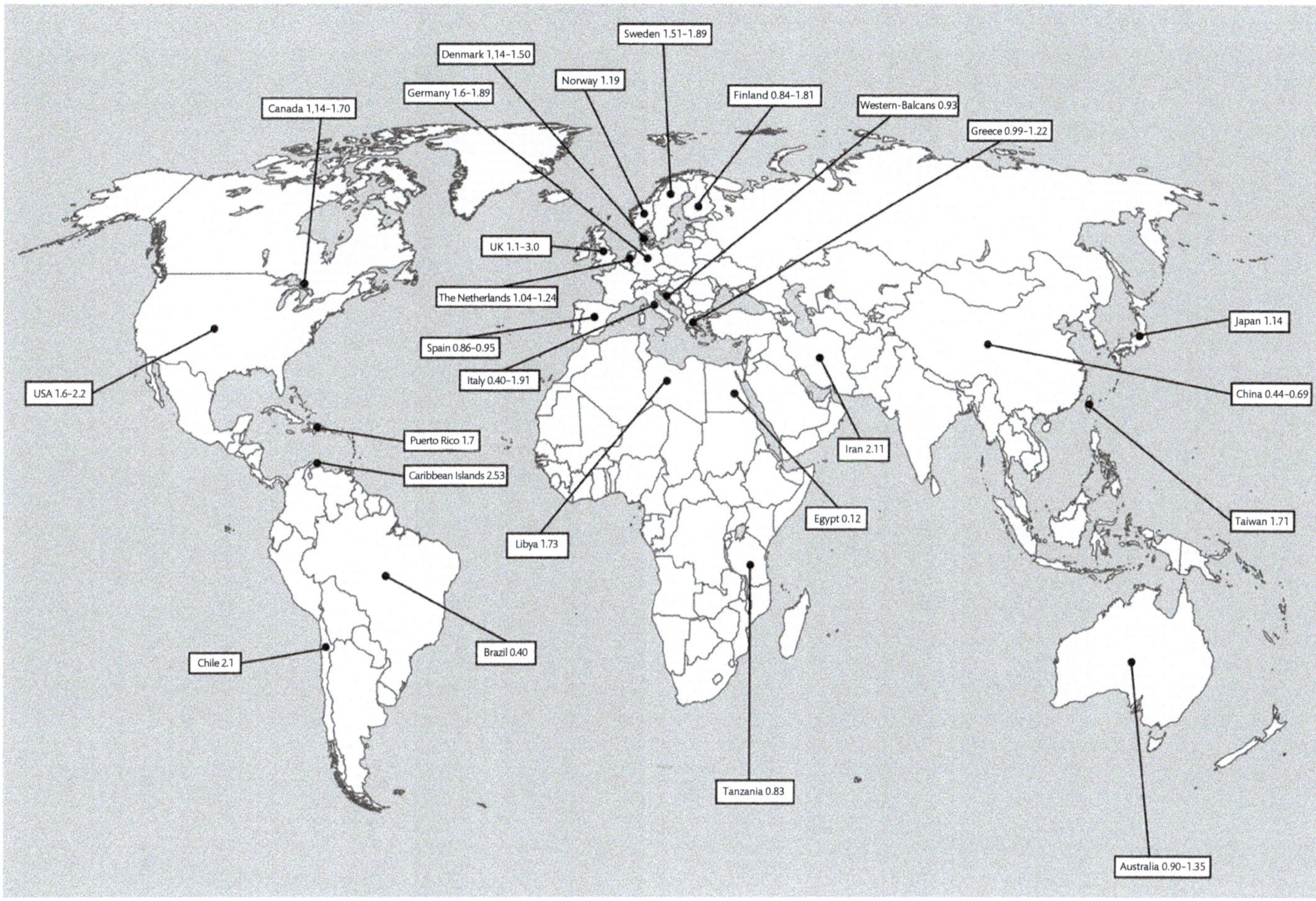

Fig. 32.1 Worldwide incidence (per 100,000/year) of Guillain-Barre syndrome.

and electrophysiological characteristics of these patients has been published.[50] Ninety-eight per cent of patients with GBS tested positive for Zika virus infection (IgG and IgM) and 100% had neutralizing antibodies against Zika virus, compared to 56% of controls.

Chronic inflammatory demyelinating polyneuropathy

Chronic inflammatory demyelinating polyneuropathy (CIDP) is a symmetric, predominantly motor, proximal and distal demyelinating peripheral neuropathy with a relapsing or a slowly progressive course.[51] CIDP subtypes include multifocal motor neuropathy (MMN) and paraproteinemic demyelinating neuropathy (PDN). Prevalence studies revealed variable rates (1–7.7 per 100,000)(see Table 32.3),[16,53–61] which may be attributed to differing case ascertainment, study methodology, and geography. A recent study on neuromuscular diseases in Ireland provided an overall prevalence of 5.87 per 100,000 (95% CI 5.06–6.68).[54] The prevalence was 0.70 per 100,000 (95% CI 0.42–0.98) for MMN and 0.32 (95% CI 0.13–0.51) for PDN. The incidence of CIDP ranged from 0.36 to 1.6 per 100,000 person-years (Table 32.3). The variable results are mostly due to the use of different diagnostic criteria.[52]

Paraneoplastic Neuropathies

Paraneoplastic neuropathies are part of a heterogeneous group of neurological disorders triggered by cancer. As with all paraneoplastic syndromes, neuropathies are caused by mechanisms other than metastases, metabolic or nutritional deficits, infections, coagulopathy, or side effects of cancer treatment such as chemotherapy. As many paraneoplastic syndromes are associated with antibodies against neural antigens expressed by the tumour (antineural antibodies), immune-mediated mechanisms have been postulated. Four diagnostic categories have been identified: (1) a classical syndrome and cancer that develops within five years of the diagnosis of the neurological disorder; (2) a non-classical syndrome that resolves or significantly improves after cancer treatment without concomitant immunotherapy, provided that the syndrome is not susceptible to spontaneous remission; (3) a non-classical syndrome with onconeural antibodies (well characterized or not) and cancer that develops within five years of the diagnosis of the neurological disorder; (4) a neurological syndrome (classical or not) with well characterized onconeural antibodies (anti-Hu, Yo, CV2, Ri, Ma2, or amphiphysin), and no cancer.[62]

The frequency of paraneoplastic neuropathies is virtually unknown for the absence of population-based studies. In a recent meta-analysis of 42 reports and 92 patients with a variety of cancers, the commonest form was pure sensory neuropathy (sensory ganglionopathy and symmetrical sensory neuropathy).[63] Axonal neuropathies were reported in 87% of cases, the most common neurophysiological type being asymmetrical sensory ganglionopathy. The commonest first manifestation of PPN was sensory loss (67.4%), followed by pain (41.3%), weakness (22.8%), and sensory ataxia (20.7%).

Table 32.3 Prevalence and incidence of chronic inflammatory demyelinating polyneuropathy

Author, year	Study area	Source of cases	Diagnostic criteria	N. of patients	Prevalence/Incidence (per 100,000)
Roy, 2015[53]	Belgium	BNMDR	Belgian NMD		P 1.1
Chiò, 2007[54]	Piemonte, Italy	Hospital records & regional archives (4,334,225)	AAN diagnostic criteria	294	P 3.58 I 0.36
Lefter, 2017[55]	Ireland	Multiple sources (4,588,252)	EFNS/PNS Task Forces	202	P 5.87
Hafsteinsdottir, 2016[56]	Iceland	Neurologists' records	EFNS/PNS Task Forces	19	I 0.3
Mahdi-Rogers, 2014[57]	South East England	Multiple sources (3,557,352)	EFNS/PNS Task Forces, and serum protein electrophoresis	101	P 2.84
Laughlin, 2009[58]	Olmsted county, MN, USA	Mayo Clinic Records Linkage System (1581)	Dyck's diagnostic criteria (course, nerve fibre class affected, distribution and symmetry of neuropathic involvement)	23	P 8.9 I 1.6
Lunn, 1999[59]	Four Thames health regions, UK	National consultant neurologist surveillance programme & personal case series (14,049,850) + 3,717,638	AAN diagnostic criteria	94	P 1 P 0.67; 0.46-1.24
McLeod, 1999[60]	New South Wales, Australia	5,995,544 + 448,663	Clinical, electrophysiological and nerve biopsy (if performed)	112	P 1.87 I 0.15
Mygland, 2001[16]	Vest-Agder, Norway	Population register (155,464, all ages)	Clinical and electrophysiological. Immunofixation electrophoresis	15	P 7.7
Iijima, 2008[61]	Japan	127,655,000	AAN diagnostic criteria	2433	P 1.61 I 0.48

NMD = Neuromuscular diseases; AAN = American Academy of Neurology; EFNS = European federation of Neurological Societies; PNS = Peripheral Nerve Society; P = Prevalence; I = Incidence.

Infectious Neuropathies

Apart from GBS, various neuropathies have been reported in association with bacterial or viral infections. In resource-poor countries leprosy remains an important cause of peripheral neuropathy. Leprosy is a chronic infection caused by *Mycobacterium leprae* leading to various clinical manifestations. The infection in humans results from the ability of this bacterial pathogen to induce severe injury of peripheral nerves (Schwann cells) and skin (keratinocytes and histiocytes).[64] Since the introduction of multi-drug therapy (MDT) in highly affected communities, the prevalence of the disease has decreased. However, new cases continue to be detected in highly endemic areas. According to the WHO, the highest prevalence of leprosy is in South-East Asia (116 per 100,000), followed by Africa (53 per 100,000) and Central and South America (46 per 100,000).[65] The mode and route of transmission of the disease has not been precisely defined. The clustering of cases of leprosy tends to occur among individuals living in resource-poor areas with favourable ecological niches for *M. leprae* to thrive. Peripheral nerve involvement occurs in all infected patients. At the time of a diagnosis of leprosy, up to 60% of cases have evidence of peripheral nerve damage.[66] Neural tropism of *M. leprae* is through its binding and entry into Schwann cells causing demyelination, manifesting clinically with decreased sensorimotor function. Damage to nerves can occur before, during, and after treatment and results in disability and long-term disfigurement. Peripheral nerve involvement is observed in 33–56% of patients at diagnosis.[7] A cohort study in Ethiopia showed that 47% of newly diagnosed cases already had established nerve function impairment and a further 8% had recent nerve damage.[67] An additional 12% of patients developed nerve damage after the start of treatment, and only 33% had no clinical evidence of nerve involvement at any time. The delay between the onset of symptoms and diagnosis is frequently years, and during this time neuropathy can develop almost unnoticed.

Peripheral neuropathy is one of the commonest complications of HIV infection. In a systematic review of 25 studies, the prevalence of HIV-related neuropathy was found to range from 1.2% to 69.4%. These estimates are undoubtedly imprecise because there are no population-based studies available. The corresponding incidence was 0.7–39.7 per 100 person-years, with an increase with age and an association with the severity of the disease.[68] Distal sensory polyneuropathy is the commonest clinical manifestation. Acute and chronic inflammatory demyelinating polyneuropathy or multifocal mononeuropathy can be also observed. Currently available reports suggest great variation in the frequency of the disease across studies, possibly explained by clinical heterogeneity, but also by the lack of standardized diagnostic criteria and the differing study designs. In addition, factors other than HIV infection must be considered, like diabetes, genetic susceptibility, use of psychoactive drugs, including alcohol, and anti-retroviral treatment (see below).

Toxic and Iatrogenic Neuropathies

Toxic neuropathies are a variety of peripheral nerve disorders involving preferably dorsal roots or peripheral sensory nerves. When involving the peripheral nerves, axonopathies are the predominant pathologic manifestations of toxic neuropathies. Clinically, toxic neuropathies are purely sensory neuropathies or mixed sensory-motor neuropathies. With few exceptions, onset is gradual and progression is slow, with recovery after removal of the toxin in most but not all cases. Toxic agents include drugs, heavy metals, chemicals, and animal and plant toxins. The association between neuropathy and toxin exposure can be confirmed when the insurgence of the disease follows the exposure; there is a correlation between the severity of the disease and the magnitude of the exposure; the removal of the toxin is followed by improvement of symptoms and signs; and there is a known biological effect of the toxic agent.[69] In the absence of population-based studies, the burden of toxic neuropathies can rely only on clinical series or reports on industrial workers. For a comprehensive review of toxic neuropathies see Feigin and Bennett (2007).[7]

Drug-induced neuropathies

Several drugs have adverse effects on the peripheral nervous system. These include, among others, antibacterial and antiparasitic agents, cardiovascular drugs, and chemotherapeutic agents. For most drugs, an association with peripheral neuropathy was found only with the use of high doses. Genetic variants of drug metabolizing enzymes and drug transporters can be also be implicated as possible biomarkers for adverse drug reactions. Here, we will discuss only drugs for which an association was documented by studies with appropriate design.

Incidence and prevalence of peripheral neuropathy have been investigated in HIV-infected patients enrolled in randomized trials of combination anti-retroviral therapy and screened for neuropathic symptoms and/or signs.[70] Prior to treatment initiation, the prevalence of peripheral neuropathy was 22.6% (95% CI 19.0–26.4%) and the prevalence of symptomatic peripheral neuropathy was 4.3% (95% CI 2.7–6.4%). Rates of symptomatic and asymptomatic peripheral neuropathy at three years were 32.1% and 8.6%, respectively. Neuropathic signs persisted despite viral control and improved immune function. Variables associated with neuropathy included older age, lower CD4+ cell counts, current antiretroviral drugs use, and non-white race.

Oral fluoroquinolones are potent antimicrobial agents. In a case-control study, cases were defined as patients with a first diagnosis of peripheral neuropathy or drug-induced polyneuropathy.[71] Compared to matched controls, current users of fluoroquinolones were at a higher risk of developing peripheral neuropathy (RR 5 1.83, 95% CI 1.49–2.27). Current new users had the highest risk (RR 5 2.07, 95% CI 1.56–2.74).

Statins are used in the primary and secondary prevention of coronary artery disease. The adverse effects of statins on the peripheral nerves are scarcely understood. Interference with cholesterol synthesis may alter nerve membrane function because cholesterol is a ubiquitous component of human cell membranes. In a Danish population-based patient registry, each first-ever case of idiopathic polyneuropathy was matched to 25 control subjects.[72] Drug exposure was assessed through a prescription register. The OR linking idiopathic polyneuropathy with statin use was 14.2 (5.3–38.0) for definite cases. The corresponding ORs in current users were 16.1 (5.7–45.4) for definite cases. For patients treated with statins for two or more years the OR was 26.4 (95% CI 7.8–45.4). In a UK study performed with general practitioners during 1991–1997, incidence of neuropathy induced by statins was 7.3/100000 person/year.[73]

Amiodarone is a highly effective antiarrhythmic agent. The drug has a number of adverse effects, including peripheral neuropathy.[74] Amiodarone-induced neuropathy is characterized by lysosomal inclusions in Schwann cells, vessels, and endothelial cells and is axonal, demyelinating, and both axonal and demyelinating.[75] In a cohort of 707 residents of Olmsted County, Minnesota, followed for 151 months, the cumulative incidence of likely amiodarone neurotoxic effects was 2.8%.[76] Exposure to long-term and/or high-dose amiodarone therapy increased the risk of neurological manifestations.

Chemotherapy-induced peripheral neuropathy is a frequent adverse effect of the most common cancer treatments. The disease is characterized by paraesthesia, dysaesthesia and often pain, primarily in the hands and feet.[2] Patients most often report sensory symptoms that may be so intense to require treatment reduction or discontinuation. Known mechanisms include irreversible DNA binding, neuronal apoptosis, and dysfunction of cellular and axonal transport. Peripheral neuropathies have been most commonly reported with cisplatin, oxaliplatin, vincristine, paclitaxel, and bortezomib. The incidence has been reported to vary from 10% to 95% of cases, depending on the drug, the dose, and the tumour severity and type.[77]

Peripheral neuropathy is a common finding in alcohol abusers. The pathophysiology of peripheral nerve dysfunction among alcohol addicts may be the result of a direct toxic effect of alcohol and/or of chronic nutritional deficiency.[78] In a cohort of 296 alcohol addicts, symptoms of polyneuropathy were present in 16.2% of cases and EMG findings compatible with polyneuropathy in 48.6%.[79] The disease was more prevalent in men, older people, individuals with prolonged exposure, and in those who were drinking wine.

Entrapment Neuropathies

The most common and best studied entrapment neuropathy is carpal tunnel syndrome. The disease is caused by the narrowing of the carpal canal or the swelling of the tendon sheaths. These abnormal findings result in constriction in the canal and produce impingement on the median nerve. Dysaesthesias and paraesthesias are the predominant symptoms that may evolve into wasting and weakness of the thenar muscles, resulting in weakened pinch grip. One of the first studies on the incidence of carpal tunnel syndrome was performed in the population of Rochester, Minnesota, from 1961 through 1980.[80] The overall incidence of the disease was 99 per 100,000 person-years. Age-adjusted rates were 52 for the men, 149 for the women, and 105 for both sexes combined. Age-adjusted incidence increased from 88 in the period 1961–1965 to 125 in the period 1976–1980, perhaps reflecting better recognition of the disease. Age-specific rates increased with age in men, whereas in women a peak was reached in the 45–54 age group. The temporal trends of carpal tunnel syndrome were assessed in 10,069 residents of Olmsted County, Minnesota, over a 25-year period.[81] The annual incidence of the disease was 491 per 100,000 in women and 258 per 100,000 in men. The rate increased from 258 in the first five years to 424 in the last five years of the study. The annual incidence of work-related carpal tunnel syndrome was 11 per 100,000. The significant increase in the incidence of carpal tunnel syndrome has been attributed by the authors to a better recognition of the disease by caring physicians, the introduction of more sensitive electrodiagnostic techniques, and a greater awareness among the general population. The predominance of the disease in women can be explained by hormonal factors, as pregnancy and breastfeeding put women at increased risk,[82] while occupational biomechanical factors play a substantial role in both sexes.[83] A number of non-occupational risk factors have been also been identified. These include inflammatory arthritis (OR 2.9; 95% CI 2.2, 3.8, corticosteroid use (OR 1.6; 95% CI 1.2, 2.1), diabetes (OR 1.4; 95% CI 1.2, 1.8), and hypothyroidism (OR 1.7; 95% CI 1.1, 2.8).[84] The incidence of the disease varies significantly depending on the sources of cases and the populations at risk (Table 32.4).[80,81,85–90]

Hereditary Neuropathies

Charcot-Marie-Tooth (CMT) disease is the most frequently inherited neuropathy and one of the commonest neurogenetic disorders. Clinical features of CMT disease include childhood onset, familial aggregation, slowly progressive weakness, and muscle atrophy in the lower extremities, followed by the involvement of the upper extremities, with reduction/loss of deep tendon reflexes and only mild to moderate distal sensory impairment. The CMT disease is subdivided in two main subgroups, a demyelinating form (CMT1) and an axonal form (CMT2). A systematic review of the epidemiology of the disease has recently been published.[91] The prevalence of CMT disease has been studied in several countries and found to range between 9.7 and 82.3 per 100,000 (Table 32.5).[92–103] The prevalence of CMT1 disease varied from 37.6% to 84% and the prevalence of CMT2 disease from 12% to 35.9%. The differences are mostly explained by the extent of case ascertainment, but the possibility cannot be excluded that the disease varies in different populations and, within countries, in different regions. With the contribution of genetic testing, an increase of the prevalence and a further complication of the genetic heterogeneity of the disease are expected.

Less frequent hereditary neuropathies include familial amyloidotic polyneuropathy and hereditary motor and sensory neuropathy (HMSN). In a study using the Data Bank of Cyprus Institute of Neurology and Genetics, the prevalence of HMSN was 3.72/100000.[104] A Spanish ten-year study conducted in the main hospital of Cantabria region[105] found the prevalence of HMSN was

Table 32.4 Prevalence of carpal tunnel syndrome in different populations

Author, year	Study area	Source of cases	Diagnostic criteria	N. of patients	Prevalence/ Incidence (per 100,000)	Risk factors
Stevens, 1988[80]	Rochester, Minnesota, US	Mayo Clinic records linkage system (94,335)	Transient or persisting numbness or paraesthesias of fingers innervated by the median nerve aggravated by activities such driving, reading, sewing	1016	I 99 (adjusted 105)	NA
Petit, 2015[85]	Loire region, France	Large working population (5.6% of French working population) (3710)	Intermittent paraesthesia or pain in at least two of the first three digits; either of these also being present at night Symptomatic CTS	59 incident cases among 1532 without CTS at baseline	I 3.9%	Female sex, increasing age
Palmer, 2000[86]	UK	National postal survey using registries of 34 GPs and pay records of the armed services (22,194)	Sensorineural symptoms attributable to hand-transmitted vibration	2607	20.2%	Work/leisure (men)
Tanaka, 1994[87]	USA	National Health Interview Survey Data, 44,233 households	Self-report	2.65 million	1.55%	Increasing age, women, white race
Mattioli, 2009[88]	Italy	13 local administrative databases and National Health Service registry records (NA)	ICD-9 codes	220, age 18–65	NA	Blue-collar/housewife status, BMI≥30, sibling history of CTS, coexistence of trigger finger, rheumatoid arthritis
Mondelli, 2002[89]	Local Health District, Siena, Italy	Electromyographic services (119,027)	Clinical history & electrophysiologic evidence	3142	I 329 I (standardized) 276	Rural, industrial areas
Gelfman, 2009[81]	Olmsted County, MN, USA	Mayo Clinic records linkage system (127,203)	ICD-9 codes (68% validated)	10,069	I 376 (2000) Trend 1981–1985: 258 to 424	Elderly subjects
Atroshi, 2011[90]	Skane County, Sweden care registry (SHCR)	Skane Health Care Registry (1,200,000)	Physician-made CTS diagnosis	14,264	I 428 (women) 182 (men)	NA

CTS = Carpal tunnel syndrome; I = Incidence; NA = Not available.

Table 32.5 Prevalence and incidence of Charcot-Marie-Tooth syndrome in different populations

Author, year	Study area	Source of cases	Diagnostic criteria	N. of patients	Prevalence (per 100,000)	Risk factors
Gudmundsson, 2010[92]	Iceland	Data from neurology departments, neurophysiology units, practicing neurologists (307,672)	Clinical features & neurophysiology tests	37	12	NA
Foley, 2012[93]	England	Neurogenetic, diagnostic and clinical neurophysiology service (2.99 million)	Clinical presentation, positive family history, electrophysiological studies, (if available) molecular genetic tests	293	9.8	NA
Kurihara, 2002[94]	Yonago and Sakainamoto, in the Tottori in western Japan	Neurology departments, questionnaires, phone contacts with patients, April 2000 (176,086)	Electrophysiological and pathological studies were performed using a standard protocol Genomic DNA	19 with CMT	10.8	-
Mladenovic, 2011[95]	Belgrade, Serbia	Neurological Institutions (1,576,124)	Clinical and CMT diagnosis established according to European CMT Consortium criteria	161	9.7	Oldest age
Mostacciuolo, 1991[96]	Padua & Rovigo, Italy	Neurology departments of two provinces & Regional Centre for Neuromuscular Disorders (1,067,130)	Nerve biopsies and EMGs	100 with HSMN1	9.37	-
Braathen, 2011, 2012[97,98]	Eastern Akershus County, Norway	Institute of Medical Genetics, Oslo, Akershus University Hospital, CMT pedigrees	Muscle weakness, age at onset, mode of inheritance	245	82.3	PMP22 duplication, mutation in Cx32, MPZ, MFN2
Holmberg, 1994[99]	Norrbotten & Vasterbotten, Northern Sweden	Departments of internal medicine, geriatrics, paediatrics and orthopaedics in the hospitals of the region and the Health Care System (518,742)	Family history, pedigree analysis, DNA analysis. CMT type 1 or 2 on the basis of median motor nerve conduction velocity, EMG	39	20.1	-
MacMillan, 1994[100]	Glamorgan, South Wales, UK	University Hospital of Cardiff (939,300)	Standard clinical electrophysiological and, wherever available, histological criteria	133	18.1	-
Morocutti, 2002[101]	Molise, Italy	All practising neurologists & neurophysiologists (332,155)	Neurological and electroneurographic evaluation and bio-molecular analysis	58	17.5	-
Nicolaou, 2010[102]	Cyprus	Clinical and neurogenetic databases of Cyprus Institute of Neurology and Genetics (794,000)	Standard motor and sensory nerve conduction studies performed on all available family members	41	16	-
Marrtila, 2017[103]	Northern Ostrobothnia, Finland	Oula University Hospital registries (329,110)	Patients with clinical and neurophysiological feature pertinent with CMT were included Molecular diagnostic if DNA available ICD-10 codes	107	34.6	CMTH

HSMN = Hereditary sensory-motor neuropathy; NA = Not available.

28.2/100000, while in an Egyptian door-to-door study in rural and urban areas, the prevalence of HMSN was 12/100000.[106]

Conclusions and Future Directions

Peripheral neuropathies continue to be a challenge for the epidemiologists because most of the available data come from selected cohorts of patients at risk who may not represent the underlying populations. The few population-based studies investigated only the commonest risk factors as the sample size was limited. Studies done in different countries cannot be compared because, with some exceptions, differing diagnostic criteria were generally used. For these reasons, the actual burden of peripheral neuropathies is still unknown. There is a need for guidelines for the diagnosis of peripheral neuropathies to be used worldwide. Standard clinical and electrophysiological criteria should be established. Shared diagnostic criteria are also needed for a proper definition of risk and aetiologic factors.

National and regional claims databases, if properly validated, are precious sources of data to investigate the toxic effects of drugs and unexpected exposures to be interpreted as risk factors. Registries can be also useful for the detection of rare neuropathies or complications of occupational and other environmental exposures. Using these sources, the incidence of selected peripheral neuropathies could be also calculated.

The GBD collaboration[107–111] can be a useful reference to assess the burden of peripheral neuropathies in the future. At present the disease burden attributable to these clinical conditions cannot be precisely calculated when they are complications of other diseases. However, while waiting for the development of methods to establish the fraction of disability attributable to peripheral neuropathies, some of these clinical conditions could be identified as separate nosographical entities and assessed in terms of premature mortality and persisting disability in survivors.

REFERENCES

1. von Hehn CA, Baron R, Woolf CJ. Deconstructing the neuropathic pain phenotype to reveal neural mechanisms. Neuron. 2012; 73(4): 638–52.
2. Boyette-Davis JA, Walters ET, Dougherty PM. Mechanisms involved in the development of chemotherapy-induced neuropathy. Pain Manag. 2015; 5(4): 285–96.
3. Hirokawa N, Niwa S, Tanaka Y. Molecular motors in neurons: transport mechanisms and roles in brain function, development, and disease. Neuron. 2010; 68(4): 610–38.
4. Martyn CN, Hughes RAC. Epidemiology of peripheral neuropathy. J Neurol Neurosurg Psychiatry. 1997; 62(4): 310–18.
5. Hanewinckel R, van Oijen M, Ikram MA, van Doorn PA. The epidemiology and risk factors of chronic polyneuropathy. Eur J Epidemiol. 2016; 31(1): 5–20.
6. Franklin GM. Peripheral neuropathy. In: Nelson LM, Tanner CM, Van Den Eeden SK, McGuire VM (eds). Neuroepidemiology. From Principles to Practice. New York: Oxford University Press, 2004. pp279–302.
7. Bharucha N, Ward CD. Peripheral neuropathy. In: Feigin VL, Bennett DA (eds). Handbook of Clinical Neuroepidemiology. New York: Nova Science Publ, 2007. pp233–300.
8. Cruz ME, Schoenberg BS, Ruales J, et al. Pilot study to detect neurologic disease in Ecuador among a population with a high prevalence of endemic goiter. Neuroepidemiology. 1985; 4(2): 108–16.
9. Osuntokun BO, Adeuja AO, Nottidge VA, et al. Prevalence of the epilepsies in Nigerian Africans: a community-based study. Epilepsia. 1987; 28(3): 272–9.
10. Cruz Gutierrez-del-Olmo M, Schoenberg BS, Portera-Sanchez A. Prevalence of neurological diseases in Madrid, Spain. Neuroepidemiology. 1989; 8(1): 43–7.
11. Longe AC, Osuntokun BO. Prevalence of neurological disorders in Udo, a rural community in southern Nigeria. Trop Geogr Med. 1989; 41(1): 36–40.
12. Bharucha NE, Bharucha AE, Bharucha EP. Prevalence of peripheral neuropathy in the Parsi community of Bombay. Neurology. 1991; 41(8): 1315–17.
13. al Rajeh S, Bademosi O, Ismail H, et al. A community survey of neurological disorders in Saudi Arabia: the Thugbah study. Neuroepidemiology. 1993; 12(3): 164–78. Review.
14. Beghi E, Monticelli ML. Diabetic polyneuropathy in the elderly. Prevalence and risk factors in two geographic areas of Italy. Italian General Practitioner Study Group (IGPSG). Acta Neurol Scand. 1997; 96(4): 223–8.
15. Beghi E, Monticelli ML. Chronic symmetric symptomatic polyneuropathy in the elderly: a field screening investigation of risk factors for polyneuropathy in two Italian communities. Italian General Practitioner Study Group (IGPST). J Clin Epidemiol. 1998; 51(8): 697–702.
16. Mygland A, Monstad P. Chronic polyneuropathies in Vest-Agder, Norway. Eur J Neurol. 2001; 8(2): 157–65.
17. Baldereschi M, Inzitari M, Di Carlo A, Farchi G, Scafato E, Inzitari D; ILSA Working Group. Epidemiology of distal symmetrical neuropathies in the Italian elderly. Neurology. 2007; 68(18): 1460–67.
18. Kruja J, Beghi E, Zerbi D, et al. High prevalence of major neurological disorders in two Albanian communities: results of a door-to-door survey. Neuroepidemiology. 2012; 38(3): 138–47.
19. Kandil MR, Darwish ES, Khedr EM, Sabry MM, Abdulah MA. A community-based epidemiological study of peripheral neuropathies in Assiut, Egypt. Neurol Res. 2012; 34(10): 960–6.
20. Hoffman EM, Staff NP, Robb JM, St Sauver JL, Dyck PJ, Klein CJ. Impairments and comorbidities of polyneuropathy revealed by population-based analyses. Neurology. 2015; 84(16): 1644– 51.
21. Hanewinckel R, Drenthen J, van Oijen M, Hofman A, van Doorn PA, Ikram MA. Prevalence of polyneuropathy in the general middle-aged and elderly population. Neurology. 2016; 87(18): 1892–8.
22. GBD 2015 DALYs and HALE Collaborators. Global, regional, and national disability-adjusted life-years (DALYs) for 315 diseases and injuries and healthy life expectancy (HALE), 1990–2015: a systematic analysis for the Global Burden of Disease Study 2015. Lancet. 2016; 388(10053): 1603–58.
23. Hanewinckel R, Ikram MA, Van Doorn PA. Peripheral neuropathies. HandbClin Neurol. 2016; 138: 263–82.
24. Vincent AM, Calabek B, Roberts L, Feldman EL. Biology of diabetic neuropathy. Handb Clin Neurol. 2013; 115: 591–606.
25. Malik RA. Pathology of human diabetic neuropathy. Handb Clin Neurol. 2014; 126: 249–59.
26. Tesfaye S, Boulton AJ, Dyck PJ, et al. Diabetic neuropathies: update on definitions, diagnostic criteria, estimation of severity, and treatments. Diabetes Care. 2010; 33(10): 2285–93.
27. Dyck PJ, Kratz KM, Karnes JL, et al. The prevalence by staged severity of various types of diabetic neuropathy, retinopathy, and nephropathy in a population-based cohort: the Rochester Diabetic Neuropathy Study. Neurology. 1993; 43(4): 817–24.
28. Palumbo PJ, Elveback LR, Whisnant JP. Neurologic complications of diabetes mellitus: transient ischemic attack, stroke, and peripheral neuropathy. Adv Neurol. 1978; 19: 593–601.
29. Franklin GM, Kahn LB, Baxter J, Marshall JA, Hamman RF. Sensory neuropathy in non-insulin-dependent diabetes mellitus. The San Luis Valley Diabetes Study. Am J Epidemiol. 1990; 131(4): 633–43.
30. Harris M, Eastman R, Cowie C. Symptoms of sensory neuropathy in adults with NIDDM in the US population. Diabetes Care. 1993; 16(11): 1446–52.
31. Savettieri G, Rocca WA, Salemi G, et al. Prevalence of diabetic neuropathy with somatic symptoms: a door-to-door survey in

two Sicilian municipalities. Sicilian Neuro-Epidemiologic Study (SNES) Group. Neurology. 1993; 43(6): 1115–20.
32. Partanen J, Niskanen L, Lehtinen J, Mervaala E, Siitonen O, Uusitupa M. Natural history of peripheral neuropathy in patients with non-insulin-dependent diabetes mellitus. N Engl J Med. 1995; 333(2): 89–94.
33. MacDonald BK, Cockerell OC, Sander JW, Shorvon SD. The incidence and lifetime prevalence of neurological disorders in a prospective community-based study in the UK. Brain. 2000; 123(Pt 4): 665–76.
34. Davies M, Brophy S, Williams R, Taylor A. The prevalence, severity, and impact of painful diabetic peripheral neuropathy in type 2 diabetes. Diabetes Care. 2006; 29(7): 1518–22.
35. Hall GC, Carroll D, Parry D, McQuay HJ. Epidemiology and treatment of neuropathic pain: the UK primary care perspective. Pain. 2006; 122(1–2):156–62.
36. Gregg EW, Sorlie P, Paulose-Ram R, et al. Prevalence of lower-extremity disease in the US adult population >=40 years of age with and without diabetes: 1999–2000 national health and nutrition examination survey. Diabetes Care. 2004; 27(7): 1591–7.
37. Daousi C, MacFarlane IA, Woodward A, Nurmikko TJ, Bundred PE, Benbow SJ. Chronic painful peripheral neuropathy in an urban community: a controlled comparison of people with and without diabetes. Diabet Med. 2004; 21(9): 976–82.
38. Willison HJ, Jacobs BC, van Doorn PA. Guillain-Barré syndrome. Lancet. 2016; 388(10045): 717–27.
39. Sejvar JJ, Baughman AL, Wise M, Morgan OW. Population incidence of Guillain-Barré syndrome: a systematic review and meta-analysis. Neuroepidemiology. 2011; 36(2): 123–33.
40. Webb AJ, Brain SA, Wood R, Rinaldi S, Turner MR. Seasonal variation in Guillain-Barré syndrome: a systematic review, meta-analysis and Oxfordshire cohort study. J Neurol Neurosurg Psychiatry. 2015; 86(11): 1196–1201.
41. McKhann GM, Cornblath DR, Griffin JW, et al. Acute motor axonal neuropathy: a frequent cause of acute flaccid paralysis in China. Ann Neurol. 1993; 33(4): 333–42.
42. McGrogan A, Madle GC, Seaman HE, de Vries CS. The epidemiology of Guillain-Barré syndrome worldwide. A systematic literature review. Neuroepidemiology. 2009; 32(2): 150–63.
43. Schonberger LB, Bregman DJ, Sullivan-Bolyai JZ, et al. Guillain-Barré syndrome following vaccination in the National Influenza Immunization Program, United States, 1976–1977. Am J Epidemiol. 1979; 110(2): 105–23.
44. Vellozzi C, Iqbal S, Broder K. Guillain-Barré syndrome, influenza, and influenza vaccination: the epidemiologic evidence. Clin Infect Dis. 2014; 58(8): 1149–55.
45. Juurlink DN, Stukel TA, Kwong J, et al. Guillain-Barré syndrome after influenza vaccination in adults: a population-based study. Arch Intern Med. 2006; 166(20): 2217–21.
46. Lasky T, Terracciano GJ, Magder L, et al. The Guillain-Barré syndrome and the 1992–1993 and 1993–1994 influenza vaccines. N Engl J Med. 1998; 339(25): 1797–802.
47. Galeotti F, Massari M, D'Alessandro R, et al. Risk of Guillain-Barré syndrome after 2010–2011 influenza vaccination. Eur J Epidemiol. 2013; 28(5): 433–44.
48. Salmon DA, Proschan M, Forshee R, et al. Association between Guillain-Barré syndrome and influenza A (H1N1) 2009 monovalent inactivated vaccines in the USA: a meta-analysis. Lancet. 2013; 381(9876): 1461–8.
49. Araujo AQ, Silva MT, Araujo AP. Zika virus-associated neurological disorders: a review. Brain. 2016; 139(Pt 8): 2122–30.
50. Cao-Lormeau VM, Blake A, Mons S, et al. Guillain-Barré Syndrome outbreak associated with Zika virus infection in French Polynesia: a case-control study. Lancet. 2016; 387(10027): 1531–9.
51. Vallat JM, Sommer C, Magy L. Chronic inflammatory demyelinating polyradiculoneuropathy: diagnostic and therapeutic challenges for a treatable condition. Lancet Neurology. 2010; 9(4): 402–12.
52. Rajabally YA, Simpson BS, Beri S, Bankart J, Gosalakkal JA. Epidemiologic variability of chronic inflammatory demyelinating polyneuropathy with different diagnostic criteria: study of a UK population. Muscle & Nerve. 2009; 39(4): 432–8.
53. Roy AJ, Van den Bergh P, Van Damme P, Doggen K, Van Casteren V, and BNMDR Scientific Committee. Early stages of building a rare disease registry, methods and 2010 data from the Belgian Neuromuscular Disease Registry (BNMDR). Acta Neurol Belg. 2015; 115(2): 97–104.
54. Chiò A, Cocito D, Bottacchi E, et al. Idiopathic chronic inflammatory demyelinating polyneuropathy: an epidemiological study in Italy. J Neurol Neurosurg Psychiatry. 2007; 78(12): 1349–53. Epub 10 May 2007.
55. Lefter S, Hardiman O, Ryan AM. A population-based epidemiologic study of adult neuromuscular disease in the Republic of Ireland. Neurology. 2017; 88(3): 304–13.
56. Hafsteinsdottir B, Olafsson E. Incidence and natural history of idiopathic chronic inflammatory demyelinating polyneuropathy: a population-based study in Iceland. Eur Neurol. 2016; 75(5–6): 263–8.
57. Mahdi-Rogers M, Hughes RA. Epidemiology of chronic inflammatory neuropathies in southeast England. Eur J Neurol. 2014; 21(1): 28–33.
58. Laughlin RS, Dyck PJ, Melton LJ 3rd, Leibson C, Ransom J, Dyck PJ. Incidence and prevalence of CIDP and the association of diabetes mellitus. Neurology. 2009; 73(1): 39–45.
59. Lunn MP, Muir P, Brown LJ, MacMahon EM, Gregson NA, Hughes RA. Cytomegalovirus is not associated with IgM anti-myelin-associated glycoprotein/sulphate-3-glucuronyl paragloboside antibody-associated neuropathy. Ann Neurol. 1999; 46(2): 267–70.
60. Iijima M, Koike H, Hattori N, et al. Prevalence and incidence rates of chronic inflammatory demyelinating polyneuropathy in the Japanese population. J Neurol Neurosurg Psychiatry. 2008; 79(9): 1040–43.
62. Graus F, Delattre JY, Antoine JC, et al. Recommended diagnostic criteria for paraneoplastic neurological syndromes. J Neurol Neurosurg Psychiatry. 2004; 75(8): 1135–40.
63. Zis P, Paladini A, Piroli A, McHugh PC, Varrassi G, Hadjivassiliou M. Pain as a first manifestation of paraneoplastic neuropathies: a systematic review and meta-analysis. Pain Ther. 2017; 6(2): 143–51.
64. Franco-Paredes C, Rodriguez-Morales AJ. Unsolved matters in leprosy: a descriptive review and call for further research. Ann Clin Microbiol Antimicrob. 2016; 15(1): 33.
65. World Health Organization. Progress towards eliminating leprosy as a public health problem. Part I. Wkly Epidemiol Rec. 1994; 69(20): 145–51.
66. Lockwood DNJ, Shetty V, Oliveira Penna G. Hazards of setting targets toeliminate disease lessons from the leprosy elimination campaign. BMJ. 2014; 348: g1136.
67. Saunderson P. The epidemiology of reactions and nerve damage. Lepr Rev. 2000; 71: S106–10.

68. Ghosh S, Chandran A, Jansen JP. Epidemiology of HIV-related neuropathy: a systematic literature review. AIDS Res Hum Retroviruses. 2012; 28(1): 36–48.
69. Schaumburg HH. Human neurotoxic disease; causation criteria for identification of neurotoxicity: cardinal tenets of neurotoxic disease. In: Spencer PS, Schaumburg HH (eds). Experimental and Clinical Neurotoxicology. New York: Oxford University Press, 2000. pp55–82.
70. Evans SR, Ellis RJ, Chen H, et al. Peripheral neuropathy in HIV: prevalence and risk factors. AIDS. 2011; 25(7): 919–28.
71. Etminan M, Brophy JM, Samii A Oral fluoroquinolone use and risk of peripheral neuropathy: a pharmacoepidemiologic study. Neurology. 2014; 83(14): 1261–3.
72. Gaist D, Jeppesen U, Andersen M, García Rodríguez LA, Hallas J, Sindrup SH. Statins and risk of polyneuropathy: a case-control study. Neurology. 2002; 58(9): 1333–7.
73. Gaist D, García Rodríguez LA, Huerta C, Hallas J, Sindrup SH. Are users of lipid-lowering drugs at increased risk of peripheral neuropathy? Eur J Clin Pharmacol. 2001; 56(12): 931–33.
74. Vassallo P, Trohman RG. Prescribing amiodarone: an evidence-based review of clinical indications. JAMA. 2007; 298(11): 1312–22.
75. Midroni G, Bilbao JM. Chapter 5, Schwann cells and myelin in the peripheral nervous system. In: Midroni G & Bilbao JM (eds). Biopsy Diagnosis of Peripheral Neuropathy. Newton: Butterworth- Heinmann, 1995. pp75–103.
76. Orr CF, Ahlskog JE. Frequency, characteristics, and risk factors for amiodarone neurotoxicity. Arch Neurol. 2009; 66(7): 865–9.
77. Zedan AH, Vilholm OJ. Chemotherapy-induced polyneuropathy: major agents and assessment by questionnaires. Basic Clin Pharmacol Toxicol. 2014; 115(2): 193–200.
78. Windebank AJ. Neuropathy due to nutritional deficiency and alcoholism. In: Dyck P, Thomas P, Lambert E, Bunge R (eds). Peripheral Neuropathy. Philadelphia: WB Saunders, 1993. pp1310–21.
79. Vittadini G, Buonocore M, Colli G, Terzi M, Fonte R, Biscaldi G. Alcoholic polyneuropathy: a clinical and epidemiological study. Alcohol and Alcoholism. 2001; 36(5): 393–400.
80. Stevens JC, Sun S, Beard CM, O'Fallon WM, Kurland LT. Carpal tunnel syndrome in Rochester, Minnesota, 1961 to 1980. Neurology. 1988; 38(1): 134–8.
81. Gelfman R, Melton LJ 3rd, Yawn BP, Wollan PC, Amadio PC, Stevens JC. Long-term trends in carpal tunnel syndrome. Neurology. 2009; 72(1): 33–41.
82. Nordstrom DL, Vierkant RA, DeStefano F, Layde PM. Risk factors for carpal tunnel syndrome in a general population. Occup Environ Med. 1997; 54(10): 734–40.
83. Kozak A, Schedlbauer G, Wirth T, Euler U, Westermann C, Nienhaus A. Association between work-related biomechanical risk factors and the occurrence of carpal tunnel syndrome: an overview of systematic reviews and a meta-analysis of current research. BMC Musculoskelet Disord. 2015; 16: 231.
84. Solomon DH, Katz JN, Bohn R, Mogun H, Avorn J. Nonoccupational risk factors for carpal tunnel syndrome. J Gen Intern Med. 1999; 14(5): 310–14.
85. Petit A, Ha C, Bodin J, et al. Risk factors for carpal tunnel syndrome related to the work organization: a prospective surveillance study in a large working population. Appl Ergon. 2015; 47: 1–10.
86. Palmer AK. Complications of endoscopic and open carpal tunnel release. J Hand Surg Am. 2000; 25(1): 185.
87. Tanaka S, Wild DK, Seligman PJ, Behrens V, Cameron L, Putz-Anderson V. The US prevalence of self-reported carpal tunnel syndrome: 1988 National Health Interview Survey data. Am J Public Health. 1994; 84(11): 1846–8.
88. Mattioli S, Baldasseroni A, Bovenzi M, et al. Risk factors for operated carpal tunnel syndrome: a multicenter population-based case-control study. BMC Public Health. 2009; 9: 343.
89. Mondelli M, Giannini F, Giacchi M. Carpal tunnel syndrome incidence in a general population. Neurology. 2002; 58(2): 289–94.
90. Atroshi I, Englund M, Turkiewicz A, Tägil M, Petersson IF. Incidence of physician-diagnosed carpal tunnel syndrome in the general population. Arch Intern Med. 2011; 171(10): 943–4.
91. Lima Santos Barreto LC, Santos Oliveira F, Santos Nunes P, et al. Epidemiologic study of Charcot-Marie-Tooth disease: a systematic review. Neuroepidemiology. 2016; 46(3): 157–65.
92. Gudmundsson B, Olafsson E, Jakobsson F, Lúthvígsson P. Prevalence of symptomatic Charcot-Marie-Tooth disease in Iceland: a study of a well-defined population. Neuroepidemiology. 2010; 34(1): 13–17.
93. Foley C, Schofield I, Eglon G, Bailey G, Chinnery PF, Horvath R. Charcot-Marie-Tooth disease in Northern England. J Neurol Neurosurg Psychiatry. 2012; 83(5): 572–3.
94. Kurihara S, Adachi Y, Wada K, Awaki E, Harada H, Nakashima K. An epidemiological genetic study of Charcot-Marie-Tooth disease in Western Japan. Neuroepidemiology. 2002; 21(5): 246–50.
95. Mladenovic J, Milic Rasic V, Keckarevic Markovic M, et al. Epidemiology of Charcot-Marie-Tooth disease in the population of Belgrade, Serbia. Neuroepidemiology. 2011; 36(3): 177–82.
96. Mostacciuolo ML, Micaglio G, Fardin P, Danieli GA. Genetic epidemiology of hereditary motor sensory neuropathies (type I). Am J Med Genet. 1991; 39(4): 479–81.
97. Braathen GJ, Sand JC, Lobato A, Høyer H, Russell MB. Genetic epidemiology of Charcot-Marie-Tooth in the general population. Eur J Neurol. 2011; 18(1): 39–48.
98. Braathen GJ. Genetic epidemiology of Charcot-Marie-Tooth disease. Acta Neurol Scand Suppl. 2012; (193): iv–22.
99. Holmberg BH, Holmgren G, Nelis E, van Broeckhoven C, Westerberg B. Charcot-Marie-Tooth disease in northern Sweden: pedigree analysis and the presence of the duplication in chromosome 17p11.2. J Med Genet. 1994; 31(6): 435–41.
100. MacMillan JC, Harper PS. The Charcot-Marie-Tooth syndrome: clinical aspects from a population study in South Wales, UK. Clin Genet. 1994; 45(3): 128–34.
101. Morocutti C, Colazza GB, Soldati G, et al. Charcot-Marie-Tooth disease in Molise, a central-southern region of Italy: an epidemiological study. Neuroepidemiology. 2002; 21(5): 241–5.
102. Nicolaou P, Zamba-Papanicolaou E, Koutsou P, et al. Charcot-Marie-Tooth disease in Cyprus: epidemiological, clinical and genetic characteristics. Neuroepidemiology. 2010; 35(3): 171–7.
103. Marttila M, Kytövuori L, Helisalmi S, et al. Molecular epidemiology of Charcot-Marie-Tooth Disease in Northern Ostrobothnia, Finland: a population-based study. Neuroepidemiology. 2017; 49(1–2): 34–9.
104. Dardiotis E, Koutsou P, Papanicolaou EZ, et al. Epidemiological, clinical and genetic study of familial amyloidotic polyneuropathy in Cyprus. Amyloid. 2009; 16(1): 32–7.
105. Combarros O, Calleja J, Polo JM, Berciano J. Prevalence of hereditary motor and sensory neuropathy in Cantabria. Acta Neurol Scand. 1987; 75(1): 9–12.

106. Kandil MR, Darwish ES, Khedr EM, Sabry MM, Abdulah MA. A community-based epidemiological study of peripheral neuropathies in Assiut, Egypt. Neurol Res. 2012; 34(10): 960–6.
107. GBD 2016 Risk Factors Collaborators. Global, regional, and national comparative risk assessment of 84 behavioural, environmental and occupational, and metabolic risks or clusters of risks, 1990–2016: a systematic analysis for the Global Burden of Disease Study 2016. Lancet. 2017; 390(10100): 1345–422.
108. GBD 2016 DALYs and HALE Collaborators. Global, regional, and national disability-adjusted life-years (DALYs) for 333 diseases and injuries and healthy life expectancy (HALE) for 195 countries and territories, 1990–2016: a systematic analysis for the Global Burden of Disease Study 2016. Lancet. 2017; 390(10100): 1260–344.
109. GBD 2016 Disease and Injury Incidence and Prevalence Collaborators. Global, regional, and national incidence, prevalence, and years lived with disability for 328 diseases and injuries for 195 countries, 1990–2016: a systematic analysis for the Global Burden of Disease Study 2016. Lancet. 2017; 390(10100): 1211–59.
110. GBD 2016 Causes of Death Collaborators. Global, regional, and national age-sex specific mortality for 264 causes of death, 1980–2016: a systematic analysis for the Global Burden of Disease Study 2016. Lancet. 2017; 390(10100): 1151–210.
111. GBD 2016 Mortality Collaborators. Global, regional, and national under-5 mortality, adult mortality, age-specific mortality, and life expectancy, 1970–2016: a systematic analysis for the Global Burden of Disease Study 2016. Lancet. 2017; 390(10100): 1084–150.

33

Sensory loss—vision

Paul J Foster, Anthony Khawaja, Lisanne J Balk, Zaynah Muthy, and Axel Petzold

Introduction

The retina and optic nerve share their embryological origin with the brain, and are widely regarded as part of the central nervous system.[1] Retinal microvasculature and neuronal components offer a unique 'window' on tissues that are closely allied to intracranial structures.[2] Consequently, the eye is vulnerable to the same processes that cause neurodegenerative diseases.[1] Axonal damage in the brain may affect the retinal nerve fibre layer (RNFL), the inner plexiform, and ganglion cell layers, halting at the level of the inner nuclear layer.[3] On this basis, it seems that it is likely that patterns and trends in the inner retinal layers mirror those in the brain, and that these patterns may reflect wider risk of neurodegenerative changes. The dementias and PD are associated with measurable changes in the retina and optic nerve. Two specific forms of degenerative optic neuropathy that deserve special consideration on the basis of their greater frequency are glaucoma and MS associated optic neuritis (MSON).

Dementias and Parkinson's Disease

The RNFL comprises the axons of retinal ganglion cells linking the neuroretina with the lateral geniculate body. Thinner RNFL and axonal degeneration within the optic nerve has been observed in post-mortem samples from people with AD.[4] Gao, et al.[5] found that patients with either established AD or MCI had a significantly thinner RNFL compared to controls using *in vivo* optical coherence tomography (OCT) imaging. Similar findings have been documented in a range of studies of retinal abnormalities in neurodegeneration, including PD,[6] MND,[7] hereditary peripheral neuropathies,[8] autoimmune encephalitis,[9] Wilson's disease,[10] and Lewy body dementia.[11] Most of these studies were limited by small sample size. A recent meta-analysis on 887 patients with AD, 216 patients with MCI and 864 control subjects, nevertheless suggests robustness of the RNFL and macular thickness data.[12] In addition, a 24-month prospective study by Shi, et al.[13] examined RNFL thickness in 78 people with normal or mildly impaired cognition. There was a general trend of attenuation in RNFL with time, but those who suffered more severe cognitive decline showed greater reduction in RNFL thickness. For the purposes of risk profiling, associations between retinal vascular abnormalities and systemic diseases, including hypertension,[14] diabetes,[15] and coronary heart disease[16] have all been validated. An association between retinopathy and cognitive impairment has been documented, particularly in people with hypertension.[2]

Multiple Sclerosis

Visual problems are frequent in MS.[17] Retinal ganglion cell and brain grey matter involvement is now considered at least as relevant as white matter disease in MS. RNFL loss can readily be quantified[18] and axonal loss is a central feature of retinal neurodegeneration.[19] Contemporary understanding is that neuro-axonal loss in the visual system occurs both secondary to demyelination, but also as part of a primary neurodegenerative process. The afferent and efferent components of the visual system are almost always affected at some stage of the disease, leading to a heterogeneous range of symptoms. An acute episode of optic neuritis is a frequent presentation for MS and may be a relapsing feature. Progressive visual loss in MSON is exceedingly rare and may represent a pure visual form of primary progressive MS which affects about 10–15% of patients.[20]

Prevalence and incidence

A recent, large population-based incidence cohort representing all 50 US states identified visual symptoms in 18% of MS patients at onset.[21] However, comprehensive data from a population-based study in the French West Indies demonstrated a prevalence of delayed visual evoked potentials (VEP) in 81% of patients with MS. Although optic neuritis often occurs in the setting of MS, it can also occur in isolation as monosymptomatic, idiopathic optic neuritis, or in cases of neuromyelitis optica (NMO). In 1971, the prevalence of optic neuritis was estimated at 5.5 cases per 100,000,[22] whereas the incidence rate of optic neuritis ranges between 0.56 and 5.1 cases per 100,000 person-years.[23] However, recent studies suggest that the incidence of optic neuritis in MS is on the rise.[23]

A population-based incidence case-control study demonstrated that the magnitude of the increase in incidence rate per higher degree of latitude was greater for optic neuritis than for spinal cord or brainstem/cerebellar syndromes.[24] There is a lack of data on the potential contribution of nutritional toxic factors to progressive optic neuritis in LICs. It is therefore likely that eye pathology in MS is under reported worldwide.

Environmental risk factors

In most populations, women are affected more often than men. The female-to-male ratio varies between 1.5:1 and 2.5:1.[25] Interestingly, there is a trend towards higher ratios in the more recent studies, which may be due to gender-specific changes in smoking behaviour. Again, there is a lack of systematic data on the detrimental effect of smoking on the prognosis of visual recovery in optic neuritis.

A potential explanation for the latitudinal variation seen in MS and therefore also MSON is solar exposure. Sunlight intensity and UV radiation are strongly related to latitude.[26,27] As MS prevalence increases with increasing latitude, this could be due to limited sun exposure and vitamin D deficiency in these areas.[28] Although sun exposure is a major source of vitamin D, intake through food or supplements is also relevant and was also inversely associated with the risk of MS. This further supports the findings of lower MS prevalence in areas with high latitude, but with high fish consumption (being an important source of vitamin D), such as coastal villages in Norway and Inuit people living in Canada's far north.[29] Because there is no epidemiological evidence to suggest a direct influence of vitamin D levels on vision,[30] the effects on the retina and optic nerve are thought to be secondary to MS pathology in general.

Optic neuritis is not only a frequent presentation in MS, but even more frequently in, NMO. The change of the incidence ratio of MS to NMO has been related to reduced immune tolerance with increased hygiene.[31] The hygiene hypothesis suggests that the lack of childhood infections in industrialized countries (as a result of improved hygiene, vaccination, and use of antibiotics) causes proinflammatory immune responses which may increase the risk of MS.[32] The implications for visual prognosis in this context can be relevant as visual outcome is poorer in NMO compared to MS. In addition, population-based data shows a higher prevalence of visual symptoms in NMO compared to MS.[33] One viral infection which is positively associated with both optic neuritis and MS risk is the Epstein-Barr virus (EBV).[34] There is evidence showing that infection with EBV is a risk factor for MS.[35] For individuals who are EBV negative, the risk of developing MS is about 15 times lower compared to individuals who are EBV positive (with no history of mononucleosis).[36,37] But patients who have MS and are EBV negative on comprehensive, state-of-the art laboratory testing do exist.

Smoking increases the risk of developing MS and this risk increases with smoking duration and intensity. Further, smoking may also influence the disease course, with faster progression seen in smokers.[38] Likewise smoking accelerates painless visual loss, typically bilaterally in toxic nutritional optic neuropathies.[39] Taken together this suggests a direct effect of smoking on progression of neurodegeneration. Another relevant environmental risk factor is childhood obesity, which increases the risk of MS two-fold in both men and women.[40,41] Although this increased MS susceptibility in obese individuals may be explained by the lower vitamin D levels, other biological mechanisms should not be ruled out.[42] Taken together, the global change of lifestyle with carbohydrate rich food, low in vitamin D, as well as living mainly indoors (house, office) and moving by car or public transport, are all likely contributors to the observed increase of MS incidence and MS associated optic neuritis.

Genetic risk factors

In addition to environmental factors, the risk for optic neuritis and MS has been associated to HLA genes.[43] Recent studies identified a modest genetic susceptibility rather than Mendelian inheritance. The strongest effect on MS susceptibility, however, remain the genes within the HLA complex. Specifically, the class II variant HLA-DRB1*15:01 is strongly associated with an increased risk of MS (odds ratio ~3), whereas the class I variant HLA-A*02 is associated with a protective effect (OR ~0.6).[44,45] In the years to come, epigenetic studies will play an important role in further unravelling potential gene-environment interactions. Epigenetic mechanisms may shed light on the effect of genetic variation in combination with environmental exposures on disease risk and variations in phenotype expression.[46]

Prognosis

Visual prognosis remains a major concern to patients and poses a considerable challenge to the treating physician. In order to improve diagnostic accuracy recent research has focused on prognostic biomarkers. This research has been particularly rewarding for the visual system in MS. Clinical markers for a good prognosis are female gender, young age at onset, presentation with optic neuritis or isolated sensory symptoms at onset, RR or benign disease course.[47] The best validated body fluid biomarkers are neurofilament proteins. The neurofilament proteins are detected in CSF or blood following axonal injury, for example in acute optic neuritis.[48] Neurofilament proteins can be used to monitor axonal loss in MS patients and are of prognostic value because in contrast to demyelination, axonal loss is irreversible.[49] Loss of axons and release of neurofilament proteins is followed by atrophy. Atrophy is best quantified with structural imaging. Both MRI and retinal OCT can demonstrate and monitor atrophy. High neurofilament protein levels and inner retinal layer atrophy in optic neuritis are related to poor visual outcome.[50]

Future directions

A large body of evidence supports the theory that sensory visual symptoms in MS are the result of a complex, multifactorial pathology with a heterogeneous aetiology, resulting from a certain genetic predisposition in combination with multiple environmental factors. Future studies on visual problems in MS should focus on the better understanding of the interaction between these genetic and environmental factors in order to better understand disease mechanisms and provide targets for effective treatment. Furthermore, unlike the genetic risk factor, many of the environmental and lifestyle factors are modifiable, providing important potential for vision preserving strategies. Another challenge is the development of reliable prognostic measures for visual recovery, given the highly heterogeneous disease course. For this purpose, new retinal imaging modalities[51] in large longitudinal studies are needed, possibly in the form of well-orchestrated collaboration and the use of big data.

Glaucoma

Introduction

Glaucoma is a chronic, progressive, degenerative disease of the optic nerve that is clinically distinguishable from other optic neuropathies by a characteristic, excavated appearance of the optic nerve head and a pattern of visual field loss which localizes damage to the prelaminar optic nerve.[52] Affecting around 65 million people worldwide, it is probably the commonest neurodegenerative condition known.[53]

Glaucoma is classified as 'primary' or 'secondary' (depending on whether there is a discernible underlying cause, such as pseudo-exfoliation or uveitis), and 'open-angle' or 'angle-closure' (dependent on whether there is obstruction of aqueous drainage at the iridocorneal angle by the iris).[54,55] While primary open-angle glaucoma (POAG) is the commonest form of glaucoma, primary angle-closure glaucoma (PACG) damages vision more rapidly and severely.[56] POAG and PACG consequently result in similar numbers of cases of blindness.[57] Most POAG is adult-onset, occurring after the age of 40 years, though juvenile forms exist (onset between 3 and 40 years of age). Developmental glaucoma includes primary congenital glaucoma and secondary congenital glaucoma associated with syndromes, such as aniridia. This description primarily concerns adult-onset glaucoma. Until 2002, there was no consensus for the definition of glaucoma in epidemiological studies and this complicated comparison of frequency estimates between studies. For example, when diagnostic criteria from different large epidemiological studies were applied to one analytical dataset, prevalence estimates varied by up to ten-fold.[58] To address this issue, the International Society for Geographical and Epidemiological Ophthalmology (ISGEO) published a consensus definition of glaucoma for epidemiological studies.[54] Box 33.1 summarizes the ISGEO criteria.

Descriptive epidemiology

Population-based studies of prevalence of adult glaucoma span a broad range of races and geographical locations.[53,59] A systematic review and meta-analysis of 50 population-based studies reported global prevalence of glaucoma as 3.5% (95% CI 2.1–5.8) in people aged 40–80 years; POAG represented 86% of all glaucoma.[59] POAG was most common in African derived people (4.2%; 95% CI, 2.1–7.4). Prevalence of PACG was highest in Asians (1.09%; 95% CI, 0.4–2.3).[59] Incidence of POAG ranges from 0.3%/year (Sweden) to 0.5%/year (Barbados).[60–63] Older age is a strong and consistent risk factor for the prevalence and incidence of POAG. The Barbados Eye Study[64] and Rotterdam Eye Study[65] reported relative risks of 1.04 and 1.06 respectively, per year of age. The strength of the relationship between age and POAG has led some to suggest that glaucoma is a form of accelerated ageing.[66]

The evidence for a gender predilection in POAG is inconsistent,[67] though two recent meta-analyses indicate higher age-adjusted risk in men.[53,59] Higher rates of incident open-angle glaucoma in men for all age groups except the oldest (80+) has been reported.[60] This may be related to a protective effect of endogenous oestrogens in pre-menopausal women, consistent with the finding that earlier menopause may be a risk factor for glaucoma.[68,69]

Box 33.1 International Society for Geographical and Epidemiological Ophthalmology criteria for diagnosis of glaucoma in cross-sectional prevalence surveys

1. Structural and functional evidence
   - CDR or CDR asymmetry ≥97.5th percentile for normal population, or rim reduced to ≤0.1 CDR between 11 to 1 o'clock or 5 to 7 o'clock *and*
   - Definite visual defect consistent with glaucoma (glaucoma hemifield test graded 'outside normal limits' and a cluster of 3 contiguous points at the 5% level on the pattern deviation plot, using the threshold test strategy with the 24-2 test pattern of the Zeiss-Humphrey field analyser 2)
2. Advanced structural damage with unproved visual field loss
   - Subject unable to satisfactorily complete visual field testing *and*
   - CDR or CDR asymmetry ≥99.5th percentile for the normal population
3. Optic disc not seen. Field test impossible
   - Visual acuity <3/60 and intraocular pressure >99.5th percentile *or*
   - Visual acuity <3/60 and eye shows evidence of previous glaucoma surgery, or access to medical records confirms previous glaucoma related visual morbidity

CDR cup-disc-ratio

Adapted with permission from Foster PJ, et al. The definition and classification of glaucoma in prevalence surveys. *Br J Ophthalmol*; 86(2): 238–242. Copyright © 2002, British Medical Journal. DOI: http://dx.doi.org/10.1136/bjo.86.2.238.

Time trends

Given the strong association between age and POAG, the number of people affected by glaucoma is expected to rise markedly due to population ageing. Projecting future numbers of glaucoma cases requires consideration of the race-specific ageing population and disease trends. A recently published 40-year forecast of the demographic shift in POAG in the USA estimated an increase in the number of people with the disease from 2.71 million in 2011 to 7.32 million in 2050.[70] The number of people aged 40–80 years with glaucoma globally was estimated to be 64.3 million in 2013; this has been projected to increase to 76.0 million in 2020 and 111.8 million in 2040.[59]

Ocular and environmental risk factors

Intraocular pressure

Raised intraocular pressure (IOP) is a strong risk factor for POAG, and remains the only consistent risk factor that is modifiable. Population-based studies have demonstrated higher IOP to be associated with both prevalent and incident POAG across different continents and ethnicities.[64,71,72] It is important to appreciate that it is not just 'raised IOP' (i.e. IOP >21 mmHg) that is associated with POAG; the increased risk is apparent across the whole range of IOP. Longitudinal studies have reported an increased risk of incident POAG of 10–18% per 1 mmHg higher IOP at baseline.[64,71–74] The traditional definition for 'raised IOP', or ocular hypertension (OHT), is based on the population mean IOP plus 2 standard deviations.[75,76] While the value of 21 mmHg may be somewhat arbitrary, this cut-off has global acceptance and is used extensively in research,[56] and reported standards of high quality clinical care.[77,78] While the *relative* risk of developing POAG is much higher for a person with OHT compared with a person with IOP <21 mmHg, since there are many more people with IOP ≤ 21 mmHg compared with OHT, the *absolute* numbers of people with glaucoma are not necessarily greater among those with baseline IOP >21 mmHg. In other words, the proportion of patients with POAG that are classified as normal tension glaucoma (IOP ≤21 mmHg) at diagnosis ranges from 20% to 90% depending on the population.[79]

Refractive error

Myopic refractive error is associated with a higher prevalence of POAG.[80] Despite this strong statistical evidence for a link between myopia and POAG, there are potential issues with POAG case differential misclassification in cross-sectional studies; that is, a participant may more likely to be misclassified as POAG if they are myopic. This is due to an overlap between myopia and POAG signs; myopic individuals can also exhibit abnormal optic discs (which may look glaucomatous, or make assessment for glaucoma difficult) and visual field defects.[81,82] To date, myopia has not been associated with glaucoma incidence in a population-based study or glaucoma progression in a large clinical trial.

Central corneal thickness

Hypothetically, a thinner central corneal thickness (CCT) reflects biomechanical properties of ocular tissues, and therefore susceptibility of the optic nerve to glaucoma. However, CCT is positively associated with measured IOP;[83] a thicker cornea is stiffer, on average, and will lead to biased higher values of 'measured IOP', whereas a thinner cornea (less stiff) will lead to biased lower values. Therefore, it remains unclear whether CCT is an *independent* risk factor for glaucoma.

Lifestyle risk factors

There is no consistent evidence that dietary factors are associated with POAG. While studies have reported a lower prevalence of glaucoma in people eating more carrots and green collards[84] and a lower risk of incident glaucoma in people with higher intake of retinol equivalents and vitamin B1[85] these findings have not been replicated. The largest study examining the link between dietary antioxidants and glaucoma was negative.[86] There is a suggestion that the balance of omega-3 and omega-6 fatty acid intake is associated with glaucoma, though in a direction that is adverse for cardiovascular health.[87,88] An increased risk of POAG with greater caffeine intake has been reported, but the association was only apparent in a post-hoc, subgroup analysis suggesting the finding may be due to chance.[89] Acutely, drinking alcohol appears to reduce IOP in a dose-dependent manner.[90] However, studies examining the association between usual alcohol intake and IOP suggest higher IOP in people drinking more alcohol.[91] Studies examining the association between alcohol intake and glaucoma have reported inconsistent results.

There are many studies demonstrating an acute reduction of IOP following exercise.[92] However, it cannot be assumed that reducing IOP by exercise reduces the risk of glaucoma. For example, exercise also reduces blood pressure, which in turn may reduce the perfusion of the optic nerve.[93] There have been few studies examining the association between physical activity and glaucoma. One study reported that the seven-year incidence of self-reported glaucoma in a group of runners was lower in those that ran further each week, and those that ran 10 km in a quicker time.[94] The potential link between physical activity and the risk of glaucoma remains under-investigated.

Genetic Epidemiology of Glaucoma

First-degree relatives of POAG patients have a 22% lifetime risk of developing glaucoma compared with a risk of 3% in those without a family history.[95] One twin study has estimated the heritability of POAG, calculated from twin concordance ratios; however, the reported heritability of 0.13 is a likely underestimate given glaucoma case ascertainment was via prescribing registries. Additionally, around half of glaucoma in the population is undiagnosed.[96] Traditional linkage analysis has identified several genes associated with glaucoma, such as *MYOC*,[97] *OPTN*,[98] and *WDR36*.[99] However, these genes appear to only be relevant in a limited number of families and explain around 6% of glaucoma cases in the general population.[100–102] More recently, GWAS have identified more loci associated with glaucoma. Results from an Icelandic population have suggested a significant locus near *CAV1* and *CAV2* (both of which are expressed in RGCs and trabecular meshwork).[103] An Australian GWAS using an enriched sample of 590 patients with advanced POAG identified two significant loci at *TMCO1* and *CDKN2B*.[104] A follow-up GWAS from the Australian group with a larger sample size including 1155 cases identified three further loci significantly associated with POAG near *ABCA1, AFAP1*, and *GMDS*.[105] The largest GWAS for POAG to date used a discovery cohort of 3853 US cases and 33,480 controls and identified a further three loci at *TXNRD2, ATXN2*, and *FOXC1*.[106] While multiple common genetic variants have now been identified as associated with POAG, these still explain only a small fraction (<5%) of the disease heritability and are currently of limited predictive value.

Glaucoma burden, prognosis, and blindness

The WHO recognizes glaucoma as the second commonest cause of blindness globally following cataract, accounting for 8% of blindness.[107] Since cataract is successfully treatable by surgery, glaucoma is considered the commonest cause of irreversible vision loss in the world. Vision impairment certification data suggests that glaucoma is the second commonest cause of blindness in the UK, following age-related macular degeneration (AMD).[108,109] Given the chronic nature of the glaucoma, lifelong follow-up is currently advised. Therefore, glaucoma patients form a large proportion of outpatient visits in the UK hospital eye service (an estimated 23% of all follow-up attendances) with over one million glaucoma-related visits per year.[110] Two retrospective studies examined rates of incident glaucoma blindness in patients over a 20-year period. Data from the Mayo Clinic, Minnesota,[111] and Skane University Hospital, Malmo, Sweden,[112] reported unilateral blindness in 27% and 38%, and for both eyes, 9% and 13%, respectively. The major risk factor for developing glaucoma-related blindness is advanced disease at presentation.[113,114] It has been reported that 39% of UK glaucoma patients present with advanced disease,[115] and those at higher risk of presenting late include people living in more deprived areas,[115] of lower social class, with higher presenting IOP, and no family history of glaucoma.[116]

Future directions

The pathophysiological mechanisms underlying POAG remain largely obscure and very little evidence exists to support appropriate lifestyle advice for glaucoma patents. Further genetic and environmental epidemiological studies are needed to better understand glaucoma aetiology and better advise patients. Large cohort studies (e.g. UK Biobank), and global consortia (e.g. the International Glaucoma Genetics Consortium) offer exciting potential to answer these important research questions.

Age-Related Macular Degeneration

Descriptive epidemiology, time trends, and visual impairment

AMD is a chronic degeneration of the central region of the retina which serves detailed, colour vision used, for example, in reading and face recognition. It affects around 196 million people (95% CrI, 140-261) worldwide currently. This number is projected to rise to 288 million (95% CrI, 205-399) in 2040.[117] It is the fourth most common cause of blindness globally (in approximately 5.8% of blind individuals) and third most common cause for moderate visual impairment (3.9%).[117] Prevalence of AMD increases with age. In a large European meta-analysis, early AMD (drusen and/or retinal pigment epithelial clumping or atrophy) increased from 3.5% (95% CI 2.1–5.0%) in those aged 55–59 years to 17.6% (95% CI 13.6–21.5%) in those aged ≥85 years; for late AMD, these figures were 0.1% (95% CI 0.04–0.3%) and 9.8% (95% CI 6.3–13.3%), respectively. However, prevalence appears to have declined over the last two decades, due to better general health and better treatments. Projections of AMD showed an almost doubling of affected persons despite a decreasing prevalence. By 2040, the number of individuals in Europe with early AMD will range between 14.9–21.5 million, and for late AMD between 3.9–4.8 million.[118]

Risk factors

The condition is classified as either 'dry' or 'wet' based on the clinical presentation. Wet AMD is characterized by sub-retinal neovascularization, exudative fluid, and subsequent scarring, whereas the dry form begins with thinning, depigmentation, and ultimately atrophy of the retinal pigment epithelium. The deposition of cellular debris related to photoreceptor metabolism (manifesting as yellow sub-retinal deposits called 'drusen') is regarded as indicating an increased risk of AMD. Immune mediators are plentiful in drusen.[119] Mutations in the complement factor H (*CFH*, 1q31.3) and complement component 3 (*C3*) genes are strongly associated with AMD.[120,121] Another important genetic risk marker localizes to *LOC387715* (10q26). A polymorphism at this site reduces the expression of *ARMS2*.[122] Although the function of *ARMS2* is not well understood, it has been implicated in energy metabolism. The presence of inclusion bodies in the retina containing amyloid-like proteins has led to AMD being called dementia of the eye.[123] Smoking is the overwhelming modifiable risk factor.

It is estimated that *CFH, ARMS2*, and cigarette smoking together explain 61% of the population-attributable risk (PAR) of AMD. The adjusted PAR percentage estimates are 20% for smoking, 36% for *ARMS2*, and 43% for *CFH*.[124] There is significant gene-environment interaction, with smoking strongly increasing the risk in those with high-risk genotypes.

AMD and Dementia

It has been suggested that AD and other forms of dementia may occur more frequently in people with AMD. In the Rotterdam Study cohort, participants with advanced age-related maculopathy at baseline showed an increased risk of incident AD (relative risk = 2.1, 95% CI: 1.1, 4.3; adjusted for age and gender), but this risk decreased after additional adjustment for smoking and atherosclerosis (relative risk = 1.5, 95% CI: 0.6, 3.5).[125] Similarly, in a large insurance database study from Taiwan using data on 29,958 people, 1589 (5.3%) were diagnosed with incident AD or senile dementia during a mean follow-up period of 4.4 years. Of these, 294 (5.9%) had AMD compared with 1295 (5.2%) without. The incidence of dementia was higher in people with AMD than in the controls (P = 0.044), with an HR of 1.44 (95% CI, 1.26–1.64) after adjusting for covariates.[126] These studies offer a plausible argument for an association between AMD and dementia. However, a very large study using data from 65,894 with AMD in the English NHS system suggested the risk of AD or dementia in people with an AMD diagnosis was not elevated. The rate ratio was 0.86 (95% CI, 0.67–1.08) for AD and 0.91 (0.79–1.04) for dementia. The likelihood of being admitted for AMD following AD or dementia was very low: the rate ratio was 0.04 (0.01–0.10) for people with AD and 0.07 (0.04–0.11) for those with dementia. The authors concluded: 'These neurodegenerative conditions may share environmental risk factors and histopathologic features. However, considering AD and other dementia after AMD, their coexistence at the individual level is no different from that expected by chance.'[127]

The biology and genetics of AMD is now relatively well understood. The mechanisms and genetics appear to be separate from those underlying AD and other dementia. AMD appears to centre on abnormalities of regulation of inflammation, whereas AD is predominantly a disease of abnormal protein folding.

Future directions

Clarifying the association between AMD and dementias is important in view of the number people affected and the significant suffering that both conditions cause. It appears that shared risk factors exist (such as smoking and dyslipidaemia), and that these should be targeted in prevention programmes.

REFERENCES

1. Whitson HE, Farsiu S, Stinnett S, et al. Retinal imaging biomarkers for early diagnosis of Alzheimer's disease. Invest Ophthalmol Vis Sci. 2015; 56: 389.
2. Liew G, Mitchell P, Wong TY, et al. Retinal microvascular signs and cognitive impairment. J Am Geriatr Soc (online serial). 2009; 57: 1892–6.
3. Martinez-Lapiscina EH, Arnow S, Wilson JA, et al. Retinal thickness measured with optical coherence tomography and risk of disability worsening in multiple sclerosis: a cohort study. Lancet Neurology. 2016; 15: 574–84.
4. Hinton DR, Sadun AA, Blanks JC, Miller CA. Optic-nerve degeneration in Alzheimer's disease. N Engl J Med. 1986; 315: 485–7.
5. Gao L, Liu Y, Li X, Bai Q, Liu P. Abnormal retinal nerve fiber layer thickness and macula lutea in patients with mild cognitive impairment and Alzheimer's disease. Arch Gerontol Geriatr (online serial). 2015; 60: 162–7.
6. Inzelberg R, Ramirez JA, Nisipeanu P, Ophir A. Retinal nerve fiber layer thinning in Parkinson disease. Vision Res (online serial). 2004; 44: 2793–7.
7. Ringelstein M, Albrecht P, Sudmeyer M, et al. Subtle retinal pathology in amyotrophic lateral sclerosis. Ann Clin Transl Neurol. 2014; 1: 290–7.

8. Brandt AU, Meinert-Bohn E, Rinnenthal JL, et al. Afferent visual pathway affection in patients with PMP22 deletion-related hereditary neuropathy with liability to pressure palsies. PLOS One. 2016; 11: e0164617.
9. Brandt AU, Oberwahrenbrock T, Mikolajczak J, et al. Visual dysfunction, but not retinal thinning, following anti-NMDA receptor encephalitis. Neurol Neuroinflammation. 2016; 3: e198.
10. Langwinska-Wosko E, Litwin T, Dziezyc K, Karlinski M, Czlonkowska A. Optical coherence tomography as a marker of neurodegeneration in patients with Wilson's disease. Acta Neurol Belg. Epub 2017.
11. Moreno-Ramos T, Benito-Leon J, Villarejo A, Bermejo-Pareja F. Retinal nerve fiber layer thinning in dementia associated with Parkinson's disease, dementia with Lewy bodies, and Alzheimer's disease. J Alzheimers Dis (online serial). 2013; 34: 659–64.
12. den Haan J, Verbraak FD, Visser PJ, Bouwman FH. Retinal thickness in Alzheimer's disease: a systematic review and meta-analysis. Alzheimer's Dement Diagnosis, Assess Dis Monit. 2017; 6: 162–170.
13. Shi Z, Wu Y, Wang M, et al. Greater attenuation of retinal nerve fiber layer thickness in Alzheimer's disease patients. J Alzheimers Dis (online serial). 2014; 40: 277–83.
14. Ikram MK, Cheung CY, Lorenzi M, Klein R, Jones TLZ, Wong TY. Retinal vascular caliber as a biomarker for diabetes microvascular complications. Diabetes Care (online serial). 2013; 36: 750–9.
15. Cheung CY, Ikram MK, Sabanayagam C, Wong TY. Retinal microvasculature as a model to study the manifestations of hypertension. Hypertension (online serial). 2012; 60: 1094–103.
16. Liew G, Wong TY, Mitchell P, Cheung N, Wang JJ. Retinopathy predicts coronary heart disease mortality. Heart. 2009; 95: 391–4.
17. Balcer LJ, Miller DH, Reingold SC, Cohen JA. Vision and vision-related outcome measures in multiple sclerosis. Brain. 2015; 138: 11–27.
18. Petzold A, de Boer JF, Schippling S, et al. Optical coherence tomography in multiple sclerosis: a systematic review and meta-analysis. Lancet Neurology. 2010; 9: 921–32.
19. Trapp BD, Peterson J, Ransohoff RM, Rudick R, Mork S, Bo L. Axonal transection in the lesions of multiple sclerosis. N Engl J Med. 1998; 338: 278–85.
20. Manfredonia F, Ciccarelli O, Khaleeli Z, et al. Normal-appearing brain T1 relaxation time predicts disability in early primary progressive multiple sclerosis. Arch Neurol (online serial). 2007; 64: 411.
21. Wallin MT, Culpepper WJ, Maloni H, Kurtzke JF. The Gulf War era multiple sclerosis cohort: 3. Early clinical features. Acta Neurol Scand (online serial). Epub 22 Aug 2017.
22. Alter M, Good J, Okihiro M. Optic neuritis in Orientals and Caucasians. Neurology (online serial). 1973; 23: 631–9.
23. Martínez-Lapiscina E, Fraga E, Pastor X, et al. Is optic neuritis incidence rising? Evidence from an epidemiological study in Barcelona, Spain 2008–2012. Neurology (online serial). 2014; 82.
24. Taylor B V, Lucas RM, Dear K, et al. Latitudinal variation in incidence and type of first central nervous system demyelinating events. Mult Scler (online serial). 2010; 16: 398–405.
25. Koch-Henriksen N, Sorensen PS. The changing demographic pattern of multiple sclerosis epidemiology. Lancet Neurology. 2010; 9: 520–32.
26. Kurtzke JF. On the fine structure of the distribution of multiple sclerosis. Acta Neurol Scand. 1967; 43: 257–82.
27. Leibowitz U, Sharon D, Alter M. Geographical considerations in multiple sclerosis. Brain. 1967; 90: 871–86.
28. Ascherio A, Munger KL, Simon KC. Vitamin D and multiple sclerosis. Lancet Neurology. 2010; 9: 599–612.
29. Milo R, Kahana E. Multiple sclerosis: geoepidemiology, genetics and the environment. Autoimmun Rev. 2010; 9: A387–94.
30. Williams KM, Bentham GCG, Young IS, et al. Association between myopia, ultraviolet B radiation exposure, serum vitamin D concentrations, and genetic polymorphisms in vitamin D metabolic pathways in a multicountry European study. JAMA Ophthalmol (online serial). American Medical Association. 2017; 135: 47.
31. Cabre P. Environmental changes and epidemiology of multiple sclerosis in the French West Indies. J Neurol Sci (online serial). 2009; 286: 58–61.
32. Fleming J, Fabry Z. The hygiene hypothesis and multiple sclerosis. Ann Neurol (online serial). 2007; 61: 85–9.
33. Cabre P, Heinzlef O, Merle H, et al. MS and neuromyelitis optica in Martinique (French West Indies). Neurology (online serial). 2001; 56: 507–14.
34. Petzold A, Wong S, Plant GT. Autoimmunity in visual loss. Handb Clin Neurol. Amsterdam: Elsevier, 2016. pp353–376.
35. Ascherio A. Environmental factors in multiple sclerosis. Expert Rev Neurother. 2013; 13: 3–9.
36. Thacker EL, Mirzaei F, Ascherio A. Infectious mononucleosis and risk for multiple sclerosis: a meta-analysis. Ann Neurol. 2006; 59: 499–503.
37. Dobson R, Kuhle J, Middeldorp J, Giovannoni G. Epstein-Barr-negative MS: a true phenomenon? Neurol Neuroinflammation. 2017; 4: e318.
38. Riise T, Nortvedt MW, Ascherio A. Smoking is a risk factor for multiple sclerosis. Neurology. 2003; 61: 1122–4.
39. Kesler A, Pianka P. Toxic optic neuropathy. Curr Neurol Neurosci Rep. 2003; 3: 410–14.
40. Munger KL. Childhood obesity is a risk factor for multiple sclerosis. Mult Scler J. Epub 2013.1352458513507357.
41. Munger KL, Chitnis T, Ascherio A. Body size and risk of MS in two cohorts of US women. Neurology. 2009; 73: 1543–50.
42. Pereira-Santos M, Costa PR, Assis AM, Santos CA, Santos DB. Obesity and vitamin D deficiency: a systematic review and meta-analysis. Obes Rev (online serial). 2015; 16: 341–9.
43. Fielder AH, Batchelor JR, Vakarelis BN, Compston DA, McDonald WI. Optic neuritis and multiple sclerosis: do factor B alleles influence progression of disease? Lancet (London, England) (online serial). 1981; 2: 1246–8.
44. International Multiple Sclerosis Genetics C, Wellcome Trust Case Control C, Sawcer S, et al. Genetic risk and a primary role for cell-mediated immune mechanisms in multiple sclerosis. Nature (online serial). 2011; 476: 214–19.
45. Moutsianas L, Jostins L, Beecham AH, et al. Class II HLA interactions modulate genetic risk for multiple sclerosis. Nat Genet (online serial). 2015; 47: 1107–13.
46. Olsson T, Barcellos LF, Alfredsson L. Interactions between genetic, lifestyle and environmental risk factors for multiple sclerosis. Nat Rev Neurol. 2017; 13: 25–36.
47. Fernandez O. Integrating the tools for an individualized prognosis in multiple sclerosis. J Neurol Sci. 2013; 331: 10–13.
48. Petzold A, Rejdak K, Plant GT. Axonal degeneration and inflammation in acute optic neuritis. J Neurol Neurosurg Psychiatry. 2004; 75: 1178–80.
49. Teunissen CE, Khalil M. Neurofilaments as biomarkers in multiple sclerosis. Mult Scler J. 2012; 18: 552–6.

50. Modvig S, Degn M, Sander B, et al. Cerebrospinal fluid neurofilament light chain levels predict visual outcome after optic neuritis. Mult Scler J (online serial). 2016; 22: 590–8.
51. Cordeiro MF, Normando EM, Cardoso MJ, et al. Real-time imaging of single neuronal cell apoptosis in patients with glaucoma. Brain (online serial). Epub 2017.
52. King A, Azuara-Blanco A, Tuulonen A. Glaucoma. BMJ (online serial). 2013; 346: f3518.
53. Kapetanakis VV, Chan MPY, Foster PJ, Cook DG, Owen CG, Rudnicka AR. Global variations and time trends in the prevalence of primary open angle glaucoma (POAG): a systematic review and meta-analysis. Br J Ophthalmol (online serial). Epub 2015. bjophthalmol-2015-307223.
54. Foster PJ, Buhrmann R, Quigley HA, Johnson GJ. The definition and classification of glaucoma in prevalence surveys. Br J Ophthalmol (online serial). 2002; 86: 238–42.
55. Quigley HA. Glaucoma. Lancet (online serial). 2011; 377: 1367–77.
56. Day AC, Baio G, Gazzard G, et al. The prevalence of primary angle closure glaucoma in European derived populations: a systematic review. Br J Ophthalmol (online serial). 2012; 96: 1162–7.
57. Quigley HA, Broman AT. The number of people with glaucoma worldwide in 2010 and 2020. Br J Ophthalmol (online serial). 2006; 90: 262–7.
58. Wolfs RC, Borger PH, Ramrattan RS, et al. Changing views on open-angle glaucoma: definitions and prevalences—the Rotterdam Study. Invest Ophthalmol Vis Sci. 2000; 41: 3309–21.
59. Tham Y-C, Li X, Wong TY, Quigley HA, Aung T, Cheng C-Y. Global prevalence of glaucoma and projections of glaucoma burden through 2040: a systematic review and meta-analysis. Ophthalmology (online serial). 2014; 121: 2081–90.
60. Mukesh BN, McCarty CA, Rait JL, Taylor HR. Five-year incidence of open-angle glaucoma: the visual impairment project. Ophthalmology (online serial). 2002; 109: 1047–51.
61. de Voogd S, Ikram MK, Wolfs RC, Jansonius NM, Hofman A, de Jong PT. Incidence of open-angle glaucoma in a general elderly population: the Rotterdam Study. Ophthalmology. 2005; 112: 1487–93.
62. Leske MC, Wu SY, Honkanen R, et al. Nine-year incidence of open-angle glaucoma in the Barbados Eye Studies. Ophthalmology. 2007; 114: 1058–64.
63. Ekström C. Incidence of open-angle glaucoma in central Sweden. Acta Ophthalmol. 2008; 86: 747–54.
64. Leske MC, Wu S-Y, Hennis A, Honkanen R, Nemesure B. Risk factors for incident open-angle glaucoma: the Barbados Eye Studies. Ophthalmology (online serial). 2008; 115: 85–93.
65. Müskens RPHM, de Voogd S, Wolfs RCW, et al. Systemic antihypertensive medication and incident open-angle glaucoma. Ophthalmology (online serial). 2007; 114: 2221–6.
66. Caprioli J. Glaucoma: a disease of early cellular senescence. Invest Ophthalmol Vis Sci (online serial). 2013; 54: ORSF60–7.
67. Vajaranant TS, Nayak S, Wilensky JT, Joslin CE. Gender and glaucoma: what we know and what we need to know. Curr Opin Ophthalmol (online serial). 2010; 21: 91–9.
68. Hulsman CA, Westendorp IC, Ramrattan RS, et al. Is open-angle glaucoma associated with early menopause? The Rotterdam Study. Am J Epidemiol (online serial). 2001; 154: 138–44.
69. Pasquale LR, Rosner BA, Hankinson SE, Kang JH. Attributes of female reproductive aging and their relation to primary open-angle glaucoma: a prospective study. J Glaucoma (online serial). 2007; 16: 598–605.
70. Vajaranant TS, Wu S, Torres M, Varma R. A 40-year forecast of the demographic shift in primary open-angle glaucoma in the United States. Invest Ophthalmol Vis Sci (online serial). 2012; 53: 2464–6.
71. Le A, Mukesh BN, McCarty CA, Taylor HR. Risk factors associated with the incidence of open-angle glaucoma: the visual impairment project. Invest Ophthalmol Vis Sci (online serial). 2003; 44: 3783–9.
72. Jiang X, Varma R, Wu S, et al. Baseline risk factors that predict the development of open-angle glaucoma in a population: The Los Angeles Latino Eye Study. Ophthalmology (online serial). 2012; 119: 1–9.
73. Sommer A, Tielsch JM, Katz J, et al. Relationship between intraocular pressure and primary open angle glaucoma among white and black Americans. The Baltimore Eye Survey. Arch Ophthalmol (online serial). 1991; 109: 1090–5.
74. Kim C, Seong GJ, Lee N, Song K. Prevalence of primary open-angle glaucoma in central South Korea the Namil study. Ophthalmology (online serial). Elsevier Inc.; 2011; 118: 1024–30.
75. Hollows FC, Graham PA. Intra-ocular pressure, glaucoma, and glaucoma suspects in a defined population. Br J Ophthalmol (online serial). 1966; 50: 570–86.
76. Leydhecker W, Akiyama K, Neumann H. Der intraokular Druck gesunder menschlicher Augen. Klin Monatsbl Augenheilkd augenarztl Fortbild. 1958; 133: 662–70.
77. National Institute for Health and Care. Diagnosis and management of chronic open angle glaucoma and ocular hypertension (NICE clinical guideline 85) (online). 2009.
78. Ophthalmology AA of. Primary open-angle glaucoma preferred practice pattern (online). 2015.
79. Iwase A, Suzuki Y, Araie M, et al. The prevalence of primary open-angle glaucoma in Japanese: the Tajimi Study. Ophthalmology (online serial). 2004; 111: 1641–8.
80. Marcus MW, de Vries MM, Junoy Montolio FG, Jansonius NM. Myopia as a risk factor for open-angle glaucoma: a systematic review and meta-analysis. Ophthalmology (online serial). 2011; 118: 1989–94. e2.
81. Brazitikos PD, Safran AB, Simona F, Zulauf M. Threshold perimetry in tilted disc syndrome. Arch Ophthalmol (online serial). 1990; 108: 1698–700.
82. Jonas JB, Gusek GC, Naumann GO. Optic disk morphometry in high myopia. Graefes Arch Clin Exp Ophthalmol (online serial). 1988; 226: 587–90.
83. Hoffmann EM, Lamparter J, Mirshahi A, et al. Distribution of central corneal thickness and its association with ocular parameters in a large central European cohort: the Gutenberg health study. PLOS One (online serial). 2013; 8: e66158.
84. Coleman AL, Stone KL, Kodjebacheva G, et al. Glaucoma risk and the consumption of fruits and vegetables among older women in the study of osteoporotic fractures. Am J Ophthalmol (online serial). 2008; 145: 1081–9.
85. Ramdas WD, Wolfs RCW, Kiefte-de Jong JC, et al. Nutrient intake and risk of open-angle glaucoma: the Rotterdam Study. Eur J Epidemiol (online serial). 2012; 27: 385–93.
86. Kang JH, Pasquale LR, Willett W, et al. Antioxidant intake and primary open-angle glaucoma: a prospective study. Am J Epidemiol (online serial). 2003; 158: 337–46.
87. Kang JH, Pasquale LR, Willett WC, et al. Dietary fat consumption and primary open-angle glaucoma. Am J Clin Nutr (online serial). 2004; 79: 755–64.

88. Pérez de Arcelus M, Toledo E, Martínez-González MÁ, Sayón-Orea C, Gea A, Moreno-Montañés J. Omega 3:6 ratio intake and incidence of glaucoma: the SUN cohort. Clin Nutr (online serial). Elsevier Ltd; Epub 2013. 3–7.
89. Kang JH, Willett WC, Rosner B a, Hankinson SE, Pasquale LR. Caffeine consumption and the risk of primary open-angle glaucoma: a prospective cohort study. Invest Ophthalmol Vis Sci (online serial). 2008; 49: 1924–31.
90. Buckingham T, Young R. The rise and fall of intra-ocular pressure: the influence of physiological factors. Ophthalmic Physiol Opt (online serial). 1986; 6: 95–9.
91. Lin H-Y, Hsu W-M, Chou P, et al. Intraocular pressure measured with a noncontact tonometer in an elderly Chinese population: the Shihpai Eye Study. Arch Ophthalmol (online serial). 2005; 123: 381–6.
92. Risner D, Ehrlich R, Kheradiya NS, Siesky B, McCranor L, Harris A. Effects of exercise on intraocular pressure and ocular blood flow: a review. J Glaucoma (online serial). 2009; 18: 429–36.
93. Leske MC. Ocular perfusion pressure and glaucoma: clinical trial and epidemiologic findings. Curr Opin Ophthalmol (online serial). 2009; 20: 73–8.
94. Williams PT. Relationship of incident glaucoma versus physical activity and fitness in male runners. Med Sci Sports Exerc (online serial). 2009; 41: 1566–72.
95. Wolfs RC, Klaver CC, Ramrattan RS, van Duijn CM, Hofman A, de Jong PT. Genetic risk of primary open-angle glaucoma. Population-based familial aggregation study. Arch Ophthalmol (online serial). 1998; 116: 1640–45.
96. Teikari JM. Genetic factors in open-angle (simple and capsular) glaucoma. A population-based twin study. Acta Ophthalmol (online serial). 1987; 65: 715–20.
97. Morissette J, Côté G, Anctil JL, et al. A common gene for juvenile and adult-onset primary open-angle glaucomas confined on chromosome 1q. Am J Hum Genet (online serial). 1995; 56: 1431–42.
98. Rezaie T, Child A, Hitchings R, et al. Adult-onset primary open-angle glaucoma caused by mutations in optineurin. Science (online serial). 2002; 295: 1077–9.
99. Monemi S, Spaeth G, DaSilva A, et al. Identification of a novel adult-onset primary open-angle glaucoma (POAG) gene on 5q22.1. Hum Mol Genet (online serial). 2005; 14: 725–33.
100. Alward WLM, Kwon YH, Kawase K, et al. Evaluation of optineurin sequence variations in 1,048 patients with open-angle glaucoma. Am J Ophthalmol (online serial). 2003; 136: 904–10.
101. Fingert JH, Héon E, Liebmann JM, et al. Analysis of myocilin mutations in 1703 glaucoma patients from five different populations. Hum Mol Genet (online serial). 1999; 8: 899–905.
102. Hauser MA, Allingham RR, Linkroum K, et al. Distribution of WDR36 DNA sequence variants in patients with primary open-angle glaucoma. Invest Ophthalmol Vis Sci (online serial). 2006; 47: 2542–6.
103. Thorleifsson G, Walters GB, Hewitt AW, et al. Common variants near CAV1 and CAV2 are associated with primary open-angle glaucoma. Nat Genet (online serial). Nature Publishing Group; 2010; 42: 906–9.
104. Burdon KP, Macgregor S, Hewitt AW, et al. Genome-wide association study identifies susceptibility loci for open angle glaucoma at TMCO1 and CDKN2B-AS1. Nat Genet (online serial). Nature Publishing Group; 2011; 43: 574–8.
105. Gharahkhani P, Burdon KP, Fogarty R, et al. Common variants near ABCA1, AFAP1 and GMDS confer risk of primary open-angle glaucoma. Nat Genet (online serial). Nature Publishing Group; 2014; 46: 1120–25.
106. Bailey JNC, Loomis SJ, Kang JH, et al. Genome-wide association analysis identifies TXNRD2, ATXN2 and FOXC1 as susceptibility loci for primary open-angle glaucoma. Nat Genet (online serial). 2016; 48: 189–94.
107. World Health Organization. Global Data on Visual Impairments 2010 (online). 2012.
108. Bamashmus MA, Matlhaga B, Dutton GN. Causes of blindness and visual impairment in the West of Scotland. Eye (online serial). 2004; 18: 257–61.
109. Bunce C, Wormald R. Leading causes of certification for blindness and partial sight in England & Wales. BMC Public Health (online serial). 2006; 6: 58.
110. Spry PG, Spencer IC, Sparrow JM, et al. The Bristol Shared Care Glaucoma Study: reliability of community optometric and hospital eye service test measures. Br J Ophthalmol (online serial). 1999; 83: 707–12.
111. Hattenhauer MG, Johnson DH, Ing HH, et al. The probability of blindness from open-angle glaucoma. Ophthalmology. 1998; 105: 2099–104.
112. Peters D, Bengtsson B, Heijl A. Lifetime risk of blindness in open-angle glaucoma. Am J Ophthalmol (online serial). 2013; 156: 724–30.
113. Kooner KS, AlBdoor M, Cho BJ, Adams-Huet B. Risk factors for progression to blindness in high tension primary open angle glaucoma: Comparison of blind and nonblind subjects. Clin Ophthalmol (online serial). 2008; 2: 757–62.
114. Rivera JL, Bell NP, Feldman RM. Risk factors for primary open angle glaucoma progression: what we know and what we need to know. Curr Opin Ophthalmol (online serial). 2008; 19: 102–6.
115. Ng WS, Agarwal PK, Sidiki S, McKay L, Townend J, Azuara-Blanco A. The effect of socio-economic deprivation on severity of glaucoma at presentation. Br J Ophthalmol (online serial). 2010; 94: 85–7.
116. Fraser S, Bunce C, Wormald R. Risk factors for late presentation in chronic glaucoma. Invest Ophthalmol Vis Sci (online serial). 1999; 40: 2251–7.
117. Jonas JB, Cheung CMG, Panda-Jonas S. Updates on the epidemiology of age-related macular degeneration. Asia-Pacific J Ophthalmol (online serial). Epub 14 Sep 2017.
118. Colijn JM, Buitendijk GHS, Prokofyeva E, et al. Prevalence of age-related macular degeneration in Europe. Ophthalmology (online serial). Epub 14 July 2017.
119. Mullins RF, Russell SR, Anderson DH, Hageman GS. Drusen associated with aging and age-related macular degeneration contain proteins common to extracellular deposits associated with atherosclerosis, elastosis, amyloidosis, and dense deposit disease. FASEB J. 2000; 14: 835–46.
120. Haines JL, Hauser MA, Schmidt S, et al. Complement factor H variant increases the risk of age-related macular degeneration. Science (80) (online serial). 2005; 308: 419–21.
121. Yates JRW, Sepp T, Matharu BK, et al. Complement C3 variant and the risk of age-related macular degeneration. N Engl J Med (online serial). 2007; 357: 553–61.

122. Fritsche LG, Loenhardt T, Janssen A, et al. Age-related macular degeneration is associated with an unstable ARMS2 (LOC387715) mRNA. Nat Genet (online serial). 2008; 40: 892–6.
123. Ratnayaka JA, Serpell LC, Lotery AJ. Dementia of the eye: the role of amyloid beta in retinal degeneration. Eye (online serial). 2015; 29: 1013–26.
124. Schmidt S, Hauser M a, Scott WK, et al. Cigarette smoking strongly modifies the association of LOC387715 and age-related macular degeneration. Am J Hum Genet (online serial). 2006; 78: 852–64.
125. Klaver CC, Ott A, Hofman A, Assink JJ, Breteler MM, de Jong PT. Is age-related maculopathy associated with Alzheimer's Disease? The Rotterdam Study. Am J Epidemiol (online serial). 1999; 150: 963–8.
126. Tsai DC, Chen SJ, Huang CC, Yuan MK, Leu HB. Age-related macular degeneration and risk of degenerative dementia among the elderly in Taiwan. A population-based cohort study. Ophthalmology. 2015; 122: 2327–35.
127. Keenan TDL, Goldacre R, Goldacre MJ. Associations between age-related macular degeneration, Alzheimer disease, and dementia: record linkage study of hospital admissions. JAMA Ophthalmol (online serial). 2014; 132: 63–8.

34

Sensory loss—hearing

Adele M Goman and Frank R Lin

Introduction

Sensorineural hearing loss (herein referred to as 'hearing loss') refers to impairments of the peripheral auditory system that affect the precise encoding of sound by the cochlea. An estimated 360 million people worldwide have a hearing loss[1] and the prevalence of hearing loss increases with age, with almost two-thirds of adults over the age of 70 having a hearing loss.[2,3] Epidemiologic factors associated with hearing loss reflect features that contribute to cochlear pathophysiology. The strongest risk factors for hearing loss in older adults include age,[3] race (darker-skinned individuals have less risk of hearing loss because of a possible protective role of melanin in the cochlea),[3,4] sex (women have less hearing loss because of a possible protective effect of oestrogen in the cochlea),[5] and noise exposure.[3,6] Intermediate risk factors include diabetes, smoking, and hypertension (likely through microvascular injury and inflammatory damage to the cochlea).[7,8] Central hearing impairment is much less common than peripheral hearing loss and refers to dysfunction in the central auditory pathways. Individuals with central hearing impairment experience difficulty understanding speech which is not explained by peripheral impairment.[9] However, research has indicated that central hearing loss may not exist in isolation; rather it may arise as a manifestation of changes in the brain and auditory system due to age or disease.[10] This section will first describe how hearing loss is defined in epidemiologic studies. Second, it will address the evidence on the association between hearing loss and cognitive function. Third, it will outline the effects of hearing amplification on neuropsychological performance.

Defining Hearing Loss in Epidemiologic Studies

When interpreting the results of epidemiologic research findings researchers should be aware of how hearing loss was measured and defined. Importantly, objective and subjective measures assess different aspects of hearing loss, with objective measures generally assessing hearing and speech understanding and self-report assessing perceived difficulties with hearing.[11] Audiometry is the most common method used to assess hearing ability, and reflects the sensitivity of the peripheral auditory system to detect pure tones. This method does not substantively depend on higher-order cortical processing and has been reliably performed in adults with early dementia and in children as young as three years of age.[12,13] Pure tones at specific frequencies are presented to each ear individually and the listener indicates when they hear a tone. The level of presentation is varied to identify the quietest level ('threshold') at which a pure tone at a given frequency is detected 50% of the time. The World Health Organization defines hearing loss as a pure tone average (PTA) of thresholds 0.5–4kHz in the better ear >25 dB hearing level (HL) although various other definitions for hearing loss are used in the literature. An alternative, or supplemental, measure of hearing loss is self-report, whereby individuals subjectively report their self-perceived difficulty with their hearing or report their current or previous hearing device use. The utilization of different testing methodologies, audiometric definitions of hearing loss, and questions can make comparisons across studies challenging.

Potential Pathways Linking Hearing Loss and Cognition

A conceptual model (Fig. 34.1) developed by Lin and Albert[14] depicts the causal mechanisms that may mediate the effects of hearing impairment on impaired cognitive functioning and dementia. Common factors that could underlie a simple correlation between hearing and cognition include age, shared pathologic aetiologies (e.g. diabetes, hypertension, neurodegenerative processes), and demographic factors (e.g. education). In contrast, mechanistic pathways through which hearing loss could contribute to poorer cognitive functioning include effects on cognitive load, brain structure/function, and decreased social engagement.

Cognitive load

Hearing loss results in poor fidelity and distorted encoding of complex sounds, such as speech, in the cochlea.[13] The effect of poor peripheral encoding of sound is demonstrated by studies in which, under conditions where the auditory signal is degraded, greater cognitive resources are required for auditory perceptual processing

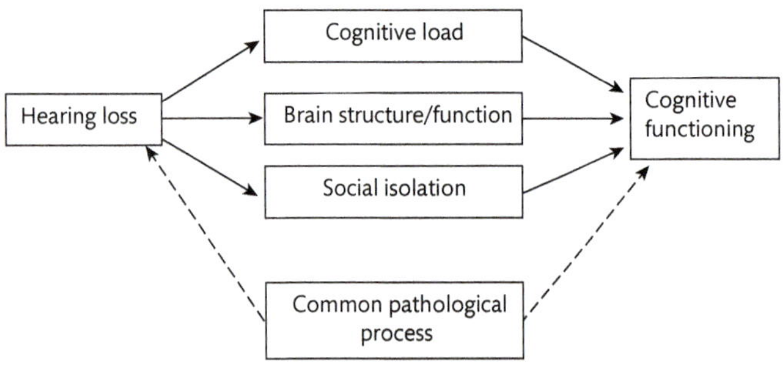

Fig. 34.1 Conceptual model of the common cause (dashed line) or mechanistic pathways (solid line) that may underlie the association between hearing loss and cognitive functioning.

Reproduced with permission from Lin F.R. and Albert M. Hearing Loss and Dementia - Who's Listening? *Aging Ment Health*. 2014;18(6): 671–673. Rights managed by Taylor & Francis. DOI: https://doi.org/10.1080/13607863.2014.915924.

to the detriment of other cognitive processes such as working memory.[15–17] These observations are consistent with resource capacity models.[18] Furthermore, these observations are supported by functional neuroimaging studies demonstrating compensatory recruitment of prefrontal regions to maintain auditory processing in older adults with hearing loss.[19–21]

Brain structure

Neuroimaging studies have demonstrated that hearing loss is associated with reduced volumes in the primary auditory cortex[20,22] and the loss of integrity of central auditory white matter tracks.[22,23] The basis of these associations remains unknown but may be related to alterations in the degree of neural activation provided by an impoverished auditory signal, with subsequent changes in cortical reorganization and brain morphometry.[20] In animal models, cochlear impairments are known to be causally associated with both tonotopic reorganization of the auditory cortex[24] and morphologic changes in central neuronal structures.[25] This observation is further supported by work in humans demonstrating that hearing loss is prospectively associated with accelerated volume declines in the right superior, middle, and inferior temporal gyri over a mean of 6.4 years of longitudinal follow-up.[26] These regions are intriguing because they are important not only for spoken language processing (and hence may be affected by impoverished/reduced auditory stimuli), [27,28] but also for semantic memory, sensory integration, and are involved in the early stages of MCI or early AD.[29,30]

Social isolation

Communication impairments caused by hearing loss can also lead to reduced social engagement and loneliness in older adults,[31,32] and epidemiologic[33,34] and neuroanatomic studies[34] have demonstrated associations of loneliness with cognitive decline and dementia. Poor social engagement could likely contribute to impaired cognitive functioning through both behavioural and psychological effects[35,36] and direct neurobiological effects from stress and inflammation.[37,38]

Multiple factors

Cognitive decline and dementias occurring in late life (i.e. affecting individuals over 70 years of age) are often multifactorial in aetiology. Hearing impairment, therefore, may act in parallel to other established risk factors for cognitive decline and dementia (e.g. AD pathology, microvascular disease) to adversely affect cognitive performance.[14]

Hearing Loss, Cognitive Decline, and Dementia

One of the earliest demonstrations of an association between hearing loss and dementia was shown in a case-control study.[12] In this study 100 adults with dementia and 100 adults without dementia, who were matched on age, sex, and education, completed a global measure of cognitive functioning: the MMSE, and pure-tone audiometry. After adjusting for potential covariates, hearing loss (defined in this study as a PTA ≥30 dB HL) was associated with 2.3 increased odds for dementia. More recently, the relationship between hearing loss and cognitive functioning has been investigated using several large-scale epidemiological datasets. These studies (Table 34.1) that have used objective audiometric assessments of hearing, as well as both auditory and non-auditory tests of cognition, and have adjusted for multiple confounders (e.g. age, vascular risk factors) have, for the most part, demonstrated strong associations between hearing and cognition in older adults both cross-sectionally and longitudinally, which is broadly consistent with prior studies.[12,39]

Cross-sectional studies

Using data from the National Health and Nutritional Examination Survey, Lin[40] examined the association between audiometrically-defined hearing loss and cognitive functioning amongst adults aged 60–69 in the USA. The analytic sample consisted of 605 participants who had completed the digit symbol substitution test. This non-verbal test assesses executive function and psychomotor processing and requires participants to match a sequence of numbers with a corresponding symbol as quickly as they can. After adjusting for multiple confounders including demographic and cardiovascular risk factors, it was found that greater hearing loss was associated with significantly poorer cognitive performance. Furthermore, the magnitude of the association of a 25 dB difference in hearing (equivalent to going from a normal to a mild hearing loss) with cognitive performance on the digit symbol test was estimated to be equivalent to nearly seven years of ageing.

In a smaller (n = 347), yet older (mean age = 71 years) sample, Lin and colleagues[41] investigated the association of hearing loss and cognitive functioning using data from the Baltimore Longitudinal Study of Aging, an ongoing prospective study of community-dwelling adults aged over 55 years. Participants completed pure-tone audiometry and a battery of cognitive tests including the MMSE, and tests of memory, executive function, attention, psychomotor and processing speed, verbal function, and language. After adjusting for potential confounders, it was found that audiometric-defined hearing loss was associated with significantly poorer performance on the MMSE and on measures of memory and executive function. Whilst the relationship between hearing loss and processing speed and psychomotor performance showed a trend towards a positive association, this was not significant in adjusted analyses and there was no significant relationship found between hearing loss and verbal function and language. Similar findings have been found in other studies using US datasets.[42,43]

Table 34.1 Summary of studies looking at the association between hearing loss and cognitive functioning

Author	Year	Country	Sample size	Age	Survey	Hearing assessment	Adjustment for covariates	Design	Outcome	Result
Lin[39]	2011	USA	605	60–69	National Health and Nutrition Examination Survey	Audiometry: 0.5,1,2,4 better ear PTA.	Age, sex, race/ ethnicity, education, income, smoking, diabetes, hypertension, stroke.	Cross-sectional.	Executive function & psychomotor processing.	Hearing loss significantly associated with poorer performance (-3.3 points per 10 dB of hearing loss on the digit symbol substitution test).
Lin, Ferrucci, Metter, Zonderman, Resnick[40]	2011	USA	347	>55; mean = 71	Baltimore Longitudinal study of aging	Audiometry: 0.5,1,2,4 better ear PTA.	Age, sex, race, education, diabetes, smoking, hypertension.	Cross-sectional.	Mental status, memory, executive function, processing and psychomotor speed, verbal function & language.	Hearing loss significantly associated with poorer mental status, memory, and executive function performance. No significant association between hearing loss and processing and psychomotor speed, verbal function and language.
Deal, Betz, Yaffe et al.[41]	2016	USA	721	72–81 at baseline	Health ABC Cognitive Vitality substudy	Audiometry, PTA (0.5,1,2,4) better ear.	Age, sex, race, education, study site, smoking, hypertension, diabetes, stroke.	Longitudinal, 7 years	Cognitive decline	No sig differences in rates of cognitive decline.
								Longitudinal, 9 years.	Incident dementia.	Moderate/severe hearing loss associated with an increased risk of incident dementia: HR = 1.55 (95% 1.09, 2.18).
Harrison Bush, Lister, Lin, Betz, Edwards[42]	2015	USA	894	mean = 73.4	Staying keen in Later Life study	Audiometry (3 frequency PTA 0.5,1,2 in better ear.	Age, sex, race, education, diabetes, heart disease, hypertension, stroke, depressive symptomology.	Cross-sectional.	Global cognitive status, speed of processing, executive function, memory.	Hearing loss accounted for a significant yet small amount of variance in processing speed, executive function, memory, global cognitive status.
Lin, Metter, O'Brien, Resnick, Zonderman, Ferrucci[43]	2011	USA	639	>55	Baltimore Longitudinal study of aging	Audiometry, PTA (0.5,1,2,4) better ear.	Age, sex, race, education, diabetes, smoking, hypertension.	Longitudinal, 11.9 years.	Incident dementia.	Hearing loss associated with an increased risk of incident dementia: HR = 1.27 (95% CI = 1.06,1.50).
Gurgel, Ward, Schwartz, Norton, Foster, Tschanz[44]	2014	USA	4463	65+ (mean age = 75.4)	Cache County study	Subjective assessment of hearing loss by the examiner.	Age, sex, education, apoe E4 status, diabetes, smoking, high cholesterol, hypertension.	Longitudinal, 4.3 years (hearing impaired) and 6.1 years (non-hearing impaired).	Dementia	Hearing loss associated with an increased risk of incident dementia: HR = 1.27 (95% CI = 1.03, 1.56). Hearing loss associated with accelerated rates of cognitive decline (54% faster).
Gallacher, Ilubaera, Ben-Shlomo et al.[45]	2012	UK	1057	Aged 44–68 at baseline. Mean age = 56.1	Caerphilly Prospective Study	Audiometry (0.5, 1,2,4) PTA.	Age, social class, anxiety, premorbid intelligence.	Longitudinal, 17 years.	Incident dementia.	Hearing loss associated with an increased risk of incident dementia: OR = 2.67, 95% CI = 1.38, 5.18.
									Cognitive decline	Hearing loss was not associated with an increased risk of cognitive decline: OR = 1.24 (95% CI = 0.77, 2.01).
Lin, Yaffe, Xia, Xue, Harris[46]	2013	USA	1984	65+	Health ABC	Audiometry, PTA (0.5,1,2,4) better ear.	Age, sex, race/ ethnicity, study site, smoking, hypertension, diabetes, stroke.	Longitudinal, 6 years.	Incident cognitive impairment.	Hearing loss associated with an increased risk of incident dementia. Per 10 dB of hearing loss: HR = 1.07 (95% CI 1.01, 1.14); For moderate or greater hearing loss: HR = 1.36 (95% CI = 1.08, 1.70).

(continued)

Table 34.1 *Continued*

Author	Year	Country	Sample size	Age	Survey	Hearing assessment	Adjustment for covariates	Design	Outcome	Result
Wu & Chiu[47]	2016	Taiwan	4707	50+	Survey of Taiwan longitudinal study of aging	Self-report 'Can you clearly hear without a hearing aid' coded as not hearing impaired ('very clearly' or 'clearly') of hearing impaired 'medium', 'unclearly' and 'very unclearly'.	Age, education, ethnicity, health status (self-rated health status, hypertension, diabetes, heart disease, stroke, cancer, lung disease, arthritis, gastric ulcer, liver disease), behavioural variables (smoking, alcohol, fruit-vegetable intake, multivitamin supplement use, physical activity).	Longitudinal, 11 years.	Memory	Rate of decline did not differ between hearing groups.
Anstey, Hofer, Luszcz[48]	2003	Australia	525	70+	Australian longitudinal study on aging	Audiometry. PTA 2,3,4 better ear	Age, sex, education, health variables.	Longitudinal, 8 years.	Verbal ability, processing speed, memory.	Declines in auditory threshold were associated with declines in memory performance.
Uchida, Nishita, Tange, et al.[49]	2016	Japan	1109	60–70 at baseline	National Institute for Longevity Sciences - Longitudinal study of aging	Audiometry (0.5– 8) PTA better ear >25	Age, sex, education, hypertension, diabetes, stroke, marital status, occupation, prior exposure to neuropsychological tests (i.e. practice effects).	Longitudinal, 12 years.	Cognitive decline on Japanese Wechsler Adult Intelligence Scale-Revised short forms.	Significantly greater decline for hearing loss individuals on factual knowledge test and digit symbol substitution test. No difference in rates of decline on logical abstract reasoning test or the picture completion test.
Valentjin, van Boxtel, van Hooren et al.[50]	2005	Netherlands	418	55+	Maastricht Aging Study	Audiometry. (1,2,4) PTA better ear	Age, sex, education, baseline cognitive performance, change in hearing, baseline hearing.	Longitudinal, 6 years.	Memory and processing speed.	Declines in auditory threshold were associated with declines in memory performance.
							Age, sex, education	Cross-sectional	Memory and processing speed.	No significant association.
Mitoku, Masaki, Ogata, Okamoto[51]	2016	Japan	1754	65+	Gujo City Long-Term Care insurance database	Self report: 'normal hearing', 'able to hear a loud conversation', 'not able to hear a loud conversation'.	Age, sex, level of dependency, diabetes, neurological disorders, hypertension, heart disease, cerebrovascular disease, respiratory disease, musculoskeletal and connective tissue disorders, and eye and ear diseases.	Longitudinal, 4.7 years.	Cognitive impairment and/or dementia as assessed by a trained investigator using the functional assessment for cognitively impaired elders.	Hearing impairment associated greater cognitive decline: OR = 1.47 (95% CI = 1.13–1.92).

Amieva, Ouvrard, Giolioli, Meillon, Rullier, Dartigues[52]	2015	France	3670 (3413 in final model)	65+	Personnes Agees QUID study	Self report 'Do you have hearing trouble?' and also asked if they had a hearing aid.	Age, sex, education, depressive symptomatology, social network, comorbidities, IADL dependency, psychotropic drug use, dementia.	Longitudinal, 25 years.	MMSE	In fully adjusted models there was no significant relationship between hearing loss and rates of cognitive decline.
Deal, Sharrett, Albert et al.[53]	2015	USA	253	mean = 76.9	Pilot study within the Atherosclerosis risk in communities study	Audiometry: 0.5,1,2,4 better ear PTA	Age, sex, education, smoking, hypertension, diabetes, depressive symptoms.	Cross-sectional	Memory, language, processing speed/ attention.	Hearing loss significantly associated with poorer memory performance. Mixed results for processing speed executive function.
								Longitudinal, 20 years	Memory, language, processing speed/ attention.	Rate of decline was accelerated for those with hearing loss.
Taljaard, Olaithe, Brennan-Jones, Eikelboom, Bucks[54]	2016	Multiple	33 studies	40 samples; 5710 participants	–	Variable	–	Meta-analysis	Attention/ processing speed, short term/working memory, long-term memory, executive function, semantic processing and word knowledge.	Poorer hearing was associated with poorer attention/processing speed, short term/working memory, long-term memory, executive function, semantic processing and word knowledge. These were small effect sizes range 0.24 through 0.64.

Central hearing impairment has also been shown to be associated with mild cognitive impairment (OR = 2.4) and AD (OR = 1.8).[9] However, while central hearing loss may be a prodromal symptom of cognitive decline it is unlikely to be a modifiable risk factor.[44]

Whilst cross-sectional designs enable the association between hearing loss and cognitive functioning to be investigated, these designs include the potential for bias by cohort effects and provide no data on the temporal relationship between hearing loss and cognitive functioning.

Longitudinal studies

Longitudinal studies have demonstrated independent associations between hearing loss and cognitive decline and dementia. Using data from 639 participants in the Baltimore Longitudinal Study of Aging with a median follow-up period of 12 years, it was found that hearing impaired individuals had an increased risk for incident dementia; with the risk being greater for those with greater levels of hearing loss.[45] These results have subsequently been replicated using other US epidemiologic datasets[42,46] and in another study of 1057 older adults followed for 17 years in the UK,[47] where every 10 dB increase in baseline PTA was associated with a 2.7 increased odds of dementia 17 years later.

Lin and colleagues[48] investigated the association between audiometric-defined hearing loss and cognitive decline in 1984 participants from the Health, Aging, and Body Composition (HealthABC) study, a prospective observational study of a random sample of Medicare beneficiaries, a national social insurance programme for US citizens aged 65 and older. Performance on cognitive tests was gathered at three, five, and six years after audiometric testing. Measures of cognitive functioning included the MMSE and the digit symbol substitution test. After adjusting for potential confounders, an accelerated rate of cognitive decline—equivalent to three years of ageing—was observed amongst individuals with hearing loss. MMSE scores declined by an average of 0.65 points per year amongst individuals with hearing loss, compared to just 0.46 points per year amongst individuals with normal hearing. Furthermore, scores on the digit symbol substitution test declined by 0.83 points per year for individuals with hearing loss compared to just 0.63 points per year for those with normal hearing. Altogether, compared to those with normal hearing, individuals with hearing loss had a 24% increased risk for incident cognitive impairment during the six-year follow-up period.

However, Deal et al.[42] found that whilst audiometric-defined hearing impaired individuals performed worse than normal hearers at baseline on a memory task, no significant differences between hearing impaired and normal hearing groups were found for rates of cognitive change over a seven-year follow-up period. Similar findings were found between self-reported hearing loss and a memory test using data from a Taiwanese population-based study of adults aged 50+.[49] Other studies with follow-up durations of two and nine years have also not found hearing loss to be independently associated with cognitive decline.[47,50] However, several studies in multiple countries with follow-up periods ranging from 5 to 12 years have found hearing loss to be significantly associated with poorer rates of decline in executive functioning and processing speed,[51] and memory.[52,53] Potential explanations for these discrepant findings include differences in methodology (e.g. different assessment tests, different definitions of hearing loss), different participant characteristics, or a lack of statistical power.

Few studies have investigated the association between hearing loss and rates of cognitive decline for longer than a 12-year period. However, the relationship between self-reported hearing loss and prospective cognitive decline over a 25-year period was investigated by Amieva et al.[54] In this study, 3670 participants aged 65+ were asked at baseline: 'Do you have hearing trouble?' In a model adjusted for age, sex, and education it was found that self-reported hearing loss was associated with faster rates of cognitive decline, as measured by the MMSE, over a 25-year follow up. However, this association did not survive correction for additional covariates. Deal et al.[55] investigated the relationship between hearing loss and retrospective 20-year cognitive decline using audiometric data from a pilot study within the Atherosclerosis Risk in Communities Study (ARIC). ARIC is a large, biracial prospective cohort study that enrolled 15,792 participants aged 45–64 years from four US communities in 1987–1989. The pilot study contained 253 white participants (mean age = 77) who received audiometric testing in 2013 and who had completed a battery of cognitive tests in the domains of memory, language, and speed of processing and attention in the preceding 20 years. It was found that moderate or greater hearing loss (>40 dB) was associated with a faster rate of prior 20-year decline in memory and global cognitive function. Although, as hearing loss was only measured in 2013, it was not possible to determine the causal relationship between hearing loss and cognitive functioning. In a systematic review[56] that included 33 studies and a meta-analysis, it was demonstrated that hearing loss is associated with poorer cognitive functioning in attention and processing speed, short-term and working memory, long-term memory, executive functioning, and language, although effect sizes were small.

Different cognitive tests, different definitions of hearing impairment, or a lack of statistical power in some studies, could explain discrepant results between studies. Known confounders such as demographic factors and cardiovascular risk factors have often been adjusted for. Whilst there is still likely to be residual confounding from unmeasured common pathologic factors (e.g. mitochondrial ageing, neuroinflammation), the association of hearing loss and cognition, particularly in the domains of memory, executive functioning, and processing speed, across multiple studies and independent datasets, strongly suggest that there are mechanistic pathways through which peripheral hearing loss contributes to cognitive decline.

A recent systematic review and meta-analysis explored the relationship between hearing loss and incident dementia.[44] This review identified three longitudinal studies[42,45,47] that had at least five years of follow-up, measured hearing loss objectively, and adjusted for age and cardiovascular risk factors. A pooled risk ratio of 1.94 (95% CI 1.38, 2.73) was observed, showing that hearing loss was a significant risk factor for dementia. In that same paper, the authors estimated that nine potentially modifiable risk factors account for 35% of dementia. Of these nine risk factors, hearing loss was estimated to have the largest contribution, accounting for 9.1%, followed by early life education (7.5%), smoking (5.5%), depression (4.0%), physical inactivity (2.6%), social isolation (2.3%), hypertension (2.0%), diabetes (1.2%), and obesity (0.8%).

The most salient and pressing public health question that arises is whether existing hearing rehabilitative therapies, which remain underutilized,[57,58] could potentially reduce cognitive decline in older adults.

Impact of Hearing Rehabilitative Therapies on Cognitive Functioning

Acute effects of hearing amplification

Many neuropsychological tests incorporate auditory stimuli or verbal instructions. Hearing amplification could affect performance in two ways: through enabling speech understanding or reducing cognitive load. On the one hand, if the hearing impairment is severe enough that instructions or verbal stimuli are not heard accurately, then the participant may not understand the task requirements or may mishear target words in a memory recall task. Hearing amplification may improve speech understanding so that the participant accurately hears verbal instructions and stimuli. Therefore, any improvement in performance is simply an artefact of the testing procedure and reflects a testing bias. On the other hand, even if there is adequate speech perception without amplification, hearing amplification can provide a clearer auditory signal. As a result, fewer cognitive resources are required to decode the auditory input, enabling more resources to be used on the neuropsychological test, which could result in better performance. However, these effects are not likely to be transferable to, or reflective of, everyday functioning if the participant does not routinely use the sensory aids.

In order to distinguish between the two possibilities outlined above, it is necessary to ensure that test performance is not confounded by a lack of audibility. If standard neuropsychological testing procedures, such as administering the test face to face in a quiet room, are followed, then inadequate speech understanding is unlikely to be an issue for those with mild-to-moderate hearing loss. However, individuals with severe-to-profound hearing loss may still have difficulty understanding verbal instructions and stimuli even when the testing environment adheres to standard neuropsychological test guidelines. As such, protocols for assessing whether the participant has accurately heard instructions and stimuli should be routinely followed when administering neuropsychological tests to individuals with hearing loss. Such a protocol could involve asking participants to repeat back spoken stimuli or instructions as well as having the tester speaking clearly and slowly.[59]

Long-term outcomes

Despite the high prevalence of hearing loss,[2] fewer than 20% of individuals with a hearing loss over the age of 70 use a hearing aid.[57] Importantly, previous studies provide proof of principle that hearing aids, or interventions that provide enhanced auditory stimuli, can engage and modify the hypothesized mechanistic pathways linking hearing and cognition (Fig. 34.1) through reducing cognitive load,[60–62] altering functional pathways and brain structure,[63–65] and improving social engagement.[66]

Results from observational epidemiologic studies of hearing aid use and cognition are difficult to interpret. Most studies have demonstrated a trend toward self-reported hearing aid use being positively associated with cognitive functioning,[40,41,45,48] and in some cases these results have reached significance.[54,55] However, data on other key variables (e.g. years of hearing aid use, adequacy of hearing aid fitting, and rehabilitation, etc.) that would affect the success of hearing loss treatment and affect any observed association have not been available in these studies. This limitation, coupled with other methodological issues (e.g. small sample), make drawing any conclusions on the impact of hearing aids on cognition premature.[67]

Results obtained from observational studies must also be interpreted with caution because individuals who choose to use a hearing aid likely differ from those individuals not using a hearing aid in both measured and unmeasured factors. In a recent meta-analysis[56] it was demonstrated that interventions for hearing loss, which included, but were not limited to, hearing aids, significantly improved cognitive functioning. However, this analysis contained just four studies, had a small effect size and there was evidence of publication bias. Consequently, determining whether hearing rehabilitative strategies could affect cognitive decline will require a randomized trial. The importance of conducting such a trial has been highlighted recently in the USA by high-profile national advisory bodies.[58] A recent pilot study[68] of a randomized controlled trial compared the impact of a successful ageing education intervention and a best practice hearing rehabilitative intervention on cognitive functioning over a six-month period. The successful ageing education intervention followed the ten keys to ageing programme and consisted of four one-hour sessions with a research nurse. During these one-on-one sessions the participant selected a 'key' topic relevant to chronic disease and disability prevention to focus on. The hearing intervention consisted of four one-hour sessions with an audiologist. During these one-on-one sessions the participant's needs were assessed, participants received bilateral hearing aids, participants were offered assistive listening devices, and rehabilitative counselling was provided. An early efficacy signal of improved cognitive function, particularly in memory, was observed after six months for the hearing group. This pilot study has demonstrated the feasibility of conducting a full-scale trial which has been planned to randomize 850 individuals who will be followed up over three years. To that end, the full-scale Aging and Cognitive Health Evaluation in Elders (ACHIEVE) study began in 2017. Trials such as this will be able to inform us whether existing hearing rehabilitative therapies could potentially reduce cognitive decline in older adults.

Conclusion

Epidemiologic studies demonstrate that peripheral hearing loss in older adults is strongly and independently associated with accelerated cognitive decline and incident dementia. Hypothesized mechanistic pathways underlying this observed association include the effects of poor hearing and distorted peripheral encoding of sound on cognitive load, brain structure/function, and reduced social engagement. Identifying interventions to reduce cognitive decline is a critical public health priority. Research thus far has suggested that interventions for hearing loss can provide benefits to cognitive functioning. Results from the ongoing ACHIEVE randomized control trial are needed to determine whether hearing rehabilitative strategies could affect cognitive decline and the risk of dementia.

REFERENCES

1. World Health Organization. WHO global estimates on prevalence of hearing loss (Internet). 2012. Available from: http://www.who.int/pbd/deafness/estimates/en/.
2. Goman AM, Lin FR. Prevalence of hearing loss by severity in the United States. Am J Public Health. 2016; 106(10): 1820–2.
3. Lin FR, Thorpe R, Gordon-Salant S, Ferrucci L. Hearing loss prevalence and risk factors among older adults in the United States. J Gerontol A Biol Sci Med Sci. 2011; 66(5): 582–90.
4. Lin FR, Maas P, Chien W, Carey JP, Ferrucci L, Thorpe R. Association of skin color, race/ethnicity, and hearing loss among adults in the USA. JARO—J Assoc Res Otolaryngol. 2012; 13(1): 109–17.
5. Charitidi K, Meltser I, Tahera Y, Canlon B. Functional responses of estrogen receptors in the male and female auditory system. Hear Res. 2009; 252(1–2): 71–8.
6. Cruickshanks KJ, Nondahl DM, Tweed TS, Wiley TL, Klein BEK, Klein R, et al. Education, occupation, noise exposure history and the 10-yr cumulative incidence of hearing impairment in older adults. Hear Res. 2010; 264(1–2): 3–9.
7. Gates GA, Cobb JL, D'Agostino RB, Wolf PA. The relation of hearing in the elderly to the presence of cardiovascular disease and cardiovascular risk factors. Arch Otolaryngol Head Neck Surg. 1993; 119(2): 156–61.
8. Cruickshanks KJ, Klein R, Klein BK, Wiley TL, Nondahl DM, Tweed TS. Cigarette smoking and hearing loss: The epidemiology of hearing loss study. JAMA. 1998; 279(21): 1715–19.
9. Quaranta N, Coppola F, Casulli M, Barulli MR, Barulli O, Panza F, et al. The prevalence of peripheral and central hearing impairment and its relation to cognition in older adults. Audiol Neurootol. 2014; 19(Suppl 1): 10–14.
10. Humes LE, Dubno JR, Gordon-Salan S, Lister JJ, Cacace AT, Cruickshanks KJ, et al. Central presbycusis: A review and evaluation of the evidence. J Am Acad Audiol. 2012; 23(8): 635–66.
11. Kiely KM, Gopinath B, Mitchell P, Browning CJ, Anstey KJ. Evaluating a dichotomized measure of self-reported hearing loss against gold standard audiometry. J Aging Health. 2012; 24(3): 439–58.
12. Uhlmann RF, Larson EB, Rees TS, Koepsell TD, Duckert LG. Relationship of hearing impairment to dementia and cognitive dysfunction in older adults. JAMA. 1989; 261(13): 1916–19.
13. Pickles JO. An Introduction to the Physiology of Hearing. Vol. 1. Bingley, West Yorks: Emerald Group Publishing, 2008.
14. Lin FR, Albert M. Hearing loss and dementia—who is listening? Aging Ment Health. 2014; 18(6): 671–3.
15. Pichora-Fuller MK, Schneider BA, Daneman M. How young and old adults listen to and remember speech in noise. J Acoust Soc Am. 1995; 97(1): 593–608.
16. McCoy SL, Tun PA, Cox LC, Colangelo M, Stewart RA, Wingfield A. Hearing loss and perceptual effort: downstream effects on older adults' memory for speech. Q J Exp Psychol A. 2005; 58(1): 22–33.
17. Wingfield A, McCoy SL, Peelle JE, Tun PA, Cox LC. Effects of adult aging and hearing loss on comprehension of rapid speech varying in syntactic complexity. J Am Acad Audiol. 2006; 17(7): 487–97.
18. Kahneman D. Attention and Effort. Englewood Cliffs, New Jersey: Prentice-Hall Inc., 1973.
19. Wingfield A, Grossman M. Language and the aging brain: patterns of neural compensation revealed by functional brain imaging. J Neurophysiol. 2006; 96(6): 2830–9.
20. Peelle JE, Troiani V, Grossman M, Wingfield A. Hearing loss in older adults affects neural systems supporting speech comprehension. J Neurosci Off J Soc Neurosci. 2011; 31(35): 12638–43.
21. Davis MH, Johnsrude IS. Hearing speech sounds: top-down influences on the interface between audition and speech perception. Hear Res. 2007; 229(1–2): 132–47.
22. Husain FT, Medina RE, Davis CW, Szymko-Bennett Y, Simonyan K, Pajor NM, et al. Neuroanatomical changes due to hearing loss and chronic tinnitus: a combined VBM and DTI study. Brain Res. 2011; 1369: 74–88.
23. Miao W, Li J, Tang M, Xian J, Li W, Liu Z, et al. Altered white matter integrity in adolescents with prelingual deafness: a high-resolution tract-based spatial statistics imaging study. Am J Neuroradiol. 2013; 34(6): 1264–70.
24. Cheung SW, Bonham BH, Schreiner CE, Godey B, Copenhaver DA. Realignment of interaural cortical maps in asymmetric hearing loss. J Neurosci Off J Soc Neurosci. 2009; 29(21): 7065–78.
25. Gröschel M, Götze R, Ernst A, Basta D. Differential impact of temporary and permanent noise-induced hearing loss on neuronal cell density in the mouse central auditory pathway. J Neurotrauma. 2010; 27(8): 1499–507.
26. Lin FR, Ferrucci L, An Y, Goh JO, Doshi J, Metter EJ, et al. Association of hearing impairment with brain volume changes in older adults. Neuroimage. 2014; 15(90): 84–92.
27. Davis MH, Gaskell MG. A complementary systems account of word learning: neural and behavioural evidence. Philos Trans R Soc B Biol Sci. 2009; 364(1536): 3773–800.
28. Adank P. Design choices in imaging speech comprehension: an Activation Likelihood Estimation (ALE) meta-analysis. NeuroImage. 2012; 63(3): 1601–13.
29. Kantarci K, Jack CR. Quantitative magnetic resonance techniques as surrogate markers of Alzheimer's disease. NeuroRx. 2004; 1(2): 196–205.
30. Chételat G, Landeau B, Eustache F, Mézenge F, Viader F, de la Sayette V, et al. Using voxel-based morphometry to map the structural changes associated with rapid conversion in MCI: a longitudinal MRI study. NeuroImage. 2005; 27(4): 934–46.
31. Weinstein BE, Ventry IM. Hearing impairment and social isolation in the elderly. J Speech Hear Res. 1982; 25(4): 593–9.
32. Sung Y, Li L, Blake C, Betz J, Lin FR. Association of hearing loss and loneliness in older adults. J Aging Health. 2015; 1–16.
33. Fratiglioni L, Wang HX, Ericsson K, Maytan M, Winblad B. Influence of social network on occurrence of dementia: a community-based longitudinal study. Lancet. 2000; 355(9212): 1315–19.
34. Bennett DA, Schneider JA, Tang Y, Arnold SE, Wilson RS. The effect of social networks on the relation between Alzheimer's disease pathology and level of cognitive function in old people: a longitudinal cohort study. Lancet Neurology. 2006; 5(5): 406–12.
35. Berkman LF, Glass T, Brissette I, Seeman TE. From social integration to health: Durkheim in the new millennium. Soc Sci Med. 2000; 51(6): 843–57.
36. Seeman TE. Health promoting effects of friends and family on health outcomes in older adults. Am J Health Promot AJHP. 2000; 14(6): 362–70.
37. Cole SW, Hawkley LC, Arevalo JM, Sung CY, Rose RM, Cacioppo JT. Social regulation of gene expression in human leukocytes. Genome Biol. 2007; 8(9): R189.
38. Seeman TE, McEwen BS. Impact of social environment characteristics on neuroendocrine regulation. Psychosom Med. 1996; 58(5): 459–71.

39. Uhlmann RF, Larson EB, Koepsell TD. Hearing impairment and cognitive decline in senile dementia of the Alzheimer's type. J Am Geriatr Soc. 1986; 34(3): 207–10.
40. Lin FR. Hearing loss and cognition among older adults in the United States. J Gerontol. 2011; 66(10): 1131–6.
41. Lin FR, Ferrucci L, Metter EJ, An Y, Zonderman AB, Resnick SM. Hearing loss and cognition in the Baltimore Longitudinal Study of Aging. Neuropsychology. 2011; 25(6): 763– 70.
42. Deal JA, Betz J, Yaffe K, Harris T, Purchase-Helzner E, Satterfield S, et al. Hearing impairment and incident dementia and cognitive decline in older adults: The Health ABC Study. J Gerontol A Biol Sci Med Sci. 2017; 72(5): 703–9.
43. Harrison Bush AL, Lister JJ, Lin FR, Betz J, Edwards JD. Peripheral hearing and cognition: evidence from the Staying Keen in Later Life (SKILL) Study. Ear Hear. 2015; 36(4): 395–407.
44. Livingston G, Sommerlad A, Orgeta V, Costafreda SG, Huntley J, Ames D, et al. Dementia prevention, intervention, and care. Lancet. 2017; 390(10113): 2673–734.
45. Lin FR, Metter EJ, O'Brien RJ, Resnick SM, Zonderman AB, Ferrucci L. Hearing loss and incident dementia. Arch Neurol. 2011; 68(2): 214–20.
46. Gurgel RK, Ward PD, Schwartz S, Norton MC, Foster NL, Tschanz JT. Relationship of hearing loss and dementia: a prospective, population-based study. Otol Neurotol Off Publ Am Otol Soc Am Neurotol Soc Eur Acad Otol Neurotol. 2014; 35(5): 775–81.
47. Gallacher J, Ilubaera V, Ben-Shlomo Y, Bayer A, Fish M, Babisch W, et al. Auditory threshold, phonologic demand, and incident dementia. Neurology. 2012; 79(15): 1583–90.
48. Lin FR, Yaffe K, Xia J, Xue Q-L, Harris TB, Purchase-Helzner E, et al. Hearing loss and cognitive decline in older adults. JAMA Intern Med. 2013; 173(4): 293–9.
49. Wu S-T, Chiu C-J. Age-related trajectories of memory function in middle-aged and older adults with and without hearing impairment. Neuroepidemiology. 2016; 46: 282–9.
50. Anstey KJ, Hofer SM, Luszcz MA. A latent growth curve analysis of late-life sensory and cognitive function over 8 years: evidence for specific and common factors underlying change. Psychol Aging. 2003; 18(4): 714–26.
51. Uchida Y, Nishita Y, Tange C, Sugiura S, Otsuka R, Ueda H, et al. The longitudinal impact of hearing impairment on cognition differs according to cognitive domain. Front Aging Neurosci. 2016; 8: 201.
52. Valentijn SAM, van Boxtel MPJ, van Hooren SAH, Bosma H, Beckers HJM, Ponds RWHM, et al. Change in sensory functioning predicts change in cognitive functioning: results from a 6-year follow-up in the Maastricht aging study. J Am Geriatr Soc. 2005; 53(3): 374–80.
53. Mitoku K, Masaki N, Ogata Y, Okamoto K. Vision and hearing impairments, cognitive impairment and mortality among long-term care recipients: a population-based cohort study. BMC Geriatr. 2016; 16: 112.
54. Amieva H, Ouvrard C, Giulioli C, Meillon C, Rullier L, Dartigues J-F. Self-reported hearing loss, hearing aids, and cognitive decline in elderly adults: a 25-year study. J Am Geriatr Soc. 2015; 63(10): 2099–104.
55. Deal JA, Sharrett AR, Albert MS, Coresh J, Mosley TH, Knopman D, et al. Hearing impairment and cognitive decline: a pilot study conducted within the atherosclerosis risk in communities neurocognitive study. Am J Epidemiol. 2015; 181(9): 680–90.
56. Taljaard DS, Olaithe M, Brennan-Jones CG, Eikelboom RH, Bucks RS. The relationship between hearing impairment and cognitive function: a meta-analysis in adults. Clin Otolaryngol. 2016; 41(6): 718–29.
57. Chien W, Lin FR. Prevalence of hearing aid use among older adults in the United States. Arch Intern Med. 2012; 172(3): 292–3.
58. NASEM (National Academies of Sciences, Engineering, and Medicine). Hearing health care: Priorities for improving access and affordability (Internet). Washington, DC: National Academies Press; 2016. Available from: doi: 10.17226/23446.
59. Lezak MD, Howieson DB, Loring DW, Hannay HJ, Fischer JS. Neuropsychological assessment (4th edition). New York: Oxford University Press, 2004.
60. Hornsby BWY. The effects of hearing aid use on listening effort and mental fatigue associated with sustained speech processing demands. Ear Hear. 2013; 34(5): 523–34.
61. Picou E, Ricketts TA, Hornsby BWY. How hearing aids, background noise, and visual cues influence objective listening effort. Ear Hear. 2013; 1–13.
62. Desjardins JL. The effects of hearing aid directional microphone and noise reduction processing on listening effort in older adults with hearing loss. J Am Acad Audiol. 2016; 27(1): 29–41.
63. Philibert B, Collet L, Vesson J-F, Veuillet E. Intensity-related performances are modified by long-term hearing aid use: a functional plasticity? Hear Res. 2002; 165(1–2): 142–51.
64. Munro KJ. Reorganization of the adult auditory system: perceptual and physiological evidence from monaural fitting of hearing aids. Trends Amplif. 2008; 12(3): 254–71.
65. Hwang J-H, Wu C-W, Chen J-H, Liu T-C. Changes in activation of the auditory cortex following long-term amplification: an fMRI study. Acta Otolaryngol (Stockholm). 2006; 126(12): 1275–80.
66. Chisolm TH, Johnson CE, Danhauer JL, Portz LJP, Abrams HB, Lesner S, et al. A systematic review of health-related quality of life and hearing aids: final report of the American Academy of Audiology Task Force on the health-related quality of life benefits of amplification in adults. J Am Acad Audiol. 2007; 18(2): 151–83.
67. Wallhagen MI, Strawbridge WJ. Association between hearing aid use and cognitive decline. J Am Geriatr Soc. 2016; 64(5): 1147–8.
68. Deal JA, Albert MS, Arnold M, Bangidwala S, Chisolm T, Davis S, et al. A randomized pilot trial of hearing treatment for reducing cognitive decline: Results from the Aging, Cognition, and Hearing Evaluation in Elders Pilot (ACHIEVE-P) study. Alzheimer's Dement Transl Res Clin Interv. 2017; 3(3): 410–15.

SECTION 7
Infections, exposures, injuries, and the brain

35

The neuroepidemiology of human prion disease

Patrick JM Urwin and Anna M Molesworth

Introduction

Prion diseases affect both humans and animals, and comprise a number of rare and ultimately fatal neurodegenerative conditions that result from the accumulation in the CNS of an abnormal form of a naturally occurring protein, called the prion protein.[1] This protein, coded for by the prion protein gene (*PRNP*), is widely expressed in many different tissues although it is predominantly found in the CNS.[2] In its normal, protease sensitive form, designated PrP^c, the prion protein is thought to be neuroprotective even though its exact function remains unclear; in disease states, PrP^c is converted to an abnormal form, designated PrP^{Sc}, following a 'seeding' event. The PrP^{Sc} is protease resistant and able to propagate through further contact with PrP^c, building up over extended incubation periods and causing pathology in the CNS tissues involved.

Prion disease in humans is characterized by prolonged incubation periods followed by a relatively rapid progressive loss of cognitive and motor functions. Case identification relies principally on the investigation of suspected cases by neurologists and neuropathologists, although other specialities, for example general and elderly medicine, and old age psychiatry may be involved. Clinical diagnostic criteria include abnormal neurological features and investigation results, the latter principally involving magnetic resonance imaging of the brain and CSF tests. Definitive diagnosis, however, requires neuropathological assessment, usually at post-mortem, where there may be evidence of aggregated PrP^{Sc}, gliosis, neuronal loss and brain tissue vacuolation, or spongiform change[3] (see also http://www.cjd.ed.ac.uk/sites/default/files/criteria_0.pdf). Currently there are no diagnostic blood tests for pre-clinical infection.

Human prion diseases can be classified as genetic, sporadic, or acquired, according to the initial PrP^{Sc} seeding event thought to have occurred (see Fig. 35.1). According to the prion hypothesis, genetic or familial prion disease in humans is associated with the presence of over 30 established *PRNP* mutations that destabilize PrP^c and cause or predispose to conversion to PrP^{Sc}. In sporadic disease, the initial seeding event is thought to be a spontaneous protein misfolding event, likely associated with a somatic mutation or chance conversion of PrP^c to PrP^{Sc} of unknown cause. Acquired disease results from exposure to exogenous PrP^{Sc}, from an animal or another human. A methionine-valine polymorphism at codon 129 of the *PRNP* gene affects disease phenotype as well as susceptibility, with methionine homozygosity at this locus predisposing to prion disease and the presence of valine generally associated with longer incubation periods and slower disease progression.[4,5]

In recent years there has been increased interest in the field of human prions, with evidence that the proteins associated with other neurodegenerative diseases, for example Aβ associated with AD, may also propagate in a prion-like manner.[6] Recent evidence of Aβ seeding in the brains of UK recipients of human pituitary derived growth hormone has also raised concerns regarding the potential for transmission through surgery and other routes.[7] Although there is no evidence to date that AD itself has been caused in this way, research into the potential transmissibility of non-prion neurodegenerative disorders will continue to be important to clarify these issues in the future. However, we have not included these other conditions in this chapter, instead focusing on the classical definition of prion disease. As detailed below, our focus is on Creutzfeldt-Jakob Disease (CJD) and variant Creutzfeldt-Jakob Disease (vCJD) although we will mention other forms of human prion disease, as well as animal prion diseases relevant to humans.

Sporadic Creutzfeldt-Jakob Disease

Clinical-pathological features

CJD was first described in 1920 by the neuropathologist Hans Creutzfeldt[8] and shortly afterwards by neurologist Alfons Jakob.[9] Although rare, the majority of CJD cases are idiopathic, occurring sporadically worldwide. Most sporadic CJD patients suffer rapidly progressive cognitive decline with myoclonus, ataxia, cortical visual impairment, pyramidal and/or extrapyramidal signs, progressing to akinetic mutism before death. Disease duration from first symptoms to death is usually short, with a median of around four months. However, there can be significant variation, with death occurring within one month of onset or after several years. Sporadic

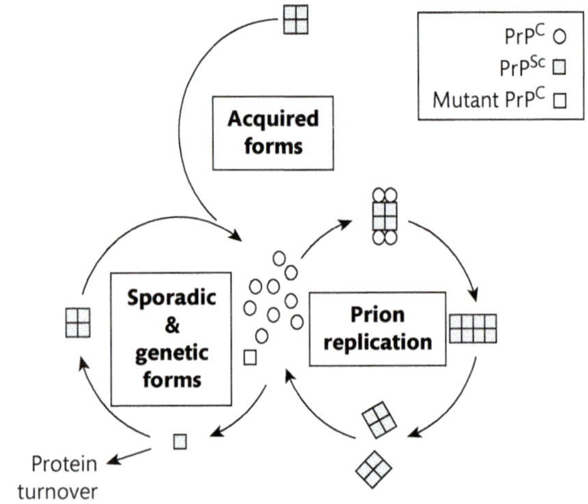

Fig. 35.1 Simplified schematic of the prion hypothesis.
Reproduced courtesy of Mark Head, NCJDRSU, Edinburgh (UK).

CJD is clinically heterogenous, with the patient's *PRNP* codon 129 methionine-valine polymorphism status and the type (type 1 or type 2) of the protease-resistant component of PrP^{Sc} found when investigating PrP^{Sc} by Western Blot, designated PrP^{res}, associated with the clinical and pathological phenotype.[4] This combination of *PRNP* codon 129 polymorphism status and PrP^{res} type is the most widely used classification system to describe the different subtypes of sporadic CJD. MM1 and MM2 are the most common and best documented forms, representing 70% of all patients, with a duration from symptom onset to death of four months. The VV2 subtype comprises 16% of all sporadic CJD, with a duration of six months, typically presenting with early cerebellar ataxia, prior to the onset of other clinical features. The MV2 subtype comprises 9% of patients, and presents similarly to VV2 but with a longer duration of 17 months.[10] The remaining subtypes of MM2-thalamic, MM2-cortical, and VV1 represent the remaining 5% of patients, and are each associated with relatively slow disease courses (15 months). There are relatively distinct neuropathological features associated with each of the subtypes. PrP^{res} 1 and 2 can coexist in a single patient, with the clinical presentation usually reflecting the dominant PrP^{res} subtype.[11] Aside from any theoretical importance, the subgroup classification is useful to clinicians in emphasizing the heterogenous clinical nature of sporadic CJD. However, while clinical investigation results may vary with subtype, in the late stages of illness the clinical picture across all subtypes becomes one of severe brain disease and often the terminal state is one of akinetic mutism.

Incidence and basic demographics

Sporadic CJD occurs at annual rates of between one and two cases per million population worldwide (see http://www.eurocjd.ed.ac.uk/surveillance data 1.html). It affects males and females approximately equally and is a disease mainly of the older population. In the UK, the median age at death is 68 (range 20–95) with a peak in mortality between 65 and 79 years of age, and fewer cases in individuals under 50 or above 80 years of age, although cases have been reported in adolescents and adults over 90.

In the UK and other countries with well-established surveillance systems, annual mortality rates for sporadic CJD have increased over time (see Fig. 35.2).[12] This may reflect better ascertainment of cases across all ages, particularly in older patients who have perhaps become better investigated as new treatments and diagnostic tools are developed for certain forms of dementia. However, the low rate of disease seen in the most elderly is noteworthy, in that perhaps more cases might be expected in this age group from a sporadic protein misfolding event. It is unclear whether this decline in incidence at older ages is real or reflects incomplete case ascertainment in the most elderly, the diagnosis perhaps being mistaken for a more common dementia, resulting in cases of prion disease being missed.[13,14]

Risk factors

Codon 129 may be regarded as a risk factor for the development of sporadic CJD, with over-representation amongst cases of the homozygote states, particularly methionine, relative to the general population.[15]

Although some exposures to sporadic CJD in medical settings have resulted in transmission from person to person, associated with the accidental transplantation of infective tissue or inoculation of small amounts of residual tissue adhering to reusable surgical instruments (see section on iatrogenic CJD below), no consistent

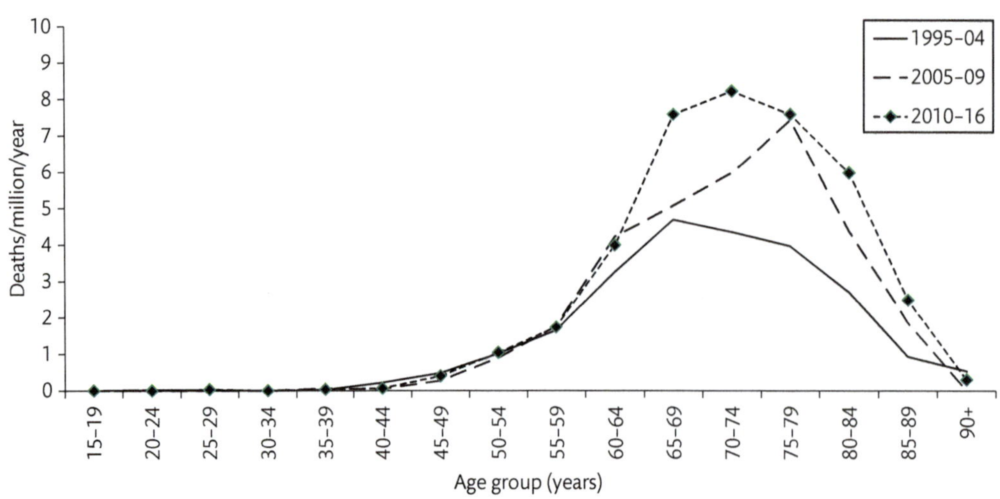

Fig. 35.2 Age-specific mortality from sporadic CJD in the UK, 1995–2016.
Reproduced courtesy of NCJDRSU, Edinburgh (UK)

risk factors for the development of sporadic CJD have been identified. Some case-control studies have identified an increased risk of sporadic CJD associated with prior surgical exposure[16–18] or through blood transfusion,[19] but this has not been convincingly demonstrated by others.[20,21] In addition, there is no evidence of an increased occupational risk,[22] even though people employed in certain professions, for example neuropathologists or neurosurgeons, might be exposed to infectivity in the course of their work. Very occasionally, sporadic CJD cases are identified who have lived close together at some point in their lives, raising the possibility that the cases may be linked, for example a husband and wife pair, both of whom developed sporadic CJD.[23] One analysis has also provided evidence of increasing geographic clustering of sporadic CJD cases with increasing time before disease onset, consistent with some sporadic CJD cases resulting from past exposure to a common external factor.[24] Identifying a common source of transmission many years after the event is difficult, however, and there are other limitations to the above studies, not least bias and confounding.[25] While it is plausible that a small number of cases classified as sporadic CJD have resulted from transmission associated with other, as yet unidentified, causative factors, the evidence for this is weak. Overall the findings are consistent with the hypothesis that sporadic CJD is not an acquired disease.

Variably Protease Sensitive Prionopathy

Recently a new disease called variably protease sensitive prionopathy (VPSPr) has been identified with distinct biochemical characteristics: the accumulating PrP^{Sc} shows a markedly different response to the proteases used in biochemical analysis from other forms of CJD, with variable sensitivity in different brain regions.[26,27] Affecting those in mid to later life, patients have a non-specific clinical profile and duration of illness ranging from under one to over five years; the pathology is atypical when compared with sporadic CJD.

Currently, the true incidence and underlying epidemiology of this novel prion disease are uncertain. Diagnosis is neuropathological and consequently case identification has been retrospective, with most cases of VPSPr worldwide having been identified in the UK (14 cases reported to date, see http://www.cjd.ed.ac.uk/sites/default/files/figs.pdf), as well the USA and other parts of Europe. Cases have been identified in all codon 129 *PRNP* polymorphism groups, but the disease has predominantly been identified in valine homozygotes, the rarest codon 129 status. Although research suggests that VPSPr has limited transmission potential,[28] its longer disease course and non-specific early clinical findings may mean VPSPr is falsely diagnosed as other forms of dementia and likely to be under-ascertained.

Variant Creutzfeldt-Jakob Disease

Clinical-pathological features

In 1996 a new disease, variant Creutzfeldt-Jakob Disease (vCJD), was identified in the UK.[29] It was differentiated from the more commonly encountered sporadic form of CJD by the young age of patients (the median age at death based on UK cases observed to date is 28, range 14–75) and unusual neuropathological and clinical features. Cases presented with a neuropsychiatric prodrome of apathy or withdrawal, early ataxia, early and prominent sensory features, and a notable absence in early stages of memory problems or dementia. Neuropathological examination identified plaques of PrP^{Sc} deposition, described as 'florid' and largely distinct from other forms of CJD, alongside the more typical features of spongiform changes, loss of neurones and astrocytosis seen in other prion disease. Cases had a longer disease duration than was typical of other forms of CJD; the median duration based on UK cases is currently 14 months (range 6–114).[12]

Incidence worldwide

Following reports of the first vCJD cases in 1996, the vCJD epidemic comprised a single wave of epidemic cases, peaking in the UK in 2000, later elsewhere, and subsequently declining to under one new diagnosis currently reported per year worldwide (see Fig. 35.3). At the time of writing, a total of 231 cases of vCJD have been

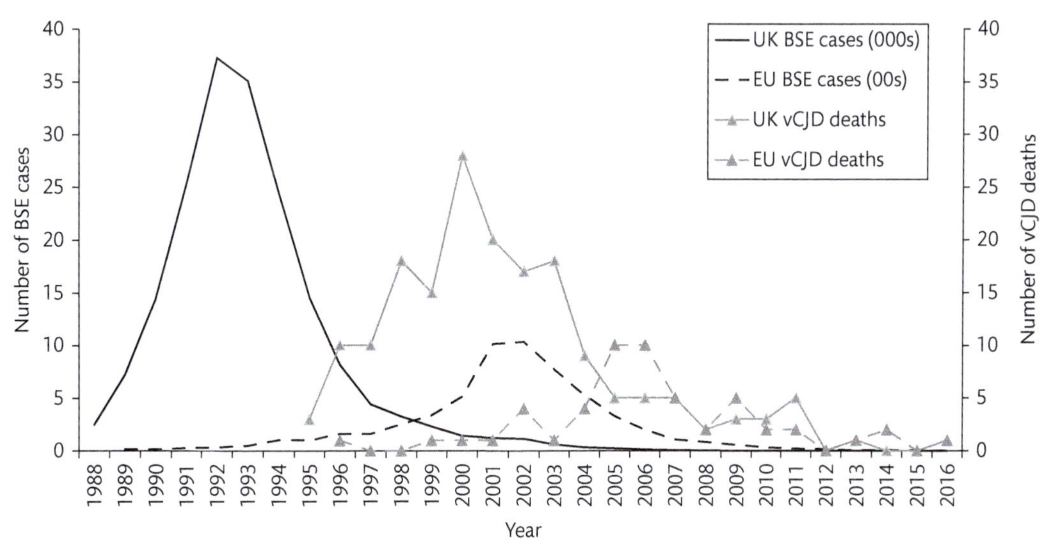

Fig. 35.3 BSE and vCJD deaths by year in the UK and other European Union (EU) countries.
Source: data from NCJDRSU, Edinburgh (UK) and World Organization for Animal Health.

identified worldwide, mostly (178, 77%) from the UK (see http://www.cjd.ed.ac.uk/sites/default/files/worldfigs.pdf). The non-UK vCJD cases have occurred mainly in France (27 cases), with no more than five cases reported in each of a small number of other countries in Europe and the rest of the world.

Biochemical similarities, transmission studies, and strong geographic and temporal associations with the animal zoonotic bovine spongiform encephalopathy (BSE) have provided strong laboratory and epidemiological evidence that vCJD and BSE are linked.[30–33] The first cases of BSE were reported in the UK in 1986.[34,35] In total, one million cattle are thought to have been infected during the ensuing BSE epidemic, with over 400,000 of these animals estimated to have entered the human food chain.[36] The epidemic peaked in 1992 and 1993 and then subsequently declined to one or two cases per year (see http://www.oie.int/en/animal-health-in-the-world/bse-specific-data/). Far fewer BSE cases have been diagnosed outside the UK.

Risk factors

The vast majority of UK vCJD cases have been attributed to transmission of the BSE agent to humans between 1980, when BSE is first thought to have been circulating, and 1996, when the final controls to protect animal and human food chains were put in place. Non-UK vCJD cases have been attributed to exposure to BSE in UK exported cattle, meat, or animal products, rather than indigenous infection, or to time spent in the UK during the period of potential BSE exposure.[37,38] The greatest risk to humans is thought to have been the dietary consumption of meat products which could have been contaminated with the BSE agent by the extraction techniques required in production of mechanically recovered meat,[39] or by contact with brain and other CNS material from infected animals during butchering,[40] particularly prior to the UK ban in 1989 of tissues of cattle, sheep, and goats (including brain, spinal cord, and other material) likely to be infective. It is certainly noteworthy that no UK cases have been born after 1989.

Other important risk factors include age. Despite the fact that most BSE exposure occurred in the UK in the late 1980s and early 1990s, the median age at onset of vCJD (26 years, range 12–74 years) has remained the same, consistent with those born in the 1980s being infected later in the BSE epidemic when they were older, rather than at the beginning (see http://www.cjd.ed.ac.uk/sites/default/files/cjdq72.pdf). This may reflect lower age-related susceptibility to infection[41] or reduced exposure to BSE in food in the very young.[42]

Codon 129 genotype is also important: until 2016, all neuropathologically confirmed cases of vCJD who were tested (119 tested of 123 confirmed cases) were found in methionine homozygous individuals; in 2016 the first pathologically confirmed case of vCJD in a methionine-valine heterozygous patient was identified.[43] Whether this case represents the beginning of a second epidemic wave of vCJD amongst other genotypes, or is an isolated case remains to be seen. The incubation period between exposure to infection and vCJD symptom onset is estimated to be 15 years; however, in non-methionine homozygous individuals this is likely to longer.[44] An earlier case of suspected vCJD has been reported in a codon 129 methionine-valine heterozygote; the patient lacked the supportive investigations to be classified, according to World Health Organization criteria, as a definite or probable case.[45]

Prevalence

Despite early fears of a very large epidemic, far fewer vCJD cases have arisen than anticipated. The reasons for this are unclear, but given the extensive exposure of the human population to BSE, it is likely that there is a substantial species barrier. Other factors may also be involved, including effect of dose, age-related and genetic susceptibility, and the presence of co-factors necessary for infection and the development of disease.[46,47]

Studies of the prevalence of PrP^{Sc} deposition in appendix tissue in the UK have, however, suggested a significant asymptomatic carrier state occurring at a frequency far higher than the observed symptomatic cases. This prevalence has been estimated at 1 in 2000 in those born 1941–85, the age group considered most exposed to BSE[48] with all codon 129 genetic subgroups affected and a higher proportion of valine homozygotes (25% of positive specimens) than would be expected in the normal population (11%). Rates of asymptomatic carriage consistent with the above have also been found in time periods outside the period 1980–1996, when the population had not previously been considered to be exposed to BSE.[49] While such asymptomatic infection is of unknown significance to the individuals' risk of developing vCJD, or as yet to interpreting the general population exposure to BSE, it is a significant public health concern.

Person-to-person spread

In vCJD, PrP^{Sc} is deposited outside the CNS at significantly higher levels compared to other forms of CJD, most likely due to the route of exposure to BSE across the gut.[50] This peripheral, predominantly lymphoreticular, pathogenesis outside the CNS in patients with vCJD has led to concerns regarding the potential for iatrogenic transmission of vCJD. This is a particular concern given the current absence in routine clinical and infection control practice, of both a decontamination method that can fully remove PrP^{Sc} from surgical instruments and a validated early blood test for pre-clinical disease.

There is no evidence of mother-to-child vertical transmission,[51] or from case-control studies of a risk of vCJD associated with occupation or past surgery.[39] Dental instruments may provide a route of transmission,[52] although no dental risk factors have been identified in UK cases.[53] Lookback studies have also not identified any associations between cases linked to tissue or organ transplantation.[54] Nonetheless such procedures may carry a risk of passing on vCJD infection if the donor were to be infective, depending on the mass of tissue transplanted, the site of transplant, and infectivity of the tissues involved.

Crucially, however, vCJD may be transmitted through blood. To date, three cases of vCJD have been identified worldwide, all occurring in the UK, where a patient received a non-leucodepleted red cell transfusion from a donor who subsequently developed vCJD.[55,56] These three cases, two of whom received blood from the same donor, became symptomatic of vCJD at 6.5, 7.8, and 8.3 years respectively after receiving the implicated transfusion. This is a shorter incubation period than is associated with dietary exposure to BSE. In addition, asymptomatic infection has been identified in the spleens of two patients who died of non-neurological illness. The first was a recipient of vCJD-implicated non-leucodepleted blood[57] and the other was treated with UK-sourced blood products, including batches of clotting factors derived from a donor who subsequently developed vCJD.[58] It is considered statistically unlikely that these splenic deposits of PrP^{Sc} were acquired through dietary means and this is supported by the absence of detectable PrP^{Sc} in their tonsils or gut associated lymphoid tissue. Both of these cases were codon 129 methionine-valine heterozygous; it is unknown whether, had they lived longer after the exposure, they might have developed clinical vCJD.

The occurrence of the blood/blood product-associated cases, together with laboratory evidence that indicates that the vCJD strain is not altered significantly following transfusion transmission,[59,60] suggest that transfusion of blood from vCJD donors may be an efficient means of transmission. To try to prevent (the at that point theoretical) transmission of vCJD through blood transfusion, leucodepletion was implemented in 1999 in the UK, based on experimental data suggesting that lymphocytes were involved in early pathogenesis, and there have been no further reports of blood or blood product associated transmission of vCJD subsequently.[61]

Kuru

Kuru was first described in western literature in 1957[62] although according to local verbal histories it may have dated back to around 1920. Originally known as the shaking palsy (the term kuru is derived from the local word meaning 'to shake with fear'), the disease was characterized by ataxia, tremor, and other movement disorders, emotional lability, and had a typical duration 4–24 months from symptom onset to death.

Kuru affected individuals in the Fore region of the eastern highlands of Papua New Guinea, disproportionately affecting women (67% of kuru patients) and children/adolescents of both sexes (23%) and was caused by ritual funeral endocannibalism. It is hypothesized that the epidemic began when an individual who died from sporadic CJD was consumed by their family members. Women were responsible for preparation for the mortuary feast, and women and children were significantly more likely to consume brain tissue during the ritual than men; furthermore, men tended not to eat materials from female relatives.[63] The incubation period for the disease has proven to be widely variable, between around 5 and 50 years, with codon 129 methionine valine heterozygotes having longer incubation periods and methionine homozygous individuals having earlier onset and more aggressive presentations.[64] Following the prohibition of cannibalism in the late 1950s, the number of cases declined steadily, first in the younger age groups born after the alteration in practice, with no new cases identified in individuals born after 1959. The last reported case died in 2005; as such kuru is now regarded as an historical disease.

A genetic polymorphism at codon 127 of the *PRNP* gene, not reported in other populations, has been identified among survivors of the kuru epidemic and appears to completely protect against prion diseases in animal studies, illustrating the very strong selection pressure exerted during the kuru epidemic.[65,66]

Iatrogenic Creutzfeldt-Jakob Disease

Incidence and sources of infection

A number of CJD cases worldwide have been acquired as a result of medical interventions, although the incidence varies from country to country, due mainly to differences in the medical practices that exposed the patients to CJD infectivity.[67,68] The main routes of transmission comprise human pituitary derived growth hormone and dura mater grafts, produced from cadaveric tissues presumed to have been sourced from cases of sporadic CJD or asymptomatic carriers who had died from an unrelated illness. There have also been a small number of CJD cases acquired through other iatrogenic routes. All these cases of secondary transmission of CJD have been associated with parenteral exposure to contaminated materials, the latter which were extracted from, or in close proximity to, brain tissue.[69]

Human pituitary derived hormones

Starting in the late 1950s, intramuscular injection of human pituitary derived growth hormone was used to treat short stature in children. By 1985, when the first related CJD cases occurred,[70–72] around 30,000 children had been treated worldwide. To date, around 240 cases have been identified in total worldwide, with deaths still occurring. More than half of these have occurred in France, where all of the cases received human pituitary derived growth hormone injections between December 1983 and July 1985, strongly suggesting that a batch of injections used in this time period was contaminated.[73] Smaller numbers have been seen in other countries, mainly the UK and USA.[67,68] Human gonadotropin was also extracted from cadavers around the same time period, and injected as a fertility treatment. There have been four cases of CJD reported among recipients of this hormone in Australia, the first reported in 1990,[74] the most recent in 1995. The production of all human pituitary derived hormones involved pooling of thousands of donated cadaveric pituitaries, increasing the potential for contamination before extraction of the relevant hormone. The use of human pituitary derived hormones was stopped in 1985 in most countries, and since then has been replaced with synthetic treatments, making new exposures through these routes unlikely to occur.

The clinical features of human pituitary derived hormone-related CJD differ from sporadic CJD cases, in that most cases typically presented with a progressive cerebellar, ataxic syndrome. In the UK, median survival has been 12 months, with dementia occurring infrequently and typically late in the illness.[69] Incubation periods made in relation to the midpoint of treatment range from 5 to 42 years worldwide, but are widely variable between countries, reflecting intercountry variation in dosage regimes and period of exposure, as well as the levels of infectivity to which cases were exposed. The estimated incubation period is 13 years in France, 20 years in the UK, and 22 years in the USA; the incubation period observed in the four recipients of gonadotrophin was from 12 to 16 years.[68] As in other human prion diseases, codon 129 polymorphisms impact upon incubation periods and susceptibility to the condition; methionine-valine heterozygosity is associated with longer incubation periods, and methionine homozygosity is more common among growth hormone iatrogenic CJD patients than the population prevalence. However differences in the codon 129 distribution of human pituitary derived growth hormone transmitted CJD have been also noted between different populations, which might be due to infection with different contaminating strains of the CJD agent.[73]

Cadaveric dura mater grafts

The dura mater is a tough membrane which surrounds and protects the brain. Until 1992, dura mater was commonly used as a patching material in neurosurgery, for example to repair cerebrospinal fluid leaks, and also in some other surgical domains. The first reported CJD death in a dura mater graft recipient occurred in 1979, and since then approximately 240 cases have been reported from 19 different countries worldwide.[67,68] The vast majority of these cases have been associated with a single brand, Lyodura®, and were treated between 1981 and 1987, when the production of Lyodura® was modified to include disinfection using sodium hydroxide. The exposure most likely resulted from cross-contamination in the production process.[69] Incubation periods for dura mater associated CJD from exposure to symptom onset have varied between 1 and 30 years, with a mean of 12. Most cases occurred during the 1990s, but small numbers continue to be reported.

Worldwide, more than 60% of dura mater graft related iatrogenic CJD has occurred in Japan, where grafts were used more frequently than in other countries, particularly for neurosurgery relating to vascular disease, hemifacial spasm, and trigeminal neuralgia.[75] Lyodura® was used predominantly, while other product brands were used with greater frequency in other countries. Codon 129 methionine homozygosity is far more common in Japan than in many other studied populations, found in 92% of the population, and appears to convey susceptibility to the development of human dura mater graft associated iatrogenic CJD. Cadaver derived dura mater usage was reduced substantially after 1991 with the development of synthetic substitutes, but may not have ceased until 1997.

Two distinct clinical and neuropathological phenotypes have been identified among the dura mater associated iatrogenic CJD patients.[76] Two-thirds of patients present similarly to sporadic CJD, but in some cases there is a prominent, isolated ataxic syndrome at onset and widespread plaque deposition. It is thought that these differences might arise from differences in the strains of sporadic CJD that contaminated the grafts. The group that mimic typical sporadic CJD presentations are suspected to have originated from methionine homozygous type 1 PrP^{res} or methionine-valine heterozygous type 1 PrP^{res} sporadic CJD donors, while those with the atypical presentation are thought most likely to have originated from a valine homozygous type 2 PrP^{res} subtype sporadic CJD donor.

Other iatrogenic risk factors

More rarely, cases of iatrogenic CJD have also been associated with corneal grafts, the use of infected neurosurgical instruments and EEG depth electrodes.[67–69] The first evidence of iatrogenic transmission of CJD was reported in 1974 in the recipient of a corneal transplant. The cornea had been sourced from the cadaver of a person subsequently found to have died from sporadic CJD.[77] The cornea recipient became symptomatic 18 months after grafting, and died 8 months later. A second case was reported in 1997, the recipient dying 30 years after the corneal graft.[78] It is likely that the implicated grafts in both these cases included small quantities of retinal tissue, which is continuous through the optic nerve with brain tissue. Other anterior eye tissues are not regarded as containing high levels of infectivity. There have also been multiple reports of death by CJD in recipients of corneal grafts where it has not been possible to identify the cause of death of the cornea donors; these cases might represent further cases of iatrogenic transmission of CJD, but more likely reflect the relatively common occurrence of corneal transplantation as an ophthalmological procedure.

There have been a small number of iatrogenic CJD cases associated with the re-use of stereotactic EEG depth electrodes (two cases, both linked to a single patient later confirmed as having died of CJD)[79] or neurosurgical instruments (four cases)[80,81] previously used on patients subsequently discovered to have CJD. The instruments were likely to have carried infectivity, allowing direct intracerebral inoculation of the infectious agent to the recipient's brain. Consequently, these procedures have been associated with shorter incubation periods than for other forms of iatrogenic CJD: 16 and 20 months for the two cases of EEG electrode transmission, and between 12 and 28 months for the four reported cases of neurosurgical instrument-related transmission.[68] Although PrP^{Sc} remains resistant to standard decontamination processes, there have been no new descriptions of surgical transmission through these routes reported since 1997.

Genetic Prion Disease

Incidence and geographic distribution

Genetic forms of prion disease account for around 10–15% of human prion disease, and are caused by over 30 known mutations within the *PRNP* prion protein gene.[82] These mutations alter the sequence of amino acids within the prion protein, resulting in an increased likelihood of conversion of PrP^{C} to PrP^{Sc}. The different mutations are associated with different clinical-pathological phenotypes of disease, for example affecting age at onset and duration of illness. There are considerable differences in the prevalence of genetic prion disease between countries and regions.[83,84]

Clinical-pathological features

There is significant variation in clinical phenotype between the different forms of genetic prion disease.[83,85] The most common genetic form of CJD is associated with the E200K mutation and may have a course indistinguishable from sporadic CJD, although it is typically associated with a younger age (30–60 years) at disease onset. Gerstmann-Sträussler-Scheinker syndrome (GSS, most frequently associated with the P102L mutation) and fatal familial insomnia (FFI, D178N 129M) usually have a slower disease course (2–5 years). GSS presents as a slowly progressive cerebellar ataxia and pyramidal syndrome, with later dementia. FFI patients present with insomnia and autonomic failure, unusual for the other human prion diseases. There is a sporadic disease, sporadic fatal insomnia (sFI), which is clinically and pathologically indistinguishable from FFI but lacks any FFI-associated *PRNP* mutation and is thought to be the rare MM2-thalamic subtype of sporadic CJD.

Risk factors

All the genetic forms of human prion disease are inherited in an autosomal dominant fashion, which means that if only one parent has the mutation there is a 50% chance of the offspring inheriting this.[83,85] However, a surprisingly high number of cases are identified in individuals with no known history in other family members (between 12% and 88%) and even in those families where the disease is known, it can appear to skip a generation. These occurrences may, to a large extent, be explained by age-dependent penetrance of the mutation, although other factors such as stigma around dementia preventing family discussion may play a role. For example, the E200K point mutation has penetrance of 0.45 by 60 years, increasing to 0.96 around 80 years, meaning that individuals may die of other causes before they develop genetic prion disease. Blood relations of patients with genetic prion disease may be eligible for pre-symptomatic testing to identify whether they carry the mutation and are at risk of developing the condition subsequently.

In the UK it is assumed that exposure in the medical setting to PrP^{Sc} in patients with or incubating pre-clinical genetic prion disease can result in a transmission risk, although no such cases are known to have arisen to date. Therefore public health precautions are taken for individuals with a recognized risk of developing genetic prion disease later in life, namely those with a known *PRNP* mutation or the presence of a *PRNP* mutation in a blood relative, or for other individuals who have not been tested, those with two or more relatives with any form of prion disease.[86]

Animal Prion Diseases

Scrapie

Scrapie cases were reported in the 1730s among sheep in England, but the disease has since been found in most countries where sheep are farmed, except Australia and New Zealand.[87] It is an acquired disease, associated with transmission through direct contact with infected animals and environmental contamination, where infectivity can persist for years. The classical form of the disease presents with intense pruritis, leading to rubbing and scraping which damages the wool, and provides the name of the disease. The disease has an incubation period of over two years and is fatal within two weeks to six months of clinical onset. Atypical scrapie differs on clinical, epidemiological, and neuropathological features and is not known to be transmissible among sheep through environmental routes. There is no evidence that scrapie, or atypical scrapie in sheep is transmissible to humans but public and veterinary health authorities remain vigilant to this possibility.[88]

Bovine Spongiform Encephalopathy

BSE was first reported as a new disease in 1986 in the UK, the first case coming to the attention of a veterinary surgeon in December 1984 and dying in early 1985, shortly before additional cows in the same herd developed similar signs.[34,35] The disease was noted to have similar neuropathological features to scrapie, kuru, and CJD, causing spongiform changes in the brain and spine of affected animals. The animals developed altered mental state, becoming fearful and aggressive, demonstrating exaggerated startling to minor stimuli and gait ataxia.

The disease is thought to have been spread among cattle through dietary supplementation (particularly given to young calves of dairy herds) using meat and bone meal (MBM), a protein rich product derived from cattle carcass waste products and used in intensive agriculture from the 1940s. The incubation period of the disease was around five years, suggesting that MBM may have been first contaminated in the late 1970s.[89,90] It is plausible that changes in the rendering process facilitated the transmission of the disease, although the initial source of contamination of MBM remains unknown. Hypotheses include contamination by scrapie material or a sporadic, atypical occurrence of BSE.

Following the identification of BSE, several steps to try to control the epidemic were introduced by the UK government and livestock farming industry. These included the withdrawal of cattle feed containing mammalian protein in 1988; the removal from animal and human food chains of tissues of cattle, sheep, and goats likely to be infective in 1989; and the ban on sale for human consumption of any cow older than 30 months in 1996. Similar measures followed worldwide and the totality of changes resulted in significant reductions in disease transmission both to animals and humans. Atypical forms of BSE in cattle (called H- and L-type BSE) have been identified. They are believed to occur sporadically, are typically found in older cattle and are associated with different clinical and neuropathological findings. They have been found in most countries with BSE surveillance and account only for a very small number of total BSE cases. They may represent a zoonotic risk to human health, although this is unclear.[91]

Chronic wasting disease

Chronic wasting disease (CWD) was first identified in north Colorado in 1967 among a captive population of a single species of deer.[92] Subsequently it has been identified in both wild and farmed animals across a number of cervid species, throughout North America and elsewhere, with cases identified in South Korea in 2002,[93] and more recently Norway in 2016[94] and Finland (see https://www.ruokavirasto.fi/en/farmers/animal-husbandry/animal-health-and-diseases/animal-diseases/wildlife/chronic-wasting-disease-cwd-in-cervids/).

Most likely initially spread through translocation of infected animals and animal products by farmers and hunters, outbreaks appear to be self-sustaining, with transmission likely to occur in the presence of live infected animals or as a result of the infectious agent persisting in the environment. The disease presents with slowly progressive weight loss, mobility, and behavioural changes (including a loss of fear of humans) and excess salivation due to difficulty swallowing and thirst, with urinary frequency. Most animals survive for a period of weeks up to four months from the point of diagnosis. PrP^{Sc} is found in high levels in animal CNS and lymphoid tissue, as well as other body tissues and fluids, even in pre-symptomatic animals. Moreover, infected animals express PrP^{Sc} in their saliva, blood, and urine, resulting in environmental contamination.[95] Once in the environment, the PrP^{Sc} binds to soil and vegetable matter and may be consumed by other animals.[96]

Concern has been raised in relation to both the impact of CWD on local ecology and the environment, and the risk CWD may pose to human health. The recent occurrence of CWD cases in Europe is a particular concern; the cases include the first instances of CWD reported in reindeer, which unlike previous naturally affected animals, live in huge herds, migrate across vast areas of land and form the staple diet of many indigenous people; there is evidence, moreover, in some of the European cervids of strain difference with North American strains. Hunting is a concern because enthusiasts may butcher and/or consume the animals they kill. It is highly likely that humans have already consumed CWD prions, and accumulated animal data suggest CWD may have zoonotic potential. This raises concern that we may witness transmission to humans in the years ahead, although to date, no such transmission to humans has been identified.[96,97] Should such transmission occur, efforts to eradicate the disease will be hampered by environmental contamination—a feature not identified in BSE.

Conclusion

Although human prion diseases are rare, their long incubation periods, transmissibility, and the risk of vCJD posed by asymptomatic carriage of PrP^{Sc} in the general population, along with the possibility that further cases of vCJD may occur in the future due to past food-borne infections in mostly unaffected codon-129 genotypes or as a result of secondary person-to-person spread, all caution against complacency.[46] Underlying these concerns is the absence of both a validated test that can be used to identify subclinical infection, and effective instrument decontamination methods that can fully remove the prion agent from instruments used in surgical practice, although progress continues to be made in both these areas. In the UK and many other countries, a range of public health measures have been put in place to protect the human and animal food chains, and to reduce the risk of person-to-person transmission in medical settings. These measures include universal precautions to better safeguard the supply of blood, organs, and tissues for transplantation, to mitigate against the risk of transmission through surgery and also potentially occupational exposure. Further precautions may be adopted for high-risk situations in relation to the handling of surgical instruments and the identification and notification of those with a specific exposure to infection through surgery, through treatment with blood or blood products or with a genetic risk.[86]

The possibility of animal sources of future human prion disease also cannot be excluded. There is no evidence that scrapie or atypical scrapie in sheep is transmissible to humans but the international CJD surveillance community remains vigilant to this possibility.[88] While the BSE epidemic is at an end, ongoing occasional atypical cases may represent a zoonotic risk to human health, although this is unclear.[91] The possibility of a widespread epidemic of CWD in cervids has elevated concerns for human health, as well as the impact this may have on the animal health and the environment.[94-97] Sporadic forms of human prion disease have varied phenotypes which, as demonstrated by VPSPr,[26] are challenging to diagnose in rarer or atypical cases. It is possible that some of these rarer forms of idiopathic origin may, in fact, reflect transmission of atypical or novel infections from an as yet unknown source, even though there is no evidence to date that this is the case.

Continued scrutiny of clinical-pathological phenotypes and epidemiological risk factors for prion disease in the general population and in those at risk, as part of national prion disease research and surveillance initiatives, is essential to help address the uncertainties and inform the subsequent management of risk.

REFERENCES

1. Prusiner SB. Novel proteinaceous infectious particles cause scrapie. Science. 1982; 216(4542): 136–44.
2. WHO. *WHO Table on Tissue Infectivity Distribution in Transmissible Spongiform Encephalopathies.* Geneva: World Health Organization, 2010.
3. WHO. *WHO Manual For Surveillance of Human Transmissible Spongiform Encephalopathies.* Geneva: World Health Organization, 2003.
4. Parchi P, Giese A, Capellari S, Brown P, Schulz-Schaeffer W, Windl O, et al. Classification of sporadic Creutzfeldt-Jakob disease based on molecular and phenotypic analysis of 300 subjects. Ann Neurol. 1999; 46(2): 224–33.
5. Bishop MT, Hart P, Aitchison L, Baybutt HN, Plinston C, Thomson V, et al. Predicting susceptibility and incubation time of human-to-human transmission of vCJD. Lancet Neurology. 2006; 5(5): 393–8.
6. Miller G. Neurodegeneration. Could they all be prion diseases? Science. 2009; 326(5958): 1337–9.
7. Ritchie DL, Adlard P, Peden AH, Lowrie S, Le Grice M, Burns K, et al. Amyloid-β accumulation in the CNS in human growth hormone recipients in the UK. Acta Neuropathologica. 2017; 134: 221–40.
8. Creutzfeldt H. Uber eine eigenartige herdformige Erkrankung des Zentralnervensystems. Gesamte Neurol. 1920; 57: 1–8.
9. Jakob A. Uber eigenartige Erkrankungen des Zentralnervensystems mit bemerkenswertem anatomishem Befunde (spastishe Pseudosklerose-Encephalomyelopathie mit disseminierten Degenerationsherden). Dtsch Nervenheilkunde. 1921; 70: 132–46.
10. Pocchiari M, Puopolo M, Croes EA, Budka H, Gelpi E, Collins S, et al. Predictors of survival in sporadic Creutzfeldt-Jakob disease and other human transmissible spongiform encephalopathies. Brain. 2004; 127(Pt 10): 2348–59.
11. Gambetti P, Kong Q, Zou W, Parchi P, Chen SG. Sporadic and familial CJD: classification and characterisation. British Medical Bulletin. 2003; 66(1): 213–39.
12. National CJD Research & Surveillance Unit. Creutzfeldt-Jakob Disease Surveillance in the UK, 27th Annual Report 2018. http://www.cjd.ed.ac.uk/sites/default/files/report27.pdf. Edinburgh: NCJDRSU, 2018.
13. El Tawil S, Mackay G, Davidson L, Summers D, Knight R, Will R. Variant Creutzfeldt-Jakob disease in older patients. J Neurol Neurosurg Psychiatry. 2015; 86(11): 1279–80.
14. Karch A, Raddatz LM, Ponto C, Hermann P, Summers D, Zerr I. Diagnostic profiles of patients with late-onset Creutzfeldt-Jakob disease differ from those of younger Creutzfeldt-Jakob patients: a historical cohort study using data from the German National Reference Center. J Neurol. 2014; 261(5): 877–83.
15. Bishop M, Pennington C, Heath C, Will R, Knight R. PRNP variation in UK sporadic and variant Creutzfeldt-Jakob disease highlights genetic risk factors and a novel non-synonymous polymorphism. BMC Medical Genetics. 2009; 10(1): 146.
16. Ward HJ, Everington D, Cousens SN, Smith-Bathgate B, Gillies M, Murray K, et al. Risk factors for sporadic Creutzfeldt-Jakob disease. Ann Neurol. 2008; 63(3): 347–54.
17. Davanipour Z, Sobel E, Ziogas A, Smoak C, Bohr T, Doram K, et al. Ocular tonometry and sporadic Creutzfeldt-Jakob Disease (sCJD): A confirmatory case-control study. British Journal of Medicine and Medical Research. 2014; 4(12): 2322–33.

18. Mahillo-Fernandez I, de Pedro-Cuesta J, Bleda MJ, Cruz M, Mølbak K, Laursen H, et al. Surgery and risk of sporadic Creutzfeldt-Jakob Disease in Denmark and Sweden: registry-based case-control studies. Neuroepidemiology. 2008; 31(4): 229–40.
19. Puopolo M, Ladogana A, Vetrugno V, Pocchiari M. Transmission of sporadic Creutzfeldt-Jakob disease by blood transfusion: risk factor or possible biases. Transfusion. 2011; 51(7): 1556–66.
20. Dorsey K, Zou S, Schonberger LB, Sullivan M, Kessler D, Notari Et, et al. Lack of evidence of transfusion transmission of Creutzfeldt-Jakob disease in a US surveillance study. Transfusion. 2009; 49(5): 977–84.
21. Molesworth AM, Mackenzie J, Everington D, Knight RS, Will RG. Sporadic Creutzfeldt-Jakob disease and risk of blood transfusion in the United Kingdom. Transfusion. 2011; 51(8): 1872–73; author reply 3–4.
22. Alcalde-Cabero E, Almazan-Isla J, Brandel JP, Breithaupt M, Catarino J, Collins S, et al. Health professions and risk of sporadic Creutzfeldt-Jakob disease, 1965– 2010. Euro Surveill. 2012; 17(15): 20144.
23. Brown P, Cervenakova L, McShane L, Goldfarb LG, Bishop K, Bastian F, et al. Creutzfeldt-Jakob disease in a husband and wife. Neurology. 1998; 50(3): 684–8.
24. Linsell L, Cousens SN, Smith PG, Knight RSG, Zeidler M, Stewart G, et al. A case-control study of sporadic Creutzfeldt-Jakob disease in the United Kingdom. Analysis of clustering. Neurology. 2004; 63(11): 2077–83.
25. de Pedro Cuesta J, Ruiz Tovar M, Ward H, Calero M, Smith A, Verduras CA, et al. Sensitivity to biases of case-control studies on medical procedures, particularly surgery and blood transfusion, and risk of Creutzfeldt-Jakob Disease. Neuroepidemiology. 2012; 39(1): 1–18.
26. Head MW, Yull HM, Ritchie DL, Langeveld JP, Fletcher NA, Knight RS, et al. Variably protease-sensitive prionopathy in the UK: a retrospective review 1991–2008. Brain. 2013; 136(4): 1102–15.
27. Zou WQ, Puoti G, Xiao X, Yuan J, Qing L, Cali I, et al. Variably protease-sensitive prionopathy: a new sporadic disease of the prion protein. Ann Neurol. 2010; 68(2): 162–72.
28. Notari S, Xiao X, Espinosa JC, Cohen Y, Qing L, Aguilar-Calvo P, et al. Transmission characteristics of variably protease-sensitive prionopathy. Emerg Infect Dis. 2014; 20(12): 2006–14.
29. Will RG, Ironside JW, Zeidler M, Cousens SN, Estibeiro K, Alperovitch A, et al. A new variant of Creutzfeldt-Jakob disease in the UK. Lancet. 1996; 347(9006): 921–5.
30. Bruce ME, Will RG, Ironside JW, McConnell I, Drummond D, Suttie A, et al. Transmissions to mice indicate that 'new variant' CJD is caused by the BSE agent. Nature. 1997; 389(6650): 498–501.
31. Collinge J, Sidle KCL, Meads J, Ironside J, Hill AF. Molecular analysis of prion strain variation and the aetiology of 'new variant' CJD. Nature. 1996; 383(6602): 685–90.
32. Hill AF, Desbruslais M, Joiner S, Sidle KCL, Gowland I, Collinge J, et al. The same prion strain causes vCJD and BSE. Nature. 1997; 389(6650): 448–50.
33. Scott MR, Will R, Ironside J, Nguyen H-OB, Tremblay P, DeArmond SJ, et al. Compelling transgenetic evidence for transmission of bovine spongiform encephalopathy prions to humans. Proceedings of the National Academy of Sciences. 1999; 96(26): 15137–42.
34. Wells GA, Scott AC, Johnson CT, Gunning RF, Hancock RD, Jeffrey M, et al. A novel progressive spongiform encephalopathy in cattle. Vet Rec. 1987; 121(18): 419–20.
35. Wilesmith JW, Wells GA, Cranwell MP, Ryan JB. Bovine spongiform encephalopathy: epidemiological studies. Vet Rec. 1988; 123(25): 638–44.
36. Anderson RM, Donnelly CA, Ferguson NM, Woolhouse MEJ, Watt CJ, Udy HJ, et al. Transmission dynamics and epidemiology of BSE in British cattle. Nature. 1996; 382(6594): 779–88.
37. Brandel JP, Heath CA, Head MW, Levavasseur E, Knight R, Laplanche JL, et al. Variant Creutzfeldt-Jakob disease in France and the United Kingdom: evidence for the same agent strain. Ann Neurol. 2009; 65(3): 249–56.
38. Sanchez-Juan P, Cousens SN, Will RG, van Duijn CM. Source of variant Creutzfeldt-Jakob disease outside United Kingdom. Emerg Infect Dis. 2007; 13(8): 1166–9.
39. Ward HJ, Everington D, Cousens SN, Smith-Bathgate B, Leitch M, Cooper S, et al. Risk factors for variant Creutzfeldt-Jakob disease: a case-control study. Ann Neurol. 2006; 59(1): 111–20.
40. Monk P, Bryant G. Final report of the investigation into the North Leicestershire cluster of variant Creutzfeldt-Jakob disease. Leicester 2001. Leicestershire NHS Health Authority. 2001: http://webarchive.nationalarchives.gov.uk/20140714084352/http://www.hpa.org.uk/web/HPAwebFile/HPAweb_C/1194947321932.
41. Boelle PY, Cesbron JY, Valleron AJ. Epidemiological evidence of higher susceptibility to vCJD in the young. BMC Infect Dis. 2004; 4: 26.
42. Cooper JD, Bird SM. UK dietary exposure to BSE in beef mechanically recovered meat: by birth cohort and gender. Journal of Cancer Epidemiology and Prevention. 2002; 7(2): 59–70.
43. Mok T, Jaunmuktane Z, Joiner S, Campbell T, Morgan C, Wakerley B, et al. Variant Creutzfeldt-Jakob disease in a patient with heterozygosity at PRNP Codon 129. New England Journal of Medicine. 2017; 376(3): 292–4.
44. Valleron AJ, Boelle PY, Will R, Cesbron JY. Estimation of epidemic size and incubation time based on age characteristics of vCJD in the United Kingdom. Science. 2001; 294(5547): 1726–8.
45. Kaski D, Mead S, Hyare H, Cooper S, Jampana R, Overell J, et al. Variant CJD in an individual heterozygous for PRNP codon 129. Lancet. 2009; 374(9707): 2128.
46. d'Aignaux JN, Cousens SN, Smith PG. Predictability of the UK variant Creutzfeldt-Jakob disease epidemic. Science. 2001; 294(5547): 1729–31.
47. Garske T, Ghani AC. Uncertainty in the tail of the variant Creutzfeldt-Jakob disease epidemic in the UK. PLOS One. 2010; 5(12): e15626.
48. Gill ON, Spencer Y, Richard-Loendt A, Kelly C, Dabaghian R, Boyes L, et al. Prevalent abnormal prion protein in human appendixes after bovine spongiform encephalopathy epizootic: large scale survey. 2013; 347: 5675.
49. Public Health England. Summary results of the third national survey of abnormal prion prevalence in archived appendix specimens. Health Protection Report. 2016; 10(26).
50. Head MW, Ironside JW, Ghetti B, Jeffrey M, Piccardo P, Will B. Prion diseases. In: Love S, Perry A, Ironside J, Budka H (eds). Greenfield's Neuropathology. 2 (9th edition). London: CRC Press, 2015. pp1197–273.
51. Murray K, Peters J, Stellitano L, Winstone AM, Verity C, Will RG. Is there evidence of vertical transmission of variant Creutzfeldt-Jakob disease? J Neurol Neurosurg Psychiatry. 2011; 82(7): 729–31.

52. Kirby E, Dickinson J, Vassey M, Dennis M, Cornwall M, McLeod N, et al. Bioassay studies support the potential for iatrogenic transmission of variant Creutzfeldt-Jakob Disease through dental procedures. PLOS One. 2012; 7(11): e49850.
53. Molesworth AM, Smith AJ, Everington D, Ord F, Watt P, Will RG, et al. Risk factors for variant Creutzfeldt-Jakob disease in dental practice: a case-control study. Br Dent J. 2012; 213(11): E19-E.
54. Molesworth A, Yates P, Hewitt PE, Mackenzie J, Ironside JW, Galea G, et al. Investigation of Variant Creutzfeldt-Jakob disease implicated organ or tissue transplantation in the United Kingdom. Transplantation. 2014; 98(5): 585–9.
55. Hewitt PE, Llewelyn CA, Mackenzie J, Will RG. Creutzfeldt-Jakob disease and blood transfusion: results of the UK transfusion medicine epidemiological review study. Vox Sang. 2006; 91(3): 221–330.
56. Llewelyn CA, Hewitt PE, Knight RS, Amar K, Cousens S, Mackenzie J, et al. Possible transmission of variant Creutzfeldt-Jakob disease by blood transfusion. Lancet. 2004; 363(9407): 417–21.
57. Peden AH, Head MW, Ritchie DL, Bell JE, Ironside JW. Preclinical vCJD after blood transfusion in a PRNP codon 129 heterozygous patient. Lancet. 2004; 364(9433): 527–9.
58. Peden A, McCardle L, Head MW, Love S, Ward HJ, Cousens SN, et al. Variant CJD infection in the spleen of a neurologically asymptomatic UK adult patient with haemophilia. Haemophilia. 2010; 16(2): 296–304.
59. Bishop MT, Ritchie DL, Will RG, Ironside JW, Head MW, Thomson V, et al. No Major Change in vCJD agent strain after secondary transmission via blood transfusion. PLOS One. 2008; 3(8): e2878.
60. Bishop MT, Diack AB, Ritchie DL, Ironside JW, Will RG, Manson JC. Prion infectivity in the spleen of a PRNP heterozygous individual with subclinical variant Creutzfeldt-Jakob disease. Brain. 2013; 36(Pt 4): 1139–45.
61. Urwin PJM, Mackenzie JM, Llewelyn CA, Will RG, Hewitt PE. Creutzfeldt–Jakob disease and blood transfusion: updated results of the UK Transfusion Medicine Epidemiology Review Study. Vox Sanguinis. 2016; 110(4): 310–16.
62. Gajdusek DC, Zigas V. Degenerative disease of the central nervous system in New Guinea; the endemic occurrence of kuru in the native population. N Engl J Med. 1957; 257(20): 974–8.
63. Alpers MP. Review. The epidemiology of kuru: monitoring the epidemic from its peak to its end. Philosophical transactions of the Royal Society of London Series B, Biological Sciences. 2008; 363(1510): 3707–13.
64. Collinge J, Whitfield J, McKintosh E, Beck J, Mead S, Thomas DJ, et al. Kuru in the 21st century—an acquired human prion disease with very long incubation periods. Lancet. 2006; 367(9528): 2068–74.
65. Asante EA, Smidak M, Grimshaw A, Houghton R, Tomlinson A, Jeelani A, et al. A naturally occurring variant of the human prion protein completely prevents prion disease. Nature. 2015; 522(7557): 478–81.
66. Mead S, Whitfield J, Poulter M, Shah P, Uphill J, Campbell T, et al. A novel protective prion protein variant that colocalizes with kuru exposure. N Engl J Med. 2009; 361(21): 2056–65.
67. Bonda DJ, Manjila S, Mehndiratta P, Khan F, Miller BR, Onwuzulike K, et al. Human prion diseases: surgical lessons learned from iatrogenic prion transmission. Neurosurgical Focus. 2016; 41(1): E10.
68. Brown P, Brandel JP, Sato T, Nakamura Y, MacKenzie J, Will RG, et al. Iatrogenic Creutzfeldt-Jakob disease, final assessment. Emerg Infect Dis. 2012; 18(6): 901–7.
69. Will RG. Acquired prion disease: iatrogenic CJD, variant CJD, kuru. British Medical Bulletin. 2003; 66(1): 255–65.
70. Gibbs CJJ, Joy A, Heffner R, Franko M, Miyazaki M, Asher DM, et al. Clinical and pathological features and laboratory confirmation of Creutzfeldt–Jakob disease in a recipient of pituitary-derived human growth hormone. New England Journal of Medicine. 1985; 313(12): 734–8.
71. Koch TK, Berg BO, De Armond SJ, Gravina RF. Creutzfeldt-Jakob disease in a young adult with idiopathic hypopituitarism. Possible relation to the administration of cadaveric human growth hormone. N Engl J Med. 1985; 313(12): 731–3.
72. Powell-Jackson J, Weller RO, Kennedy P, Preece MA, Whitcombe EM, Newsom-Davis J. Creutzfeldt-Jakob disease after administration of human growth hormone. Lancet. 1985; 2(8449): 244–6.
73. Brandel JP, Preece M, Brown P, Croes E, Laplanche JL, Agid Y, et al. Distribution of codon 129 genotype in human growth hormone-treated CJD patients in France and the UK. Lancet. 2003; 362(9378): 128–30.
74. Cochius JI, Burns RJ, Blumbergs PC, Mack K, Alderman CP. Creutzfeldt-Jakob disease in a recipient of human pituitary-derived gonadotrophin. Australian and New Zealand Journal of Medicine. 1990; 20(4): 592–3.
75. Hamaguchi T, Sakai K, Noguchi-Shinohara M, Nozaki I, Takumi I, Sanjo N, et al. Insight into the frequent occurrence of dura mater graft-associated Creutzfeldt-Jakob disease in Japan. J Neurol Neurosurg Psychiatry. 2013; 84(10): 1171–5.
76. Kobayashi A, Matsuura Y, Mohri S, Kitamoto T. Distinct origins of dura mater graft-associated Creutzfeldt-Jakob disease: past and future problems. Acta Neuropathol Commun. 2014; 2: 32.
77. Duffy P, Wolf J, Collins G, DeVoe AG, Streeten B, Cowen D. Letter: Possible person-to-person transmission of Creutzfeldt-Jakob disease. N Engl J Med. 1974; 290(12): 692–3.
78. Heckmann JG, Lang CJ, Petruch F, Druschky A, Erb C, Brown P, et al. Transmission of Creutzfeldt-Jakob disease via a corneal transplant. J Neurol Neurosurg Psychiatry. 1997; 63(3): 388–90.
79. Bernoulli C, Siegfried J, Baumgartner G, Regli F, Rabinowicz T, Gajdusek DC, et al. Danger of accidental person-to-person transmission of Creutzfeldt-Jakob disease by surgery. Lancet. 1977; 1(8009): 478–9.
80. Nevin S, McMenemey WH, Behrman S, Jones DP. Subacute spongiform encephalopathy—a subacute form of encephalopathy attributable to vascular dysfunction (spongiform cerebral atrophy). Brain. 1960; 83(4): 519–64.
81. el Hachimi KH, Chaunu MP, Cervenakova L, Brown P, Foncin JF. Putative neurosurgical transmission of Creutzfeldt-Jakob disease with analysis of donor and recipient: agent strains. Comptes rendus de l'Academie des sciences Serie III, Sciences de la vie. 1997; 320(4): 319–28.
82. Mead S. Prion disease genetics. Eur J Hum Genet. 2006; 14(3): 273–81.
83. Kovács GG, Puopolo M, Ladogana A, Pocchiari M, Budka H, van Duijn C, et al. Genetic prion disease: the EUROCJD experience. Human Genetics. 2005; 118(2): 166–74.
84. Ladogana A, Puopolo M, Croes EA, Budka H, Jarius C, Collins S, et al. Mortality from Creutzfeldt-Jakob disease and related disorders in Europe, Australia, and Canada. Neurology. 2005; 64(9): 1586–91.

85. Knight R, Will R. Prion diseases. Journal of Neurology, Neurosurgery, and Psychiatry. 2004; 75(Suppl 1): i36–42.
86. UK Advisory Committee on Dangerous Pathogens TSE Subgroup. Minimise transmission risk of CJD and vCJD in healthcare settings. London: Department of Health, 2015.
87. Fast C, Groschup MH. Classical and Atypical Scrapie in Sheep and Goats. In: Zou W-Q, Gambetti P (eds). Prions and Diseases Volume 2: Animals, Humans and the Environment. 2. New York: Springer, 2013. pp15–44.
88. Cassard H, Torres JM, Lacroux C, Douet JY, Benestad SL, Lantier F, et al. Evidence for zoonotic potential of ovine scrapie prions. Nat Commun. 2014; 5: 5821.
89. Smith PG, Bradley R. Bovine spongiform encephalopathy (BSE) and its epidemiology. British Medical Bulletin. 2003; 66(1): 185–98.
90. Stevenson MA, Wilesmith JW, Ryan JB, Morris RS, Lockhart JW, Lin D, et al. Temporal aspects of the epidemic of bovine spongiform encephalopathy in Great Britain: individual animal-associated risk factors for the disease. Vet Rec. 2000; 147(13): 349–54.
91. Zanusso G, Monaco S. Bovine spongiform encephalopathy. In: Zou W-Q, Gambetti P (eds). Prions and Diseases Volume 2: Animals, Humans and the Environment. 2. New York: Springer; 2013. pp1–13.
92. Williams ES, Young S. Chronic wasting disease of captive mule deer: a spongiform encephalopathy. Journal of Wildlife Diseases. 1980; 16(1): 89–98.
93. Sohn HJ, Kim JH, Choi KS, Nah JJ, Joo YS, Jean YH, et al. A case of chronic wasting disease in an elk imported to Korea from Canada. Journal of Veterinary Medical Science. 2002; 64(9): 855–8.
94. Benestad SL, Mitchell G, Simmons M, Ytrehus B, Vikøren T. First case of chronic wasting disease in Europe in a Norwegian free-ranging reindeer. Veterinary Research. 2016; 47: 88.
95. Mathiason CK, Hays SA, Powers J, Hayes-Klug J, Langenberg J, Dahmes SJ, et al. Infectious prions in pre-clinical deer and transmission of chronic wasting disease solely by environmental exposure. PLOS One. 2009; 4(6): e5916.
96. Saunders SE, Bartelt-Hunt SL, Bartz JC. Occurrence, transmission, and zoonotic potential of chronic wasting disease. Emerg Infect Dis. 2012; 18(3): 369–76.
97. Barria MA, Balachandran A, Morita M, Kitamoto T, Barron R, Manson J, et al. Molecular barriers to zoonotic transmission of prions. Emerging Infectious Diseases. 2014; 20(1): 88–97.

36

Epidemiology of bacterial and parasitic infections of the central nervous system

Charles R Newton

Introduction

Bacteria and parasites are important infections of the CNS, but the epidemiology has changed significantly over the last few decades with the introduction of vaccines, appearance of organisms resistant to antimicrobial and anti-parasitic drugs, increase in number of immunocompromised people from human immunodeficiency virus (HIV) and oncological conditions, and increased movement of people throughout the world.

The CNS infections present with a multitude of symptoms and signs, which often overlap, making case definitions for epidemiological studies difficult. The main syndromes of CNS infections are outlined in Table 36.1.

Bacteria

Most bacteria gain access to the CNS via blood, although scalp, ear, and oropharyngeal infections are possible routes of infection. The bacteria usually produce meningitis, with direct invasion of the brain parenchyma causing brain abscesses and bacterial infection of the ventricular system as ventriculitis.

Acute Bacterial Meningitis

The introduction of vaccines has had a major impact on the epidemiology of acute bacterial meningitis (ABM), particularly in children.[1] Most epidemiological studies rely on confirmation of the diagnosis in health facilities, since the diagnosis depends upon detection of bacteria in the CSF. The clinical features lack sensitivity (particularly in neonates and infants) and specificity. Thus, the reported incidences generally under-report the incidence, as the diagnosis of ABM is not made since a lumbar puncture is not performed or people may die before diagnosis is made.

The diagnosis, and thus case definition depends upon obtaining a CSF sample. The appearance, cell count, and protein concentration are suggestive of ABM, but it is the detection of the bacteria which confirms the diagnosis for the case definition. Detection of the bacteria can be obtained by microscopy (Gram stains), culture or detection of bacterial antigens, or more recently nucleic acids. The sensitivity and specificity of these methods varies considerably, not only between the methods, but also with the laboratories, immune status of the patient, and organism (Table 36.2).

Prior to the advent of the vaccines against the major causes of ABM, the annual incidence of ABM was reported up to 11 per 100,000. The best epidemiological data comes from the USA, where the reported annual incidence during 1964–1971 varied from 6.7 to 10.6 per 100,000.[2,3,4,5] Haemophilius meningitis was the most common, with an annual incidence of 2.8 to 4.3 per 100,000, followed by pneumococcal meningitis 1.1 to 2.6 per 100,000.

The epidemiology of ABM has changed significantly with the introduction of vaccines. In the USA, there was significant reduction in the annual incidence from 1986 to 1995 of bacterial meningitis cause by *H. influenzae* from 2.9 to 0.2 per 100.000 (94% reduction) and *N. meningitidis* 0.9 to 0.6 (33% reduction) with the introduction of the haemophilus and meningococcal vaccines.[6] The

Table 36.1 Clinical syndromes associated with bacterial and parasitic infections on the central nervous system

Syndrome	Pathology	Clinical manifestations	Aetiological agents
Meningitis	Inflammation of meninges of the brain	Headache, photophobia, neck stiffness, fever	Bacteria, virus, parasites
Encephalitis	Inflammation of the brain and spinal cord parenchyma	Impaired consciousness, fever	Virus
Epilepsy	Focal lesions	Generalized, focal, and/or focal becoming generalized seizures	Parasites, bacteria
Paralysis	Myelitis	Weakness of limbs	Bacteria, virus

Table 36.2 The major causes of ABM vary with age

Age group	Most common organisms
Newborns	Group B *Streptococcus, Strepyococcus pneumoniae, Listeria monocytogenes, Escherichia coli*
Infants and children	*Streptococcus pneumoniae, Neisseria meningitidis, Haemophilus influenzae* type b (Hib), group B *Streptococcus*
Adolescents and young adults	*Neisseria meningitidis, Streptococcus pneumoniae*
Older adults	*Streptococcus pneumoniae, Neisseria meningitidis, Haemophilus influenzae* type b (Hib), group B *Streptococcus, Listeria monocytogenes*

incidence of group B Streptococcus meningitis also decreased from 0.4 to 0.3 (25%) and suggesting more widespread use of antibiotics. The median age of patients with ABM increased from 15 months in 1986 to 25 years in 1995, driven by the reduction in haemophilius meningitis.[6]

The introduction of the PCV-7 and MCV4 vaccines were associated with significant declines in the pneumococcal and meningococcal meningitis respectively, although the annual incidences appeared to be decreasing prior to the introduction of these vaccines, and the meningitis caused by serogroups not covered by the vaccines also decreased (Fig. 36.1).

Data from other parts of the world is less robust, since many countries do not have the facilities for the diagnosis or the epidemiological framework (accurate denominators and case ascertainment) to provide accurate measures. Areas such as those in Africa have high incidences, with reported annual incidences of 46 (31–52) per 100,000 for haemophilius and 38 (11–48) for pneumococcal meningitis, compared to Europe 16 (12–22) and 6 (5–9) per 100,000.[1] The incidence of meniningococcal meningitis is estimated to be 1–2, increasing to 2–10 during epidemics in Europe. Epidemics of meningococcal meningitis occur in a region stretching across Africa from Ethiopia to Senegal. The annual incidence reaches over 1000 per 100,000 during epidemics, usually caused by serogroup A.[1] In 2012, a vaccination programme in Chad reduced the incidence in by 94% with the incidence in three regions of 2.48 per 100 000 compared to 43.8 per 100 000.[7]

The risk factors for the development of ABM varies according to the organism, the age, and immune competency of the patient. For neonatal meningitis the risk factors are premature rupture of membranes, prolonged rupture of membranes (>18 h), maternal colonization with group B Streptococcus (GBS), maternal chorioamnionitis, low socioeconomic status, low birth weight, and prematurity.[8] The common risk factors for community acquired pneumococcal, meningococcal, and haemophilius meningitis in older children and adults include living in crowded conditions, smoking, splenectomy (including splenic atrophy as in sickle cell disease), and HIV infection.[9] Specific risk factors for pneumococcal meningitis include B-cell dysfunction, complement deficiencies, haematological cancer and cochlear implants, and older patients (>65 years). For meningococcal meningitis risk factors are late complement deficiency and complement inhibitor treatment, and for haemophilius meningitis risk factors are diminished humoral immunity.

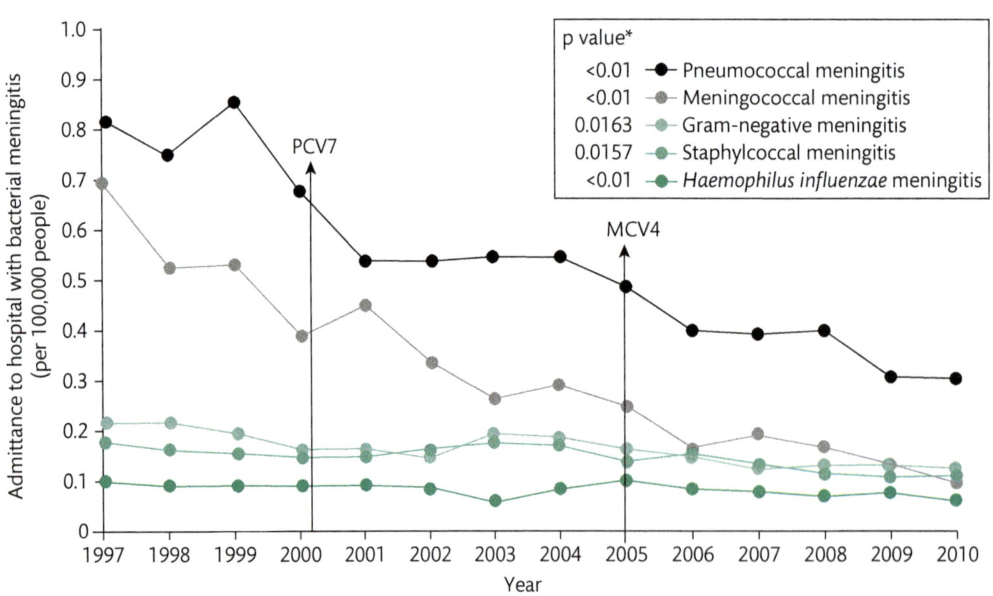

Fig. 36.1 Meningitis trends for different bacteria, 1997–2010.

Case estimation based on total number of cases per 100,000 people by international Classification of Diseases code (320 0, 320 1, 320 3, 320 82, and 036) from hospital discharges across the USA with the nationwide inpatient sample Healthcare Cost and Utilization Project net database. * p values calculated on the basis of the comparison between 1997 and 2010.

Reproduced with permission from Castelblanco R.L. et al.Epidemiology of bacterial meningitis in the USA from 1997 to 2010: a population-based observational study. *The Lancet: Infectious Diseases*, 14(9):813–819. DOI:https://doi.org/10.1016/S1473-3099(14)70805-9.

The outcome of ABM is determined by the aetiological organism, age of the patient, and their immune competency. In neonates ABM is associated with a poor outcome. In areas of low incidence the mortality is about 4 per 100,000 per year from haemophilius and pneumococcal meningitis, compared to about 30 per 100,000 per year in Africa.[1] The proportion of those with long-term sequelae for meningitis caused by haemophilius is 9.5% (95% CI: 7.1–15.3), pneumococcus is 24.7% (16.2–35.3) and meningococcus is 7.2% (4.3–11.2).[1]

Brain Abscesses

Brain abscesses are focal infections of the brain parenchyma, caused by a variety of organisms, mainly bacteria. The clinical features depend upon the location, size, growth rate of abscess, aetiological agent and number of abscesses, and the immunocompetency of the host. Thus, the case definition is not well defined, and epidemiology is not well described. The classical triad of headache, fever, and focal neurological deficits is not sufficiently sensitive or specific for epidemiological studies.

The few recent population based studies provide annual incidence estimates per 100,000 of 1.3 in Minnesota (USA) in 1981,[10] 0.3 in Helsinki (Finland) between 1970 and 2012,[11] and 0.4 in Copenhagen (Denmark) between 1994 and 2007.[11] These studies demonstrated a decline in the annual incidence, for example from 2.7/100,000 in 1935 to 0.9/100,000 in 1984 the Minnesota study.[10] All these studies reported a male predominance.[12] However, there have been no studies reported from LMIC nor in immunocompromised individuals, in whom the incidence would be higher.

Overall an aetiological agent could be identified in 68% of cases, with 23% having multiple organisms.[13] The most common pathogens identified are *Streptococcus sp.* and *Staphylococcus sp.* However, most studies were conducted on bacteria, and thus other organisms may have been under-reported.

Most patients (86%) with brain abscesses have readily identifiable risk factors,[13] which are associated with specific pathogens. These risk factors include: immunodeficiency, penetration of the blood brain barrier, or haematogenous spread from distant infections.[12] More recently, genetic susceptibility was suggested, with increased risk of developing brain abscesses in subjects with specific polymorphisms of the intercellular adhesion molecule-1 (ICAM-1, K469E/E) and monocyte chemoattractant protein-1 (MCP-1, -2518 ANG/G).[14] The abscesses in HIV infected patients are most often caused by *Toxoplasmosis gondii, Mycobacterium sp.*, and *Nocardia sp.* The abscesses that occur in patients with solid-organ or haematopoietic cancers, stem-cell transplantation, or neutropaenia following chemotherapy are caused usually by fungi such as *Aspergillus, Candida sp., Mucorales*, and *Scedosporium* species, or bacteria such as *Escherichia coli, Enterobacter, Klebsiella, Proteus*, and *Salmonella species*. The organisms identified following penetrating trauma, neurosurgery, or infections of the ear and paranasal sinuses are *Staphylococcus aureus*, anaerobic and aerobic Streptococcus species, but also enterobacteria, Klebsiella, Proteus, and Salmonella species. Haematogenous spread can occur from endocarditis, congenital heart disease, pulmonary or dental infections, endocarditis, congenital heart disease, lung infections, or dental infections. *S. aureus* and *Streptococcus spp.* are the organisms most commonly found with endocarditis, whilst a mixture of organisms including *Fusobacterium, Prevotella, Actinomyces, Bacteroides*, and *Haemophilus* species are found following dental infections.

Ventriculitis

Ventriculitis occurs most commonly after invasive procedures such external ventricular drainage or ventriculo-shunts for hydrocephalus. There is little data on the incidence of this infection, although it is reported that 8% of people who have external ventricular drainage[15] develop ventriculitis.[16] The most common organisms are *Staphlycoccus aureus* or *S. epidermis*, but other organisms such as enterobacteriaceae and *Pseudomonas spp., Acinetobacter spp.* and *Candidia spp.* are also isolated.

Tuberculosis Meningitis

It was estimated that in 2015, 10.2 million (95% UI, 9.2–11.5 million) tuberculosis incident cases occurred, with 10.1 million (9.2–11.1 million) prevalent cases and 1.3 million (1.1–1.6 million) deaths.[15] The age-standardized tuberculosis incidence rate (per 100000 people) was 154.4 (140.0–172.2) in men and 86.3 (78.0–97.4) in women. Mortality was double in men (21.9 (16.5–29.5)) versus women (10.8 (8.5–13.1)). Since 1990, the incidence has decreased by about 2%, with more rapid decreases in the last ten years.[15] The changes in the epidemiology are influenced by the rolling out of the BCG vaccine and introduction of isonazid prophylaxis (both of which are particularly effective in preventing tuberculosis meningitis) and the advent of HIV and multi-drug resistant organisms.

The major CNS manifestations of *Mycobacterium tuberculosis* infection are meningitis and tuberculoma. Tuberculosis meningitis (TBM) occurs in about 1% of the tuberculosis cases, accounts for 94% of the CNS manifestations,[17] and is associated with significant mortality and morbidity. It occurs most commonly in children, who have the highest mortality and most severe morbidity. Diagnosis of TBM is often difficult since it has an insidious course and is often diagnosed late. The clinical features are not specific, and the diagnosis from the CSF are hampered by poor sensitivity of the tests or slow growth of the organism. Attempts are being made to improve the consistency of the definitions used.[18] The definitive diagnosis is made by identifying *M. tuberculosis* from the CSF either by microscopy or culture. Thus, the sensitivity of microscopy of the CSF stained with Ziehl-Neelson stain and conventional PCR is about 60%. Real time PCR increased the sensitivity to about 80%, but interferon release assays still only have a sensitivity of 50–70%. In a recent multi-centre study, of 506 TBM patients the sensitivities of interferon-c release assay (Quantiferon) was 90%, automated culture systems 82%, Lowenstein Jensen medium 73%, and Ziehl-Neelson stain 27%.[19]

The risk factors for developing TBM include young age (particularly under five years), HIV infection, immune suppression, and diabetes. In a study of children with CNS tuberculosis in the USA,[20] risk factors identified in multivariate analysis were age <5 years (adjusted odds ratio (aOR): 3.3 (95% CI: 2.0–5.4)), birth in the USA (aOR: 1.8 (1.2–2.7)), and Hispanic origin (aOR: 1.5 (1.1–2.1)). There is little recent comparable data from adults. There are differences in the propensity of the *M. tuberculosis* strains to cause TBM, with those of the Indo-Oceanic or East Asian Beijing lineages more likely to cause meningitis than the Euro-American strains.

The mortality from TBM occurs in up to 88%.[21] In a recent review of children with TBM, the mortality was 19.3% (95% CI 14.0–26.1), with neurological sequelae found in 53.9% (95% CI 42.6–64.9) of the survivors.[22] Corticosteroids reduce mortality by about 25%, with a pooled analysis finding a relative risk of 0.75 (95% CI 0.65–0.87); based upon 1337 participants.[23] The median mortality in those without corticosteroids was 41% in this meta-analysis. This review did not find a significant effect on neurological sequelae.

Malaria

Malaria is caused by *Plasmodium* species transmitted by *Anopheles sp.* mosquitos. There are five species of *Plasmodium* known to infect humans: *P. falciparum, P. vivax, P. ovale, P. malariae*, and *P. knowlesi*. Most of these parasites cause an acute infection, characterized by fever, headaches, and gastrointestinal symptoms. *P. falciparum* is responsible for the most deaths and it is associated with most of the neurological complications. It can cause seizures, psychosis, and an encephalopathy (cerebral malaria), as well as post-malaria syndromes. *P. vivax* was not thought to be associated with neurological complications, but there have been recent reports of severe vivax malaria with encephalopathy and seizures, although the most common manifestations are severe anaemia, thrombocytopenia, and hepatic dysfunction.[24] *P. ovale* and *P. malariae* do not appear to have neurological complications. *P. knowlesi* is a relatively recently described infection of humans (2004) restricted to South East Asia, but is not usually associated with neurological complications.[25]

There are significant problems in studying the epidemiology of malaria infections. First, in malaria endemic areas, a significant proportion of the population may be infected with the parasites but not have any clinical symptoms. Thus, when a person develops symptoms such as headache, seizures, or coma, there may be causes other than the malaria infection. Exclusion of these causes is important, but rarely possible in malaria endemic areas because of lack of laboratory and neuroimaging facilities. Thus, models are developed to determine the malarial attributable fraction. So for example, Kariuki et al. used logistic regression to model malaria-attributable fractions for seizures (the proportion of seizures caused by malaria) in a malaria endemic area.[26] Second, a person may be infected with more than one species of *Plasmodium*, and thus it is difficult to attribute the infection to one particular species of malaria. Third, the surveillance systems in many LMICs do not capture all malaria cases, since there is inconsistent reporting, with under-reporting or reporting cases which have not been confirmed by diagnostic tests, the cases treated by private health institutions are not captured. Methods such as the Malaria Atlas Project (https://map.ox.ac.uk/) model the parasite prevalence measured in cross-sectional surveys and the incidence to determine the burden of malaria. Despite these reservations the burden of malaria has been reported and tracked over the last few decades.

In 2016, the WHO estimated that there were 216 million cases of malaria in the world.[27] Over 90% of the cases were in sub-Saharan Africa, where children in malaria endemic areas bear the brunt of infections, and 7% in South East Asia. *P. vivax* was estimated to cause 4% of the infections, mainly in South East Asia, Eastern Mediterranean, and South American regions. The number of cases has dropped from 237 million in 2010, possibly due improved preventative measures such as insecticide spraying, insecticide treated bed nets, and more effective treatment. However, the estimated number of cases has increased from a nadir in 2013 and 2014, when there were an estimated 210 million cases.

The proportion of neurological and psychiatric conditions that can be attributed to malaria infections is difficult to determine for the reasons outlined above. In malaria endemic areas of sub-Saharan Africa, where children have most symptomatic malaria infections, nearly 48% of children admitted to hospital have neurological features such as seizures, prostration, coma, and agitation.[28] With the decrease in malaria between 2002 and 2008, the incidence of all acute symptomatic seizures decreased by 69%, with 93% of this decrease in malaria-associated seizures.[26] The adjusted malaria-attributable fractions for seizures with falciparum parasitaemia were 93% (95% CI 90–95%) for all acute symptomatic seizures, 92.9% (95% CI 89–96%) for convulsive status epilepticus, 94% (95% CI 91–96%) for repetitive seizures, and 92% (95% CI 86–96%) for focal seizures.[26]

The mortality in patients with cerebral malaria is determined by the age of the patient, affected organ systems, and antimalarial and supportive treatment used. In the large SEAQUAMAT trial in Asian adults with severe malaria, overall mortality of cerebral malaria was 34%, whereas mortality was 17% in comatose patients without other organ involvement. In comatose patients with concomitant metabolic acidosis and renal impairment, mortality increased to 70%.[29] Using similar definitions in the large AQUAMAT trial in African children with severe malaria, overall mortality of cerebral malaria was 6% without other organ involvement, increasing to 43% with concomitant metabolic acidosis and renal impairment.[30] The reported case fatality of cerebral malaria in the USA is 18%[31] and France of 25%.[32]

Neurological sequelae are rare in adults (<3%) and include psychiatric sequelae, persisting problems with balance, and hemiparesis.[30] Sequelae are more common in children following cerebral malaria, with up to 11% of African children with persistent deficits and up to 25% with neurocognitive deficits.[33]

Cysticercosis

Taenia solium is an intestinal tapeworm that is ubiquitous.[34] The infection of the intestine is known as taeniasis, but it is the larval forms that cause cysticercosis, which involves the CNS and the eye. Humans can be definitive or intermediate hosts of *T. solium*, with pigs acting as intermediate hosts. Eating raw or undercooked pork containing cysticeri leads to adult *T. solium* worms in the small intestine (definitive host), which is usually asymptomatic. If eggs from the adult worm, found in food or water contaminated by human faeces, are ingested (including self-infection), the eggs will develop into oncospheres which penetrate that intestinal wall, enter the circulation and lodge as cysticerci in tissues such as the muscles, brain, eye, and lung (intermediate host). It is the cysticerci that give rise to the neurological complications of *T. solium*, that is, neurocysticercosis.

Box 36.1 Diagnostic criteria for neurocysticercosis

Absolute
- Histological proof (biopsy of a brain or spinal cord lesion)
- Cystic lesions with scolex on neuroimaging
- Retinal cysticercosis visible on fundoscopic examination

Major
- Lesions highly suggestive of neurocysticercosis on neuroimaging
- Positive serum antibodies on enzyme-linked immunoelectrotransfer blot (EITB)
- Cyst resolution after antiparasitic treatment
- Single brain enhancing lesion spontaneously resolved

Minor
- Suggestive lesions on neuroimaging
- Suggestive clinical manifestations
- Positive CSF antigen or antibodies on ELISA
- Extraneural cysticercosis

Epidemiological
- From or living in an endemic region
- Frequently travels to disease-endemic areas
- Household contact with taeniasis

Reproduced with permission from Garcia H.H. Clinical symptoms, diagnosis, and treatment of neurocysticercosis. *Lancet Neurol*; 13(12): 1202–1215. DOI:https://doi.org/10.1016/S1474-4422(14)70094-8.

Neurocysticercosis can be asymptomatic (cysticerci found on CT scans or at post-mortem) or classified as one or more of the following clinical syndromes: parenchymal, subarachnoid, intraventricular, spinal, or ocular. Single enhancing nodules are more frequent in younger people (<30 years) and subarachnoid neurocysticercosis in older age groups. The main presenting symptoms are headache (23–98%), seizures (37–92%), papilloedema (48–94%), meningism (29–33%), nausea and vomiting (74–80%).[35] Other less common presentations include dementia, psychosis, focal neurological deficits, cranial nerve palsies, visual disturbances, ataxia, and rarely spinal cord compression. The clinical syndromes are determined by the burden and location of cysts, whether the organisms are alive, dying, or dead, and host response to the cysts. The peak incidence of cysticercosis is 20–50 years, although the clinical manifestations are different between children and adults.

The diagnosis of neurocysticercosis is based upon clinical examination, neuroimaging, and serology, since the manifestations are protean, and few patients have pathognomonic features. Criteria have been developed to aid the diagnosis (Box 36.1):

Blood serological tests for neurocysticercosis are problematic since there is a high frequency of false positives, as the parasites may be present in sites outside the CNS, or low sensitivity in people with one lesion in the brain or calcified lesions. CSF serology is more sensitive and specific for neurocysticercosis. Antibody detection by enzyme-linked immunoelectrotransfer blot (EITB) is the most reliable, with a sensitivity of nearly 100% and specificity of 98% in blood for cysticercosis. It has low sensitivity in people with one lesion in the brain or calcified lesions.[36] The sensitivity is 80% and 100% specificity in CSF. Likewise, ELISA for IgG antibodies have sensitivities of >80% and specificity of nearly 100% in CSF.

Although *T. solium* is widely distributed through the world, most of the neurological complications occur in Latin America, Asia and Africa (Fig. 36.2).

The prevalence of cysticercosis detected by various methods ranges up to 24% in endemic areas. Most of these studies have used serological diagnosis, which is not specific for active symptomatic disease.

Neurocysticercosis has many manifestations, but it is the seizures and epilepsy which is focus of most epidemiological research. Now there is compelling evidence from case control studies that cysticercosis is associated with epilepsy in South and Central America, Africa, and Asia. A recent meta-analysis found that the OR ranged from 0.2 to 25.4, with a common OR of 2.7 (95% CI 2.1–3.6) from a random effects model.[37] Three subgroup analyses performed gave OR of 2.2 (95% CI 1.6–3.0) for EITB-based studies, 3.2 95% CI 2.5–4.1) for CT-based studies and 1.9 (95% CI 1.2–3.0) for neurologist-confirmed epilepsy following a door-to-door survey. There did not appear to be any difference between the regions of the world, although there was considerable heterogeneity (I^2 78%, $p<0.0001$) between the studies. This meta-analysis was similar to another one where the OR calculated from a random effects model was 2.76 (95% CI: 2.19–3.48),[38] but also had considerable heterogeneity. In the same paper, the authors estimated that proportions of neurocysticercosis in people with epilepsy ranged from 10% (95% CI: 6–15) to 56% (45–67), with results from a random effects model estimating that 32% (95% CI: 27–36) of people with epilepsy had neurocysticercosis.

However, people in endemic areas have cysticerci detected at post-mortem (up to 4% in subjects without pre-morbid neurological symptoms dying in endemic areas) or on neuroimaging, who are asymptomatic or do not develop epilepsy. Thus, determination of the casual pathway is problematic. One study in Honduras has shown that a reduction in transmission of *T. solium*,[39] and large-scale studies in Peru have demonstrated a reduction in transmission of *T. solium*,[40] but it is too early to assess the impact on epilepsy. However, there is a lack of longitudinal studies to examine the incidence of epilepsy following infection.

Onchocerciasis

Onchocerca volvulus causes onchocerciasis, which manifests river blindness and it is associated with epilepsy and cognitive impairment. It is transmitted by the black fly, *Simulium sp.*, which lives near fast-flowing streams and is endemic in some parts Africa and to a lesser extent in Latin America and the Arabian peninsula.

Onchocerciasis usually presents with eye or skin involvement. The eye involvement includes keratitis (which may lead to sclerosing keratitis and corneal scars), iritis, choroio-retinitis, and optic neuropathy. These are thought to be caused by the localized host inflammatory responses to dead or dying microfilariae.

Diagnosis is confirmed by finding onchocercial microfilaria from skin biopsies, although serology tests and PCR tests of parasite DNA and recombinant antigen-based enzyme-linked immunoassays have been developed.[41] The microfilaria are rarely found in the CSF.

The association onchocerciasis and epilepsy has been difficult to establish, partly because the putative mechanisms of epileptogenesis are unclear. Systematic reviews have demonstrated that prevalence of epilepsy increased on by 0.4% for each 10% increase in onchocerciasis prevalence.[42] A study of active convulsive epilepsy conducted in several countries of sub-Saharan Africa found an OR of 2.2 (CI 95%: 1.6–3.2)

Endemicity of *Taenia solium*, 2015

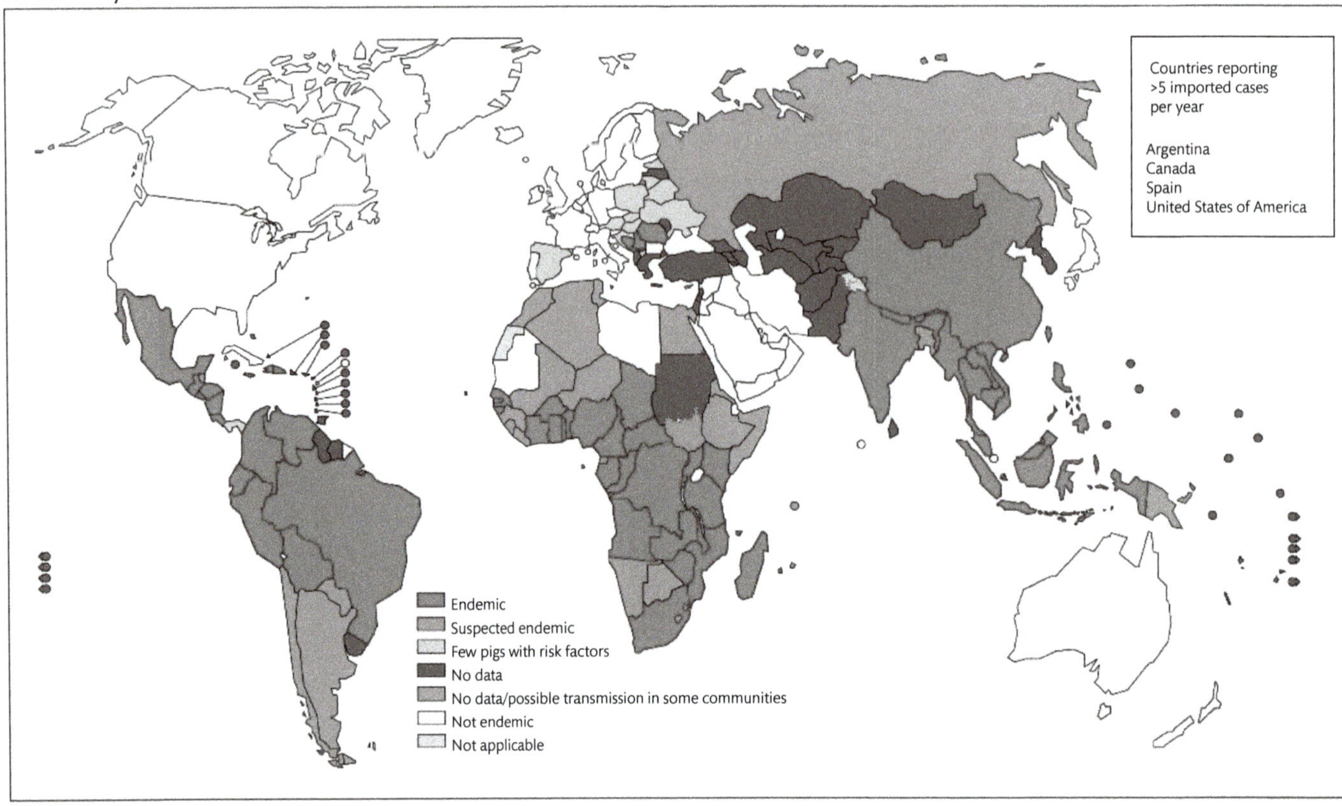

The boundaries and names shown and the designations used on this map do not imply the expression of any opinion whatsoever on the part of the World Health Organization concerning the legal status of any country, territory, city or area or of its authorities, or concerning the delimitation of its frontiers or boundaries. Dotted lines on maps represent approximate border lines for which there may not yet be full agreement.

Data Source: World Health Organization
Map Production: Control of Neglected TropicalDiseases (NTD)
World Health Organization

Fig. 36.2 Endemicity of Taenia solium 2015.

Reproduced with permission from World Health Organization. Taeniasis/cysticercosis. https://www.who.int/news-room/fact-sheets/detail/taeniasis-cysticercosis. Copyright © WHO 2016 (Accessed: 16 July 2019).

using serology.[43] A systematic review of 11 studies which used skin biopsies for diagnosis, found a pooled OR of 2.49 (95% CI: 1.61–3.86).[44] Presence of nodules for diagnosis of onchocerciasis analysed in four studies found an OR of 1.74; 95% CI: 0.94–3.20).

More recently *O. vulva* is being implicated in the pathogenesis of 'nodding syndrome' (NS) an epileptic encephalopathy found in isolated regions of Africa.[45] This syndrome usually presents in children and young adults, with myoclonic seizures, wasting, and cognitive impairment.

Sparganosis and Paragonimiasis

Sparganosis and paragonimiasis are caused by *Spirometra mansoni* and *Paragonimus sp.*, respectively. They are similar in that they have two intermediate hosts, with humans infected by drinking contaminated water, eating raw chicken or fish (sparganosis); or crabs (paragonimiasis), with the definitive hosts as cats and dogs. The CNS involvement is relatively uncommon. In both infections there may be an initial meningoencephalitis, followed by the development of the granulomata. In sparganosis the granulomas often become calcified (small punctuate calcification best seen on CT scan), whilst in paragonimiasis the granulomas evolve into encapsulated abscesses, developing into cystic lesions, which infrequently become calcified.[46] Seizures are common CNS manifestations of paragonimiasis, but they are usually acute symptomatic seizures, and epilepsy may develop in association with the chronic lesions.

Seizures are common CNS manifestations of paragonimiasis, but they are usually acute symptomatic seizures, and epilepsy may develop in association with the chronic lesions.

These are uncommon infections, mostly reported from South East Asia, China, Korea, and Japan, with sporadic cases reported from the rest of the world. Individual species vary across continents.

Conclusion

Infections of the CNS are a considerable burden in the world, with the epidemiology determined by the organisms, age, immune status, and geographical region. The incidence of CNS infections has decreased with the introduction of more effective antimicrobial and anti-parasitic agents, reduction in the transmission of vectors (e.g. malaria) and vaccines (meningitis). However, the development of antimicrobial resistance, HIV epidemic, and increase travel has increased the burden.

REFERENCES

1. McIntyre PB, O'Brien KL, Greenwood B, van de Beek D. Effect of vaccines on bacterial meningitis worldwide. *Lancet*. 2012; 380(9854): 1703–11.
2. Fraser DW, Geil CC, Feldman RA Bacteri.al meningitis in Bernalillo County, New Mexico: a comparison with three other American populations. Am J Epidemiol. 1974; 100(1): 29–34.
3. Fraser DW, Henke CE, Feldman RA. Changing patterns of bacterial meningitis in Olmsted County, Minnesota, 1935–1970. *J Infect Dis*. 1973; 128(3): 300–7.
4. Fraser DW, Mitchell JE, Silverman LP, Feldman RA. Undiagnosed bacterial meningitis in Vermont children. *Am J Epidemiol*. 1975; 102(5): 394–9.
5. Wenger JD, Hightower AW, Facklam RR, Gaventa S, Broome CV. Bacterial meningitis in the United States, 1986: report of a multistate surveillance study. The Bacterial Meningitis Study Group. *J Infect Dis*. 1990; 162(6): 1316–23.
6. Schuchat A, Robinson K, Wenger JD, Harrison LH, Farley M, Reingold AL, et al. Bacterial meningitis in the United States in 1995. Active Surveillance Team. *N Engl J Med*. 1997; 337(14): 970–6.
7. Daugla DM, Gami JP, Gamougam K, Naibei N, Mbainadji L, Narbé M, et al. Effect of a serogroup A meningococcal conjugate vaccine (PsA–TT) on serogroup A meningococcal meningitis and carriage in Chad: a community study. *Lancet*. 2014; 383(9911): 40–7.
8. Furyk JS, Swann O, Molyneux E. Systematic review: neonatal meningitis in the developing world. *Trop Med Int Health*. 2011; 16(6): 672–9.
9. Lundbo LF, Benfield T. Risk factors for community-acquired bacterial meningitis. *Infect Dis (Lond)*. 2017; 49(6): 433–44.
10. Nicolosi A, Hauser WA, Musicco M, Kurland LT. Incidence and prognosis of brain abscess in a defined population: Olmsted County, Minnesota, 1935–1981. *Neuroepidemiology*. 1991; 10(3): 122–31.
11. Laulajainen-Hongisto A, Lempinen L, Farkkila E, Saat R, Markkola A, Leskinen K, et al. Intracranial abscesses over the last four decades; changes in aetiology, diagnostics, treatment and outcome. *Infect Dis (Lond)*. 2016; 48(4): 310–16.
12. Brouwer MC, Tunkel AR, McKhann GM 2nd, van de Beek D. Brain abscess. *N Engl J Med*. 2014; 371(5): 447–56.
13. Brouwer MC, Coutinho JM, van de Beek D. Clinical characteristics and outcome of brain abscess: systematic review and meta-analysis. *Neurology*. 2014; 82(9): 806–13.
14. Mishra P, Prasad KN, Singh K, Sahu RN, Ojha BK. Association of ICAM-1 (K469E) and MCP-1 -2518 A>G gene polymorphism with brain abscess. *J Neuroimmunol*. 2016; 292: 102–7.
15. Kyu HH, Maddison ER, Henry NJ, Mumford JE, Barber R, Shields C, et al. The global burden of tuberculosis: results from the Global Burden of Disease Study 2015. *Lancet Infectious Diseases*. 2018; 18(3): 261–84.
16. Beer R, Lackner P, Pfausler P, Schmutzhard E. Nosocomial ventriculitis and meningitis in neurocritical care patients. *J Neurol*. 2008; 255(11): 1617–24.
17. Erdem H, Inan A, Guven E, Hargreaves S, Larsen L, Shehata G, et al. The burden and epidemiology of community-acquired central nervous system infections: a multinational study. Eur J Clin Microbiol Infect Dis. 2017; 36(9): 1595–611.
18. Marais S, Thwaites G, Schoeman JF, Torok ME, Misra UK, Prasad K. Tuberculous meningitis: a uniform case definition for use in clinical research. *Lancet Infect Dis*. 2010; 10(11): 803–12.
19. Erdem H, Ozturk-Engin D, Elaldi N, Gulsun S, Sengoz G, Crisan A. The microbiological diagnosis of tuberculous meningitis: results of Haydarpasa-1 study. *Clin Microbiol Infect*. 2014; 20(10): O600–8.
20. Duque-Silva A, Robsky K, Flood J, Barry PM. Risk factors for central nervous system tuberculosis. *Pediatrics*. 2015; 136(5): e1276–84.
21. Woldeamanuel YW, Girma B. A 43-year systematic review and meta-analysis: case-fatality and risk of death among adults with tuberculous meningitis in Africa. *J Neurol*. 2014; 261(5): 851–65.
22. Chiang SS, Khan FA, Milstein MB, Tolman AW, Benedetti A, Starke JR and B. MC. Treatment outcomes of childhood tuberculous meningitis: a systematic review and meta-analysis. *Lancet Infect Dis*. 2014; 14: 947–57.
23. Prasad K, Singh MB, Ryan H. Corticosteroids for managing tuberculous meningitis. *Cochrane Database Syst Rev*. 2016 (4): CD002244.
24. Khan W, Zakai HA, Umm EA. Clinico-pathological studies of *Plasmodium falciparum* and *Plasmodium vivax*—malaria in India and Saudi Arabia. *Acta Parasitol*. 2014; 59(2): 206–12.
25. Cox-Singh J, Singh B. Knowlesi malaria: newly emergent and of public health importance? *Trends in Parasitology*. 2008; 24(9): 407–10.
26. Kariuki SM, Ikumi M, Ojal J, Sadarangani M, Idro R, Olotu A, et al. Acute seizures attributable to falciparum malaria in an endemic area on the Kenyan coast. *Brain*. 2011; 134(5): 1519–28.
27. WHO (2017). *World Malaria Report 2017*. Geneva: World Health Organization, 2017.
28. Idro R, Ndiritu M, Ogutu B, Mithwani S, Maitland K, Berkley J, et al. Burden, features, and outcome of neurological involvement in acute falciparum malaria in Kenyan children. *JAMA*. 2007; 297(20): 2232–40.
29. Dondorp A, Nosten F, Stepniewska K, Day N, White N. Artesunate versus quinine for treatment of severe falciparum malaria: a randomised trial. *Lancet*. 2005; 366(9487): 717–25.
30. Dondorp A, Fanello CI, Hendriksen IC, Gomes E, Seni A, Chhaganlal KD, and group. Artesunate versus quinine in the treatment of severe falciparum malaria in African children (AQUAMAT): an open-label, randomised trial. *Lancet*. 2010; 376(9753): 1647–57.
31. Tan KR, Wiegand RE, Arguin PM. Exchange transfusion for severe malaria: evidence base and literature review. *Clin Infect Dis*. 2013; 57(7): 923–8.
32. Bruneel F, Hocqueloux L, Alberti C, Wolff M, Chevret S, Bedos JP, et al. The clinical spectrum of severe imported falciparum malaria in the intensive care unit: report of 188 cases in adults. *Am J Respir Crit Care Med*. 2003; 167(5): 684–9.
33. Idro R, Marsh K, John CC, Newton CR. Cerebral malaria: Mechanisms of brain injury and strategies for improved neurocognitive outcome. *Pediatric Research*. 2010; 68(4): 267–74.
34. Garcia HH, Nash TE, Del Brutto OH. Clinical symptoms, diagnosis, and treatment of neurocysticercosis. *Lancet Neurology*. 2014; 13(12): 1202–15.
35. Scheld WM, Whitley RJ, Durack DT. *Infections of the Central Nervous System*. Philadelphia: Lippincott-Raven, 1997.
36. Carpio A, Romo ML. State of the art in neurocysticercosis: Imaging and epidemiology. *Asian Pac J Trop Med*. 2016; 9(8): 821–2.
37. Debacq G, Moyano LM, Garcia HH, Boumediene F, Marin B, Ngoungou EB, et al. Systematic review and meta-analysis

estimating association of cysticercosis and neurocysticercosis with epilepsy. *PLOS Negl Trop Dis.* 2017; 11(3): e0005153.

38. Gripper LB, Welburn SC. The causal relationship between neurocysticercosis infection and the development of epilepsy—a systematic review. *Infect Dis Poverty.* 2017; 6(1): 31.
39. Medina MT, Aguilar-Estrada RL, Alvarez A, Duron RM, Martinez L, Dubon S, et al. Reduction in rate of epilepsy from neurocysticercosis by community interventions: the Salama, Honduras study. *Epilepsia.* 2011; 52(6): 1177–85.
40. Garcia HH, Gonzalez AE, Tsang VC, O'Neal SE, Llanos-Zavalaga F, Gonzalvez G, et al., and Cysticercosis Working Group. Elimination of *Taenia solium* transmission in Northern Peru. *N Engl J Med.* 2016; 374(24): 2335–44.
41. Udall DN. Recent updates on onchocerciasis: diagnosis and treatment. *Clin Infect Dis.* 2007; 44(1): 53–60.
42. Pion SD, Kaiser C, Boutros-toni F, Cournil A, Taylor MM, Meredith SE, et al. Epilepsy in onchocerciasis endemic areas: systematic review and meta-analysis of population-based surveys. *PLOS Negl Trop Dis.* 2009; 3(6): e461.
43. Ngugi AK, Bottomley C, Kleinschmidt I, Wagner RG, Kakooza-Mwesige A, Ae-Ngibise K, et al. Prevalence of active convulsive epilepsy in sub-Saharan Africa and associated risk factors: cross-sectional and case-control studies. *Lancet Neurology.* 12(3): 253–63.
44. Kaiser C, Pion SD, Boussinesq M. Case-control studies on the relationship between onchocerciasis and epilepsy: systematic review and meta-analysis. *PLOS Negl Trop Dis.* 2013; 7(3): e2147.
45. Colebunders R, Njamnshi AK, van Oijen M, Mukendi D, Kashama JM, Mandro M, et al. Onchocerciasis-associated epilepsy: From recent epidemiological and clinical findings to policy implications. *Epilepsia Open.* 2017; 2(2): 145–52.
46. Chen JZ, Chen J, Lin G, Zhu H, Meng G, Cui N, et al. Cerebral paragonimiasis: a retrospective analysis of 89 cases. Clin Neurol Neurosurg, 2013; 115(5): 546–51.

37

Infection, other than bacterial, including HIV

Inès Yoro-Zohoun, Jaime Luna, Salmane Amidou, and Pierre-Marie Preux

CNS Parasitic Infections

Parasitic infections are common causes of neurological disorders in the tropics, especially in the poorest areas of America, Africa, and Asia. In developed countries, they are uncommon except in immunocompromised patients. The WHO considers several parasite infections as neglected tropical diseases. They prevail in tropical and subtropical conditions and can cause severe illness, but limited resources have been devoted to better understanding their impact and burden.[1] Parasites can invade the central and peripheral nervous system, directly or by other mechanisms (immunological in particular) and cause neurological symptoms.

Human parasites are classified in helminthiases and protozoans. Helminthiases include the nematodoses (roundworms), cestodoses (flat—tapeworms) and trematodoses (flat—flukes). Protozoans include the amoebas, flagellates, foraminiferans, and ciliates.

Helminthiasis

Taenia solium

Approximately 50 million people worldwide are estimated to have cysticercosis infection, although estimates are probably low since many infections are subclinical and there are relatively few population-based data on prevalence.[2]

The larval stage infection of the pork tapeworm *Taenia solium* in the nervous system known as neurocysticercosis (NCC) is considered an important cause of neurologic diseases in Latin America, Africa, and Asia.[3–5] Active transmission does not seem to occur nowadays in Europe or North America, although clinical cases are seen because of immigration and travel.[6] Multiple factors, such as conditions of hygiene, breeding, and slaughtering of pigs, cooking habits, and absence or poor efficiency of wastewater network, maintain the cycle of contamination.[7] Severity and clinical manifestations depend on number, size, and location of cysts and intensity of the host's immune response.[8]

Epidemiological studies have found that NCC is associated with 30–50% of all epilepsy in endemic zones, such as Peru, where nearly half of the population lives under conditions in which *Taenia solium* transmission is an everyday occurrence.[9] In rural Tanzania more than half of people with epilepsy and abnormalities on CT scan had lesions related to NCC.[10] NCC lesions on CT was significantly more common in people with epilepsy than in controls (OR 4.1, 95%, CI 2.0–8.5, $p<0.0001$).[11] A recent meta-analysis assessing the association between cysticercosis and epilepsy across Latin America, Asia, and sub-Saharan Africa found an overall OR estimated of 2.7 (95% CI 2.1–3.6).[12] NCC offers an excellent opportunity to study prospectively the natural history of the genesis of seizures and epilepsy in a human population. This is due to its unique epidemiology and timing of seizures associated with increased inflammation, a predictable occurrence of seizures in the treatment of parenchymal disease, and subsequent development of epilepsy.[13]

Diagnostic criteria for NCC have been set up and the most important issue is neuroimaging. The most common neuroimaging examination available in endemic areas is CT scan.[14] Serological detection of anti-cysticercal antibodies or cysticercal antigen could help to assess the prevalence of human cysticercosis, but is only the marker of the presence (active or inactive) of the parasite.[15] Therapeutic measures include anti-parasitic drugs, corticosteroids, surgery, and symptomatic medication (anti-epileptic drugs). Anti-parasitic drugs help to reduce the recurrence of seizures. Treatment of NCC must be individualized in terms of number and location of lesions, as well as based on the viability of the parasites within the nervous system.[16]

Onchocerca volvulus

Onchocerca volvulus is a filarial nematode transmitted by the blackfly *Simulium spp.*, which causes river blindness and acute, as well as chronic, dermatitis.

The main burden is in 30 countries in sub-Saharan Africa, though the parasite is found in limited areas in the Americas and in Yemen in the Middle East. The number of infected people worldwide was estimated in 2006 to be 37 million, with 90 million at risk in Africa.[17]

Onchocerca volvulus has drawn attention in recent years due to the controversial epidemiological evidence of its association with epilepsy and NS. NS is an emerging or re-emerging epilepsy disorder that mainly affects children and has been confirmed in only three African regions so far: northern Uganda, South Sudan, and southern Tanzania. NS was first described and classified in Tanzania, where it has been reported endemic for many decades.[18,19] To date, high numbers are still reported from South Sudan.[20]

The Centers for Disease Control and Prevention (CDC) and the Ugandan Ministry of Health conducted a single-stage cluster survey to perform the first systematic assessment of prevalence of NS in Uganda using a new consensus case definition.[21] Based on the modified definition, a prevalence of 6.8 (95% CI 5.9–7.7) probable NS cases per 1000 children aged 5–18 years was found in the three districts.[22]

The characteristic clinical feature of NS is a paroxysmal spell where the head nods forward repeatedly in a seemingly unresponsive affected child.[23] These nodding episodes represent a form of epilepsy during which generalized electrodecrement is seen on electroencephalography and paraspinal dropout on electromyography.[24] NS leads to physical and cognitive decline as well as behavioural problems in the majority of patients, if left untreated.[25]

A positive onchocerciasis serology association with NS has been reported (age-adjusted OR: 14.4, 95% CI 2.7–78.3).[26] However, onchocerciasis has long been endemic in large parts of western and central Africa, as well as parts of central and South America, but NS has been reported only in small localized areas.[27]

Researchers hypothesize that NS may be an autoimmune-mediated disease. People with NS have higher levels of antibodies against a protein called leiomodin-1 than do healthy people from the same village. These antibodies were found to be neurotoxic. This protein is structurally similar to those made by *O. volvulus*, and antibodies that react against *O. volvulus* do the same against leiomodin-1, suggesting that NS is an autoimmune disease triggered by the parasite.[28]

Further investigation of NS is needed to identify the causes, preventive measures, and treatments.

Toxocara

Human toxocariasis is a parasitic zoonosis caused by the larval stages of the ascarids *Toxocara canis* (*T. canis*), the common roundworm of dogs, and by the roundworm of cats, *Toxocara cati* (*T. cati*).[29] The reported prevalence of soil contamination with *Toxocara spp.* eggs goes from 6.6 to 87.1%.[30] Therefore, toxocariasis is one of the most prevalent zoonotic helminth infections. High seroprevalence rates of *Toxocara spp.* have been found in tropical countries, where the humid climate favours the survival of parasite eggs in the soil, and in rural settings, where the poor hygiene and the rare administration of anthelmintic treatments to animals increase the probability of human infection.[31,32]

The clinical manifestations of human toxocariasis vary from asymptomatic infection to severe organ injury, depending on the parasite load, the sites of larval migration, and the host's inflammatory response.[33] The CNS migration may lead to a variety of neurological disorders,[34,35] such as meningoencephalitis, myelitis, cerebral vasculitis, optic neuritis,[30] and probably cognitive[36] and behavioural disorders.[37]

An association between toxocariasis and epilepsy has been discussed.[31] A recent meta-analysis showed a positive association with an OR of 1.7 (95% CI 1.4 –2.0).[30] The meta-analysis included studies across different populations in disparate geographic locations and socioeconomic climates. However, further research is needed to clarify this association, mainly population-based studies.

Protozoans

Plasmodium

Malaria is a protozoan disease caused by *Plasmodium* transmitted by Anopheles mosquitoes in tropical and sub-tropical areas of the world. Of the four species of the parasite (*P. vivax, P. ovale, P. malariae, P. falciparum*) that are responsible for disease, *P. falciparum* and *P. vivax* are most common, with widespread distribution throughout the world. Although globally distributed, the highest levels of endemicity have been documented in the sub-Saharan Africa and parts of South and South East Asia and South America.[38]

The WHO reported in 2015, an estimated 212 million cases of malaria occurring worldwide, resulting in 429,000 deaths from malaria globally, 92% of them in the African region. Most of deaths (70%) were among African children aged under five years.

Cerebral malaria (CM) is a febrile encephalopathy responsible for the majority of deaths related to malaria.[39]

An epidemiological study in Cameroon reported a prevalence of 7.1% for cerebral malaria. The highest prevalence of these infections occurred in the 0–5 years age group, dropping in people aged 16 years and above.[40] Mortality approaches 20% in children and most of those who die do so within the first 24 hours.[41]

CM is characterized anatomo-pathologically by the sequestration of infected red cells in the cerebral microvasculature and clinically by impaired consciousness or coma with repetitive and focal seizures.[42] CM is a medical emergency. Complications of CM, such as convulsions, hypoglycaemia, and hyperpyrexia should be prevented or detected and treated early.[38]

CM is a potential cause of epilepsy in malaria endemic regions of the world, primarily for the most part of sub-Saharan Africa. A cross-sectional study among children demonstrated a significantly increased prevalence of epilepsy with prior CM (OR: 4.4; 95% CI: 1.4–13.7; p = 0.01) and acute symptomatic seizures (OR: 6.1; 95% CI: 2.0–18.3; p = 0.001) in comparison to unexposed children.[43] A hospital-based, matched, case-control study found a risk of developing epilepsy of 3.9 (95% CI: 1.7–8.9; p <0.001) times greater among those with prior exposure to CM than unexposed people.[44] A cohort study reported a higher incidence rate of epilepsy in the CM group (17.0/1000 person years) compare to the unexposed group (1.8/1000 person-years). The age-adjusted relative risk for developing epilepsy after exposure to CM was 14.3 (95% CI: 1.6–132.0; p = 0.01).[45] The studies establish temporal plausibility of the association between CM and epilepsy, implying, thereby, that epilepsy followed the occurrence of CM. Furthermore, a recent meta-analysis found that CM was associated with an increased risk of epilepsy (OR 4.7, 95% CI 2.5–8.7), an increased risk of intelligence quotient (IQ) impairment (OR 4.7, 95% CI 0.8–28.5), an increased risk of neurodisabilities (OR 16.2, 95% CI 1.3–195.4), and an increased risk of behavioural disorder (OR 8.5, 95% CI 2.7–26.0).[46] All of these provide reasonable ground for inferring a causal association between CM and epilepsy.[38]

Specific antimalarial treatment, if promptly instituted, unequivocally reduces mortality due to acute severe malaria but its impact on long-term neurological sequelae including epilepsy has not been studied.[47]

Toxoplasma

Toxoplasmosis is a food-borne disease caused by *Toxoplasma gondii*, a ubiquitous protozoan parasite. While usually asymptomatic, *T. gondii* infection can cause severe disease, including encephalitis, retinochoroiditis, or multi-visceral dissemination especially in congenitally infected foetuses, newborns, and immunocompromised patients, particularly those with acquired immune-deficiency syndrome (AIDS).[48]

T. gondii prevalence has significantly decreased in the USA and Europe during the past decades, but remains high (>50%) in many tropical countries.[49] In Brazil, a high prevalence has been reported in the general population, as high as 78% in some areas, which maintains a high rate of toxoplasmic encephalitis in HIV-infected patients.[50] In sub-Saharan Africa, toxoplasmic encephalitis is a leading cause of hospitalization and mortality in patients infected with HIV.[51] Congenital infections can result in miscarriage or a child born with signs of toxoplasmosis (e.g. jaundice, macrocephaly, microcephaly, seizures).[52] The chronic infection in immunocompetent patients, usually considered as asymptomatic, is now suspected to be a risk factor for various neurological disorders, including epilepsy.[53]

Other parasitic diseases

Chagas disease is a parasitic illness caused by the flagellate protozoan *Trypanosome cruzi*.

An estimated eight million people are infected with *T. cruzi*, mainly in Latin America. It has been a neglected tropical disease and an important health problem in endemic regions for many decades. Around 95% of untreated patients advance into the chronic stage of the disease; at least 30% then develop chagasic cardiomyopathy and up to 10% can develop digestive, neurological, or mixed alterations.[54] Furthermore, Chagas disease is an independent risk factor for ischaemic stroke and a major cause of cardioembolic stroke.[55]

Human African trypanosomiasis, also called sleeping sickness, is a chronic form of the disease present in Western and Central Africa. It is caused by the protozoan *Trypanosome brucei*, and transmitted to human beings by the blood-sucking tsetse fly (genus: *Glossina*).[56] This important disease in sub-Saharan Africa is responsible for a considerable degree of suffering and mortality in countries where it is endemic.[57] The annual incidence of the disease is decreasing.[58] As well as multiple systemic features seen in the early (haemolymphatic) stage of disease, the late (encephalitic) stage, is associated with a wide range of other neurological features, including neuropsychiatric, motor, and sensory abnormalities.[59]

Many other parasites could lead to neurological disorders, in particular convulsions and epilepsy like gnathostomiasis, paragonimiasis, etc.

CNS Fungal infections

Fungal diseases are a public health problem. There are mainly seen in immunocompromised individuals. Their global mortality is expected to reach 1,500,000 per year[60] and 50% of deaths are related to AIDS.[61] Fungal meningitis is responsible for 500,000 deaths each year among persons living with AIDS.[62] More than 90% of all reported fungal-related deaths result from species that belong to one of the following four: *Cryptococcus, Candida, Aspergillus*, and *Pneumocystis*.[60]

Up to 1,500,000 fungal species exist and nearly 300 species have been associated with human infection, there are about a dozen yeasts and about 30 moulds that are commonly identified as human pathogens. The main routes of acquisition are respiratory or traumatic inoculation with subsequent spread, haematogenous or contiguous. Pathogens encountered in the CNS include yeasts (*Candida, Cryptococcus*), moniliaceous molds (*Aspergillus, Fusarium*), dimorphic fungi (*Blastomyces, Coccidioides, Histoplasma*), zygomycetes (Mucorales, *Rhizopus*) and dematiaceous fungi (*Pseudallescheria*).[63] The main aetiologies of CNS fungal infections include *Aspergillus* species, *Cryptococcus neoformans, Candida* species, Mucorales, Zygomycetes, melanized fungi and others.[64]

Aspergillus and *Cryptococcus* in the immunosuppressed are the most common baseline aetiologies.[65] In this part, we will discuss these CNS fungal infections.

Cryptococcus

Cryptococcus neoformans (C. neoformans) is an opportunistic human pathogen. There are two varieties of *C. neoformans var. neoformans* (Serotype A and D) and *var. gatti* (Serotype B and C). Serotype A is distributed worldwide and is most associated with pigeon droppings.[66]. Serotype D is isolated in Europe with heterogeneous distribution and serotype B is originally associated with vicinity of Eucalyptus trees.[67]

Cryptococcosis is an invasive fungal infection that is usually manifested as meningoencephalitis mainly in immunocompromised patients. However, recent studies show that the clinical presentation of cryptococcal meningitis (CrM) in both immunocompetent and immunocompromised patients is similar.[68] *Cryptococcus* has higher incidence among AIDS patients in developing countries in Africa and South East Asia than in the USA.[69]

CrM is a neglected tropical disease that is responsible for a high mortality of approximately 20% in immunosuppressed patients.[70] The risk factors identified in the studies are AIDS, decompensated liver cirrhosis, and cell-mediated immunity-suppressive regimens without calcineurin inhibitors.[71,72] In a more recent study in 2016, the OR for developing CrM was 42.9 (95% CI: 3.3–555.5, p = 0.0055) in patients with positive serum cryptococcal antigens.[72]

Worldwide, the yearly global burden of CrM is estimated to nearly one million cases.[62]

According to recent data, among HIV/AIDS-patients the global incidence of CrM was 223,100 cases in 2014 and the mortality was estimated at 181,100 annual global deaths, with 135,900 (75%) deaths in sub-Saharan Africa. Globally, CrM was responsible for 15% of AIDS-related deaths (95% CI 10–19) in 2014.[73]

This mortality rates in AIDS patients are estimated to range from 15 to 20% in the USA and 55–70% in Latin America and sub-Saharan Africa, despite treatment.[62]

Aspergillus

Aspergillus is a ubiquitous fungus that lives in soil and decaying vegetation. *A. fumigatus* is the most common species of *Aspergillus* family, others being *A. niger* and *A. flavus*.[74] Aspergillosis is a filamentous fungal infection caused of the genus *Aspergillus*.[74]

This disease develops primarily in immunocompromised patients and may progress to disseminated aspergillosis, defined by the infection of at least two non-contiguous organs. The incidence of invasive aspergillosis in HIV/AIDS patients varies between 0% and 12%.[75] The risk factors for aspergillosis were bone marrow transplantation and haematologic malignancy, but patients had a variety of underlying conditions, including solid organ transplants, AIDS, and pulmonary diseases.[76]

Aspergillosis of the CNS is rare. CNS involvement is mainly due to haematogenous spread rather than via direct spread of infection from sinus, orbit, nose, and ear. *Aspergillus* targets blood vessels and invades them, producing a thrombus, haemorrhage, or, rarely, mycotic aneurysm. Haemorrhagic infarct is the most common pathologic finding on autopsy. Cerebral aspergillosis (CA) is the worst clinical form, accounting for 5–10% of all intracranial fungal pathology[77] with a 85–100% mortality rate.[78,79] CA is mainly reported with recipients of immunosuppressive disorders such as HIV/AIDS, solid organ transplants, patients on chemotherapy, diabetes, heroin abuse, long-term steroid or broad-spectrum antibiotics use, neutropenia, history of opportunistic infection, and use of ganciclovir/valacyclovir.[75,80,81] CA is uncommon among immunocompetent patients.[82]

CNS Viral infections

Several viruses can infect the CNS. The most common include:

- Human herpes viruses (herpes simplex viruses: HSV, Varicella-Zoster virus: VZV, Epstein-Barr virus: EBV, cytomegalovirus: CMV).
- Arboviruses such as the flaviviruses: dengue virus, yellow fever virus, West Nile virus, Japanese encephalitis virus (JEV), and tick-borne encephalitis (TBE) virus, the alphavirus (chikungunya virus), the rhabdovirus (rabies virus), the bunyavirus.
- Retrovirus: HIV.
- Other virus: polyomavirus (JC virus), adenovirus, Coxsackie viruses, echoviruses, enteroviruses, arenavirus.

CNS viral infections present mostly clinically with meningitis and encephalitis.

Herpes viruses

Herpes simplex encephalitis (HSE) is a potentially lethal viral infection of the brain parenchyma caused by HSV type 1 and 2 (HSV1 and HSV2). Despite being a rare disease, HSE is the most common form of sporadic encephalitis worldwide and the commonest cause of viral encephalitis in HMICs. Most studies reported incidence rates ranging from 1 to 4.64 cases per million population per year without seasonal or sex-related variability.[83–86]

Untreated, HSE is associated with 70% mortality. This mortality decreased to 15–20% with the advent of acyclovir treatment and improvements in diagnostic techniques.[84,87]

About 90% of HSE cases in adults, children, and patients with a healthy immune system are due to HSV1, while HSV2 is associated with HSE in neonates, inducing disseminated infection, and in immunocompromised patients.[88–90] There are two peaks of morbidity: one under the age of 20 and the other in the mid-sixties.[91] Nevertheless, patients in immuno-suppression are at risk of a less favourable and atypical course of the infection.[89]

HSE is a medical emergency. The signs of HSE are those of a non-specific meningoencephalitis. The EEG is invariably abnormal. Non-specific slowing of electrical activity may be the only characteristic at the onset of the disease and usually involves a temporal lobe. Then, as the disease progresses, this slowing spreads in the contralateral temporal lobe, usually for a period of 7–10 days. Focal changes in the EEG are characterized by spike, slow-wave activity, and periodic lateralized epileptiform discharges at the temporal lobe.

Arbovirus

In travellers, arthropod-borne encephalitis viruses (arboviruses) are important causative agents in those returning from endemic areas. These viruses are transmitted to human beings by the bites of arthropods (particularly mosquitos and ticks) and are a leading cause of encephalitis globally. Arboviruses, such as West Nile virus and JEV, have spread to new areas, and West Nile virus has caused outbreaks in the Americas and southern Europe.[92] Worldwide, rabies and JEV are responsible for an estimated annual mortality of 60,000 and 17,000 people respectively.[93,94] Cases of JEV encephalitis are restricted to Asia, whereas rabies is a scourge throughout South East Asia, Africa, and Latin America and occurs, although less frequently, in other areas worldwide. JEV has variable mortality, depending, in part, on the infected individual's age. Among survivors, long-term cognitive or neurological impairment is present in as many as 70% of those with HSV encephalitis.[95]

There is little data on dengue and chikungunya viruses in Low and Middle Income Countries (LMICs), but they will probably become global causes of arboviral encephalitis in the next decade.[93,96,97] Although encephalitis is present in only a fraction of those infected with dengue virus, the large number of dengue infections worldwide could lead to hundreds of thousands of encephalitis cases.

Dengue is the second most common mosquito-borne disease affecting humans after malaria.[96] Neurological complications of dengue virus infection can be categorized into dengue encephalopathy, encephalitis, immune-mediated syndromes, dengue muscle dysfunction, and neuro-ophthalmic disorders. CNS manifestations or complications include dengue encephalopathy, encephalitis, immune complex-mediated syndromes, and dengue muscle dysfunction.[98] An estimated 390 million dengue infections occur annually.[99] Some 3.9 billion people are at risk of dengue worldwide.[96]

Outbreaks of chikungunya virus have been reported in several African countries, the Indian subcontinent, and South East Asia,[33] and an outbreak was recently reported in Italy.[34]

Sporadic cases of Zika virus (ZIKV), an emerging flavivirus were reported worldwide. In 2016, the link between Zika virus and microcephaly in foetuses born to mothers infected with ZIKV was confirmed.[100,101]

TBE caused by a TBE virus, is prevalent in forested areas of moderate climate across a large geographical area spanning from northern China and Japan through far-eastern Russia and into Europe. TBE is a serious cause of acute CNS disease, which may result in death or long-term neurological sequelae. The risk for travellers of acquiring TBE is increasing with the rise in tourism to areas of endemicity during spring and summer.[102] TBE is transmitted from the saliva of an infected tick. TBE can occasionally be transmitted after an intake of non-pasteurized milk products from viraemic livestock. Single cases of TBE after slaughter of probably viraemic goats, blood transfusions, breastfeeding, and laboratory investigations have also been described.[103]

According to the official data, there are about 10,000–15,000 cases of TBE per year worldwide, Russia alone accounting for nearly half to two-thirds of this number.[104] Reported incidence rates vary greatly between and within countries, from 0.7/100,000 in Austria to 55/100,000 in some regions of Latvia, and 76/100,000 in Koroska region of Slovenia or similarly in Tomsk region of Russia.[104] In prospective studies, a predominance of infection in men is usually seen in all age groups. TBE has recently joined the diseases under surveillance in the EU.[105]

The disease burden is attributed mainly to resulting long-term disability, especially in individuals over 50 years of age. Currently, there is no causative treatment, but a very effective vaccination is available with a good safety profile. The vaccination requires three basic doses to be fully effective and regular boosters afterwards.

Retrovirus: HIV

HIV is transmitted through contaminated blood or blood products, by use of contaminated needles or surgical instruments, via sexual contact, and from mother-to-child. In 2016, an estimated 36.7 million people were living with HIV worldwide.[106] Most of the morbidity and mortality about HIV infections result from secondary infections due to the immunodeficiency. But the CNS can be directly affected, with a great variability in manifestations. A standardized diagnostic classification of HIV-Associated Neurocognitive Disorders (HAND) have been provided.[107] This covers neurocognitive disorders as much as functional decline and other HIV associated conditions.

Indeed, the CNS is the second target of HIV after the immune system.[108] CNS attack can occur at all stages of HIV infection, and especially during the early and later stage of HIV infection when HIV viral load is high. AIDS, a clinical syndrome associated with a progressive deterioration of the immune status of the individual, is characterized by the progressive depletion of the CD4+ T-lymphocyte population. HIV enters the brain at the time of the primary HIV infection. On crossing the barrier monocytes may become activated perivascular macrophages. HIV replicates in these cells, as well as in microglia and astrocytes. More than 20% of HIV infected persons die from opportunistic infections of the CNS and CNS malignancy which were common prior to the use of antiretroviral therapy. But since the increased access to antiretroviral therapy less than 5% of HIV infected persons are affected and HIV encephalitis has become exceptional.[109]

Antiretroviral therapy is the main treatment for prevention and cure of CNS from HIV.

CMV

Human CMV is a strictly human virus, which infects 40–70% of the population in industrialized countries.[110,111] The prevalence increases with population and low socio-economic level. It can reach 90% or even 100% in some populations, especially in developing countries, or highly populated areas of Asia.[112,113] Transmission of CMV occurs through biological fluids like saliva, urine, blood, and sperm. CMV retinitis is the most frequent localization. The other localizations are rare (about 15%) and concern lungs, oesophagus, and CNS. In immunocompetent patients, CMV infection is most of the time asymptomatic or with an influenza-like syndrome, particularly in children. In adults, there may be an infectious mononucleosis-like syndrome with abnormal lymphocytes, thrombopenia splenomegaly, and impaired liver function. However, CNS diseases (encephalitis, myelitis, myeloradiculitis) may sometimes arise in immunocompetent patients, more often in middle-aged or elderly people.[114] Serological diagnosis is based on the dosage of the IgG and IgM. In case of primary infection, IgG and IgM are both detected in most cases, but the best proof of primary infection is the seroconversion between two sera. Indeed, IgM can be detected during a reactivation.

Actually, detection of CMV DNA has to be performed by real-time PCR in blood when there is a suspicion of CMV infection and in CSF when signs of CNS infection are present. Quantification of CMV DNA is used to follow the efficacy of antiviral treatment.

First therapeutic line against CMV is ganciclovir administered intravenously, or valganciclovir, given orally, until symptom resolution and negativation of the DNAemia with monitoring of side effects. Drug-resistant CMV is a therapeutic challenge. The first alternative is foscarnet but a high level of renal toxicity is associated with the use of this drug. The nucleoside analog cidofovir may be used in case of foscarnet toxicity or resistance.[115] Immune reconstitution, through reduction in immunosuppression contributes to viral control. Despite a lot of vaccinal trials, no CMV vaccine is available to prevent infection.

JC virus

Progressive multifocal leukoencephalopathy (PML) is an opportunistic demyelinating infection of the CNS caused by the JC virus (JCV), a ubiquitous polyoma virus which is found in approximately 50–86% of the adult population worldwide.[116–118] Prevalence of PML increased significantly during the last century in conjunction with the AIDS epidemic, with approximately 5% of patients developing the complications resulting in PML being considered among the disease-defining illnesses.[119,120]

In immunocompetent individuals, JCV infection remains a latent asymptomatic infection of the kidneys.[116,121] However, in immunocompromised individuals, it can cause a rapidly progressive and often fatal CNS infection which was first described in the setting of Hodgkin's disease and chronic lymphocytic leukaemia in 1958.[122] PML remained rare until the HIV epidemic when it was seen in the context of AIDS with 1.3 cases per 1000 HIV + person-years.[123] In recent years, PML has also increased in incidence in HIV-uninfected persons with the rise of immunomodulatory and immunosuppressive agents, including chemotherapies, rheumatologic disease-modifying therapies, and MS treatments, which result in decreased immune surveillance in the CNS and increased risk of PML. In most cases, the disease results in a fatal outcome within a few months. Antiretroviral therapy is currently considered to be the only method for the prevention and treatment of PML in HIV-infected patients.

Limitations and Issues of Epidemiological Studies

Epidemiological evidence concerning non-bacterial CNS infections is still limited. Methodological heterogeneities between the studies (case-control or cohort, hospital-based or population-based) and the lack of use of standardized definitions weaken firm conclusions.

Different studies consist in the heterogeneity of techniques to determine an agent exposure/infection (e.g. NCC prevalence: EITB assay or CT scan; *Toxocariasis*: Ab-ELISA or WB). Using gold standard methods is essential for accurate conclusions.

The lack of trained healthcare personnel, inadequate tools, and equipment to perform diagnosis, especially in LMICs could lead to a lack of availability of epidemiological data in several regions. Establishing causality between a specific pathogen and a disease is challenging on this context.

Conclusion

Viruses, fungi, and parasites lead to many neurological diseases and carry a high burden especially in LMICs. CNS attempt is a particularly severe form of those infections. Most of the non-bacterial CNS infections are considered neglected diseases and need more attention from the international community. Some of these infections have become rare due to access to effective treatment, thus modifying their epidemiological distribution. Others are emerging because of their association with HIV/AIDS especially in LMICs, in spite of access to antiretroviral therapy.

The heterogeneity of the existing literature and lack of standardized methodology limits comparisons, establishment of causality, and epidemiological conclusions. Use of standardized methods, the inclusion of incident cases, population-based studies, training of healthcare personnel, and providing access to adequate tools especially in LMICs are the challenges to provide accurate epidemiological evidence of non-bacterial CNS infections.

REFERENCES

1. World Health Organization. Investing to Overcome the Global Impact of Neglected Tropical Diseases: Third WHO Report on Neglected Tropical Diseases 2015. Geneva: World Health Organization, 2015. p211.
2. Ndimubanzi PC, Carabin H, Budke CM, Nguyen H, Qian Y-J, Rainwater E, et al. A systematic review of the frequency of neurocyticercosis with a focus on people with epilepsy. PLOS Negl Trop Dis (Internet). 2010; 4(11). Available from: https://www.ncbi.nlm.nih.gov/pmc/articles/PMC2970544/.
3. Ba-Diop A, Marin B, Druet-Cabanac M, Ngoungou EB, Newton CR, Preux PM. Epidemiology, causes, and treatment of epilepsy in sub-Saharan Africa—Lancet Neurology. Lancet Neurology. 2014; 1029–44.
4. Pal DK, Carpio A, Sander JW. Neurocysticercosis and epilepsy in developing countries. J Neurol Neurosurg Psychiatry. 2000; 68(2): 137–43.
5. White AC. Neurocysticercosis: a major cause of neurological disease worldwide. Clin Infect Dis Off Publ Infect Dis Soc Am. 1997; 24(2): 101–13; quiz 114–15.
6. Singh G, Prabhakar S. Taenia Solium Cysticercosis: From Basic to Clinical Science. Wallingford: CABI, 2002. p480.
7. Quet F, Guerchet M, Pion SDS, Ngoungou EB, Nicoletti A, Preux P-M. Meta-analysis of the association between cysticercosis and epilepsy in Africa. Epilepsia. 2010; 51(5): 830–7.
8. Garcia HH, Nash TE, Del Brutto OH. Clinical symptoms, diagnosis, and treatment of neurocysticercosis. Lancet Neurology. 2014; 13(12): 1202–15.
9. Bhalla D, Godet B, Druet-Cabanac M, Preux P-M. Etiologies of epilepsy: a comprehensive review. Expert Rev Neurother. 2011; 11(6): 861–76.
10. Winkler AS, Kerschbaumsteiner K, Stelzhammer B, Meindl M, Kaaya J, Schmutzhard E. Prevalence, incidence, and clinical characteristics of epilepsy-a community-based door-to-door study in northern Tanzania. Epilepsia. 2009; 50(10): 2310–3.
11. Winkler AS, Blocher J, Auer H, Gotwald T, Matuja W, Schmutzhard E. Epilepsy and neurocysticercosis in rural Tanzania—an imaging study. Epilepsia. 2009; 50(5): 987–93.
12. Debacq G, Moyano LM, Garcia HH, Boumediene F, Marin B, Ngoungou EB, et al. Systematic review and meta-analysis estimating association of cysticercosis and neurocysticercosis with epilepsy. PLOS Negl Trop Dis. 2017; 11(3): e0005153.
13. Nash TE, Mahanty S, Loeb JA, Theodore WH, Friedman A, Sander JW, et al. Neurocysticercosis: a natural human model of epileptogenesis. Epilepsia. 2015; 56(2): 177–83.
14. Garcia HH, Del Brutto OH. Cysticercosis Working Group in Peru. Neurocysticercosis: updated concepts about an old disease. Lancet Neurology. 2005; 4(10): 653–61.
15. Winkler AS, Blocher J, Auer H, Gotwald T, Matuja W, Schmutzhard E. Anticysticercal and antitoxocaral antibodies in people with epilepsy in rural Tanzania. Trans R Soc Trop Med Hyg. 2008; 102(10): 1032–8.
16. García HH, Evans CAW, Nash TE, Takayanagui OM, White AC, Botero D, et al. Current consensus guidelines for treatment of neurocysticercosis. Clin Microbiol Rev. 2002; 15(4): 747–56.
17. Basáñez M-G, Pion SDS, Churcher TS, Breitling LP, Little MP, Boussinesq M. River blindness: a success story under threat? PLOS Med (Internet). 2006; 3(9). Available from: https://www.ncbi.nlm.nih.gov/pmc/articles/PMC1576321/.
18. Winkler AS, Friedrich K, Meindl M, Kidunda A, Nassri A, Jilek-Aall L, et al. Clinical characteristics of people with head nodding in southern Tanzania. Trop Doct. 2010; 40(3): 173–5.
19. Winkler AS, Wallner B, Friedrich K, Pfausler B, Unterberger I, Matuja W, et al. A longitudinal study on nodding syndrome-a new African epilepsy disorder. Epilepsia. 2014; 55(1): 86–93.
20. Centers for Disease Control and Prevention (CDC). Nodding syndrome—South Sudan, 2011. MMWR Morb Mortal Wkly Rep. 2012; 61(3): 52–4.
21. World Health Organization. *International Scientific Meeting on Nodding Syndrome. Meeting report.* Kampala, Uganda: World Health Organization, 2012.
22. Iyengar PJ, Wamala J, Ratto J, Blanton C, Malimbo M, Lukwago L, et al. Prevalence of nodding syndrome—Uganda, 2012–2013. MMWR Morb Mortal Wkly Rep. 2014; 63(28): 603–6.
23. Colebunders R, Post R, O'Neill S, Haesaert G, Opar B, Lakwo T, et al. Nodding syndrome since 2012: recent progress, challenges and recommendations for future research. Trop Med Int Health TM IH. 2015; 20(2): 194–200.
24. Sejvar JJ, Kakooza AM, Foltz JL, Makumbi I, Atai-Omoruto AD, Malimbo M, et al. Clinical, neurological, and electrophysiological features of nodding syndrome in Kitgum, Uganda: an observational case series. Lancet Neurology. 2013; 12(2): 166–74.
25. Winkler AS, Friedrich K, König R, Meindl M, Helbok R, Unterberger I, et al. The head nodding syndrome-clinical classification and possible causes. Epilepsia. 2008; 49(12): 2008–15.
26. Foltz JL, Makumbi I, Sejvar JJ, Malimbo M, Ndyomugyenyi R, Atai-Omoruto AD, et al. An epidemiologic investigation of potential risk factors for nodding syndrome in Kitgum District, Uganda. PLOS One. 2013; 8(6): e66419.

27. Dowell SF, Sejvar JJ, Riek L, Vandemaele KAH, Lamunu M, Kuesel AC, et al. Nodding syndrome. Emerg Infect Dis. 2013; 19(9): 1374–84.
28. Johnson TP, Tyagi R, Lee PR, Lee M-H, Johnson KR, Kowalak J, et al. Nodding syndrome may be an autoimmune reaction to the parasitic worm Onchocerca volvulus. Sci Transl Med. 2017; 9(377).
29. Rubinsky-Elefant G, Hirata CE, Yamamoto JH, Ferreira MU. Human toxocariasis: diagnosis, worldwide seroprevalences and clinical expression of the systemic and ocular forms. Ann Trop Med Parasitol. 2010; 104(1): 3–23.
30. Luna J, Cicero CE, Rateau G, Quattrocchi G, Marin B, Bruno E, et al. Updated evidence of the association between toxocariasis and epilepsy: Systematic review and meta-analysis. PLoS Negl Trop Dis. 2018;12(7):e0006665.
31. Lynch NR, Eddy K, Hodgen AN, Lopez RI, Turner KJ. Seroprevalence of Toxocara canis infection in tropical Venezuela. Trans R Soc Trop Med Hyg. 1988; 82(2): 275–81.
32. Magnaval JF, Michault A, Calon N, Charlet JP. Epidemiology of human toxocariasis in La Réunion. Trans R Soc Trop Med Hyg. 1994; 88(5): 531–3.
33. Gavignet B, Piarroux R. Toxocariasis in humans: clinical expression and treatment dilemma. J Am Acad Dermatol. 2008; 59(6): 1031–42.
34. Finsterer J, Auer H. Neurotoxocarosis. Rev Inst Med Trop Sao Paulo. 2007; 49(5): 279–87.
35. Bächli H, Minet JC, Gratzl O. Cerebral toxocariasis: a possible cause of epileptic seizure in children. Childs Nerv Syst ChNS Off J Int Soc Pediatr Neurosurg. 2004; 20(7): 468–72.
36. Richartz E, Buchkremer G. Cerebral toxocariasis: a rare cause of cognitive disorders. A contribution to differential dementia diagnosis. Nervenarzt. 2002; 73(5): 458–62.
37. Vidal JE, Sztajnbok J, Seguro AC. Eosinophilic meningoencephalitis due to Toxocara canis: case report and review of the literature. Am J Trop Med Hyg. 2003; 69(3): 341–3.
38. Ngoungou EB, Preux P-M. Cerebral malaria and epilepsy. Epilepsia. 2008; 49 (Suppl 6): 19–24.
39. Snow RW, Craig M, Deichmann U, Marsh K. Estimating mortality, morbidity and disability due to malaria among Africa's non-pregnant population. Bull World Health Organ. 1999; 77(8): 624–40.
40. Ikome LE, Ndamukong KJN, Kimbi H. Prevalence and case-control study of cerebral malaria in Limbe of the South-West Cameroon. Afr J Health Sci. 2002; 9(1–2): 61–7.
41. Molyneux ME, Taylor TE, Wirima JJ, Borgstein A. Clinical features and prognostic indicators in paediatric cerebral malaria: a study of 131 comatose Malawian children. Q J Med. 1989; 71(265): 441–59.
42. Newton CR, Hien TT, White N. Cerebral malaria. J Neurol Neurosurg Psychiatry. 2000; 69(4): 433–41.
43. Carter JA, Neville BGR, White S, Ross AJ, Otieno G, Mturi N, et al. Increased prevalence of epilepsy associated with severe falciparum malaria in children. Epilepsia. 2004; 45(8): 978–81.
44. Ngoungou EB, Koko J, Druet-Cabanac M, Assengone-Zeh-Nguema Y, Launay MN, Engohang E, et al. Cerebral malaria and sequelar epilepsy: first matched case-control study in Gabon. Epilepsia. 2006; 47(12): 2147–53.
45. Ngoungou EB, Dulac O, Poudiougou B, Druet-Cabanac M, Dicko A, Mamadou Traore A, et al. Epilepsy as a consequence of cerebral malaria in area in which malaria is endemic in Mali, West Africa. Epilepsia. 2006; 47(5): 873–9.
46. Christensen SS, Eslick GD. Cerebral malaria as a risk factor for the development of epilepsy and other long-term neurological conditions: a meta-analysis. Trans R Soc Trop Med Hyg. 2015; 109(4): 233–8.
47. Van der Torn M, Thuma PE, Mabeza GF, Biemba G, Moyo VM, McLaren CE, et al. Loading dose of quinine in African children with cerebral malaria. Trans R Soc Trop Med Hyg. 1998; 92(3): 325–31.
48. Jones JL, Dubey JP. Foodborne toxoplasmosis. Clin Infect Dis Off Publ Infect Dis Soc Am. 2012; 55(6): 845–51.
49. Pappas G, Roussos N, Falagas ME. Toxoplasmosis snapshots: global status of Toxoplasma gondii seroprevalence and implications for pregnancy and congenital toxoplasmosis. Int J Parasitol. 2009; 39(12): 1385–94.
50. Coelho L, Cardoso SW, Amancio RT, Moreira RI, Campos DP, Veloso VG, et al. Trends in AIDS-defining opportunistic illnesses incidence over 25 years in Rio de Janeiro, Brazil. PLOS One. 2014; 9(6): e98666.
51. Lewden C, Drabo YJ, Zannou DM, Maiga MY, Minta DK, Sow PS, et al. Disease patterns and causes of death of hospitalized HIV-positive adults in West Africa: a multicountry survey in the antiretroviral treatment era. J Int AIDS Soc. 2014; 17: 18797.
52. Woodhall D, Jones JL, Cantey PT, Wilkins PP, Montgomery SP. Neglected parasitic infections: what every family physician needs to know. Am Fam Physician. 2014; 89(10): 803–11.
53. Ngoungou EB, Bhalla D, Nzoghe A, Dardé M-L, Preux P-M. Toxoplasmosis and epilepsy—systematic review and meta analysis. PLOS Negl Trop Dis. 2015; 9(2): e0003525.
54. Liu Q, Zhou X-N. Preventing the transmission of American trypanosomiasis and its spread into non-endemic countries. Infect Dis Poverty (Internet). 2015; 4. Available from: https://www.ncbi.nlm.nih.gov/pmc/articles/PMC4693433/.
55. Carod-Artal FJ, Vargas AP, Horan TA, Nunes LGN. Chagasic cardiomyopathy is independently associated with ischemic stroke in Chagas disease. Stroke. 2005; 36(5): 965–70.
56. Kennedy PG. Clinical features, diagnosis, and treatment of human African trypanosomiasis (sleeping sickness). Lancet Neurology. 2013; 12(2): 186–94.
57. Hide G. History of Sleeping Sickness in East Africa. Clin Microbiol Rev. 1999; 12(1): 112–25.
58. WHO. Trypanosomiasis, human African (sleeping sickness) (Internet). WHO. 2017. Available from: http://www.who.int/mediacentre/factsheets/fs259/en/.
59. Kennedy PGE. Human African trypanosomiasis—neurological aspects. J Neurol. 2006; 253(4): 411–16.
60. Brown GD, Denning DW, Gow NAR, Levitz SM, Netea MG, White TC. Hidden killers: human fungal infections. Sci Transl Med. 2012; 4(165): 165rv13-165rv13.
61. Armstrong-James D, Meintjes G, Brown GD. A neglected epidemic: fungal infections in HIV/AIDS. Trends Microbiol. 2014; 22(3): 120–7.
62. Park BJ, Wannemuehler KA, Marston BJ, Govender N, Pappas PG, Chiller TM. Estimation of the current global burden of cryptococcal meningitis among persons living with HIV/AIDS. AIDS Lond Engl. 2009; 23(4): 525–30.
63. Redmond A, Dancer C, Woods ML. Fungal infections of the central nervous system: A review of fungal pathogens and treatment. Neurol India. 2007; 55(3): 251–9.
64. Zarrin M, Zarei Mahmoudabadi A. Central nervous system fungal infections; a review article. Jundishapur J Microbiol. 2010; 3(2): 41–7.
65. Murthy JMK, Sundaram C. Fungal infections of the central nervous system. Handb Clin Neurol. 2014; 121: 1383–401.

66. Majid Z, Masoomeh J, Nasrin A, Morad R. Isolation of Cryptococcus neoformans from pigeon droppings in Ahwaz, Iran. Turk J Med Sci. 2010; 40(2): 313–16.
67. Ito-Kuwa S, Nakamura K, Valderrama B, Aoki S, Vidotto V, Osafune T. Diversity of laccase among Cryptococcus neoformans serotypes. Microbiol Immunol. 2008; 52(10): 492–8.
68. Koshy JM, Mohan S, Deodhar D, John M, Oberoi A, Pannu A. Clinical diversity of CNS Cryptococcosis. J Assoc Physicians India. 2016; 64(10): 15–19.
69. Koshy JM, Deodhar D, Brar I, Pandian J, John M, Oberoi A, et al. Central nervous system manifestations in human immunodeficiency virus patients in the antiretroviral therapy era—Scenario from a developing country. CHRISMED J Health Res. 2015; 2(3): 245–50.
70. Brizendine KD, Baddley JW, Pappas PG. Predictors of mortality and differences in clinical features among patients with Cryptococcosis according to immune status. PLOS One (Internet). 2013; 8(3). Available from: https://www.ncbi.nlm.nih.gov/pmc/articles/PMC3608592/.
71. Lin Y-Y, Shiau S, Fang C-T. Risk factors for invasive Cryptococcus neoformans diseases: a case-control study. PLOS One. 2015; 10(3): e0119090.
72. Henao-Martínez AF, Gross L, Mcnair B, McCollister B, DeSanto K, Montoya JG, et al. Risk factors for Cryptococcal meningitis: A single United States center experience. Mycopathologia. 2016; 181(11–12): 807–14.
73. Rajasingham R, Smith RM, Park BJ, Jarvis JN, Govender NP, Chiller TM, et al. Global burden of disease of HIV-associated cryptococcal meningitis: an updated analysis. Lancet Infect Dis. 2017; 17(8): 873–81.
74. Nadkarni T, Goel A. Aspergilloma of the brain: an overview. J Postgrad Med. 2005; 51(5): 37.
75. Vidal JE, Dauar RF, Melhem MSC, Szeszs W, Pukinskas SRBS, Coelho JFGS, et al. Cerebral aspergillosis due to Aspergillus fumigatus in AIDS patient: first culture—proven case reported in Brazil. Rev Inst Med Trop São Paulo. 2005; 47(3): 161–5.
76. Patterson TF, Kirkpatrick WR, White M, Hiemenz JW, Wingard JR, Dupont B, et al. Invasive aspergillosis. Disease spectrum, treatment practices, and outcomes. I3 Aspergillus Study Group. Medicine (Baltimore). 2000; 79(4): 250–60.
77. Ellenbogen JR, Waqar M, Cooke RPD, Javadpour M. Management of granulomatous cerebral aspergillosis in immunocompetent adult patients: a review. Br J Neurosurg. 2016; 30(3): 280–5.
78. Balasubramaniam P, Madakira PB, Ninan A, Swaminathan A. Response of central nervous system aspergillosis to voriconazole. Neurol India. 2007; 55(3): 301.
79. Phuttharak W, Hesselink JR, Wixom C. MR Features of cerebral aspergillosis in an immunocompetent patient: correlation with histology and elemental analysis. Am J Neuroradiol. 2005; 26(4): 835–8.
80. Denning DW. Invasive aspergillosis. Clin Infect Dis Off Publ Infect Dis Soc Am. 1998; 26(4): 781–803; quiz 804–5.
81. Pongbhaesaj P, Dejthevaporn C, Tunlayadechanont S, Witoonpanich R, Sungkanuparph S, Vibhagool A. Aspergillosis of the central nervous system: a catastrophic opportunistic infection. Southeast Asian J Trop Med Public Health. 2004; 35(1): 119–25.
82. Bao Z-S, You G, Li W-B, Jiang T. A single aspergillus fumigatus intracranial abscess in an immunocompetent patient with parietal lobe tumorectomy. World J Surg Oncol. 2014; 12: 181.
83. Whitley RJ. Herpes simplex encephalitis: Adolescents and adults. Antiviral Res. 2006; 71(2–3): 141–8.
84. Hjalmarsson A, Blomqvist P, Sköldenberg B. Herpes simplex encephalitis in Sweden, 1990-2001: incidence, morbidity, and mortality. Clin Infect Dis Off Publ Infect Dis Soc Am. 2007; 45(7): 875–80.
85. Jouan Y, Grammatico-Guillon L, Espitalier F, Cazals X, François P, Guillon A. Long-term outcome of severe herpes simplex encephalitis: a population-based observational study. Crit Care. 2015; 19(1): 345.
86. Barbadoro P, Marigliano A, Ricciardi A, D'Errico MM, Prospero E. Trend of hospital utilization for encephalitis. Epidemiol Infect. 2012; 140(4): 753–64.
87. Raschilas F, Wolff M, Delatour F, Chaffaut C, De Broucker T, Chevret S, et al. Outcome of and prognostic factors for herpes simplex encephalitis in adult patients: results of a multicenter study. Clin Infect Dis Off Publ Infect Dis Soc Am. 2002; 35(3): 254–60.
88. Arciniegas DB, Anderson CA. Viral encephalitis: neuropsychiatric and neurobehavioral aspects. Curr Psychiatry Rep. 2004; 6(5): 372–9.
89. Meyding-Lamadé U, Strank C. Herpesvirus infections of the central nervous system in immunocompromised patients. Ther Adv Neurol Disord. 2012; 5(5): 279.
90. Kennedy PGE, Chaudhuri A. Herpes simplex encephalitis. J Neurol Neurosurg Psychiatry. 2002; 73(3): 237–8.
91. Steiner I, Kennedy PG, Pachner AR. The neurotropic herpes viruses: herpes simplex and varicella-zoster. Lancet Neurology. 2007; 6(11): 1015–28.
92. Solomon T, Hart IJ, Beeching NJ. Viral encephalitis: a clinician's guide. Pract Neurol. 2007; 7(5): 288–305.
93. LaBeaud Ad, Bashir F, King CH. Measuring the burden of arboviral diseases: the spectrum of morbidity and mortality from four prevalent infections. Popul Health Metr. 2011; 9(1): 1.
94. Fooks AR, Banyard AC, Horton DL, Johnson N, McElhinney LM, Jackson AC. Current status of rabies and prospects for elimination. Lancet. 2014; 384(9951): 1389–99.
95. McGrath N, Anderson NE, Croxson MC, Powell KF. Herpes simplex encephalitis treated with acyclovir: diagnosis and long-term outcome. J Neurol Neurosurg Psychiatry. 1997; 63(3): 321–6.
96. Bhatt S, Gething PW, Brady OJ, Messina JP, Farlow AW, Moyes CL, et al. The global distribution and burden of dengue. Nature. 2013; 496(7446): 504–7.
97. Robin S, Ramful D, Le Seach' F, Jaffar-Bandjee M-C, Rigou G, Alessandri J-L. Neurologic manifestations of pediatric chikungunya infection. J Child Neurol. 2008; 23(9): 1028–35.
98. Carod-Artal FJ, Wichmann O, Farrar J, Gascón J. Neurological complications of dengue virus infection. Lancet Neurology. 2013; 12(9): 906–19.
99. WHO | *Dengue and severe dengue* (Internet). WHO. Available from: http://www.who.int.gate2.inist.fr/mediacentre/factsheets/fs117/en/
100. Cauchemez S, Besnard M, Bompard P, Dub T, Guillemette-Artur P, Eyrolle-Guignot D, et al. Association between Zika virus and microcephaly in French Polynesia, 2013–15: a retrospective study. Lancet Lond Engl. 2016; 387(10033): 2125–32.
101. WHO. *WHO Director-General summarizes the outcome of the Emergency Committee regarding clusters of microcephaly and Guillain-Barré syndrome*. WHO. Available from: http://

www.who.int/mediacentre/news/statements/2016/emergency-committee-zika-microcephaly/en/.
102. Chrdle A, Chmelik V, Ruzek D. Tick-borne encephalitis: what travellers should know when visiting an endemic country. Hum Vaccines Immunother. 2016; 2694–9.
103. Lindquist L, Vapalahti O. Tick-borne encephalitis. Lancet. 2008; 371(9627): 1861–71.
104. Amicizia D, Domnich A, Panatto D, Lai PL, Cristina ML, Avio U, et al. Epidemiology of tick-borne encephalitis (TBE) in Europe and its prevention by available vaccines. Hum Vaccines Immunother. 2013; 9(5): 1163–71.
105. Amato-Gauci A, Zeller H. Tick-borne encephalitis joins the diseases under surveillance in the European Union. Euro Surveill Bull Eur Sur Mal Transm Eur Commun Dis Bull. 2012; 17(42).
106. Fact sheet: Latest statistics on the status of the AIDS epidemic | UNAIDS (Internet). Available from: http://www.unaids.org/en/resources/fact-sheet.
107. Antinori A, Arendt G, Becker JT, Brew BJ, Byrd DA, Cherner M, et al. Updated research nosology for HIV-associated neurocognitive disorders. Neurology. 2007; 69(18): 1789–99.
108. Girard P-M, Katlama C, Pialoux G. VIH 2011. 8th ed. DOIN; 2011. 840 p.3.
109. Kolson D. Neurologic complications in persons with HIV infection in the era of antiretroviral therapy. Top Antivir Med. 2017; 25(3):97–101.
110. Kenneson A, Cannon MJ. Review and meta-analysis of the epidemiology of congenital cytomegalovirus (CMV) infection. Rev Med Virol. 2007; 17(4):253–76.
111. Ludwig A, Hengel H. Epidemiological impact and disease burden of congenital cytomegalovirus infection in Europe. Euro Surveill Bull Eur Sur Mal Transm Eur Commun Dis Bull. 2009;14(9): 26–32.
112. Cannon MJ, Schmid DS, Hyde TB. Review of cytomegalovirus seroprevalence and demographic characteristics associated with infection. Rev Med Virol. 2010; 20(4): 202–13.
113. Manicklal S, Emery VC, Lazzarotto T, Boppana SB, Gupta RK. The 'silent' global burden of congenital cytomegalovirus. Clin Microbiol Rev. 2013; 26(1): 86–102.
114. Studahl M, Hagberg L, Rekabdar E, Bergström T. Herpesvirus DNA detection in cerebral spinal fluid: differences in clinical presentation between alpha-, beta-, and gamma-herpesviruses. Scand J Infect Dis. 2000; 32(3): 237–48.
115. Tan BH. Cytomegalovirus Treatment. Curr Treat Options Infect Dis. 2014; 6(3): 256–70.
116. White MK, Khalili K. Pathogenesis of progressive multifocal leukoencephalopathy—revisited. J Infect Dis. 2011; 203(5): 578–86.
117. Bozic C, Subramanyam M, Richman S, Plavina T, Zhang A, Ticho B. Anti-JC virus (JCV) antibody prevalence in the JCV Epidemiology in MS (JEMS) trial. Eur J Neurol. 2014; 21(2): 299–304.
118. Miskin DP, Koralnik IJ. Novel syndromes associated with JC virus infection of neurons and meningeal cells: no longer a gray area. Curr Opin Neurol. 2015; 28(3): 288.
119. Vennegoor A, Van Rossum JA, Polman CH, Wattjes MP, Killestein J. Longitudinal JCV serology in multiple sclerosis patients preceding natalizumab-associated progressive multifocal leukoencephalopathy. Mult Scler. 2015; 21(12): 1600–3.
120. Calic Z, Cappelen-Smith C, Hodgkinson SJ, McDougall A, Cuganesan R, Brew BJ. Treatment of progressive multifocal leukoencephalopathy—immune reconstitution inflammatory syndrome with intravenous immunoglobulin in a patient with multiple sclerosis treated with fingolimod after discontinuation of natalizumab. J Clin Neurosci. 2015; 22(3): 598–600.
121. Egli A, Infanti L, Dumoulin A, Buser A, Samaridis J, Stebler C, et al. Prevalence of polyomavirus BK and JC infection and replication in 400 healthy blood donors. J Infect Dis. 2009; 199(6): 837–46.
122. Astrom KE, Mancall EL, Richardson EP. Progressive multifocal leuko-encephalopathy; a hitherto unrecognized complication of chronic lymphatic leukaemia and Hodgkin's disease. Brain J Neurol. 1958; 81(1): 93–111.
123. Engsig FN, Hansen A-BE, Omland LH, Kronborg G, Gerstoft J, Laursen AL, et al. Incidence, clinical presentation, and outcome of progressive multifocal leukoencephalopathy in HIV-infected patients during the highly active antiretroviral therapy era: a nationwide cohort study. J Infect Dis. 2009; 199(1): 77–83.

38

Traumatic brain and spinal cord injury

Alice Theadom and Kelly M Jones

What Is a Traumatic Brain Injury?

According to the World Health Organisation (WHO), traumatic brain injury (TBI) are defined as damage to the brain resulting in an altered mental state (e.g. dizziness, confusion and/or not remembering what happened) caused by external forces.[1] This may include a direct hit by a person or object, rapid acceleration or deceleration, a penetrating object (e.g. gunshot), or blast waves from an explosion. This definition of TBI stipulates that a person does not need to have experienced loss of consciousness to have sustained a TBI. Indeed loss of consciousness only occurs in just over half of TBI cases.[2] Concussions resulting in an altered state of consciousness are now considered to be a form of mild TBI.[3] The term TBI does not include injuries to the brain caused by internal factors (i.e. stroke, asphyxiation, medication, or drowning)[1] or broader 'head injuries' (i.e. injuries to the bones, muscles, or skin of the head). A diagnosis of TBI should informed by the description of the accident, symptomatology, and imaging if available.

Traumatic Brain Injury Incidence

Findings from current reviews on the incidence of TBI have been problematic to interpret. This is due to the inclusion of studies focusing on specific populations (e.g. older adults or just those experiencing moderate and severe TBI). Examinations limited to specific population groups can skew the findings when applied to the general population. Looking specifically at studies that encompass all ages, ethnicities, mechanisms, and severities of injury in a well-defined population, crude incidence rates have been found to vary widely even within continents. In Europe, incidence ranges between 45–546 per 100,000.[4,5] In Asia, average incidence is 181 per 100,000 ranging between 44–318 per 100,000.[6,7] In Australasia only one study[8] has been identified, reporting an incidence rate of 790 per 100,000. In North America average incidence ranges between 69–558 per 100,000.[9,10] The wide variation in incidence is likely to reflect first, the use of different definitions of TBI (e.g. some studies included self-harm and suicide in their estimates, which are excluded in other studies) and second, the use of different methods of case ascertainment (e.g. incidence rates are higher when sources beyond hospital admission and discharge records are included). Age-adjusted incidence rates are important to account for different population age distributions. For example, countries with a high proportion of very young or elderly people can skew the findings. However, at the time of writing this chapter only been reported in three studies, with estimates ranging widely between 69.7–811.[8,11,12]

Findings from studies conducted over the last 20 years have revealed that incidence appears to have remained relatively stable, and in Europe even to have decreased slightly. However, few longitudinal studies based on the same population and methodology have been conducted to date. These observations contrast with findings from the longitudinal TBI incidence surveillance project being run by the Centers for Disease Control and Prevention (CDC). The CDC project has revealed that in the USA, rates of TBI have been found to have steadily increased from 521 per 100,000 in 2001 to 824 per 100,000 in 2010.[13] Whilst the trend has steadily increased over time, declines in incidence were observed between 2005 and 2007, before inclining sharply again in 2008. The sharp increase in incidence at this time may reflect, at least in part, in public awareness of TBI, through increased media attention, particularly within the sports context.

Given more than a third of those with TBI do not present at hospital, current estimates, predominantly based on hospitalization data, may be significantly underestimating the actual burden.[8,14] Coding errors, duplicates, discounting pre-hospital deaths, and undiagnosed cases that may be overlooked due to being masked by other injuries also present major challenges to accurately determining the true incidence and nature of TBI. Given the diversity in methodology applied across studies, several reviews have called for the reporting of TBI incidence studies to be standardized to facilitate data comparison.[15–18]

Traumatic Brain Injury Prevalence

On review of the literature, very few studies of TBI prevalence currently exist. Those studies that have been undertaken are often limited by short follow-up periods, and inconsistent reporting, with loss to follow-up often relatively high in TBI cohorts.[17–20] A further limitation is that prevalence studies have tended to focus on specific populations such as war veterans, athletes, or prisoners and therefore it is difficult to generalize the findings. Nevertheless, a recent meta-analysis of prevalence studies[19] revealing prevalence range between 6–60 per 100,000 revealed combined prevalence of 12% of adults reported having experienced at least one TBI with loss of consciousness in their lifetime. This figure is likely to be much higher given just over half of TBI cases experience loss of consciousness. Indeed one study conducted in New Zealand revealed that over 30% of people had experienced at least one TBI before the age of 25 years.[21] Prevalence is an important aspect of TBI to be explored, with emerging evidence revealing links between early childhood TBI and later life antisocial/criminal behaviour and psychiatric symptoms.[22,23]

Severity of traumatic brain injury

TBIs are most commonly referred to as being mild, moderate, or severe. There are numerous classification systems available to define TBI severity, typically based on the duration of post-traumatic amnesia (state of confusion and disorientation), loss of consciousness and/or presence of injury on brain imaging. For example, the Glasgow Coma Scale (GCS)[24] is widely used to assess level of consciousness by observing verbal, motor, and eye responses post-injury. For individual clinical assessment of severity, the three components should be reported separately. However, for classification in research, calculating the sum score across the three domains has greater utility (Table 38.1). Given GCS scores can change over time due to the amount of time since injury, the worst GCS score recorded is most commonly used to determine severity where multiple scores are available.

Post-traumatic amnesia (PTA), referring to a state of confusion that occurs immediately following brain injury, can also be used to assess severity. The most common measure to assess PTA is the 12-item Revised Westmead PTA Scale[25] that assesses orientation to person, place, and time and the ability to retain new information from one day to the next. Until a person passes the PTA Scale for three consecutive days or more they are considered 'in PTA'. Typically used as an adjunct to the GCS, 80–95% of all TBIs are considered to be in the mild severity range.[8] While any discrepancies in ratings typically lead to the more severe category being assigned, this approach is limited given measurement difficulties within the context of alcohol or substance use, sedation, paralysis, and dementia.[26] Scores can also be influenced by the training and approach of the assessor. Additional to mild, moderate, and severe classifications of injury, sub-concussive injuries occur when an external force causes the brain to move around and against the hard skull, but may not lead to acute symptoms. It is proposed that the damage caused by sub-concussive injuries may accumulate over time.[27] Emerging research indicates a need to also consider the impact of sub-concussive injuries. The severity of TBI and the experience of symptoms is outlined in Fig. 38.1.

Table 38.1 Assessing the severity of TBI

Measurement tool	TBI severity category		
	Mild	Moderate	Severe
Glasgow Coma Score	13–15	9–12	3–8
Revised Westmead Post-traumatic Amnesia Scale—days 'in PTA'	0–1 days	1–7 days	7 + days
Loss of consciousness	<30 minutes	>30 minutes–24 hours	24 hours +
Abbreviated injury scale	1–2	3	4–6
Injury severity score	1	2–3	4–6

Adapted with permission from Corrigan J.D. The epidemiology of traumatic brain injury. *J Head Trauma Rehabil*; 25(2):72–80. Copyright © 2010 Lippincott Williams. DOI: 10.1097/HTR.0b013e3181ccc8b4.

Challenges remain in differentiating between those who will go on to experience persistent symptoms and will need active treatment and those who are likely to recover naturally. Some mild subclassification scales have been proposed over the last few decades to try and identify patients most at risk of long-term difficulties, but these have been found to have low clinical utility.[28] Additionally, prognostic models found to be predictive of outcome for moderate and severe TBI have had low value for mild TBI.[29] There is a clear need to develop new ways of classifying mild TBI that are more meaningful and have greater prognostic value.

Mechanisms of injury

The main causes of TBI are falls, assaults, and motor vehicle accidents, although there is variation between countries and continents (Fig. 38.2). In westernized countries, the most common mechanism of TBI has changed from motor vehicle accidents (MVA) to falls.[8,30] In other countries such as Asia, motor vehicle accidents remain the most common mechanism of injury, particularly involving pedestrians, cyclists, and motorcyclists.[6,7] This trend may reflect the need for increased traffic safety awareness, high traffic volume, motor vehicle minimum safety requirements, road and vehicle maintenance, and enforcement of traffic rules.[31] Neither of the two studies conducted in Asia classified mechanism of injury by assault and so these cases are likely to be embedded within the 'other' category.

Recurrent Traumatic Brain Injury

After a TBI, the brain remains vulnerable to further damage as it needs time to recover and repair itself.[32] Sustaining a recurrent (repeated) TBI before the brain has healed can result in far more serious consequences for the affected person, than if the second injury was sustained in isolation.[33] The timeframe within which the brain remains vulnerable is currently unclear. It was initially believed that people should be careful not to sustain another injury within several weeks or months of their initial injury.[34,35] However, more recent evidence has highlighted that this 'vulnerability period' may be even longer.[36] For example, prior injuries sustained many years previously have been linked to poorer increased symptoms, low mood, cognitive impairment, and life satisfaction following a TBI.[37,38] The link between TBI and outcome appears cumulative, with higher numbers of prior TBI linked to increased cognitive impairment,[33–35] and persistent symptoms (e.g. dizziness and headache).[33] However, there has been some inconsistency in findings to date.[39] Given up to one in ten people experience more than one TBI in a given year, with the majority of injuries caused by the same mechanism (i.e. repeated falls),[36] further research is urgently needed to better understand the impact of recurrent injuries on functioning.

Traumatic Brain Injury Mortality

Despite observed increases in people with TBI presenting for medical treatment over the years, the CDC reveals that mortality rates have remained stable.[13,40] Mortality rates from epidemiological

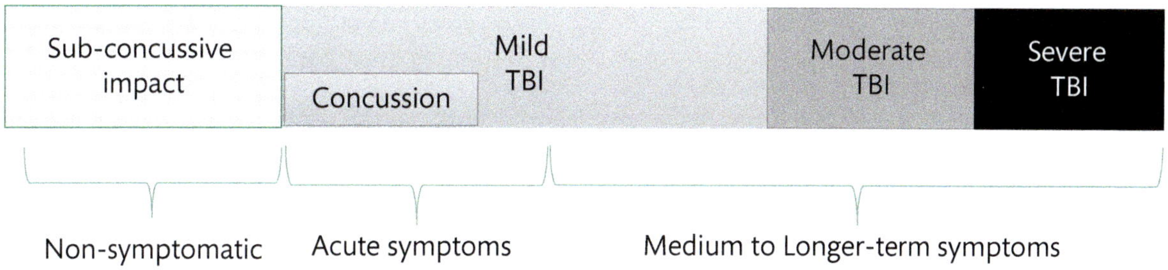

Fig. 38.1 Severity of traumatic brain injury.

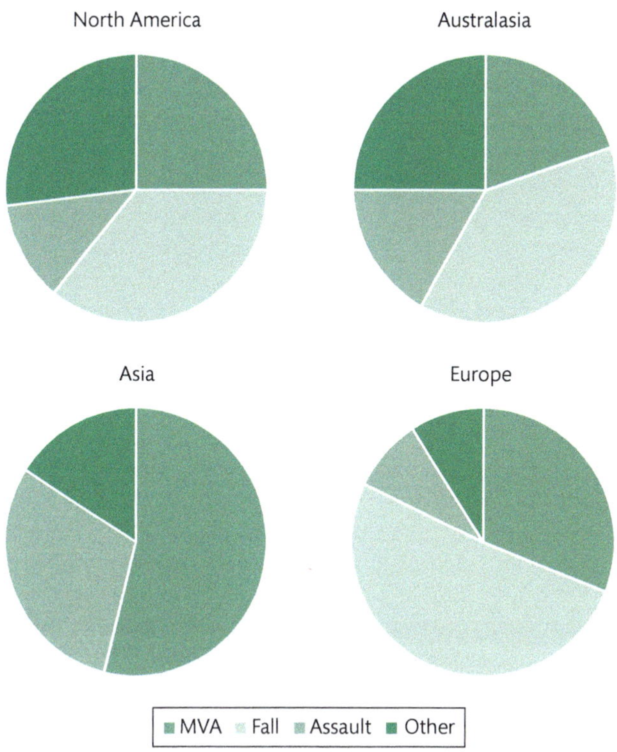

Fig. 38.2 Mechanism of injury by continent.

studies vary widely, with figures ranging from 0.3 (Spain) to 39.3 (Brazil) per 100,000 person-years. In the western world patterns of TBI mortality by injury mechanism appear to be changing, with declining rates of traffic-related TBI deaths and an increase in deaths due to falls.[41] Highest rates of mortality are observed in older adults. A recent meta-analysis of 24 studies in moderate and severe TBI in people aged 60 years or above, revealed an overall in-hospital mortality of 57.2% (95% confidence intervals (CI) = 42.6–70.6) and six-month mortality of 74.7% (CI = 62.1–84.1).[42] It is difficult to determine whether a death occurred directly due to the TBI or from other complications. Increased mortality may also be a consequence of the ageing process, complications arising from existing or concurrent comorbidities and their treatment, and/or inappropriately conservative management approaches.[42]

Risk Factors for Sustaining Traumatic Brain Injury

Efforts to prevent TBI and to deliver effective interventions to optimize recovery highlight the need to identify associated risk factors, especially those that are modifiable. Those at highest risk of sustaining TBI are males aged 15–34 years with a history of alcohol/drug use and of low socioeconomic status.[43] A recent TBI incidence study found that children (aged 0–14 years, especially those aged 0–4 years), adolescents, and young adults (aged 15–34 years) constituted almost 70% of all TBI cases.[44] In older adults (aged >65 years), chronic health conditions, greater frailty, and the effects of taking multiple medications concurrently were attributed to increased risk of fall-induced TBI.[45] Walking on stairs and outside activities have been found to be particularly associated with risk of falls and TBI in the elderly.[45] Such findings clearly highlight the value of identifying TBI risk factors in subgroups to determine preventative opportunities. While much effort has been made to reduce the burden of motor-vehicle-related TBI, prevention programmes aimed at reducing fall-induced TBI, especially amongst high-risk groups should be promoted.

Acute and Long-term Complications

TBI can result in long-term cognitive, emotional, and behavioural difficulties that persist for many years. Even following a mild TBI nearly 50% of cases go on to experience persistent symptoms one year later.[37,46] Additionally, adults with a history of TBI have been found to be at increased risk for the development of a number of neurological and psychiatric diseases, including but not limited to, Parkinson's disease, stroke, epilepsy, and earlier onset of cognitive impairment/dementia.[47–50] Caplan et al. revealed statistically significant associations between epilepsy and prior TBI diagnosis (penetrating TBI: adjusted odds ratio (OR) = 18.77 (95% CI, 9.21–38.23); other TBI: adjusted OR = 1.64 (1.43–1.89)).[51] Links between TBI and chronic traumatic encephalopathy (CTE) (previously known as dementia pugilistica or 'punch-drunk' syndrome) have received considerable media attention. Studies propose evidence of a unique type of aggregation of tau protein in the brains of deceased athletes is associated with neuropsychiatric symptoms, behavioural changes, and cognitive deficits believed to result from repetitive mild TBI.[52] However, these studies are limited by selection bias and lack of control of potential influencing factors such as substance use and psychiatric history. It is also not clear how the proposed abnormal tau protein deposition differs from that observed as part of the normal ageing process. Consequently, CTE is not universally accepted as a distinct pathology.[53,54]

In terms of affective outcomes, TBI has been associated with an elevated risk of both bipolar disorder (Hazard Ratio (HR) = 1.42, 95% CI = (1.26, 1.59)) and major depression (HR = 1.41, 95%

CI = (1.28, 1.54)).[55] More severe injury has been associated with greater risk. The first year following the injury has been identified as the highest risk period for major depression, while the highest risk period for bipolar disorder was delayed until 2–4 years following the injury. Evidence in adults suggests that environmental factors interact with injury severity to significantly influence outcome, with severe TBI coupled with social disadvantage associated with poorest functional outcomes.[56]

While much of the focus is on longer-term complications for adults, children and adolescents potentially face the greatest risk of longer-term implications over the lifespan.[8] TBI has the potential to significantly and permanently derail ongoing neurological maturational processes during childhood. This can lead to long-term, complex, and comorbid neurodevelopmental impairments,[57] particularly in the context of rapid brain development. Chronic sequelae of childhood TBI include deficits in cognitive and executive function, social difficulties, inattention, and conduct disorders,[58,59] with poor outcomes most often apparent in infants and young children.[60] Whilst deficits are well documented following moderate and severe TBI, there is little evidence of persistent problems beyond the acute and subacute period following mild TBI in children and adolescents.[61] However, the current literature has been limited by a lack of comparisons to non-TBI injured controls and challenges associated with a typical lack of availability of information concerning child functioning (i.e. behaviour, social competence, cognitive function) prior to sustaining a TBI.

Cost of Traumatic Brain Injury

In the USA, costs of TBI totalled $76.3 billion in 2010, including $11.5 billion in direct medical costs and $64.8 billion in indirect costs (e.g. lost wages, lost productivity, and non-medical expenditures).[62] However, it has been acknowledged that these data underestimate the true national burden of TBI, given a focus on TBI managed within hospital settings and the exclusion of military personnel treated within military services.[63] In a recent New Zealand study, the average cost per new TBI case during the first 12 months and over a lifetime varied between US $4636 (95% CI $3756–5561) for mild cases to US $36,648 (95% CI $16,348–65,350) for moderate/severe cases.[64] Whilst the cost per mild brain injury cases is lower, due the high frequency of mild TBIs the total cost is estimated at nearly three times that of moderate/severe TBI. Alongside the personal costs of TBI, the health economic costs of TBI further highlight an urgent need to develop effective preventative strategies to prevent both mild and moderate/severe injuries.

What is Traumatic Spinal Cord Injury?

Traumatic injury to the spinal cord (SCI) refers to damage arising from external forces. This excludes injury to the spinal cord caused by another medical condition or degeneration such as spina bifida (referred to as non-traumatic spinal cord injury). Damage can occur to any part of the spinal cord, including the nerves at the end of the spinal canal. Injury usually results in either temporary or permanent motor, sensory, and autonomic dysfunction. The location of the injury is described by the area of the spinal cord where the injury occurred, for example cervical (C), thoracic (T), lumbar (L), and sacral (S) area, and the segment of that area (ranging between 1 and 12) as shown in **Fig. 38.3**. Injuries to the thoracic, lumbar, or sacral spine result in paraplegia (loss of use of lower limbs), whereas injuries to the cervical spine result in tetraplegia or quadraplegia (loss of use of both upper and lower limbs).

Spinal Cord Injury Incidence

Five systematic reviews on the incidence of spinal cord injury have recently been published.[20,65–68] Globally, traumatic spinal cord injury is estimated to affect nearly 200,000 people every year, with a projected incidence rate of 23 cases per million.[20] There is wide between-country variance in incidence of SCI. Incidence is lowest in Finland at 9.2 per million and up to 49.1 per million in New Zealand.[65] It is not clear if these variations reflect actual country-specific distinctions in SCI incidence or differences in research methodologies used, for example whether deaths prior to hospital admission are included or excluded. Some studies also include non-traumatic causes of SCI and rates therefore need to be considered in light of the reported methods used. Little is known about SCI rates in developing and low income countries. A recent systematic review found epidemiologic data was available for only 41 countries in the world, being mostly European and high-income.[68]

Evidence indicates that ethnic minority populations have a higher incidence than Caucasians, although more research exploring the impact of ethnicity on risk of injury is needed to confirm this finding.[69] While SCI is less common in children than adults, differences are also evident in stratification by race and sex. In the USA, the examination of discharge records from public databases revealed African Americans had a significantly higher rate of SCI (1.53 cases per 100,000 children) compared to native Americans (1.00) and Asians (0.36). Boys were also found to be at a more than two-fold risk for SCI (2.79) than girls (1.15).[70] As shown in Fig. 38.4 from data extracted from the study by Martins et al.[71] there are peaks in incidence between 15–30 years and in older adults over 55 years of age. It has been difficult to identify any age disparities across countries due to inconsistencies in reporting, highlighting the need for standardized reporting of epidemiological studies to facilitate comparison.

In adults, SCIs are most commonly sustained in the cervical area of the spine, accounting for 54% of injuries.[66] This is a trend that appears to be increasing. For example, in Finland cervical injuries increased from 48% in 1976 to 57% in 2005.[72] Thoracic injuries account for 24%, lumbar 19%, and sacral are least common, affecting only 1% of cases.[66] In children, SCI is relatively rare. In the USA the incidence of SCI in those aged <18 years is estimated at 17.5 per million.[73] In European countries, it is estimated that 0.9–21.2 children sustained SCI per million children.[74]

Whilst assessing trends in the severity of injury over time can be challenging, given changing definitions of SCI and research methodologies used, there does appear to be an increasing trend that less complete injuries (grades B–D) are being sustained.[75] This trend may reflect an increase in injuries sustained by older adults and through falls, with the ageing of the population, but may also reflect improvements in acute care at the scene, reducing the risk of further damage to the spinal cord.[66,75] It should

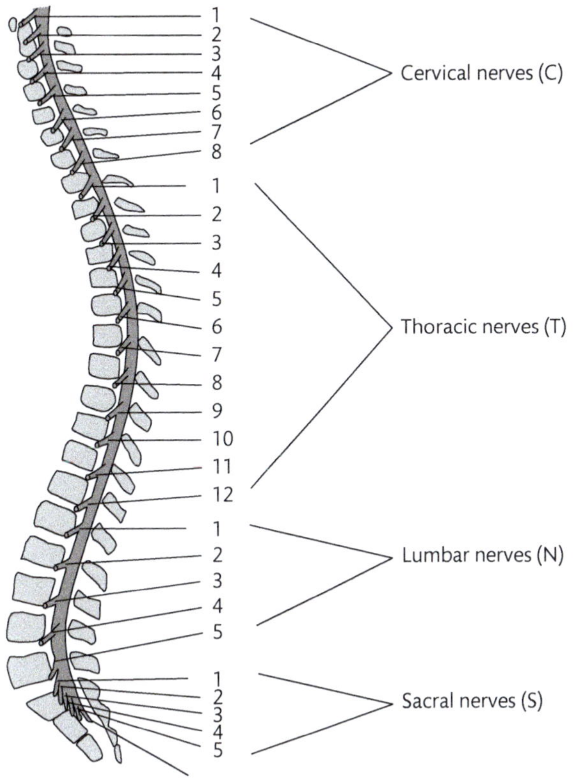

Fig. 38.3 Assessing location of spinal cord injury.

be noted that multi-level injuries can also occur, which can make recording of level of injury challenging. This is particularly the case following natural disasters, where up to 29% of injuries were found to be multi-level.[76]

Spinal Cord Injury Prevalence

Estimating prevalence for SCI is challenging because a large sample is needed to determine prevalence of a relatively rare condition.[75] Consequently, few prevalence studies of SCI currently exist. From the studies that have been completed, prevalence has been found to vary widely. Prevalence estimates range between 250 per million in France and 906 per million in the USA.[65] Prevalence rates are on the increase, particularly in developed countries, due to lower mortality rates and increased ageing of the population.[75] In order to access large populations feasibly and economically, prevalence studies may rely on self-reported SCI and therefore prevalence figures do need to be interpreted with caution. For example, prevalence may include SCI from non-traumatic causes or that do not meet some diagnostic criteria.

Severity of injury

The American Spinal Injury Association (ASIA) Impairment Scale is typically used to determine the extent and severity of a patient's SCI. This system of tests is ideally completed within 72 hours following the initial injury. Each patient's resulting grade is based on the level of sensation that can be felt at multiple points in the body, along with tests of motor function. Injuries are graded from A (most severe) to E (normal functioning).[77]

- A = Complete: no sensory or motor function is preserved in sacral segments S4–5
- B = Incomplete: sensory, but not motor, function is preserved below the neurologic level and extends through sacral segments S4–5
- C = Incomplete: motor function is preserved below the neurologic level, and most key muscles below the neurologic level have a muscle grade of less than 3
- D = Incomplete: motor function is preserved below the neurologic level, and most key muscles below the neurologic level have a muscle grade that is greater than or equal to 3
- E = Normal: Sensory and motor functions are normal

Mechanisms of injury

In western countries the most common mechanism of SCI is motor vehicle accidents, whereas in the eastern world the most common mechanism of SCI is falls (e.g. falls from trees, balconies, roofs, and construction sites). However, there is an increasing trend in the eastern world with regards to traffic related accidents, particularly

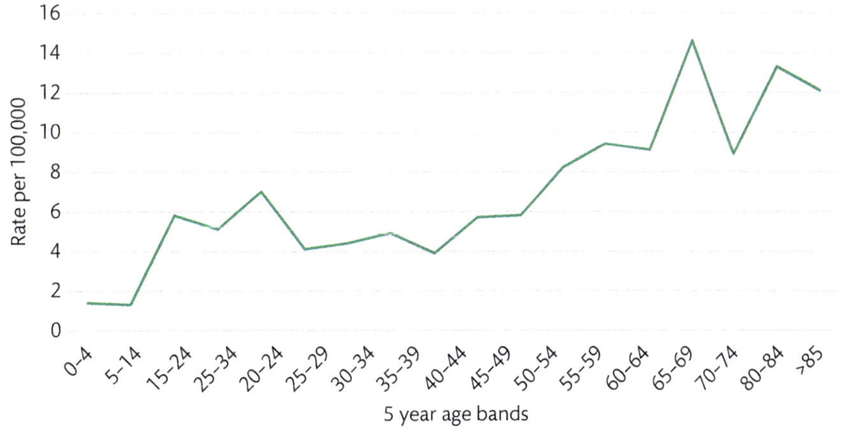

Fig. 38.4 Incidence of SCI across the lifespan per 100,000.[71]

with two-wheeled vehicles such as bikes and motorcycles.[20] Rates of injury caused by violence and self-harm are noticeably higher in the USA and sub-Saharan Africa, which may reflect increased access to firearms in these areas. Although rates of gunshot related SCI do appear to be on the decrease in the USA.[75] Within the context of paediatric SCI, there appear to be age-related differences in the leading causes of injury. Motor vehicle accidents typically affect younger children, while adolescents face greater risks of sustaining a SCI while participating in sporting activities.[78] As is the case with other traumatic injuries, such as TBI, the context of the injury such as sports and work-related injuries is not always presented in epidemiological studies. For studies that have reported on the context of injury, the highest rates of work-related injuries occur in Western Europe, Asia, and Africa.[20] In the context of sports and recreational activities, the risk of SCI has been reduced over time through injury prevention strategies, particularly relating to injuries resulting from trampolines and American football.[75] However, a recent systematic review highlights that high rates of SCI occur from diving, skiing, rugby, and equestrian activities, where more focus on injury prevention is needed.[79]

Spinal Cord Injury Mortality

Studies have revealed that approximately 16% of SCI cases die before admission to hospital.[71] Whilst there have been significant improvements in pre-admission mortality rates since the 1940s, acute in-hospital/rehabilitation mortality rates have remained relatively stable since the 1980s.[80] A recent meta-analysis has revealed that in-hospital mortality across countries ranges between 1.1–15.9% in Europe and 10.8–34.6% in Africa.[81] Higher rates of early mortality in developed countries may reflect that it is rare for patients to be immobilized and transferred to hospital by trained healthcare personnel, which may exacerbate existing injuries. Additionally there is often limited access to specialist spinal care clinicians and facilities, negatively impacting on recovery.[82]

In the longer term, survival rates have been found to range between 79–100% at one year, 85–96% at five years, and 81–93% at ten years.[81] Evidence suggests that those who have experienced a SCI are 2–5 times more likely to die prematurely than people without SCI. Increasing age, complete injuries, and being of male gender have been linked to higher risk of mortality.[81] Complications arising from the SCI, including pneumonia, heart disease, and urogenital disease have been identified as the main causes of death in the post-acute phase following injury.[81] Those injured before age 16 years face higher annual odds of dying compared to those injured at an older age, and those who survive face reduced life expectancies compared to the general population and those sustaining SCI after age 16 years,[83] perhaps due to longer exposure to SCI and secondary complications.

Risk Factors for Sustaining Spinal Cord Injury

Males are more at risk of SCI than females, with male to female ratios ranging between 2.5:1 in Canada and up to 7.1:1 in Greece.[65] Similarly, most studies report a predominance of males compared to females with SCI in childhood.[78] There are indications that this gender disparity may be decreasing over time.[75] Decreasing gender disparity may be reflective of the increase in injuries sustained in older adults, where there is a lower male:female risk ratio. The mean age that SCIs are sustained has increased from 28 years in the 1970s to 37 years in the 2000s.[80] However, the majority of injuries are sustained in young to mid adulthood. Engagement in risky behaviours such as violence, risky driving, and substance use have also been linked to increased risk of SCI. Indeed, one study of people who had sustained a SCI at an acute inpatient rehabilitation programme revealed that 38% had significant lifetime alcohol-related problems and 33% reported illicit pre-injury drug use.[84]

Acute and Long-term Complications from Spinal Cord Injury

Sustaining a SCI can have a profound impact on a person's life and on those around them. Not only are the restrictions with physical mobility challenging, but people can experience a myriad of symptoms and medical complications. More than half of those affected by SCI report leg spasms, constipation, and back and lower limb pain.[69] Pressure sores, and bladder control can also be highly problematic, particularly in LICs, where the resources needed to manage these issues are less widely available.[82] Indeed, a study in Sierra Leone revealed that 47% of SCI cases died in the community following hospital discharge, with severe pressure sores.[85] This study highlights the difficulties in providing the necessary nutrition, hygiene, wound care, and access to medical follow-up to adequately manage pressure sores associated with SCI in LICs.[85]

In addition to the physical impact, SCI can have a profound psychological impact. A study of adults who had experienced a SCI found 13.3% reported experiencing suicidal ideation within the past two weeks, with 7.4% reporting a suicide attempt.[86] Suicidal ideation does not appear to be a reaction to the acute event given that the risk of suicidal ideation increases with time since injury. Engagement in the community, spiritual well-being, sense of personal control, self-worth, hope, and having a purpose in life have all been found to be linked to improved quality of life amongst those with SCI.[86,87] Re-engaging in employment remains a challenge for many following a SCI, with relatively stable estimates suggesting that only 40% of those affected are in employment at one year post-injury. This low rate of employment has remained quite consistent since the mid-1990s.[88] It is becoming increasing recognized that more needs to be known about employment post-SCI, beyond 'return to employment' rates. Whilst SCI can place a strain on close personal relationships, as those involved adjust to injury and find ways to adapt to the person's needs and changes in sense of self and social roles, over time many people describe that the injury has strengthened their relationships.[89]

For children with SCI, several studies have shown good neurological recovery in children following injury, especially for those sustaining incomplete lesions.[90] Compared to adults, children with SCI face unique secondary complications, including scoliosis, especially when injury is sustained at a younger age, and due to poor bone health.[91] Of 130 children who sustained SCI aged 0–21 years, 97% of those injured before the adolescent growth spurt developed scoliosis (a lateral curvature in the normally vertical line of the spine) compared to 52% of those injured after their growth spurt.[92] This

Table 38.2 Range of the incidence, prevalence and mortality for TBI and SCI

	Incidence per 100,000	Prevalence per 100,000	In-hospital mortality
Traumatic brain injury	45–790	6–60	1–22%
Spinal cord injury	1–6	3--9	1–35%

finding did not appear to be related to the level of injury. Evidence also suggests that long-term life satisfaction in adults who sustained SCI during childhood is not primarily driven by injury severity but more widely influence by psychosocial factors (i.e. education, employment satisfaction, income, and social opportunities).[93]

Cost of Spinal Cord Injury

Surprisingly few studies on the health economic costs of SCI have been published. Those that currently exist have revealed that the overall economic costs associated with people with SCI are extremely high, ranging between US $131 million and $302 million. Costs have been found to be affected by the level and severity of the injury as well as the injury mechanism.[94,95] Indirect costs, such as productivity losses due to sick leave and loss of earnings, have been found to be high following a SCI and generally exceed the direct costs such as emergency transport and hospital care.[95] Total cost per injured person has been estimated at between US $200,000–213,000.[95] Research has been restricted to the USA, Europe, and Australia, and so the economic costs for developing countries remains unknown. An overall summary of the epidemiology of TBI and SCI is presented in Table 38.2.

Concurrent Traumatic Brain Injury and Spinal Cord Injury

Whilst TBI and SCI are distinct diagnoses that can occur in isolation, they frequently co-occur. Estimates suggest that up to 70% of people experiencing a SCI also experience a TBI.[96] Co-occurrence has been found to place greater challenges and time demands on health professionals, which is likely to increase cost estimates. For example, the cognitive and behavioural challenges experienced following a TBI can make it more difficult for patients to engage in their rehabilitation to increase mobility following the SCI. Indeed it has been found that those experiencing both a TBI and SCI experience poorer recovery at two years compared to those experiencing a SCI in isolation.[97] The recovery process consequently appears more complex when multiple injuries are sustained.

Conclusion

Epidemiological studies of TBI and SCI have revealed wide differences in the incidence and prevalence of these conditions between and within countries. A greater focus on population-based epidemiological studies is needed. Differences in definitions and inclusion criteria and case identification sources make comparisons between studies difficult and there is a need for agreed standards to facilitate future work. There is also a need for clear reporting and guidelines such as the STROBE, https://www.strobe-statement.org/index.php?id=strobe-home) to ensure that studies are interpreted accurately. Overall it appears that the burden of TBIs and SCIs are substantial and given the increased risk of injury among young adults, with increased lifetime burden, there is a need for targeted injury prevention programmes.

REFERENCES

1. Carroll LJ, Cassidy JD, Holm L, Kraus J, Coronado VG. Methodological issues and research recommendations for mild traumatic brain injury: the WHO Collaborating Centre Task Force on Mild Traumatic Brain Injury. J Rehabil Med. 2004 (43 Suppl):113–25.
2. Theadom A, Starkey NJ, Dowell T, Hume P, Kahan M, McPherson K, et al. Sports-related brain injury in the general population: an epidemiological study. J Sci Med Sport. 2014; 17(6): 591–6.
3. Menon DK, Schwab K, Wright DW, Maas AI. Position statement: definition of traumatic brain injury. Arch Phys Med Rehabil. 2010; 91: 1637–40.
4. Andersson EH, Bjorklund R, Emanuelson I, Stalhammar D. Epidemiology of traumatic brain injury: a population based study in western Sweden. Acta Neurologica Scandinavica. 2003; 107(4): 256–9.
5. El-Menyar A, Mekkodathil A, Al-Thani H, Consunji R, Latifi R. Incidence, demographics and outcome of traumatic brain injury in the Middle East: a systematic review. World Neurosurg. 2017; 107: 6–21. doi: 10.1016/j.wneu.2017.07.070.
6. Bener A, Omar AO, Ahmad AE, Al-Mulla FH, Abdul Rahman YS. The pattern of traumatic brain injuries: a country undergoing rapid development. Brain Inj. 2010; 24(2): 74–80.
7. Chiu WT, Huang SJ, Tsai SH, Lin JW, Tsai MD, Lin TJ, et al. The impact of time, legislation, and geography on the epidemiology of traumatic brain injury. J Clin Neuroscience. 2007; 14(10): 930–5.
8. Feigin VF, Theadom A, Barker-Collo SL, Starkey N, McPherson K, Kahan M, et al. Incidence of traumatic brain injury in New Zealand: a population-based study. Lancet Neurology. 2013; 12(1): 53–64.
9. Langlois JA, Kegler SR, Butler JA, Gotsch KE, Johnson RL, Reichard AA, et al. Traumatic brain injury-related hospital discharge. MMWR Surveill Summ. 2003; 52(4): 1–20.
10. Leibson CL, Brown AW, Ransom JE, Diehl NN, Perkins PK, Mandrekar J, et al. Incidence of traumatic brain injury across the full disease spectrum: a population-based medical record review study. Epidemiol. 2011; 22(6): 836–44.
11. Koskinen S, Alaranta H. Traumatic brain injury in Finland 1991–2005: A nationwide register study of hospitalized and fatal TBI. Brain Inj. 2008; 22(3): 205–14.
12. Thurman DJ, Jeppson L, Burnett CL, Beaudoin DE, Rheinberger MM, Sniezek JE. Surveillance of traumatic brain injuries in Utah. West J Med. 1996; 165(4): 192–6.

13. Centers for Disease Control. Report to Congress on Traumatic Brain Injury in the United States: Epidemiology and Rehabilitation. Atlanta, GA: Centers for Disease Control, 2015.
14. Whiteneck GG, Cuthbert JP, Corrigan JD, Bogner JA. Prevalence of self-reported lifetime history of traumatic brain injury and associated disability: a statewide population-based survey. J Head Trauma Rehabil. 2016; 31(1): 55–62.
15. Brazinova A, Rehorcikova V, Taylor MS, Buckova V, Majdan M, Psota M, et al. Epidemiology of traumatic brain injury in Europe: a living systematic review. J Neurotrauma. 2018: doi: 10.1089/neu.2015.4126.
16. Corrigan JD, Selassie AW, Orman JA. The epidemiology of traumatic brain injury. J Head Trauma Rehabil. 2010; 25(2): 72–80.
17. Hyder AA, Wunderlich CA, Puvanachandra P, Gururaj G, Kobusingye OC. The impact of traumatic brain injuries: a global perspective. NeuroRehabil. 2007; 22(5): 341–53.
18. Roozenbeek B, Maas AI, Menon DK. Changing patterns in the epidemiology of traumatic brain injury. Nat Rev Neurol. 2013; 9(4): 231–6.
19. Frost RB, Farrer TJ, Primosch M, Hedges DW. Prevalence of traumatic brain injury in the general adult population: a meta-analysis. Neuroepidemiol. 2013; 40(3): 154–9.
20. Lee BB, Cripps RA, Fitzharris M, Wing PC. The global map for traumatic spinal cord injury epidemiology; update 2011, global incidence rate. Spinal Cord. 2014; 52: 110–16.
21. McKinlay A, Grace RC, Horwood LJ, Fergusson DM, Ridder EM, MacFarlane MR. Prevalence of traumatic brain injury among children, adolescents and young adults: prospective evidence from a birth cohort. Brain Inj. 2008; 22(2):175–81.
22. McKinlay A, Grace R, Horwood J, Fergusson D, MacFarlane M. Adolescent psychiatric symptoms following preschool childhood mild traumatic brain injury: evidence from a birth cohort. J Head Trauma Rehabil. 2009; 24(3): 221–7.
23. McKinlay A, Corrigan J, Horwood LJ, Fergusson DM. Substance abuse and criminal activities following traumatic brain injury in childhood, adolescence, and early adulthood. J Head Trauma Rehabil. 2014; 29(6): 498–506.
24. Teasdale G, Jennett B. Assessment of coma and impaired consciousness. A practical scale. Lancet. 1974; 2(7872): 81–4.
25. Marosszeky NEV, Ryan L, Shores EA, Batchelor J, Marosszeky JE. The PTA protocol: guidelines for using the Westmead Post-Traumatic Amnesia (PTA) scale. Sydney: Wild & Wooley, 1997.
26. Matis G, Birbilis T. The Glasgow Coma Scale—a brief review of past, present, future. Acta Neurol Belg. 2008; 108: 75–89.
27. Broglio SP, Eckner JT, Paulson HL, Kutcher JS. Cognitive decline and aging: the role of concussive and subconcussive impacts. Exerc Sport Sci Rev. 2012; 40(3): 138–44.
28. Theadom A, Barker-Colllo SL, Greenwood A, et al. Do mild traumatic brain injury severity sub-classification systems help to identify people who go on to experience long-term symptoms? Brain impairment. 2018; 19(2): 119–32. doi: 10.1017/BrImp.2017.11
29. Lingsma H, Yue JK, Maas A, Steyerberg EW, Manley GTMDPD, Cooper SR, et al. Outcome prediction after mild and complicated mild traumatic brain injury: external validation of existing models and identification of new predictors using the TRACK-TBI Pilot Study. J Neurotrauma. 2014; 32(2): 83–94.
30. Centers for Disease Control and Prevention. Incidence rates of hospitalization related to traumatic brain injury—12 states, 2002. MMWR Surveill Summ. 2006; 55(8): 201–4.
31. Yattoo GH, Tabish A. The profile of head injuries and traumatic brain injury deaths in Kashmir. J Trauma Manag Outcomes. 2008; 2(1): 5.
32. Cantu RC. Posttraumatic retrograde and anterograde amnesia: pathophysiology and implications in grading and safe return to play. J Athl Train. 2001; 36(3): 244–8.
33. Guskiewicz KM, Marshall SW, Bailes J, McCrea M, Cantu RC, Randolph C, et al. Association between recurrent concussion and late-life cognitive impairment in retired professional football players. Neurosurg. 2005; 57(4): 719–26.
34. Wall SE, Williams WH, Cartwright-Hatton S, Kelly TP, Murray J, Murray M, et al. Neuropsychological dysfunction following repeat concussions in jockeys. J Neurol, Neurosurg Psychiatr. 2006; 77(4): 518–20.
35. Iverson GL, Echemendia RJ, Lamarre AK, Brooks BL, Gaetz MB. Possible lingering effects of multiple past concussions. Rehabil Res Pract. 2012; 316575.
36. Theadom A, Parmar P, Jones K, Barker-Collo S, Starkey NJ, McPherson KM, et al. Frequency and impact of recurrent traumatic brain injury in a population-based sample. J Neurotrauma. 2015; 32(10): 674–81.
37. Theadom A, Parag V, Dowell T, McPherson K, Starkey N, Barker-Collo S, et al. Persistent problems 1 year after mild traumatic brain injury: a longitudinal population study in New Zealand. BJGP. 2016; 66(642): e16–23.
38. Dams-O'Connor K, Spielman L, Singh A, Gordon WA, Lingsma HF, Maas AI, et al. The impact of previous traumatic brain injury on health and functioning: a TRACK-TBI study. J Neurotrauma. 2013; 30(24): 2014–20.
39. Belanger HG, Spiegel E, Vanderploeg RD. Neuropsychological performance following a history of multiple self-reported concussions: a meta-analysis. J Int Neuropsychol Soc. 2010; 16(2): 262–7.
40. Stein SC, Georgoff P, Meghan S, Mizra K, Sonnad SS. 150 years of treating severe traumatic brain injury: a systematic review of progress in mortality. J Neurotrauma. 2010; 27(7): 1343–53.
41. Steudel WI, Cortbus F, Schwerdtfeger K. Epidemiology and prevention of fatal head injuries in Germany—trends and the impact of the reunification. Acta Neurochir (Wien). 2005; 147(3): 231–42.
42. McIntyre A, Mehta S, Aubut J, Dijkers M, Teasell RW. Mortality among older adults after a traumatic brain injury: a meta-analysis. Brain Inj. 2013; 27(1): 31–40.
43. Bruns J, Jr, Hauser WA. The epidemiology of traumatic brain injury: a review. Epilepsia. 2003; 44(Suppl 10): 2–10.
44. Feigin VL, Theadom A, Barker-Collo S, Starkey NJ, McPherson K, Kahan M, et al. Incidence of traumatic brain injury in New Zealand: a population-based study. Lancet Neurology. 2013; 12(1): 53–64.
45. Krishnamoorthy V, Distelhorst JT, Vavilala MS, Thompson H. Traumatic brain injury in the elderly: burden, risk factors, and prevention. J Trauma Nurs. 2015; 22(4): 204–8.
46. McMahon P, Hricik A, Yue JK, Puccio AM, Inoue T, Lingsma HF, et al. Symptomatology and functional outcome in mild traumatic brain injury: results from the prospective TRACK-TBI Study. J Neurotrauma. 2014; 31(1): 26–33.
47. Walsh S, Donnan J, Fortin Y, Sikora L, Morrissey A, Collins K, et al. A systematic review of the risk factors associated with the onset and natural progression of epilepsy. Neurotoxicol. 2017; 61: 64–77.
48. Liao CC, Chou YC, Yeh CC, Hu CJ, Chiu WT, Chen TL. Stroke risk and outcomes in patients with traumatic brain injury: 2 nationwide studies. Mayo Clin Proc. 2014; 89(2): 163–72.

49. Gardner RC, Burke JF, Nettiksimmons J, Goldman S, Tanner CM, Yaffe K. Traumatic brain injury in later life increases risk for Parkinson disease. Ann Neurol. 2015; 77(6): 987–95.
50. Li W, Risacher SL, McAllister TW, Saykin AJ. Traumatic brain injury and age at onset of cognitive impairment in older adults. J Neurol. 2016; 263(7): 1280–5.
51. Caplan B, Bogner J, Brenner L, Pugh MJV, Orman JA, Jaramillo CA, et al. The prevalence of epilepsy and association with traumatic brain injury in veterans of the Afghanistan and Iraq Wars. J Head Trauma Rehabil. 2015; 30(1): 29–37.
52. Kiernan PT, Montenigro PH, Solomon TM, McKee AC. Chronic traumatic encephalopathy: a neurodegenerative consequence of repetitive traumatic brain injury. Semin Neurol. 2015; 35(1): 20–28.
53. Hornbeck K, Walter K, Myrvik M. Should potential risk of chronic traumatic encephalopathy be discussed with young athletes? AMA J Ethics. 2017; 19(7): 686–92.
54. Perrine K, Helcer J., Tsiouris AJ, Pisapia DJ, Stieg P. The current status of research on chronic traumatic encephalopathy. World Neurosurg. 2017; 102: 533–44.
55. Chi YC, Wu HL, Chu CP, Huang MC, Lee PC, Chen YY. Traumatic brain injury and affective disorder: A nationwide cohort study in Taiwan, 2000–2010. Journal of Affective Disorders, 2016; 191: 56–61. DOI:10.1016/j.jad.2015.11.035.
56. Escalona S. Babies at double hazard: Early development of babies at biologic and social risk. Pediatrics. 1982; 70(5): 670–6.
57. Donders J, Warschausky S. Neurobehavioral outcomes after early versus late childhood traumatic brain injury. J Head Trauma Rehabil. 2007; 22: 296–302.
58. Gerrard-Morris A, Taylor HG, Yeates KO, Chertkoff N, Stancin T, Minich N, et al. Cognitive development after traumatic brain injury in young children. J Int Neuropsycol Soc. 2010; 16: 157–68.
59. Taylor HG, Yeates KO, Wade SL, Drotar D, Stancin T, Minich N. A prospective study of short- and long-term outcomes after traumatic brain injury in children: behavior and achievement. Neuropsychol. 2002; 16: 15–27.
60. Yeates K, Taylor HG, Rusin J, Bangert B, BDietrich A, Nuss K, et al. Longitudinal trajectories of post-concussive symptoms in children with mild traumatic brain injuries and their relationship to acute clinical status. Pediatrics. 2009; 123(3): 735–43.
61. Emery CA, Barlow KM, Brooks BL, Max JE, Villavicencio-Requis A, Gnanakumar V, et al. A systematic review of psychiatric, psychological, and behavioural outcomes following mild traumatic brain injury in children and adolescents Can J Psychiatry. 2016; 61(5): 259–69.
62. Finkelstein ES, Corso PS, Miller TR. The Incidence and Economic Burden of Injuries in the United States. Oxford: Oxford University Press, 2006.
63. Champion HR, Holcomb JB, Young LA. Injuries from explosions: physics, biophysics, pathology, and required research focus. J Trauma. 2009; 66(5): 1468–77.
64. Te Ao B, Brown P, Tobias M, Ameratunga S, Barker-Collo S, Theadom A, et al. Cost of traumatic brain injury in New Zealand: evidence from a population-based study. Neurology. 2014; 83(18): 1645–52.
65. Singh A, Tetreault L, Klasi-Ryan S, Nourian A, Fehlings MG. Global prevalence and incidence of traumatic spinal cord injury. Clinical Epidemiology. 2014; 6: 309–31.
66. Van den Berg MEL, Castellote JM, Mahillo-fernandez I, De Pedro-Cuesta J. Incidence of spinal cord injury worldwide: A systematic review. Neuroepidemiology. 2010; 34(3): 184–92.
67. Rahimi-Movaghar V, Sayyah MK, Akbari H, Khorramirouz R, Rasouli MR, Moradi-Lakeh M, et al. Epidemiology of traumatic spinal cord injury in developing countries: a systematic review. Neuroepidemiology. 2013; 41: 65–85.
68. Jazayeri SB, Beygi S, Shokraneh F, Hagen EM, Rahimi-Movaghar V. Incidence of traumatic spinal cord injury worldwide: a systematic review. European Spine Journal. 2015; 24(5): 905–18.
69. Derrett S, Beaver C, Sullivan MJ, Herbison GP, Acland R, Paul C. Traumatic and non-traumatic spinal cord impairment in New Zealand: incidence and characteristics of people admitted to spinal units. Injury Prevention. 2012; 18(5): 343–6.
70. Vitale MG, Goss JM, Matsumoto H, Roye DP. Epidemiology of pediatric spinal cord injury in the United States: Years 1997 and 2000. Journal of Pediatric Orthopaedics. 2006; 26(6): 745–9.
71. Martins F, Freitas F, Francois J, Barat M. Spinal cord injuries—epidemiology in Portugal's central region. Spinal Cord. 1998; 36: 574–8.
72. Ahoniemi E, Alaranta H, Hokkinen EM, Valtonen K, Kautiainen H. Incidence of traumatic spinal cord injuries in Finland over a 30-year period. Spinal Cord. 2008; 46: 781–4.
73. Selvarajah S, Schneider EB, Becker D, Sadowsky C, Haider AH, Hammond ER, et al. The epidemiology of childhood and adolescent traumatic spinal cord injury in the United States: 2007–2010. Journal of Neurotrauma. 2014; 31(18): 1548–60.
74. Augutis M, Abel R, Levi R. Pediatric spinal cord injury in a subset of European countries. Spinal Cord. 2006; 44(2): 106–12.
75. DeVivo MJ. Epidemiology of traumatic spinal cord injury: trends and future implications. Spinal Cord. 2012; 50: 365–72.
76. Chen R, Song Y, Kong Q, Zhou C, Liu L. Analysis of 78 patients with spinal injuries in the 2008 Sichuan, China, earthquake. Orthopedics. 2009; 32(5): 322. PubMed PMID: 19472966.
77. American Spinal IA. *International Standards for Neurological Classification of Spinal Cord Injury, revised 2000*. Atlanta: GA Reprinted, 2008.
78. Brown RL, Brunn MA, Garcia VFJPS. Cervical spine injuries in children: a review of 103 patients treated consecutively at a level 1 pediatric trauma center. Journal of Pediatric Surgery. 2001; 36(8): 1107–14.
79. Chan CW, Eng JJ, Tator CH, Krassioukov A, Spinal cord injury RET. Epidemiology of sport-related spinal cord injuries: a systematic review. Journal of Spinal Cord Medicine. 2016; 18: 1–10.
80. DeVivo MJ, Chen Y. Trends in new injuries, prevalent cases and aging with spinal cord injury. Archives of Physical Medicine & Rehabilitation. 2011; 92: 332–8.
81. Chamberlain JD, Meier S, Mader L, von Groote PM, Brinkhof MWG. Mortality and longevity after a spinal cord injury: systematic review and meta-analysis. Neuroepidemiology. 2015; 44: 182–98.
82. Burns AS, O'Connell C. The challenge of spinal cord injury care in the developing world. Journal of Spinal Cord Medicine. 2012; 35(1): 3–8.
83. Shavelle R, Stauss D, Brooks J. Discrepancies in the estimates of life expectancy after SCI. Spinal Cord. 2013; 51(12): 937.
84. Stroud MW, Bombardier CH, Dyer JR, Rimmele CT, Esselman PC. Preinjury alcohol and drug use among persons with spinal cord injury: implications for rehabilitation. Journal of Spinal Cord Medicine. 2011; 34(5): 461–72.

85. Gosselin RA, Coppotelli C. A follow-up study of patients with spinal cord injury in Sierra Leone. International Orthopedics. 2005; 29(5): 330–2.
86. McCullumsmith CB, Kalpakjian CZ, Richards JS, Forchheimer M, Heinemann AW, Richardson EJ, et al. Novel risk factors associated with current suicidal ideation and lifetime suicide attempts in individuals with spinal cord injury. Archives of Physical Medicine & Rehabilitation. 2015; 96(5): 799–808.
87. van Leeuwen CM, Kraaijeveld S, Lindeman E, Post MW. Associations between psychological factors and quality of life ratings in persons with spinal cord injury: a systematic review. Spinal Cord. 2012; 50(3): 174–87.
88. Young AE, Murphy GC. Employment status after spinal cord injury (1992– 2005): a review with implications for interpretation, evaluation, further research, and clinical practice. International Journal of Rehabilitation Research. 2009; 32(1): 1–11.
89. Pearcey TE, Yoshida KK, Renwick RM. Personal relationships after a spinal cord injury. International Journal of Rehabilitation Research. 2007; 30(3): 209–19.
90. Dickman CA, Zabramski JM, Hadley MN, Rekate HL, Sonntag VK. Pediatric spinal cord injury without radiographic abnormalities: report of 26 cases and review of literature. J Spinal Dis. 1991; 4(3): 296–305.
91. Osorio M, Reyes MR, Massagli TL. Pediatric Spinal Cord Injury. Curr Phys Med Rehabil Rep. 2014; 2: 158–68.
92. Dearolf WW, Betz RR, Vogel LC, Levin J, Clancy M, Steel HH. Scoliosis in pediatric spinal cord-injured patients. Journal of Pediatric Orthopaedics. 1990; 10(2): 214–18.
93. Vogel LC, Klaas SJ, Lubicky JP, Anderson CJ. Long-term outcomes and life satisfaction of adults who had pediatric spinal cord injuries. Archives of Physical Medicine & Rehabilitation. 1998; 79(12): 1496–503.
94. World Health Organization. *International Perspectives on Spinal Cord Injury*. Geneva: World Health Organization, 2013.
95. García-Altés A, Pérez K, Novoa A, Suelves JM, Bernabeu M, Vidal J, et al. Spinal cord injury and traumatic brain injury: a cost-of-illness study. Neuroepidemiology. 2012; 39(2): 103–8.
96. Bradbury CL, Wodchis WP, Mikulis DJ, Pano EG, Hitzig SL, McGillivray CF, et al. Traumatic brain injury in patients with traumatic spinal cord injury: clinical and economic consequences. Arch Phys Med Rehabil. 2008; 89(12 Suppl): S77–84. PubMed PMID: 19081445.
97. Richards JS, Osuna FJ, Jaworski TM, Novack TA, Leli DA, Boll TJ. The effectiveness of different methods of defining traumatic brain injury in predicting post-discharge adjustment in a spinal cord injury population. Arch Phys Med Rehabil. 1991; 72(5): 275–9. PubMed PMID: 2009041.

39

Electromagnetic fields

Joachim Schüz and Maria Feychting

Introduction

Like naturally occurring electric and magnetic fields, exposure to man-made electric (EF), magnetic (MF) and electromagnetic fields (EMF) (in this chapter in the frequency range from 0 to 300 gigahertz (GHz)) has become ubiquitous in modern times, on a global scale, related to electrification, broadcasting, medical examinations, and industrial and domestic appliances. While therefore virtually everyone is exposed to some background level of exposure, populations still show some variation and gradient in exposure, although exposures distinctly above those background levels often affect only small proportions in the population and perhaps less people than commonly assumed. Situations of relatively continuous elevated exposures are seen in residents living close to high-voltage power lines or electrical installations, those working permanently in electrical occupations, or residents living close to strong TV or radio broadcast transmitters, but much less so living close to mobile phone base stations. Even higher but intermittent exposures are experienced with the use of some domestic devices, such as hair dryers or vacuum cleaners, but due to the only occasional use cumulative exposures remain very low. The prominent exception is mobile phones where the source of EMF is held directly to the head and emissions from early generations of mobile phones were substantial, so that frequent use of these devices led to the presumably most prevalent EMF exposure in the general population.

Given the widespread exposure and known interactions of EF, MF, and EMF with the human body, there was interest in investigating possible adverse health effects related to exposure. Protection guidelines were defined to protect the public from these frequency-specific known biological effects, namely electric stimulation at low and tissue heating at high frequencies, and many countries have a legal framework in place adopting the guidelines proposed by the International Commission on Non-Ionizing Radiation Protection.[1,2] There remains scientific uncertainty about possible effects below those established guidelines, caused by yet unknown biological mechanisms, and concerns are related to chronic disease after longer term exposures. Here it is, in particular, diseases of the nervous system that have been studied. Research into the possible brain tumour risk related to occupational exposures to low frequency EF and MF, as well as residential exposures from high-voltage power lines started in the 1970s and has continued until now. More recently, studies investigated a possible association between occupational exposures to low frequency fields and the risk of neurodegenerative disease, especially ALS and AD. A large number of studies were conducted looking at a possible increase in brain tumour risks related to the use of mobile phones and large-scale epidemiological studies are still ongoing.

In this chapter, first, a more detailed characterization of exposure will be given, along with measurement of exposure in epidemiological studies. Second, the body of literature on low frequency EF and MF will be reviewed, followed by high frequency EMF (mobile phone) evidence. Lastly, the particular challenges of conducting epidemiological studies on these EMF exposures will be highlighted.

Exposure to Electric, Magnetic, and Electromagnetic Fields

Electromagnetic spectrum

Electromagnetic fields are characterized by their frequency and wavelength, with the product of frequency (in Hertz, Hz) and wavelength (in metres, m) always equalling the speed of light, hence their inverse relationship (Fig. 39.1). Extremely low-frequency (ELF) EF and MF are related to the production, transmission, and use of electricity (usually at 50–60 Hz depending on the country). At higher frequencies, EF and MF are not separated but occur as EMF in the radiofrequency (RF) and microwave range (frequencies from 3 kHz to 300 GHz), related to radio and television, mobile telephony, and microwave heating. At higher frequencies follow infrared, visible, and ultraviolet light. In the frequency range of ELF, RF and light the EMF do not carry enough energy to ionize atoms or molecules.[3] Hence, this part of the EMF spectrum is called non-ionizing radiation in contrast to ionizing radiation such as gamma and X-rays at frequencies above several PHz and wavelengths shorter than several nm (Fig. 39.1). While practically the entire non-ionizing frequency range is used for man-made fields, common exposures to the general public occur mainly at certain frequencies and consequently the research on potential adverse health effects focused on those exposures.

ELF-MF are measured as the magnetic flux density in Tesla (T). The magnetic field passes through the body, thus the interaction with the human body is the induction of electric current. In contrast to

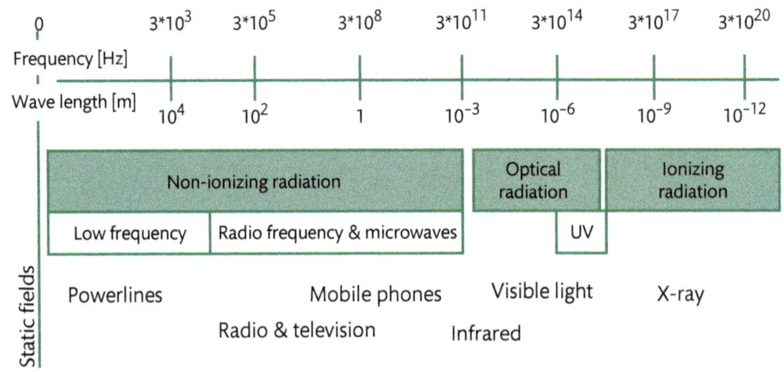

Fig. 39.1 Electromagnetic spectrum.

ELF-MF, ELF-EF—measured in volts per metre (V/m)—are shielded by most materials and hardly penetrate the human body, although if strong enough they can also induce internal electric currents. Human exposure to RF-EMF is characterized by the absorbed energy, measured in Watt per body mass (W/kg), also expressed as specific absorption rate (SAR); as the SAR cannot be directly measured in real life, exposure is mostly expressed as energy per unit area (W/m^2). Except for when it is very close to the source there is a direct relationship between the power density, the EF, and the MF, hence measurement of either EF or MF is sufficient to estimate the other quantities. At these frequencies energy is deposited and can cause heating (as used for instance with microwave ovens or dielectric heating).

Extremely low-frequency magnetic and electric fields

Typical daily average background exposures to ELF-MF from the use of electricity are usually less than 0.05 μT, but slightly higher in more densely populated urban areas.[3–5] Main sources of higher than background exposures (e.g. exceeding 0.2 μT) are related to either the transmission or distribution of power (ELF-MF from high voltage power lines, lower voltages distribution lines, underground cables, transformers, indoor wiring); the use of electrical devices; or working in electrical occupations (such as electricians, welders). ELF-MF are determined by the current and distance to the source. Electric devices may emit ELF-MF of several mT in their immediate vicinity, but only during use; therefore they are sources of intermittent very short-term exposure. In certain occupations, when working close to electric motors for example, average exposures of 1–10 μT are possible and exposure may span over the whole working day.[6] ELF-MF of >0.2 μT to few μT in residences may be reached within distances of less than 50–200 m to nearby high voltage power lines (>200 kV, depending on their power load), distances of less than 20–50 m to medium voltage power lines or other installations (>10 kV), less than 5–10 m to low voltage power lines, their roof connections to buildings, or to transformers (<1 kV), or in homes with unbalanced currents in indoor wiring.[5] Even taken together, these exposure situations are rather uncommon. Only few per cent (1–3%) of Europeans and potentially slightly more (1–10%) North Americans have average residential exposures exceeding 0.2 μT, with a scarcity of representative data from most low to middle income countries.[3,4] ELF-EF are produced wherever there is electric potential and are directly related to the voltage. Normally, ELF-EF in homes are few V/m, but can become as high as several kV/m in homes in close vicinity and with an unobstructed path to high-voltage power lines and in certain occupational situations.

Radiofrequency electromagnetic fields

Although RF-EMF has only recently received broad attention as to whether it is associated with adverse health effects, mainly motivated by the widespread use of mobile phones, RF-EMF exposure has been ubiquitous through radio and television broadcasting for about one century. It was not uncommon that these analogue transmitters had output power of several MW, resulting in exposure in the closer few km of the transmitters of several tenths of V/m, and often RF-EMF exposures still exceeding 1 V/m in 10–20 km distance.[7] Radio and broadcast reception was intended to cover entire countries, at the same time, meaning there was a guaranteed background exposure for every inhabitant. Some military installations or broadcast transmitters intended to cross borders (e.g. to deliver propaganda news during times of the Cold War) had even higher output power than civil broadcasting. In comparison, RF-EMF from mobile phone base stations normally exceed 1 V/m only in its direct vicinity of few metres, are between 0.1 V/m and 1 V/m of up to 100 m within the main beam from the antenna, but much lower otherwise.[8]

The major source of localized RF-EMF exposure is the handset, as the mobile phone is directly held to the head during transmission, although now that smart phones have other uses making calls may not be the dominant use. Handheld mobile phones were introduced in the mid-1980s but because of high costs they were used only by a minority. With the first boom of private customers occurring in the early to mid-1990s, by 2010 in many developed countries more phones were registered than the size of the population. But also, in developing countries where previously no communication was possible due to lack of landline phones, mobile technology is virtually used by everyone. From the first to the third generation of mobile technology the output power of handsets decreased dramatically, with emissions in the Watts range for the first generation, on average up to 250 mW with the second generation (Global System for Mobile Communications, GSM), to on average few mW or less in the third and fourth generation (Universal Mobile Telecommunications System, UMTS; Long Term Evolution, LTE). Consequently, even with increasing usage time due to lower costs, the cumulative exposure from mobile phone use is expected to have substantially declined; however, the number of individuals being exposed went from few per cent to almost 100% in a short time period of only around 15 years.[3] The RF-EMF exposure decreases rapidly with distance to the exposure source; thus, use of a wired hands-free device reduces the exposure to the head by approximately 90%. Another source of exposure from devices is cordless phones used within homes, with Digital Enhanced Cordless Telecommunications (DECT) phones being the most successful technology. As the DECT phone only transmits to a base station that is a few metres away, exposure was considerably lower compared to the second generation of mobile phones, but as older types of cordless phones do not have adaptive power control, as mobile phones do, to downregulate output power to have the lowest power to keep the connection, these types of cordless phones may lead to higher exposures than mobile phones. All technologies comply with the protection guidelines suggested to limit RF-EMF exposure.[2]

More recent sources of environmental exposure include mobile phone base stations, DECT phone base stations, and Wi-Fi, giving rise to exposures that are only a fraction of the exposure guidelines.[2,3] Similarly, devices such as baby monitors and smart meters, used to measure electricity consumption, also generate very low RF-EMF. Broadcasting technologies have also changed over time, with analogue radio and television having been replaced by digital broadcasting, which has mostly resulted in decreased total output power but an increase in the number of transmitters.

Occupational settings with high RF-EMF exposure are dielectric heaters or induction heaters, operators of surgical and other medical diathermy devices or magnetic resonance imaging (MRI), workers near radar equipment, or those involved in the maintenance of transmitters.[6] Applications with sometimes intentionally relatively high RF-EMF exposures are anti-theft or body scanning devices, but the time that humans stay close to those sources is usually very short.

Extremely Low-frequency Electric and Magnetic Fields and Risk of Neurological Disease

Childhood brain tumours

In 2008, Mezei et al. published a literature-based meta-analysis including results from 13 studies on residential exposure to ELF-MF and the risk of brain tumours in children.[9] The summary relative risk estimates were 1.14 (95% confidence interval (CI) 0.78–1.67) for calculated or measured MF above 0.2 μT and 1.68 (CI 0.83–3.43) for fields above 0.3 or 0.4 μT, with no indication of publication bias. With the aim of better harmonization of exposure data a pooled analysis was carried out later and it was possible to include ten studies.[10] The pooled relative risk estimate in exposure categories of 0.1–<0.2 μT, 0.2–<0.4 μT, and ≥0.4 μT were 0.95 (CI 0.65–1.41), 0.70 (CI 0.40–1.22), and 1.14 (CI 0.61–2.13), respectively, in comparison with <0.1 μT (Fig. 39.2). Employing alternate cut-off points and other sensitivity analyses did not show evidence of an increased childhood brain tumour. In summary, there is little evidence supporting an association between ELF-MF exposure and the risk of childhood brain tumours.

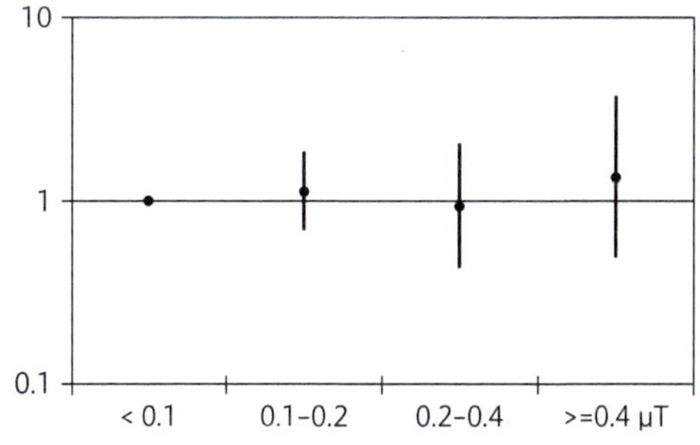

Fig. 39.2 Pooled odds ratios from combining four case-control studies on residential exposure to ELF magnetic fields and the risk of brain tumours in children,[10] using studies with long term >24 hours field measurements in the child's home.

Adult brain tumours

Although some studies on residential exposures were also conducted in adults, the vast majority of evidence on adult brain tumours comes from occupational EMF studies. In a literature-based meta-analysis, Kheifets et al. combined results from 48 studies resulting in a summary relative risk estimate of 1.14 (CI 1.07–1.22).[11] Individual study-specific estimates varied between 0.6 and 4.88, with most studies showing weak associations just above 1. There was a tendency for individual study estimates to be lower in the more recent studies. This was most strongly observed for gliomas, the most common subtype of adult brain tumours, when the summary relative risk estimate of 1.39 (CI 1.07–1.82) dropped to 1.16 (CI 1.09–1.25), albeit both estimates showed a significant positive association. Main limitations in the interpretation were that for studies that reported risks by exposure level, no clear exposure-response pattern could be seen, and many studies used rather crude exposure measurements preventing firm conclusions. In a recent multi-centre case-control study in seven countries (InterOcc study) involving 1939 cases of glioma, 1822 cases of meningioma, and 5404 controls, in which a job-exposure-matrix (JEM) based on workplace EMF surveys was applied,[7] no association was seen overall between the ELF magnetic fields and brain tumour risk (for cumulative exposure in μT-years in the highest exposure category, the OR were 0.80 (CI: 0.63–1.00) for glioma and 0.89 (CI: 0.70–1.12) for meningioma).[12] Looking at different time windows of exposure, there was an increased risk of glioma with a dose-response trend for exposures 1–4 years before diagnosis, while there was no association in both the 5–9 years before diagnosis or 10+ years before diagnosis time windows. This may suggest a role of ELF-MF in tumour promotion, but too little data are available yet to draw firm conclusions. No interactions between occupational ELF-MF and chemical exposures at the workplace were found.[13]

Neurodegenerative diseases

Over 40 studies of occupational EMF exposure and neurodegenerative diseases have been published (using a broad definition that also includes analyses of single job titles), several of them covering more than one neurodegenerative disease outcome. In addition, several reviews and meta-analyses have been conducted.[14–17] Early studies of neurodegenerative diseases mainly defined exposure as individual job titles, or used a crude categorization of job titles into 'electrical occupations' based on expert judgement, whereas later studies took advantage of JEMs based on workday measurements of ELF-MF in various occupations, which provided a quantitative assessment of the magnetic field level.

Overall, the evidence from the epidemiological studies does not support a risk increase associated with EMF exposure for PD (based on nearly 20 studies) or multiple sclerosis (a handful of studies).[15,17] For AD there is weak evidence suggesting an increased risk associated with ELF-MF exposure, both in JEM-based studies and those relying on 'electrical occupations'. The findings are, however, inconsistent, with the strongest associations found in studies with a high potential for bias, while several studies reported no association or found association only in subgroup analyses.[15,16] In a recent meta-analysis, Vergara and colleagues reported an overall pooled risk estimate of 1.27 (CI 1.15–1.40), but with considerable heterogeneity between studies, and some evidence of reporting and publication bias. Only two studies have focused on residential magnetic field exposure; a Swiss study reported an increased risk of AD among persons who had lived at least ten years within 50 metres of a high voltage power line,[18] while a Danish study could not confirm this finding.[19]

Results for ALS were initially regarded as more consistently showing a modest risk increase associated with EMF exposure, but with a growing number of studies, a pattern emerged where increased risks were observed primarily in studies that estimated exposure through the crude categorization of job titles as 'electrical occupations', while findings were generally close to unity for JEM-based studies with quantitative assessment of the magnetic fields.[16,17] None of the studies of residential magnetic field exposure have found association with ALS.[18–20] Exposure to electric shocks has been discussed as one alternative explanation for the increased risk associated with 'electric occupations', and JEMs focused on electric shocks were developed. Later studies that have estimated both exposures to ELF-MF and to electric shocks based on the available JEMs did not, however, observe an increased risk associated with work in occupations classified as having more prevalent exposure to electric shocks.[21–23] Another potential confounding factor that has been discussed is exposure to welding fumes, but this is unlikely to explain the entire risk increase associated with 'electric occupations'. The two most recent cohort analyses from 2017 from the Netherlands and Denmark do provide further support for an association between ELF-MF and ALS.[24,25]

In conclusion, there is some weak evidence of an association between ELF-MF exposure and AD, but bias cannot be ruled out as an alternative explanation. For ALS the evidence is controversial regarding an association with ELF-MF exposure, whereas there is quite consistent evidence of an association between work in 'electrical occupations' and ALS risk. It is still unclear which exposures in these occupations may be the causative agents.

Radiofrequency Electromagnetic Fields and Risk of Neurological Disease

Brain tumours

Systematic reviews of the scientific evidence on the association between use of mobile phones and the risk of brain tumours have continuously been conducted by international and national bodies such as the Scientific Committee on Emerging and Newly Identified Health Risks (SCENIHR) of the European Commission,[3] the International Agency for Research on Cancer (IARC) within their Monograph programme on the identification of carcinogenic hazards to humans,[26] as well as several national radiation protection authorities or the European Code against Cancer expert group.[27] All reviews identify considerable methodological limitations and inconsistencies in the available epidemiological studies, which prevent firm conclusions. In 2011, the IARC classified RF fields as possibly carcinogenic to humans, based on limited evidence in humans and from animal studies. Based on even more recent data, the SCENIHR review concludes that the evidence for an effect on glioma has become weaker since the IARC evaluation. It was noted in all those assessments that conclusions could not be drawn about longer latencies than up to 15 years since first mobile phone use.

Only two longer term cohort studies are available, with large sample sizes but limited information on exposure. In a nationwide study of all Danish adults, ~4 million, the brain tumour incidence among early subscribers of a mobile phone (from start to 1995) was compared to the incidence in the rest of the adult population, and in the last update until 2007 no association was seen with either short-term or long-term (≥13 years) mobile phone subscription for any type of brain tumour in men or women (e.g. the risk of glioma in men was 0.98 (CI 0.70–1.36)).[28,29] In the UK Million Women study (actual sample for the mobile phone analysis was 791,710 women), there was also no association for glioma, meningioma, or acoustic neuroma with duration of use or for daily users of mobile phones as assessed prospectively by questionnaires at two points in time.[30,31] Results from case-control studies were inconsistent, but many of them were rather small and therefore not reviewed here.[3,26] The largest one was Interphone, a 13-country case-control study including 2708 glioma, 2409 meningioma, and 1105 acoustic neuroma cases, matched to about one or two (acoustic neuroma) controls.[32,33] Mobile phone use history was assessed with face-to-face interviews, hence there was much more detail available than in the cohorts, but one had to rely on recall abilities of participants (including sometimes very sick cases) and response rates particularly in controls were low, around 50%. While the overall OR for ever regular versus never regular use were reduced for glioma (0.81, CI 0.70–0.94), for meningioma (0.79, CI 0.68–0.91), and slightly so for acoustic neuroma (0.95 (CI 0.77–1.17), and no associations were seen among the longest term users of ten years or more, with OR of 0.96 (CI 0.71–1.31), of 0.80 (0.55–1.17), and of 0.83 (CI 0.58–1.19), for glioma, meningioma, and acoustic neuroma, respectively, the increased OR in the highest decile of cumulative use for glioma (1.40 (CI 1.03–1.89)) and for acoustic neuroma (2.79 (CI 1.55–5.16)), but lesser so meningioma (1.15 (CI 0.81–1.62)), received some attention. In a series of case-control studies from the Örebro region in Sweden, researchers repeatedly found elevated risks already in association with low and short duration of use of mobile phones;[3,34–36] while this was alarming in the early years it was only indicative of serious bias later because if those risks were true a large epidemic of brain tumours would have emerged by today, which is clearly not the case. Only one case-control study is so far available on children and adolescents, with the main result showing an OR of 1.36 (CI 0.92–2.02) for ever regular use of mobile phones.[37] Table 39.1 gives an overview on the methodologies used.

The few reported risk increases appear to be implausible when comparing with time trends in brain tumour incidence rates over the same time period that the cohort and case-control studies covered. Glioma incidence time trends have been stable since the introduction of mobile phone technologies, as shown in incidence studies from many parts of the world, most extensively done in the

Table 39.1 Overview of epidemiological study designs used to investigate the association between use of mobile phones and the risk of brain tumours

Study	Country references	Design (D) strengths (S)/weaknesses (W) main outcome (O)
Cohort studies		
Danish Subscriber Cohort	Denmark[28, 29, 46]	D: Registry-based retrospective cohort study linking subscriber information (yes or no before 1995) with cancer registry and compare with expected rates in rest of the Danish population S: Entire adult population of country included (~4 million), objective and complete information from registers, no active participation required W: Misclassification if subscriber was not user or the user not among subscribers, no information on amount of use O: No association between ever subscription of mobile phone before 1995 and risk of any type of brain tumour
UK Million Women Study	UK[30,31]	D: Prospective questionnaire-based cohort study in approximately 800,000 women in UK S: Very large cohort, prospectively asked questions, detailed information on various potential confounders W: crude information on use and no details on cumulative use O: No association between long-term use or daily use of mobile phones with any type of brain tumour
Case-control studies		
Interphone Study	13 countries[32,33]	D: Population based case-control study with detailed face-to-face interviews and several validation studies S: Large sample size, common protocol in 13 countries, detailed information on mobile phone use, detailed information on potential confounders, validation studies allow sensitivity analyses on robustness of results W: Low participation in control subjects, validation studies show major challenges in people recalling their contemporary and past mobile phone use O: Inverse association with moderate mobile phone use most likely explained by selection bias, modest association with heavy mobile phone use; unclear whether causal or attributable to reporting bias
Case-control study series, Örebro region	Sweden[34–36]	D: Series of population-based case-control studies in the Örebro region of Sweden with similar methodology utilizing complete Swedish cancer and population registers S: Large sample size, detailed information on mobile phone use from self-administered questionnaires and phone calls, detailed information on potential confounders, good participation W: Lack of validation studies to assess quality of questionnaire data, lack of detailed reports on methodology and used procedures O: Association between mobile phone use and (most strongly) two types of brain tumours (glioma, acoustic neuroma); risk seen already with very modest use that, if true, would lead to major epidemic of tumours that did not occur; consequently association at least heavily inflated by bias
Cefalo Study	Denmark, Norway, Sweden, Switzerland[37]	D: Population-based case-control study on 7–19-year-olds with face-to-face interviews of children and their parents S: Detailed information on use and confounders, good participation, validation study with operator traffic records W: Rare disease hence smaller numbers, challenge to recall mobile phone use as illustrated by comparison with operator data O: Very modest non-significant association but without any indication of dose-response relationship
Ecological: time trend analyses quantitatively comparing with scenarios under hypothetical risks		
Nordic countries	Nordic countries[38]	D: Incidence rates from complete cancer registries of four Nordic countries, compared with how incidence would change under different risk scenarios S: High quality cancer registries, objective nationwide data W: no individual data on mobile phone use, only able to detect risks big enough that would change the incidence rate O: Incompatible with any major increase in brain tumour incidence related to mobile phone use
USA	USA[39]	D, S, W: Similar to above but using data from the USA O: Similar conclusions to above

Inclusion: for this methodological comparison only large cohorts (>100,000 population), case-control studies with large case numbers (>1000) or in children, and ecological studies with quantitatively contrasting time trends with prediction models are shown.

Nordic countries[38] and in the USA;[39] this was particularly so for middle-aged and younger men, which is the most relevant population group in relation to mobile phone use. Incidence increases are indeed seen in the elderly, but that was observed to start even before the introduction of mobile phone technologies and is believed to be due to improved and more readily available diagnostic imaging techniques. Simulation studies based on the observed incidence rates have demonstrated that risk increases after short duration of mobile phone use are incompatible with the observed incidence trends (Fig. 39.3).[38,39] Also for acoustic neuroma, incidence time trends do not support an effect of mobile phone use,[40,41] although less data are available.

In all, there is convincing evidence that moderate use of mobile phones does not pose an increased risk of brain tumours. For heavy use, without much hard data to quantify what this means as definitions have been inconsistent across studies, there is the possibility of a modest risk increase for glioma and for acoustic neuroma, although it is becoming less likely with accumulating years of not

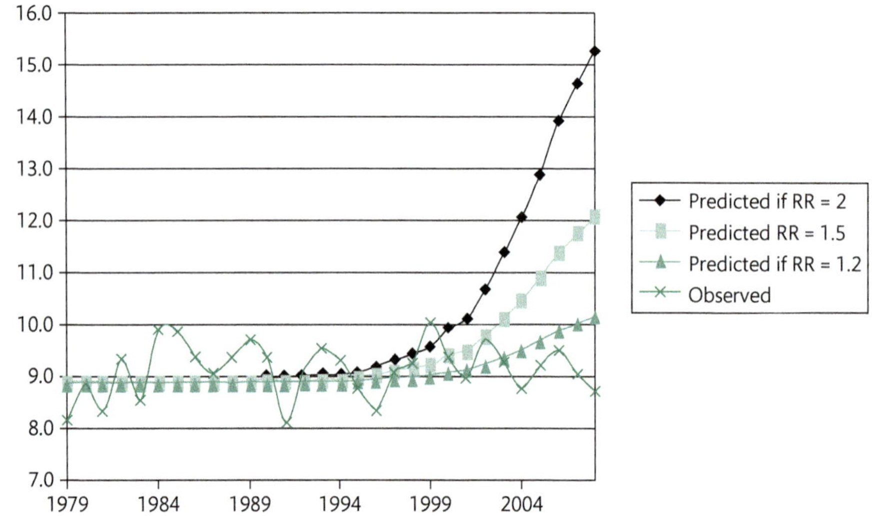

Fig. 39.3 Observed incidence rates (per 100,000) in the Nordic countries (Denmark, Finland, Norway, Sweden) of glioma in men aged 30–59 years compared to scenarios of how the incidence rates would be expected to look like when 10+ years of regular mobile phone use was associated with a 20%, 50%, and 100%, respectively, increase in risk.
Reproduced courtesy of Dr Deltour, IARC.

seeing any incidence rate increase for the two tumour types. For glioma, seen as aggressive and fast-growing cancer, observation time is believed to be sufficiently long. Acoustic neuroma is a slow-growing tumour, and one would not expect an effect on the tumour occurrence after a short latency period.

Neurodegenerative diseases

Risk of neurodegenerative disease was studied in the same nationwide Danish retrospective cohort study as adult brain cancer.[41,42] For neurodegenerative disease, hospitalizations for a variety of diseases occurring before the end of 2002 among 420,000 subscribers of a mobile phone were compared to the number of hospitalizations observed in the remaining general public (approximately 3.6 million Danes) during the same time period. Overall, the number of hospitalizations for AD was statistically significantly lower than expected from the respective rates of the general population. No association was seen for ALS. Significantly lower rates of hospitalizations were also observed for vascular dementia and PD. The reduced rates of patients with AD or PD seen following a short subscription time is likely to be due to reverse causation, in other words, persons with early symptoms of those diseases were less likely to subscribe for a mobile phone. Interestingly, a reduced relative risk estimate for AD but not PD was also seen among those subscribers who had their mobile phone for 10+ years, which is unlikely to be solely attributable to such prodromal symptoms.[41] No association was seen with MS, but presenting symptoms differed between mobile phone subscribers and the comparison group.[42] Mobile phone subscribers had more hospitalizations for migraine, but reverse causation may be an explanation.[41]

Challenges in Epidemiological Studies of Electromagnetic Fields

Bias is inherent in observational studies irrespective of the exposure of interest. In the following, some specific features of bias commonly observed in epidemiological studies on EMF are addressed, to illustrate why this is a challenging field for epidemiologists.

Selection bias

Selection bias from unrepresentative samples occurs when selection probabilities into the study are influenced by exposure or disease status, commonly at the stage of recruitment of participants and often more pronounced through voluntary participation in studies. On first thought one may assume the risk of selection bias is small in EMF studies as people are normally not aware of their exposure status, other than assuming exposure when, for instance, living close to a power line or being heavy mobile phone user. There is often some disagreement between perceived EMF exposure and real EMF exposure, and in some studies this discrepancy has even been utilized by investigating outcomes related to four exposure categories, namely those who correctly assumed their exposure, those who incorrectly assumed exposure, those who incorrectly assumed no exposure, and those truly not exposed. In a German study on symptoms related to RF-EMF from mobile phone base stations the relationship between perceived exposure and symptoms was in fact stronger than between measured exposure and symptoms,[43] providing some evidence of a nocebo effect.

When evaluating the potential for selection bias in EMF studies it was shown that it is in fact a serious concern, both for ELF and RF studies. In studies measuring residential ELF-MF there was no direct link, but an indirect link between exposure and participation probability, as best illustrated for studies on childhood leukaemia, but equally applicable to other cancers.[44] Among non-diseased, participation was higher in the more affluent, who at the same time more often lived in houses and apartment types that had lower chances of being affected by elevated ELF-MF, resulting in a possible inflation of the observed effect estimates. In RF-EMF studies, and here in particular in the largest case-control study on mobile phones and brain tumours (Interphone)—the only study with a systematic assessment of potential selection bias through non-responder questionnaires—mobile phone use was more common among those participating than non-participating, leading to a spurious protective effect in the risk estimation.[45]

In summary, state-of-the-art EMF studies would provide an assessment of potential selection bias, ideally based on supplementary data such as from non-responder information although at least through sensitivity analyses modelling various bias scenarios, but studies simply dismissing selection bias on theoretical considerations are not acceptable.

Confounding

For residential ELF-MF exposure, some potential confounders were suggested, for instance based on the observation that in some countries high-voltage power lines often run in parallel to roads with heavy car traffic. Therefore ELF-MF exposure may correlate with higher air pollution, but actually no strong correlations for air pollution or any other factor were observed to substantially affect effect estimation.[44] This is different for mobile phone studies where the early mobile phone users were commonly more affluent and had lower smoking rates and in general a healthier lifestyle than the rest of the population. Consequently, cohort studies of mobile phone users observed, for example, decreased occurrence of lung cancers among the early users.[30,46] Lifestyle factors such as smoking and alcohol use have not, however, been linked with an increased risk of brain tumours. Further, the healthy worker effect is a concern in mobile phone cohorts, as again in the early mobile phone users occupational use was most common due to the high costs.

In summary, while for ELF no general recommendations on adjustment for confounding can be given, for RF and, in particular, studies on mobile phone users it is important to adjust for lifestyle-related risk factors if they are associated with the outcome under investigation, as longer-term mobile phone use is correlated with less smoking and other lifestyle choices of a more affluent population.

Disease misclassification

In studies of neurodegenerative diseases, case ascertainment is a particular challenge. Many studies have relied on information from death certificates, which are known to under report, for example, AD. Many clinically based studies have included prevalent cases. There is a possibility that case ascertainment is not independent of the exposure, as completeness of ascertainment may be related to factors such as survival, age, place of residence, and socioeconomic status.[47] Indeed, results from a recent meta-analysis showed that studies relying on prevalent disease reported considerably higher risk estimates than studies based on incidence, which is believed to be more reliable.[17] Studies using screening for morbidity or relying on hospital discharges had, with a few exceptions, limited statistical power.

Exposure misclassification

In residential ELF-MF studies stationary measurements over one or few days in the bedroom or time-weighted average over several rooms in the apartment have shown to be the most accurate predictor of past individual exposure.[3,47] Personal dosimetry, which is also available, sounds more appealing as it takes the individual's behaviour during the day into account, but as the vast majority of studies were of case-control design, the impact of diagnosis on daily behaviour leads to severe error in predicting pre-diagnostic exposures. In addition, behaviour changes with age, and rapidly so in children. Personal dosimetry is accurate for immediate outcomes, however, such as headache. Distance to power lines has also been used as exposure metric but leads to both false negatives (neglecting of other sources than power lines) and false positives (power lines with insufficient power load to produce elevated MF), making it a poor predictor of individual exposure.[47] An exception to this is countries having historic information on the power load of power lines. By using this information, the false positives are virtually eliminated, leading to high specificity of the exposure classification, whereas sensitivity remains low. Because of the overall low prevalence of ELF-MF the low sensitivity and high specificity combination leads to loss of statistical power that can be compensated by increasing the sample size, but there is hardly any bias in estimating the magnitude of effect.

In occupational ELF and RF studies measurements were usually too laborious, so surrogate exposures were used. As is common in occupational epidemiology, in the simpler scenarios this was an expert ranking of job titles according to exposure. More sophisticated were quantitative job-exposure-matrices (JEM) based on workplace measurements, although those were not done individually for study participants, but again for typical jobs. A JEM has been developed based on workplace measurements for ELF MF,[6] but how much exposure misclassification occurs in an individual study is difficult to judge. An additional challenge is that in many jobs with elevated EMF exposures other work exposures also occur.

Studies on mobile phones mainly relied on the study participants' recall of past mobile phone use. This is challenging in studies on neurological disease as many of them affect memory capabilities, so it is likely that studies of case-control design suffer from recall bias. In the largest case-control study on mobile phones and brain tumours (Interphone), several validation studies were done by comparing self-reported amount of mobile phone use with traffic records from mobile phone operators.[49,50] Those showed a high random error in reporting, both among cases and controls, as it is apparently difficult to recall mobile phone use of ten or more years ago. It also showed systematic reporting bias as occasional users tended to even underestimate their real use while heavy users tended to overestimate it. While the former error would most likely lead to an attenuation of an association, the latter could inflate an association. When comparing cases and controls, more implausible values of use were reported in cases (possibly leading to a spurious association). These errors in the same study leading to both upward and downward trends make it difficult to interpret the observed results described above. In cohort studies, recall bias is not an issue as exposure is assessed before the occurrence of disease, but the potential for random error remains. In addition, cohort studies enrol huge populations and therefore exposure assessment is often very crude. A validation study of the Danish nationwide cohort study of mobile phone subscribers showed that exposure misclassification would lead to an attenuation of any risk, but increases >50% were still well detectable.[46] The main disadvantage was that no information was available on amount of use.

In summary, the accuracy of exposure assessment varies by study setting and research hypothesis, and therefore each state-of-the-art study should make an attempt to collect supplementary data to estimate the magnitude of exposure misclassification. This can be done by means of validation studies, including cross-comparisons of different

Table 39.2 Synthesis of the epidemiological evidence on exposure to electromagnetic fields and the risk of neurological disease

	Residential exposures to ELF	Occupational exposures to EMF	Exposures to RF (mobile phones)
Brain tumours in children	Studies suggesting no association	Few studies on parental occupational exposures, no clear associations	Only one study, no association
Brain tumours in adults	Few studies but no suggestion of association	Suggestion of weak association, but limitations prevent firm conclusions	No evidence except weak association for glioma with very heavy use; potentially caused by recall bias; observation time perhaps too short for some benign tumours
Alzheimer's disease	Few studies	Suggestion of weak association, but limitations prevent firm conclusions	Few studies, perhaps inverse association
ALS	Few studies	Suggestions of increased risk in electrical occupations, but less related to EMF	Few studies
Multiple sclerosis	No studies	Few studies	Few studies, indication that symptoms of presentations may be different
Other neurodegenerative disease	Few studies	Few studies but suggesting no association	Few studies
Migraine	No studies	No studies	Few studies, indication of positive association, perhaps reverse causation

Legend: ELF (extremely low-frequency electric or magnetic fields), EMF (electric, magnetic or electromagnetic fields of all frequencies), RF (radiofrequency electromagnetic fields), ALS (amyotrophic lateral sclerosis).

exposure assessment methods or repeated measurements, and the results of these validations should be used to estimate the impact of the exposure misclassification on the effect estimation. As validation studies are often costly, they are not routinely done. But given how many EMF studies have been done in the past decades, further studies with too many uncertainties in exposure measures will not be informative. Equally, studies without proper validation or at least reasonable impact analyses of exposure misclassification should receive less weight in synthesizing the overall scientific evidence.

Conclusion

Exposures to ELF-EF and ELF-MF related to the production, transmission, and use of electricity, as well as to RF-EMF mainly related to mobile communication and broadcasting are ubiquitous in modern times. Although protection limits prevent from known biological effects, such as induction of electric currents and tissue heating, those guidelines are challenged by several decades of research of whether adverse effects exist below those protection limits, including studies on neurological diseases. Synthesizing the evidence for brain tumours, suggests that there is no association between residential ELF fields and the risk of brain tumours in children. Occupational ELF fields and adult brain tumour studies are less consistent, some suggesting a weak positive association, but limitations in study methodology prevent firm conclusions. Most studies do not show an increased risk of adult brain tumours with RF-EMF emitted from mobile phones, but a modestly increased risk of glioma with very heavy mobile phone use cannot be excluded and for some slowly growing benign tumours observation time may still be too short to detect any effect. A weak association between occupational exposure to ELF-MF and the risk of AD has been observed in several studies, but with large heterogeneity, and bias remains a concern. An increased risk in electrical occupations was seen for ALS but not with ELF-MF, so that it is likely that other exposures than EMF in those jobs are relevant. For RF-EMF there are only a few studies on neurodegenerative disease, but the evidence for any positive association is weak. Table 39.2 gives an overview of the authors' assessment of the scientific evidence. Although most of the evidence is negative, given the widespread exposure and potentially new features in new generations of mobile technologies, monitoring studies, such as the multinational prospective cohort studies of mobile phone users,[51] as well as consistency checks with incidence rates are merited.

REFERENCES

1. International Commission on Non-Ionizing Radiation Protection. Guidelines for limiting exposure to time-varying electric and magnetic fields (1 Hz to 100 kHz). Health Phys. 2010; 99: 818–36.
2. International Commission on Non-Ionizing Radiation Protection. Guidelines for Limiting Exposure to Electromagnetic Fields (100 kHz to 300 GHz). Health Phys. 2020; 118:483–524.
3. Scientific Committee on Emerging and Newly Identified Health Risks (SCENIHR). Potential Health Effects of Exposure to Electromagnetic Fields (EMF). European Commission, 2 January 2015. http://ec.europa.eu/health/scientific_committees/emerging/docs/scenihr_o_041.pdf.
4. International Agency for Research on Cancer (IARC). IARC Monographs on the Evaluation of Carcinogenic Risks to Humans, Volume 80. Non-Ionizing Radiation, Part 1: Static and extremely low-frequency (ELF) electric and magnetic fields. Lyon, France: IARC Press. http://monographs.iarc.fr/ENG/Monographs/vol80/mono80.pdf.
5. Schüz J, Grigat JP, Störmer B, Rippin G, Brinkmann K, Michaelis J. Extremely low frequency magnetic fields in residences in Germany. Distribution of measurements, comparison of two methods for assessing exposure, and predictors for the occurrence of magnetic fields above background level. Radiat Environ Biophys. 2000; 39: 233–40.

6. Vila J, Bowman JD, Richardson L, et al. and INTEROCC Study Group. A Source-based measurement database for occupational exposure assessment of electromagnetic fields in the INTEROCC Study: a literature review approach. Ann Occup Hyg. 2016; 60: 184–204.
7. Schmiedel S, Brüggemeyer H, Philipp J, Wendler J, Merzenich H, Schüz J. An evaluation of exposure metrics in an epidemiologic study on radio and television broadcast transmitters and the risk of childhood leukemia. Bioelectromagnetics. 2009, 30: 81–91.
8. Schüz J, Mann S. A discussion of potential exposure metrics for use in epidemiological studies on human exposure to radiowaves from mobile phone base stations. J Exp Anal Env Epidemiol. 2000; 10: 600–5.
9. Mezei G, Gadallah M, Kheifets L. Residential magnetic field exposure and childhood brain cancer: a meta-analysis. Epidemiology. 2008; 19: 424–30.
10. Kheifets L, Ahlbom A, Crespi CM, et al. A pooled analysis of extremely low-frequency magnetic fields and childhood brain tumors. Am J Epidemiol. 2010; 172: 752–61.
11. Kheifets L, Monroe J, Vergara X, Mezei G, Afifi AA. Occupational electromagnetic fields and leukemia and brain cancer: an update to two meta-analyses. J Occup Environ Med. 2008; 50: 677–88.
12. Turner MC, Benke G, Bowman JD, et al. Occupational exposure to extremely low frequency magnetic fields and brain tumour risks in the INTEROCC study. Cancer Epidemiol Biomarkers Prev. 2014; 23: 1863–72.
13. Turner MC, Benke G, Bowman JD, et al. Interactions between occupational exposure to extremely low frequency magnetic fields and chemicals for brain tumour risk in the INTEROCC study. Occup Environ Med. 2017; 74(11): 802–9.
14. Garcia AM, Sisternas A, Hoyos SP. Occupational exposure to extremely low frequency electric and magnetic fields and Alzheimer disease: a meta-analysis. Int J Epidemiol. 2008; 37: 329–40.
15. Huss A, Koeman T, Kromhout H, Vermeulen R. extremely low frequency magnetic field exposure and Parkinson's disease—a systematic review and meta-analysis of the data. Int J Environ Res Public Health. 2015; 12: 7348–56.
16. Kheifets L, Bowman JD, Checkoway H, et al. Future needs of occupational epidemiology of extremely low frequency electric and magnetic fields: review and recommendations. Occup Environ Med. 2009; 66: 72–80.
17. Vergara X, Kheifets L, Greenland S, Oksuzyan S, Cho YS, Mezei G. Occupational exposure to extremely low-frequency magnetic fields and neurodegenerative disease: a meta-analysis. J Occup Environ Med. 2013; 55: 135–46
18. Huss A, Spoerri A, Egger M, Röösli M. Residence near power lines and mortality from neurodegenerative diseases: longitudinal study of the Swiss population. Am J Epidemiol. 2009; 169: 167–75.
19. Frei P, Poulsen AH, Mezei G, et al. Residential distance to high-voltage power lines and risk of neurodegenerative diseases: a Danish population-based case-control study. Am J Epidemiol. 2013; 177: 970–8.
20. Seelen M, Vermeulen RC, van Dillen LS, et al. Residential exposure to extremely low frequency electromagnetic fields and the risk of ALS. Neurology. 2014; 83: 1767–9.
21. Fischer H, Kheifets L, Huss A, et al. Occupational exposure to electric shocks and magnetic fields and amyotrophic lateral sclerosis in Sweden. Epidemiology. 2015; 26: 824–30.
22. Huss A, Spoerri A, Egger M, Kromhout H, Vermeulen R. Occupational exposure to magnetic fields and electric shocks and risk of ALS: the Swiss National Cohort. Amyotroph Lateral Scler Frontotemporal Degener. 2015; 16: 80–5.
23. Vergara X, Mezei G, Kheifets L. Case-control study of occupational exposure to electric shocks and magnetic fields and mortality from amyotrophic lateral sclerosis in the US, 1991–1999. J Expo Sci Environ Epidemiol. 2015; 25: 65–71.
24. Koeman T, Slottje P, Schouten LJ, et al. Occupational exposure and amyotrophic lateral sclerosis in a prospective cohort. Occup Environ Med. 2017; 74: 578–85.
25. Pedersen C, Poulsen AH, Rod NH, et al. Occupational exposure to extremely low-frequency magnetic fields and risk for central nervous system disease: an update of a Danish cohort study among utility workers. Int Arch Occup Environ Health. 2017; 90(7): 619–28.
26. International Agency for Research on Cancer (IARC). IARC Monographs on the Evaluation of Carcinogenic Risks to Humans, Volume 102. Non-Ionizing Radiation, Part 2: Radiofrequency electromagnetic fields. Lyon, France: IARC Press. https://monographs.iarc.fr/ENG/Monographs/vol102/mono102.pdf.
27. McColl N, Auvinen A, Kesminiene A, et al. European Code against Cancer, 4th edition: ionising and non-ionising radiation and cancer. Cancer Epidemiol. 2015; 39(Suppl 1): S93–100.
28. Frei P, Poulsen AH, Johansen C, Olsen JH, Steding-Jessen M, Schüz J. Use of mobile phones and risk of brain tumours: update of Danish cohort study. BMJ. 2011; 343: d6387.
29. Schüz J, Steding-Jessen M, Hansen S, et al. Long-term mobile phone use and the risk of vestibular schwannoma: a Danish nationwide cohort study. Am J Epidemiol. 2011; 174: 416–22.
30. Benson VS, Pirie K, Schüz J, Reeves GK, Beral V, Green J; for the Million Women Study Collaborators. Mobile phone use and risk of brain neoplasms and other cancers: prospective study. Int J Epidemiol. 2013; 42: 792–802.
31. Benson VS, Pirie K, Schüz J, Reeves GK, Beral V, Green J. Authors' response to: the case of acoustic neuroma: comment on mobile phone use and risk of brain neoplasms and other cancers. Int J Epidemiol. 2014; 43: 275.
32. The Interphone Study Group. Brain tumour risk in relation to mobile telephone use: results of the INTERPHONE international case-control study. Int J Epidemiol. 2010; 39: 675–94.
33. The INTERPHONE Study Group. Acoustic neuroma risk in relation to mobile telephone use: Results of the INTERPHONE international case-control study. Cancer Epidemiol. 2011; 35: 453–64.
34. Hardell L, Carlberg M. Mobile phone and cordless phone use and the risk for glioma—analysis of pooled case-control studies in Sweden, 1997–2003 and 2007–2009. Pathophysiology. 2015; 22: 1–13.
35. Carlberg M, Hardell L. Pooled analysis of Swedish case-control studies during 1997–2003 and 2007–2009 on meningioma risk associated with the use of mobile and cordless phones. Oncol Rep. 2015; 33: 3093–8.
36. Hardell L, Carlberg M, Söderqvist F, Mild KH. Pooled analysis of case-control studies on acoustic neuroma diagnosed 1997–2003 and 2007–2009 and use of mobile and cordless phones. Int J Oncol. 2013; 43: 1036–44.
37. Aydin D, Feychting M, Schüz J, et al. Mobile phone use and brain tumors in children and adolescents: a multicenter case-control study. J Natl Cancer Inst. 2011; 103: 1264–76.

38. Deltour I, Auvinen A, Feychting M, et al. Mobile phone use and incidence of glioma in the Nordic countries 1979–2008: consistency check. Epidemiol. 2012; 23: 301–7.
39. Little MP, Rajaraman P, Curtis RE, et al. Mobile phone use and glioma risk: comparison of epidemiological study results with incidence trends in the United States. BMJ. 2012; 344: e1147.
40. Larjavaara S, Feychting M, Sankila R, et al. Incidence trends of vestibular schwannomas in Denmark, Finland, Norway and Sweden in 1987–2007. Br J Cancer. 2011; 105: 1069–75.
41. Schüz J, Waldemar G, Olsen JH, Johansen C. Risk for central nervous system diseases among mobile phone subscribers: a Danish retrospective cohort study. PLOS One. 2009; 4: e4389.
42. Poulsen AH, Stenager E, Johansen C, Bentzen J, Friis S, Schüz J. Mobile phones and multiple sclerosis—a nationwide cohort study in Denmark. PLOS One. 2012; 7: e34453.
43. Blettner M, Schlehofer B, Breckenkamp J, et al. Mobile phone base stations and adverse health effects: a population-based cross-sectional study in Germany. Occup Environ Med. 2009; 66: 118–23
44. Schüz J. Implications from epidemiologic studies on magnetic fields and the risk of childhood leukemia on protection guidelines. Health Phys. 2007; 92: 642–8.
45. Vrijheid M, Richardson L, Armstrong BK, et al. Quantifying the impact of selection bias caused by nonparticipation in a case-control study of mobile phone use. Ann Epidemiol. 2009; 19: 33–41.
46. Schüz J, Jacobsen R, Olsen JH, Boice JD Jr, McLaughlin JK, Johansen C. Cellular telephone use and cancer risk: an update of a nationwide Danish cohort. J Natl Cancer Inst. 2006; 98: 1707–13.
47. Röösli M. Commentary: epidemiological research on extremely low frequency magnetic fields and Alzheimer's disease—biased or informative? International Journal of Epidemiology. 2008; 37: 341–3.
48. Maslanyj M, Simpson J, Roman E, Schüz J. Power frequency magnetic fields and risk of childhood leukaemia: misclassification of exposure from the use of the 'distance from power line' exposure surrogate. Bioelectromagnetics. 2009; 30: 183–8.
49. Vrijheid M, Cardis E, Armstrong BK, et al. Validation of short-term recall of mobile phone use for the Interphone study. Occup Environ Med. 2006, 63: 237–43.
50. Vrijheid M, Armstrong BK, Bédard D, et al. Recall bias in the assessment of exposure to mobile phones. J Expo Sci Environ Epidemiol. 2009; 19: 369–81.
51. Schüz J, Elliott P, Auvinen A, et al. An international prospective cohort study of mobile phone users and health (Cosmos): design considerations and enrolment. Cancer Epidemiol. 2011; 35: 37–43.

40

Metals and neurodegeneration

Susan Peters, Anne E Visser, Marc Weisskopf, Marianthi-Anna Kioumourtzoglou, and Roel Vermeulen

Metals and the Risk of Neurodegeneration

Neurotoxicants

Exposure to a toxic agent can result in neurotoxicity, which is characterized by adverse changes in the structure or function of the nervous system. Several metals and metalloids have been identified as such neurotoxicants, including aluminium (Al), manganese (Mn), arsenic (As), mercury (Hg), and lead (Pb).[1] Also cadmium (Cd) and selenium (Se) have shown toxic effects on nerve cells.[1] While excessive exposure to manganese and selenium are known to cause neurotoxicity, these metals are also nutritionally essential in the human body.[2] No beneficial effects are known for aluminium, arsenic, cadmium, lead, and mercury.[2]

Roughly, neurotoxicity can be grouped into acute and chronic effects. Acute effects occur shortly after exposure, whereas chronic effects may become apparent many months, years, or even decades later and generally result from repeated exposures at lower levels. Neurodegenerative disorders are an example of such chronic effects. It has been suggested that neurodegenerative diseases are partly caused by occupational and environmental exposures,[3] which may include exposures to metals. Early life environmental exposures have also been implicated in neurodegeneration.[4,5] Evidence of possible associations between exposure to metals and the onset of neurodegenerative disorders is very limited. Here we summarize what is known to date.

Alzheimer's disease and other dementias

The largest epidemiological literature relates to aluminium and AD, which is suggestive of an association, but not at all conclusive.[6,7] The emphasis has been on aluminium exposure through drinking water, which is not likely to be the primary source of exposure (see section on Aluminium below). Moreover, most of these studies derived exposure estimates in an ecological design, that is, assigning exposures at a group level rather than individually. Killin et al.[8] reviewed the literature regarding environmental risk factors for dementia, not limited to AD, and concluded that there is moderate evidence for aluminium exposure leading to increased dementia risk. This positive association was mainly observed in the larger and better quality studies. Large, prospective longitudinal studies with a robust measure of exposure at baseline and a clinical diagnosis of dementia were considered of highest quality.

Cadmium has also been associated with AD, but results are as yet not conclusive.[9] Likewise, mercury has been suggested to have a role in the aetiology of AD.[10] Occupational studies showed that chronic exposure to mercury affected memory and attention, which are relevant to AD. No studies reporting on an association between mercury exposure and AD have specifically been published. Results from autopsies have been inconclusive with regards to accumulation of mercury in the brains of Alzheimer patients.[10] Six epidemiological studies have explored the association between lead exposure and AD,[11–16] without finding an association. However, these studies all suffered from important limitations in exposure assessment.

Consistent positive associations between occupational metal exposure and non-vascular dementia have been found in a large prospective cohort study in the Netherlands.[17] No distinction between specific metals could be made, however, hindering identification of which metal could be accountable for the observed association.

Amyotrophic lateral sclerosis and motor neuron diseases

The association between lead exposure and ALS risk has been studied in various case-control studies and most report a positive relationship, up to over a four-fold increase.[18,19] However, these studies were predominantly reliant on self-reported exposure. One of those studies additionally presented risk estimates based on exposure assessment by (blinded) industrial hygienists, showing no association.[20] The latter exposure assessment method was considered more reliable, minimizing possible recall bias, which occurs when the diagnosis affects reporting of exposure by cases. Therefore, the observed increased risk of ALS due to lead exposure may have been influenced by this bias, whereas possibly no real association exists.

Roos et al.[21] analysed metal concentrations in cerebrospinal fluid and blood plasma of ALS patients and compared these with controls. Concentrations of aluminium, cadmium, manganese, and lead in cerebrospinal fluid of ALS patients appeared to be significantly higher. Such increases were not observed for blood plasma levels, suggesting accumulation of metals in cerebrospinal fluid.[21] Other studies have reported elevated levels of lead in both blood and bone among ALS cases,[22–24] but a causal relation has not yet been established.

Similar to lead, McGuire et al.[20] revealed no significant associations with ALS for exposure to aluminium, cadmium, manganese, or mercury in their US case-control study when based on expert assessment of occupational exposures. With regards to selenium, an increased risk of ALS with increasing levels of selenium intake through drinking water was reported in an Italian case-control study.[25]

Sutedja et al.[26] applied strict quality criteria to the methodology when reviewing epidemiological studies that looked into the association between metal exposure and ALS risk. Only studies based on objective exposure assessments (i.e. not self-reports) for full job histories or monitoring results collected repeatedly were considered sufficiently reliable. When these criteria were applied, no significant results were revealed for unspecified metals.[26] Overall, evidence about association between metal exposure and the risk of ALS is yet inconclusive.

Parkinson's disease and parkinsonism

Chronic exposure to manganese is known to cause 'manganism', which is a form of parkinsonism.[27] Exposure to welding fumes has been associated with parkinsonism and suggested as risk factor for PD, possibly due to manganese in welding fumes.[28–30] However, welding fume can contain many other metals,[31] and these other metals may also have added to the observed risks among welders.[30]

Positive associations between bone lead levels and PD were observed in US case-control studies.[32,33] The relevant exposure window was possibly many years or decades before the onset of disease. This conclusion was drawn because the association with PD was found for lead levels in the more compact cortical bone, representing cumulative exposure to lead over many years, whereas no association was observed for lead levels in the less dense cancellous bone tissue.[33] Among female nurses an association has been reported between airborne mercury exposure and risk of PD, whereas no evidence was found for any association with other airborne metals.[34]

Other neurodegenerative disorders

For MS no evidence has been reported with regards to metals specifically.[27]

Occurrence of Metal Exposure

We will here describe the occurrence of metal exposure, focusing on the metals and metalloids that have been identified as neurotoxicants, as described in the first section of this chapter and summarized in Table 40.1.

Aluminium

Occupational exposure to aluminium and its compounds predominantly occurs among workers in industries producing or using aluminium.[35] Another major intake source of aluminium is chronic use of aluminium-containing antacids, buffered aspirin, and other medical preparations. Food and drinking water can also contain aluminium and air pollution is another possible source of exposure.[35]

Arsenic

Arsenic is ubiquitously distributed in the environment, for example in geothermal waters, weathering of rocks, and forest fires. In addition to natural sources, humans encounter arsenic from man-made sources through soil, water, air, and food.

Occupational exposure to arsenic may occur in pesticide manufacturing and application, wood preservation, smelting and refining metallic ores, semiconductor manufacturing, and glassmaking.[36,37] Non-occupational exposure to arsenic mainly occurs via food, with intake from air, water, and soil being less substantial. However, exposure from water and soil may become significant in areas of arsenic contamination as a result of natural mineral deposits or mining sites, pesticide application, or industrial waste disposal.[37]

Cadmium

Cadmium is used in several applications, including nickel-cadmium batteries; pigments used in plastics, ceramics, and glass; stabilizers for polyvinyl chloride (PVC); engineering coatings on steel and non-ferrous metals; and as a component of various specialized alloys. The largest consumers of cadmium are Japan, the USA, Belgium, the UK, France, and Germany. Occupational exposure to cadmium may occur during production processes related to the aforementioned products.[38]

After occupational settings, cigarette smoke and contaminated food are the main sources of exposure.[37] About 10–15% of cadmium in the atmosphere originates from natural sources, predominantly from volcanic activity,[38] but most result from emissions from human sources. Cadmium levels in the air are higher in the proximity of cadmium-related industries.

Lead

Multiple sources can cause human exposure to lead. Its abundance and widespread usage makes lead a well-recognized environmental and occupational toxicant, particularly in the urban environment. Lead has been used in car batteries, gasoline, paints, ceramics, ammunition, pipes, solders, cosmetics, shielding for X-rays, and in corrosion and acid resistant materials.[39] Inhalation of contaminated dust particles or aerosols, and ingestion of contaminated food or water are the major routes of human exposure to lead.[37]

Elimination of lead in gasoline and the reduction of lead levels in paints, pipes, and food and drink cans has significantly decreased lead exposure since the 1970s.[37] However, human exposure continues from deteriorating household paint in older homes, contaminated soil and drinking water, and from lead used in industrial processes or hobbies.[37,39] Occupational exposures to lead may occur in a wide range of workplaces, such as in construction, printing, ceramic, glass making, primary and secondary metal manufacturing, electric and electronic industries, as well as through welding, firing ranges, and waste incineration.[40]

Manganese

Manganese is a nutritionally essential metal and diet is the major route of exposure for most people. The highest concentrations can be found in grains, rice, and nuts, but manganese can also be a component of dietary supplements.[41] Common sources of occupational exposure to manganese include welding processes, power plant, and coke oven combustion and steel production.[1,30,41] Manganese exposure may also result from the fuel additive methylcyclopentadienyl manganese tricarbonyl (MMT), which has been used to enhance the octane in gasoline in many countries, including the USA and Canada.[42]

Table 40.1 Overview of metals that have been identified as neurotoxicants

Metal	Evidence of association with neurodegenerative disorders		Major sources of human exposure
	Suggested	Established	
Aluminium (Al)	AD, dementia (ns)	–	Contaminated drinking water or food, medication or supplements, industrial processes (production and use of aluminium), air pollution
Arsenic (As)	AD, dementia (ns)	–	Contaminated drinking water or food, industrial processes (e.g. pesticide manufacturing and application, smelting and refining, semiconductor manufacturing, glassmaking)
Cadmium (Cd)	AD	–	Tobacco smoking, plastic stabilizers, pigments, batteries, industrial processes (e.g. welding, plating)
Lead (Pb)	AD, dementia (ns), ALS, PD	–	Contaminated drinking water or food, tobacco smoking, paint, gasoline, industrial processes (e.g. ceramics, soldering, plumbing, firing ranges)
Manganese (Mn)	AD, dementia (ns), PD	Parkinsonism	Food, gasoline, pesticides, industrial processes (e.g. steel factories, welding, mining plants)
Mercury (Hg)	AD, PD	–	Dental amalgams, contaminated fish, industrial processes (e.g. chlorine-alkaline and thermometer factories, mercury extraction plants), volcanic activity and coal combustion
Selenium (Se)	ALS	–	Food

AD = Alzheimer's disease; ALS = amyotrophic lateral sclerosis; PD = Parkinson's disease; ns =not specified

Mercury

Occupational exposure may occur in chlorine-alkaline factories, thermometer factories, and mercury extraction plants, as well as among dental care workers.[10] The latter is due to the application of dental amalgam fillings, containing mercury. People carrying such fillings, consisting of 50% of mercury, are also exposed. Mercury from fillings evaporates at a slow rate, but its release is faster when the fillings are put in place or removed.[10] Environmental exposure to mercury may result from volcanic activity, coal combustion, and other industrial processes.[43]

Organic mercury, methylmercury, accumulates in the aquatic food chain through waste water due to human activities.[44] Fish is the major contributor to mercury exposure through people's diet, so populations relying on fish diets can be exposed to high levels of organic mercury.[10]

Selenium

Environmental selenium can occur both in organic and inorganic form. Selenium in food is essential in the organic form, whereas inorganic selenium can be found in drinking water and occupational settings.[25] Occupational exposure to selenium has been described sparsely and can, together with drinking water, be considered only a minor source of exposure. Large regional differences exist in the selenium concentrations in food systems, as the concentration is highly dependent on the soil selenium. Soil selenium is influenced by weathering of selenium containing rocks, volcanic activity, and vicinity of coal burning.[45] Cereal grains, meats, and fish are the largest contributors to the selenium content in most diets and food is also being enriched in selenium in some places.[45]

Mechanisms of Chronic Neurotoxicity

Neurotoxicity is influenced by age and genetics: certain gene variants affect an individual's ability to respond to metals.[46] Major mechanisms are shared between virtually all neurodegenerative diseases and involve initiation or potentiation by neurotoxicants: BBB disruption, protein aggregation, oxidative stress, and mitochondrial dysfunction leading to neuroinflammation. Lipid soluble neurotoxicants can easily move across the biological membranes of the BBB by simple diffusion. Neurotoxicants that share chemical structures with endogenous molecules, but are not lipid soluble, can enter through carrier-mediated transport. If not lipophilic or mimicking a biological entity, access to the central nervous system is not gained. However, in the majority of neurodegenerative diseases, the BBB is disrupted. Whether BBB disruption contributes to the pathogenic mechanism or is part of the pathology remains to be determined. In addition to BBB disruption, protein aggregation is a major unifying mechanistic theme in neurodegenerative diseases, each disease producing a characteristic aggregation pattern. Mostly cytoplasmic protein aggregation is a pathological feature observed in many neurodegenerative diseases. Oxidative stress (i.e. having too many reactive species for available antioxidants) results in biomolecular damage caused by an attack of these reactive species upon the constituents in living organisms. The last major feature of neurodegenerative diseases is mitochondrial dysfunction which typically occurs early in the disease process. Environmental toxicants that affect mitochondrial function have been linked to various degrees epidemiologically to neurodegenerative diseases and have shown in animals to elicit neurodegeneration.[27]

Aluminium

Aluminium sensitive areas are the frontal cortex and the hippocampus.[47] Aluminium has no physiological role, but toxic consequences are thought to be related to dysregulation of other essential metals or ions:[47] increase in iron accumulation, the production of oxygen reactive species and induction of the formation of neurofibrillary tangles, and a pro-inflammatory response.[47,48,49] Aluminium has mostly been studied in relation to AD and mainly *in vitro*, where cultured rat cortical neurons show conformational changes in amyloid ß and enhanced aggregation with the formation of fibrillary deposits on the cultured neurons.[48]

Arsenic

Arsenic is thought to influence cognitive function by alternating the amyloid pathway.[48] Exposure to arsenic has been associated with brain inflammatory responses and oxidative stress through impaired cellular protein degradation and autophagy leading to intracellular protein aggregation and neurofibrillary tangle formation, extracellular accumulation of amyloid ß, reticulum endoplasmic stress, and mitochondrial dysfunction.[48,50]

Cadmium

For cadmium there is also evidence linking exposure with amyloid ß overproduction and increased size and number of senile plaques in the cerebral cortex and hippocampus. It was suggested that both the non-amyloidogenic pathway as well as degradation of amyloid ß are targets of cadmium exposure. *In vitro,* cadmium causes self-aggregation of a Tau peptide leading to astrocyte and neural cell toxicity.[48,49]

Lead

Many mechanisms have been described by which lead could result in neurotoxicity. The absorption of lead depends on the specific compound to which an individual is exposed. Lead exposure targets various voltage and ligand-gated ionic channels, such as the N-methyl-D-aspartic acid (NMDA) receptor, subtypes of the voltage and calcium-gated potassium channels, cholinergic receptors, and voltage-gated calcium channels, altering the cellular excitability and mainly resulting in an increase of the cytoplasmic calcium concentration.[51,52] Mechanisms described for nervous-system damage more specifically include lipid peroxidation, excitotoxicity, alterations in neurotransmitter synthesis, storage and release, interference with second-messenger systems, and damage to the astroglia and oligodendroglia.[51] Histologically, myelin loss and axonal degeneration have been described.[52] Furthermore, lead is thought to alter the ability of astrocytes to regulate the excitotoxic glutamate levels.[53]

Manganese

Chronic manganese intoxication gives symptoms similar to PD. Manganese increasing the dopamine autoxidation seems one of the mechanisms behind the clinical picture of parkinsonism. Manganese toxicity causes a reduction in striatal concentrations of dopamine due to accumulation in the mitochondria.[27,41,52] Elevated intra-mitochondrial manganese interferes with oxidative respiration, leading to excessive production of redox oxidative species and consequently mitochondrial dysfunction. Lastly, astrocytes function as major homeostatic regulators and as storage site for manganese. Increased accumulation of manganese in astrocytes has been shown to alter glutamate homeostasis and elicit neurotoxicity. It decreases astrocytic glutamate uptake and reduces the expression of the astrocytic glutamate-aspartate transporter leading to increased extracellular glutamate levels and neuronal excitability.[41]

Mercury

In contrast to elementary mercury, of which only a certain amount passes the BBB where it is oxidated to mercury ions, organic mercury, mostly targets the central nervous system. Brain regions that are most severely affected by organic mercury toxicity are the cerebral and cerebellar cortices. Crucial events are the interaction of mercury with sulfhydryl-containing proteins (i.e. neurotransmitter receptors, transporters, antioxidant enzymes, etc.), as well as with non-protein thiols (i.e. glutathione, cysteine). These events alter protein function and lead to disturbed proper homeostasis of neuronal and glial cells. Mercury toxicity results in glutamate dyshomeostasis, namely extracellular glutamate levels are increased. Consequently, there is calcium influx leading to oxidative stress and mitochondrial collapse.[41,54]

Selenium

The differential toxicity and metabolism of various organic and inorganic selenium forms makes it improper to generalize the term 'selenium neurotoxicity', whereas each neurotoxic effect should be referred to as a specific poisoning by a specific selenium compound. However, the neurotoxicity of inorganic selenium is shown to exceed that of the organic form. In general, the neurotoxic effects inducible by selenium compounds include, among others: an increase of central nervous system dopamine levels and metabolites; alteration of cholinergic signalling and degeneration of cholinergic neurons; inhibition of glutamate uptake and prostaglandin D synthase; decrease of total antioxidant status, gangliosides, and sulphydryl groups; activity of adenosine deaminase, succinic dehydrogenase, and acetylcholine esterase; and finally increase of thiobarbituric acid reactive substances and lipid peroxidation.[55]

Interaction between heavy metals

Metal mixtures are believed to play a role in the development of neurodegenerative diseases, potentially acting synergistically rather than displaying simple, additive effects.[49] Various metals share transporters or are controlled by overlapping signalling pathways. Neurotoxicity of perinatal and childhood mixed exposure to lead and other metals is well studied: lead and arsenic appear to have a synergistic effect on cognition and behaviour, whereas lead with cadmium, mercury, or manganese seems to work in an antagonistic way.[43] As stated previously, the toxic consequences of aluminium exposure are generally caused by the disruption of homeostasis of essential metals such as magnesium, calcium, and iron. Aluminium can mimic the biological functions of these metals, triggering biochemical alterations.[47] Cadmium interacts with iron leading to decreased haemoglobin and haematocrit concentrations[56] and selenium is thought to counteract neurotoxicity of other elements, for example mercury, cadmium, and aluminium. The ability to form complexes might also induce a longer persistence of the elements, which possibly leads to long-term release of these heavy metals in the brain.[25]

Challenges in Metal Exposure and Neurodegeneration Epidemiology

Epidemiological evidence of associations between metal exposure and neurodegenerative disorders is scarce. There are several challenges impeding the investigation of these associations, which are addressed below.

Case ascertainment

Registration of neurodegenerative disorders at a national level is not yet common practice, although more and more registrations are being established.[3] Also, neurodegenerative disorders are largely under-reported on death certificates, although registration is generally better for ALS, due to its poor prognosis, than for PD and AD. Lack of registration may result in case-ascertainment bias. For example, if only the more severe cases are being registered or only cases in a specific area, the selection of cases in the analyses is not a random sample. The results from an epidemiological study based on such data may therefore not be translatable to all cases of that particular disease.

Diagnosis of neurodegenerative disorders is largely symptom-based, which complicates accurate diagnosis. Moreover, overlap between the various disorders exists.[3,48] Studies often report on different disorders combined, for example PD with parkinsonisms together, AD with other dementias, or MND as one group. However, such grouping could obscure existing associations for one of the specific diseases, since the disease aetiologies may be different. Grouping may also hinder comparison between studies.

Disease mechanisms

Although the disease mechanism of neurodegenerative disorders is still poorly understood,[3,57] they are considered to be multifactorial and to follow a multistep process.[57,58] Interactions between genetic factors and environmental risk factors, such as metals, may play a role and strictly dividing cases into genetic and sporadic therefore seems too simplistic.[27] Besides, studying one factor at a time may be insufficient to identify possible risk factors. In a multi-step model, the same step might result from different agents, suggesting different possible pathways and therefore reducing the statistical power to identify a specific risk factor.[57] Moreover, there is experimental evidence that PD and other neurologic diseases related to ageing may be determined by exposures occurring early in the development (i.e. prenatal or in early life),[5] further complicating identifying causal risk factor(s).

Retrospective assessment of exposure

Neurodegenerative disorders typically have very long latency periods and the exact onset is usually unknown. Many studies use onset of symptoms as onset of disease, but the disease process may well have started much earlier. It is nearly impossible to know at which point to assess exposure. Furthermore, the desired time resolution may not be available.

In addition to long latency, neurodegenerative disorders are relatively rare, making it harder to include sufficient cases in a population. For rare diseases and diseases with long latency, the case-control design is therefore generally the only way to investigate potential risk factors. Where cohort studies suffer from insufficient numbers of cases or long duration before the disease develops, the statistical power of case-control studies is optimized by focusing on including cases and matching controls. Limiting analyses to a certain health outcome offers the opportunity to study a wide range of risk factors. Because subjects are identified at time of disease diagnosis for the cases, information about exposures, lifestyle factors, and other determinants can be collected for their full lifetime up to the time of the disease onset. The collection of information on medical and lifestyle factors is important because these factors may confound or modify an exposure-disease association and should be controlled for.[59]

Such lifetime information is crucial, but the inevitable retrospective character makes exposure assessment the most difficult part in case-control studies. Gaining accurate information on the early life environment can be particularly problematic. Many studies rely on self-reported exposures, as these are fairly easy to collect via interviews or questionnaires. However, metals are amongst the most difficult exposures for cases and controls to recognize and report in questionnaires.[58] Additionally, self-reports are prone to recall bias, because exposures are generally reported after cases have been diagnosed.[60] Knowledge of disease diagnosis may improve memory or provoke false memories and as such affect the reporting of exposure. The disease itself may also affect memory of patients, which may particularly be true for Alzheimer and other dementias, but also for Parkinson or ALS patients with co-existing dementias. McGuire et al.[20] showed associations between occupational exposure and ALS, both based on self-reported exposure and exposure assessment by an expert panel that was unaware of the subjects' disease status. Very different conclusions were drawn on the two approaches for lead, warranting caution for the interpretation of studies fully relying on self-reported exposures.

Expert assessments are often considered the best exposure assessment method in occupational settings.[59] However, experts may also be hindered by insufficient information to reliably assess exposure. Exposure to metals is highly task-specific and therefore very detailed information is needed to distinguish levels of metal exposure between workers with the same job title. Job-specific modules (asking questions about tasks, work conditions, and other exposure determinants) could offer such detailed information rather than simply job titles.[61]

On the other hand, occupational exposure to metals may be uncommon among study participants, as was the case in a recent ALS case-control in the USA,[62] making it inevitable to treat metals as one group. Another complication is disentangling the risks following exposure to the different metals, because exposures to metals are often correlated[34,63] and synergistic effects between metals may exist. Since humans may be exposed to a variety of metals it would be interesting to explore the combined effect of specific metal exposures, which would require large cohorts and detailed exposure assessment.

Biomarkers of exposure

Biomarkers of exposure provide the option to assess the internal concentration of a specific metal. Internal concentrations best reflect the actual exposure, capturing all sources of exposure, that is, occupationally, environmentally, and diet.[2] Ideally, a biomarker of exposure can be measured in samples that are easily collected, analyses are sensitive and reliable, and the marker is specific for a particular metal, providing information about level of exposure.[2] Concentrations highly depend on elimination half-lives and where the metal accumulates in the body. For example, recent exposure to lead is reflected in blood, while bone lead levels are considered more useful for cumulative lifetime exposure assessment.[18] Biomarkers may not be appropriate if metals do not accumulate in tissue, and suitable biomarkers have not been identified for all metals. To assess exposure to inorganic selenium, for example, available biomarkers are not able to reliably reflect exposure.[25]

When comparing biomarkers for metal exposure between cases and controls, one has to be aware of possible reverse causality. The disease may have changed the way the body metabolizes or reacts to metals. If samples are measured after disease onset, levels may have been affected by the disease process, resulting in significant bias.

Future Directions

In comparison with cancer and respiratory diseases, associations with environmental or occupational exposures have not been investigated as extensively for neurodegenerative disorders.[3] With regards to metals, research has mainly been focused on neurodevelopmental disorders, rather than neurodegenerative outcomes. Armon[64] described criteria for studies to classify the evidence of risk factors for ALS, which are also applicable to other neurodegenerative disorders. The best evidence comes from either prospective or retrospective cohort studies with parallel controls, or population-based case-control studies.[64] To be informative, such studies should include large numbers and should be well-performed. Quality studies include the assessment of exposure before disease onset, preferably quantifying exposure, and sources of biases and confounding are identified and accounted for.[64] To date, not many studies on metal exposure and neurodegenerative disorders meet these criteria.

Future research should also be focused on understanding the role of metals in the pathology of neurodegenerative disorders. Is there actually a causal relationship between metal exposure and the disease? Are metals accumulated as a result of the disease? What are the mechanisms? What are the critical time windows in the lifespan? Levels of metals in stored tissue of patients collected before their disease onset may provide more insights when compared with tissue from control subjects. Another way to limit reverse causality is the approach of Mendelian randomization studies. Such studies randomize groups based on genetic variants that influence the risk factor of interest, as a marker for lifelong exposure.[65] Large cohort studies, with a comprehensive description of the lifelong exposure history (the 'exposome'), sufficient time of follow-up, and a biobank are needed to study such questions. Such large cohorts provide the framework to study environment, lifestyle, genetic variations, and chronic disease.[66]

A multidisciplinary approach could help improve future studies. Gorell et al.[67] suggested collaboration between occupational toxicologists, industrial hygienists, neurologists, (environmental) epidemiologists, and statisticians. Combining strengths could ensure the best assessments of the disease under study, case and control ascertainment and enrolment from suitable population bases, and measurement of occupational and/or environmental metal exposure.[67]

In conclusion, future epidemiological studies should be large and high-quality studies, utilizing better quality exposure assessment to provide the crucial evidence on metal exposures as possible risk factors for neurodegenerative disorders.

REFERENCES

1. Klaassen CD. *Caserett and Doull's Toxicology. The Basic Science of Poisons* (7th edn). New York: McGraw-Hill, 2008. p1309.
2. Goyer R, Golub M, Choudhury H, Hughes M, Kenyon E, Stifelman M. *Issue Paper on the Human Health Effects of Metals.* Washington DC: US Environmental Protection Agency, 2004.
3. Pearce N, Kromhout H. Neurodegenerative disease: the next occupational disease epidemic?' *Occup Environ Med.* 2014; 71(9): 594–5.
4. Landrigan PJ, Sonawane B, Butler RN, Trasande L, Callan R, Droller D. Early environmental origins of neurodegenerative disease in later life. *Environ Health Perspect.* 2005; 113(9): 1230–3.
5. Logroscino G. The role of early life environmental risk factors in Parkinson disease: what is the evidence? *Environ Health Perspect.* 2005; 113(9): 1234–8.
6. Miu AC, Benga O. Aluminum and Alzheimer's disease: a new look. *J Alzheimer's Dis.* 2006; 10(2–3): 179–201.
7. Tomljenovic L. Aluminum and Alzheimer's disease: after a century of controversy, is there a plausible link? *J Alzheimer's Dis.* 2011; 23(4): 567–98.
8. Killin LO, Starr JM, Shiue IJ, Russ TC. Environmental risk factors for dementia: a systematic review. *BMC Geriatr.* 2016; 16(1): 175.
9. Peng Q, Bakulski KM, Nan B, Park SK. Cadmium and Alzheimer's disease mortality in US adults: updated evidence with a urinary biomarker and extended follow-up time. *Environ Res.* 2017; 157: 44–51.
10. Mutter J, Curth A, Naumann J, Deth R, Walach H. Does inorganic mercury play a role in Alzheimer's disease? A systematic review and an integrated molecular mechanism. *J Alzheimer's Dis,* 2010; 22(2): 357–74.
11. Chandra V, Philipose V, Bell PA, Lazaroff A, Schoenberg BS. Case-control study of late onset 'probable Alzheimer's disease'. *Neurology.* 1987; 37(8): 1295–300.
12. French LR, Schuman LM, Mortimer JA, Hutton JT, Boatman RA, Christians B. A case-control study of dementia of the Alzheimer type. *Am J Epidemiol.* 1985; 121(3): 414–21.
13. Gun RT, Korten AE, Jorm AF, et al. Occupational risk factors for Alzheimer disease: a case-control study. *Alzheimer Dis Assoc Disord.* 1997; 11(1): 21–7.
14. Heyman A, Wilkinson WE, Stafford JA, Helms MJ, Sigmon AH, Weinberg T. Alzheimer's disease: a study of epidemiological aspects. *Ann Neurol.* 1984; 15(4): 335–41.
15. O'Flynn RR, Monkman SM, Waldron HA. Organic solvents and presenile dementia: a case referent study using death certificates. *Br J Ind Med.* 1987; 44 (4): 259–62.
16. Shalat SL, Seltzer B, Baker EL, Jr. Occupational risk factors and Alzheimer's disease: a case-control study. *J Occup Med.* 1988; 30(12): 934–6.
17. Koeman T, Schouten LJ, van den Brandt PA, et al. Occupational exposures and risk of dementia-related mortality in the prospective Netherlands Cohort Study. *Am J Ind Med.* 2015; 58(6): 625–35.
18. Kamel F, Umbach DM, Hu H, et al. Lead exposure as a risk factor for amyotrophic lateral sclerosis. *Neurodegener Dis.* 2005; 2(3–4): 195–201.
19. Wang MD, Gomes J, Cashman NR, Little J, Krewski D. A meta-analysis of observational studies of the association between chronic occupational exposure to lead and amyotrophic lateral sclerosis. *J Occup Environ Med.* 2014; 56 (12): 1235–42.
20. McGuire V, Longstreth WT, Jr., Nelson LM, et al. Occupational exposures and amyotrophic lateral sclerosis. A population-based case-control study. *Am J Epidemiol.* 1997; 145(12): 1076–88.
21. Roos PM, Vesterberg O, Syversen T, Flaten TP, Nordberg M. Metal concentrations in cerebrospinal fluid and blood plasma

from patients with amyotrophic lateral sclerosis. *Biol Trace Elem Res.* 2013; 151(2): 159–70.
22. Fang F, Kwee LC, Allen KD, et al. Association between blood lead and the risk of amyotrophic lateral sclerosis. *Am J Epidemiol.* 2010; 171(10): 1126–33.
23. Garzillo EM, Lamberti M, Genovese G, et al. Blood lead, manganese, and aluminum levels in a regional Italian cohort of ALS patients: does aluminum have an influence? *J Occup Environ Med.* 2014; 56(10): 1062–6.
24. Kamel F, Umbach DM, Munsat TL, Shefner JM, Hu H, Sandler DP. Lead exposure and amyotrophic lateral sclerosis. *Epidemiology.* 2002; 13(3): 311–19.
25. Vinceti M, Bonvicini F, Bergomi M, Malagoli C. Possible involvement of overexposure to environmental selenium in the etiology of amyotrophic lateral sclerosis: a short review. *Ann Ist Super Sanita.* 2010; 46(3): 279–83.
26. Sutedja NA, Veldink JH, Fischer K, et al. Exposure to chemicals and metals and risk of amyotrophic lateral sclerosis: a systematic review. *Amyotroph Lateral Scler.* 2009; 10(5–6): 302–9.
27. Cannon JR, Greenamyre JT. The role of environmental exposures in neurodegeneration and neurodegenerative diseases. *Toxicol Sci.* 2011; 124(2): 225–50.
28. Antonini JM. Health effects of welding. *Crit Rev Toxicol.* 2003; 33(1): 61–103.
29. Racette BA, Criswell SR, Lundin JI, et al. Welding-related parkinsonism: clinical features, treatment, and pathophysiology. *Neurology.* 2001; 56(1): 8–13.
30. Racette BA, McGee-Minnich L, Moerlein SM, Mink JW, Videen TO, Perlmutter JS. Increased risk of parkinsonism associated with welding exposure. *Neurotoxicology.* 2012; 33(5): 1356–61.
31. IARC. Chromium, nickel and welding. *IARC Monographs on the Evaluation of Carcinogenic Risks to Humans.* Volume 49. Lyon: International Agency for Research on Cancer, 1990.
32. Coon S, Stark A, Peterson E, et al. Whole-body lifetime occupational lead exposure and risk of Parkinson's disease. *Environ Health Perspect.* 2006; 114(12): 1872–6.
33. Weisskopf MG, Weuve J, Nie H, et al. Association of cumulative lead exposure with Parkinson's disease. *Environ Health Perspect.* 2010; 118(11): 1609–13.
34. Palacios N, Fitzgerald K, Roberts AL, et al. A prospective analysis of airborne metal exposures and risk of Parkinson disease in the nurses' health study cohort. *Environ Health Perspect.* 2014; 122(9): 933–8.
35. Krewski D, Yokel RA, Nieboer E, et al. Human health risk assessment for aluminium, aluminium oxide, and aluminium hydroxide. *J Toxicol Environ Health B Crit Rev.* 2007; 10(Suppl 1): 1–269.
36. Burgess WA. *Recognition of Health Hazards in Industry: a Review of Materials and Processes* (2nd edn). New York: Wiley-Interscience, 1995. p538.
37. Tchounwou PB, Yedjou CG, Patlolla AK, Sutton DJ. Heavy metal toxicity and the environment. *EXS*, 2012; 101: 133–64.
38. IARC. Beryllium, cadmium, mercury and exposures in the glass manufacturing. *IARC Monographs on the Evaluation of Carcinogenic Risks to Humans.* Volume 58. Lyon: International Agency for Research on Cancer, 1993.
39. Sanders T, Liu Y, Buchner V, Tchounwou PB. Neurotoxic effects and biomarkers of lead exposure: a review. *Rev Environ Health.* 2009; 24(1): 15–45.
40. Koh DH, Bhatti P, Coble JB, et al. Calibrating a population-based job-exposure matrix using inspection measurements to estimate historical occupational exposure to lead for a population-based cohort in Shanghai, China. *J Expo Sci Environ Epidemiol.* 2014; 24(1): 9–16.
41. Farina M, Avila DS, da Rocha JB, Aschner M. Metals, oxidative stress and neurodegeneration: a focus on iron, manganese and mercury. *Neurochem Int.* 2013; 62(5): 575–94.
42. Davis JM. Methylcyclopentadienyl manganese tricarbonyl: health risk uncertainties and research directions. *Environ Health Perspect.* 1998; 106(Suppl 1): 191–201.
43. Chen P, Miah MR, Aschner M. Metals and neurodegeneration. *F1000Res.* 2016; 5.
44. Hong YS, Kim YM, Lee KE. Methylmercury exposure and health effects. *J Prev Med Public Health.* 2012; 45(6): 353–63.
45. Combs GF, Jr. Selenium in global food systems. *Br J Nutr.* 2001; 85(5): 517–47.
46. Caito S, Ascher M. Handbook of Clinical Neurology. *Occupational Neurology*, 2015: 169–89.
47. Maya S, Prakash T, Madhu KD, Goli D. Multifaceted effects of aluminium in neurodegenerative diseases: a review. *Biomed Pharmacother.* 2016; 83: 746–54.
48. Chin-Chan M, Navarro-Yepes J, Quintanilla-Vega B. Environmental pollutants as risk factors for neurodegenerative disorders: Alzheimer and Parkinson diseases. *Front Cell Neurosci*, 2015; 9: 124.
49. Yegambaram M, Manivannan B, Beach TG, Halden RU. Role of environmental contaminants in the etiology of Alzheimer's disease: a review. *Current Alzheimer Research.* 2015; 12: 116–46.
50. Escudero-Lourdes C. Toxicity mechanisms of arsenic that are shared with neurodegenerative diseases and cognitive impairment: role of oxidative stress and inflammatory responses. *Neurotoxicology.* 2016; 53: 223–35.
51. Garza A, Vega R, Soto E. Cellular mechanisms of lead neurotoxicity. *Med Sci Monit.* 2006; 12(3): RA57–65.
52. Wennberg A. Neurotoxic effects of selected metals. *Scand J Work Environ Health.* 1994; 20(Spec No): 65–71.
53. Struzynska L. A glutamatergic component of lead toxicity in adult brain: the role of astrocytic glutamate transporters. *Neurochem Int.* 2009; 55(1–3): 151–6.
54. Tasleem Jan A, Azam M, Siddiqui K, Ali A, Choi I, Haq QM. Heavy metals and human health: mechanistic insight into toxicity and counter defense system of antioxidants. *Int J Mol Sci.* 2015; 16(12): 29592–630.
55. Vinceti M, Mandrioli J, Borella P, Michalke B, Tsatsakis A, Finkelstein Y. Selenium neurotoxicity in humans: bridging laboratory and epidemiologic studies. *Toxicol Lett.* 2014; 230(2): 295–303.
56. Jaishankar M, Tseten T, Anbalagan N, Mathew BB, Beeregowda KN. Toxicity, mechanism and health effects of some heavy metals. *Interdiscip Toxicol.* 2014; 7(2): 60–72.
57. Al-Chalabi A, Calvo A, Chio A, et al. Analysis of amyotrophic lateral sclerosis as a multistep process: a population-based modelling study. *Lancet Neurology.* 2014; 13(11): 1108–13.
58. Lai BC, Marion SA, Teschke K, Tsui JK. Occupational and environmental risk factors for Parkinson's disease. *Parkinsonism Relat Disord.* 2002; 8(5): 297–309.
59. Teschke K, Olshan AF, Daniels JL, et al. Occupational exposure assessment in case-control studies: opportunities for improvement *Occup Environ Med.* 2002; 59(9): 575–93; discussion 94.
60. Rothman KJ, Greenland S, Lash TL. *Modern Epidemiology* (3rd edn). Philadelphia: Lippincott Williams & Wilkins, 2008. p758.
61. Stewart PA, Stewart WF, Siemiatycki J, Heineman EF, Dosemeci M. Questionnaires for collecting detailed occupational

information for community-based case control studies. *Am Ind Hyg Assoc J.* 1998; 59(1): 39–44.
62. Yu Y, Su FC, Callaghan BC, Goutman SA, Batterman SA, Feldman EL. Environmental risk factors and amyotrophic lateral sclerosis (ALS): a case-control study of ALS in Michigan. *PLOS One.* 2014; 9(6): e101186.
63. Sadetzki S, Chetrit A, Turner MC, et al. Occupational exposure to metals and risk of meningioma: a multinational case-control study. *J Neurooncol.* 2016; 130(3): 505–15.
64. Armon C. An evidence-based medicine approach to the evaluation of the role of exogenous risk factors in sporadic amyotrophic lateral sclerosis. *Neuroepidemiology.* 2003; 22(4): 217–28.
65. Brennan P. Commentary: Mendelian randomization and gene-environment interaction. *Int J Epidemiol.* 2004; 33(1): 17–21.
66. Wild CP. Complementing the genome with an 'exposome': the outstanding challenge of environmental exposure measurement in molecular epidemiology. *Cancer Epidemiol Biomarkers Prev.* 2005; 14(8): 1847–50.
67. Gorell JM, Rybicki BA, Cole Johnson C, Peterson EL. Occupational metal exposures and the risk of Parkinson's disease. *Neuroepidemiology.* 1999; 18(6): 303–8.

SECTION 8
Global health and public health

41

Estimating the global burden of stroke

Methods and challenges

Thomas Truelsen, Catherine Johnson, Mohsen Naghavi, Theo Vos, Valery L Feigin, and Gregory Roth

Introduction

The Global Burden of Disease (GBD) study dates from the early 1990s.[1–3] The first publications of estimates for 107 diseases and 483 sequelae had a marked impact on international health policy,[4] highlighting that non-communicable diseases were the leading causes of death in both developed and developing regions and that combined estimates of mortality *and* disability showed that non-communicable diseases constituted more than one-third of the disease burden in developing regions.[5,6] The GBD has been updated regularly with the publication of major GBD estimates in 2000,[7] 2010,[8–11] 2013,[12,13] and 2015.[14] The GBD has expanded into an international consortium of more than 1800 researchers globally involved in GBD 2015.

Stroke has consistently ranked as one of the leading causes of death and a leading cause of lost disability adjusted life years (DALYs).[13–17] The burden of stroke is particularly high in many low and middle income countries (LMICs). This burden is expected to increase in the future as a result of longer life expectancy, and continuous exposure to established vascular disease risk factors.[18,19] Data on stroke incidence, prevalence, and mortality continues to be limited for large parts of the global population, especially in LMICs where the burden is often high. Estimates from the GBD are particularly important for these large regions of the world where stroke surveillance systems are limited,[20] as they enable policymakers, public health professionals, and donor organizations and countries to better understand the health risks facing these populations and direct resources accordingly.[21]

Overview of the Global Burden of Disease

The GBD study provides a standard method for comparing health and disease burden within and between geographic locations. The annual updates include all available data on death and non-fatal events for thousands of health states. The GBD study produces a summary metric known as DALYs. These represent a measure of health lost due to both premature death and prevalent disease within a given population. The DALYs enable uniform comparison between geographies and across disease categories. Each new iteration of the GBD provides an updated and internally consistent time series by re-estimating disease burden starting in 1990. The GBD estimates rely on statistical models and country-level information known to be associated with stroke incidence and mortality, such as established cardiovascular risk factors, to produce estimates of stroke when data is limited. The current stroke estimates include incidence, prevalence, DALYs, and death (rates and absolute numbers) due to ischaemic stroke and haemorrhagic stroke, the two main subtypes of cerebrovascular disease, and all pathological types of stroke combined.

Estimating the Global and National Burden of Stroke

GBD applies a consistent case definition for stroke following the universal definition developed by the World Health Organization (WHO). Stroke is defined as rapidly developing clinical signs of focal disturbance of cerebral function lasting more than 24 hours or leading to death with no apparent cause other than that of vascular origin.[22] Each update to the GBD study has improved the methods used to estimate loss of health due to stroke but this case definition has remained the standard across all versions. A diagram of the key steps involved in modelling fatal and non-fatal stroke is shown in Fig. 41.1.

Estimating deaths due to stroke

GBD 2015 estimates on fatal stroke are based on all available data from vital registration systems, studies using verbal autopsy (VA), and redistribution of the so-called 'garbage codes'. All available data on stroke as a cause of death, stroke incidence, prevalence, case fatality, and excess mortality in stroke survivors are collected from vital registration systems, published data, and unpublished stroke registries.

Verbal autopsy

VA is a method used for assigning the most likely cause of death in regions where more complete medical information is unavailable. VA tools are based on structured interview forms which ask the respondents, most often surviving family members, about the circumstances of the subject's death.[23] These questions can be closed,

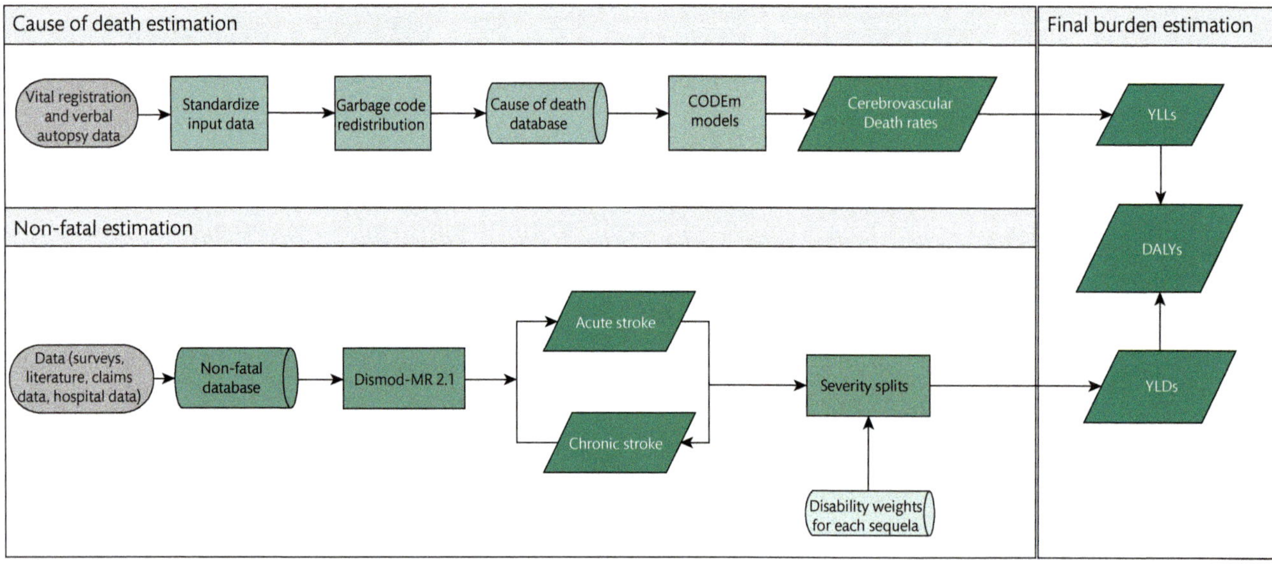

Fig. 41.1 Key steps involved in estimating health loss due to stroke for the GBD 2015 study. Cause of Death Ensemble model, CODEm; Years of Life Lost (YLL); Disability Adjusted Life Years (DALYs); Years Lived with Disability (YLD)

open-ended, or a combination; the intent is to collect sufficient information to allow the underlying cause of death to be appropriately assigned. A survey can be comprehensive across all causes of death or specific to a disease of interest like stroke.[24] The usual method for validating a VA tool is to apply it to hospital-based deaths where a physician's assessment or autopsy can serve as a "gold standard". Even in these validation studies, results will reflect local health practices, including patterns of care-seeking that may be biased by attributes of those who are hospitalized. For example, a large-scale VA study from China including 378 stroke deaths according to medical records, reported 398 stroke deaths based on VA with a specificity of 93.6 and a sensitivity of 81.5.[25] Specificity of a VA will increase as more rigid definitions of stroke as a cause of death are adopted. VA validation studies from populations in Vietnam, India, Philippines, Tanzania, and Mexico have suggested that 'sudden onset of one-sided paralysis' or 'sudden onset of coma', preferably combined with CT scan/MR imaging, should be considered key clinical characteristics before assigning stroke as the likely cause of death.[24,26]

In the GBD 2015 for cerebrovascular disease the total number of site years from VA studies was 691, thereby constituting approximately 6.5% of mortality data used for estimating the global stroke mortality. VA data included stroke deaths in the following locations: Bangladesh, Burkina Faso, Ethiopia, Ghana, India, Indonesia, Lebanon, Malawi, Mozambique, Myanmar, Nairobi, Pakistan, South Africa, Thailand, Turkey, Vietnam, and Zambia.

Vital registration stroke data for Global Burden of Disease

For GBD 2015, the total number of site years for vital registration used to estimate cerebrovascular disease reached 10,660. Data was obtained from the WHO Mortality Database as well as directly from some countries' mortality databases.

Vital registration data use the International Classification of Diseases (ICD). ICD version 9[27] and 10[28] (ICD-9 and 10) specific stroke codes used to define ischaemic and haemorrhagic or other stroke are shown in Box 41.1. Ischaemic stroke codes include the highly specific codes i63.0–i63.9 for cerebral infarction. Events also included as ischaemic stroke were stenosis or occlusion of cerebral or precerebral arteries not resulting in infarction (i.65–i.66.9), cerebral atherosclerosis (I67.2), progressive leukoencephalopathy (I67.5), moya-moya (I67.5), and sequelae of cerebrovascular disease (i.69.3–i69.398). Haemorrhagic stroke events include subarachnoid haemorrhage (I60.0–I60.9), intracerebral haemorrhage (I61.0–I61.9), subdural haemorrhage (I62.0), non-ruptured dissection of cerebral arteries (I67.0), and non-ruptured cerebral aneurysms (I67.1). Some deaths are coded to ICD-10 codes G45–G46.8 defined as 'transient cerebral ischaemic attacks and related syndromes' and 'vascular syndromes of brain in cerebrovascular diseases'. 'Transient ischaemic attack' should never be a cause of death as part of the case definition of stroke is that the symptoms last less than 24 hours and clinically the patient recovers completely.[29] As the codes obviously relate to ischaemic stroke, they are redistributed onto ischaemic stroke.

Vital registration data (ICD-9 and ICD-10) can also be coded as 'unspecified stroke' which then interferes with the direct estimation of subtypes of stroke.[30] The GBD study reassigns these events to stroke subtype proportionately by age, sex, and region. Globally,

Box 41.1 ICD-9 and ICD-10 codes used for cause of death estimation GBD 2015

Cerebrovascular disease

ICD-10: G45–G46.8, I60–I61.9, I62.0–I62.03, I63–I63.9, I65–I66.9, I67.0–I67.3, I67.5–I67.6, I68.1–I68.2, I69.0–I69.398

ICD-9: 430–435.9, 437.0–437.2, 437.5–437.8

Ischaemic stroke

ICD-10: I63–I63.9, I65–I66.9, I67.2–I67.3, I67.5–I67.6, I69.3–I69.398, G45–G46.8

ICD-9: 433–435.9, 437.0–437.1, 437.5–437.8

Haemorrhagic stroke

ICD-10: I60–I61.9, I62.0–I62.03, I67.0–I67.1, I68.1–I68.2, I69.0–I69.298

ICD-9: 430–432.9, 437.2

Source: data from *International Classification of Diseases*, Ninth Revision, Clinical Modification (ICD-9-CM). CDC. 2015; data from https://icd.who.int/browse10/2016/en#!/X

30.8% of 'unspecified' stroke events were redistributed to haemorrhagic stroke, 64.7% to ischaemic stroke, and 4.5% to subarachnoid haemorrhage in the GBD 2013 study.

While the ICD coding system provides standards on how to diagnose cerebrovascular diseases, the use of specific codes for stroke and stroke subtypes is known to vary between countries.[31] Vital registration systems also vary to the degree that they cover an entire population, ranging from the comprehensive systems found in Europe, Australia, New Zealand, and North America, to incomplete systems being developed in many LMICs.[20]

Redistribution of deaths coded to non-specific and intermediate causes

Death data must be corrected to account for the frequent use of intermediate, indeterminate, or non-specific codes certified as the underlying cause in vital records, sometimes referred to as 'garbage codes'. GBD redistributes these codes to an actual underlying cause so that mortality can be compared across geographies. GBD applies a consistent statistical method across all data sources using a regression model approach.[32] The proportion of all-cause routine mortality codes that are non-specific has remained constant at 29–33% at the global level since the launch of the GBD but varies markedly between countries.[33] Current 'garbage codes' include deaths coded to such causes as hemiplegia, atherosclerosis, and age-related senility. Completely ambiguous codes are redistributed to all causes, whereas intermediate codes that are likely secondary to a more specific underlying cause or group of causes are redistributed onto those specific cause(s). For example, deaths coded to hypertension are considered secondary to cardiovascular and cerebrovascular disease and redistributed only to these causes. The reassignment of codes to target codes is done based on ICD classification and the pathology behind each "garbage code". Depending on the type of garbage code, proportional or regression-model-based methods of redistribution are used.[12,34]

The redistribution varies between GBD regions as exemplified by Fig. 41.2, which shows the fraction of unspecified stroke redistributed onto each stroke subtype among men aged 50–69 years by GBD region. Other 'garbage codes' that were redistributed to overall cerebrovascular disease, and the three main stroke subtypes, are listed in Table 41.1. The fractions of death that have been added to each of the categories of ischaemic stroke, haemorrhagic stroke, and subarachnoid haemorrhage are listed in Table 41.2. The underlying algorithm for redistributing deaths assigned to these codes has been reported in detail.[34] Garbage code redistribution remains one of the most important steps for improving comparability of global death data.

Modelling: Cause of Death Ensemble model

With limited vital statistics data from many countries, GBD estimates mortality due to stroke using an ensemble modelling approach (Cause of Death Ensemble model, CODEm). CODem runs hundreds of separate statistical models (geospatial mixed effects or space-time Gaussian Process Regression models) for each five-year age, sex, and country strata. This method enables integration of all available data on

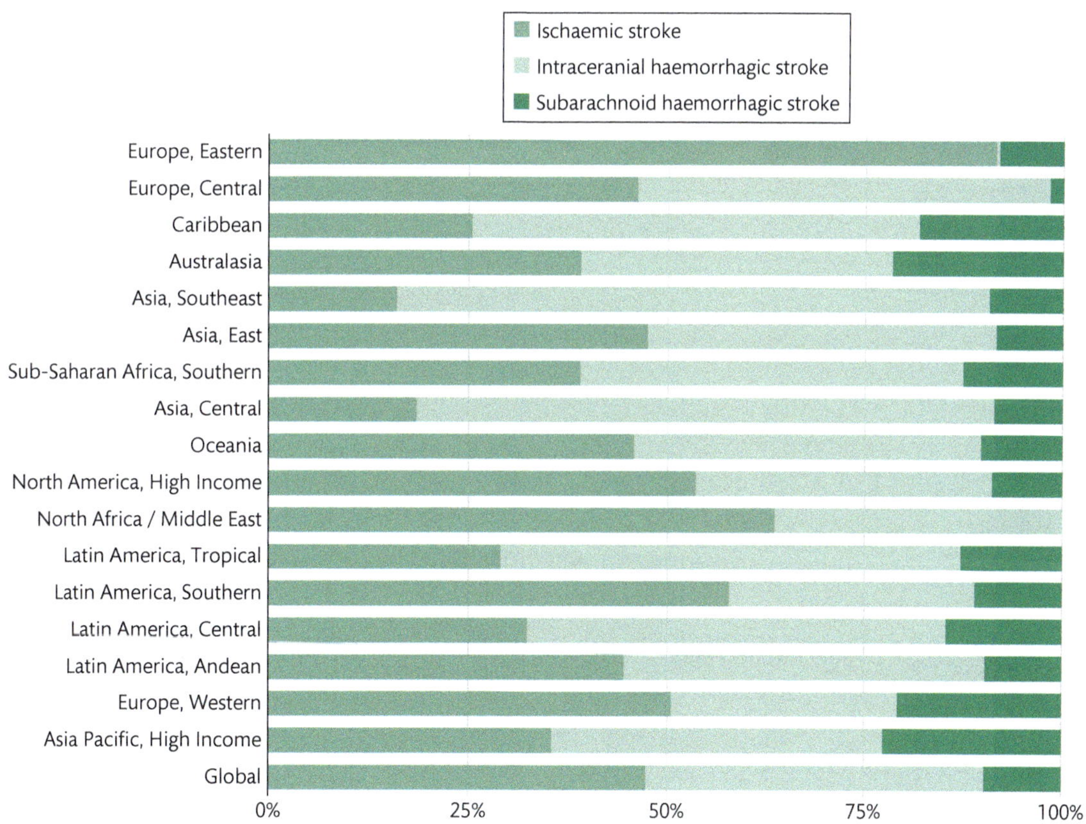

Fig. 41.2 Fraction of 'unspecified stroke' assigned to the 3 types of stroke by GBD region, men aged 50–69 years, GBD 2013.

Reproduced from Truelsen T. Causes of Death Data in the Global Burden of Disease Estimates for Ischemic and Hemorrhagic Stroke. *Neuroepidemiology.* 2015; 45(3): 152–60. Courtesy of S Karger, AG Basel. DOI: https://doi.org/10.1159/000441084.

Table 41.1 Fraction of deaths coded to each category of 'garbage codes' that have been redistributed to each type of stroke, men and women combined, all ages, ICD-10

Different group of garbage codes	Intracranial haemorrhagic stroke	Ischaemic stroke	Subarachnoid haemorrhagic stroke
Stroke unspecified	30.8%	64.7%	4.5%
No traumatic extradural haemorrhage	74.3%	0.0%	25.7%
Hemiplegia	29.9%	54.6%	9.5%
Unspecified disorders of circulatory system in diseases	46.3%	18.5%	22.7%
Compression of brain	33.1%	0.0%	31.8%
Somnolence, stupor, and coma	31.7%	27.3%	5.6%
Hypertensive encephalopathy	17.7%	27.4%	13.5%
Atherosclerosis	0.0%	50.5%	0.0%
Other and unspecified encephalopathy	0.0%	0.0%	38.3%
Pneumonitis due to solids and liquids	23.6%	14.7%	0.0%
Cerebral oedema	0.0%	35.9%	0.0%
Primary and secondary hypertension	6.7%	29.0%	0.0%

stroke as a cause of death even when data completeness is not ideal or derived from different kinds of sources.[35]

Models include country-level covariates associated with disease risk. The covariates included for stroke in the GBD2015 study are shown in Box 41.2.[36] The term 'ensemble' is used because final estimates are produced by combining the weighted results of best-performing models based on out-of-sample predictive validity statistics. The ensemble approach for cause of death estimation is superior to alternative single component models.[35] Cause-specific CODEm stroke estimates are scaled to all-cardiovascular and all-cause mortality in order to ensure that cause-specific estimates, as a fraction, are consistent with the number of total deaths.[14]

Table 41.2 Fraction of death that have been added to each type of stroke after redistribution of 'garbage codes', men and women combined, all ages, year 2008, ICD-10

Different groups of garbage codes	Intracranial haemorrhagic stroke	Ischaemic stroke	Subarachnoid haemorrhagic stroke
Stroke unspecified	88.6%	162.8%	46.1%
Primary and secondary hypertension	4.7%	17.7%	0.0%
Atherosclerosis	0.0%	21.6%	0.0%
Non traumatic extradural haemorrhage	6.0%	0.0%	7.4%
Age-related physical debility(senility)	4.9%	6.3%	2.0%

Box 41.2 Country-level data included in the final CODEm models

Tobacco use

Smoking prevalence
Cumulative cigarette consumption

Metabolic

Mean body mass index
Mean systolic blood pressure

Socioeconomic

Years of educations per capita
Income per capita
Health system access summary score
Sociodemographic index (combining fertility rate, education level, and income per capita)
Summary exposure variable (summary value between 0–1 representing level of all causal exposure risks collected by GBD study)

Dietary

Alcohol intake in litres per capita
Nut and seed consumption in kilocalories per capita
Pulse and legume consumption in kilocalories per capita
Omega 3 polyunsaturated fat consumption in kilocalories per capita
Milk consumption in kilocalories per capita
Animal fat consumption in kilocalories per capita
Fruit consumption in kilocalories per capita
Omega 6 polyunsaturated fat consumption in kilocalories per capita
Whole grain consumption in kilocalories per capita
Red meat consumption in kilocalories per capita

Estimating stroke incidence, prevalence, and survival

A large-scale systematic review of published and unpublished data on stroke incidence, prevalence, and survival was performed for the GBD 2015 study. There were 53 studies on stroke prevalence, 71 studies on stroke incidence, and mortality risk in patients with cerebrovascular disease was based on 8 studies, whereas 45 studies addressed mortality risk specifically for ischaemic stroke and 34 for haemorrhagic or other types of stroke.[36] Other inputs included inpatient hospital data from multiple countries and population-based health surveys. Ideally, data would come from gold-standard studies but the availability of population-based stroke studies is very limited and mostly from populations in high income countries (HICs).[37] Available stroke data differ in terms of volume of data and methods used to collect data, such as data sampling design and case definitions. These differences can contribute to non-sampling error. The GBD study applies statistical methods to adjust, or 'cross-walk', a broad range of data source results towards a consistent case definition.

In the GBD 2015 study, acute stroke was defined as first-ever stroke events, while chronic stroke was defined as the sequelae of a first-ever acute stroke event including any recurrent stroke events an individual might experience. In this modelling scheme, once a person has had a stroke, it is not possible to re-enter the pool of 'healthy' subjects. There are two possible outcomes after the initial event: (1) early death from stroke, defined as death occurring within the first 28 days after onset of stroke symptoms, or (2) contributing to the pool of 'chronic stroke subjects' who have survived at least 28 days. The overall prevalence of acute stroke was calculated taking into account the average duration from incidence to death in fatal cases and a 28-day duration in survivors. The short period of prevalence associated with an acute stroke was used to capture the higher level of disability associated with this time immediately following an incident stroke event. The prevalence of chronic stroke was determined by integrating the incidence of stroke survivors with the excess risk of dying over the remaining lifespan. The degree of disability in stroke survivors was estimated for both acute and chronic stroke subjects using five levels of severity and these results were used to generate the estimates for years lived with disability (YLD).

Modelling the epidemiology of stroke using DisMod-MR software

DisMod-MR is a software tool that considers the relations between disease incidence, prevalence, remission, case fatality, and excess mortality rates in persons with and without a disease, sometimes referred to as an epidemiologic state-transition model.[38] The DisMod-MR software is developed to allow the combination of diverse data and calculate an internally consistent description of stroke epidemiology for a given geography. Key components of DisMod-MR include the inclusion of country characteristics as model covariates and random effects for different geographies. If no country data are available a country estimate reflects the average for a world region or the globe. Meta-regression (hence the suffix MR) is performed to include data collected across varying age groupings. All data are evaluated through a geographical cascade of four levels: global, super-region, region, and country. Initially all available global data are evaluated to estimate the fixed effect on age, sex, study level, and country level covariates and a first estimation of the random effects for countries, regions, and super-regions. The results of these analyses are then used as Bayesian priors for the super-region level of the cascade. After the global level fit the default option is to only adjust the data by the sex and study-level covariates. At each successive level of the cascade, the fixed effects on country-level covariates are re-evaluated and centred on the average of values for the countries that make up a super-region or region. No fixed or random effects are re-evaluated at the country level. DisMod-MR also includes tools for transforming data in various ways, integrating the 'cross-walking' required for data collected with different case definitions.

In the GBD 2015, DisMod-MR 2.1, the latest version, was used to model acute stroke using all available data on acute stroke incidence and one-month excess mortality. Data reported as a case-fatality proportion were transformed into excess mortality rates using the following equation:

Incidence was multiplied by 1—(first month case fatality proportion) estimated from the excess mortality output of the model to provide an estimate of the incidence of chronic stroke (e.g. survivors of acute stroke). This measure of chronic stroke was used in a second model along with prevalence data from surveys and published literature and excess mortality data from published literature to model the prevalence of chronic stroke.

Disability weights

The GBD study reports YLD and Years of Life Lost (YLLs) prematurely for all geographies. These two parameters are summed to calculate DALYs.[1] In order to estimate disability, causes of disease are matched with a health state and associated levels of disability (disability weights) derived from population surveys. Disability weights are on a scale from 0 (no health loss) to 1 (complete health loss and equivalence to death).[39] The product of prevalence of the sequelae of stroke and the disability weight makes up the YLD and after aggregation gives the YLD due to stroke (Table 41.3).

For the Global Burden of Disease 1990, disability weights for 483 sequelae of 131 diseases and injuries were based on the judgements of a small group of healthcare professionals.[6] A major advancement in disability weights was introduced with the GBD 2010 when disability weights were updated based on the results of large-scale multinational surveys. The surveys reported perceived health loss based on simple paired comparison questions, with a major emphasis on surveying respondents from the general public.[9] The lay descriptions for health states associated with stroke were categorized into six levels, ranging from no disability to severe disability with cognition problems (Box 41.2). The household surveys were performed in Bangladesh, Indonesia, Peru, Tanzania, and the USA.[40] A web-based open-access survey was also performed in English, Spanish, and Mandarin. A total of 13,902 persons participated in the household surveys and 16,328 in the web survey. Updates to this study have included new data from Hungary, Italy, the Netherlands, and Sweden,[41] raising the total number of respondents to over 60,000 persons. The distribution of severity of stroke by the five levels was based on an analysis of the US Medical Expenditure Panel Survey, the only available population-based survey that links a validated quality of life tool (the EQ-5D) with comprehensive inpatient and outpatient medical records.[32]

The Global Burden of Stroke: Selected Results of the GBD 2015 Study

Death due to stroke

In GBD 2015 the number of deaths from stroke increased 5.1% globally, from 6.0 million in 2005 to 6.3 million in 2015. During

Table 41.3 Disability weights for stroke

Disability after stroke	Disability weight (95% uncertainty intervals)
No disability	0
Mild: has some difficulty in moving around and some weakness in one hand, but is able to walk without help.	0.019 (0.010–0.032)
Moderate: has some difficulty in moving around and in using the hands for lifting and holding things, dressing and grooming.	0.070 (0.046–0.099)
Moderate + cognition problems: has some difficulty in moving around, in using the hands for lifting and holding things, dressing and grooming, and in speaking. The person is often forgetful and confused.	0.316 (0.206–0.437)
Severe: is confined to bed or a wheelchair, has difficulty speaking and depends on others for feeding, toileting and dressing.	0.552 (0.377–0.707)
Severe + cognition problems: is confined to bed or a wheelchair, depends on others for feeding, toileting, and dressing, and has difficulty speaking, thinking clearly, and remembering things.	0.588 (0.411–0.744)

the same period the age-standardized stroke mortality rate decreased 21% from 127.9 to 101.0 per 100,000.[14] The increase in absolute numbers of stroke deaths is due to population ageing and population growth outpacing the decline in rates.[14,42–44] Stroke mortality rates vary considerably between countries, with the highest rates in Asia and Eastern Europe (Fig. 41.3). Age-adjusted stroke mortality rates were consistently higher in men compared to women.

Incidence and prevalence of stroke

Incident cases of first-ever ischaemic stroke increased from 4.7 million in 2005 to 5.4 million in 2015 and from 3.1 million to 3.6 million for haemorrhagic stroke during the same period.[45] There were 42.4 million prevalent cases of stroke in 2015, which was an absolute increase of 21% compared to 2005, while the age-standardized prevalence rate decreased by 4.4%. The total number of YLDs was 6.5 million, which was 20.7% higher than in 2005, again with a small decrease in the age-standardized rate of YLD by 4.2%.[36] Country YLD rates for men and women are shown in Fig. 41.4.

Disability adjusted life years due to stroke in the GBD 2015

Stroke is the second leading cause of DALYs in the GBD 2015 after ischaemic heart disease.[45] In absolute numbers there has been no detectable change during the years from 2005 to 2015 (118.6 million DALYs) the age-standardized rate of stroke DALYs has decreased from 2.3/1.000 to 1.8/1.000, a decrease of 22.2%. The geographic distribution of stroke DALYs varies between regions as shown in Fig. 41.5. High rates are found in Eastern Europe and South East Asia, with higher rates for men compared to women.

Challenges for the Future of Global Stroke Metrics

During the past 25 years the GBD study has advanced our understanding of the global burden of stroke, confirming it as a leading cause of premature death and disability. The study, while complex, provides a consistent analysis based on available empirical data and statistical methods enabling estimation of stroke burden for regions with no or limited data as well as estimates of uncertainty that can guide their interpretation. Stroke continues to be an area with ongoing advances in methods for modelling disease burden.[46] Annual updates to the GBD study now ensure that the latest data are integrated into its estimates. Despite these advances, many challenges remain for the measurement of disease burden due to stroke.

Limited data availability

Vital registration is an essential tool when estimating the burden of stroke. Many countries have established vital registration systems, but the completeness varies, with generally better coverage in HICs and some MICs, while less resourced regions have fewer and less comprehensive systems. VA is an important methodology for providing cause of death data from regions with no established vital registration systems. The WHO has supported the development of standardized VA tools in order to gain insight into disease patterns in data sparse regions.[47]

Stroke registries are available for some populations, allowing tracking of incidence and case fatality for stroke subtypes.[32] However, hospital-based registries (as opposed to community-based registries) reflect only those individuals that can reach a health facility. Continuous and complete registration of all stroke events, including fatal and non-hospitalized stroke events, is an important goal for future registries if they are to reflect the true burden of the disease.

Data quality and trends in data quality

Accurate diagnosis of stroke depends on access to health facilities and availability of CT/MRI imaging which is of particular importance when estimating stroke subtypes (ischaemic and haemorrhagic stroke).[48,49] Improvements in ICD coding practice will lead to more specific data on stroke subtypes.[50] Increasing access to healthcare facilities and health technology such as brain imaging may change our understanding of local disease patterns. However, improvements in stroke surveillance will occur at different paces as countries invest in their health surveillance systems. Variation between country coding practices and completeness of disease registration impact comparability of health data, and adjustment to account for these differences remains a key step in the GBD study.[51] Perhaps the most important step in this process is the redistribution of non-specific and intermediate 'garbage codes' on death certificates to more likely 'target' conditions. In the GBD study, redistribution is based on review of medical literature, knowledge of local disease patterns, and regression-based statistical methods. Further research is needed, both into local variation in death coding practices and the development of more robust methods for redistribution of 'garbage codes'.

The validity of data from VA studies require a correct evaluation of reported symptoms and their duration, which then leads to the selection of the correct underlying disease. Recall bias, in which a survey respondent provides information biased away from what would have been reported immediately at the time of death, remains a challenge to accurate VA reporting. Despite this, VA is an important source for regions without a functional vital registration system. The current research area to improve VA includes computer-based algorithms that may prove to be a more consistent and cost-effective instrument for coding survey responses than physician review.[26,52]

Burden estimation methods

Stroke data is heterogeneous, of low quality, or unavailable for many world regions. Modelling tools, such as those used by the GBD study, can produce consistent estimates, despite limited data, by leveraging information across age groups, sex categories, time, and geography. The CODEm and DisMod software are advanced analytical methods that have now been refined over almost three decades. The GBD results offer a global standard that can help guide the implementation of health interventions targeting stroke, with the long-term goal of reducing the global health burden due to this disease.

Methods for attributing stroke severity and disability remain an important step in producing an accurate assessment of health loss due to stroke. The GBD 2015 disability weights reflect highly consistent choices around perceived disability among the general population of multiple countries. The severity distributions for

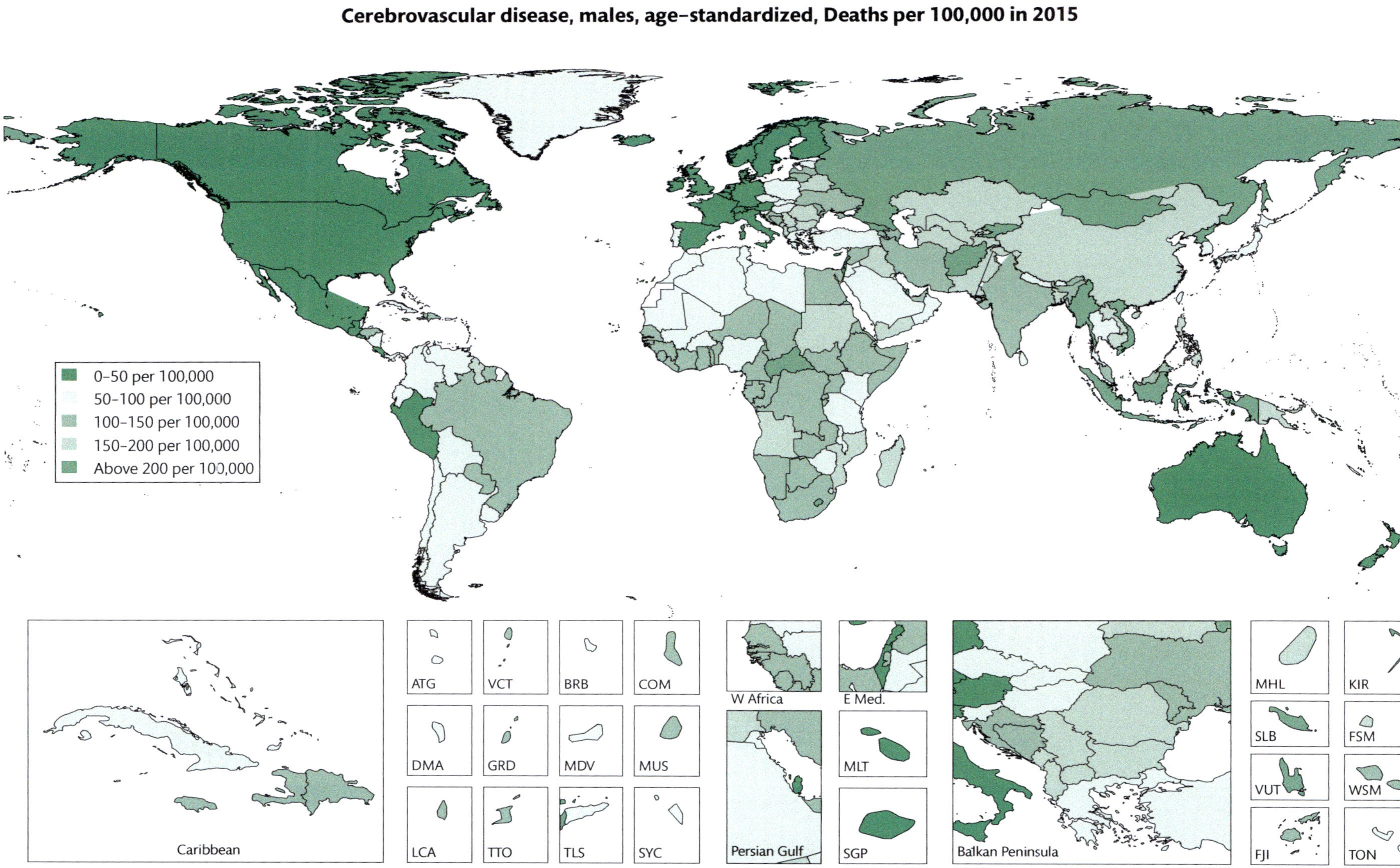

Fig. 41.3 Global rates of stroke mortality for men and women, all ages, per 100,000, GBD 2015 study.

Cerebrovascular disease, females, age-standardized, Deaths per 100,000 in 2015

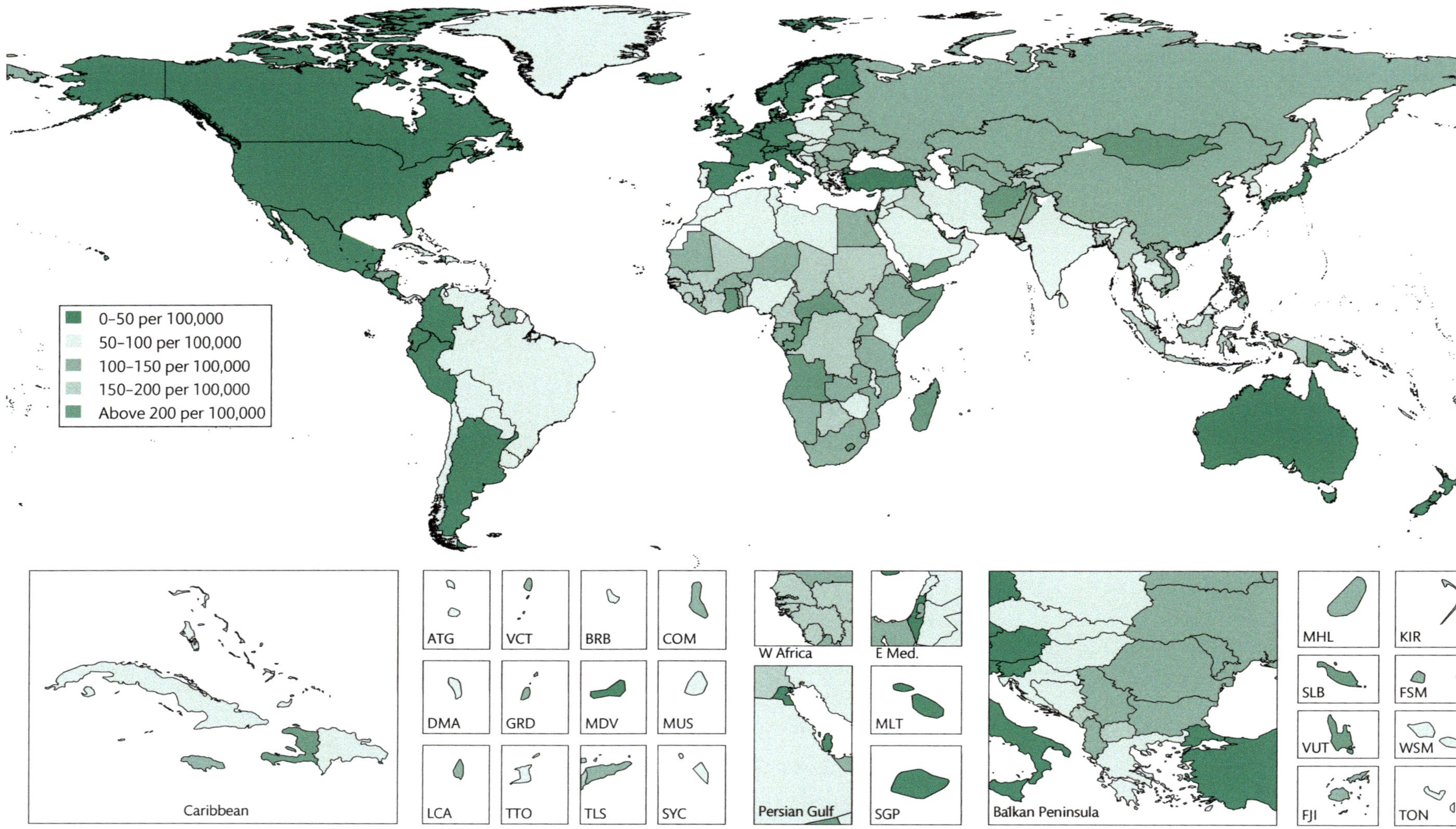

Fig. 41.3 Continued

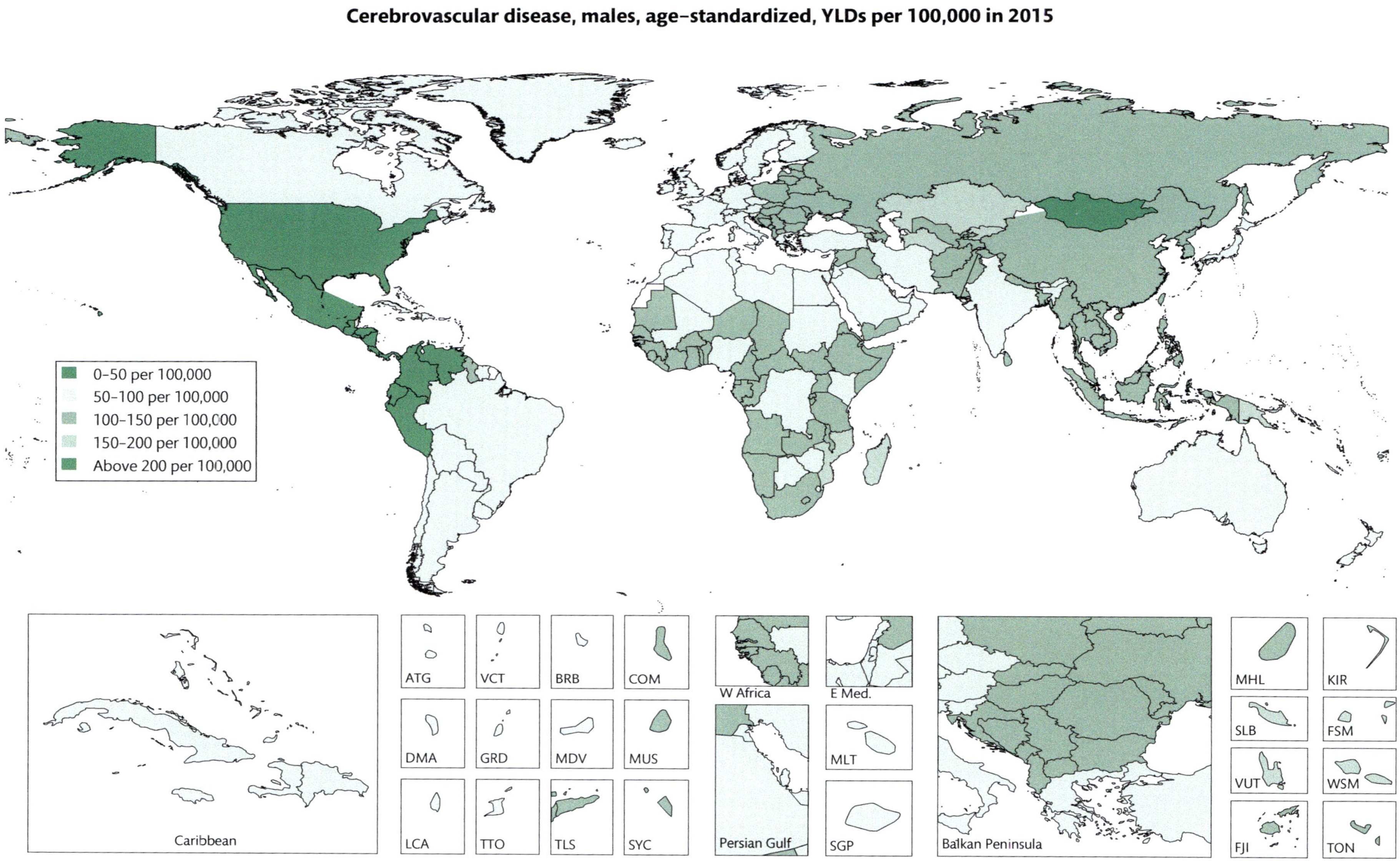

Fig. 41.4 Global rates of years lived with disability (YLD) for men and women, all ages, per 100,000, GBD 2015 study.

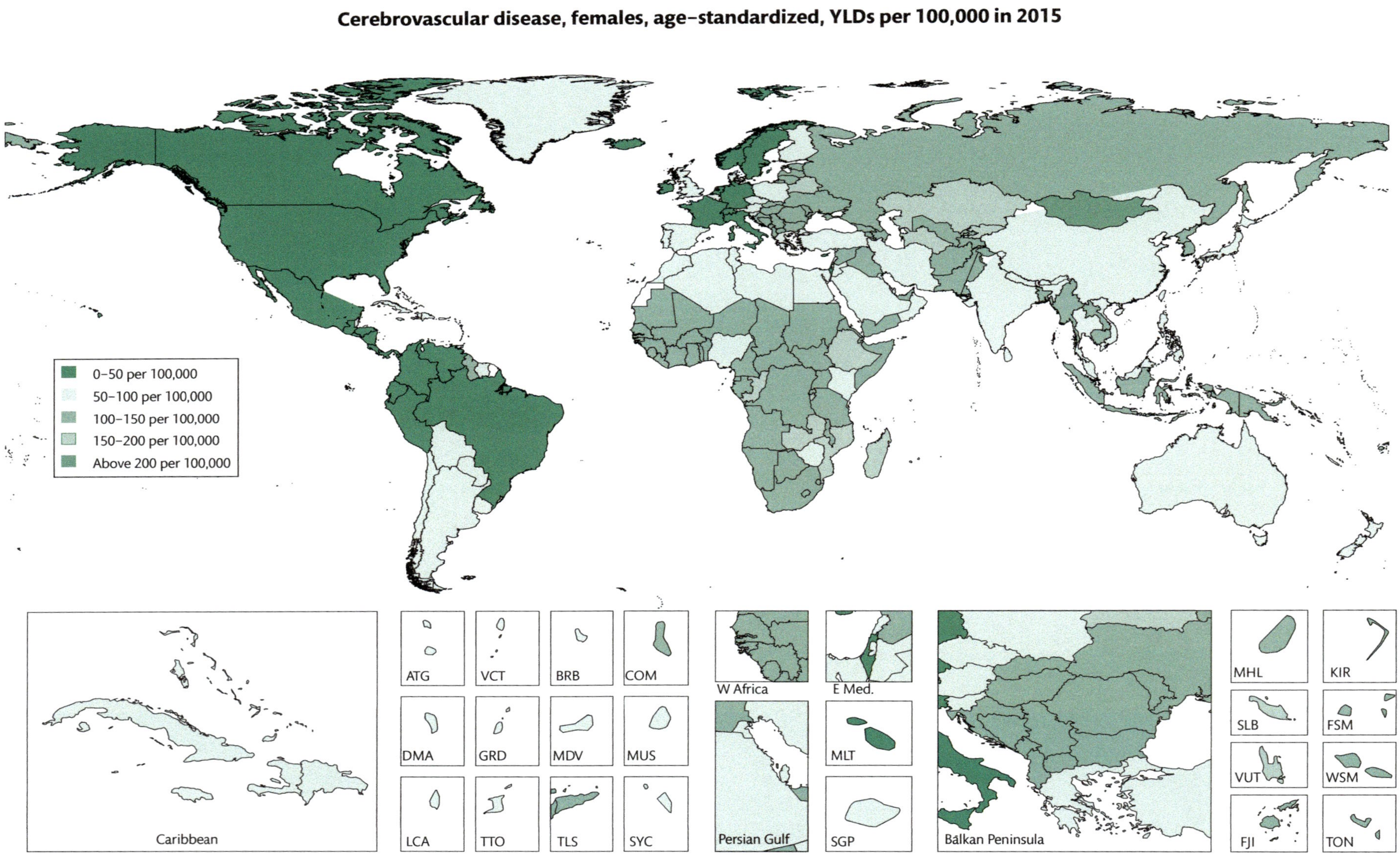

Fig. 41.4 Continued

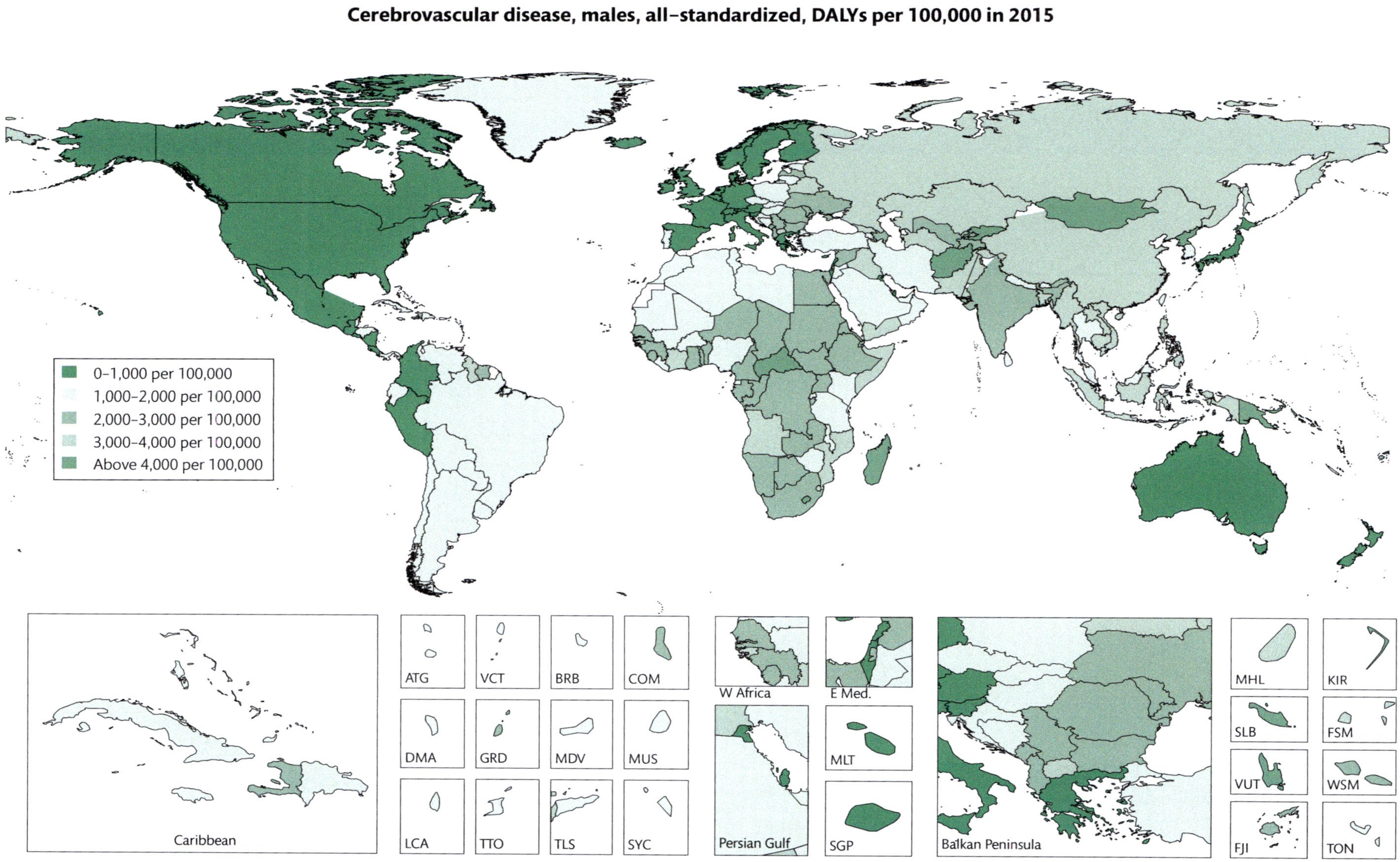

Fig. 41.5 Global rates of disability adjusted life years (DALY) for men and women, all ages, per 100,000, GBD 2015 study.

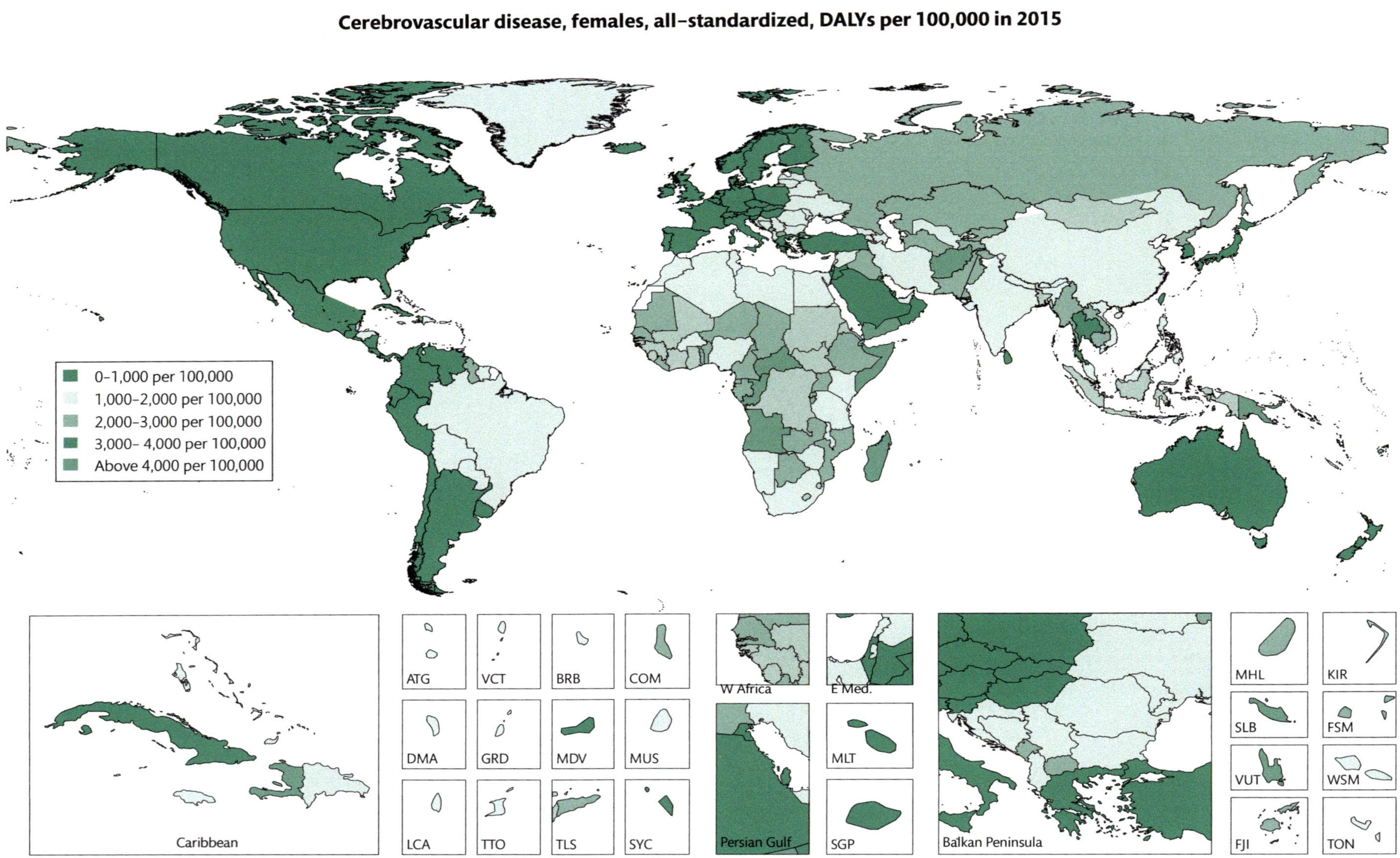

Fig. 41.5 Continued

stroke outcomes have been based on the US Medical Expenditure Panel Survey applied globally. In recognition of the limited generalizability of this data, new, more empiric methods will be needed that incorporate Rankin scores, the standard measure for stroke disability.

Conclusions

The GBD study is a major effort to improve public health by measuring the health of all populations. This large-scale epidemiologic study continues to advance knowledge related to the global burden of stroke. These estimates are only as good as real-life data permits—more and better data on stroke will lead to more accurate estimates over time. Methods that allow for the integration of all available data and software tools that handle sparse and heterogeneous data are likely to remain an important component of global population-based estimation of stroke burden. The absolute number of stroke patients is increasing and even the age-standardized stroke incidence rate may be increasing in rapidly developing regions such as South Asia. Stroke remains a leading cause of death and disability around the world and its accurate measurement will be important for future efforts to appropriately prioritize investments that can reduce the resulting health burden due to stroke.

REFERENCES

1. Murray CJ. Quantifying the burden of disease: the technical basis for disability-adjusted life years. *Bull World Health Organ.* 1994; 72(3): 429–45.
2. Murray CJ, Lopez AD. Global and regional cause-of-death patterns in 1990. *Bull World Health Organ.* 1994; 72(3): 447–80.
3. Murray CJ, Lopez AD. Quantifying disability: data, methods and results. *Bull World Health Organ.* 1994; 72(3): 481–94.
4. Murray CJ, Lopez AD. Evidence-based health policy—lessons from the Global Burden of Disease Study. *Science.* 1996; 274(5288): 740–43.
5. Murray CJ, Lopez AD. Mortality by cause for eight regions of the world: Global Burden of Disease Study. *Lancet.* 1997; 349(9061): 1269–76.
6. Murray CJ, Lopez AD. Global mortality, disability, and the contribution of risk factors: Global Burden of Disease Study. *Lancet.* 1997; 349(9063): 1436–42.
7. World Health Organization. *The World Health Report 2000: Health Systems: Improving Performance.* Geneva: World Health Organization, 2000.
8. Murray CJ, Vos T, Lozano R, Naghavi M, Flaxman AD, Michaud C, et al. Disability-adjusted life years (DALYs) for 291 diseases and injuries in 21 regions, 1990–2010: a systematic analysis for the Global Burden of Disease Study 2010. *Lancet.* 2012; 380(9859): 2197–223.
9. Vos T, Flaxman AD, Naghavi M, Lozano R, Michaud C, Ezzati M, et al. Years lived with disability (YLDs) for 1160 sequelae of 289 diseases and injuries 1990-2010: a systematic analysis for the Global Burden of Disease Study 2010. *Lancet.* 2012; 380(9859): 2163–96.
10. Lozano R, Naghavi M, Foreman K, Lim S, Shibuya K, Aboyans V, et al. Global and regional mortality from 235 causes of death for 20 age groups in 1990 and 2010: a systematic analysis for the Global Burden of Disease Study 2010. *Lancet.* 2012; 380(9859): 2095–128.
11. Wang H, Dwyer-Lindgren L, Lofgren KT, Rajaratnam JK, Marcus JR, Levin-Rector A, et al. Age-specific and sex-specific mortality in 187 countries, 1970–2010: a systematic analysis for the Global Burden of Disease Study 2010. *Lancet.* 2012; 380(9859): 2071–94.
12. Global, regional, and national age-sex specific all-cause and cause-specific mortality for 240 causes of death, 1990–2013: a systematic analysis for the Global Burden of Disease Study 2013. *Lancet.* 2015; 385(9963): 117–71.
13. Murray CJ, Barber RM, Foreman KJ, Abbasoglu OA, Abd-Allah F, Abera SF, et al. Global, regional, and national disability-adjusted life years (DALYs) for 306 diseases and injuries and healthy life expectancy (HALE) for 188 countries, 1990–2013: quantifying the epidemiological transition. *Lancet.* 2015; 386(10009): 2145–91.
14. Global, regional, and national life expectancy, all-cause mortality, and cause-specific mortality for 249 causes of death, 1980–2015: a systematic analysis for the Global Burden of Disease Study 2015. *Lancet.* 2016; 388(10053): 1459–544.
15. Murray CJ, Lopez AD, Jamison DT. The global burden of disease in 1990: summary results, sensitivity analysis and future directions. *Bull World Health Organ.* 1994; 72(3): 495–509.
16. Feigin VL, Forouzanfar MH, Krishnamurthi R, Mensah GA, Connor M, Bennett DA, et al. Global and regional burden of stroke during 1990–2010: findings from the Global Burden of Disease Study 2010. *Lancet.* 2014; 383(9913): 245–54.
17. Feigin VL, Mensah GA, Norrving B, Murray CJ, Roth GA. Atlas of the Global Burden of Stroke (1990–2013): The GBD 2013 Study. *Neuroepidemiology* 2015; 45(3): 230–6.
18. Krishnamurthi RV, Feigin VL, Forouzanfar MH, Mensah GA, Connor M, Bennett DA, et al. Global and regional burden of first-ever ischaemic and haemorrhagic stroke during 1990–2010: findings from the Global Burden of Disease Study 2010. *Lancet Glob Health.* 2013; 1(5): e259–e281.
19. Lim SS, Vos T, Flaxman AD, Danaei G, Shibuya K, Adair-Rohani H, et al. A comparative risk assessment of burden of disease and injury attributable to 67 risk factors and risk factor clusters in 21 regions, 1990–2010: a systematic analysis for the Global Burden of Disease Study 2010. *Lancet.* 2012; 380(9859): 2224–60.
20. Mathers CD, Fat DM, Inoue M, Rao C, Lopez AD. Counting the dead and what they died from: an assessment of the global status of cause of death data. *Bull World Health Organ.* 2005; 83(3): 171–7.
21. Mensah GA, Sacco RL, Vickrey BG, Sampson UK, Waddy S, Ovbiagele B, et al. From data to action: neuroepidemiology informs implementation research for global stroke prevention and treatment. *Neuroepidemiology.* 2015; 45(3): 221–9.
22. Hatano S. Experience from a multicentre stroke register: a preliminary report. *Bull World Health Organ.* 1976; 54(5): 541–53.
23. Chandramohan D, Maude GH, Rodrigues LC, Hayes RJ. Verbal autopsies for adult deaths: issues in their development and validation. *Int J Epidemiol.* 1994; 23(2): 213–22.
24. Gupta S, Khieu TQ, Rao C, Anh N, Hoa NP. Assessing the quality of evidence for verbal autopsy diagnosis of stroke in Vietnam. *J Neurosci Rural Pract.* 2012; 3(3): 267–75.
25. Yang G, Rao C, Ma J, Wang L, Wan X, Dubrovsky G, et al. Validation of verbal autopsy procedures for adult deaths in China. *Int J Epidemiol.* 2006; 35(3): 741–48.

26. Murray CJ, Lopez AD, Black R, Ahuja R, Ali SM, Baqui A, et al. Population Health Metrics Research Consortium gold standard verbal autopsy validation study: design, implementation, and development of analysis datasets. *Popul Health Metr.* 2011; 9: 27.
27. International Classification of Diseases 9. http://wwwcdcgov/nchs/icd/icd9 htm 2016.
28. International Classification of Diseases 10. *www who int* 2016. https://icd.who.int/browse10/2016/en#/I60-I69
29. Caplan LR. Transient ischemic attack: definition and natural history. *Curr Atheroscler Rep.* 2006; 8(4): 276–80.
30. Truelsen T, Krarup LH, Iversen HK, Mensah GA, Feigin VL, Sposato LA, et al. Causes of death data in the Global Burden of Disease estimates for ischemic and hemorrhagic stroke. *Neuroepidemiology.* 2015; 45(3): 152–60.
31. World Health Organization. *WHO Mortality Database.* Available at: URL: https://www.who.int/healthinfo/mortality_data/en/
32. Roth GA, Johnson CO, Nguyen G, Naghavi M, Feigin VL, Murray CJ, et al. Methods for estimating the global burden of cerebrovascular diseases. *Neuroepidemiology.* 2015; 45(3): 146–51.
33. Murray JL, Lopez AD. *Global Burden of Disease and Injury Series. The Global Burden of Disease: A Comprehensive Assessment of Mortality and Disability from Diseases, Injuries, and Risk Factors in 1990 and Projected to 2020.* Boston: Harvard School of Public Health, World Health Organization and the World Bank, 1996.
34. Naghavi M, Makela S, Foreman K, O'Brien J, Pourmalek F, Lozano R. Algorithms for enhancing public health utility of national causes-of-death data. *Popul Health Metr.* 2010; 8: 9.
35. Foreman KJ, Lozano R, Lopez AD, Murray CJ. Modeling causes of death: an integrated approach using CODEm. *Popul Health Metr.* 2012; 10: 1.
36. Global, regional, and national incidence, prevalence, and years lived with disability for 310 diseases and injuries, 1990–2015: a systematic analysis for the Global Burden of Disease Study 2015. *Lancet.* 2016; 388(10053): 1545–602.
37. Feigin VL, Lawes CM, Bennett DA, Barker-Collo SL, Parag V. Worldwide stroke incidence and early case fatality reported in 56 population-based studies: a systematic review. *Lancet Neurology.* 2009; 8(4): 355–69.
38. Barendregt JJ, Van Oortmarssen GJ, Vos T, Murray CJ. A generic model for the assessment of disease epidemiology: the computational basis of DisMod II. *Popul Health Metr.* 2003; 1(1): 4.
39. Salomon JA, Haagsma JA, Davis A, de Noordhout CM, Polinder S, Havelaar AH, et al. Disability weights for the Global Burden of Disease 2013 study. *Lancet Glob Health.* 2015; 3(11): e712–23.
40. Salomon JA, Vos T, Hogan DR, Gagnon M, Naghavi M, Mokdad A, et al. Common values in assessing health outcomes from disease and injury: disability weights measurement study for the Global Burden of Disease Study 2010. *Lancet.* 2012; 380(9859): 2129–43.
41. Haagsma JA, Maertens de NC, Polinder S, Vos T, Havelaar AH, Cassini A, et al. Assessing disability weights based on the responses of 30,660 people from four European countries. *Popul Health Metr.* 2015; 13: 10.
42. Salomon JA, Wang H, Freeman MK, Vos T, Flaxman AD, Lopez AD, et al. Healthy life expectancy for 187 countries, 1990–2010: a systematic analysis for the Global Burden Disease Study 2010. *Lancet.* 2012; 380(9859): 2144–62.
43. GBD 2013 DALYs and HALE Collaborators. Global, regional, and national disability-adjusted life years (DALYs) for 306 diseases and injuries and healthy life expectancy (HALE) for 188 countries, 1990–2013: quantifying the epidemiological transition. *Lancet.* 2015; 386: 2145–91.
44. Roth GA, Forouzanfar MH, Moran AE, Barber R, Nguyen G, Feigin VL, et al. Demographic and epidemiologic drivers of global cardiovascular mortality. *N Engl J Med.* 2015; 372(14): 1333–41.
45. Global, regional, and national disability-adjusted life-years (DALYs) for 315 diseases and injuries and healthy life expectancy (HALE), 1990–2015: a systematic analysis for the Global Burden of Disease Study 2015. *Lancet.* 2016; 388(10053): 1603–58.
46. Naghavi M, Makela S, Foreman K, O'Brien J, Pourmalek F, Lozano R. Algorithms for enhancing public health utility of national causes-of-death data. *Popul Health Metr.* 2010; 8: 9.
47. World Health Organization. Verbal Autopsy Standards. The 2012 WHO Verbal Autopsy Instrument. http://wwwwhoint/healthinfo/statistics/WHO_VA_2012_RC1_Instrument pdf 2016.
48. Krarup LH, Boysen G, Janjua H, Prescott E, Truelsen T. Validity of stroke diagnoses in a National Register of Patients. *Neuroepidemiology.* 2007; 28(3): 150–4.
49. Jones SA, Gottesman RF, Shahar E, Wruck L, Rosamond WD. Validity of hospital discharge diagnosis codes for stroke: the Atherosclerosis Risk in Communities Study. *Stroke.* 2014; 45(11): 3219–25.
50. Demant MN, Andersson C, Ahlehoff O, Charlot M, Olesen JB, Gjesing A, et al. Temporal trends in stroke admissions in Denmark 1997–2009. *BMC Neurol.* 2013; 13: 156.
51. Jougla E, Pavillon G, Rossollin F, De SM, Bonte J. Improvement of the quality and comparability of causes-of-death statistics inside the European Community. EUROSTAT Task Force on 'causes of death statistics'. *Rev Epidemiol Sante Publique.* 1998; 46(6): 447–56.
52. Flaxman AD, Vahdatpour A, Green S, James SL, Murray CJ. Random forests for verbal autopsy analysis: multisite validation study using clinical diagnostic gold standards. *Popul Health Metr.* 2011; 9: 29.

42

What is the role of trials and other 'well-designed' studies in the understanding of neurological and neuropsychiatric conditions

Carol Brayne

Introduction

Neurological and neuropsychiatric conditions have been defined by societies in the context of their cultures and history. Since the Enlightenment and the Industrial Revolution scientific methods have contributed to these definitions and shaped them too. From any given society's perspective the ability to provide individuals and their families with a diagnosis has had a particular assumed value. This value can be viewed from different perspectives and sectors of any particular society. The way disorders or deviance from what is assumed to be the functional healthy state of an individual within their context are defined and reported has led to them being seen by contemporary society as fixed in nature.

This is not, however, necessarily the case for all disorders as described in detail within other chapters. It can vary substantially across time due to changes in our understanding of their biologies and natural histories. Thus, there have been major changes to the definitions of many, if not most, disorders and diseases affecting human populations, not least with relatively regular changes in the classification systems such as ICD (WHO) and the DSM of the American Psychiatric Association. As a consequence, the meaning of these disorders within changing societies is a moving feast. This then has knock-on effects on the epidemiological descriptors, which then leads us back to interrogation of the purpose of a diagnosis and the impact of any particular disorder on relevant societies.

In very recent years, partly due to the emphasis within current research on neuroscience and new methods for investigation, this change has accelerated for the many disorders covered by this textbook with the emergence of new categories of disorder linked to new measurement methods. Much of this has been driven by the new techniques of measurement of body materials (-omics) and imaging.

In this chapter we consider the role of our current paradigms of medical research, including methodologies, and its relationship with societal meaning and prioritization. This includes how we define diseases, disorders, and outcomes including the measurement of their impact and thus the way that society prioritizes these. The chapter draws on a small number of disorders to illustrate the points made.

Basic Understanding of 'Burden'

In the understanding of a given disorder the first port of call for an epidemiologist is the definition of the disorder, and how has this been arrived at. For many disorders, including those outside the neurological and neuropsychiatric fields, such enquiry leads to the revelation that the disorder does not have clear boundaries, that the distinction between normal and abnormal is not entirely clear and that there is limited knowledge in populations of the prevalence of the disorder if different criteria are used. Many of the chapters in this book provide evidence of how such work is changing our understanding of the epistemology of neurological and neuropsychiatric disorders and this is set to have dramatic influences on our definitions of disorders in the future. From the point of view of epidemiology this is very important and underpins the importance of being able to anchor such changes to what implications they have for our understanding of any particular disorder within defined populations. It is this understanding that allows us to appreciate how to balance our investments into research of different types and also societal responses to the disorder.

How do societies assess the importance of a condition and the appropriate response from organized efforts? This is key for policymakers and depends on basic research to inform such activities. Peacetime civic societies, particularly those of HMICs, have infrastructures which collect data on a range of conditions. However, for different neurological and neuropsychiatric conditions it isn't as clear cut as for many other conditions. Many have a range of severities which include undetected and not presented to services (MS) to rapidly fatal (ALS). Sequelae of such conditions are often profound and interfere with ability to function as well as affecting quality of life.

The way in which we define what services and support we need also depends on context and the evidence available for capacity to benefit. An example is provided from the domain of public health on how to define the challenging area of need and demand, often confusingly and interchangeably used.

Need—'felt' need—what people consider and/or say they need

Demand—'expressed need'—needs expressed by action, such as seeking a service

'Normative need'—what health professionals define as need

There are three complementary approaches and methods developed within the UK's public health system to inform policy and service development. These are: epidemiologically based needs assessment; contextual needs assessment; and a third comparative needs assessment. Each is important, requiring different 'research' approaches and brings different perspectives that are important in decision making. The first is the most detailed and requires wider literature evidence synthesis as well as grey literature. The second and third require detailed work either with the relevant population or relevant wider geography/population such as nations. Research approaches and rigour are required for all of these, and all require synthesis of a variety of evidence sources whether nationally stated norms (e.g. how many psychiatrists does the national body representing this group per head of population need?). Together they form a powerful evidence base to guide societal action for disorders and particular focused work for age groups or communities. Such evidence synthesis is also a powerful way to identify research gaps.

The first will be described in detail, and the second and third more briefly (for further details see handbooks on public health in practice).

Epidemiologically Based Needs Assessment

EBNAS is defined as: 'Health care needs assessment is a systematic method of identifying unmet health and health care needs of a population and making changes to meet these unmet needs. Health needs assessment is used to improve health and other service planning, priority setting, and policy development'.[1]

This is developed with a logical sequence as follows: framing the statement of a problem, that is, understanding of health needs requires clear definition of need. This can be defined as capacity to benefit from an intervention. 'To speak of a need is to imply a goal, a measurable deficiency from the goal, and a means of achieving the goal. This differs from the description of a population health state such as prevalence or incidence, although this is key background information if known. This is because it incorporates the concept of capacity to benefit, in other words, there are many conditions in which there is no known intervention that is effective. There might be a need to do research to find an intervention that can address what is a different type of need, an unmet need but not one which can be addressed through any current provision. This definition is there to avoid provision of services from health systems that are ineffective or identification of individuals whose need cannot be met. This definition, which is clearly a refinement of the usual accepted meaning of need, combines knowledge of a population and disorder(s) with knowledge of potential for primary, secondary, and tertiary prevention. It therefore has to incorporate clinical effectiveness, costs effectiveness, and patient perspectives.

Further Approaches

The second approach is called 'comparative', which compares levels of service receipt between populations, and the third is 'corporate', which canvasses the demands and wishes of professionals, patients, politicians, and other interested parties. Combining these provides a powerful overview of a particular disorder and its place in contemporary society.

This whole approach involves active, explicit, and systematic identification of needs rather than passive and implicit response to demand. The needs include wider social and environmental determinants of health care need—deprivation, housing, diet, education and employment.

This approach, if systematically applied, provides the basis for monitoring, understanding population perceptions and relationship to evidence base, assists priorities, assists effective working with communities to set these, and addresses inequity and inequality.

What Evidence is Synthesized Using this Approach? An Illustration Using Dementia

The problem and its subcategories, dementia, must be defined, along with current understanding of its subcategories. The evidence base for knowledge of its occurrence in the population must be interrogated, including changes in definitions across time, and shifting boundaries of intermediate conditions, as well as new methods of diagnosis. The strength of the potential primary prevention and protection factors is brought together, along with knowledge of interventions that have the potential to change natural history whether they are applied before 'usual' presentation to services or at that time (secondary and tertiary prevention). Mortality relationships and the nuances of the occurrence of the disorder, along with comorbidities must be understood—in this case the challenge of creating services and population understanding for a condition as diverse as dementia, which is closely linked to age itself and to death. It can easily be seen that this exercise requires routine data, research data preferably from the populations of interest as well as clinical research data, but placed in population context. This requires mapping of service provision, and activity across the life course relating to early risk reduction, midlife risk reduction, and later life health and interventions. It includes mapping early responses, assessment and treatment, community support, long-term conditions, specialist services and service groupings, norms, average costings, actual in relation to recommended level of service provision (this also fits with the second two exercises). Often there are huge missing areas in such a distillation of research knowledge and gaps must be filled with assumptions or imperfect data. Such work is often linked to modelling for the future as well.

Evidence from each of these is rigorously reviewed, including the evidence base for effectiveness. An example of this would be the performance of diagnostic tests through Cochrane systematic reviewing. Early detection would require systematic review of the evidence for populations on what difference this makes to the individuals screened, including their characteristics, to assess the relevance of the particular evidence base to the population of interest. Then assessment methods, effectiveness of drug treatments for the individual, and the population impact are assessed. The natural history, including the evidence base on where individuals are during their natural history and how they track through services and into long-term care as well as their care at death is also part of this. The system element of the work includes models and organization of care, community resources, case management, quality, constraints on service, how outcome is measured, and for whom. In the case of dementia this would include individual, family and carers, system, community, society, and commercial sector. These are all needed to understand how research and services interact to provide the best possible care that is affordable for whole populations in the contexts of many other demands and helps to reduce waste through ineffective treatments and over treatment.

If done for an age group, such as the older old, it clearly becomes apparent that any disorder cannot be seen in isolation and that a single-disorder, epidemiologically-based assessment must be placed in its population context. For example, a dementia exercise will quickly identify the challenges present in defining what dementia is, the spectrum condition, and the changes in cognition seen across all older people in populations, including in those with multiple morbidities or close to death. It also naturally raises the question about the purpose of a diagnosis for individuals and communities. This means that exercises for individual disorders must be integrated along with the most relevant others. Such a holistic approach is rarely used and is challenging. International and research priorities tend to simplify neuropsychiatric disorders, although public mental health is emerging as a more nuanced area of attention.

Conclusion

This integrative population approach supports much that is presented in other chapters of this book, the need to generate evidence that really makes a difference to individual lives, the need to do trials that lead to benefits for lives rather than measured metrics. This is an important focus to maintain in the context of an increasingly measured life through biomarkers and behavioural indicators that might be used in artificial intelligence, early detection methodologies. Alongside the work above we must have ethical considerations and societal impact work with legal implications.

Our approaches to integration are limited at present and must include narrative approaches. However, governments and international consortia have worked for many years to produce metrics that might be useful for risk and disease measurement approaches that move beyond the focus on single disorders. The most well known of these is the Global Burden of Health for populations; however, another often used by governments for comparisons across regions and nations is the health life expectancy approach. This uses the methodology of life expectancy to extend this to life expectancy lived in particular states.[2,3] An illustration of this for PD provided by data from a long-standing population based PD cohort is to provide data on life expectancy with and without dementia in the context of overall life expectancy.[4] Such approaches can be done with cross-sectional data but are better estimated using longitudinal data.

Such exercises cannot be static. There is a need to constantly update our knowledge so we need the range of research and evidence that feeds into these synthetic approaches to be updated at appropriate intervals. For dementia we know that over the last two decades age specific dementia rates have reduced dramatically in some countries[5] and that risk factor profiles for successive generations are changing. To understand the clinical manifestations, therefore, we need to constantly check whether the disorder itself is changing, as for heart attacks and stroke over the last decades. Neuropsychiatric disorders are also changing, with new risk factors playing prominent roles as noted in earlier chapters with the change of diagnostic practice leading away from specific psychiatric disorders (schizophrenia, schizoaffective disorder, bipolar) to first episode psychosis. This includes the enormous change in exposure to risk factors such as the forms of cannabis associated with psychosis being widely available to young adults and children in many communities.

We also need to examine the absolute number of people affected by, dying from, or remained disabled by a particular disorder, as well as their trends over time. This information is very important for healthcare planning and resource allocation as well as for the determination of the effectiveness of the currently used preventative and treatment strategies. For example, in the GBD study, rates of many non-communicable disorders, including neurological and psychiatric disorders, have reduced in almost all countries in the world, but the absolute number of people affected by these disorders has increased dramatically over the last few decades.

The approaches outlined in this chapter would, if systematically applied at local population levels, lead to a transformation of the way we assess research gaps and provide services to create a truly evidence-based approach to care for those with neurological and neuropsychiatric disorders within our communities. The gap between those who must provide and plan services for whole communities and those with a special, sometimes vested, interest (including clinicians, drug developers, business sectors, ministers, charities) must be bridged in a transparent manner. For the latter, more resources are always demanded, often bringing in patients as the medium, but not always in an evidence-based or creating manner. These approaches can also be adapted for many different settings, allowing evidence to be applied appropriately in resource limited environments and systems.

REFERENCES

1. Pencheon D, Gray M, Melzer D (eds). *Oxford Handbook of Public Health Practice.* New York: Oxford University Press, 2006.
2. Jagger C, Matthews R, Matthews F, Robinson T, Robine JM, Brayne C. The burden of diseases on disability-free life expectancy in later life.

Journals of Gerontology Series A: Biological Sciences and Medical Sciences. 2007; 62(4): 408–14.
3. Jagger C, Matthews FE, Wohland P, Fouweather T, Stephan BC, Robinson L, et al., and Medical Research Council Cognitive Function and Ageing Collaboration, 2016. A comparison of health expectancies over two decades in England: results of the Cognitive Function and Ageing Study I and II. Lancet. 2016; 387(10020): 779–86.
4. Aarsland D, Andersen K, Larsen JP, Lolk A. Prevalence and characteristics of dementia in Parkinson disease: an 8-year prospective study. Archives of Neurology. 2003; 60(3): 387–92.
5. Wu Y-T, Beiser AS, Breteler MMB, Fratiglioni L, Helmer C, Hendrie HC, et al. The changing prevalence and incidence of dementia over time—current evidence. Nat Rev Neurol. 2017; 13(6): 327–39. doi: 10.1038/nrneurol.2017.63. Epub. 12 May 2017.

43

Research and methodologic opportunities and challenges conducting research among US military personnel

Ann I Scher, David W Niebuhr, and Darrell Singer

Introduction

The US military represents a unique opportunity for neurological and neuropsychiatric epidemiology. Comprised of a subset of the US population, military service members (SMs) represent an open cohort who are exposed to a variety of occupational, physical, and psychological environments. These environments, as well as associated outcomes experienced by SMs, include common to rare conditions and exposures not necessarily specific to the military as well as those that are more clearly related to combat or deployment. Robust databases are available and a range of study designs from 'hypothesis generating' to randomized clinical trials have been supported. While pre-accession socioeconomic status of individual SMs may vary, once in service, employment benefits and social support, including healthcare, are highly standardized. These attributes offer both strengths and constraints when conducting epidemiologic research among the military.

Challenges (or possibly opportunities) associated with studying military populations include demographics, the 'healthy warrior' effect, and access. The active duty population is made up predominantly of young men of above average physical and psychological fitness at the time of accession to military service. Accession medical and fitness standards may preclude important pre-existing health conditions. Retention in service requires maintaining ability to perform occupational skill and includes specific fitness and weight standards. Disability may incur a discharge from service. Conducting epidemiologic research in this population can be challenging due to difficulties in gaining access, recruitment, and maintaining contact—particularly in a war environment and particularly for a population that is highly mobile due to deployments and changes in duty station. While information on medical care may be accessed while the SM remains on active duty, and follow-up care is typically provided by the Veterans Administration (VA), the active duty medical records are not linked to those in the VA which makes long-term follow up more difficult.

Opportunities include capture of medical encounter data in a standardized way as well as the size of the population, which makes it feasible to study relatively rare conditions. The economic and ethnic diversity of the US military enhances the ability to study population subgroups. While the military population is predominantly young men, this is also a strength as young men are often under-represented in civilian population studies. Conditions that are more common in women or for which women are more likely to seek care, such as depression for example, are readily studied in military cohorts.

In this chapter, we focus on opportunities for neuroepidemiologic research in the US military. We describe demographic and other characteristics of this unique population. We present an overview of the military health system including data sources for surveillance and original research including the Department of Defense Serum Repository. We present recent surveillance data on the highest impact conditions based on healthcare utilization and medical discharge from service. In the Appendix we list resources for key data sources, publications, and studies that may be of interest to neuroepidemiologists.

Overview of the US Active Duty Military Population

The US has had an all-volunteer military since conscription ended in 1973. DoD-wide and individual service eligibility standards exist primarily in the health and education levels of recruits. Events such the 9/11 attacks and downturns in the economy typically produce increases in the numbers of recruits, allowing for higher selectivity. Requirements for an increased size of the force in the face of prolonged wars during periods of the economic prosperity of the mid 2000s led to decreased numbers of recruits and forced an increase in waivers of these standards, particularly in the areas of health and education.

SMs are individually trained in a broad range of military occupational specialties (MOS) and assigned to three basic types of military units. ‘Combat’ units are those engaged in direct combat, such as infantry or armour units; ‘combat support’ units provide specialized support to combat units and include chemical warfare, combat engineering, intelligence, security, and communications units. Combat service support units provide logistics, personnel/administrative support, and healthcare. SMs, regardless of MOS or assigned unit, may operate in a wide range of environments, from battlefields in international conflict/combat zones to general garrison assignments in the US, and are subject to a range of physical and psychological stressors commensurate with the rigour of the assigned activity. The military maintains databases that capture most of this information, including dates and locations of assignments, diagnoses, and some healthcare provided.

Detailed reports are available on the demographic representation of the force, offering researchers accurate denominator data with which to calculate descriptive epidemiologic information. Based on the 2016 Department of Defense (DoD) demographics report (Appendix: Demographics),[1] the US active duty population includes approximately 1.3 million members of the Army (471,271), Navy (320,101), Air Force (313,723), and Marines (183,501). In addition, there are 39,597 Department of Homeland Security Active Duty Coast Guard, DoD Ready Reserve, and DHS Coast Guard reserve members (1,085,109), 213,405 Retired Reserve, and 7,870 Standby Reserve.

The great majority of active duty service members are young men (Table 43.1: 84% male; mean age 29). The ratio of enlisted personnel to officers is 4.6 to 1 (82% vs 18%). About half (54%) are married and 40% have children. There are some demographic differences between the active duty population and the 18–44-year-old civilian population (using 2014 United States Census figures for comparison). Compared to the civilian population, active duty service members are more likely to have completed high school or some college (76% vs 60%) and are more likely to have attained a bachelor’s degree or advanced degree (22% vs 19%). Those of Hispanic ancestry (14% vs 17%) and whites (69% vs 78%) are under-represented, while blacks (17% vs 13%) and ‘unknown/other’ races are over-represented (7% vs 1%) relative to the civilian population. Excluding the ‘unknown/other’ group reduces some of these differences.

Table 43.1 Demographic characteristics of the United States military active duty population

Total		1.3 million
Rank	Enlisted	82%
	Officer	18%
Sex	Male	84%
	Female	16%
Age (years)	Enlisted	27
	Officer	35
	Total	29
Married		54%
Race	White	69%
	Black	17%
	Asian	4%
	Multiple	3%
	Other/unknown	7%
Hispanic ethnicity		14%
Educational level (Officers)	<High school	<1%
	High school or some college	6%
	Bachelor's degree	43%
	Advanced degree	42%
	Unknown	9%
Educational Level (Enlisted)	<High school	<1%
	High school or some college	91%
	Bachelor's degree	7%
	Advanced degree	1%
	Unknown	<1.0%
Families/dependants		**1.7 million**
Spouses		624,000
With children		40%
Adult dependants		9500

Source: data from 2016 Demographics: Profile of the Military Community. US Department of Defense. 2016.

The services have detailed criteria for medical and fitness eligibility for enlistment and retention, although waivers are considered in certain circumstances (Appendix: Army Standards for Physical Fitness for example). Specific fitness standards are provided for accession, retention, and periodic health assessments. Some special populations (Special Forces, divers, etc.) have different requirements. As an example, Table 43.2 shows the Army’s minimum fitness standards for maintenance of service in terms of sit-ups, running, and push-ups. Standards are shown for men and women by age categories. Population representation is produced and published routinely (Appendix: Demographics).[2]

The medical standards for enlistment and retention in the Armed Services are informed by evidence collected by the Accession Medical Standards Analysis and Research Activity (Appendix: AMSARA). In addition to fitness recommendations, AMSARA analyses the likelihood of attrition and disability discharges based on whether a service member received a medical waiver at accession as well as other predictors.[3] AMSARA also reports on reasons for evaluation for medical disability or retirement by body system categories and specific diagnoses.[4] Neurological conditions are the third most common body system category of unfitting conditions (after musculoskeletal or psychiatric conditions) in individuals with a disability discharge in 2016.[4] Non-specific lower back pain would be included in the musculoskeletal category. The most common specific unfitting neurological conditions associated with disability discharge are paralysis, residuals of TBI, and migraine (Army and Marine Corps) and paralysis, migraine, and epilepsy (Navy, Air Force). The most common unfitting psychiatric conditions in all services are post-traumatic stress disorder (PTSD), mood disorder, and anxiety disorder. It is possible to have more than one unfitting condition.

Table 43.2 Minimum physical fitness standards for men and women by age, United States Army

Age	Push-ups		Sit-ups	Two-mile run	
Group	(Male)	(Female)	(Male and female)	(Male)	(Female)
17-21	42	19	53	15:54	18:54
22-26	40	17	50	16:36	19:36
27-31	39	17	45	17:00	20:30
32-36	36	15	42	17:42	21:42
37-41	34	13	38	18:18	22:42
42-46	30	12	32	18:42	23:42
47-51	25	10	30	19:30	24:00
52-56	20	9	28	19:48	24:24
57-61	18	8	27	19:54	24:48
62+	16	7	26	20:00	25:00

* Push-ups and sit-ups in two minutes (minimum number), two-mile run (maximum minutes: seconds)

Source: data from DA 705. US Department of Defense. 2010.

Research in the Military Healthcare System

Active duty military personnel receive medical care in the Military Healthcare System (MHS), which includes treatment at military treatment facilities such as the Walter Reed National Military Medical Center in Bethesda, Maryland, and at civilian treatment facilities through TRICARE. Since service members share the same healthcare system, this reduces disparities in healthcare access and provides opportunities for medical encounter data collected in a consistent manner across treatment facilities. More than nine million individuals are eligible for TRICARE coverage, making it one of the largest healthcare systems in the USA. This number is substantially larger than the active duty population since dependents, survivors, and certain retired personnel and their families and survivors are also eligible for TRICARE coverage.

Medical encounter data from military and civilian treatment facilities is curated by the Armed Forces Health Surveillance Branch (Appendix: AFHSB; Fig. 43.2). Surveillance of selected health conditions in the active duty population is published by the peer-reviewed Medical Surveillance Monthly Report (Appendix: MSMR). A subset of these data is searchable online by registered users of DMED (Appendix: DMED), through which it is possible to calculate the number and rate of ambulatory or inpatient medical encounters for specific ICD9/ICD10 diagnoses by demographic categories and over time. Fig. 43.1 shows the number and rate of ambulatory encounters with a primary diagnosis of migraine/other headache disorders and schizophrenic conditions as examples. The top ten ambulatory diagnoses in ICD10 category 'Diseases of the nervous system' are shown in Table 43.3.

The MSMR reports on the epidemiology of militarily-relevant conditions using surveillance case definitions based on medical encounter data (Appendix: AFHSB). Relevant surveillance definitions are provided for epilepsy, Guillain-Barré, migraine, MS, TBI, adjustment, alcohol-related, substance-related, anxiety, bipolar, depressive, eating, factitious, mental health-related and personality disorders, psychoses, PTSD, schizophrenia, suicidal and homicidal ideation, and suicide.

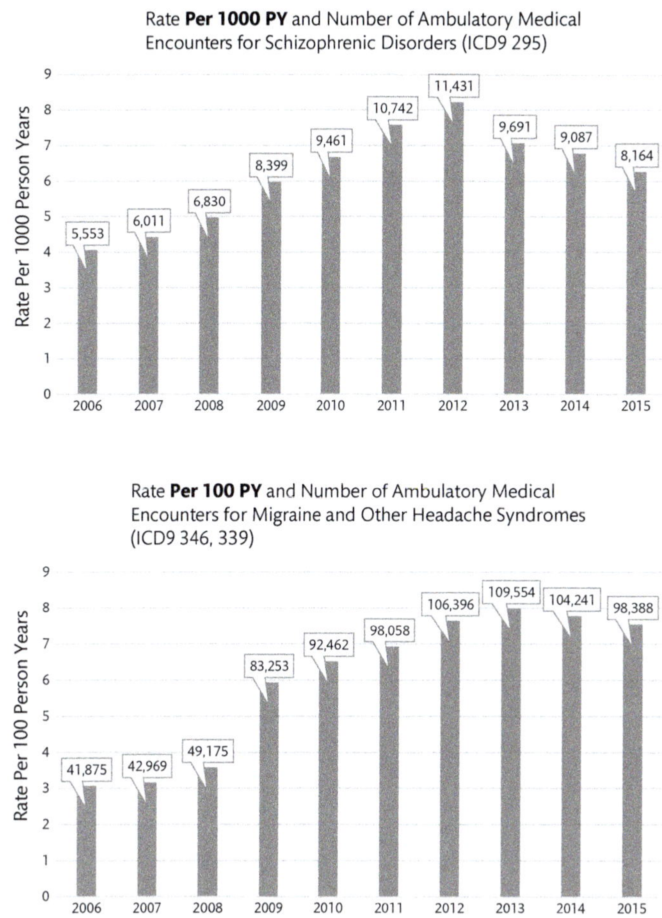

Fig. 43.1 Example DMED charts of medical encounters for schizophrenic disorders and headache/migraine from 2006 through 2015.

Table 43.3 Top ten ambulatory encounter diagnoses in 2016, ICD10 G00-G99 Diseases of the Nervous System

	Diagnosis	Description	Count	Rate*
1	G47	Sleep disorders	523,934	40.65
2	G89	Pain, not elsewhere classified	84,785	6.58
3	G43	Migraine	64,115	4.97
4	G56	Mononeuropathies of upper limb	32,655	2.53
5	G44	Other headache syndromes	27,013	2.10
6	G57	Mononeuropathies of lower limb	11,748	0.91
7	G40	Epilepsy and recurrent seizures	5924	0.46
8	G54	Nerve root and plexus disorders	4845	0.38
9	G25	Other extrapyramidal and movement disorders	4044	0.31
10	G93	Other disorders of brain	3954	0.31

*Rate per 100 person-years

Source: data from Defense Medical Epidemiology Database. US Department of Defense.

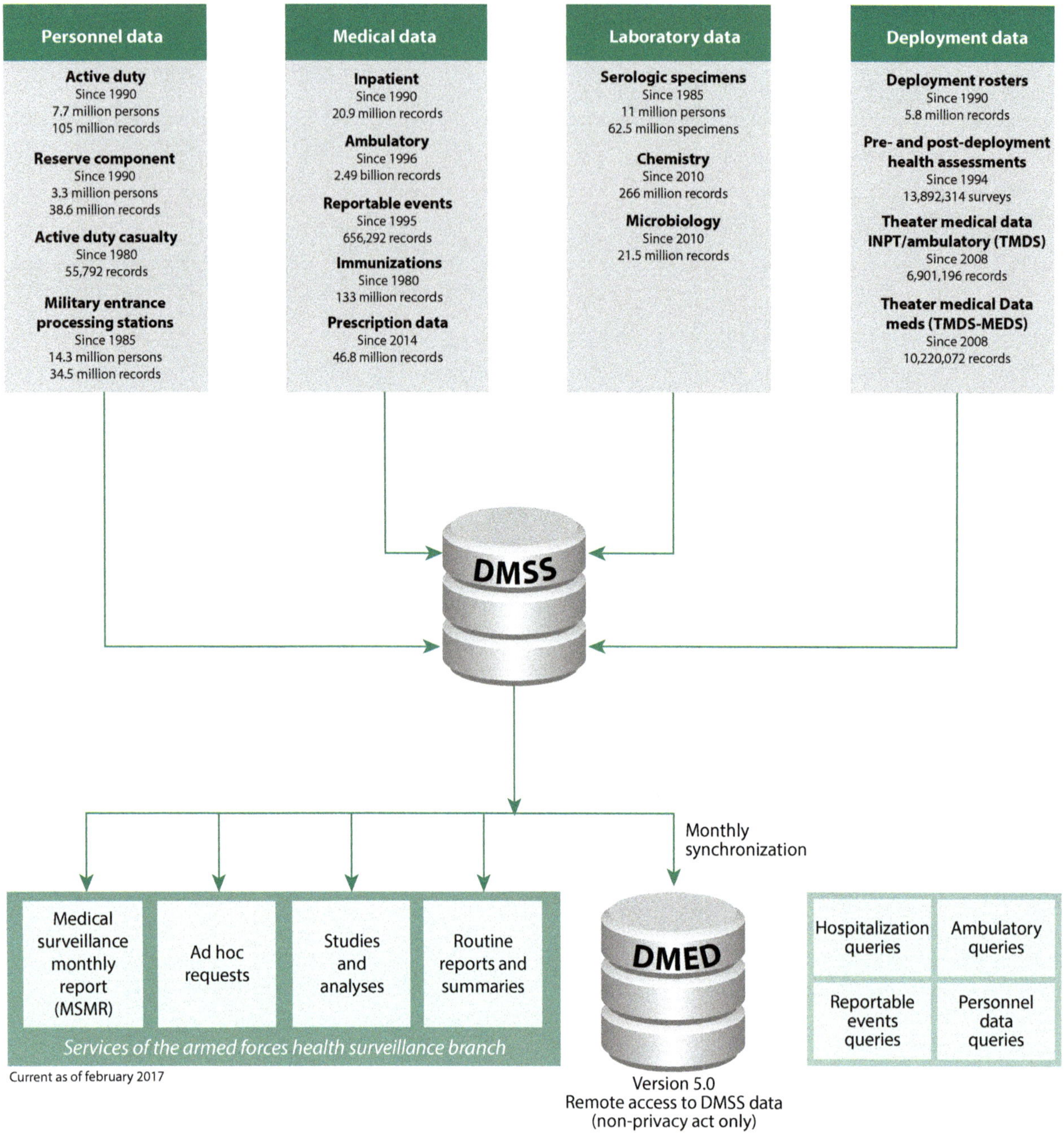

Fig. 43.2 Defense Medical Surveillance System.

Reproduced from https://health.mil/Military-Health-Topics/Combat-Support/Armed-Forces-Health-Surveillance-Branch/Data-Management-and-Technical-Support/Defense-Medical-Surveillance-System. The appearance of US Department of Defense (DoD) visual information does not imply or constitute DoD endorsement.

Surveillance of TBI has received substantial attention during the current conflicts in Afghanistan and Iraq and the surveillance case definition for TBI has been refined during this period (Box 43.1).[5,6] The cumulative incidence of a post-deployment TBI diagnosis was recently estimated as 9.46 per 100 deployments. The authors also considered the impact of secular trends on post-deployment TBI incidence during 2003–2013. Post-deployment TBI was defined as a TBI diagnosis occurring within 24 months of returning from deployment. Secular trends impacting TBI incidence were attributed to three factors: (1) the background (e.g. non-deployment related) incidence of TBI occurring within 24 months of deployment—estimated at 4.2%; (2) enhanced diagnosis over this time period; and (3) risk associated with active war service.

The proportion of TBI diagnoses thus attributed to background risk decreased from about 80% (2003–2005) to about 35% (2009–2013). However, the proportion attributed to enhanced ascertainment increased from about 9% (2003–2005) to about 35% (2009–2013). Thus, at the end of the surveillance period, the proportion of TBI attributable to active war service was approximately equal to the proportion attributable to enhanced diagnosis.

Box 43.1 TBI surveillance case definition based on ICD9 diagnoses

ICD-9 codes
310.2 (post-conscussion syndrome)
800.0x-800.9x (fracture of vault of skull)
801.0x-801.9x (fracture of base of skull)
803.0x-803.9x (other and unqualified skull fractures)
804.0x-804.9x (multiple fractures involving skull or face with other bones)
850.x (concussion)
851.0x-851.8x (cerebral laceration and contusion)
852.0x-852.5x (subarachnoid, subdural, and extradural haemorrhage, following injury)
853.0x-853.1x (other and unspecified intracranial haemorrhage following injury)
854.0x-854.1x (intracranial injury of other and unspecified nature)
907.0 (late effect of intracranial injury without skull or facial fracture)
950.1-950.3 (injury to optic chiasm/pathways or visual cortex)
959.01 (head injury, unspecified)
Personal history of TBI
V15.52 (no extenders); V15.52_0-V15.52_9; V15.52_A-V15.52_F (currently only codes in use)
V15.5_1-V15.5_9; V15.5_A-V15.5_F
V15.59_1-V15.59_9; V15.59_A-V15.59_F

Reproduced with permissionfrom Brundage J.F. et al. Whither the "signature wounds of the war" after the war: estimates of incidence rates and proportions of TBI and PTSD diagnoses attributable to background risk, enhanced ascertainment, and active war zone service, active component, U.S. Armed Forces, 2003-2014. *MSMR.* 2015, 22(2):2-11. The appearance of U.S. Department of Defense (DoD) visual information does not imply or constitute DoD endorsement.

The Department of Defense Serum Repository

The DoDSR contained more than 62 million frozen serum specimens (2020) and grows by an estimated two million specimens per year (Appendix: DoDSR).[7] Most DoDSR samples are the residual sera from mandatory periodic HIV testing (typically every two years) that was initiated in the 1980s for active duty personnel. After 1994, when responsibility for maintaining the repository was transferred to the Army Medical Surveillance Activity (Appendix: AMSA), samples were linked with demographic data, deployment histories, and medical encounter data, among other records. Access to specimens is strictly controlled through the Armed Forces Health Surveillance Branch (Appendix: AFHSB), which ensures separation of potentially identifying information from the requestor. The current policy limits specimen access to studies with at least one DoD principal investigator.[7] It is believed that the DoDSR is the largest bank of human serum in the world.[8]

Some features of this repository make it very attractive for epidemiologic biomarker research. Since an individual service member might have contributed specimens spanning a period of years or decades depending on length of military service, there is the opportunity to analyse preclinical and post-diagnosis, or pre-deployment and post-deployment, specimens. The size of the repository makes it feasible to study relatively rare conditions. Limitations are that this repository contains only serum at this time, storage at -30°C, variability in collection protocols, and the relatively young age of the study population.

Perdue et al.[8] described the utilization and composition of DoDSR specimens in 2012. The DoDSR at this time contained specimens taken at an average age of 27.7, with an average of 3.9 specimens per contributor.[8] However, only 0.42% of samples had been accessed thus far[8] and some have argued that this extraordinary resource has been under-utilized.[9] Table 43.4 lists 22 studies of neurologic or psychiatric conditions that used DoDSR samples, including PTSD, suicide, schizophrenia, bipolar disorder, MS, and epilepsy. A few of these studies have demonstrated that it is possible to extract sufficient genetic material from the serum samples for genetic studies.[10–12]

Appendix: Resources for Military Epidemiology in the United States Armed Forces

AFHSB: Armed Forces Health Surveillance Branch https://health.mil/afhsb

Main epidemiologic resource for the United States Armed Services. Activities under this branch include the Medical Surveillance Monthly Report (MSMR), Defense Medical Epidemiology Database (DMED), the DoD Serum Repository (DoDSR), and Defense Medical Surveillance System (DMSS) (below). The AFHSB also defines surveillance case definitions for militarily-relevant conditions. https://health.mil/Military-Health-Topics/Combat-Support/Armed-Forces-Health-Surveillance-Branch/Epidemiology-and-Analysis/Surveillance-Case-Definitions

Also see **MHS**: Military Health System Data Repository https://health.mil/Military-Health-Topics/Technology/Clinical-Support/Military-Health-System-Data-Repositor

AMSARA: Accession Medical Standards Analysis & Research Activity http://www.amsara.amedd.army.mil/

The AMSARA performs analysis and research in support of evidence-based recommendations for medical eligibility criteria for enlistment to the Armed Services. Other activities include epidemiologic research and statistics related to enlistment, medical waivers, medical encounters, attrition, and disability evaluation.

Army Standards for Medical Fitness, Army Publication AR50-501

https://armypubs.army.mil/epubs/DR_pubs/DR_a/pdf/web/ARN8673_AR40_501_FINAL_WEB.pdf

Demographics: Demographic Profiles of Military Community

http://download.militaryonesource.mil/12038/MOS/Reports/2018-demographics-report.pdfwww.cna.org/research/pop-rep

DMED: Defense Medical Epidemiology Database

https://health.mil/Military-Health-Topics/Combat-Support/Armed-Forces-Health-Surveillance-Branch/Data-Management-and-Technical-Support/Defense-Medical-Epidemiology-Database

Table 43.4 Biomarker studies of neurological/neuropsychiatric conditions using the Department of Defense Serum Repository

Year	Condition	Publication
2004[13]	Multiple sclerosis	Munger KL et al. A prospective study of Chlamydia pneumonia infection and risk of MS in two US cohorts. Neurology. 2004; 62(10): 1799–803.
2005[14]	Multiple sclerosis	Levin LI et al. Temporal relationship between elevation of Epstein-Barr virus antibody titers and initial onset of neurological symptoms in multiple sclerosis. JAMA. 2005; 293(20): 2496–500.
2006[15]	Multiple sclerosis	Munger KL et al. Serum 25-hydroxyvitamin D levels and risk of multiple sclerosis. JAMA. 2006; 296(23): 2832–8.
2008[16]	Schizophrenia	Niebuhr DW et al. Selected infectious agents and risk of schizophrenia among US military personnel. Am J Psychiatry. 2008; 165(1): 99–106.
2008[17]	Multiple sclerosis	Wang H et al. Myelin oligodendrocyte glycoprotein antibodies and multiple sclerosis in healthy young adults. Neurology. 2008; 71(15): 1142-6.
2008[18]	Schizophrenia	Niebuhr DW et al. Results from a hypothesis generating case-control study: herpes family viruses and schizophrenia among military personnel. Schizophr Bull. 2008; 34(6): 1182–8.
2009[19]	Multiple sclerosis	Massa J et al. Serum titers of IgG antibodies against tetanus and diphtheria toxoids and risk of multiple sclerosis. J Neuroimmunol. 2009; 208(1–2): 141–2.
2010[20]	Schizophrenia	Schwarz E et al. Validation of a blood-based laboratory test to aid in the confirmation of a diagnosis of schizophrenia. Biomark Insights. 2010; 5: 39–47.
2010[21]	Multiple sclerosis	Levin LI et al. Primary infection with the Epstein-Barr virus and risk of multiple sclerosis. Ann Neurol. 2010; 67(6): 824–30.
2011[22]	Schizophrenia	Niebuhr DW et al. Association between bovine casein antibody and new onset schizophrenia among US military personnel. Schizophr Res. 2011; 128(1–3): 51–5.
2011[10]	Epilepsy, post-traumatic epilepsy	Scher AI et al. MTHFR C677T genotype as a risk factor for epilepsy including post-traumatic epilepsy in a representative military cohort. J Neurotrauma. 2011; 28(9): 1739–45.
2011[23]	Multiple sclerosis	Munger KL et al. Anti-Epstein-Barr virus antibodies as serological markers of multiple sclerosis: a prospective study among United States military personnel. Mult Scler. 2011; 17(10): 1185–93.
2011[24]	Suicide	Lewis MD et al. Suicide deaths of active-duty US military and omega-3 fatty-acid status: a case-control comparison. J Clin Psychiatry. 2011; 72(12): 1585–90.
2012[12]	Post-traumatic stress disorder	Rusiecki JA et al. DNA methylation in repetitive elements and post-traumatic stress disorder: a case-control study of US military service members. Epigenomics. 2012; 4(1): 29–40.
2012[25]	Schizophrenia, bipolar disorder	Schwarz E et al. Identification of a blood-based biological signature in subjects with psychiatric disorders prior to clinical manifestation. World J Biol Psychiatry. 2012; 13(8): 627–32.
2013[11]	Post-traumatic stress disorder	Rusiecki JA et al. PTSD and DNA Methylation in Select Immune Function Gene Promoter Regions: A Repeated Measures Case-Control Study of U.S. Military Service Members. Front Psychiatry. 2013; 4: 56.
2013[26]	Suicide	Umhau JC et al. Low vitamin D status and suicide: a case-control study of active duty military service members. PLoS One. 2013; 8(1): e51543.
2013[27]	Schizophrenia	Li Y et al. Association between antibodies to multiple infectious and food antigens and new onset schizophrenia among US military personnel. Schizophr Res. 2013; 151(1–3): 36–42.
2015[28]	Multiple sclerosis	Wallin MT et al. Serum proteomic analysis of a pre-symptomatic multiple sclerosis cohort. Eur J Neurol. 2015; 22(3): 591–9.
2015[29]	Schizophrenia	Weber NS et al. Predictors of the onset of schizophrenia in US Military personnel. J Nerv Ment Dis. 2015; 203(5): 319–24.
2015[30]	Schizophrenia	Chan MK et al. Development of a blood-based molecular biomarker test for identification of schizophrenia before disease onset. Transl Psychiatry. 2015; 5: e601.
2016[31]	Bipolar disorder	Haenisch F et al. Towards a blood-based diagnostic panel for bipolar disorder. Brain Behav Immun. 2016; 52: 49–57.

Adapted from Perdue C.L., Cost, A. A. E., Rubertone, M. V., LindLer, L. E., Ludwig, S. L (2015). Description and utilization of the United States department of defense serum repository: a review of published studies, 1985–2012. *PLoS One*, 10(2): e0114857. Distributed under the Creative Commons Universal Public Domain Dedication (CC0 1.0). https://creativecommons.org/publicdomain/zero/1.0/

DMED provides web access to a subset of DMSS inpatient and ambulatory medical encounter data, searchable by ICD9/ICD10 codes.

DMSS: Defense Medical Surveillance System

https://health.mil/Military-Health-Topics/Combat-Support/Armed-Forces-Health-Surveillance-Branch/Data-Management-and-Technical-Support/Defense-Medical-Surveillance-System

DMSS is the central data repository for military medical surveillance data.

DoDSR: Department of Defense Serum Repository

https://health.mil/Military-Health-Topics/Combat-Support/Armed-Forces-Health-Surveillance-Branch/Data-Management-and-Technical-Support/Department-of-Defense-Serum-Repository

The DoDSR is believed to be the largest bank of human serum samples in the world, containing over 62 million specimens. This unique specimen repository is linked to medical encounter and other data. Access at present it is limited to research protocols with at least one DoD Principal Investigator.

DoDTR: DoD Trauma Registry
https://jts.amedd.army.mil/
Formerly Joint Theater Trauma Registry (JTTR), the DoDTR collects data on combat and non-combat related injuries for the Armed Services.

Fitness Standards (Army)
https://usarmybasic.com/army-physical-fitness/apft-standards
https://usarmybasic.com/army-physical-fitness/army-height-weight-standards

MSMR: Medical Surveillance Monthly Report
https://health.mil/MSMR

DVBIC: The Defense and Veterans Brain Injury Center conducts epidemiologic research related to TBI.
https://dvbic.dcoe.mil/

REFERENCES

1. 2016 Demographics Profile of the Military Community: Department of Defense, 2016. https://download.militaryonesource.mil/12038/MOS/Reports/2016-Demographics-Report.pdf
2. Population Representation in the Military Services, 2015: Office of the Under Secretary of Defense, Personnel and Readiness, 2015. https://www.cna.org/pop-rep/2015/
3. AMSARA. Attrition and Morbidity Data for 2015 Accessions Annual Report 2016: Walter Reed Army Institute of Research, 2016. https://www.amsara.amedd.army.mil/Documents/AMSARA_2016%20Report/AMSARA%20AR%202016.pdf
4. AMSARA. Disability Evaluation Systems Analysis and Research Annual Report 2016: Walter Reed Army Institute of Research, 2016. https://www.amsara.amedd.army.mil/Documents/DES_2016/DES%20AR%202016.PDF
5. Medical Surveillance Monthly Report. Notice to readers: New surveillance case definition for traumatic brain injury (TBI). MSMR 2008;15.
6. Brundage JF, Taubman SB, Hunt DJ, Clark LL. Whither the 'signature wounds of the war' after the war: estimates of incidence rates and proportions of TBI and PTSD diagnoses attributable to background risk, enhanced ascertainment, and active war zone service, active component, US. Armed Forces, 2003–2014. MSMR. 2015; 22: 2–11.
7. Perdue CL, Eick-Cost AA, Rubertone MV. A brief description of the operation of the DoD Serum Repository. Mil Med. 2015; 180: 10–12.
8. Perdue CL, Cost AA, Rubertone MV, Lindler LE, Ludwig SL. Description and utilization of the United States department of defense serum repository: a review of published studies, 1985–2012. PlOS One. 2015; 10: e0114857.
9. Baird CP. Maximizing the utility of the serum repository with current technologies and recommendations to meet future needs: report of the technical panel. Mil Med. 2015; 180: 25–33.
10. Scher AI, Wu H, Tsao JW, et al. MTHFR C677T genotype as a risk factor for epilepsy including post-traumatic epilepsy in a representative military cohort. J Neurotrauma. 2011; 28(9): 1739–45.
11. Rusiecki JA, Byrne C, Galdzicki Z, et al. PTSD and DNA methylation in select immune function gene promoter regions: a repeated measures case-control study of US Military Service Members. Frontiers in Psychiatry. 2013; 4: 56.
12. Rusiecki JA, Chen L, Srikantan V, et al. DNA methylation in repetitive elements and post-traumatic stress disorder: a case-control study of US military service members. Epigenomics. 2012; 4(1): 29–40.
13. Munger KL, DeLorenze GN, Levin LI, et al. A prospective study of Chlamydia pneumoniae infection and risk of MS in two US cohorts. Neurology. 2004; 62: 1799–803.
14. Levin LI, Munger KL, Rubertone MV, et al. Temporal relationship between elevation of Epstein-Barr virus antibody titers and initial onset of neurological symptoms in multiple sclerosis. JAMA. 2005; 293(20): 2496–500.
15. Munger KL, Levin LI, Hollis BW, Howard NS, Ascherio A. Serum 25-hydroxyvitamin D levels and risk of multiple sclerosis. JAMA. 2006; 296(23): 2832–8.
16. Niebuhr DW, Millikan AM, Cowan DN, Yolken R, Li Y, Weber NS. Selected infectious agents and risk of schizophrenia among US military personnel. American Journal of Psychiatry. 2008; 165: 99–106.
17. Wang H, Munger KL, Reindl M, et al. Myelin oligodendrocyte glycoprotein antibodies and multiple sclerosis in healthy young adults. Neurology. 2008; 71(15): 1142–6.
18. Niebuhr DW, Millikan AM, Yolken R, Li Y, Weber NS. Results from a hypothesis generating case-control study: herpes family viruses and schizophrenia among military personnel. Schizophrenia Bulletin. 2008; 34(6): 1182–8.
19. Massa J, Munger KL, O'Reilly EJ, Levin LI, Ascherio A. Serum titers of IgG antibodies against tetanus and diphtheria toxoids and risk of multiple sclerosis. Journal of Neuroimmunology. 2009; 208 (1–2): 141–2.
20. Schwarz E, Izmailov R, Spain M, et al. Validation of a blood-based laboratory test to aid in the confirmation of a diagnosis of schizophrenia. Biomarker Insights. 2010; 5: 39–47.
21. Levin LI, Munger KL, O'Reilly EJ, Falk KI, Ascherio A. Primary infection with the Epstein-Barr virus and risk of multiple sclerosis. Ann Neurol. 2010; 67(6): 824–30.
22. Niebuhr DW, Li Y, Cowan DN, et al. Association between bovine casein antibody and new onset schizophrenia among US military personnel. Schizophr Res. 2011; 128(1–3): 51–5.
23. Munger KL, Levin LI, O'Reilly EJ, Falk KI, Ascherio A. Anti-Epstein-Barr virus antibodies as serological markers of multiple sclerosis: a prospective study among United States military personnel. Mult Scler. 2011; 17(10): 1185–93.
24. Lewis MD, Hibbeln JR, Johnson JE, Lin YH, Hyun DY, Loewke JD. Suicide deaths of active-duty US military and omega-3 fatty-acid status: a case-control comparison. J Clin Psychiatry. 2011; 72(12): 1585–90.
25. Schwarz E, Guest PC, Rahmoune H, et al. Identification of a blood-based biological signature in subjects with psychiatric disorders prior to clinical manifestation. World Journal of Biological Psychiatry: the official journal of the World Federation of Societies of Biological Psychiatry. 2012; 13(8): 627–32.
26. Umhau JC, George DT, Heaney RP, et al. Low vitamin D status and suicide: a case-control study of active duty military service members. PLOS One. 2013; 8(1)1: e51543.
27. Li Y, Weber NS, Fisher JA, et al. Association between antibodies to multiple infectious and food antigens and new onset schizophrenia among US military personnel. Schizophr Res. 2013; 151(1–3): 36–42.

28. Wallin MT, Oh U, Nyalwidhe J, et al. Serum proteomic analysis of a pre-symptomatic multiple sclerosis cohort. Eur J Neurol. 2015; 22(3): 591–9.
29. Weber NS, Larsen RA, Yolken RH, Cowan DN, Boivin MR, Niebuhr DW. Predictors of the onset of schizophrenia in US military personnel. J Nerv Ment Dis. 2015; 203(5): 319–24.
30. Chan MK, Krebs MO, Cox D, et al. Development of a blood-based molecular biomarker test for identification of schizophrenia before disease onset. Translational Psychiatry. 2015; 5: e601.
31. Haenisch F, Cooper JD, Reif A, et al. Towards a blood-based diagnostic panel for bipolar disorder. Brain, Behavior, and Immunity. 2016; 52: 49–57.

44

Global evidence generation

Adesola Ogunniyi

Introduction

Neuroepidemiology is the study of the distribution (descriptive epidemiology) and the determinants (analytic epidemiology) of neurological diseases.[1] Since diseases neither know geographic boundaries nor respect persons, neuroepidemiology enables us to tease out the variables that predispose to diseases and such information is useful in planning preventive strategies for reducing disability as well as for improving quality of life. The epidemiological indices to be used for generating evidences are: prevalence (number of individuals affected by a neurological disease encountered in a community), incidence (the number of new cases diagnosed in a period of time), and case fatality (the proportion of individuals affected by a disease that die in a given time period).

DALY is a more-recently introduced measure of disease burden which provides information on the useful years of life lost from an earlier than expected death and healthy years of life lost from disability weighted by severity of the disability.[2] DALY is useful for quantifying the health gap between current and ideal health status. One DALY is equivalent to one lost year of healthy life. DALY will be used for most of the neurological and mental health disorders (NMHD) discussed in this chapter.

The 2010 GBD publication showed that NMHD contributed significantly to morbidity and mortality.[3] Mental health disorders (MHD) accounted for 7.4% of GBD while neurological disorders (excluding meningitis, encephalitis, HIV/AIDS), stroke, chronic pain, head and spinal cord injury) contributed 3%. Stroke alone accounted for 4.1% of the global burden of disease.[3] Thus, if all these other neurological diseases were included, NMHD would constitute more than 15% of the total GBD. Migraine, epilepsy, dementias, and PD collectively accounted for 72% of the burden of neurological disorders.[4] In monetary terms, the global cost of mental health conditions was estimated at US$ 2.5 trillion in 2010 and projected to increase to over US$6 trillion by 2030.[4] Thus, the economic burden of NMHD is enormous.

This chapter will highlight evidence for the peculiar global distribution of the disorders as well as the factors associated with their pathogenesis and observed peculiarities. It will not be possible to cover all the diseases, but emphasis will be placed on common neurological diseases namely: stroke, epilepsy, dementia, PD, and tropical myelopathies in the first part. Mood disorders and psychosis are the MHD that will be focused on in the second part. Evidence will be derived from meta-analyses, systematic reviews, large cohort studies (both prospective and retrospective), and from animal experiments.

Stroke

Stroke occurs worldwide and is the most important neurological cause of disability. According to the WHO, stroke is the second leading cause of cardiovascular deaths after ischaemic heart disease and is responsible for about 5.7 million deaths annually, with 87% of these occurring in LMIC.[5,6] In 2005, it was reported that 40% of deaths due to stroke occurred in individuals less than 70 years of age.[6] This overall number of deaths is projected to increase to 7.8 million by 2030 if preventive efforts are not instituted particularly in LMICs.[6]

Stroke is currently defined as sudden global or focal neurological deficit resulting from spontaneous haemorrhage or infarction of the central nervous system with objective evidence of infarction/haemorrhage irrespective of duration of clinical symptoms.[7] The old definition required that the diagnosis be made after disability had resulted in death or lasted for 24 hours or longer. The new definition requires the utilization of imaging and tissue pathology in making diagnosis. Thus, there may be disparity between high and low-income countries with respect to the extent of case ascertainment and diagnostic specificity.

The prevalence estimates of stroke in LMIC range between 15 and 1230 per 100,000 individuals while the rates in western countries range between 400 and 800/100,000.[8–10] The lowest estimate was from a study in rural Ethiopia,[8] while the highest figure was obtained from a study in the oil-rich Kegbara-Dere District of Rivers State, Nigeria.[9] The low rates could be due to high case fatality and missed diagnosis. The higher prevalence estimates in more recent studies are indicative of rising stroke incidence due to changing lifestyles, ineffective action against the risk factors, and socioeconomic factors. Adeloye, in a meta-analysis of stroke incidence in sub-Saharan Africa (SSA), reported a 10.8% increase in incidence and 9.6% rise in survivorship.[11] The previous impression that stroke was uncommon in developing countries is therefore not supported by current evidence. Feigin et al.[12] had documented that air pollution is a risk factor for stroke and that could be a contributory factor to the very high prevalence in Kegbara-Dere.

With regards to global stroke incidence, the crude rates ranged between 25 and 223 per 100,000 individuals in Lagos, Nigeria, and Estonia, respectively.[13,14] A comparative analysis of the average annual incidence according to economic categorization of countries yielded the following rates (per 100,000): 70 for high and low income, but for emerging/transitional countries (Estonia, Brazil, India) a much higher value of 135 was obtained.[14] The highest incidence in emerging economies would suggest increasing affluence with changing lifestyles, stress, and environmental pollution. Countries in that category would need to redouble efforts at stroke prevention. In a systematic review of stroke incidence in sub-Saharan Africa in 2013,

With regards to DALY for stroke, a comparison is made between the figures for the years 2000 and 2012 in different WHO regions to highlight time trends in Table 44.1.

Table 44.1 Comparison of Stroke DALYS for the years 2000 and 2012 in WHO regions

WHO Region	2000	2012	% change
West Pacific	43,421,595	55,121,610	27.0
South East Asia	28,358,339	33,993,970	19.9
Europe	27,959,064	23,032,796	-17.6
Africa	9,173,325	11,562,808	26.1
Regions of America	9,438,417	9,601,613	1.7
East Mediterranean	6,095,034	7,659,589	25.7
World	**141,348,082**	**141,333,193**	**0.01**

Reproduced with permission from Global Health Observatory Visualizations. Disability Adjusted Life Year (DALY) rates. DALY rates by WHO Regions. http://apps.who.int/gho/data/node.wrapper.YLDYLLDALY/lang=en. © World Health Organization 2018. Source: Global Health Observatory (http://www.who.int/gho)

In both time periods, the highest stroke burden was in the West Pacific region and lowest in the East Mediterranean region. The factors responsible for this observation are likely to be environmental. The reversal of the values for Europe (17.6% reduction) and virtually unchanged value in the Americas would be in keeping with reduced stroke disability most likely due to less useful years lost. This is corroborated by the review of DALYs for four selected countries (USA, UK, South Africa, and Nigeria) in 2000 and 2012 as presented in Fig. 44.1 and 44.2. The graphs showed that individuals who suffered stroke lived longer (reduction in YLL and increase in YLD) in the selected HICs, unlike the situation in the LMICs. Reductions in the DALY associated with ischaemic and haemorrhagic stroke in HICs were also reported in the analysis by Krishnamurthi and colleagues based on 2010 GBD data.[16]

Risk factors for stroke

The INTERSTROKE study that recruited about 27,000 participants from 32 (initially 22) countries has provided the most comprehensive information on the risk factors for stroke.[17,18] Hypertension remains the most dominant risk factor, with almost three-fold increase in risk (OR 2.98 and attributable risk of 47.9%), while regular physical activity and healthy diet each conferred 40% protection against stroke. Apolipoprotein (Apo) B/ApoA1 ratio increases stroke risk by 84% for the highest vs lowest tertile. The other risk factors are: psychosocial factors (OR = 2.20); current smoking (OR = 1.67), cardiac causes (OR = 3.17), alcohol consumption (OR = 2.09 for high or heavy episodic intake vs never or former drinker), waist-to-hip ratio (OR = 1.44 for highest vs lowest tertile), and diabetes mellitus (OR = 1.16). These variables collectively accounted for over 90% of all the attributable stroke risk globally.

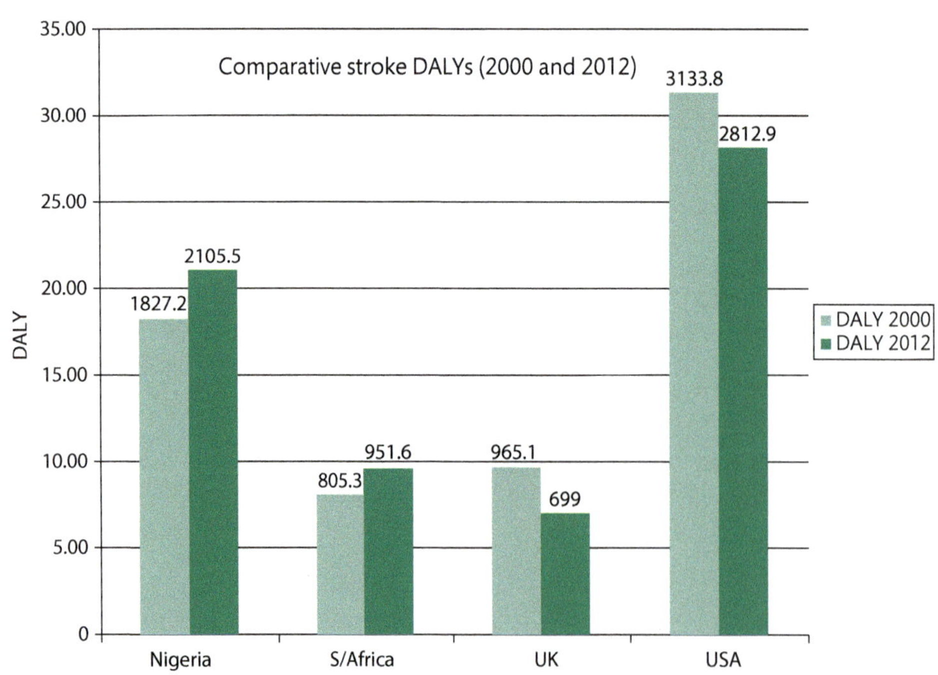

Fig. 44.1 Comparison of DALYs due to stroke in four selected countries in years 2000 and 2012.

Reproduced with permission from Global Health Observatory Visualizations. Disability Adjusted Life Year (DALY) rates. DALY rates by WHO Regions. http://apps.who.int/gho/data/node.wrapper.YLDYLLDALY/lang=en. © World Health Organization 2018. Source: Global Health Observatory (http://www.who.int/gho).

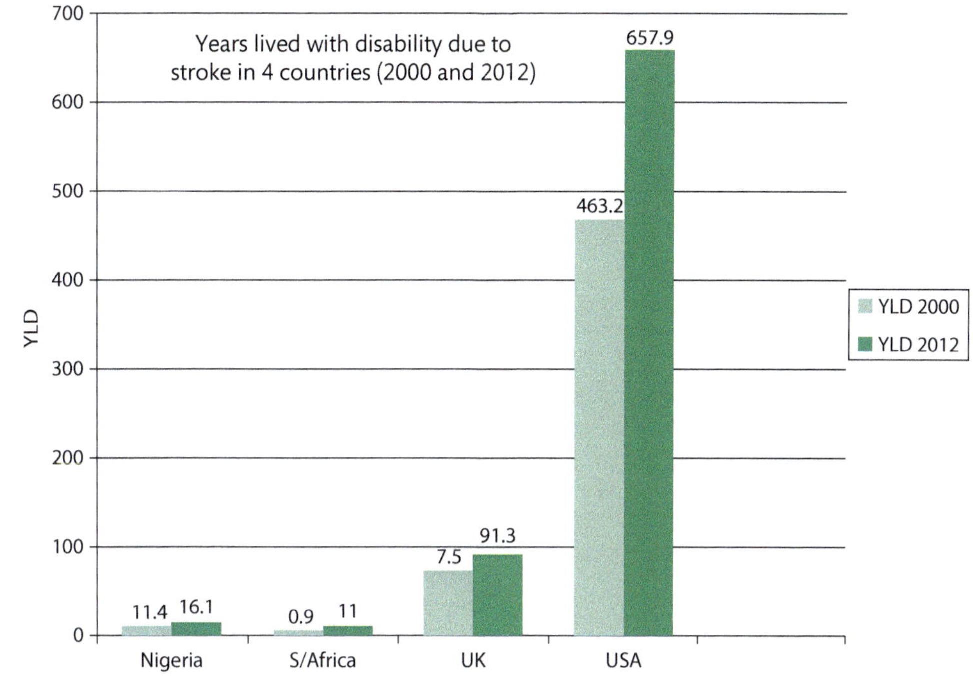

Fig. 44.2 Comparison of years of life lost due to stroke in four selected countries in years 2000 and 2012.

Regional variations in the magnitude of risks for the various factors were also evident. For instance, hypertension was associated with almost five-fold increased risk in Africa, compared to three times increase in HICs. The reverse was observed for waist-hip ratio with the risk being higher in HICs.[17] The situation may, however, change with the obesity paradox being experienced in LMIC. Hypertension increases the risk of intracerebral haemorrhage, while current smoking, diabetes, apolipoproteins, and cardiac causes are associated with ischaemic stroke.[18] The INTERSTROKE authors advocated development of region-specific programmes for stroke prevention. The change in DALY for HICs would be in line with effective measures against stroke risk factors. Therefore, paying attention to the control of hypertension through public education and provision of cheaper drugs with good drug adherence will go a long way in reducing stroke burden in LMIC, particularly Africa.

A much larger modelling data on the risk factors for stroke was provided in the 2013 GBD study, which involved 188 countries and compared risks between 1990 and 2013. Using Bayesian meta-regression analysis, Feigin and associates determined PAF for the various risk factors and showed that modifiable risk factors accounted for over 90% of stroke risk.[12] They grouped the risk factors into three: behavioural (smoking, poor diet, and lack of physical activity), metabolic (systolic blood pressure, diabetes, dyslipidemia, and renal impairment), and environmental (air pollution and lead exposure). Behavioural factors accounted for 74.2% PAF; metabolic for 72.4%, and environmental for 33.4%. The authors calculated that air pollution accounted for 29.2% of global stroke burden. Thus, pollution is emerging as an important risk factor for stroke, particularly in emerging economies and LMIC. Emulation of HICs by promoting the use of clean energy and emission control in LMIC will go a long way in reducing stroke burden.

Stroke is a major cause of mortality worldwide and the case fatality rate varied between 8% for France and 30% in India.[14] The rates seem to tally with the incidence rates. Decline in stroke mortality had been observed in the western world for over 60 years. The first observation was made by Whisnant, who reported a decline in stroke mortality by 76% between 1950 and 1984.[19] This was observed to be more in women. It was concluded at that time that the decline resulted from better control of hypertension. Quite unlike the experience in western countries, mortality due to stroke appeared to be on the increase in LMIC. Walker reported very high stroke case fatality in Gambia and at a relatively younger age. In that study, 61% of the patients died and the mean age at death was 58 years which was about a decade earlier than the age at death from stroke in western countries.[20] The predictors of mortality in Gambia were: incontinence in the first 24 hours, sensory inattention, and impaired gag reflex. Thus, stroke patients should be managed in a stroke unit for better outcome. The World Stroke Organization recently rolled out global stroke care guidelines and an action plan which advocates a three-tier approach to stroke care with huge possibility of reducing stroke deaths, especially in LMIC, if rigorously adhered to.[21]

Epilepsy

This is the most prevalent paroxysmal neurological disorder and a highly stigmatizing disorder. Both the sufferer and his/her family are discriminated against for employment, marriage, and job opportunities. The social consequences make life unbearable for the sufferer and suicidal thoughts are not uncommon. For over three decades, the WHO has advocated urgent control because of its high prevalence and potentially severe consequences in developing countries.[22] Discrimination against epilepsy sufferers was associated with short interval between attacks, long duration of seizures, and family history.[23] Epilepsy affects all age groups but predominantly children and young adults. In Africa, more than 80% of sufferers are below 30 years of age. Epilepsy of late onset is more common in western countries and the important aetiologic factors are cerebrovascular diseases, neurodegenerative diseases, traumatic brain injuries, brain tumours, and metabolic abnormalities.[24]

The 2005 ILAE defined epilepsy as a disorder of the brain characterized by an enduring predisposition to generate epileptic seizures, and by the neurobiologic, cognitive, psychological, and social consequences of this condition. This was modified with more specificity in 2014 as follows: 'Epilepsy is a disease of the brain defined by any of the following conditions: (1) at least two unprovoked (or reflex) seizures occurring greater than 24 hours apart; (2) one unprovoked (or reflex) seizure and at least 60% probability of further seizures occurring over the next ten years; (3) diagnosis of an epilepsy syndrome.'[25]

Lifetime prevalence rates of epilepsy are used for comparison between HICs and LMICs. Active epilepsy implies that the affected individuals continue to have seizures, at least in the previous 12 months and/or continue to use antiepileptic medications. Overall, the prevalence rates varied between 5 and 74 per 1000, with higher rates in LMIC.[26] The lifetime prevalence of epilepsy is about seven times higher in developing countries and the lifetime burden of active epilepsy is 2–3 times higher in developing countries. Even within LMIC, the lifetime prevalence is much higher in rural than in urban communities.[27] According to the WHO, the DALY associated with epilepsy is highest in Africa (7.4 million +) followed by South East Asia (4.8 million +) and least for Europe (1.5 million +).[15]

The following reasons can be adduced for the high epilepsy prevalence and disability in developing countries:

(1) the huge treatment gap, particularly in Africa. A value of 56% was determined by Mbuba et al.[28] although it is believed that it could be as high as 90% in some communities. The implication is that more than half the cases are not on treatment and thus would have recurrent attacks. The phrase 'seizures beget seizures' would seem relevant in this situation.

(2) Malnutrition is rife in these countries and can predispose to epilepsy in two ways. One is through compromised immunity with proneness to infection and the other is because of the resulting low serum protein which can affect pharmacokinetics of antiepileptic drugs. Since many of these medications are protein-bound, toxicity is likely to occur if there is abundant free drug in circulation, unbound to protein. This can affect medication adherence. The frequency of malnutrition was reported to be two times higher in people with epilepsy (22.1%) than in non-epileptic matched controls in one study (9.4%).[29] The situation is further compounded by unjustified forceful restraint of affected individuals during an attack with insertion of sharp or hard objects into the mouth. These objects cause bruises and lacerations which in turn make eating difficult.

(3) Traumatic brain injuries either from vehicular accidents or missile injuries contribute to the high prevalence of epilepsy in developing countries. Poorly maintained highways, some of which are death traps, poor maintenance of old dilapidated vehicles, alcohol abuse by commercial drivers, and non-compliance with traffic regulations contribute to such accidents. Missile injuries occur in soldiers and civilians in war-ravaged areas and have been documented to predispose to epilepsy.[30] Another important cause of traumatic brain injury is fall from heights in certain occupations. In a prospective study of 520 individuals with head injury in India who were followed for one year, 11.2% of them developed epilepsy. The risk factors were severity of head injury (Glasgow Coma Score <9), falls from height, and concomitant medical problems.[31]

(4) Poor obstetric care as reflected in high maternal and infant mortality rates in most LMIC serves as a pointer to high frequencies of perinatal factors that can result in early brain damage and subsequent epilepsy.

Infection deserves special attention. The heavy burden of communicable diseases, including HIV infection in developing countries, contributes significantly to the high prevalence of epilepsy. Epilepsy is a known sequel of meningitis, encephalitis, and cerebral abscess. Healing of the infective focus by fibrosis (gliosis) results in electrical disturbances with generation of excitatory potentials and epilepsy. The role of HIV as a cause of epilepsy has been studied in South Africa. HIV infection was associated with 3–11% of new onset seizures.[32] The seizures result from opportunistic infections, neoplasia, cerebrovascular disease, drug toxicity, and metabolic derangements. With regards to non-intracranial infections in children, febrile convulsions have been reported in many studies to increase epilepsy risk particularly if they are recurrent, multiple, and associated with focal neurologic deficits. Malaria is a culprit here and studies in African children have documented acute seizure, status epilepticus, and various neurological sequelae associated with *Plasmodium falciparum* infection.[33–35]

NCC is another important parasitic disease that causes epilepsy. It accounts for up to 29% of acquired epilepsy in endemic countries, particularly in adults.[36] In many Latin American countries, Asia, and in parts of sub-Saharan Africa, notably Zimbabwe, Tanzania, Togo, Cameroon, and Burundi, NCC is an important aetiologic agent. Inflammatory responses to degenerating and later calcified cysts result in seizures and epilepsy. Neuroimaging shows features of hippocampal sclerosis/atrophy.[37] Animal models for NCC have been developed and have facilitated the study of pathogenesis of seizures associated with the infestation.[38] The Peru MIGRANT study provided data linking NCC with increased prevalence of epilepsy. Epilepsy prevalence (per 1000 people) was 15.3 in the urban group, 35.6 in migrants, and 25 in rural inhabitants.[39]

Onchocerciasis is another parasitic infestation that has been associated with epilepsy in studies from Central African Republic, West Uganda, and Nigeria. In a meta-analysis, Pion et al. reported that the prevalence of epilepsy increased on the average by 0.4% for each 10% increase in onchocerciasis prevalence.[40] Though not a direct cause and effect relationship, the association raises the possibility of increased epilepsy burden with onchocerciasis endemicity. Nodding syndrome, a peculiar form of encephalopathy reported in Uganda and parts of Southern Sudan, appears to be related to *Onchocerca* infestation.[41] It is, however, not clear at this stage whether nodding syndrome is a type of epileptic syndrome or just an encephalopathy. The other parasitic diseases that have been reported to increase epilepsy risk are: toxocariasis, ascariasis, paragonimiasis, trypanosomiasis, hydatid cyst, and sparganosis.[42,43] Interested readers may consult reviews on the link between parasitism and epilepsy.

Epilepsy is a recurrent condition and with good treatment, up to 70% of the affected individuals enter into remission.[44] The factors associated with seizure intractability in children include: presence of neurologic impairment (OR = 12.25; 95% CI 3.58–41.89), age at onset of seizure less than 1 year (OR 11.70; 95% CI 2.95–46.43), myoclonic seizure/infantile spasm (OR 10.36; 95% CI 2.39–44.93), and remote symptomatic epilepsy (OR 2.9; 95% CI1.13–7.43) according to Chawla et al.[45]

Neurodegenerative Diseases

Dementia

Dementia, a clinical syndrome characterized by cognitive decline and impairment in the performance of the activities of daily living in the alert state, is the most common neurodegenerative disease. It has been described as a public health priority because of the rapid increase in the number of cases especially in LMICs.[46] The rapid increase is due to demographic transition, with increasing numbers of individuals reaching old age and at risk of developing dementia. Like epilepsy, dementia is a stigmatizing neurological condition. Affected individuals are prone to injuries, maltreatment, and even accidental death due to misconceptions. Their forgetfulness can result in various domestic accidents. The cost of managing affected cases is enormous and beyond the capability of most developing countries.[47] Promoting preventive strategies is therefore of paramount importance.

AD is the most common type of dementia and a major cause of disability and death. The other common types are: vascular dementia, FTD, DLB, and dementia in PD and HD. Dementia associated with prion diseases, particularly CJD, is well documented. Dementia affects 5–11% of the population above the age of 65 years and could be as high as 30% in persons older than 85 years. AD accounts for 50–75% of the cases.[46] At present, it is estimated that about 40 million people worldwide have dementia and the number is projected to reach over 130 million by the year 2050.[48] Variation in dementia burden is evident from GBD and WHO data from different world regions. The highest DALYs are encountered in Europe and the Americas, with much lower DALYs from Africa and South East Asia.[15]

The prevalence of dementia is influenced by the age group studied, with much lower rates reported in relatively young populations. It is also dependent on the diagnostic criteria used. Studies whose rate estimations were based on the DSM fourth edition of the American Psychiatric Association appear to report lower figures than those that utilized the 10/66 algorithm.[49] The lowest rate of dementia of 0.3% was reported in rural India, which contrasted with 6.3% reported from Cuba.[50] In general, rates in India and rural China were 25–50% of the rates in Europe, while rates in Latin America were about 80% of European figures. A meta-analysis of global prevalence rates of dementia in the population aged 60 years and over by Prince and associates reported that the values ranged between 5–7% with South America, averaging 8.5%, and SSA countries having lowest rate of 2–4%.[51]

With regards to Africa, there has been a rapid increase in the number of studies of dementia from about 3 in 1995 to almost 41 in 2014 but about a third were hospital based.[52] The rates of dementia in Africa ranged between 2.29–21.60%, with AD being the most prevalent type, as in other regions of the world. Thus, the initial impression that dementia is rare in Africa has been challenged by findings from some studies that have come up with rates similar to those in western countries. The note of caution is that direct comparison may be fraught with errors because of methodologic issues. The reasons adduced for the hitherto lower prevalence of dementia in earlier studies included young age of the population, concealment within families and high mortality of the cases.[53] Community-based studies using door-to-door and face-to-face interviews, and age standardization and cross-cultural study design involving simultaneous comparison of data in two disparate populations (Indianapolis-Ibadan Study), have provided useful baseline data for rate comparison with the rest of the world.[54] Determination of ages of study participants using culturally-relevant historical events is a well-tested and validated method for less literate populations with no birth records.[55]

The mechanisms of neurodegeneration leading to dementia provide a pathway for identifying the risk factors. These include apoptosis, neuro-inflammation, excitotoxicity, oxidative stress, ischaemia, and more recently, autophagy as shown in Fig. 44.3. Age is by far the most important risk factor for dementia and female gender is associated with increased risk due to their longer lifespan. The older population in Europe and America would be one reason for the higher prevalence of dementia in those regions, unlike Africa. In western countries and many parts of the world, education is protective against dementia, although this has not been found in all studies.

Although AD is primarily a neurodegenerative disease, vascular factors are increasingly being implicated in its pathogenesis. Apolipoprotein E (APOE), which is linked with cholesterol transport, increases the risk of sporadic AD particularly in individuals with the homozygous ε4 allele. However, despite the high frequencies of APOE in some communities in Africa, no association with AD risk was reported.[56] The association between APOE homozygous ε4 allele and AD in the Yoruba seems to have been reversed in a recent data analysis which reported increased risk of cognitive decline and AD.

Homocysteine is another vascular risk factor that has been extensively investigated for association with AD. Elevated homocysteine induces atherogenesis through oxidative mechanisms and also promotes platelet aggregation.[57] It increases stroke risk and is associated with increased cortical and hippocampal atrophy. Thus, homocysteine increases stroke risk and may be neurotoxic via apoptosis. Homocysteine has also been shown to be associated with cognitive functioning in older persons.[57] The association of homocysteine with AD was first reported in the Framingham cohort by Seshadri and associates[58] and this had also been confirmed in African Americans and Yoruba.[59] Remethylation of homocysteine to methionine requires the enzyme 5,10-methylenetetrahydrofolate reductase (MTHFR) and mutations in the gene (C-to-T substitution at codon 677) has been investigated in studies in Egypt and linked to increased AD risk.[60]

Prospective studies have shown that midlife obesity increases the risk of dementia and the risk estimates were reversed for late-life

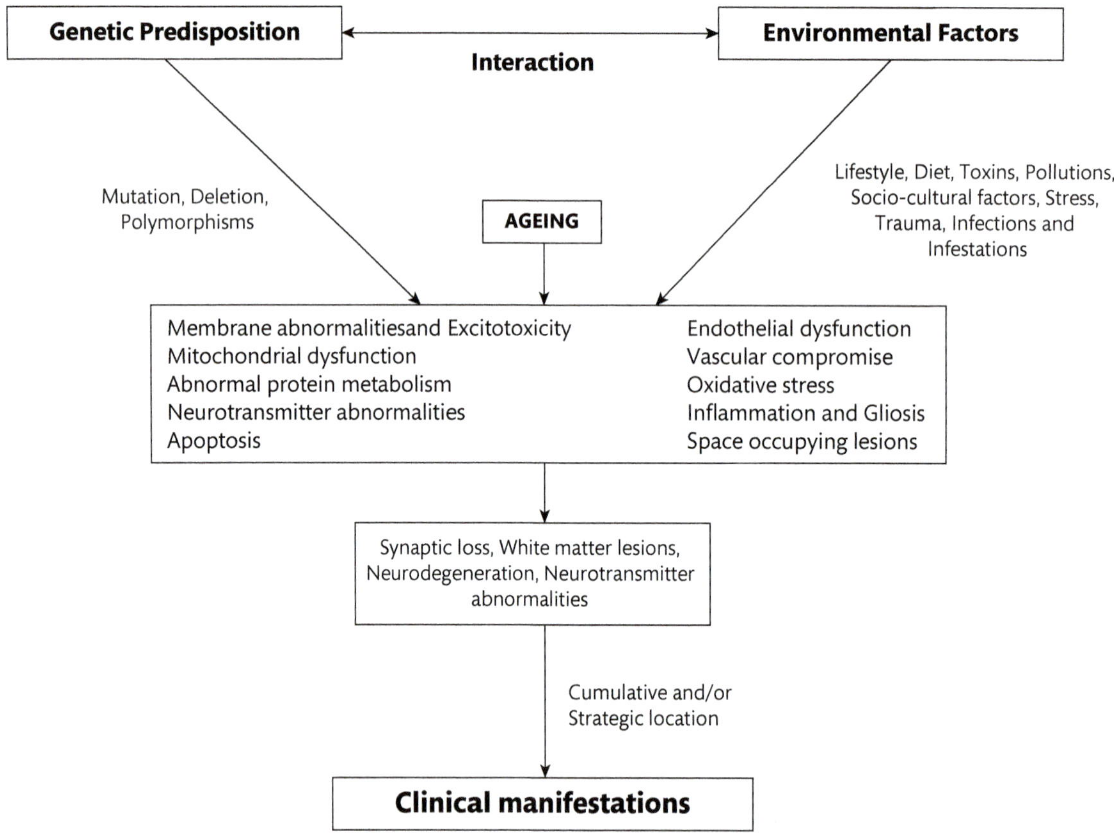

Fig. 44.3 Pathogenesis of neurological and mental health disorders.

BMI measurements with low BMI (<20) increasing dementia risk.[61] Up to 40% of AD patients may present with weight loss. The obesity paradox across time was considered to be consistent with physical changes in the trajectory towards disability. Low BMI had been reported to be associated with dementia in some African studies as well.[52,56,62] Unintentional weight loss in dementia may suggest affectation of the feeding/appetite control centre in the brain, poor feeding habit, forgetfulness to eat, nutritional deprivation, and effect of hormones like leptin. Weight loss does not only occur in AD, it seems to be a characteristic feature of other neurodegenerative diseases like PD and HD.[63]

Longitudinal studies of dementia in the USA, Rotterdam (Netherlands), Stockholm (Sweden), and England (CFAS I and II) have reported recent decrease in prevalence and incidence rates. The reasons adduced for the observations include better prevention/control of vascular diseases, higher education, decline in stroke incidence, and healthier lifestyles.[64] This underscores the importance of vascular factors in the pathogenesis of dementia. LMICs would need to adopt measures aimed at controlling vascular factors in order to stem the looming dementia epidemic predicted.

Severe traumatic brain injury is a risk factor for many neurodegenerative diseases like AD, PD, and ALS, as well as epilepsy.[65] Dementia pugilistica, described in association with boxing, is well known and more recently attention has been drawn to concussion associated with contact sports. Thus, mild traumatic brain injury, also referred to as CTE, is a possible risk factor for dementia since it results in a form of tauopathy. More studies are, however, required on the mechanisms involved in the pathogenesis to dementia.

Parkinson's disease

PD is the second most common neurodegenerative disease affecting the elderly, and the most common movement disorder. It is an akinetic rigid syndrome due to dopamine deficiency in the nigro-striatal system and the hallmark is the presence of intra-cytoplasmic eosinophilic inclusions, called Lewy bodies, in neurons. Clinically PD is characterized by poverty of movement, rest tremors, postural instability, and rigidity. PD constitutes just about 1% of DALYs due to neurological diseases in the WHO estimation.[15] The prevalence varies between 7–659 per 100,000 individuals, with both extreme figures coming from studies carried out in Ethiopia and Egypt.[8,66] Schoenberg and others had reported a prevalence of 341/100,000 in Copiah County, Mississippi, USA.[67] Like dementia, the presumed lower prevalence in developing countries, which was initially ascribed to the relatively young age of the population and lower health-seeking behaviour is no longer tenable.

PD has a strong genetic basis, and positive family history is present in 15–20% of the cases.[68,69] Five genes are associated with PD. Two are autosomal dominant: α-synuclein (SNCA), leucine-rich repeat kinase 2 (LRRK2), while three are autosomal recessive: Parkin (PARK2), P-TEN-induced putative kinase 1 (PINK1), and PARK7 or DJ1. Their putative roles are in the control of neurotransmitter release, maintenance of mitochondrial functions, and response to oxidative stress. Thus, mutations in these genes cause various neuronal dysfunctions leading to degeneration.[69] It has also been hypothesized that selective vulnerability of the neurons to calcium channels could also add to the pathogenesis.[70] With regards to the LRRK2 gene, variations in the frequencies of the G2019S mutation in sporadic and familial PD cases have been reported. The frequencies vary from 36% in North Africa, 10% in Ashkenazi Jews to between 1–4% for other world regions and the lowest value of <1% in Asia.[71] Carriers of the gene were reported to be 22.6 times more likely to be affected by PD according to Hulihan and associates.[72] Although no pathogenic genetic mutations were reported in a cohort of Nigerian patients studied by Okubadejo et al., other workers in Africa have reported novel LRRK2 misense variant in Zambia and mutation in Parkin gene in South Africa.[73–75] Neurodegenerative diseases thus provide immense opportunities for studying interactions between inheritance and environmental factors with regards to disease phenotypes.

Numerous environmental risk factors have been reported in meta-analyses and systematic reviews to contribute to the development of PD. Boxing stood out clearly as being associated the disease apart from its link with dementia. Rural living, drinking well water, proximity to cultivated agricultural fields, exposure to wood pulp, and working in paper and steel industries are some of the risk factors for PD.[76–78] It is believed that these risk factors serve as surrogate for exposure to heavy metals and pesticides which could be neurotoxic. In a study in Nigeria, welding was associated with development of PD.[79] Obstructive sleep apnoea (OSA), which is associated with various cardiovascular diseases, has been reported to predispose to the development of PD. One study reported 37% increased risk of OSA and PD particularly in the setting of ischaemic heart disease, stroke, and old age.[80] Inconsistent association of PD with smoking, cancer, and chronic inflammatory diseases had been reported. Low PD risk was reported in patients diagnosed with rheumatoid arthritis and systemic lupus erythematosus, although there was increased risk in psoriasis.[81–84] In the FINRISK study that involved over 50,000 participants, above-optimal blood pressure level in women was associated with increased PD risk.[85] It is opined that some of these risks may reflect reverse causation, residual confounding, or bias in research methodology.

Of particular interest is the link between essential tremor (ET) and PD. The two conditions are common causes of rest tremor in the elderly and ET cases may also present with rigidity and slowness. It had also been reported that a few individuals progressed from ET to PD after some years.[86] It is not clear whether this link is just coincidental or may have a biologic basis. Unal Gulsuner and associates studied mitochondrial serine protease HTRA2 p.G399S mutation in a Turkish kindred with ET and PD.[87] They showed that in some families, HTRA2 p.G399S was responsible for hereditary essential tremor and that homozygotes for this allele developed PD. Another mutation of interest is the leucine-rich repeat and Ig domain containing 1 gene (LINGO1) which has been reported to increase the risk of ET as well as being linked with PD.[88] Researchers continue to use various methods, including genome wide association studies to tease out the relationship between ET and PD, but there is no firm conclusion at present.

Myelopathies

Tropical spastic paraparesis (TSP) deserves special consideration because of advances in the understanding of its pathogenetic mechanism. TSP is characterized by abrupt onset of symmetrical, spastic weakness in the lower limbs that is non-progressive and leaves permanent damage including cognitive impairment. TSP predominantly affects children and young adults. More women are affected than men. Clusters of the disease have been described in Seychelles, Zaire, Côte d'Ivoire, South Africa, and Zimbabwe.[89] TSP is associated with the consumption of poorly-processed cassava especially during periods of severe food shortage. Deficiency of sulphur amino acids in the diet had been reported, which should normally protect against oxidative stress. Kimani and others have demonstrated that carbamoylation may be involved in the process of neurotoxicity,[90] and prevention of this process might protect against the neuropathic effects of cyanate. Intense research on the prevention of neurotoxic damage is associated with this important dietary staple of many indigenous populations of the world.

Mental Health Disorders

Mental health is a pervasive global problem and there is 'no health without mental health'. According to a survey in the UK, one in four adults and one in ten children are likely to be affected by MHD in a year.[91] MHD is stigmatizing and the resulting discrimination and neglect result in many affected individuals not seeking appropriate care, and on time. MHDs are characterized by a combination of abnormal thoughts, perceptions, emotions, behaviour, and relationships with others. They include: depression, bipolar affective disorder, schizophrenia and other psychoses, dementia, intellectual disabilities, and developmental disorders, including autism. The others are anxiety, and drug and alcohol use disorders. Dementia had already been discussed under neurodegenerative diseases and will be omitted in this section.

Disability associated with mental health disorders

The important MHD constituted 76% of the GBD and overall they accounted for 183,912,000 DALYs globally in 2010 or approximately 2.7% DALYs.[3–5] Depression is the only MHD that was listed in the first ten causes of DALYs, although stroke accounted for a higher DALY. Comparing the GBD data between the years 2000–2012, there were increases in the ranking and proportion of DALYs associated with unipolar depressive disorders, rising from 2.2% and occupying the eleventh position in the year 2000 to 2.8% and ninth position in 2012.[15] The trend was observed in all the WHO regions, but was marked in the Americas, Europe, Mediterranean, and West Pacific regions. Much lower DALYs were calculated for the African region and South East Asia. This peculiar global distribution could be explained by the influence and effects of social factors. The other mental disorders listed among the top 20 in the HICs in 2012 were: alcohol use disorders (seventh), anxiety disorders (fifteenth), and drug use disorders (eighteenth).[3] The increasing trend of disability associated with MHD could suggest stress and changing lifestyles. The reasons for the low burden in South East Asia are not fully explained but are probably cultural.

Prevalence of mental health disorders

A meta-analysis and systematic review on the global prevalence of common MHD between 1980–2013 was published by Steel and associates.[92] The group reviewed data from 174 surveys across 63 countries; 26 were in the HIC category and included 829,673 persons. They reported a prevalence of 17.6% for common MHD within the past 12 months and a lifetime prevalence of 29.2%. Female individuals were found to have higher frequencies of mood and/or anxiety disorders while males were more prone to alcohol and other substance use disorder. The lowest prevalence rates were found in North and South East Asia countries.

The WHO Mental Health survey (WMH) that was carried out in 28 countries also provided data on the prevalence and correlates of common mental health disorders.[93,94] The survey consistently utilized the WHO CIDI,[95] a structured, diagnostic interview designed to be used by trained lay interviewers. The survey showed that MHD started quite early, between late teenage years and early 20s. Phobias were the earliest, followed by impulse-control disorders. Of later onset were anxiety disorders, mood disorders, and substance disorders in that order. If any MHD started later, it was likely to be secondary.[93] MHD were reported to be quite common in all the countries studied, with interquartile range (IQR) of 18.1–36.1% for the 25–75th percentiles across countries of lifetime prevalence estimates of any DSM-V disorder.

Anxiety disorders were consistently found to be the most prevalent mental disorder in the general population, with estimated lifetime prevalence of any anxiety disorder of 16% and 12-month prevalence averaging approximately 11% across surveys. The prevalence estimates were generally higher in HICs than in LMICs. Mood disorders with a lifetime prevalence of 12% were next in frequency and the 12-month prevalence estimates averaged 6%. Like anxiety disorders, the estimates were higher in developed countries. The 12-month prevalence estimates for any mood disorder averaged 5.1%, with an IQR of 3.4–6.8%. It was inferred that mental disorders were not only common in the general population, but had early age of onset, and were often associated with significant adverse societal costs.[91] Seedat and associates[96] confirmed the gender differences in anxiety-mood disorders that was reported by Steel et al.,[92] but reported a narrowing of the frequencies due to changes in gender roles as female individuals now seek gainful employment.

Risk factors for mental health disorders

MHDs result from complex interactions of social, psychological, environmental, and biological factors. According to the WHO, stress, genetics, nutrition, perinatal infections, and exposure to environmental hazards contribute to mental disorders.[6,15] However, risk factors must be differentiated from causative factors, since the former when present would only increase the likelihood of development of MHD. HIV infection was significantly associated with the diagnosis of common mental disorders and depression in a study in Zimbabwe.[97] The authors also reported negative life events as being associated with these diagnoses.

WMH data revealed that MHD is linked with poverty. Kawakami et al. showed that early-onset mental disorders were associated with reduced family income in high and upper-middle income countries after adjusting for education.[98] The population attributable risk proportions varied between 1.0–1.4% of gross household income in these countries. Tampubolon and Hannandita[99] reported that a 1% increase in per capita household expenditure in Indonesia was associated with a 0.05% decrease in depression score using the Centre for Epidemiological Studies Depression scale. This implied that even in LMICs, improved household income could reduce the incidence of depression. Lund therefore called for the study of social determinants of mental health in LMIC settings which would include the facilitators, mediators, and social drift factors.[100]

Low IQ has been reported to be linked with psychotic disorders. Data from the Danish Psychiatry Central Register incorporating the Copenhagen Perinatal Cohort published by Mortensen and colleagues showed a significant association between low IQ and the following: schizophrenia and schizotypal disorders, other psychotic disorders, adjustment disorders, personality disorders, alcohol-related and substance use disorders.[101] The association remained significant after adjusting for comorbid diagnoses. The conclusion was that low IQ may either be the consequence or a causal factor in psychotic and non-psychotic disorders. Low IQ can result from perinatal injuries, congenital malformations affecting the brain, traumatic brain injuries, metabolic brain diseases including kernicterus, and chromosomal abnormalities (Down's syndrome).

Vascular factors have been implicated in the pathogenesis of MHD particularly depression. There is the vascular depression hypothesis that links vascular disease with depression.[102] It is postulated that vascular damage (focal lesions damage, white matter lesions, hypoperfusion, and inflammatory changes) result in a neural disconnection leading to clinical symptomatology. The white matter hyperintensities on MRI are usually located in the frontal and temporal lesions in individuals with depression, unlike the periventricular region in non-depressed persons. Another vascular factor that had been implicated is physical inactivity. Reduced physical activity was associated with higher depression scores in a Swedish cohort of women who were followed up for 32 years.[103] It must be emphasized however, that reduced physical activity could itself be a manifestation of depression, so the data must be interpreted with caution.

Genetic factors also have a role to play in the burden of MHD. Based on the amine theory, the BDNF (brain derived neurotrophic factor) and the COMT (cathecol-O methyl transferase) genes as well as GABAergic neurotransmission received initial attention in mood disorders.[104] For schizophrenia, the following genes have been implicated: NRG1 (neuregulin 1) 8p12-p21; DTNBP1 (dysbindin) 6p22; G72 13q34; DAAO (D-aminoacid oxidase) 12q24; RGS4 (regulator of G-protein signaling-4) 1q21-22; COMT22q11; and PRODH (proline dehydrogenase) 22q11.[105] Another group of researchers investigated genetic predisposition to schizophrenia, bipolar affective disorders, depression, and autism spectrum disorders. They reported linkage with chromosomes 3p21, 10q24, and SNPs within two L-type voltage-gated calcium channel subunits of CACNA1C and CACNB2.[106] The similarities in the genetic underpinning of these independent disorders suggested that their pathogenesis may be related. While genetic factors may have some role to play in the pathogenesis of MHD, the total contribution is small compared to environmental factors.

Conclusion

Interesting differences are evident in the distribution and disabilities associated with neurological and mental health disorders in different geographic regions of the world. Evidence has been adduced to show that the burden of stroke is decreasing in the HICs and this has contributed to the fall in dementia incidence in such countries. Huge treatment gap and the parasitic infestations contribute to the high prevalence of epilepsy in LMICs. Neurotoxins of dietary origin predominantly damage the spinal cord in tropical regions, but better understanding of the pathogenesis can make cassava a safe staple diet in such communities. Environmental factors appear to play an exceedingly important role in the development of MHDs, including poverty, stress, and socio-cultural factors. Appropriate culturally-relevant interventions will go a long way in reducing the burden and disabilities associated with neurological and mental health disorders for better quality of life.

REFERENCES

1. Schoenberg BS. The scope of neuroepidemiology: from stone age to Stockholm. Neuroepidemiology. 1982; 1: 1–16.
2. Lopez AD, Mathers CD, Ezzati M, Jamison DT, Murray CJL. Measuring the global burden of disease and risk factors, 1990–2001. In: Lopez AD, Mathers CD, Ezzati M, Jamison DT, Murray CJL (eds). *Global Burden of Disease and Risk Factors*. New York: Oxford University Press/World Bank, 2006. Ch 1, pp1–11.
3. Whiteford HA, Degenhardt L, Rehim J, et al. Global burden of disease attributable to mental and substance use disorders: an analysis from the Global Burden of Disease Study 2010. PLOS One 2015; 10(2): e0116820. Doi:10.1371/journal.pone.0116820.
4. Global Burden of Neurological and Mental Disorders. http://www.BrainFacts.org.
5. Murray CJ, Vos T, Lozano R, et al. Disability-adjusted life years (DALYs) for 291 diseases and injuries in 21regions, 1990–2010: a systematic analysis for the Global Burden of Disease Study 2010. Lancet. 2012; 380(9859): 2197–223. doi: 10.1016/S0140-6736(12)61689-4.
6. World Health Organization. Global Burden of Disease (GBD) 2002 estimates. *World Health Report 2004*. Geneva, Switzerland: WHO, 2004.
7. Sacco RL, Kasner SE, Broderick JP, et al. An updated definition of stroke for the 21st century: a statement for healthcare professionals from the American Heart Association/American Stroke Association. Stroke. 2013; 44(7): 2064–89.
8. Tekle-Haimanot R. Neurological disorders in Ethiopia: a community-based study on pattern and prevalence. Umea University Medical Dissertations, New series No. 291: Umea, Sweden, 1990.
9. Onwuchekwa AC, Tobin-West C, Babatunde S. Prevalence and risk factors for stroke in an adult population in a rural community in the Niger Delta, south-south Nigeria. J Stroke Cerebrovasc Dis. 2014; 23(3): 505–10.
10. Wolf PA, Kannel WB, Verter J. Current status of risk factors for stroke. Neurology Clinics. 1983; 1: 317–43.
11. Adeloye D. An estimate of the incidence and prevalence of stroke in Africa: a systematic review and meta-analysis. PLOS One. 2014; 9(6): e100724.
12. Feigin VL, Roth GA, Naghavi M, et al. Global burden of stroke and risk factors in 188 countries, during 1990–2013: a systematic analysis for the Global Burden of Disease Study 2013. Lancet Neurology. 2016. Published online 9 June 2016. http://dx.doi.org/10.1016/S1474-4422(16)30073-4 1.
13. Danesi MA, Okubadejo NU, Ojini FI, Ojo OO. Incidence and 30-day case fatality rate of first-ever stroke in urban Nigeria: the prospective community based Epidemiology of Stroke in Lagos (EPISIL) phase II results. J Neurol Sci. 2013; 331: 43–7.
14. Feigin VL, Lawes CM, Bennett DA, Barker-Collo SL, Parag V. Worldwide stroke incidence and early case fatality reported in 56 population-based studies: a systematicreview. Lancet Neurology. 2009; 8: 355–69.
15. Global Health Observatory Visualizations. Disability Adjusted Life Year (DALY) rates. DALY rates by WHO Regions. http://apps.who.int/gho/data/node.wrapper.YLDYLLDALY/lang=en.
16. Krishnamurthi RV, Feigin VL, Forouzanfar MH, et al. Global and regional burden of first-ever ischaemic and haemorrhagic stroke during 1990–2010: findings from the Global Burden of Disease Study 2010. Lancet Glob Health. 2013; 1(5): e259–81. doi:10.1016/S2214-109X(13)70089-5.
17. O'Donnell MJ, Xavier D, Liu L, et al. Risk factors for ischaemic and intracerebral haemorrhagic stroke in 22 countries (the INTERSTROKE study): a case-control study. Lancet. 2010. Published online 18 June 2010. DOI:10.1016/S0140-6736(10)60834-3.
18. O'Donnell MJ, Chin SL, Rangarajan S, et al. Global and regional effects of potentially modifiable risk factors associated with acute stroke in 32 countries (INTERSTROKE): a case-control study. Lancet. 2016; 388(10046): 761–75. doi: 10.1016/S0140-6736(16)30506-2.
19. Whisnant JP. The decline of stroke. Stroke. 1984; 15: 160–8.
20. Walker RW, Rolfe M, Kelly PJ, George MO, James OFW. Mortality and recovery after stroke in the Gambia. Stroke. 2003; 34: 1604–9.
21. Lindsay P, Furie KL, Davis SM, Donnan GA, Norrving B. World Stroke Organization Global Stroke Services Guidelines and Action Plan. Int. J Stroke. 2014; 9(Suppl. A100): 4–13.
22. World Health Organization. Global burden of epilepsy and the need for coordinated action at the country level to address its health, social and public knowledge implications. Document EB136.R8. Agenda item 6.6 2 February 2015.
23. Nuhu FT, Fawole JO, Babalola OJ, Ayilara OO, Sulaiman ZT. Social consequences of epilepsy: a study of 231 Nigerian patients. Ann Afr Med. 2010; 9(3): 170–5.
24. Leppik IE, Birnbaum AK. Epilepsy in the elderly. Ann N Y Acad Sci. 2010; 1184: 208–24.
25. Fisher RS, Acevedo C, Arzimanoglou A, et al. A practical clinical definition of epilepsy. ILAE Special Report. Epilepsia. 2014; 55(4): 475–82. doi: 10.1111/epi.12550.
26. Preux P-M, Druet-Cabanac M. Epidemiology and aetiology of epilepsy in sub-Saharan Africa. Lancet Neurology. 2005; 4: 21–31.
27. Ngugi AK, Bottomley C, Kleinschmidt I, Sander JW, Newton CR. Estimation of the burden of active and life-time epilepsy: a meta-analytic approach. Epilepsia. 2010; 51(5): 883–90.
28. Mbuba CK, Ngugi AK, Newton CR, Carter JA. The epilepsy treatment gap in developing countries: a systematic review of the magnitude, causes, and intervention strategies. Epilepsia. 2008; 49(9): 1491–503.
29. Crepin S, Houinato D, Nawana B, Avode GD, Preux PM, Desport JC. Link between epilepsy and malnutrition in a rural area of Benin. Epilepsia. 2007; 48(10): 1926–33.
30. Adeloye A, Odeku EL. Epilepsy after missile wounds of the head. J Neurol Neurosurg Psychiatry. 1971; 34(1): 98–103.
31. Thapa A, Chandra SP, Sinha S, Sreenivas V, Sharma BS, Tripathi M. Post-traumatic seizures—a prospective study from a tertiary

level trauma center in a developing country. Seizure. 2010; 19(4): 211–16.
32. Bhigjee AI. Seizures in HIV/AIDS: a South African perspective. Acta Neurol Scand Suppl. 2005; 181: 4–7.
33. Oluwayemi IO, Brown BJ, Oyedeji OA, Oluwayemi MA. Neurological sequelae in survivors of cerebral malaria. Pan African Medical Journal. 2013; 15: 88. doi:10.11604/pamj.2013.15.88.1897.
34. Kariuki SM, Abubakar A, Newton CRJC, Kihara M. Impairment of executive function in Kenyan children exposed to severe falciparum malaria with neurological involvement. Malaria Journal. 2014, 13: 365.
35. Ngugi AK, Bottomley C, Fegan G, et al. Prevalence and factors associated with convulsive status epilepticus in Africans with epilepsy. Neurology. 2015; 84: 1838–45.
36. Nash TE, Garcia HH. Diagnosis and treatment of neurocysticercosis. Nature Reviews Neurology. 2011; 7: 584–94.
37. Del Brutto OH, Salgado P, Lama J, et al. Calcified neurocysticercosis associates with hippocampal atrophy: a population-based study. Am J Trop Med Hyg. 2015; 92(1): 64–8. doi: 10.4269/ajtmh.14-0453.
38. Nash TE, Mahanty S, Loeb JA, et al. Neurocysticercosis: a natural human model of epileptogenesis. Epilepsia. 2015; 56(2): 177–83. doi:10.1111/epi.12849.
39. Gonzales I, Miranda JJ, Rodriguez S, et al., Seizures, cysticercosis and rural-to-urban migration: the PERUMIGRANT study. Trop Med and Inter Health. 2015; 10: 546–52.
40. Pion SDS, Kaiser C, Boutros-Toni F, et al. Epilepsy in onchocerciasis endemic areas: systematic review and meta-analysis of population-based surveys. PLOS Neglected Tropical Diseases. 2009; 3 (6): e461.
41. Colebunders R, Post R, O'Neill S, et al. Nodding syndrome since 2012: recent progress, challenges and recommendations for future research. Trop Med Int Health. 2015; 20(2): 194–200. doi: 10.1111/tmi.12421.
42. Nash TE. Parasitic diseases that cause seizures. Epilepsy Currents. 2014; 14(1 Suppl.): 29–34.
43. Kamuyu G, Bottomley C, Mageto J, et al. Exposure to multiple parasites is associated with the prevalence of active convulsive epilepsy in sub-Saharan Africa. PLOS Neglected Tropical Diseases. 2014; 8(5): e2908.
44. World Health Organization. Epilepsy. Fact sheet No 999. January 2009.
45. Chawla S, Aneja S, Kashyap R, Mallika V. Etiology and clinical predictors of intractable epilepsy. Pediatr Neurol. 2002; 27(3): 186–91.
46. World Health Organization. *Dementia: a Public Health Priority*. Geneva: World Health Organization, 2012.
47. Wimo A, Winblad B, Jonsson L. An estimate of the total worldwide societal cost of dementia in 2005. Alz. & Dem. 2007; 3: doi:1-.1016/j.jalz.2007.02.001.
48. Alzheimer's Disease International. World Alzheimer Report 2015. The global impact of dementia: an analysis of prevalence, incidence, cost and trends. www.alz.co.uk/worldreport2015.
49. Paddick S, Longdon AR, Kisoli A, et al. Dementia prevalence estimates in sub-Saharan Africa: comparison of two diagnostic criteria. Global Health Action. 2013; 6: doi: 10.3402/gha.v6i0.19646.
50. Rodriguez JJL, Ferri CP, Acosta D, et al. Prevalence of dementia in Latin America, India and China: a population-based cross-sectional survey. Lancet. 2008; 372: 464–74.
51. Prince M, Bryce R, Albanese E, Wimo A, Ribeiro W, Ferri CP. The global prevalence of dementia: a systematic review and metaanalysis. Alzheimer's Dement. 2013; 9(1): 63–75. e2. doi: 10.1016/j.jalz.2012.11.007.
52. Olayinka OO, Mbuyi NN. Epidemiology of dementia among the elderly in sub-Saharan Africa. Int J Alz Dis. 2014. Article ID 195750. Doi.org/10.1155/2014/195750.
53. Ineichen B. The geography of dementia: an approach through epidemiology. Health & Place. 1998; 4(4): 383–94.
54. Hendrie HC, Ogunniyi A, Hall KS, et al. Incidence of dementia and Alzheimer disease in 2 communities: Yoruba residing in Ibadan, Nigeria and African Americans residing in Indianapolis, Indiana. JAMA. 2001; 285: 739–47.
55. Ogunniyi A, Osuntokun BO. Determination of ages of elderly Nigerians through historical events: validation of the Ajayi-Igun 1963 listing. West Afr J Med. 1993; 12: 189–90.
56. Kalaria RN, Meastre GE, Arizaga R, et al. Alzheimer's disease and vascular dementia in developing countries: prevalence, management, and risk factors. Lancet Neurology. 2008; 7: 812–26.
57. Garcia A, Zanibbi K. Homocysteine and cognitive function in elderly people. Can Med Assoc J. 2004; 171(8): 897–904.
58. Seshadri S, Beiser A, Selhub J, et al. Plasma homocysteine as a risk factor for dementia and Alzheimer's disease. N Eng J Med. 2002; 346: 476–83.
59. Kim S, Nho K, Ramanan VK, et al. Genetic influences on plasma homocysteine levels in African Americans and Yoruba Nigerians. J Alzheimer's Dis. 2016; 49(4): 991–1003. doi: 10.3233/JAD-150651.
60. Elhawary NA, Hewedi D, Arab A, et al. The MTHFR 677T allele may influence the severity and biochemical risk factors of Alzheimer's disease in an Egyptian population. Dis Markers. 2013; 35(5): 439–46. doi: 10.1155/2013/524106.
61. Kivipelto M, Ngandu T, Fratiglioni L, et al. Obesity and vascular factors at midlife and risk of dementia and Alzheimer's disease. Arch Neurol. 2005; 62: 1556–60.
62. Ogunniyi A, Gao S, Unverzagt FW, et al. Weight loss and incident dementia in elderly Yoruba Nigerians: a 10-year follow-up study. Int Psychogeriatr. 2010; 25: 1–8.
63. Aziz NA, van der Marck, Pijl H, OldeRikkert MGM, Bloem BR, Roos RAC. Weight loss in neurodegenerative disorders. J Neurol. 2008; 255: 1872–80.
64. Larson EB, Yaffe K, Langa KM. New insights into the dementia epidemic. N Engl J Med. 2013; 369(24): 2275–7. doi: 10.1056/NEJMp1311405.
65. Gardner RC, Yaffe K. Epidemiology of mild traumatic brain injury and neurodegenerative disease. Mol Cell Neurosci. 2015; 66(Pt B): 75–80. doi:10.1016/j.mcn.2015.03.001.
66. Khedr EM, Al Attar GS, Kandil MR, Kamel NF, Abo Elfetoh N, Ahmed MA. Epidemiological study and clinical profile of Parkinson's disease in the Assiut Governorate, Egypt: a community-based study. Neuroepidemiology. 2012; 38(3): 154–63. doi: 10.1159/000335701.
67. Schoenberg BS, Osuntokun BO, Adeuja AOG et al. Comparison of the prevalence of Parkinson's disease in black populations in the rural United States and in rural Nigeria: door-to-door community studies. Neurology. 1988; 38: 645–6.
68. Hardy J, Cookson MR, Singleton A. Genes and Parkinsonism. Lancet Neurology. 2003; 2: 221–8
69. Nuytemans K, Theuns J, Cruts M, Van Broekhoven C. Genetic etiology of Parkinson disease associated with mutations in the SNCA, PARK2, PINK1, PARK7, and LRRK2 Genes: a mutation update. Human Mutation. 2010; 31: 763–80.

70. Surmeier DJ. Calcium, ageing, and neuronal vulnerability in Parkinson's disease. Lancet Neurology. 2007; 6: 933–8.
71. Bardien S, Lesage S, Brice A, Carr J. Genetic characteristics of leucine-rich repeat kinase 2 (LRRK2) associated Parkinson's disease. Parkinson and Related Disorders. 2011; 17: 501–8.
72. Hulihan MM, Ishihara-Paul L, Kachergus J, et al. LRRK2 Gly2019Ser penetrance in Arab-Berber patients from Tunisia: a case-control genetic study. Lancet Neurology. 2008; 7(7): 591–4. doi: 10.1016/S1474-4422(08)70116-9.
73. Okubadejo NU. An analysis of genetic studies of Parkinson's disease in Africa. Parkinsonism Related Dis. 2008; 14: 177–82.
74. Yonova-Doing E, Atadzhanov M, Quadri M, et al. Analysis of LRRK2, SNCA, Parkin, PINK1, and DJ-1 in Zambian patients with Parkinson's disease. Parkinsonism Relat Disord. 2012; 18(5): 567–71. doi: 10.1016/j.parkreldis.2012.02.018.
75. Blanckenberg J, Bardien S, Glanzmann B, Okubadejo NU, Carr JA. The prevalence and genetics of Parkinson's disease in sub-Saharan Africans. J Neurol Sci. 2013; 335(1–2): 22–5. doi: 10.1016/j.jns.2013.09.010.
76. Sade MY, Zlotnik Y, Kloog I, Novack V, Peretz C, Ifergane G. Parkinson's disease prevalence and proximity to agricultural cultivated fields. Parkinson's Disease. 2015. Article ID 576564. http://dx.doi.org/10.1155/2015/576564.
77. Ascherio A, Schwarzschild MA. The epidemiology of Parkinson's disease: risk factors and prevention. Lancet Neurology. 2016; 15(12): 1257–72. doi: 10.1016/S1474-4422(16)30230-7.
78. Rajput AH, Uitti RJ, Stern W, et al. Geography, drinking water chemistry, pesticides and herbicides and the etiology of Parkinson's disease. Can J Neurol Sci. 1987; 14(3 Suppl): 414–8.
79. Falope ZF, Osuntokun BO, Ogunniyi AO. Risk factors for Parkinson's disease in Nigerians: a case-control study. J Trop and Geogr Med. 1992; 2: 177–80.
80. Yeh NC, Tien KJ, Yang MC, Wang JJ, Weng SF. Increased risk of Parkinson's disease in patients with obstructive sleep apnea: a population-based, propensity score-matched, longitudinal follow-up study. Medicine. 2016; 95(2): e2293. DOI: 10.1097/MD.0000000000002293.
81. Feng DD, Cai W, Chen X, et al. The associations between Parkinson's disease and cancer: the plot thickens. Transl Neurodegener. 2015; 4: 20. doi: 10.1186/s40035-015-0043-z.eCollection 2015.
82. Sung YF, Liu FC, Lin CC, et al. Reduced risk of Parkinson disease in patients with rheumatoid arthritis: a nationwide population-based study. Mayo Clin Proc. 2016; 91: 1346–53. doi: 10.1016/j.mayocp.2016.06.023.
83. Ungprasert P, Srivali N, Kittanamongkolchai W. Risk of Parkinson's disease among patients with psoriasis: a systematic review and meta-analysis. Indian J Dermatol. 2016; 61(2): 152–6. doi: 10.4103/0019-5154.177771.
84. Liu FC, Huang WY, Lin TY, et al. Inverse association of Parkinson disease with systemic lupus erythematosus: a nationwide population-based study. Medicine (Baltimore). 2015; 94(46): e2097. doi: 10.1097/MD.0000000000002097.
85. Qiu C, Hu G, Kivipelto M, et al. Association of blood pressure and hypertension with the risk of Parkinson disease: the National FINRISK Study. Hypertension. 2011; 57(6): 1094–100. doi: 10.1161/HYPERTENSIONAHA.111.171249.
86. Jiménez-Jiménez FJ, Alonso-Navarro H, García-Martí E, Agúndez JAG. The relationship between Parkinson's disease and essential tremor: review of clinical, epidemiologic, genetic, neuroimaging and neuropathological data, and data on the presence of cardinal signs of parkinsonism in essential tremor. Tremor and Other Hyperkinetic Movements.2012; 2: http://tremorjournal.org/article/view/75.
87. Unal Gulsuner H, Gulsuner S, Mercan FN, et al. Mitochondrial serine protease HTRA2 p.G399S in a kindred with essential tremor and Parkinson disease. Proc Natl Acad Sci USA. 2014; 111(51): 18285–90. doi:10.1073/pnas.1419581111.
88. Deng H, Gu S, Jankovic J. LINGO1 variants in essential tremor and Parkinson's disease. Acta Neurol Scand. 2012; 125(1): 1–7. doi: 10.1111/j.1600-0404.2011.01516.x.
89. Tshala-Katumbay DD, Spencer PS. Toxic disorders of the upper motor neuron system. In: Eisen A, Shaw P (eds). Handbook of Clinical Neurology. 2007; Vol. 82 (3rd series). Ch. 18, pp361–81.
90. Kimani S, Moterroso V, Lasarev M, et al. Carbamoylation correlates of cyanate neuropathy and cyanide poisoning: relevance to the biomarkers of cassava cyanogenesis and motor system toxicity. SpringerPlus. 2013, 2: 647. http://www.springerplus.com/content/2/1/647.
91. Mental Health Foundation. Fundamental facts about mental health. 2015.
92. Steel Z, Marnane C, Iranpour C. The global prevalence of common mental disorders: a systematic review and meta-analysis 1980–2013. International Journal of Epidemiology. 2014; 476–93. doi: 10.1093/ije/dyu038.
93. Kessler RC, Amminger GP, Aguilar-Gaxiola S, Alonso J, Lee S, Ustun TB. Age of onset of mental disorders: A review of recent literature. Curr Opin Psychiatry. 2007; 20(4): 359–64.
94. Kessler RC, Aguilar-Gaxiola S, Alonso J, et al. The global burden of mental disorders: An update from the WHO World Mental Health (WMH) Surveys. Epidemiol Psychiatr Soc. 2009; 18(1): 23–33.
95. Kessler RC, Üstün TB. The World Mental Health (WMH) Survey Initiative Version of the World Health Organization (WHO) Composite International Diagnostic Interview (CIDI). International Journal of Methods in Psychiatric Research. 2004; 13: 93–121.
96. Seedat S, Scott KM, Angermeyer MC, et al. Cross-national associations between gender and mental disorders in the WHO World Mental Health Surveys. Arch Gen Psychiatry. 2009; 66(7): 785–95. doi:10.1001/archgenpsychiatry.2009.36.
97. Chibanda D, Cowan F, Gibson L, Weiss HA, Lund C. Prevalence and correlates of probable common mental disorders in a population with high prevalence of HIV in Zimbabwe. BMC Psychiatry. 2016; 16: 55. doi: 10.1186/s12888-016-0764-2.
98. Kawakami N, Abdulghani EA, Alonso J, et al. Early-life mental disorders and adult household income in the World Mental Health Surveys. Biol Psychiatry. 2012; 72(3): 228–37. doi:10.1016/j.biopsych.2012.03.009.
99. Tampubolon G, Hanandita W. Poverty and mental health in Indonesia. Soc Science & Med. 2014; 106C: 20–7.
100. Lund C. Poverty and mental health: towards a research agenda for low and middle income countries. Commentary on Tampubolon and Hanadita (2014). Soc Sc & Med. 2014; 111: 134–6.
101. Mortensen EL, Sorensen HJ, Jensen HH, Reinisch JM, Mednick S. IQ and mental disorder in young men. Brit. J Psychiatry. 2005; 187: 407–15.
102. Taylor WD, Aizenstein HJ, Alexopoulos GS. The vascular depression hypothesis: mechanisms linking vascular disease with depression. Mol. Psychiatry. 2013; 18(9): 963–74. Doi. 10.1038/mp.2013.20.

103. Gudmundsson P, Lindwall M, Gustafon DR, et al. Longitudinal associations between physical activity and depression scores in Swedish women followed 32 years. Acta Psychiatr Scand. 2015; 132(6): 451–458. Doi. 10.1111/acps.12419.
104. Brambilla P, Perez J, Barale F, Schettini G, Soares JC. GABAergic dysfunction in mood disorders. Molecular Psychiatry. 2003; 8, 721–37.
105. Harrison PJ, Owen MJ. Genes for schizophrenia? Recent findings and their pathophysiological implications. Lancet. 2003; 361: 417–19.
106. Zhang C. Genetic findings are challenging the symptom-based diagnostic classification system of mental disorders. Shanghai Archives of Psychiatry. 2016; 28(1): 42–4.

45

The role of prevention in common neurological disorders

Giancarlo Logroscino, Carol Brayne, and Rosanna Tortelli

Prevention, Public Health, and Neurology

Prevention is at the heart of medicine for populations, aiming to both reduce the number of people with disorder and those at risk. A balance between tertiary, secondary, and primary prevention should be based on current knowledge of potential for each to contribute to population health and well-being. Tertiary prevention is intervention aimed at mitigating the impacts of the disorder once present, whether through pharmaceutical agents or other types of intervention. Secondary prevention is early detection, which can be through intense case identification including population level screening. Current research suggests the target populations for secondary prevention will become those with biological manifestations years before any clinical outcomes would become manifest. Primary prevention is true prevention of the disorder being initiated and would be through eradication of known closely linked risk factors, and increasingly discussed could be pharmaceutical intervention to stop a pathological process ever occurring. The broad population-based perspective with elimination or reduction of risk factors needs to be closely linked to the therapeutic intervention of clinical medicine.[1]

The diseases that are suitable for the implementation of preventive strategies in populations are common diseases with high incidence and prevalence. Increasing evidence on the risk factors and natural history of common neurological disorders, neuropathology at different disease stages, and pathogenic pathways are now being interpreted as justifying a different approach for diagnosis, classification, and also the targeting of new therapies. The main thrust of recent research, due largely to changes in our ability to measure biological materials likely to be associated with generally accepted pathological processes through invasive investigations, has emerged as a pivotal change in the diagnostic process used in tertiary and leading research settings. Application of these methods in such settings has led to industry, media researcher, government, and therefore a societally endorsed goal of shifting diagnosis to what is assumed to be a preclinical phase or, at least, a very early phase of the clinical manifestations. This research approach is transforming our understanding of the novel measures and their performance in particular populations recruited to volunteer or clinical studies. These methods have started to leak into the usual clinical settings of selected institutions. The risk is that these new methods have been adopted before they have been fully evaluated. The major problem in assessing the value of these approaches is that the studies are conducted in tertiary referral centres which cannot provide evidence on their performance in usual clinical or indeed population settings. Such evidence has not been collected as yet and there has been insufficient investment and effort into understanding what are the differences and disconnections in several domains between research and clinical practice. This includes age and sociodemographic and comorbidity profiles of those seen in tertiary referral centres when compared with the usual incident dementias seen in primary care or social care settings. The clinical part with minimal symptoms (minimal cognitive symptoms) will be part of the same natural history with a previous preclinical stage with presence of neuropathological changes and an antecedent part without neuropathology but with possible risk factors. However, and extremely importantly, unanswered questions also include, even within the published studies (as evidenced in numerous Cochrane reviews), substantial inaccuracy in prediction of change of disease status or staging. A further major concern that remains mostly ignored, attracting very little investment and capacity building, is consideration of societal implications. Outstanding ethical issues include communication of a pathological condition, without any certain prognosis for that individual and no effective treatment. These gaps stem from a systemic failure to understand that in parallel with the biomedical and technological advances society needs a range of other types of research, drawing on ethics, law, history, public understanding of science, and more. Society also needs public health analysis to provide the full narrative about uncertainty and what choices there might be, with the possible impact of each in terms of cost, environment, and inequalities.

Thus, the major and urgent challenge for society is a woefully inadequate evidence base to examine the public health consequences of labelling people possibly years before onset of a disorder, including a substantial chance of not in their lifetime, as diseased 'patients' but without clinical symptoms, who would in all probability live an additional unknown number of years without any clinical manifestation.[1] This situation has parallels with hypertension and preclinical diabetes, where we are treating increasing proportions of ageing populations with resulting polypharmacy. The issue of differences between subjects with and without clinical symptoms is particularly relevant for older people because an increasing proportion of older people with subclinical disease will die of other causes without developing clinical manifestations of the disease of interest. As noted above, those interventions being developed, including secondary and tertiary prevention, are driven by the perspective of specialized clinical setting research based on smaller highly selected clinical samples, distant from any source population. Further, a robust public health approach for common neurological diseases needs to be placed in context of the rapidly changing demographics, economics, and disease epidemiology experienced by global societies in the last few decades. These are intimately connected and cannot be divorced from the research response to the global challenge that neurodegeneration represents, particularly important when prevention strategies are planned and subsequently implemented. Many examples in this chapter are drawn from the dementia field, because this is the critical area where most of the questions related to prevention of common neurological diseases have been posed and remain largely unanswered.

Common Neurological Diseases Around the World

Life expectancy, as estimated within the 2015 GBD exercise, has increased from 62 years in 1980 to almost 72 years. This represents an increase of approximately 3.5 months per calendar year since 1980.[2] The total number of deaths went up from 2005 to 2015 by 4.1%, but the age-standardized death rates dropped by 17%, indicating an exceptional improvement in life expectancy and consequently mortality over a remarkably short time period.[3] These phenomena are deeply linked to the increase in the world population (about 7.6 billions in 2018) (http://www.worldometers.info/world-population/).

The percentage of deaths explained by NCDs is roughly 71% against 20% explained by communicable/maternal/neonatal/nutritional and 9% by violent deaths and injuries.[3] The proportion of deaths attributed to neurological diseases rose by 36.7% from 1990 to 2015.[4] The years lost for death or DALY due to neurological diseases went up by the 7.4% in the same period.[4] There are now more cases of several common NCDs, including dementia, in LMICs than in HICs, due, in part, to rapid ageing and population growth of these countries (including China, India, Indonesia, and Brazil). Chronic diseases and disabilities define health status in these ageing populations. A significant proportion of the years will be lived with disabilities, with an important load due to neurological diseases, particularly to dementias and stroke.[3]

Thus there will be a rapid expansion in the absolute numbers of neurological disorders and consequent strain on societies, and health and welfare systems of all countries, rich and poor.[4]

Prevention: Controlling Diseases and Risk Factors

Many risk factors are associated with many NCD outcome disorders, including dementia and stroke. The GBD study indicates that risk factors of NCD are responsible for more deaths and disabilities than any single disease. Hypertension ranks first, and then tobacco, physical inactivity, diabetes, obesity, and alcohol follow.[5] GBD provides further evidence that approaches to the prevention of individual and combined risk factors themselves can play a key role in addressing the burden of all NCDs including common neurological diseases.

Framingham is historically considered the landmark study to establish risk factors for cardiovascular diseases.[6] Successive studies, such as the Karelia programme in Finland, linked risk factor assessments to prevention programmes in a particularly high-risk area for cardiovascular diseases. The Karelia programme demonstrated a dramatic reduction of all cause deaths in this area, with a major drop in cardiovascular disease incidence and improvement of general health, as well as an impact on cancer.[7] The Karelia programme is one of the best examples in medicine in which identification of risk factors has been linked to implementation of an effective programme of prevention in a population. A medically informed intervention can therefore produce a favourable change in incidence of diseases when changing the prevalence of established risk factors in a population. This demonstrates that medical management of conditions that are established risk factors of another medical condition can work. Stroke is a good example. The GBD reported a 12% decrease in the age-standardized incidence of overall stroke in HIC.[8] This temporal trend has been explained with the efficiency of therapeutic management of hypertension and diabetes, even in the presence of increasing prevalence of these diseases. The increases in incidence of many chronic diseases are at least in part due to changes in definition and boundaries.[9,10]

Recent evidence from Europe and the USA reveals reduction in age-specific dementia incidence.[11] The Framingham study shows a declining trend in the incidence of dementia of more than 40% over three recent decades.[12] Similarly, a decline in dementia incidence has been shown in the multicentre population representative study Cognitive Function and Ageing in the UK[13] and a decline in dementia prevalence in the Health and Retirement Study in the USA.[14] These figures are probably explained, at least partially, by the better management of vascular risk factors over the last decades.

Beyond medical risk factors there are social and behavioural determinants that play an important role in NDD. Increased years spent in education and better general living conditions, including household economic situations,[15] may also play a protective role.

In cardiovascular diseases, reduction in the risk factors has been proven particularly more efficacious than secondary and tertiary prevention in several studies.[16,17] In this complex context, a linked hypothesis has been recently proposed. In the most recent periods, partly because of better treatment, a decline of diseases or component of diseases related to vascular mechanisms (including AD and vascular dementia as well), has been observed.[18] In contrast, the other two more common NDD, PD and ALS have shown an increase in incidence over time.[19,20] These incidence changes may be at least in part due to earlier detection of diseases over time as first symptom-diagnosis interval show and inclusion of milder forms.[21] Dementia due to AD is based on both vascular and neurodegenerative mechanisms. It is possible that the risk factors connected to vascular mechanisms are, at least in part, declining (better management even in presence of higher prevalence of several risk factors) while risk factors connected directly to neurodegeneration are stable or possibly increasing over time. Determinants can therefore go in both directions.[18] The situation is therefore complex, even without considering the methodologies such as the use of record-based studies with changes in both diagnostic practices and population awareness of these conditions. As yet there is no simple interpretative model that can explain the observed trends for dementias of neurodegenerative and vascular origin. The role of education, better nutrition in the early phase of life, and better general conditions of life (all modifiable risk factors) in the last decades remains to be fully investigated. Even after including in dementia risk reduction models all known risk factors, most of the reduction remains unexplained.[22] The general decline of stroke and dementia highlights that diseases are modifiable and can change rapidly across time. Reductions in disease burden are therefore achievable, and large effects through preventive intervention aimed at causative risk are central to this. Intervention to remove or reduce the prevalence of modifiable risk factors should be the primary focus of epidemiological research in NDD drawing on both current individually based approaches, but more critically and effectively on population-wide strategies given the latter's larger impact for whole populations in the future.

The Role of Prevention

In the early 1980s dementia in the elderly was described as the 'silent epidemic', underlying its high prevalence in later life. Prevention has been demonstrated repeatedly as the key instrument to control epidemics of infectious diseases in the last century. Since development of an effective and efficient cure for NDD, deliverable to large populations is unlikely in the near future, prevention is the most effective approach towards delaying dementia onset. Prevention in turn should reduce the number of new dementia cases as long as life expectancy does not increase the number of cases at the same or at a higher rate.

During the G8 (later G7 for implementation) dementia summit in London in December 2013, international experts in dementia called upon governments of the G8 countries to make prevention one of the major health aims[23] and encouraged an increase in research funding on prevention of dementia, as well as shifting the direction of research towards dementia prevention.[23]

In the following three paragraphs a model with an integrated life-course approach is suggested with three possible strategic axes for observational and intervention studies, and for public health policies on dementia. This can be applied to other chronic common neurological diseases.

The Three Axes of the Prevention Paradigm

Vertical (from health to disease 'accumulation')

The concept of disease has changed during the last 50 years, largely due to advances in scientific understanding of pathways, mechanisms, and technologies to investigate these. Although it was already known and is similar to CVD, these methods have reinforced the fact that neurological disorders and for NDD in particular, pathophysiological process, starts decades before the clinical manifestations of these disorders. The current paradigm, widely although not universally accepted, is that intracellular and extracellular protein aggregates accumulate over time in the brain until a threshold level is reached for that individual, at which point clinical manifestation of the disorder occurs (see Fig. 45.1).[24]

AD provides an illustration of contemporary thinking. The pathological changes observed alongside brain degeneration and cognitive loss, assumed to have a causal link, seen in patients with AD occur at least 20 years prior to dementia clinical onset.[25] Aβ and tau, markers of AD pathology, have been recently identified and quantified *in vivo* both in cognitively normal and impaired individuals. Imaging and CSF biomarkers have been therefore introduced in the National Institute of Aging[26,27] and in the International Working Group[28] new diagnostic criteria, increasing the diagnostic accuracy and enabling an early diagnosis.

In this scenario, the 'starting point' of the disease has been completely redefined. The start of the disease is defined by the early pathophysiological changes (protein deposition, largely because it is now measurable) instead of the first time at which an individual would meet the complex diagnostic criteria that define the dementia syndrome.[22] This is also happening with other neurodegenerative diseases and stroke. A possible parallel between stroke and AD has been proposed, describing an asymptomatic phase, an early symptomatic phase (TIA/MCI), and a symptomatic phase (stroke/dementia) for both.[29] This is happening in dementia research many years after this had been clearly described both in cancer and CVD with recognition that there is a variable and sometimes long silent period. Neuropathological studies from more than 60 years ago had already demonstrated the presence of plaques and tangles in unselected post-mortem series from the fifth decade onwards. The dementia research field has not drawn sufficiently strongly on the expertise and experience of other major areas that could have informed its own approaches, and indeed avoided many of the pitfalls of biased designs and thus interpretation described here. The dementia research needs to rediscover what is already well known for other chronic diseases, trying to avoid further repetition of mistakes from the past, and blind alleys.

It would be bizarre if neurological disorders did not start with their pathophysiological mechanisms, but clinical manifestation and current investigative methodologies now allow us to examine how these previously unknown natural histories unfold. With these changes the concept of primary and secondary prevention have been left-shifted to take into account the measurement of how neurobiological and assumed neuropathologies changes across preclinical time, as illustrated in Fig. 45.2

In the old scenario ('disorder/syndrome starts with clinical symptoms at level meeting diagnostic criteria') *primary prevention* refers to prevention aimed at asymptomatic as well as to pre-symptomatic individuals, *secondary prevention* to early disease manifestations which may be clinically silent, but before individuals meet diagnostic criteria, and *tertiary prevention* to reduction of disability associated with the clinical syndrome. In this new scenario ('disease starts with neuropathological changes'), primary prevention refers to individuals without any of the neuropathological processes associated with dementia only, secondary prevention to those who are pre-symptomatic or early symptomatic with minimal clinical signs (in which the pathophysiological process has already started and puts individuals at greater risk than those without), and tertiary

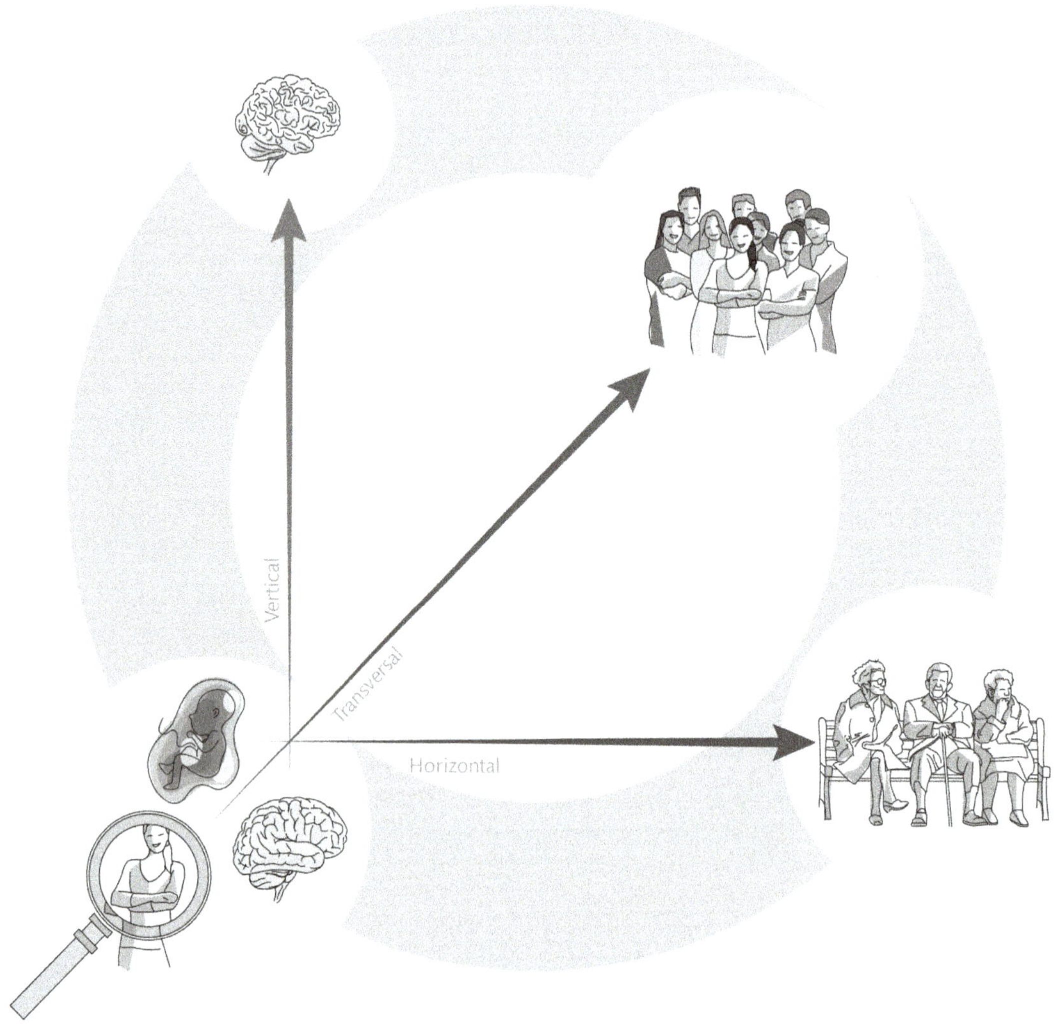

Fig. 45.1 Three axes of the prevention paradigm.

prevention encompasses both early clinical disease manifestations and more advanced phases of the disease with reduction of disease burden and disability. The new definition of primary, secondary, and tertiary prevention also reduces the separation between prevention and treatment strategies.[30] In the new scenario the target of different forms of preventions would be the whole natural history of the disease. In this perspective, RCTs with anti-amyloid compounds target asymptomatic individuals with evidence of amyloid deposition (asymptomatic), or PSEN1, PSEN2, and APP mutation carriers (pre-symptomatic AD) have been indicated in the new scenario as secondary prevention trials.[31]

Horizontal (from the intrauterine conception to late life)

Most cases of NDD, as for conditions apart from those that are purely genetic, will be the result of interactions between genetic and environmental factors that may have a beneficial or detrimental effect over the whole lifetime. This life-course approach is central to the epidemiology of chronic disorders.[32,33]

Over the last 40 years the window of interest for studying modifiable risk factors for NCDs has progressively moved back in time to include the prenatal period. This shift started with the original observation that English regions with the highest rates of infant mortality due to low birthweight in the early twentieth century followed the same pattern, decades later, in mid to late life, for mortality due to coronary heart disease.[34] The resulting hypothesis was that low birthweight babies who survived might be at increased risk of coronary heart disease later in life. This was then supported by other larger observational studies confirming that low birthweight, BMI, and head circumference were independent predictors of death for coronary heart disease.[35–37] Furthermore, maternal obesity has been showed to be associated with increased risk of obesity, diabetes, and coronary heart disease in adult offspring.[38–40] These findings are relevant for NDD considering that cardiovascular risk factors and metabolic syndromes are recognized risk factors for all-cause dementia. This also suggests a possible link between maternal obesity and increased risk of dementia later in life.[41]

The Dutch famine study has been key in understanding the relationships of prenatal exposures to vascular and metabolic diseases.[42] Furthermore, prenatal famine exposure has now been linked to specific unhealthy behaviours in later life such as smoking and physical inactivity.[43] In another study, participants exposed to famine in

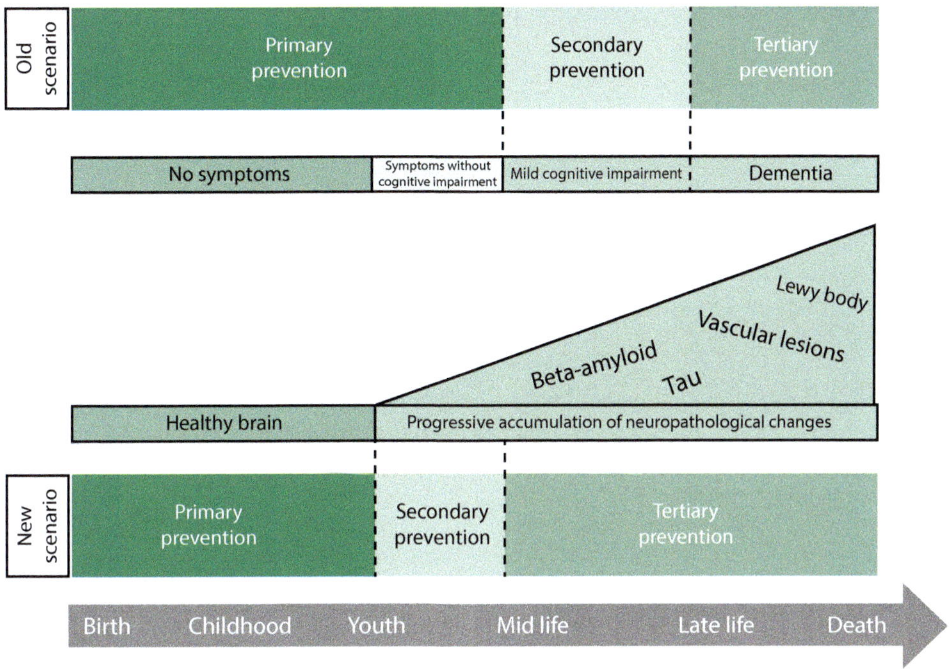

Fig. 45.2 Prevention: old and new scenario.
Legend: SCC = subjective cognitive complaints without any impairment at neuropsychological test; MCI = mild cognitive impairment.

the early period of pregnancy (gestational weeks 1–10) had a global cognitive functioning index at the age of 59 more than four points lower than those without this exposure on a mean score global cognitive functioning of one hundred.[44]

Childhood and early adulthood factors have also been associated with high risk of developing late-life chronic disorders.[45] Indicators of disadvantage, socioeconomic position in childhood (place of birth and literacy), and in adulthood (occupation and income), increased the risk of dementia later in life.[46] Cumulative unfavourable conditions are associated across the life course with dementia. Childhood and adulthood socioeconomic status are associated with occurrence of cardiovascular events. Low childhood and adulthood socioeconomic status increase the risk of stroke later in life, interacting with other vascular risk factors, such as diabetes and hypertension.[47] It is likely that these cumulative unfavourable conditions operate through both biological mechanisms and social opportunities.[46]

There are two main life course models for causation of chronic diseases: (1) accumulation of risk (exposures); (2) a critical period model.[48] The first model relies on the additive effect of adverse exposures in different life periods and applies to general outcomes as all-cause mortality, overall measures of self-perceived mortality,[49] or a broad cause-of-death group, such as cardiovascular mortality.[50] The adverse exposures can be independent or correlated (clusters or chains of risks).

The second model is based on the 'window of exposure' concept, according to which the effects of an exposure depend on the action of that exposure in a defined period of vulnerability ('critical periods'). The ultimate effect of an exposure experienced at critical periods depends on the action of other later-life risk factors or disease modifiers. It is clear that specific patterns of life-course exposure are related to specific diseases. For example, stroke seems to be particularly dependent on deprivation in early life,[51,52] and similarly PD may be determined by exposures in very early periods of life.[53] Family clusters of several chronic conditions, described initially as genetic, need to be re-examined.[54,55] PD data collected in Iceland show clearly that the presence of horizontal clustering in one generation is indicative of a strong environmental influence, while vertical clustering in families is more indicative of genetic causation.[48,49]

The two models are not mutually exclusive as it is possible that both mechanisms could be important for different outcomes.

The application of a life-course perspective when examining risk factors and planning preventive interventions is also based on the observation that several exposures can have both a harmful or a beneficial effect on an outcome depending on timing of exposure. For instance, high cholesterol levels and obesity increase dementia risk when present in midlife.[56–58] On the other hand, high total cholesterol levels and a high BMI in late life have been shown to be associated with a reduced risk of dementia.[59,60] Similarly, a systematic review of observational population-based studies and RCTs on the effect of blood pressure/hypertensive drugs and cognitive function/dementia, proposed that long-standing high blood pressure in midlife can lead to dementia in an age-dependent manner throughout atherosclerosis and, in the presence of atherosclerosis, low blood pressure in late-life can contribute to dementia manifestation with a mechanism of cerebral hypoperfusion.[58]

The dynamic model of interaction between different exposures in populations should include both the models of exposure: the accumulation of risk model and the critical period model in which critical events (famine, wars, and traumatic injuries) acting in a short timeframe are very important.[61]

This approach has only relatively recently gained traction in relation to NDDs closely related to ageing. All these observations have contributed to the opinion among scientists that it is extremely important to apply a life-course perspective when considering risk (and protective) factors and in planning preventive interventions.[62] Addressing risk factors in early life again highlights the importance not only of biological and medical factors, but also of social and economic determinants.

Moving from individuals to populations

Research on prevention of common neurological disorders should explore ways of reducing risk factors at both societal and individual levels. Integrating these implies both a population approach and a high-risk approach.[63]

Starting with the high-risk approach in which there is a need to identify individuals for intervention, several stroke and dementia risk scores have been developed. These scores were designed and investigated starting with the Framingham general cardiovascular disease risk score, a multivariable risk algorithm which has been shown to accurately predict the occurrence of ischaemic attacks and cardiovascular events.[64,65] The Framingham Heart Study population was used to derive the first individual risk score for stroke prediction over the next ten years.[66] Since then several dementia risk scores have been proposed, considering different theoretical models and risk factors. These include those based on routine data in primary care, such as Q-RISK in the UK, with the development and validation of risk prediction algorithms to estimate future risk of cardiovascular disease.[67] An analogous approach for predicting dementia in primary care would be helpful and such work is underway.

In 2006 the first dementia risk score was created using data from 1449 Finnish participants of the CAIDE (Cardiovascular risk factors, Aging and Dementia) study, to predict 20-years dementia risk among middle-age people.[68] The CAIDE risk score, based on age, education, hypertension, obesity, hyperlipidaemia in midlife, and APOE genotype, predicts the onset of dementia 20 years later with an area under the receiver operating characteristic (ROC) curve of 78%.[68] Three more late-life dementia risk scores focusing on shorter term (4–6 years) prediction in the elderly have been published.[69–71] Age is, unsurprisingly, the most important predictor within both in midlife and late-life risk scores, but cannot be modified, while other factors differ. Consistent with a lifetime course view, it is extremely important to consider the time of assessment in the exposure-outcome relationship.[72–74] This is the reason why the CAIDE risk score focused on prediction in midlife, incorporates primarily cardiovascular risk factors. On the other hand, late-life scores evaluate cumulative long-term impact on the brain of vascular and non-vascular risk factors including data from neuroimaging and neuropsychological evaluations. Such scores can be useful in clinical settings to predict evolution of the disease process in short time periods for people who already have preclinical stages or early clinical phase of dementia. The main limitation is that these types of scores do not provide known estimation for particular individuals, with uncertainty boundaries for that individual. The cardiovascular ones are far more robust, although also do not provide uncertainty. A comparison in predicting cognitive decline of CAIDE, CVD, and stroke Framingham risk scores has been conducted in the Whitehall cohort in UK.[75] CVD and stroke risk scores were associated with more cognitive decline than CAIDE. New Framingham Risk scores for dementia, including new items such as the presence of history of cancer and marital status, have been recently proposed. New tools have been proposed for GPs and lay people in primary care and community settings.[76]

Both in mid and late life, non-invasive, cheap, and easily attainable predictors may be useful in population-based settings, but if applied to populations in an individualized manner they are likely to be taken up in a preferential way by those who are already advantaged. Individual prevention strategies are known to increase inequalities in health.[77] Midlife risk scores are valid tools for individually based primary prevention strategies (primary risk scores); late-life risk scores as constructed so far, may be useful to implement secondary prevention (secondary risk scores), and for studies in the area of tertiary prevention, including stratification in randomized clinical trials. Timing of exposure needs to be carefully considered when constructing risk scores in mid and late life.

Individual risk scores allow identification of high-risk patients and are thought to motivate patients for intervention. However, the evidence that behaviour changes based on communication of risk scores is not strong. These risk scores are often used as an indication for pharmaceutical treatment in primary and secondary prevention. There is no strong evidence that people with high-risk genetic profile change their behaviour after hearing DNA-based risk estimates.[78] Assessment of absolute risk for coronary heart diseases and cardio-vascular diseases has become an accepted basis for the use of cholesterol-lowering drugs and the use of antihypertensive agents.[79,80] Absolute risk assessment is also needed to calculate the NNT, to evaluate the cost-effectiveness of treatment, and to assess the population implications of treatment policies based on RCT evidence.[81]

Absolute risk predictions can be translated to other settings beyond those in which they were developed. However, to assess the transportability of risk predictions to other populations is a complex task. It is important to look at the distribution, incidence, and impact of contributing risk factors and the incidence of endpoints. Possible variations of prevalence and impact of risk factors across different populations must be examined and taken into account.[82]

Projection models are built on the assumption from observational studies that primary prevention strategies are likely to delay dementia onset, and therefore to reduce the future prevalence of dementia at particular ages.[83] There is a wide range of potentially modifiable risk factors for dementia, including cardiovascular, psychosocial, and behavioural factors.[84] A substantive question is what is the number of cases that could be avoided if the prevalence of modifiable risk factors was changed. Barnes and Yaffe reviewed evidences from other meta-analysis of seven potentially modifiable risk factors for AD that had been identified to have sufficient evidence of association: diabetes, midlife hypertension, midlife obesity, physical inactivity, depression, smoking, and low education level.[85] The population attributable risk was calculated (i.e. the percentage of cases of a disease attributable to a given risk factor in a given population) for each risk factors and the potential positive effect of prevention. Based on an additive model of risk prevention, almost a half of AD cases were estimated to be preventable assuming a relationship with no interaction between the risks. In a subsequent study, the introduction of an adjustment for non-independence in the model reduced the preventable fraction to about 30% of AD cases worldwide with substantial reduction of the prevalence of AD worldwide by 2050.[86] This is a more realistic prediction, suggesting a huge number of avoidable cases as well. No therapy could produce a positive effect of such dimension on the health of populations in the foreseeable future.

Common neurological disorders are multifactorial and interventions targeting several risk factors simultaneously are likely to produce the largest preventive effect.[87] The role of public health research is to implement large-scale prevention strategies that impact on populations targeting simultaneously many people with a modest or no increased risk.[86]

In summary, an integrated prevention approach that balances the targeting of both individuals and populations, with a life course approach could delay the onset of many chronic neurological disorders as well as enhancing health in older age. The population strategy in which the incidence curve is shifted to older ages is preferable to a high-risk strategy, particularly when thinking about resource allocation for intervention.[88] A combined approach has been successful for reduction of cardiovascular disease and stroke in many countries. Greater emphasis on population prevention in the context of chronic neurological diseases, as for cardiovascular diseases, is clearly indicated.

Challenges in Prevention

Challenge 1—prevention of dementia in the community: the role of macrosocial determinants

Most medical research has been based on biological risk factors, with an acceleration of a reductionist approach since the molecular revolution. In the real world, however, determinants of diseases can be seen at many levels, from the individual to the societal. The distribution of health and disease cannot be examined without considering societies.[89] This is particularly highlighted by dementia research and is true for all most common neurological diseases. Risk factors include economic factors and social connections. Social relationships are particularly relevant for cognitive function during ageing. This has been shown using both objective measures of social networks and measures of the social network perception by the single subject, such as loneliness. These characteristics can be measured in a very simple way as in recent data from the English Longitudinal Study of Ageing. In this study a considerable increase in dementia risk has been reported in presence of loneliness, while a protective effect is determined by the numbers of close relationships.[90]

A major contribution in this area has been provided by the Rush Memory and Aging Project in Chicago. This study has had a major focus on the psychosocial aspects of experience across the whole life course, including social connectedness, personality, and psychological traits.[91] This study has provided strong evidence that frequent participation in late-life social activities is associated with reduced risk of dementia.[92] Conversely, loneliness was again associated with an increased risk of dementia in late life. The relevant characteristic of the Rush Memory and Aging study is that neuropathological examination was included. No pathological changes typical of dementia were associated with loneliness.[93] In contrast, in a more recent finding from the Harvard Aging Study, based on the participation of elderly volunteers, loneliness was found to be associated with amyloid deposition.[94]

Data from the HRS, a nationally representative, population-based longitudinal survey of individuals in the USA 65 years or older (survey in two waves of about 20,000 subjects) show that more years of education has been associated with a lower risk for dementia, and average years of education increased significantly during recent years. In the same study annual income was directly associated with decreased risk of dementia, while increased risk was present for blacks and Hispanics.[22] More detailed analysis indicated that clinically diagnosed AD is more common among blacks and Latinos. However, the reason for disparity in estimates for clinically diagnosed AD in different ethnic groups remains a subject of controversy.[95]

In the Rush Memory and Aging Study, with the exception of low purpose in life and cerebral infarction, no clear association between any psychosocial measures and neuropathological traits typical of late onset dementia was found.[91] These findings exclude reverse causation and strengthen the importance of socio-psychological factors in the manifestation of dementia. The underlying biological and neuropathological features and pathways of these traits still need much clarification. The likely role of social determinants as causes or modifiers in the dementia causal pathways highlight the compelling need for more studies on determinants for possible intervention in this area.

Also, macrosocial factors need to be taken into consideration. These factors include social networks, migration and ethnicity patterns, regional income, and social inequities and disparities. Small changes in these factors may determine extensive changes in the health of populations because they are ubiquitous.[61] This is extraordinarily important for prevention in large populations.

There is a further layer to be added to these already complex patterns. When we deal with health and prevention in large populations, such as the whole population of a country, the strategies and policies that local and national governments implement beyond health areas have consequences on population health status and frequency of diseases. Dementia offers again a possible example. In recent years many European governments have launched national dementia plans. The first was launched by the UK government in 2009 with a campaign to enhance dementia awareness.[96] From data of the national health system the number of dementia cases and the quality of diagnosis, including shorter time from concern to diagnosis, has increased substantially since 2009.[97] The timing of diagnosis has substantial consequences on preventive strategies. The UK plan, therefore, has considerable effects on the population and changes its profiles. Improvement of diagnosis and timing of diagnosis may be more relevant for older populations where the quality of dementia diagnosis was reported as particularly low.[98] Plans at city level may have an impact, especially in communities with low socioeconomic status. Institutional policies could also have effects on secondary prevention when targeted at particular groups (the time of diagnosis changes and earlier diagnosis will be easier) and tertiary prevention (cases are more likely to be more numerous but many patients will be in a milder stage of disease).

Such considerations suggest a multilayer approach, again akin to that implemented for vascular disease vascular should be considered for NDD prevention (Fig. 45.3).

Challenge 2—the best study designs: observational and intervention studies in prevention

Prevention strategies and interventions do not always produce their expected results;[99] increasing the number of people labelled as diseased without any benefit is not necessarily a positive outcome.[100]

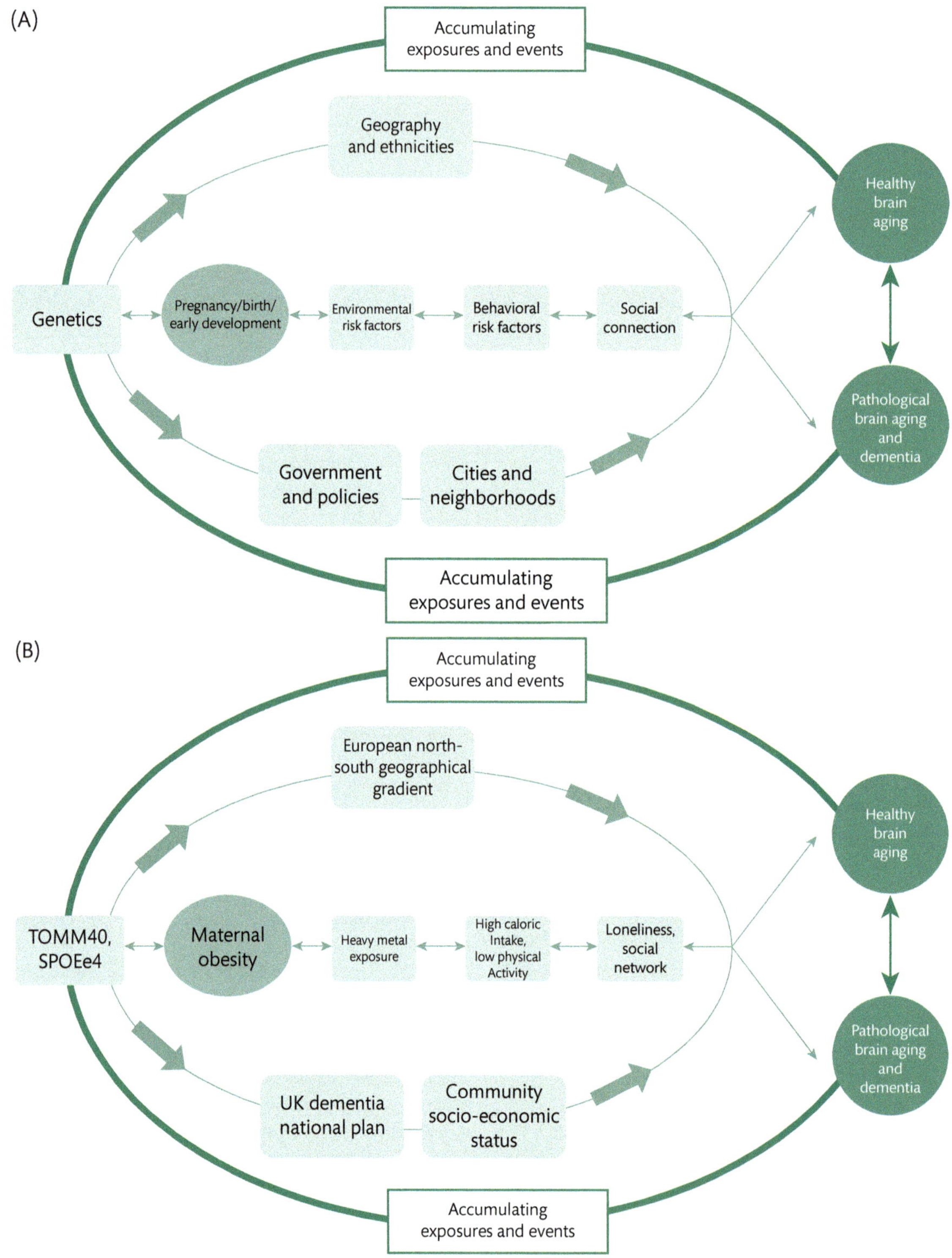

Fig. 45.3 (A) A complex approach to causation of chronic diseases over lifetime: the multilayer Causal Network model. (B) Application of the Multilayer Causal Network model to determine causes over lifetime in dementia.

From a global prospective it is now clear that complex factors have to be taken into account to reach efficacy in the field of prevention of neurodegenerative disorders.

The low efficacy of prevention strategies will have many explanations, within three main categories: (1) uncertain and undefined characterization of risk factors; (2) incorrect design of the intervention strategies; (3) timing and type of intervention.

Uncertain characterization of risk factors

Preventive interventions target risk factors identified from observational studies, which are prone to systematic errors, such as outcome misclassification, selection, and confounding, leading to uncertainty about the real importance of the proposed risk factors. To avoid this methodological limitation, alternative approaches, which aim to test more fully for the biases that can arise when risk factors are identified, should be explored. For example, in a recent review Deckers and colleagues used a mixed-method approach, integrating findings from a systematic literature review on the available evidence from observational epidemiological studies, and a Delphi consensus study, to identify the major modifiable risk factors for dementia.[101]

Second, given that neuropathological changes start many years before manifestation of the clinical syndrome, researchers should focus also on risk factors responsible for particular neuropathologies. These risk factors are not necessarily the same as risk factors for clinical manifestations of the disease. Furthermore, the interpretation of epidemiological studies can be sometimes confusing. In observational studies conducted in older populations, there will be recruitment of healthy participants with neuropathological changes, with subclinical and/or not detected early clinical manifestations of the disease and many of these will go on to live and die without the clinical manifestation of the disorder.[25]

An additional issue is the quantification of different types of damage both in normal and affected individuals. The presence of multi-morbidities, disabilities, and cognitive impairment at the same time makes the clinical and epidemiological scenario in the elderly much more challenging.[1]

Data on possible effects of primary prevention strategies do not exist and will take many years, given the recentness of the techniques to look at neuropathological indicators *in vivo*. A more realistic strategy has been, to date, targeting individuals with minimal symptoms and signs (MCI in the early stages, incident TIA) to test a secondary prevention strategy.

Design of intervention strategies: population-wide approach/high-risk individuals

Prevention strategies can be conducted at a population level (prevention-wide strategies) or target high-risk individuals (high-risk strategies). Population-wide prevention strategies, suggested by Geoffrey Rose in 1985 as the most effective approach to cardiovascular disease prevention,[63] are essential for most of common NCDs because even small changes in the distribution of risk factors could lead to major reductions in NCD incidence. Population-wide approaches target several behavioural and lifestyle risk factors common to most NCDs and over the last 20 years this approach has been included in all major NCD prevention guidelines. Nevertheless, this strategy has not yet been implemented at a national level by any country, probably because of costs (increasing the presence of physical activity facilities and healthy food stores), and because of competing economic interests by the private sector (reduction of salt consumption or exposure to smoking, alcohol, and unhealthy food). There is also a strong national and international media and political rhetoric about the undesirability of a state or national agency's role in determining some types of exposure ('nanny state'). On the contrary, the high-risk approach is based on the identification of high-risk individuals and is a highly intuitive and attractive approach for many sectors of the population, through the calculation of absolute risks of developing the disease at different time points (personalized risk score). In this approach, low and intermediate risk groups are excluded from prevention strategies and probably less motivated to control lifestyle risk factors, but in fact these groups, because they are the largest, lead to the greatest number of incident cases. The high-risk approach has been used in prevention of cardiovascular diseases and stroke and is strongly based often on pharmacological interventions (e.g. statins use). This strategy is strongly limited by the access to medical care and the adherence to therapies (such as anti-hypertensive drugs), and requires a tight collaboration between individuals and the healthcare system, including, but not limited to, doctors. Translating the theoretical chance of disease into realistic conceivable realities for the patient is often one of the most important practical problems faced by physicians. As the simplicity and quality of individual risk calculation methods increase, treatment implementation becomes more efficient. Furthermore, new generation technology could allow individuals to directly calculate and monitor their own risk profile. There has been the publication of a self-reported index score for dementia: the Australian National University AD Risk Index (the ANU_ADRI) with a good prediction based on the evaluation of 15 risk factors.[102]

There are limitations in these risk profiles, particularly for the older age groups and there are concerns that a single disease secondary prevention model leads to considerable polypharmacy in the older old.

The ideal preventive intervention should target social, behavioural, lifestyle, and environmental risk factors in whole populations with the integrated and inclusive intervention of government bodies, non-governmental organizations, and the health sector in all its components.

Timing and type of intervention

Preventive intervention strategies have been conducted to date in later life, mainly as secondary or tertiary prevention in individuals. These interventions are likely to be outside the window of intervention and characterized by short duration and period of follow up. More sustained interventions could result in greater effects. A challenge to observing outcomes is attrition because it is inversely related to the duration of the intervention and can influence the results of clinical trials and preventive interventions. Longer interventions are time consuming and can be cost ineffective. The optimal duration of a preventive intervention is unknown and we do not have a valuable idea of the best window of intervention for the majority of the recognized risk factors. Most prevention studies for NDD have been conducted in older people. It is now largely accepted that midlife, or even earlier life periods, are likely to be the optimal windows of intervention for primary prevention, especially for lifestyle, behavioural, and social prevention strategies. On the contrary secondary prevention is likely to play a role both in middle age and in later life.

The use of unimodal interventions (e.g. diet or exercise), seem unlikely to adequately target the multiple interacting risk factors for multifactorial diseases. Over the last ten years multimodal preventive interventions have been accepted as the optimal approach for prevention of neurological disorders and chronic NCD in general. Several multi-domain RCTs with a multimodal approach are ongoing or recently concluded for prevention of cognitive impairment. Three from Europe are combined into the European Prevention of Dementia Initiative: the Finnish Geriatric Intervention Study to Prevent Cognitive Impairment and Disability (FINGER), the Multidomain Alzheimer Prevention Trial (MAPT), and the PreDIVA are examples of important multidomain RCTs in Europe.[103–105] Table 45.1 summarizes the principal characteristics and the main results of these studies.

Table 45.1 Principal characteristics of the cited three multi-domain intervention trials (Finger, MAPT, PreDIVA)

	FINGER	MAPT	PreDIVA
Study design	Double blind multicentre randomized clinical trial	Multicentre, randomized, placebo-controlled trial	Multisite, open, cluster-randomized, parallel group trial
Study location	Six cities in Finland (Helsinki, Vantaa, Kuopio, Oulu, Seinajoki, Turku)	Toulouse (7 university hospital centres, and 6 memory clinics around Toulouse Gerontopole/Alzheimer Disease research clinical centre	The Netherlands
No. of enrolled subjects	1260 (631 intervention group; 629 control group)	1680 frail elderly people (420 for each group)	3526 (1890 vascular care; 1636 standard care)
Inclusion criteria	60–77 years of age; recruited from previous random, population-based, non-intervention surveys (i.e. FINRISK); at least 6 points at the CAIDE Dementia Risk Score; Word List Memory Task (10 words x 3) 19 words; Word List Recall 75% or MMSE 26/30 points	70 years and over; independent living; good functional and cognitive status; presence of frailty	70–78 years of age; registration with a GP
Exclusion criteria	Malignant diseases; major depression; dementia/substantial cognitive decline; MMSE <20; symptomatic cardiovascular disease; revascularization within 1 year; severe loss of vision, hearing, or communicative ability; conditions preventing cooperation as judged by the study physician; coincident participation in any intervention trial	Dementia (DSM-IV criteria); MMSE score lower than 24/30; ADL score lower than 6/6; depression (GDS score over 15); visual or hearing impairments, or other disorders that could interfere with the interpretation of the study	Prevalent dementia; disorders or circumstances expected to interfere with successful long-term follow-up
Outcome measures	**Primary outcome:** cognitive performance **Secondary outcomes:** incidence of dementia and AD; vascular risk factors; cardiovascular and cerebrovascular morbidity and mortality; dietary intake; dietary markers and other biomarkers; disability; falls; cardiorespiratory fitness; depressive symptoms; health-related quality of life; utilization of health resources; individuals' experience of participation in the study	**Primary outcome:** change from baseline to 36 months in a composite Z score combining four cognitive tests **Secondary outcomes:** individual components of the composite score, scores on other cognitive tests; scores on the Short Physical Performance Battery and the Alzheimer's disease Cooperative Study—Activities of Daily Living Prevention Instrument; Clinical Dementia Rating—Sum of Boxes; Fried's frailty criteria; Geriatric Depression Scale	**Primary outcomes:** incident dementia and the change from baseline in disability as measured by the ALDS **Secondary outcomes:** mortality, incidence of vascular events including myocardial infarction, stroke, and peripheral vascular disease
Groups of intervention	1. intensive multi-domain intervention; 2. regular health advice (control group)	3 treatment groups and 1 control group (placebo group)	1 treatment group and 1 control group
Type of intervention	**1. Regular health advice:** healthy diet and level of physical, cognitive, and social activities beneficial for vascular risk factors management and disability prevention; **2. Intensive multi-domain intervention:** a. nutritional guidance; b. physical exercise; c. cognitive training and social activity; d. intensive monitoring and management of metabolic and vascular risk factors	1. omega 3 alone; 2. multi-domain intervention alone; 3. omega 3 plus multi-domain intervention	1. nurse-led multicomponent intervention directed at vascular care; 2. standard care
Time of intervention	2 years	3 years	6 years
Main results	A multi-domain intervention could improve or maintain cognitive functioning in at-risk elderly people from the general population.	The multi-domain intervention and polyunsaturated fatty acids, either alone or in combination, had no significant effects on cognitive decline over 3 years in elderly people with memory complaints.	A nurse-led, multi-domain intervention did not result in a reduced incidence of all-cause dementia in an unselected population of older people. This absence of effect might have been caused by modest baseline cardiovascular risks, and high standards of usual care.

FINGER: Finnish Geriatric Intervention Study to Prevent Cognitive Impairment and Disability; MAPT: Multidomain Alzheimer Preventive Trial; PreDIVA: Prevention of Dementia by Intensive Vascular Care; CAIDE: Cardiovascular Risk Factors, Aging and Dementia; MMSE: Mini Mental State Examination; AD: Alzheimer's disease; ADL: Activities of Daily Living; GDS: Geriatric Depression Scale; GP: general practitioner; ALDS: Academic Medical Centre Linear Disability Scale.

It is not yet clear what should constitute 'sufficient evidence' for prevention recommendations.[106] Observational studies are prone to biases and uncontrolled confounders. RCTs are generally thought to give the best evidence of efficacy but are not realistic in this field because of the costs, difficulties in randomization related to the study question, small sample size, uncertainty about window of opportunity, length and scale of interventions, and outcome measurement. Finally, and significantly, those who take part in clinical trials have characteristics that are often very different from the target population (selective sampling of participants).

Conclusion

Epidemiology should be at the heart of the definition of the practice of healthcare in populations.[107] Prevention of chronic diseases should start early in life and continue through all the lifespan. The best model of intervention to modify risk factors and disease frequencies should be identified at community level. In this context, the intervention should focus on modifiable risk factors: biomedical, environmental, and social. The medical approach in connected and resilient communities[108] has a specific role in the prevention of chronic diseases. Secondary and tertiary prevention should complement primary intervention strategies. Furthermore, social policies should have a key role in reducing socioeconomic adversities, in changing lifestyle towards healthier population behaviour.

There is a clear urgency for action. The promotion of brain health and healthy ageing should be established as one of public health priority by national and international governmental bodies both in HICs and LMICs, possibly through connected and integrated programmes. The heterogeneity of risk factor prevalence and role across different populations in different geographic areas should be carefully considered.

Recently the special 'Lancet Health Commission for Global Health' has endorsed a grand convergence for disease prevention and control of non-communicable diseases, highlighting the importance of governmental and societal plans. The Commission recommendation included free access to healthcare as part of the intervention to improve public health.[109] The 'grand convergence in health' within one generation should help to implement common and diverse international policies to implement prevention (taking into account regional diversities and specificities).[109]

At the same time, there is a continuous call for initiative that is labelled as 'precision medicine' involving big data, biomarkers, genomics, and new techniques from system biology in several chronic diseases including NDD as AD.[110] The role of precision medicine should be carefully evaluated for its ability to deliver true benefits for populations beyond tertiary advanced research centres.

Population science is part of a unified and combined approach of innovation in biomedicine with public health and health policies. In this complex scenario, epidemiology has a specific role as a pragmatic discipline with the double aim of identification and removal of causes of diseases through intervention.[61,107]

In a rapidly changing scenario, with the world population increasing and ageing by the week, prevention is the inevitable and probably the only choice to reduce the load of chronic neurological diseases globally.

REFERENCES

1. Brayne C. The elephant in the room—healthy brains in later life, epidemiology and public health. Nature Reviews Neuroscience. 2007; 8(3): 233–9.
2. Global, regional, and national life expectancy, all-cause mortality, and cause-specific mortality for 249 causes of death, 1980–2015: a systematic analysis for the Global Burden of Disease Study 2015. Lancet. 2016; 388(10053): 1459–544.
3. Global, regional, and national burden of neurological disorders during 1990–2015: a systematic analysis for the Global Burden of Disease Study 2015. Lancet Neurology. 2017; 16(11): 877–97.
4. Global, regional, and national incidence, prevalence, and years lived with disability for 310 diseases and injuries, 1990–2015: a systematic analysis for the Global Burden of Disease Study 2015. Lancet. 2016; 388(10053): 1545–602.
5. Global, regional, and national comparative risk assessment of 79 behavioural, environmental and occupational, and metabolic risks or clusters of risks, 1990–2015: a systematic analysis for the Global Burden of Disease Study 2015. Lancet. 2016; 388(10053): 1659–724.
6. Kannel WB, Dawber TR, Kagan A, Revotskie N, Stokes J, 3rd. Factors of risk in the development of coronary heart disease—six-year follow-up experience. The Framingham Study. Annals of Internal Medicine. 1961; 55: 33–50.
7. Puska P. From Framingham to North Karelia: from descriptive epidemiology to public health action. Progress in Cardiovascular Diseases. 2010; 53(1): 15–20.
8. Feigin VL, Forouzanfar MH, Krishnamurthi R, Mensah GA, Connor M, Bennett DA, et al. Global and regional burden of stroke during 1990–2010: findings from the Global Burden of Disease Study 2010. Lancet. 2014; 383(9913): 245–54.
9. Wang Y, Wang QJ. The prevalence of prehypertension and hypertension among US adults according to the new joint national committee guidelines: new challenges of the old problem. Archives of Internal Medicine. 2004; 164(19): 2126–34.
10. Yudkin JS, Montori VM. The epidemic of pre-diabetes: the medicine and the politics. BMJ (Clinical research ed). 2014; 349: g4485.
11. Wu YT, Beiser AS, Breteler MMB, Fratiglioni L, Helmer C, Hendrie HC, et al. The changing prevalence and incidence of dementia over time—current evidence. Nature Reviews Neurology. 2017; 13(6): 327–39.
12. Satizabal CL, Beiser AS, Chouraki V, Chene G, Dufouil C, Seshadri S. Incidence of dementia over three decades in the Framingham Heart Study. New England Journal of Medicine. 2016; 374(6): 523–32.
13. Matthews FE, Stephan BC, Robinson L, Jagger C, Barnes LE, Arthur A, et al. A two decade dementia incidence comparison from the Cognitive Function and Ageing Studies I and II. Nature Communications. 2016; 7: 11398.
14. Langa KM. Is the risk of Alzheimer's disease and dementia declining? Alzheimer's Research & Therapy. 2015; 7(1): 34.
15. Jones DS, Greene JA. Is Dementia in decline? Historical trends and future trajectories. New England Journal of Medicine. 2016; 374(6): 507–9.
16. Mytton OT, Jackson C, Steinacher A, Goodman A, Langenberg C, Griffin S, et al. The current and potential health benefits of the National Health Service Health Check cardiovascular disease prevention programme in England: A microsimulation study. PLOS medicine. 2018; 15(3): e1002517.

17. Wong ND. Epidemiological studies of CHD and the evolution of preventive cardiology. Nature Reviews Cardiology. 2014; 11(5): 276–89.
18. Rocca WA. Time, sex, gender, history, and dementia. Alzheimer disease and associated disorders. 2017; 31(1): 76–9.
19. Chio A, Mora G, Moglia C, Manera U, Canosa A, Cammarosano S, et al. Secular Trends of amyotrophic lateral sclerosis: the Piemonte and Valle d'Aosta register. JAMA Neurology. 2017; 74(9): 1097–104.
20. Savica R, Grossardt BR, Bower JH, Ahlskog JE, Rocca WA. Time trends in the incidence of Parkinson disease. JAMA Neurology. 2016; 73(8): 981–9.
21. Logroscino G, Traynor BJ, Hardiman O, Chio A, Mitchell D, Swingler RJ, et al. Incidence of amyotrophic lateral sclerosis in Europe. Journal of Neurology, Neurosurgery, and Psychiatry. 2010; 81(4): 385–90.
22. Langa KM, Larson EB, Crimmins EM, Faul JD, Levine DA, Kabeto MU, et al. A comparison of the prevalence of dementia in the United States in 2000 and 2012. JAMA Internal Medicine. 2017; 177(1): 51–8.
23. Smith AD, Yaffe K. Dementia (including Alzheimer's disease) can be prevented: statement supported by international experts. Journal of Alzheimer's Disease. 2014; 38(4): 699–703.
24. Jellinger KA. Recent advances in our understanding of neurodegeneration. J Neural Transm (Vienna). 2009; 116(9): 1111–62.
25. Bennett DA, Schneider JA, Arvanitakis Z, Kelly JF, Aggarwal NT, Shah RC, et al. Neuropathology of older persons without cognitive impairment from two community-based studies. Neurology. 2006; 66(12): 1837–44.
26. Albert MS, DeKosky ST, Dickson D, Dubois B, Feldman HH, Fox NC, et al. The diagnosis of mild cognitive impairment due to Alzheimer's disease: recommendations from the National Institute on Aging-Alzheimer's Association workgroups on diagnostic guidelines for Alzheimer's disease. Alzheimer's & Dementia: the journal of the Alzheimer's Association. 2011; 7(3): 270–9.
27. McKhann GM, Knopman DS, Chertkow H, Hyman BT, Jack CR Jr, Kawas CH, et al. The diagnosis of dementia due to Alzheimer's disease: recommendations from the National Institute on Aging-Alzheimer's Association workgroups on diagnostic guidelines for Alzheimer's disease. Alzheimer's & Dementia: the journal of the Alzheimer's Association. 2011; 7(3): 263–9.
28. Dubois B, Feldman HH, Jacova C, Hampel H, Molinuevo JL, Blennow K, et al. Advancing research diagnostic criteria for Alzheimer's disease: the IWG-2 criteria. Lancet Neurology. 2014; 13(6): 614–29.
29. Bu XL, Jiao SS, Lian Y, Wang YJ. Perspectives on the tertiary prevention strategy for Alzheimer's disease. Current Alzheimer Research. 2016; 13(3): 307–16.
30. Solomon A, Mangialasche F, Richard E, Andrieu S, Bennett DA, Breteler M, et al. Advances in the prevention of Alzheimer's disease and dementia. Journal of Internal Medicine. 2014; 275(3): 229–50.
31. Carrillo MC, Brashear HR, Logovinsky V, Ryan JM, Feldman HH, Siemers ER, et al. Can we prevent Alzheimer's disease? Secondary 'prevention' trials in Alzheimer's disease. Alzheimer's & Dementia: the journal of the Alzheimer's Association. 2013; 9(2): 123–31.e1.
32. Kuh D, Ben-Shlomo Y. *A Life Course Approach to Chronic Disease Epidemiology*. Oxford: Oxford University Press, 2004.
33. Kuh D, Hardy R, Richards M, Ben-Shlomo Y. A Life Course Approach to Healthy Ageing. Oxford: Oxford University Press, 2013.
34. Barker DJ, Osmond C. Infant mortality, childhood nutrition, and ischaemic heart disease in England and Wales. Lancet. 1986; 1(8489): 1077–81.
35. Barker DJ, Osmond C, Simmonds SJ, Wield GA. The relation of small head circumference and thinness at birth to death from cardiovascular disease in adult life. BMJ (Clinical research ed). 1993; 306(6875): 422–6.
36. Frankel S, Elwood P, Sweetnam P, Yarnell J, Smith GD. Birthweight, body-mass index in middle age, and incident coronary heart disease. Lancet. 1996; 348(9040): 1478–80.
37. Stein CE, Fall CH, Kumaran K, Osmond C, Cox V, Barker DJ. Fetal growth and coronary heart disease in south India. Lancet. 1996; 348(9037): 1269–73.
38. Huda SS, Brodie LE, Sattar N. Obesity in pregnancy: prevalence and metabolic consequences. Seminars in Fetal & Neonatal Medicine. 2010; 15(2): 70–6.
39. Parlee SD, MacDougald OA. Maternal nutrition and risk of obesity in offspring: the Trojan horse of developmental plasticity. Biochimica et Biophysica Acta. 2014; 1842(3): 495–506.
40. Reynolds RM, Allan KM, Raja EA, Bhattacharya S, McNeill G, Hannaford PC, et al. Maternal obesity during pregnancy and premature mortality from cardiovascular event in adult offspring: follow-up of 1,323,275 person years. BMJ (Clinical research ed). 2013; 347: f4539.
41. Lahiri DK, Zawia NH, Greig NH, Sambamurti K, Maloney B. Early-life events may trigger biochemical pathways for Alzheimer's disease: the 'LEARn' model. Biogerontology. 2008; 9(6): 375–9.
42. van Abeelen AF, Elias SG, Bossuyt PM, Grobbee DE, van der Schouw YT, Roseboom TJ, et al. Famine exposure in the young and the risk of type 2 diabetes in adulthood. Diabetes. 2012; 61(9): 2255–60.
43. Fransen HP, Peeters PH, Beulens JW, Boer JM, de Wit GA, Onland-Moret NC, et al. Exposure to famine at a young age and unhealthy lifestyle behavior later in life. PLOS One. 2016; 11(5): e0156609.
44. de Groot RH, Stein AD, Jolles J, van Boxtel MP, Blauw GJ, van de Bor M, et al. Prenatal famine exposure and cognition at age 59 years. International Journal of Epidemiology. 2011; 40(2): 327–37.
45. Kivimaki M, Smith GD, Elovainio M, Pulkki L, Keltikangas-Jarvinen L, Talttonen L, et al. Socioeconomic circumstances in childhood and blood pressure in adulthood: the cardiovascular risk in young Finns study. Annals of Epidemiology. 2006; 16(10): 737–42.
46. Scazufca M, Seabra CA. Sao Paulo portraits: ageing in a large metropolis. International Journal of Epidemiology. 2008; 37(4): 721–3.
47. Liu L, Xue F, Ma J, Ma M, Long Y, Newschaffer CJ. Social position and chronic conditions across the life span and risk of stroke: a life course epidemiological analysis of 22,847 American adults in ages over 50. International Journal of Stroke: official journal of the International Stroke Society. 2013; 8(Suppl A100): 50–5.
48. Ben-Shlomo Y, Kuh D. A life course approach to chronic disease epidemiology: conceptual models, empirical challenges and interdisciplinary perspectives. International Journal of Epidemiology. 2002; 31(2): 285–93.

49. Power C, Manor O, Matthews S. The duration and timing of exposure: effects of socioeconomic environment on adult health. American Journal of Public Health. 1999; 89(7): 1059–65.
50. Smith GD, Hart C. Life-course socioeconomic and behavioral influences on cardiovascular disease mortality: the collaborative study. American Journal of Public Health. 2002; 92(8): 1295–8.
51. Leon DA, Davey Smith G. Infant mortality, stomach cancer, stroke, and coronary heart disease: ecological analysis. BMJ (Clinical research ed). 2000; 320(7251): 1705–6.
52. Hart CL, Davey Smith G. Relation between number of siblings and adult mortality and stroke risk: 25-year follow-up of men in the Collaborative study. Journal of Epidemiology and Community Health. 2003; 57(5): 385–91.
53. Rajput AH, Uitti RJ, Stern W, Laverty W. Early onset Parkinson's disease in Saskatchewan—environmental considerations for etiology. The Canadian Journal of Neurological Sciences. 1986; 13(4): 312–16.
54. Sveinbjornsdottir S, Hicks AA, Jonsson T, Petursson H, Gugmundsson G, Frigge ML, et al. Familial aggregation of Parkinson's disease in Iceland. New England Journal of Medicine. 2000; 343(24): 1765–70.
55. de la Fuente-Fernandez R, Calne DB. Familial aggregation of Parkinson's disease. New England Journal of Medicine. 2001; 344(15): 1168.
56. Kivipelto M, Helkala EL, Laakso MP, Hanninen T, Hallikainen M, Alhainen K, et al. Apolipoprotein E epsilon4 allele, elevated midlife total cholesterol level, and high midlife systolic blood pressure are independent risk factors for late-life Alzheimer disease. Annals of Internal Medicine. 2002; 137(3): 149–55.
57. Kivipelto M, Ngandu T, Fratiglioni L, Viitanen M, Kareholt I, Winblad B, et al. Obesity and vascular risk factors at midlife and the risk of dementia and Alzheimer disease. Archives of Neurology. 2005; 62(10): 1556–60.
58. Qiu C, Winblad B, Fratiglioni L. The age-dependent relation of blood pressure to cognitive function and dementia. Lancet Neurology. 2005; 4(8): 487–99.
59. Mielke MM, Zandi PP, Sjogren M, Gustafson D, Ostling S, Steen B, et al. High total cholesterol levels in late life associated with a reduced risk of dementia. Neurology. 2005; 64(10): 1689–95.
60. Atti AR, Palmer K, Volpato S, Winblad B, De Ronchi D, Fratiglioni L. Late-life body mass index and dementia incidence: nine-year follow-up data from the Kungsholmen Project. Journal of the American Geriatrics Society. 2008; 56(1): 111–16.
61. Katherine M. Keyes SG. Population Health Science. New York: Oxford University Press, 2016.
62. Sindi S, Mangialasche F, Kivipelto M. Advances in the prevention of Alzheimer's Disease. F1000prime reports. 2015; 7: 50.
63. Rose G. Sick individuals and sick populations. International Journal of Epidemiology. 1985; 14(1): 32–8.
64. Anderson KM, Odell PM, Wilson PW, Kannel WB. Cardiovascular disease risk profiles. American Heart Journal. 1991; 121(1 Pt 2): 293–8.
65. Kannel WB, McGee D, Gordon T. A general cardiovascular risk profile: the Framingham Study. American Journal of Cardiology. 1976; 38(1): 46–51.
66. Wolf PA, D'Agostino RB, Belanger AJ, Kannel WB. Probability of stroke: a risk profile from the Framingham Study. Stroke; a Journal of Cerebral Circulation. 1991; 22(3): 312–18.
67. Hippisley-Cox J, Coupland C, Brindle P. Development and validation of QRISK3 risk prediction algorithms to estimate future risk of cardiovascular disease: prospective cohort study. BMJ (Clinical research ed). 2017; 357: j2099.
68. Kivipelto M, Ngandu T, Laatikainen T, Winblad B, Soininen H, Tuomilehto J. Risk score for the prediction of dementia risk in 20 years among middle aged people: a longitudinal, population-based study. Lancet Neurology. 2006; 5(9): 735–41.
69. Barnes DE, Covinsky KE, Whitmer RA, Kuller LH, Lopez OL, Yaffe K. Predicting risk of dementia in older adults: the late-life dementia risk index. Neurology. 2009; 73(3): 173–9.
70. Reitz C, Tang MX, Schupf N, Manly JJ, Mayeux R, Luchsinger JA. Association of higher levels of high-density lipoprotein cholesterol in elderly individuals and lower risk of late-onset Alzheimer disease. Archives of Neurology. 2010; 67(12): 1491–7.
71. Jessen F, Wiese B, Bickel H, Eifflander-Gorfer S, Fuchs A, Kaduszkiewicz H, et al. Prediction of dementia in primary care patients. PLOS One. 2011; 6(2): e16852.
72. Qiu C, Kivipelto M, Aguero-Torres H, Winblad B, Fratiglioni L. Risk and protective effects of the APOE gene towards Alzheimer's disease in the Kungsholmen project: variation by age and sex. Journal of Neurology, Neurosurgery, and Psychiatry. 2004; 75(6): 828–33.
73. Kloppenborg RP, van den Berg E, Kappelle LJ, Biessels GJ. Diabetes and other vascular risk factors for dementia: which factor matters most? A systematic review. European Journal of Pharmacology. 2008; 585(1): 97–108.
74. Gustafson D. A life course of adiposity and dementia. European Journal of Pharmacology. 2008; 585(1): 163–75.
75. Kaffashian S, Dugravot A, Elbaz A, Shipley MJ, Sabia S, Kivimaki M, et al. Predicting cognitive decline: a dementia risk score v. the Framingham vascular risk scores. Neurology. 2013; 80(14): 1300–6.
76. Li J, Ogrodnik M, Devine S, Auerbach S, Wolf PA, Au R. Practical risk score for 5-, 10-, and 20-year prediction of dementia in elderly persons: Framingham Heart Study. Alzheimer's & Dementia: the journal of the Alzheimer's Association. 2018; 14(1): 35–42.
77. Capewell S, Graham H. Will cardiovascular disease prevention widen health inequalities? PLOS Medicine. 2010; 7(8): e1000320.
78. Hollands GJ, French DP, Griffin SJ, Prevost AT, Sutton S, King S, et al. The impact of communicating genetic risks of disease on risk-reducing health behaviour: systematic review with meta-analysis. BMJ (Clinical research ed). 2016; 352: i1102.
79. Ramsay LE, Haq IU, Jackson PR, Yeo WW, Pickin DM, Payne JN. Targeting lipid-lowering drug therapy for primary prevention of coronary disease: an updated Sheffield table. Lancet. 1996; 348(9024): 387–8.
80. Ramsay LE, Wallis EJ, Haq IU, Jackson PR. Coronary risk assessment methods and cholesterol lowering. Lancet. 1999; 353(9158): 1095; author reply 6–7.
81. Haq IU, Wallis EJ, Jackson PR, Yeo WW, Ramsay LE. Implication of recent trials with b-hydroxy-b-methylglutaryl coenzyme A reductase inhibitors for hypertension management. Journal of Hypertension. 1999; 17(11): 1641–6.
82. Justice AC, Covinsky KE, Berlin JA. Assessing the generalizability of prognostic information. Annals of Internal Medicine. 1999; 130(6): 515–24.
83. Norton S, Matthews FE, Brayne C. A commentary on studies presenting projections of the future prevalence of dementia. BMC Public Health. 2013; 13: 1.
84. Daviglus ML, Bell CC, Berrettini W, Bowen PE, Connolly ES Jr, Cox NJ, et al. National Institutes of Health State-of-the-Science

Conference statement: preventing Alzheimer disease and cognitive decline. Annals of Internal Medicine. 2010; 153(3): 176–81.
85. Barnes DE, Yaffe K. The projected effect of risk factor reduction on Alzheimer's disease prevalence. Lancet Neurology. 2011; 10(9): 819–28.
86. Norton S, Matthews FE, Barnes DE, Yaffe K, Brayne C. Potential for primary prevention of Alzheimer's disease: an analysis of population-based data. Lancet Neurology. 2014; 13(8): 788–94.
87. Richard E, Andrieu S, Solomon A, Mangialasche F, Ahtiluoto S, Moll van Charante EP, et al. Methodological challenges in designing dementia prevention trials—the European Dementia Prevention Initiative (EDPI). Journal of the Neurological Sciences. 2012; 322(1–2): 64–70.
88. Geoffrey Rose K-TK, *Michael Marmot. Rose's Strategy of Preventive Medicine.* New York: Oxford University Press, 2008.
89. Krieger N. *Epidemiology and the People's Health: Theory and Context.* New York: Oxford University Press. 2011.
90. Rafnsson SB, Orrell M, d'Orsi E, Hogervorst E, Steptoe A. Loneliness, social integration, and incident dementia over 6 years: prospective findings from the English Longitudinal Study of Ageing. Journals of Gerontology Series B, Psychological Sciences and Social Sciences. 2017; 75(1): 114–24.
91. Wilson RS, Bennett DA. How does psychosocial behavior contribute to cognitive health in old age? Brain Sciences. 2017; 7(6): ii, E56.
92. Barnes LL, Mendes de Leon CF, Wilson RS, Bienias JL, Evans DA. Social resources and cognitive decline in a population of older African Americans and whites. Neurology. 2004; 63(12): 2322–6.
93. Wilson RS, Schneider JA, Arnold SE, Bienias JL, Bennett DA. Conscientiousness and the incidence of Alzheimer disease and mild cognitive impairment. Archives of General Psychiatry. 2007; 64(10): 1204–12.
94. Donovan NJ, Okereke OI, Vannini P, Amariglio RE, Rentz DM, Marshall GA, et al. Association of higher cortical amyloid burden with loneliness in cognitively normal older adults. JAMA Psychiatry. 2016; 73(12): 1230–7.
95. Vega IE, Cabrera LY, Wygant CM, Velez-Ortiz D, Counts SE. Alzheimer's Disease in the Latino community: intersection of genetics and social determinants of health. Journal of Alzheimer's Disease. 2017; 58(4): 979–92.
96. Department of Health Working Group. Living with dementia: a national Dementia Strategy. London: Department of Health, 2009.
97. Mukadam N, Livingston G, Rantell K, Rickman S. Diagnostic rates and treatment of dementia before and after launch of a national dementia policy: an observational study using English national databases. BMJ Open. 2014; 4(1): e004119.
98. Rait G, Walters K, Bottomley C, Petersen I, Iliffe S, Nazareth I. Survival of people with clinical diagnosis of dementia in primary care: cohort study. BMJ (Clinical research ed). 2010; 341: c3584.
99. Chiolero A, Paradis G, Paccaud F. The pseudo-high-risk prevention strategy. International Journal of Epidemiology. 2015; 44(5): 1469–73.
100. Chiolero A, Paccaud F. Prediabetes and the risk of diabetes. Lancet. 2012; 380(9849): 1225; author reply 6.
101. Deckers K, van Boxtel MP, Schiepers OJ, de Vugt M, Munoz Sanchez JL, Anstey KJ, et al. Target risk factors for dementia prevention: a systematic review and Delphi consensus study on the evidence from observational studies. International Journal of Geriatric Psychiatry. 2015; 30(3): 234–46.
102. Anstey KJ, Cherbuin N, Herath PM, Qiu C, Kuller LH, Lopez OL, et al. A self-report risk index to predict occurrence of dementia in three independent cohorts of older adults: the ANU-ADRI. PLOS One. 2014; 9(1): e86141.
103. Ngandu T, Lehtisalo J, Solomon A, Levalahti E, Ahtiluoto S, Antikainen R, et al. A 2-year multidomain intervention of diet, exercise, cognitive training, and vascular risk monitoring versus control to prevent cognitive decline in at-risk elderly people (FINGER): a randomised controlled trial. Lancet. 2015; 385(9984): 2255–63.
104. Moll van Charante EP, Richard E, Eurelings LS, van Dalen JW, Ligthart SA, van Bussel EF, et al. Effectiveness of a 6-year multidomain vascular care intervention to prevent dementia (preDIVA): a cluster-randomised controlled trial. Lancet. 2016; 388(10046): 797–805.
105. Andrieu S, Guyonnet S, Coley N, Cantet C, Bonnefoy M, Bordes S, et al. Effect of long-term omega 3 polyunsaturated fatty acid supplementation with or without multidomain intervention on cognitive function in elderly adults with memory complaints (MAPT): a randomised, placebo-controlled trial. Lancet Neurology. 2017; 16(5): 377–89.
106. Williams JW, Plassman BL, Burke J, Benjamin S. Preventing Alzheimer's disease and cognitive decline. Evidence Report/Technology Assessment. 2010(193): 1–727.
107. Miettinen OS, Karp, I. Epidemiological Research: An Introduction. New York: Springer, 2012.
108. Marmot M. The Health Gap. The Challenge of an Unequal World. London: Bloomsbury Publishing, 2015. pp22–48.
109. Jamison DT, Summers LH, Alleyne G, Arrow KJ, Berkley S, Binagwaho A, et al. Global health 2035: a world converging within a generation. Lancet. 2013; 382(9908): 1898–955.
110. Hampel H, O'Bryant SE, Durrleman S, Younesi E, Rojkova K, Escott-Price V, et al. A precision medicine initiative for Alzheimer's disease: the road ahead to biomarker-guided integrative disease modeling. Climacteric: the journal of the International Menopause Society. 2017; 20(2): 107–18.

Index

Note: tables, figures, and boxes are indicated by *t*, *f*, and *b* following the page number.